Please
affix
postage
stamp
here

D0300272

The Editorial Board

Medicines for Children

ROYAL COLLEGE OF PAEDIATRICS AND CHILD HEALTH

50 Hallam Street

London

W1N 6DE

The editorial board of the *Medicines for Children* formulary would welcome any corrections, amendments or suggestions on how the formulary could be improved. Please do not expect an immediate or individual reply, although you views will be very welcome.

Corrections/amendments: _____

_____

_____

Comments for improvement: _____

_____

_____

New developments in treatment and drug usage: _____

_____

_____

NAME AND ADDRESS (optional)

Name: _____

Address: _____

Postcode: _____

Please tick here if you would use a CD ROM version of the formulary. ☐

If you would like to send more detailed information regarding the formulary, please write to the address listed overleaf.

2003

Medicines for Children

75 Years of Service to Children · BPA · RCPCH ·

PATRON
HRH The Princess Royal

RCPCH

Royal College of Paediatrics and Child Health

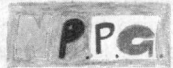

Neonatal and Paediatric Pharmacists Group

Published by RCPCH Publications Limited
50 Hallam Street, London W1W 6DE
Tel: 020 7307 5600
Fax: 020 7307 5601

© 1999, 2003 RCPCH Publications Limited

First published July 1999
This second edition published August 2003

ISBN 190095468 0

1 2 3 4 5 6 7 8 9

Produced by Chamberlain Dunn Associates,
Gothic House, 3 The Green, Richmond TW9 1PL
Tel: 020 8334 4500
Fax: 020 8332 7201
email: mail@chamberdunn.co.uk

Printed by Hobbs the Printers Limited, Southampton, England

A catalogue record for this book is available from
the British Library.

Copies may be obtained direct from:

Direct Books,
PO Box 4995,
Poole,
Dorset BH12 3WF
Tel: 01202 712937
Fax: 01202 712930
email: rcpch@bebc.co.uk
web: www.directbooks.uk.com

Not for sale in the United States of America or Canada

Notice

Medicines for Children is an independently written publication
designed as a guide to those who prescribe and dispense
medicines for children. Out of date copies should not be used.
The contributors, reviewers, editorial board, publishers, and
printers cannot accept liability for any errors or omissions.

Every effort has been made to ensure that the contents herein
are accurate and in accord with the standards accepted at the
time of publication. As new research and experience broaden
our knowledge, changes in treatment and drug therapy occur.
The reader is advised to check the product information sheet
(if available) included in the package of each product he or
she plans to prescribe or dispense. This is of particular
importance for new or infrequently used products. The use of
unlicensed medicines and of licensed medicines for unlicensed
applications is explained on pages xvi to xviii. Those who
prescribe or dispense remain responsible for what they are doing.

Contents

Four years have elapsed since the first edition of *Medicines for Children* was published. The format of the new edition will be familiar but the contents have changed. All clinical guidelines have been reviewed and updated. New drug monographs have been introduced, many at the suggestion of readers.

The partnership between the Royal College of Paediatrics and Child Health and the Neonatal and Paediatric Pharmacists Group is the foundation stone on which *Medicines for Children* is built and gives the formulary its extra value. It remains relevant to daily practice and the welfare of children by giving statements of best practice even when the evidence base remains imperfect. The necessity of prescribing licensed medicines for unlicensed applications and unlicensed medicines to children remains a constant concern and awaits the active participation of Government. By highlighting such areas *Medicines for Children* is a stimulus for debate, research and future improvement.

In 1999 the Formulary Committee, a subcommittee of the RCPCH/NPPG Standing Committee on Medicines, was replaced by an Editorial Board comprising of paediatric pharmacists, paediatricians, a dietitian and nurse. Over that time the first edition was reprinted with some revision in 2000 and *Pocket Medicines for Children* was published in 2001. In preparation for the second edition, Mrs Carol Jackson was appointed as the key position of co-ordinating paediatric pharmacist to oversee the project. Through her pharmaceutical and administrative skills, Carol has performed an exceptional job. Although such a complex undertaking cannot be achieved by one person alone, the completion of this book owes more to Carol's energy and dedication than any other individual. RCPCH and NPPG also gratefully acknowledge the support received from Mrs Regina Brophy, head of pharmacy at the Royal United Hospital, Bath who generously supported Carol's secondment from the Trust to carry out this work. Special thanks also goes to the Bath Unit for Research in Paediatrics for supplying essential equipment and office space to house the nerve centre of a truly national effort.

A book as detailed and complex as *Medicines for Children* requires wide collaboration between colleagues. There lies not only the difficulty but also the strength of the publication. The second edition was compiled by 75 contributors and scrutinised by 60 reviewers from both RCPCH and NPPG, many continuing their involvement from the first edition. All have given generously of their time. Their experience and expertise gives authority to the book and provides a unique resource for future development.

Members of the Editorial Board took on the role of editor for sections of the book. Some require a special mention. Dr Anita McDonald continued to review and update the nutrition tables, which were published as a separate booklet, *Special Foods for Children* for the first time in 2002 and has proved extremely popular with paediatric dietitians throughout the United Kingdom. Catherine Hall not only fulfilled her role on the Editorial Board but also wrote some sections and reviewed others. Anne Burns took on the responsibility of preparing a second edition of *Pocket Medicines for Children* to accompany and complement this publication. Linda Haines, principal research officer of RCPCH, was a constant source of sound advice and was influential in securing the invaluable assistance of Nancy Elder and Morwenna Stewart who assisted with the enormous administrative task.

Medicines for Children has achieved much success and recognition through the hard work and goodwill of RCPCH and NPPG colleagues. However, developments will have continued which were unknown when the volume went to press. Those who prescribe, dispense or administer medicines remain responsible for taking all necessary precautions. For genuine oversights and errors we ask our readers' forgiveness. In keeping with the first edition, we invite feedback to correct our mistakes, share ideas, offer criticism and, when deserved, words of encouragement.

Dennis Carson.

Dennis Carson
Chair of Editorial Board

Acknowledgements

Contributors

Mrs Anita Aindow
Dr Richard Appleton
Mr Nigel Ballantine
Mrs Jennifer Bartlett
Dr Helen Bedford
Ms Amanda Bevan
Dr Lynda Brook
Dr Andrew Bush
Mrs Fiona Clark
Mr Michael Patrick Clarke
Mrs Sharon Conroy
Ms Judith Cope
Mr Ian Costello
Dr Brian Coulter
Dr Brian Craig
Mr Peter Crawford
Mr Philip Dale
Professor Timothy David
Dr Mark Dalzell
Dr Julie Edge
Dr David Elliman
Dr Paul Eunson
Dr Rupert Evans
Mr Nigel Gooding
Dr James Gray

Dr Richard Hain
Dr Ann Hall
Miss Catherine Hall
Ms Paula Hayes
Dr Martin Hewitt
Professor Peter Hill
Mrs Vicky Holden
Ms Alison Hole
Miss Rhian Isaac
Dr Adam Jaffe
Dr Satbir Jassal
Dr Derek Johnston
Dr Anita MacDonald
Ms Sukeshi Makhecha
Dr Katherine Martin
Miss Helen Martin
Dr Patrick McKiernan
Dr Neil McLellan
Dr Andrew Morris
Dr Neil Morton
Dr Celia Moss
Mrs Julie Mycroft
Dr Simon Newell
Mrs Veronica Newland
Mr Clive Newman

Ms Claire Norton
Professor June Nunn
Mr Antony Nunn
Professor Chris O'Callaghan
Mrs Katherine O'Donnell
Ms Funmi Peters
Ms Liza Pickrell
Professor Ross Pinkerton
Dr John Puntis
Dr Sam Richmond
Ms Cathy Sedgeworth
Mr Ian Sharkey
Dr Nick Shaw
Dr Roderick Skinner
Dr Graham Smith
Dr Stephanie Smith
Professor Rosalind Smyth
Professor Terence Stephenson
Dr Graham Taylor
Mr Steve Tomlin
Dr Helen Venning
Dr Kate Verrier-Jones
Mr James Wallace
Miss Lynn Williams
Mr Vincent Yeung

Reviewers

Dr Mario Abinun
Ms Annette Adams
Mr David Adams
Ms Elke Albert
Ms Sharon Andrew
Dr Eileen Baildam
Mr Nigel Ballentine
Dr Kathleen Berry
Ms Amanda Bevan
Ms Soni Bhatt
Dr Paula Bolton-Maggs
Ms Vicky Bradnam
Ms Teresa Brooks
Dr Michael Burch
Ms Amanda Clarkson
Mr Niall Corry
Dr Helen Cross
Mr Mike Dunn
Dr Theo Fenton
Professor Adam Finn

Dr Martha Ford-Adams
Dr Ann Goldman
Dr Helen Goodyear
Mr Terry Gregg
Miss Catherine Hall
Ms Yolande Hanssens
Mr David Harris
Professor Peter Helms
Ms Sarah Irwin
Ms Sue Jarvis
Mrs Tasneem Khalid
Dr Daphne Keen
Dr Christopher Kelnar
Professor Bryan Lask
Mr Jimmie Latona
Dr Eleanor Magill
Dr Anthony McCarthy
Mr Gerry McGinnity
Dr Mary McGraw
Ms Kate Niland

Ms Penny North-Lewis
Mrs Kate Pine
Dr John Puntis
Dr Martin Richardson
Mr Neil Richardson
Dr Andrew Riordan
Dr Peter Robinson
Mr Craig Rore
Ms Vanessa Shaw
Mrs Julia Simmons
Mrs Elish Smith
Dr David Spencer
Dr Bob Taylor
Ms Sarah Templeman
Mr John Timmins
Dr Peter Weller
Dr William Whitehouse
Dr Ian Wong
Mrs Elizabeth Worthing

Editorial Board Members

Mrs Anita Aindow
Miss Liesa Barr
Mrs Anne Burns
Dr Dennis Carson
Professor Imti Choonara

Ms Helena Dunbar
Mrs Linda Haines
Miss Catherine Hall
Mrs Carol Jackson
Dr Warren Lenney

Dr Anita MacDonald
Mrs Rowena McArtney
Dr George Rylance
Professor Terence Stephenson

Medicines for Children was first published in 1999 and has quickly become the authoritative reference for prescribing, dispensing and administering medicines to children. The first edition was followed by *Pocket Medicines for Children* to assist the junior doctor, nurse or pharmacist working on the wards. In this second edition of *Medicines for Children*, the guidelines section makes recommendations on which medicines to use. The second section contains information on the individual drugs; these are listed in alphabetical order. The information is what we think those who prescribe or dispense for children should know about the drugs they use. These drugs are listed as monographs. Further information, for example on rare side-effects, should be sought from other sources such as the Summary of Product Characteristics. The nutrition section gives the ingredients of special foods.

The data on individual drugs includes the licensed status for the usage recommended. To market a product in the UK, a pharmaceutical company must obtain a licence from the Licensing Authority (UK Health Ministers) which is guided by the Medicines Control Agency (MCA) or the European Medical Evaluation Agency (EMEA). The MCA or EMEA have to be assured of the safety, quality and efficacy of the medicinal product and this requires data from large trials.

Because there are fewer trial data from children, many drugs do not have a licence to be promoted by a pharmaceutical company for use in childhood. This does not mean it is illegal or necessarily dangerous to use these drugs in children. It is a doctor's duty, as it is for all health professionals, to act as best they can for the benefit of their patients. Hence, many drugs given to children are used outside the conditions of the product licence. The product licence specifies which diseases the company can promote the drug for, in which age groups, at what dose etc. The diseases for which they are prescribed in children may be different from those in adults. The formulation of the drug may have to be changed, for example, tablets may be crushed and suspended to enable young children to swallow them, or liquids licensed for injection may be given orally. The dosage recommended for adults will be different from the child's requirements. One of the main reasons for producing *Medicines for Children* was the need to have a single authoritative consensus source which would provide a defence for practising paediatricians and avoid the need for individual prescribers to find the dose from a multitude of possible sources. In *Medicines for Children*, we have given dosages in the age bands proposed in *Licensing Medicines for Children* (RCPCH publications 1996), and which are now in the European Union guidance on *Clinical Investigation of Medicinal Products in Children* (1997).

The introduction to the first edition closed with the statement that 'There is much to do by all concerned if children are to get the full benefit of modern medicines'. Even in the short time since 1999, much progress has been made. The first step has been to increase awareness of the problems of prescribing for children and the disadvantage children may suffer. *Medicines for Children* has helped highlight these problems. The UK Committee on Safety of Medicines now has a paediatric working group, training posts in paediatric clinical pharmacology have been established and the Medicines Control Agency is developing a paediatric strategy, and looking at ways of enhancing pharmacovigilance in children. The Council of the European Union has resolved 'to ensure that new medicinal products for children and medicinal products already on the market, are fully adapted to the specific needs of that population group'.

However, much more still needs to be done. The major obstacle remains the dearth of good data in children on the pharmacokinetics ('what the child does to the drug'), pharmacodynamics ('what the drug does to the child') and safety of many drugs. Whilst the first aim of this book is to present current practice based on the authority of experts, a second and equally important objective is to identify those medicines which need further evaluation. The recent RCPCH statement on research ethics clarifies that children can participate in studies not of direct benefit to themselves and the European Parliament have supported this position.
http://www.rcpch.ac.uk/publications/BPSU/Ethics_Advice_summary_May_2001.pdf

There is some evidence that children enrolled into trials have better outcomes, irrespective of which arm of the trial they are randomised to, and many paediatricians would argue that it is unethical not to undertake drug trials in children. It is not acceptable that children require medicines which have not been properly tested. Sadly, when research in children exists, paediatricians do not always follow the recommendations. Doctors and others who prescribe medicines for children must be familiar with current opinion on their effectiveness and safety. The second edition of *Medicines for Children* helps address this need.

Introductory notes

DRUG MONOGRAPHS

The drug monographs are (with a few exceptions) presented in alphabetical order by generic name and are indexed and cross referenced. Dosage information in the majority of monographs is presented in tabular form using age bands as recommended in *Licensing Medicines for Children* 1996, a joint report of the British Paediatric Association (BPA) and the Association of the British Pharmaceutical Industry (ABPI), namely: newborn (birth to 1 month), 1 month-2 years, 2-12 years and 12-18 years. The dose may be stated on a dose per weight basis (generally in the younger age groups) or by dose per age band (more commonly in the older age groups). Occasionally, the dose is stated in a dose per surface area basis.

An example of a monograph table is given. The actual dose to be prescribed/administered is stated in the shaded part of the table followed by the frequency of dosing in a separate column. This method is chosen in preference to stating the total daily dose which requires further calculation to derive the actual dose to be prescribed/administered. Occasionally, if appropriate, a maximum total daily dose is given for some medications in the 'Notes' column.

Route	Age				Frequency	Notes
	birth–1 month	1 month-2 years	2–12 years	12–18 years	(times daily)	
Oral	1mg/kg	← 2mg/kg →		20mg	4	
IV bolus	← 300–400 microgram/kg →			10–15mg	single dose	

A small number of tables will state a dose to be prescribed/administered on the basis of both weight and age within the same age band, e.g. clonazepam. The table below shows how this is clearly marked with a warning to avoid a dosage error.

Route	Age				Frequency	Notes
	birth–1 month	1 month-2 years	2–12 years	12–18 years	(times daily)	
Oral	–	**DOSE BY WEIGHT** ← 25 microgram/kg →		–	1	Starting dose. May be given at night.
		DOSE BY AGE <5 years 250 microgram		1mg	1	Higher, divided doses have been used (up to 100 microgram/kg/day).
		5–12 years 500 microgram			1	

GOOD PRESCRIBING PRACTICE

☐ Ensure that all relevant patient details, including full name, address/hospital number, age and current weight (in kg) are included on the prescription

☐ Ensure that a child's allergy status is known before prescribing, dispensing or administering any medication

☐ Take care to establish a full medication history

☐ Medicines should be prescribed by their approved name in full, printed clearly in block capitals, dated and signed

☐ The dosage of single medicine preparations, whether in liquid or solid form, should be prescribed as a weight, i.e. gram (g), milligram (mg), microgram, nanogram or unit

☐ The dosage of a preparation containing two or more medicines should be prescribed using the proprietary name and quantity required, e.g. Ketovite® liquid 5mL once daily

☐ It is not acceptable to write prn alone after a medicine. The clinical indication (e.g. pyrexia, pain relief), minimum time interval, dose and route of administration must be specified

☐ Cancellation of a prescription should be carried out by drawing a line distinctly through the entry to be cancelled. The date of cancellation and signature should be recorded

☐ For hospital in-patients the nurse in charge must be informed of any change in prescription

☐ Medicines dispensed from wards and A&E should be provided in child resistant containers with the following information:
   a) patient name
   b) date of issue
   c) name of medicine
   d) dosage (for patient information this should also be recorded as a volume for liquid preparations, number of tablets or capsules, etc.)
   e) route of administration
   f) frequency of administration
   g) duration of course

☐ Professional pharmaceutical advice should be sought before making modifications to medications, e.g. crushing tablets.

AVOIDING MEDICATION ERRORS

Children are at increased risk of medication errors. This is due to a combination of factors including the need for calculations to be performed at all stages of the process. Calculations are required in the prescribing, dispensing and administration of medicines because drug doses tend to vary with the age and weight of the child. The lack of suitable dosage formulations also means that it is necessary to use vials, tablets and oral liquids that have been designed for adults.

One of the most common errors seen is the ten-fold dosing error. Errors can also be generated because children and their carers tend to remember doses in mL rather than mg. Oral liquids may be available in a variety of strengths sometimes with a ten-fold difference in concentration.

☐ Take care with calculations - use your head as well as a calculator
☐ If possible, always obtain a second independent check of a calculation of dosage
☐ Avoid the use of decimal points by prescribing in whole units, i.e. 100 microgram rather than 0.1mg
☐ If a decimal point is required always use a leading zero, i.e. 0.5mg
☐ Never use a trailing zero, i.e. state 5mg and not 5.0mg as the latter can lead to a ten-fold overdose
☐ There is no accepted abbreviation for microgram, nanogram or unit. Replacing unit by 'U' can be misinterpreted as a zero causing a ten-fold overdose
☐ Remember to take account of any administration issues such as displacement volume for IV medicines, the correct diluent and administration method.

REGIONAL MEDICINES INFORMATION SERVICES

Information about all aspects of drug therapy can be obtained from Regional Medicines Information Services which can be contacted by telephoning the following numbers:

England

Birmingham	(0121) 311 1974
Bristol	(0117) 928 2867
Ipswich	(01473) 704430/1
Leeds	(0113) 245 0530
	(0113) 392 3547
Leicester	(0116) 255 5779
	(0116) 258 6491
Liverpool	(0151) 794 8117
	(0151) 794 8206

Introductory notes

London

Guy's	(020) 7955 5000 Ext. 3594/5892
Northwick Park	(020) 8869 3973/2763
Newcastle	(0191) 232 1525
Southampton	(023) 8079 6908/9

Wales

Cardiff	(029) 2074 2979/2251

Scotland

Aberdeen	(01224) 552316
Dundee	(01382) 632351
Edinburgh	(0131) 536 2843
Glasgow	(0141) 211 4407

Northern Ireland

Belfast	(028) 9063 2032

Republic of Ireland

Dublin	(003531) 473 0589

DRUG INFORMATION ADVISORY LINE (DIAL)

DIAL is a paediatric medicines information service based in the Medicines Information Unit of the Pharmacy Department at the Royal Liverpool Children's NHS Trust (Alder Hey), Liverpool. The service is available to healthcare professionals working in the UK and Ireland. It supports and complements local services, rather than replaces them.

In the first instance, enquiries should usually be directed to the local Medicines Information Service or the Regional Medicines Information Service (listed above). Poisoning enquiries should be directed to the Poisons Information Service (0870 600 6266).

DIAL: Paediatric Drug (Medicines) Information Advisory Line

Tel: 0151 252 5837

Email: info@dial.org.uk

FURTHER INFORMATION

Further to the information given by the Regional Medicines Information Services, general advice on the prescribing of medicines to children can be sought from Professor Imti Choonara, Academic Division of Child Health, Derbyshire Children's Hospital.

Tel: 01332 625635.

Email: Imti.Choonara@nottingham.ac.uk

USE OF RECOMMENDED INTERNATIONAL NON-PROPRIETARY NAMES (rINN) AND BRITISH APPROVED NAMES (BAN).

As directive 92/27EEC requires the use of rINN for medicinal substances, this nomenclature has been adopted as standard throughout the second edition of *Medicines for Children*. In most cases the rINN is exactly the same as the BAN. Where they differ the rINN is followed by the BAN in brackets, e.g. furosemide (frusemide). This is a change from the first edition. The only exception to this rule is in the case of adrenaline where the BAN is used in preference to the rINN which appears in brackets i.e. adrenaline (epinephrine).

GLOSSARY OF TERMS

Product licence (PL)
A licence to market a particular drug product, granted by the Licensing Authority of the MCA. A licence is issued on application when the Licensing Authority is satisfied regarding the product's inherent safety, quality and efficacy for the indicated purpose or purposes. Enables a product to be placed on the market for its licensed use.

Manufacturers licence (ML)
Issued when the Licensing Authority is satisfied that an applicant can manufacture and/or assemble medicinal products to acceptable standards so as to ensure the safety, quality and efficacy of those products.

Licensed medicinal products
Products in respect of which a PL has been granted and which have been manufactured and assembled by the holder of a ML.

'Specials'
Medicinal products in respect of which a PL is not in existence but which have been made by the holder of a special manufacturers licence to the order of a practitioner for administration to a particular patient. Practitioners who order 'specials' should be aware that they have a responsibility for the safety and efficacy of that product for their particular patient. Pharmacists who procure and sell or supply 'specials' have a responsibility for the inherent quality and safety of the product being sold or supplied.

Extemporaneously prepared medicinal products
These are products which are prepared in a registered pharmacy, hospital or health centre by or under the supervision of a pharmacist in accordance with a prescription given by a practitioner or in anticipation of such a prescription and with a view to dispensing the product.

Prepared products have a similar status to that of 'specials'. The preparing or supervising pharmacist has a professional responsibility for the inherent quality and safety of the product supplied. These products are not, however, subjected to full quality assurance.

Central Intravenous Additive Service (CIVAS)
A hospital pharmacy service which provides, for example, reconstituted antibiotic injections in individual doses, in a ready to administer form, in accordance with a prescription from a doctor.

Unlicensed, 'off-label', 'off-licence'
Many drugs used for children are used outside the specification of the PL, i.e. are 'unlicensed'. The drug itself may be unlicensed, i.e. an unlicensed medicine, or it may be given by an unlicensed route of administration or for an unlicensed indication or at an unlicensed dose. There may be age limits on its use or it may be unlicensed for use in children. Sometimes the terms 'Off-label' or 'Off-licence' may be used to describe a medicine which is being used outside the specifications of the PL.

Named patient basis
When a commercial company supplies a product for which no PL exists, it is supplied on a named patient basis. The company will generally require a consultant's name, patient name and details of the condition which the drug will be used to treat.

Excipient
A substance that is added to a dosage form in order to facilitate the preparation, patient acceptability and functioning of that dosage form as a drug delivery system. Excipients include diluents, lubricants, suspending agents, flavouring agents etc. They should have no pharmacological action themselves. Those excipients which may potentially cause a problem for certain groups of patients, for example, sugar for patients with diabetes and aspartame for those with phenylketonuria, have been listed in the drug monographs.

Borderline substances
These are products (foods or toilet preparations) which the Advisory Committee on Borderline Substances (ACBS) have stated can be regarded as drugs for the management of specified conditions, e.g. Aminogran® for phenylketonuria.

Summary of product characteristics (SPC)
These are information sheets for medicinal products produced by pharmaceutical companies. SPCs are prepared by the individual companies concerned and, in consequence, vary somewhat in style, but all follow the European Commission's Committee for Proprietary Medicinal Products (CPMP) *Note for Guidance (for SPCs)*.

ABBREVIATIONS

AIDS	acquired immune deficiency syndrome
AUC	area under the curve
CNS	central nervous system
CSF	cerebral spinal fluid
DNA	deoxyribonucleic acid
ECG	electrocardiogram
EEG	electroencephalogram
ETT	endotracheal tube
FBC	full blood count
G6PD	glucose 6-phosphate dehydrogenase
GFR	glomerular filtration rate
HIV	human immunodeficiency virus
IM	intramuscular
INR	international normalised ratio
IP	intraperitoneally
ITU	intensive therapy unit
IV	intravenous
LFT	liver function test
MAOI	monoamine-oxidase inhibitor
NaCl	sodium chloride
NSAID	non-steroidal anti-inflammatory drug
PN	parenteral nutrition
RNA	ribonucleic acid
SC	subcutaneous
SPC	summary of product characteristics
U&E	urea and electrolytes
UK	United Kingdom

Units of measurement

g	gram
hr(s)	hour (s)
kg	kilogram
kJ	kilojoules
dL	decilitre
L	litre
mg	milligram
min(s)	minute (s)
mL	millilitre
mmol	millimole
mth	month
mOsm/L	milliosmols per litre
ppm	parts per million
yr(s)	year (s)

The abbreviations yr(s), hr(s) and min(s) have only been used when absolutely necessary. Whenever possible these have not been abbreviated.

Symbols

$\geq$	greater than or equal to
$>$	greater than
$\leq$	less than or equal to
$<$	less than
$\equiv$	equivalent to

Age-mean weight and surface area for age-dose percentages

Age	Mean weight for age		Height		Body surface area	% Adult dose
	kg	lb	cm	inches	m²	
Newborn*	3.5	7.7	50	20	0.23	12.5
1 month	4.2	9	55	22	0.26	14.5
3 months	5.6	12	59	23	0.32	18
6 months	7.7	17	67	26	0.40	22
1 year	10	22	76	30	0.47	25
3 years	15	33	94	37	0.62	33
5 years	18	40	108	42	0.73	40
7 years	23	50	120	47	0.88	50
12 years	39	86	148	58	1.25	75
Adult male	68	150	173	68	1.8	100
Adult female	56	123	163	64	1.6	100

*Full term newborn infant

The percentage adult dose method should not be used to calculate doses if paediatric doses in mg/kg or mg/m² are available. Newborn and preterm newborn infants may need reduced dosage.

USING WEIGHT ALONE TO CALCULATE BODY SURFACE AREA

The United Kingdom Children's Cancer Study Group (UKCCSG) Chemotherapy Standardisation group 1998 have produced tables for estimation of body surface area (based on body weight only) in infants and children. They have also produced recommendations of what percentage of calculated dose by body surface area (of cytotoxic drugs) to give to infants (≤1 year or ≤10kg). These tables and dosage recommendations can be obtained from UKCCSG or any regional paediatric cancer treatment centre.

An alternative method of calculating surface area based on body weight only is:

$$\text{Surface area (m}^2) \quad = \quad \frac{4 \times \text{Weight (kg)} + 7}{\text{Weight (kg)} + 90}$$

Many nomograms underestimate the body surface area in infants and small children, therefore separate nomograms for infants (fig 1) and children (fig 2) have been included (Reprinted from *The Journal of Pediatrics*, Vol 93, Haycock *et al*, "Geometric method for measuring body surface area: A height-weight formula validated in infants, children and adults", pages 62-66, copyright 1978, with permission from Elsevier Science).

Calculation of body surface area

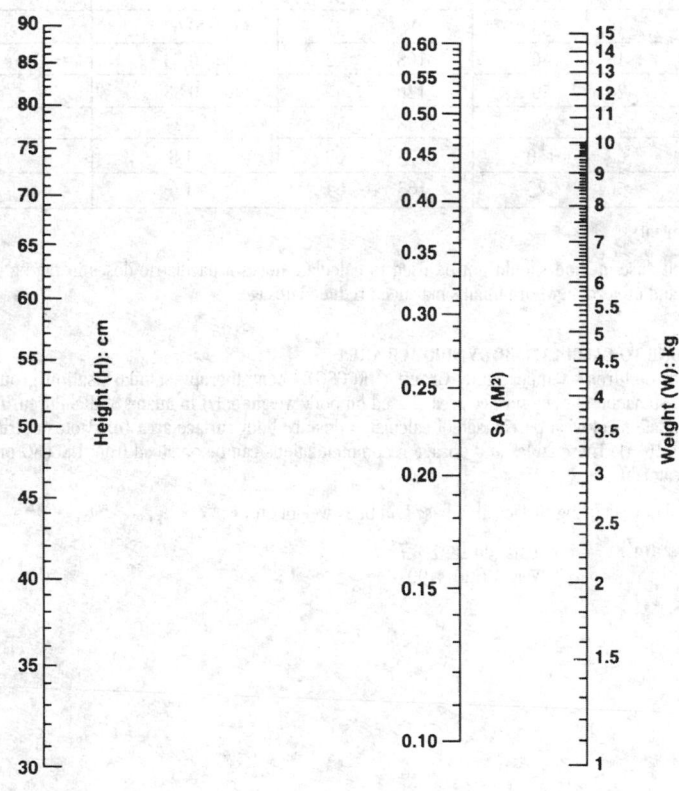

$$SA = W^{0.5378} \times H^{0.3964} \times 0.024265$$

Fig 1. Nomogram representing the relationship between height, weight and body surface area in infants.

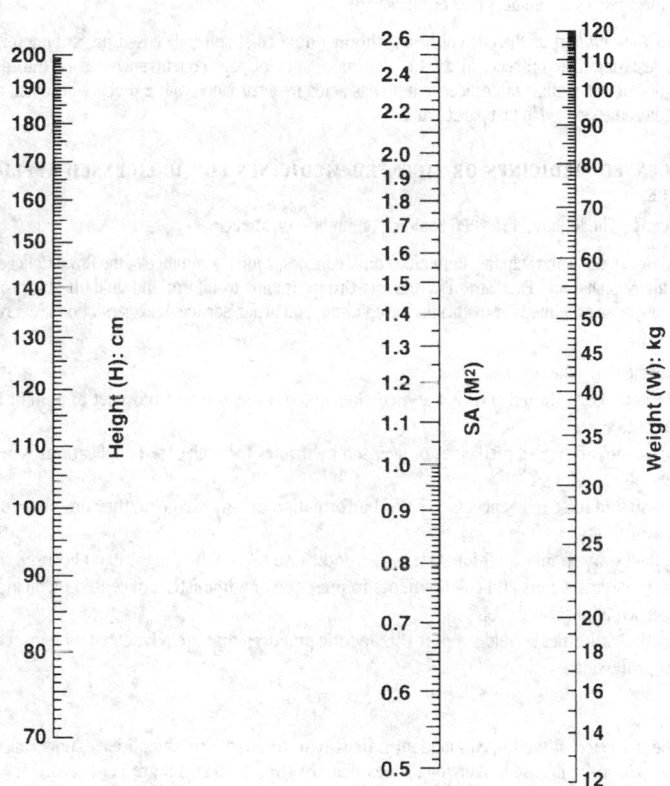

$$SA = W^{0.5378} \times H^{0.3964} \times 0.024265$$

Fig 2. Nomogram representing the relationship between height, weight and body surface area in children and adults.

THE LICENSING OF MEDICINES

Before a pharmaceutical company can promote a drug, it must obtain a licence. The company must demonstrate the safety, quality and efficacy of the drug when given in the dose and for the disease and age group recommended in the Summary of Product Characteristics (SPC). In the UK, doctors can legally prescribe drugs without a licence (unlicensed) or outside the terms of the licence (off-label) (e.g. in a different dose, as a different formulation or for a different disease or age group). Prescribing outside the licence is relatively common for children. As many as 90% of infants on a neonatal intensive care unit receive unlicensed or off-label drugs and in primary care, up to one third of prescriptions for children are unlicensed/off-label. The Joint Standing Committee on Medicines of the Royal College of Paediatrics and Child Health and the Neonatal and Paediatric Pharmacists Group has produced a position statement on the use of unlicensed medicines in children and the current updated version follows on the succeeding pages. This explains the anomalous position of drugs used for children (about which hospital managers, lawyers and therapeutics committees may be unaware).

The status of *Medicines for Children* as the current best authority on off-label and unlicensed prescribing for children may assist paediatricians in justifying their practice. In the UK, the importance of peer concurrence can be traced to the Bolam judgement of 1957: 'A doctor is not guilty of negligence if he has acted in accordance with a practice accepted as proper by a responsible body of medical men skilled in that particular art'.

THE USE OF UNLICENSED MEDICINES OR LICENSED MEDICINES FOR UNLICENSED APPLICATIONS IN PAEDIATRIC PRACTICE

Policy statement produced by The Joint RCPCH/NPPG Standing Committee on Medicines

This statement has been drawn up by the Standing Committee on Medicines, a joint committee of the Royal College of Paediatrics and Child Health and the Neonatal and Paediatric Pharmacists Group. It aims to inform and guide health professionals and parents who prescribe, dispense or administer medicines for children, and health service managers who have a responsibility to support them.

The recommendations of the Committee are that:

☐ Those who prescribe for a child should choose the medicine which offers the best prospect of benefit for that child, with due regard to cost.

☐ The informed use of some unlicensed medicines or licensed medicines for unlicensed applications is necessary in paediatric practice.

☐ Health professionals should have ready access to sound information on any medicine they prescribe, dispense or administer, and its availability.

☐ In general, it is not necessary to take additional steps, beyond those taken when prescribing licensed medicines, to obtain the consent of parents, carers and child patients to prescribe or administer unlicensed medicines or licensed medicines for unlicensed applications.

☐ NHS Trusts and Health Authorities should support therapeutic practices that are advocated by a respectable, responsible body of professional opinion.

LICENSING

1. For a medicine to be marketed in the United Kingdom it must have received a product licence, now called a marketing authorisation. It is then said to be licensed. Many medicines that are given to children are not licensed for the particular indication, age of the child, suitable formulation, or route of administration. This position arises when a pharmaceutical company has made an application to the Licensing Authority for a marketing authorisation for use of the medicine in adults, but chooses not to make an application for the use of that medicine in particular ways in children. Certain medicines that are given to children have not received a licence for any indication, and are said to be unlicensed.

2. The use of unlicensed medicines or licensed medicines for unlicensed applications is necessary in paediatric practice when there is no suitable alternative. Such uses are informed and guided by a respectable and responsible body of professional opinion.

3. The Medicines Act and Regulations (which incorporate the relevant EC directives) provide exemptions which enable doctors to:

☐ Prescribe unlicensed medicines

☐ Use in particular (named) patients, unlicensed products specially prepared, imported or supplied

☐ Use medicines which are not authorised to be marketed, in clinical trials, after approval of the trial by the Medicines Control Agency (MCA) either through the Doctors and Dentists Exemption Scheme or, in the case of pharmaceutical industry sponsorship, through the Trials Certificate (Exemption) Scheme

☐ Use or advise the use of licensed medicines for indications, or in doses, or by routes of administration, outside the recommendations of the licence

☐ Override the warnings and the precautions given in the licence.

4. In each case, the doctor has to be able to justify the action taken as being in accordance with a respectable, responsible body of professional opinion.

The informed use of unlicensed medicines or of licensed medicines for unlicensed applications is necessary in paediatric practice.

SOURCES OF INFORMATION

5. Although the choice of a medicine is not necessarily determined by its licence status, it will take account of information made available as a consequence of licensing and contained in the marketing authorisation. When the product licence does not include indications for use in children, the marketing authorisation is of limited help. When the medicine is unlicensed, the necessary information must be sought elsewhere. It often is available, though might not be readily accessible.

6. To meet the need for accessible sound information and guidance the Committee has undertaken the preparation of a new formulary, *Medicines for Children*. The standing of its contributors and of those who undertake independent review will ensure that it is an authoritative statement of paediatric therapeutic practice in the UK.

INFORMATION FOR OTHER HEALTH PROFESSIONALS AND THE PUBLIC

7. Parents, patients and teachers, and others in *loco parentis*, require information about medicines from health professionals, including general practitioners, paediatricians, nurses, health visitors, and pharmacists. The information must be given in a way they can understand, and be accurate and consistent. This is particularly important when the specialist who has advised the use of unlicensed medicines or licensed medicines for unlicensed applications, hands over the care of the patient and responsibility for the administration of the medicine to someone else. Given the complexity of therapeutic and pharmacological information, and the burdens upon those giving and receiving it, the need is for sound, practical and sensible arrangements for communication, supplemented by readily available sources of reference.

It is essential that health professionals should have ready access to sound information on any medicine they prescribe, dispense or administer, and on its availability.

CONSENT OF PARENTS, CARERS AND PATIENTS

8. Health professionals must respect the right of child patients and their parents to participate in decisions on the health care of the child, and seek to ensure that those decisions are properly informed. In normal paediatric practice no additional steps, beyond those taken when prescribing licensed medicines, are required to obtain the consent of patients and parents/carers for the use of unlicensed medicines.

9. Clinicians are anxious that the licence status of a drug should not be perceived as reflecting what is or is not best for the child. They are mindful of a possible impact upon the confidence of parents and patients who might then be reluctant to accept advice, with consequences for a child who might not receive a medicine that offers benefit.

10. Most licensed medicines are dispensed in standard packages together with a Patient Information Leaflet (PIL) approved by the Licensing Authority. When the licence does not include indications for children, the PIL may caution against such use. Naturally, this may undermine confidence in the advice given by health professionals, besides provoking a call for explanation. The Committee has produced two generic PILs, for patients and parents/carers respectively, which explains why it may be necessary to prescribe unlicensed medicines or to use licensed medicines for unlicensed applications. This leaflet will be made widely available to hospitals and pharmacies and may be of practical value in such situations.

11. There are circumstances when a clinician will decide to give fuller information than is usually judged necessary. These may arise when a medicine is new or experimental; or carries known or possible risks of harm, even if those risks are small in relation to the disorder to be treated; or when the concerns of some parents, carers or patients generate a need for more detailed discussion and explanation on the medicines that are prescribed. In each instance, practice is guided by clinical judgement.

We consider that in general it is not necessary to take additional steps, beyond those taken when prescribing licensed medicines, to obtain the consent of parents, carers and child patients to prescribe or administer unlicensed medicines or licensed medicines for unlicensed applications.

POLICIES OF NHS TRUSTS

12. Some NHS Trusts have suggested that a clinician should not use an unlicensed medicine, or a licensed medicine for unlicensed application. In 1993 the Department of Health stated that it would not expect that a health authority would seek to fetter a clinician's freedom to prescribe by expressly directing its medical staff against prescribing unlicensed products or licensed products for unlicensed purposes. The Department of Health's lawyers also stated that, should a health authority so direct its medical staff, a court would be reluctant to support the authority in those circumstances.

13. However, the emphasis on risk management and evidence based medicine in the clinical governance framework implies that Trusts may be encouraged to introduce systems and protocols to monitor, and even direct, the use of both licensed and unlicensed medicines. We understand that, because the Medicines Act's (1968) exemptions remain current, the courts would not hold the prescription of an unlicensed medicine to be a breach of the duty of care, if that treatment was supported by a respected body of medical opinion. The best evidence available should always inform the prescription of medicines for children.

We consider that NHS Trusts should support therapeutic practices that are advocated by a respectable, responsible body of professional opinion.

REFERENCES

British Paediatric Association. *A Paediatrician's Guide to the UN Convention on the Rights of the Child.* London: British Paediatric Association, 1995.

A Report of the Joint Working Party of the British Paediatric Association and the Association of the British Pharmaceutical Industry. *Licensing Medicines for Children.* London: Royal College of Paediatrics and Child Health, 1996.

The General Medical Council. *Good Medical Practice.* London: The General Medical Council, 1998.

The General Medical Council. *Seeking Patients' Consent: The Ethical Considerations.* London: The General Medical Council, 1999.

Department of Health. *Letter to the President, British Paediatric Association*, 3 November 1993. Department of Health, London.

Nurse prescribing

In October 2000, proposals for the extension of nurse prescribing were published for consultation. The outcome of this process was that other groups of nurses (i.e. not just those with a district nurse and health visitor qualification) will be eligible to become independent nurse prescribers. DNs and HVs who are already nurse prescribers will continue to prescribe from the current Nurse Prescribers' Formulary (NPF). Once trained the new independent nurse prescribers will be able to prescribe from a wider range of medicines. These will include all General Sale List (GSL) and pharmacy medicines (P). They will also include a list of Prescription only Medicines (PoM) linked to specified medical criteria in four areas:- minor injuries, minor ailments, health promotion, and maintenance and palliative care. The list of medicines and clinical areas is available on the Department of Health website www.doh.gov.uk/nurseprescribing/pomlist.htm Those nurses and midwives who successfully complete the **extended independent prescribing** course will be responsible for the assessment of patients with undiagnosed conditions and for decisions about the clinical management required including prescribing.

In addition, consultation is underway to allow **supplementary prescribing**. Following clinical assessment and once a diagnosis has been established or a treatment plan prepared, responsibility for clinical management including prescribing could pass to another health professional.

Other nurses and midwives may also continue to use **patient group directions (PGD)**. This is a written instruction relating to the supply and/or administration of a PoM in an identified clinical situation. It applies to groups of patients or other service users who may not be individually identified before presentation for treatment. When drafting a PGD it is imperative to follow not only the guidance laid down by Crown (DoH, 1998) but the information which is dictated necessary by the NHS Executive and required by statutory law (NHS Executive, 2000).

DoH (1998) *Review of Prescribing, Supply and Administration of Medicines. Report on the Supply & Administration of Medicines under Group Protocols.* London, HMSO.

NHS Exec (2000) *Patient Group Directions [England only] Health Service Circular* 2000:026. Leeds, NHSE.

ADVERSE DRUG REACTIONS IN CHILDREN
Any medicine may produce an unwanted or unexpected adverse drug reaction (ADR). Detection and recording of these is of vital importance. ADR is not synonymous with 'drug side-effect'. It is not necessary for you to be certain that the drug caused the reaction. Spontaneous reporting of suspected reactions is particularly valuable for recognising possible new hazards rapidly.

The Yellow Card Scheme
Doctors, dentists, coroners, pharmacists and nurses are urged to help by reporting adverse reactions to:
MHRA
CSM Freepost
London SW8 5BR
info@mhra.gsi.gov.uk
(0800 731 6789)
Alternatively, reporters within the regions listed at the end of this section may report to their local Regional Monitoring Centre.

Prepaid yellow cards for reporting are available from the above address and are also bound in this book (inside back cover). For on-line reporting, please see the Medicines and Healthcare products Regulatory Agency (MHRA) (formerly the Medicines Control Agency (MCA)) website www.mca.gov.uk/yellowcard. The reporting of all suspected adverse drug reactions in children is strongly encouraged through the yellow card scheme even if the intensive monitoring symbol (▼) has been removed, because experience in children may still be limited. The Committee on Safety of Medicines (CSM) recommends that those using medicines in children should report all suspected ADRs which occur in children, regardless of whether the medicines are licensed for use in children.

The Black Triangle Scheme
A black triangle printed next to the name of a medicine indicates that MCA/CSM are closely monitoring the product (usually for a minimum of 2 years) because:
☐ It contains a new active substance
☐ It requires administration through a new route
☐ It uses a novel drug delivery system
☐ It is given for significant new indications which may alter the established risks and benefits of the drug.

The MHRA asks that the black triangle is used in the Summary of Product Characteristics (SPC), British National Formulary (BNF), Monthly Index of Medical Specialities (MIMS) and advertisements. Doctors, dentists, coroners, pharmacists and nurses should report all suspected ADRs involving black triangle drugs. For non-black-triangle products, reports are sought only for reactions in adults that are severe or unusual but MHRA/CSM recommends that all reactions in children are reported as mentioned previously.

Suspected adverse reactions to any therapeutic agent should be reported, including drugs (*self-medication* as well as *prescribed* ones), blood products, vaccines, X-ray contrast media, dental or surgical materials, intra-uterine devices, herbal products and contact lens fluids.

The identification and reporting of ADRs in children is particularly important because:
☐ The action of the drug and its disposition in children (especially in the very young) may be different from that in adults
☐ Drugs may be less intensively tested in children
☐ Many drugs are not specifically licensed for use in children and are used 'off-label'
☐ Suitable formulations may not be available to allow precise dosing in children
☐ The nature and course of illnesses and ADRs may differ between adults and children.

Further information on adverse reactions to drugs
A 24-hour Freefone service is available to all parts of the UK for advice and information on suspected ADRs: contact the National Yellow Card Information Service at the MHRA on 0800 731 6789. Outside office hours a telephone answering machine will take messages.

Adverse drug reactions

The following regional centres also collect data:

CSM Mersey
Freepost
Liverpool L3 3AB
0151 794 8206

CSM Wales
Freepost
Cardiff CF14 1ZZ
029 2074 4181

CSM Northern and Yorkshire
Freepost 1085
Newcastle-upon-Tyne NE1 1BR
0191 232 1525

CSM West Midlands
Freepost SW2991
Birmingham B18 7BR
0121 507 5672

CSM Scotland
FREEPOST
SCO7777
Edinburgh
EH3 0BR
0131 242 2919

More detailed information on reporting can be found on the MHRA website www.mca.gov.uk

Giving medicines

Medicines vary in form and are given by different routes.

Route		Form
By mouth	Liquid	solutions, suspensions, syrups, elixirs, emulsions, oils.
	Solid	tablets, capsules, granules, lozenges, beads.
Inhaled		metered dose inhalers, powder devices, compressed air nebulisers.
Into the ear		solutions, suspensions, drops.
Into the eye		solutions, suspensions, drops, ointments.
Into the nose		solutions, suspensions, drops, ointments, sprays.
On the skin		solutions, suspensions, ointments, sprays, creams, lotions, pastes, powders, shampoos and soaps.
In the mouth		lozenges, chewing gum, sublingual tablets (rarely).
Injected Subcutaneous Intramuscular Intravenous Intrathecal Intraosseous		water solutions, suspensions, and oil in water emulsions, depending on the route.
Into the rectum		enemas – large and small – water solutions, suspensions, oils, suppositories, ointments.

If possible, children should know why they need a medicine and be shown how they can take it. Young children and infants who cannot understand will usually take medicine from someone they know and trust – a parent or main carer.

It is important that those who give medicines know about the medicine and how to give it. Occasionally a medicine has to be disguised. Rarely, a child has to be restrained for the medicine to be administered. Then, especially, the child should be comforted and reassured. They must not be left with the impression that being given medicine is a punishment for being sick.

The approach depends on the child's understanding and the circumstances:
- □ *Under 2 years.* Administration by parents if possible, using an approach which they believe is most likely to succeed.
- □ *2–5 year olds* need a calm, gentle, firm and efficient approach after they have been told what is happening. Play and acting out may help them understand. Rewards and an acceptable 'chaser' (drink) encourage further collaboration.
- □ *5–12 year olds* also need encouragement, respect for their trust, and an explanation attuned to their understanding.
- □ *Over 12 years.* At this age children must have a proper understanding of what is happening and share in the decision making as well as the responsibility. They must feel in control.

BY MOUTH
Liquids. Children under 5 years are unlikely to accept tablets, though they may well swallow whatever they find in the medicine cabinet, or indeed in any other place. Older children also often prefer liquids. Liquid formulations sometimes have the disadvantage of an unpleasant taste and the accuracy of the dose may be less. The taste of medicines may be disguised by flavouring or by mixing them with, or following them immediately by, favourite foods or drinks. Mixing the drugs with food may cause dosage problems and influence absorption. Guidance is given with the individual drugs.

□ Do NOT mix medicines in a baby's bottle.

Liquid medicines may contain 'excipients' which enhance stability and acceptability. It may be important to know what they are, for example sugar, sodium and alcohol content. Some medicines may be held in solution by oils to which the child may be sensitive. Sugar-free medicines should be dispensed whenever possible.

Domestic teaspoons vary in size and are not a reliable measure. Users need to be shown how the administering device works, including the 5mL medicine spoon! Often they are not interchangeable. Plastic oral syringes are a welcome development, for they avoid the need to dilute liquids to a 5mL dose with the consequent effects on stability and can deliver volumes accurately into the mouth. They are available from pharmacists.

Tablets. Tablets are convenient, compact, stable, portable and relatively cheap. A liquid 'chaser' should follow the tablet down. Most tablets can be crushed and most capsules emptied to make a suspension in something acceptable to the child.

□ Do NOT break slow release or enteric coated tablets.

Down a feeding tube. Children with feeding tubes in place should be encouraged to take medicines by mouth. This may not be possible if, for example, the tube is in place because of a problem with swallowing. Liquid medicines can be given via the tube, provided special precautions are taken to avoid the tube being blocked by the medicine. The liquid formulation should flow easily down the tube and the medicine should be 'washed' through with warm water.

□ If medicines are given to a newborn infant via a nasogastric tube, then sterile water must be used.

Medicines may be mixed with enteric feeds provided the two are compatible. In general, continuous feeding should be discontinued for 15 minutes before giving a medicine down the tube, unless otherwise specified.

Evening doses of oral medicines are given about half an hour before bedtime.

INHALED
Giving drugs by inhalation for respiratory conditions delivers the medicine to where it is most needed, uses a lower dose and has fewer side-effects. Allowing the child a say in the choice of device to be used improves the chances of success. Inhalation therapy is least reliable when the child is not co-operative or very distressed.

The teaching of technique and good care of the devices is essential for success. Regular review is necessary to ensure that the devices remain effective and that the child uses the system most appropriate to their ability. Because products and delivery systems vary, it is important that the manufacturers directions are followed precisely.

Spacers with metered dose inhalers (MDI). The child breathes in and out of a reservoir filled with an aerosol from an MDI. It does not require 'hand-lung' co-ordination. A mouth piece or facemask may be used. The inspiratory breath must be sufficient to visibly or audibly open the valve. A tidal volume of 10mL/kg can be used to estimate the number of breaths required to empty the spacer. If necessary the child should be supine and the inhaler and spacer held at 90° (vertical) in order to keep the valve open. Spacers should be cleaned weekly by washing, and standing in air to dry but they should not be wiped. They should be replaced annually.

Dry powder inhalers. To use these correctly children need to be able to take a good deep breath in, to draw the powder into the airways. They need to be able to hold their breath and not to blow out first.

Nebulisers can be used in children of all ages. The child breathes an aerosol through a facemask or preferably, a mouthpiece. A mouthpiece gives better deposition.

Breath–activated inhalers do not require co-ordination but the child must be able to take a deep breath.

Metered dose inhalers require a child to press and breathe in at the same time. Most school children cannot manage them and their use without spacers is not encouraged. A spacer should always be used if a corticosteroid is being administered via a metered dose inhaler.

INTO THE EYE
Medicines should be kept sterile. The ideal is to drop the solution or squeeze the ointment into a gully formed by gentle pressure of a finger on the lower lid. Tilt the head back or lie the child down and direct the gaze of the child upwards. Avoid touching the eye. Alternatively, lie the infant on his or her back, drop the solution or ointment into the corner, wait until the infant's eyes open and then gently mop away the excess. Gentle finger pressure on the inner corner of the eye to occlude the tear duct enhances the effect of the eye drop. Massage the ointment into the upper and lower conjunctival sacs with finger massage on the upper and lower lids.

INTO THE EAR
This is to treat conditions of the external auditory canal, which is not sterile. To administer ear drops, place the head on one side and pull the ear back and down for the infant, and back and up for the older child.

INTO THE NOSE
The lining of the nose is very vascular, so the intranasal route offers an alternative to an injection to achieve a systemic effect. This is the chosen route for some peptides (e.g. desmopressin). Currently however, most nose drops are given for the treatment of local conditions. Lie the child on his or her back with neck extended and instil the drops, then sit him or her up, and tilt the head forward.

ON TO THE SKIN
Topical application is mainly directed at treating disorders of the skin. However, it can be used as a route for drugs with systemic effect, and it must always be remembered that topical drugs may cause systemic toxicity, particularly if applied to damaged skin or to preterm infants. Generally the skin is left exposed, but a wet dressing may facilitate absorption, and a dry dressing may be used for protection.

BY INJECTION
Drugs may be injected into most of the body spaces. The drugs must be sterile and pyrogen free. The skin may be washed and then cleaned with antiseptic (70% isopropyl alcohol) or in children not sensitive to iodine, an iodophor (e.g. Betadine®). If the alcohol is not allowed to evaporate, this may add to the pain of injection. A topical anaesthetic cream may also be used (Emla® or Ametop®). Neither is common practice when insulin is self-administered or vaccines are given.

Children under 5 years should be held firmly; 5 to 12 year olds should be well supported but not overpowered; those over 12 years of age, like many adults, may be frightened of needles and their feelings need to be recognised and addressed. Many parents are a great help and will assist with restraining and comforting their child, but others find the experience upsetting and should not be forced to hold their child during the procedure, but encouraged to comfort afterwards.

Subcutaneous (SC). Small volumes (under 2mL) of isotonic solutions are usually given into the subcutaneous tissue using short needles with narrow bore and regular bevel. The subcutaneous route is used for insulin self-injection and although fat atrophy or hypertrophy can occur, this can be minimised by rotating injection sites, including the outer aspect of the upper arm, the anterior or lateral thigh, and the abdomen. In thinner children it may help to pick up the skin gently between the fingers to create a pocket in which to inject vertically.

Intramuscular (IM). Most drugs can be injected into muscle but the IM route should be avoided if at all possible. In practice the route is used for concentrated and irritating solutions which may cause local pain if injected subcutaneously and which cannot be given other ways. In a child who has already received several days of intravenous antibiotics and in whom cannulation has become difficult, two or three days of a once a day IM injection to complete the course may be preferable to multiple intravenous cannulation attempts. Thin infants may be given 1-2mL and bigger children 1-5mL, using needles of appropriate length for the site chosen. The shorter and the narrower the needle, the less pain it will cause. Some draw up the fluid with one needle and inject with another, to avoid the solution on the wet needle irritating the needle track. Using a single needle saves time and for most drugs leads to no extra reaction. Before injecting the solution, the plunger should be slightly withdrawn to check whether the needle has entered a blood vessel. If blood is withdrawn, another site must be chosen. IM injections should not be given to children on anticoagulants or to those with thrombocytopenia. As IM injections can damage muscles and leave deep scars, injection sites should be regularly inspected, particularly in the immobile and very sick.

The injection is vertical, and it may help to lift the muscle gently between the fingers. In children less than 5 years old, the muscle in the middle and outside of the thigh is used (vastus lateralis); the muscle in the front of the thigh (rectus femoris) is an alternative. For older children the upper outer quadrant of the buttock (dorsogluteal site) is safe, provided care is taken to avoid the sciatic nerve. The deltoid muscle is small in infants and is best avoided if possible, but can be used in older children and adolescents.

Creating a Z track may avoid irritation and discolouration due to injected solutions leaking back up the path of the needle.

In summary:

☐ Avoid IM injections if possible

☐ Never give IM injections if there is a bleeding problem

☐ The front or lateral thigh is safest.

Intravenous (IV). In hospital practice medicinal drugs not given orally are usually given IV rather than SC or IM, as the effect is quicker and more predictable, the pain of multiple injections is avoided and larger volumes can be given. The delivery systems are improving with sharp but short bevel needles and catheters that reduce the risk of damage to the vessel. Central venous access is used for children who need irritant or inotropic drugs, the administration of medicines over long periods and for home therapy with IV drugs. Aseptic technique is essential. The intrathecal, epidural and intraosseous routes should only be used by staff who have been trained in their use and who have had appropriate experience.

INTO THE RECTUM
This route is indicated for local treatments and when the oral and IV routes are not available – when the child is unconscious, vomiting or on continuous suction. Conscious children and adolescents may find insertion embarrassing, difficult and distasteful. These sensitivities should be sought and addressed. The modesty of the child should be respected with appropriate drapes and a lubricant used to ease the insertion. Splitting suppositories is not recommended.

INTO THE VAGINA
Rarely, children and adolescents need vaginal drugs to treat local infections. Creams, foams, tablets and pessaries are dispensed with applicators; medical douches and irrigations are also available. A gynaecologist's advice should be sought for any treatment other than topical creams and ointments.

Giving medicines

Prescribing information for children and families

Children and their carers need to know how to use medicines safely and effectively. All concerned have a responsibility to give appropriate information. This should be done in full open discussion in a clear unambiguous way. The prescribing doctor, carers and child should together plan the best and most convenient way of ensuring medicines achieve their optimum effect. The following check list may prove helpful.

WHAT THE PRESCRIBER NEEDS TO KNOW

☐ What is the medicine used for?

☐ How does it work?

☐ What dose formulations, amounts and concentrations/volumes are available?

☐ Dose according to age band or weight (or, if necessary, surface area) and to what extent rounding up or down of dose is expected to be safe and effective?

☐ Whether dose modification is needed (and, if so, by how much) according to underlying disease (e.g. renal insufficiency, liver problems)?

☐ Are there any contra-indications to its use or special precautions that may be needed?

☐ Are there any possible interactions with other medicines and what are the effects?

☐ What are the signs of poisoning and how should they be managed?

☐ Are there any contra-indications to breast-feeding or special precautions that may be needed?

☐ Are there any drug handling characteristics that need to be considered when using the medicine?

WHAT CHILDREN AND CARERS NEED TO KNOW

☐ The name of the medicine

☐ The reason for using it

☐ When and how to take it

☐ How to know if it is effective, and what to do if it is not

☐ What to do if one or more doses are missed

☐ How long to continue taking it

☐ The risks of stopping it

☐ The most likely adverse effects; those unlikely, but important; and what to do if they occur

☐ Whether other medicines can be taken at the same time

☐ Whether other remedies alter the medicine's effect.

Patient information leaflets

Currently, manufacturers Patient Information Leaflets (PIL) are enclosed with medicines. However, the law dictates that these must concur with the information in the manufacturers Summary of Product Characteristics. Therefore, if the drug is not licensed for children the PIL will indicate this, even if the drug is widely used in paediatric practice. To help communication with parents and children, and to try and avoid misunderstandings and complaints, the Joint RCPCH/NPPG Committee on Medicines has produced a generic PIL for parents and a modified version for older children. These can be included with all paediatric prescriptions and clarify the current position. The advice of consumer groups has been incorporated and the text has a reading age of 13 years as recommended for public information documents. Copies are available on the website: http://www.rcpch.ac.uk/publications/formulary_medicines.html

Most medicines given to a mother cause no harm to breast-fed babies and there are few contra-indications to breast-feeding when maternal medicines are necessary. The risks have frequently been overstated, leading to avoidance of a necessary drug or the interruption or prevention of breast-feeding.

Allergic reaction in a baby due to a maternal drug in breast milk is extremely rare.

Some babies in the first week of life, for example preterm and jaundiced babies, are at slightly greater than normal risk. Infants with G6PD deficiency and infants with an allergic tendency may be at increased risk, although these conditions are not usually known at the time. Idiosyncratic reactions, not related to dose and blood concentration, may theoretically occur even with low milk concentrations of the drug, but these are seldom of clinical importance.

Medicines which should not be given to breast-feeding mothers.

Medicine	Reason	Special consideration
Abuse drugs – cocaine, marijuana	Cocaine (CNS irritation); marijuana (may delay motor development)	Methadone is safe at 20mg/day and probably also up to 80mg/day. Monitor concentration in doses above 20mg/day.
Cytotoxic agents	Immediate and delayed toxicity e.g. methotrexate once weekly	Use in rheumatic disease is safe.
Ergot alkaloids e.g. bromocriptine, ergotamine	Suppress lactation, 'ergotism'	Short-term use – less than three days is safe.
Gold	Heavy metal poisoning	(controversial)
Iodine	Induces a goitre	
Phenindione	Bleeding tendency	Warfarin and heparin are safe alternatives.
Radio-iodine	Hypothyroidism Hyperthyroidism	Temporary cessation only, half-life determines length of breast-feeding interruption required.

Medicines that require more careful assessment of risk than usual

Category	Medicine	Considerations
Aminosalicylates	5-aminosalicylic acid; sulfasalazine (sulphasalazine)	May cause bloody diarrhoea.
Analgesic	Oxycodone	Neurobehavioural disturbance. Use morphine cautiously for severe pain. Paracetamol and NSAIDs for lesser pain.
Antidepressants	Doxepin, fluoxetine, lithium	Cautious use. Doxepin (sedation); fluxetine (colic); lithium (near to therapeutic concentrations).
Antiepileptics	Ethosuximide, phenobarbital (phenobarbitone)	Sedation. Carbamazepine, phenytoin, sodium valproate preferred.
Antimicrobials	Chloramphenicol, tetracyclines	Alternatives preferred. Chloramphenicol (idiopathic aplastic anaemia); tetracyclines (bone and teeth concerns).
Cardioactives and blood pressure lowering medicines	Amiodarone, atenolol, nadolol, sotalol	Labetalol and propranolol are safe and preferred. These others produce relatively high concentrations.
Combined oral contraceptives	Oestrogen and progesterone	Combined oral contraceptives can suppress lactation. Progesterone-only pills are preferred as these do not affect lactation.

Breast feeding *(side tab)*

GOOD PRACTICE

☐ Review safety of medicine

☐ If significant doubt, select alternative

☐ Give advice on risk, possible symptoms and signs of action and known adverse effects

☐ Give drug to mother immediately after breast-feeding where possible

☐ Watch baby for symptoms and signs of possible adverse effects and pharmacological effects

For further information on medicines and breast feeding please refer to www.ukmicentral.nhs.uk

Interactions

An interaction is said to occur when the effects of one drug are changed by the presence of another drug or food. The outcome may be harmful if the interaction causes an increase in the toxicity or a reduction in efficacy of the drug. Food interactions, whereby the presence of food in the stomach or intestine affects the rate or extent of absorption, are uncommon and generally unimportant. There are relatively few combinations of drugs which should be avoided and a substantial number of interacting drugs can be given together safely if the appropriate precautions are taken. Medicines interact with other medicines in two ways.

PHARMACODYNAMIC INTERACTIONS

Pharmacodynamic interactions are where the effects of one drug are changed by the presence of another drug at its site of action. Medicines may increase the effect of other medicines, which act on the same physiological system; sedative drugs affecting brain function and respiration are common examples. Alternatively, medicines may reduce the effect of other medicines by competing for the same receptor site. It is unusual for these interactions to be clinically important.

PHARMACOKINETIC INTERACTIONS

Pharmacokinetic interactions are those which can affect the processes by which drugs are absorbed, distributed, metabolized, and excreted.

Drug absorption interactions can decrease the rate of absorption or alter the total amount absorbed. For drugs which are given chronically on a multiple dose regimen, (e.g. oral anticoagulants) the rate of absorption is usually unimportant provided the total amount of drug absorbed is not markedly altered. A reduction in the rate of absorption of drugs, which are given as single doses intended to be absorbed rapidly and produce rapid high concentration, may be a problem.

Competition for protein binding sites. Only medicines more than 90% protein bound with a low apparent volume of distribution will be affected. The increased effect of one drug displaced by another is transient and rarely of clinical importance.

Influence on the rate of metabolism of other medicines. Enzyme inducing agents accelerate the metabolism of other medicines, causing a reduction in their clinical effect. Examples of enzyme inducing drugs include carbamazepine, phenytoin and rifampicin. Except in the management of epilepsy, problems due to enzyme induction are uncommon and can be managed by careful monitoring and dose adjustment.

Enzyme inhibiting medicines such as cimetidine, erythromycin, clarithromycin and sodium valproate reduce the rate of metabolism of other medicines thereby causing an increase in effect. The clinical relevance of many enzyme inhibition interactions depends on the extent to which the serum levels of the drug rise. The interaction only becomes adverse if serum levels climb into the toxic range.

In the drug monographs, only those interactions considered to be clinically important have been included.

Kidney disease
This may lead to reduced clearance of drugs and metabolites primarily excreted by the kidney. Problems with metabolites usually only occur when these are pharmacologically active.

Dose modifications are only necessary for drugs or metabolites which are more than 90% excreted by the kidney.
☐ Drugs with wide safety margins, a wide difference between doses causing clinically beneficial effects and toxicity, are generally safe even in relatively severe renal impairment
☐ Drugs which are nephrotoxic are more likely to exert this effect in children with kidney disease.

Modification of dose depends on the degree of renal impairment. Measures of creatinine clearance are frequently not available, but plasma creatinine concentrations can be used. There are two possible approaches:
☐ Lengthening the interval between the doses
☐ Reduction of dose but maintaining usual recommended dose interval.

Consideration of dose modification in kidney disease is discussed in the individual drug monographs where appropriate.

Where applicable, the monographs contain dosage adjustments for renal function based on normalised clearance of creatinine. Adjustments should be made using the glomerular filtration rate (GFR), if determined, or by calculating the estimated creatinine clearance, see below.

Use the equation, calculated by Morris *et al* (1982), for children aged 1-18 years. This equation may be used for infants although it is not a reliable method.

$$\text{'Estimated' Clcr (mL/minute/1.73m}^2) = \frac{40 \times ht}{Scr}$$

Where Clcr	=	Creatinine clearance in mL/minute/1.73m^2
Scr	=	Serum creatinine in micromol/litre
ht	=	Height in cm

Calculated creatinine clearances are not reliable below 1 year of age, however, the following equation may be of some value as a guide to dosage adjustments in neonates.

$$\text{'Estimated' Clcr (mL/minute/1.73m}^2) = \frac{30 \times L}{Scr}$$

Where Clcr	=	Creatinine clearance in mL/minute/1.73m^2
Scr	=	Serum creatinine in micromol/litre
L	=	Length in cm

(Adapted from Schwartz *et al*) Reproduced from Guy's Hospital Formulary, with kind permission.

Liver disease
Modification of the choice and dosage of drugs is usually unnecessary in children with liver disease. This is because there is a relatively large reserve of function of the liver metabolism even when liver disease appears to be severe. The following situations are those for which special consideration is required:
☐ Liver failure: children who have severely deranged liver enzymes and profound jaundice
☐ Coagulation impairment: increased response to oral anticoagulants
☐ Hypoproteinaemia: drugs which are highly protein bound like phenytoin and the benzodiazepines may have increased effect
☐ Hepatotoxic drug use: regardless of whether their effects are dose related or idiosyncratic, hepatotoxic drugs are more likely to cause toxicity in children with liver disease. These drugs should be avoided if at all possible.

Where special care is needed for a particular drug this will be indicated in the drug monograph.

Renal and liver disorders

ANAEMIA

Haemoglobin values vary with age and results should be checked with the appropriate reference range. Haemoglobin levels are high at birth and reach a nadir at 9-12 weeks of life. The World Health Organisation makes a practical definition of anaemia as a haemoglobin value less than 11g/dL (= 110g/L). Persistent anaemia is associated with poor growth, developmental delay, poor school performance and recurrent infections.

Iron deficiency anaemia. Confirm iron status by testing levels of serum ferritin. A positive response to treatment with oral iron is demonstrated by a rise in haemoglobin of at least 1g/100mL over a month. The maximum reticulocyte count is seen at 5-7 days. After a normal haemoglobin level is reached, iron treatment should continue for at least 12 more weeks to replace depleted body stores. Clinicians should become familiar with one cost-effective ferrous preparation. Failure to respond to oral iron is an indication to check compliance and to further investigate (the commonest reason for non-response is because the child is not taking the iron). There are few indications for a combined preparation in children. Parenteral iron is rarely necessary and should only be considered in proven iron deficiency where oral therapy has failed. The risks of blood transfusion outweigh the short-term advantages and should be reserved for children who are symptomatic.

Iron overload. Certain haematological conditions require long-term transfusion therapy as part of their management, and this will lead to iron overload if uncorrected. Desferrioxamine is an iron-chelating agent approved for clinical use and is administered as an 8-10 hour subcutaneous infusion in those children who are transfusion-dependent. The use of subcutaneous bolus injections has recently been reported. The oral iron chelator is deferiprone but it has significant side-effects and should only be given in specialist units.

Megaloblastic anaemia is very rare in childhood and is treated with folic acid or hydroxocobalamin (vitamin B12) according to the cause.

Haemolytic anaemia. Hereditary spherocytosis is the commonest cause of haemolytic anaemia in children. Some children with moderate or severe disease will benefit from splenectomy. *Haemophilus influenzae* type b (Hib), meningococcal and polyvalent pneumococcal vaccines should all be given prior to splenectomy. For children 2 months to 2 years of age, the polyvalent (7-valent) pneumococcal polysaccharide conjugated vaccine (Prevenar® in the UK) should be used. For children over 2 years, the polyvalent (23-valent) unconjugated pneumococcal polysaccharide vaccine (Pneumovax® II or Pnu-Imune® in the UK) should be given (ref: Update on Immunisation Issues – pneumococcal conjugate vaccine for children under 2 years of age, Dept of Health, August 2002). This is followed by oral phenoxymethylpenicillin (penicillin V) to reduce the risk of overwhelming infection following splenectomy. An influenza vaccination schedule should form part of continued care of all children with asplenia or splenic dysfunction (Ref: *Update on Immunisation Issues – Influenza Immunisation Programme 2002/2003*, Dept of Health, August 2002).

Renal anaemia. Erythropoietin has a place in management of the anaemia of chronic renal failure. Dietary factors can contribute and therefore iron and folate studies should be undertaken.

Neutropenia. Recombinant granulocyte colony stimulating factors (G-CSF) are used in children with aplastic anaemia, following chemotherapy for malignant disease, during bone marrow transplantation, and as part of stem cell harvesting protocols. Current evidence suggests that routine use cannot be justified. G-CSF is however used in patients with a high risk of overwhelming sepsis, and may support severely ill patients with febrile neutropenia. Children with congenital neutropenia respond to G-CSF but not to granulocyte macrophage-colony stimulating factors (GM-CSF).

Thrombocytopenia. Idiopathic thrombocytopenic purpura (ITP) is mainly benign and self-limiting and platelet counts alone should not dictate treatment. Consider treatment if active bleeding. Treatment may be with prednisolone, intravenous immunoglobulin (IVIG) or anti-D (for those who are rhesus D positive).

Coagulation. Thrombotic episodes are uncommon in childhood. Prevention of thrombus in high-risk patients and limitation of extension of clot is usually undertaken with heparin. Surgery or thrombolytic agents may be necessary if there is obstruction of major vessels. Due to the rapid clearance of heparin, any induced bleeding will usually be corrected by stopping the infusion. Protamine may also have a role in this situation. Duration of heparin treatment may be 5-10 days, depending upon the underlying thrombotic condition. Heparin is a rapidly acting inhibitor of clotting and is therefore started as soon as the diagnosis of thrombosis is considered. Warfarin acts by preventing the activation of vitamin K-dependent factors (II, VII, IX and X) and is usually started once the diagnosis of thrombosis has been confirmed, often within 24 hours of heparin therapy. Duration of treatment and desirable International Normalised Ratio (INR) range depends upon the underlying condition. Ensure INR is monitored. Induced haemorrhage can be corrected by vitamin K and plasma concentrate containing vitamin K-dependent factors II, IX and X but a full dose of vitamin K (300 microgram/kg) will make re-introduction of warfarin difficult for up to 2 weeks. Low molecular weight heparins may have a role. They are given subcutaneously and do not require routine monitoring in older children. Low molecular weight heparins, however, do require monitoring in young children because the dosage schedules are not established. Low molecular weight heparins have a longer half-life, which can present problems if surgery is anticipated.

Anti-platelet drugs. Aspirin has been implicated in the aetiology of Reye syndrome in children and therefore its use in those under 16 years (NEW GOVERNMENT GUIDELINE) is limited to conditions where a therapeutic advantage is clearly present. Children with Kawasaki disease should be treated with intravenous immunoglobulin and aspirin. Dipyridamole may have a role but no formal trial results are available.

Anti-fibrinolytic drugs. Tranexamic acid inhibits plasminogen activity and thereby limits fibrin dissolution. It is therefore useful in low-grade haemorrhage.

Blood products. Children with haemophilia A should receive recombinant factor VIII, and children with haemophilia B should receive recombinant factor IX. These are used in factor-deficiency states. Administration should ideally be under the control of a haematologist in a haemophiliac centre.

Cardiac

ARRHYTHMIA – EMERGENCY MANAGEMENT
Supraventricular tachycardia (SVT). In infancy this presents with pallor and irritability and in older children with palpitations. Usually there is a regular narrow complex tachycardia with a rate greater than 220 beats/minute (bpm).

SVT in infancy (<1 year)
If hypotensive or if severe congestive cardiac failure is present, proceed immediately to direct current cardioversion (0.5 joule/kg body weight).
If normotensive and not in major congestive cardiac failure then:
☐ First attempt to induce vagal tone by applying ice pack to face (diving reflex)
☐ Then try adenosine intravenously by rapid bolus, increasing the dose every 2 minutes. If adenosine is effective in restoring sinus rhythm, digitalise intravenously or orally (digoxin loading regimen) to maintain sinus rhythm.
☐ Although oral digitalisation is safer, the intravenous route is preferred here because of the urgency
☐ Then try IV propranolol
☐ Finally try synchronised direct current cardioversion (0.5 joule/kg body weight).

SVT in older child (>1 year)
☐ First try vagal manoeuvres – Valsalva or one-sided carotid sinus massage
☐ Then give intravenous adenosine by rapid bolus, increasing the dose every 2 minutes
☐ Then try flecainide intravenously slowly over 10 minutes and finally direct current cardioversion 0.5 joule/kg body weight
☐ In resistant cases consider amiodarone slowly IV over 30 minutes.

Ventricular tachycardia
This is defined as greater than 3 ectopic ventricular beats occurring consecutively. The tachycardia is described as sustained if lasting longer than 30 seconds. This is an uncommon arrhythmia in children. The rate is usually between 120-250 bpm and the ECG demonstrates a broad complex tachycardia which is almost regular but with minor variation in R-R interval. This arrhythmia may be associated with myocarditis, cardiomyopathy, congenital heart disease, prolonged QT interval, drug overdose (e.g. tricyclic antidepressants) and hypokalaemia.

If hypotensive:
☐ Proceed immediately to synchronised direct current cardioversion at a starting energy dose of 1 joule/kg followed by a bolus and infusion of lidocaine (lignocaine).

If normotensive:
☐ First administer bolus of lidocaine (lignocaine) followed by an infusion of lidocaine (lignocaine). Then, if this is not effective after 5 minutes:
☐ Amiodarone IV over 30 minutes. If this is not effective then:
☐ Propranolol IV over 10 minutes.

If ventricular tachycardia is secondary to tricyclic antidepressant overdose, try phenytoin IV as the second-line drug after lidocaine (lignocaine).

Bradycardia may take the form of sinus or nodal bradycardia or varying degrees of atrioventricular block. In paediatric practice bradycardia is usually secondary to respiratory or circulatory insufficiency and is related to myocardial hypoxia.

In this situation the management is:
☐ Secure the airway and administer 100% oxygen
☐ Commence basic life support including cardiac compressions is if there is clinical evidence of a reduced cardiac output and the heart rate is less than 80 bpm in an infant and less than 60 bpm in an older child
☐ Adrenaline (epinephrine) may be given IV
☐ If bradycardia persists despite adequate oxygenation, administer atropine IV.

Acute atrioventricular block or nodal bradycardia may occur in congenital heart disease or cardiomyopathy. The dysrhythmia may be precipitated by cardiac surgery or cardiac catheterisation. Atrioventricular block is particularly common in children with anatomically corrected transposition of the great arteries and in children with atrioventricular septal defect. If cardiac output is compromised the treatment is as follows:
☐ Protect airway and administer 100% oxygen
☐ Administer atropine IV
☐ Commence isoprenaline infusion.

If symptomatic bradycardia persists, insert transvenous pacing catheter for temporary pacing.

CYANOTIC SPELLS
An acute cyanotic spell in congenital heart disease is a medical emergency and potentially life threatening. Most cases, however, will respond to the prompt administration of oxygen and adoption of the knee/chest position. Cyanotic spells are usually a complication of Tetralogy of Fallot or complex congenital heart disease with reactive sub-pulmonary stenosis. They present with an acute increase in cyanosis associated with tachycardia, hyperpnoea and decrease in outflow tract murmur. They occur commonly in early morning or they are precipitated by dehydration or general anaesthesia.

To treat, give 100% oxygen via face-mask and place the child on his or her side in the knee/chest position. If cyanosis persists, gain IV access and administer propranolol by slow infusion over 10 minutes. The starting dose is 10 microgram/kg body weight increasing to a maximum of 100 microgram/kg. Then administer sodium bicarbonate intravenously after checking an arterial blood gas, or empirically in a dosage of 1mmol/kg body weight if the spell becomes prolonged (>10 minutes). Use 4.2% sodium bicarbonate solution in infants less than 1 year and 8.4% in older children. If the capillary blood glucose reading is less than 3mmol/L give 10% glucose intravenously (2mL/kg over 10 minutes), then administer morphine 100 microgram/kg intravenously or intramuscularly.

CARDIAC FAILURE
Administer oxygen via face-mask, tilt incubator floor to head up position in the newborn and nurse older infant and child in propped up position and restrict fluid intake. Try to avoid restricting calorie intake in infants. Nasogastric tube feeding may be necessary if very breathless. Administer dinoprostone (prostaglandin E2) IV in a duct-dependent systemic circulation and give furosemide (frusemide) IV. Digitalise intravenously or orally (digoxin loading regimen). The use of digoxin is controversial in high-output cardiac failure. Consider vasodilators such as oral captopril.

DUCT-DEPENDENT CONGENITAL HEART DISEASE
In the newborn with congenital heart disease it is often necessary to maintain patency of the ductus arteriosus using a prostaglandin E2 infusion. The structural heart defects amenable to this form of therapy fall into three main categories:

Duct-dependent pulmonary circulation. In this group of defects, maintaining patency of the ductus promotes pulmonary blood flow by left to right shunting through the vessel. In the event of ductal closure the pulmonary circulation becomes severely reduced with increasing central cyanosis. Examples of such defects include:
☐ Pulmonary atresia
☐ Tetralogy of Fallot
☐ Critical pulmonary valve stenosis

☐ Tricuspid atresia with hypoplastic right ventricle or pulmonary stenosis
☐ Hypoplastic right heart syndrome
☐ Univentricular heart with pulmonary atresia or stenosis.

Duct-dependent systemic circulation. In this group of defects the systemic circulation is partially or completely supported by right-to-left shunting through the ductus arteriosus. In the event of ductal closure these infants may become rapidly hypotensive with a low cardiac output. Examples of such defects include:
☐ Coarctation of the aorta
☐ Interrupted aortic arch
☐ Aortic atresia
☐ Critical aortic stenosis
☐ Hypoplastic left heart syndrome
☐ Univentricular heart with systemic outflow obstruction.

Transposition of the great arteries with intact ventricular septum. In this defect patency of the ductus arteriosus encourages mixing of the systemic and pulmonary circulations not only at ductal level but also across the foramen ovale by increasing pulmonary venous return to the left atrium. Ductal patency may also improve systemic saturation in the related defects of transposition of the great arteries with ventricular septal defect, double outlet right ventricle with a subpulmonary ventricular septal defect, and univentricular heart with malposed great vessels.

Treatment. The starting dose of a dinoprostone (prostaglandin E2) infusion in the newborn period is 5 nanogram/kg/minute. This infusion rate can be titrated against clinical effect up to an infusion rate of 20 nanogram/kg/minute. During dinoprostone infusion the newborn requires careful monitoring of heart rate, blood pressure, respiratory rate and core body temperature. In the event of a major complication such as apnoea, profound bradycardia or severe hypotension the infusion should be temporarily discontinued and appropriate intervention instituted. After resolution of the complication the infusion should be recommenced at a lower dose. Recurrent or prolonged apnoea may require ventilatory support in order that the dinoprostone infusion may be continued.

Chemotherapy

Children presenting with solid tumours or leukaemia in the UK receive most of their treatment at one of the 22 specialist paediatric oncology regional centres affiliated to the United Kingdom Children's Cancer Study Group (UKCCSG). Children treated at such centres on national protocols have been shown to have higher survival rates than those treated exclusively elsewhere. The information in the drug monographs concurs with that produced by the UKCCSG Chemotherapy Standardisation Committee.

The management of most solid tumours involves multimodality treatment, including surgery and/or radiotherapy in addition to chemotherapy. Cytotoxic drugs are used in well-defined protocols for all of the common (and many of the rarer) solid malignancies and are the principal component of treatment for leukaemia in children. Such protocols are usually part of trials or studies performed on behalf of national or international organisations such as the UKCCSG, the MRC (Medical Research Council), or SIOP (the International Society of Paediatric Oncology), with specified entry and diagnostic criteria, detailed treatment guidelines, and careful data registration and collection, including long-term follow-up. Due to the very rapid advances in treatment, such protocols should only be used by, or under the overall direction of, a UKCCSG centre, to ensure that patients may receive both the maximum benefit from the correct protocol, and expert supportive care in the event of treatment-related complications. Although some cytotoxic drugs given to children may not be licensed for each tumour for which they are used, their administration is usually within the context of a formal national or international study or trial protocol.

Particular care must be taken in the treatment of infants, and drug doses are often modified. Where specified, pharmacokinetic data apply to reported values from paediatric studies and may differ significantly from adult values.

CYTOTOXIC DRUGS
Some cytotoxic drugs display 'selectivity', whereby tumour cells are preferentially targeted by a variety of biochemical mechanisms. However, the therapeutic index of cytotoxic drugs is narrow, and acute and chronic adverse effects are

common. Combination chemotherapy, incorporating two or more cytotoxic drugs with complementary mechanisms of action but non-overlapping toxicities, aims to achieve improved cytotoxic action with less toxicity, and to reduce the risk of drug resistance. Combination chemotherapy protocols generally incorporate repeated treatment courses at defined intervals (usually 2-3 weekly) with clear criteria (e.g. adequate bone marrow, renal or cardiac function) for starting each course.

High-dose chemotherapy (e.g. cyclophosphamide, melphalan or busulfan (busulphan)), often in combination with radiotherapy (e.g. cyclophosphamide with total body irradiation), is used as myeloablative and immunosuppressive conditioning treatment prior to allogeneic bone marrow transplantation for haematological malignancies. Such conditioning protocols are increasingly complex and may include monoclonal or polyclonal anti-lymphocyte antibodies, or highly lymphosuppressive cytotoxics (e.g. fludarabine), to facilitate donor engraftment. Post-transplant immunosuppression is usually achieved with ciclosporin (cyclosporin), whilst methotrexate or corticosteroids may be added in some situations. High-dose chemotherapy (e.g. melphalan ± busulfan) is also used as consolidation treatment prior to autologous bone marrow or peripheral stem cell transplantation for certain solid tumours.

The major classes of cytotoxic drugs used in paediatric cancer include:
☐ Alkylating agents (e.g. cyclophosphamide) which interfere with DNA replication by formation of covalent intercalating cross-links between DNA strands
☐ Platinum agents (e.g. cisplatin) which bind with DNA, interfering with its replication
☐ Antibiotics which interfere with DNA replication and transcription (e.g. doxorubicin) or cause DNA strand breaks (e.g. bleomycin)
☐ Epipodophyllotoxins (e.g. etoposide) which inhibit topoisomerase II during DNA replication and transcription
☐ Vinca alkaloids (e.g. vincristine) which block formation of the mitotic spindle
☐ Antimetabolites (e.g. methotrexate, cytarabine, mercaptopurine) which inhibit biochemical mechanisms involved in cell division.

SIDE-EFFECTS / TOXICITY
Cytotoxic drugs damage rapidly dividing cells such as those in bone marrow (leading to myelosuppression), the gastrointestinal tract and mucous membrane (causing enteritis and mucositis), and skin and hair follicles (causing alopecia), but these effects are usually reversible. Other acute and usually temporary side-effects include nausea and vomiting, and organ-specific toxicity (e.g. vincristine neurotoxicity, dactinomycin hepatotoxicity, ifosfamide urotoxicity). These are usually managed with supportive care (see below), although methylthioninium chloride (methylene blue) may be used to reverse ifosfamide encephalopathy. Chronic toxicity due to chemotherapy is also often organ-related (e.g. doxorubicin cardiotoxicity, cisplatin and ifosfamide nephrotoxicity, bleomycin pulmonary toxicity and methotrexate neurotoxicity). Such toxicity may develop months or even years after treatment, and may cause substantial morbidity, or even, rarely, threaten life. Careful follow-up is therefore necessary, particularly in certain high-risk groups of patients (such as those receiving high cumulative doses of doxorubicin). Gonadal toxicity may be caused by several cytotoxic drugs, especially alkylating agents. In adolescent males, sperm storage before starting gonadotoxic chemotherapy may be considered. The harvesting and cryopreservation of ovarian cortical strips has been performed within research protocols in a few centres, in the (as yet unproven) hope that ovarian tissue autotransplantation may allow return of ovarian function with ovulatory cycles in adult females treated previously with gonadotoxic chemotherapy. Both alkylating agents and epipodophyllotoxins are particularly implicated in the development of secondary malignant neoplasms.

All cytotoxic drugs should be regarded as teratogenic, or potentially so. They should not normally be administered during pregnancy (especially the first trimester), so contraceptive advice should be offered (where appropriate) to older girls with reproductive potential. Breast-feeding should also be avoided in those receiving cytotoxic drugs. Overdosage with a cytotoxic drug is a very serious and potentially life-threatening event. Unfortunately, few specific antidotes are available (but see methotrexate monograph), though full supportive care (which may include specific therapies such as plasmapheresis for platinum overdosage) should be provided.

PREPARATION/ADMINISTRATION
Prescriptions for chemotherapy should be written by, or under the careful supervision of, experienced medical staff with a detailed knowledge of the drugs and protocols by which they are used. This is important to avoid confusion and potential drug errors, caused for example by the use of very similar drugs at different stages of the same protocol (e.g. up to three different preparations of asparaginase are used in the current protocol for acute lymphoblastic leukaemia).

Cytotoxic drugs should be reconstituted in dedicated pharmacy units, with adequate facilities and written procedures for chemotherapy preparation and for disposal of cytotoxic waste, in view of their potential carcinogenicity. They should be administered only by experienced medical or nursing staff, using careful guidelines to ensure both their patients' and their own safety. In particular, great care should be taken in the use of intrathecal chemotherapy, and clear documentation should be employed to prevent the inadvertent administration of drugs not intended for intrathecal use (e.g. vincristine). The necessary equipment and clear protocols should be available to manage spillage and extravasation episodes.

SUPPORTIVE CARE

There are many important components of supportive care that are crucial for the successful outcome of children treated with chemotherapy. Complications may also result from either radiotherapy or surgery, and in some cases these may interact with chemotherapy-related toxicity, e.g. sensitisation by recently administered doxorubicin may greatly increase acute tissue damage due to radiotherapy. A limited number of specific 'protective' drugs are used alongside particular cytotoxic drugs as part of well-defined protocols. The two major examples are mesna, which is used with both cyclophosphamide and ifosfamide to reduce the risk of haemorrhagic cystitis, and folinic acid (given as calcium folinate), which is used to rescue normal somatic cells from the folate antagonism of methotrexate. The use of dexrazoxane as a cardioprotectant in children receiving anthracyclines is under investigation.

Most cytotoxic drugs, particularly cisplatin, cause nausea and vomiting. Exceptions include vincristine, asparaginase, bleomycin, mercaptopurine, tioguanine (thioguanine), and low dose methotrexate. Anti-emetic drugs ameliorate or prevent most of the emesis associated with chemotherapy. $5HT_3$ receptor antagonists (e.g. ondansetron or granisetron) are particularly effective, but other agents, including metoclopramide, phenothiazines, dexamethasone, lorazepam and nabilone, may also be used individually or in combination. Infection is a very frequent and potentially life-threatening complication of chemotherapy, and may be due to a variety of organisms, including bacteria, fungi, viruses, and protozoa. Therefore, appropriate powerful and broad-spectrum antibacterial, antifungal, antiviral and antiprotozoal drugs are used frequently in a variety of prophylactic and treatment regimens in children treated with chemotherapy based on a local sensitivity audit. Colony stimulating factors (CSFs) such as G-CSF may, in limited circumstances, be used to accelerate recovery from myelosuppression, both prophylactically and therapeutically. G-CSFs are also used routinely in the mobilisation of peripheral blood stem cells for transplantation. Blood products, principally red blood cells and platelets, are used extensively to support the other haematological complications of cytotoxic drugs.

Maintenance of gastrointestinal integrity and function is an important component of supportive care in children receiving chemotherapy, and may involve the use of H2-receptor antagonists, antacids and proton pump inhibitors to protect gastric mucosa, laxative agents to treat constipation, and nutritional support, both enterally and parenterally. Many other classes of drugs may be used in children during or after treatment for malignancies, including analgesics, antihypertensives, and hormone replacement therapy.

A few aspects of supportive care are largely confined to children with CNS tumours, including the use of dexamethasone to reduce cerebral (or spinal) oedema in newly diagnosed tumour (especially to achieve stabilisation prior to and after neurosurgery), and the use of appropriate antibiotics, administered either intravenously (e.g. cefotaxime or meropenem, both of which have good CNS penetration) or directly into the cerebrospinal fluid, usually intraventricularly (e.g. vancomycin or gentamicin). Anticonvulsant drugs are necessary in many children with CNS tumours, both in the acute treatment of status epilepticus and in longer term prevention and treatment of convulsions which may occur as a consequence of the tumour itself or of its surgical treatment. The management of status epilepticus in children with CNS tumours follows similar overall principles to its treatment in other children, but the possibility of cerebrospinal fluid infection (especially in the presence of a ventriculo-peritoneal/atrial shunt or external ventricular drain) may need to be investigated and treated with appropriate antibiotic therapy, and the potential presence of raised intracranial pressure, which may necessitate urgent IV treatment with dexamethasone and /or mannitol, should be suspected.

Children who have received a bone marrow (or peripheral blood stem cell) transplant are at risk of more frequent and serious complications, including some only seen occasionally in other patients (e.g. hepatic veno-occlusive disease, severe cases of which may be treated with specialised investigational protocols).

Drugs commonly used in the United Kingdom in combination chemotherapy protocols for children.

NB Different cytotoxic agents may be used in the treatment of relapsed disease.

INDICATION	FIRST-LINE DRUGS
Acute lymphoblastic leukaemia (ALL)	Asparaginase (including PEG asparaginase), cyclophosphamide, cytarabine, daunorubicin, dexamethasone, doxorubicin, etoposide, mercaptopurine, methotrexate, prednisolone, tioguanine (thioguanine), vincristine
Acute myeloid leukaemia (AML)	Amsacrine, cytarabine, daunorubicin, fludarabine, etoposide, mitoxantrone (mitozantrone)
B-cell non-Hodgkin lymphoma (NHL). Note that T-cell NHL is treated by an ALL-type protocol	Cyclophosphamide, cytarabine, doxorubicin, etoposide, methotrexate, prednisolone, vincristine
Ependymoma	Etoposide, cyclophosphamide
Ewing sarcoma	Busulfan (busulphan), cyclophosphamide, dactinomycin, doxorubicin, etoposide, ifosfamide, melphalan, vincristine
Germ cell tumour (intra- and extra-cranial)	Bleomycin, carboplatin, cisplatin, cyclophosphamide, etoposide, ifosfamide
Hepatoblastoma and hepatocellular carcinoma	Carboplatin, cisplatin, doxorubicin
Hodgkin disease	Bleomycin, chlorambucil, dacarbazine, doxorubicin, prednisolone, procarbazine, vinblastine, vincristine
Infant brain tumour (applicable to many but not all types of CNS tumour in children <36 months of age)	Carboplatin, cisplatin, cyclophosphamide, methotrexate, vincristine
Low-grade glioma (including astrocytoma)	Carboplatin, vincristine
Neuroblastoma	Busulfan, carboplatin, cisplatin, cyclophosphamide, etoposide, melphalan, vincristine
Neuroectodermal tumour (including medulloblastoma)	Cisplatin, lomustine, vincristine, carboplatin
Osteosarcoma	Cisplatin, doxorubicin, methotrexate
Retinoblastoma	Carboplatin, etoposide, vincristine
Rhabdomyosarcoma and soft tissue sarcoma	Carboplatin, cyclophosphamide, dactinomycin, epirubicin, etoposide, ifosfamide, vincristine
Wilms tumour	Dactinomycin, doxorubicin, vincristine
Haematopoietic stem cell transplantation	Busulfan, cyclophosphamide, fludarabine, melphalan

Chemotherapy

Dental

Sugar-free medicine. If possible, all liquid oral medicines prescribed for children or available over the counter should be sugar-free. This is particularly important for children who are intellectually, physically or medically compromised and for whom oral and dental disease (or its treatment) poses a significant threat to their life.

Fluoride. Regular administration of fluoride to the teeth reduces the prevalence of tooth decay. Systemic administration of fluoride is achieved by daily doses of fluoride drops or tablets during the period of tooth formation if the water supply is not optimally fluoridated (1mg/L in temperate climates = 1ppm). The daily use of a fluoride supplement (drops or tablets depending upon age) has in addition a topical effect on the teeth once they have erupted. Prescription is age and risk related and should be under the supervision of a dental surgeon familiar with current published guidelines. An alternative in children over 6 years old is the daily or fortnightly use of fluoride mouthwash at home. At this age it is judged that a child is capable of rinsing and spitting out reliably, since fluoride mouthwash should not be swallowed.

Caries-preventing agents. Fluorides are routinely used by dentists to prevent the onset of dental caries ('decay') as well as reversing the development of very early caries. They are available as supplements, mouthwashes, and toothpastes – and are more effective if used on a more regular, frequent basis at home but in a controlled way.

Treatment of caries. Where decay has advanced to involve the pulp of the tooth, antibiotics may be required in the acute phase to control the associated infection. Treatment of such conditions will require the use of medicaments such as formocresol and calcium hydroxide, confined to the pulp chamber. Appropriate analgesics, acting peripherally rather than centrally, should be used for effective pain management.

Sensitive teeth. Apply topical fluoride and home use of a desensitising toothpaste which should also contain fluoride.

Sore mouth. Treat with chlorhexidine as a mouthwash or gel 2–3 times daily, or 'TePe Select Special Care®' toothbrushes if the gingivae are very sore. For mucositis not of viral origin, a beclometasone (beclomethasone) inhaler (used as a topical mouthspray) or alternatively, betamethasone soluble tablets (as a mouthwash), may give some relief. These two agents may be used together in severe cases. If the mucosa is too sore for toothbrushing then chlorhexidine can be applied on mouth sponges or gauze. Alternatively, benzydamine hydrochloride can be sprayed onto sore areas in the under 6 year old or given as a mouth rinse in older children. A dentist should be consulted if the soreness persists.

Dry mouth. Consider the use of sugarless gum to stimulate saliva flow. Damage or disease of the salivary glands from radiotherapy and/or chemotherapy, primary salivary gland pathology or the effect of drugs with an anticholinergic effect (e.g. antispasmodics, tricyclic antidepressants, and antipsychotics) may necessitate the use of saliva substitutes. To be beneficial the agents should mimic saliva, with adequate levels of fluoride to prevent dental caries. Local measures such as frequent sips of water and sucking sugar-free sweets or ice-cubes can also bring some relief.

Drooling. In children with dysfunctional swallowing (e.g. severe cerebral palsy) pharmacological control of salivary flow is preferable to surgical correction to avoid the likely sequelae of rampant dental caries.

Erosion. Some medicines with a low pH predispose the teeth to acid erosion. Inhalers used for asthma control may also pose a risk for erosion children should be encouraged to rinse out their mouth with water after using an inhaler.

Ear, nose and throat

Diseases of the ear, nose and throat (ENT) are common in childhood. Children inhale a wide variety of pathogens and allergens, which cause inflammation and oedema of the mucosa, vascular congestion, increased mucus secretion and alterations to ciliary function as well as a systemic response. Many conditions present in a similar way making precise diagnosis and therefore treatment difficult. Illness involving the ear, nose and throat in young children is more likely to present in a non-specific way and before localising signs become apparent. Antibiotic therapy should, if required, cover the likely respiratory pathogens including *Haemophilus influenzae*, *Streptococcus pneumoniae*, *Moraxella catarrhalis* and *Staphylococcus aureus*. An appropriate analgesic/antipyretic is usually indicated for the discomfort and fever associated with ENT inflammation.

THE EAR

Diseases of the ear often cause earache (otalgia). Although this is commonly associated with inflammation of the external and/or middle ear, it may also arise secondary to problems in the temporomandibular joint, the teeth or the pharynx. Purulent otorrhoea in children is a sign of otitis media with perforation of the tympanic membrane. It can occasionally be bloodstained. A clear discharge would be more suggestive of a CSF leak. Swelling around the ear at such times may represent cellulitis or, more commonly, associated lymphadenopathy. If the mastoid is swollen and tender or the pinna displaced forward mastoiditis should be considered. Other symptoms and signs relating to disease of the ear include nystagmus, loss of hearing, tinnitus or vertigo. Symptoms may be vague and not necessarily related to any labyrinthine dysfunction.

Wax. Examination of the ear is often difficult in young children, not only because of lack of cooperation but also because of the sensitivity and smaller dimensions of the external auditory meatus. Obstructing cerumen (ear wax) can be an additional nuisance. Impaction through attempts at cleansing using such things as cotton buds is not uncommon. Physical removal of the wax may be difficult. Children often find irrigation of the ear canal distressing. Softening of the wax with olive oil or almond oil often aids removal. Commercial preparations are also available, although without clear advantages. Softening agents may need to be used for a couple of days if the wax is particularly hardened. Care should be taken when irrigating the external ear, especially if there is a possibility of a perforation of the tympanic membrane.

Otitis externa, although not common, is usually associated with an underlying seborrhoeic dermatitis or eczema. This can be secondarily infected with *Pseudomonas aeruginosa*, *Enterobacter aerogenes*, *Proteus mirabilis*, *Klebsiella pneumoniae*, *Streptococcus* species, *Staphylococcus epidermidis* and occasionally fungi such as *Candida* or *Aspergillus*. Herpes (simplex and zoster) may affect the ear canal. Irrigation is best avoided in otitis externa. Local toilet using suction under a microscope is preferable. Topical treatments with an astringent such as aluminium acetate may be helpful. If infection is present, a preparation containing an antibiotic and steroid is often used e.g. flumetasone (flumethasone) and clioquinol, or hydrocortisone with gentamicin or neomycin.

Otitis media has a peak incidence in young children and often complicates even minor upper respiratory tract infections (URTIs). The acute presentation is characterized by otalgia and fever; localising symptoms may be absent or inapparent in infants. Although amoxicillin (amoxycillin) and erythromycin are the first-line antibiotics in use, the increasing resistance to amoxicillin of *Haemophilus influenzae* and *Moraxella catarrhalis* indicate the use of co-amoxiclav, particularly in the younger child and when there is a history of recurrent otitis media. However, a recent meta-analysis suggests that for many children, the symptoms of otitis media remit adequately with the use of simple analgesics/antipyretics and without long-term sequelae. It may be appropriate to restrict the use of antibiotics to the younger more systemically unwell child with a history of previous infection/hospital admissions. In such cases there is no evidence that prolonged courses of antibiotics provide greater benefit.

Otitis media with effusion (OME). This usually presents with hearing loss and is associated with recurrent URTIs as well as other factors such as parental smoking. Although systematic reviews have shown that prolonged courses of antibiotics speed resolution there is no good evidence of long-term benefit and they are probably best avoided. An increased incidence of adverse effects such as nausea and diarrhoea are reported associated with antibiotic usage. Oral steroids, antihistamines, and decongestants have not shown any clear benefits in randomised controlled trials.

Labyrinthitis is usually associated with acute or chronic bacterial or viral infections. Symptoms include vertigo, often accompanied by nausea and vomiting, and sensorineural hearing loss. Acute otitis media and other potential local causes should be looked for. Treatment includes anti-emetics, antihistamines and occasionally sedatives.

Benign paroxysmal vertigo is rare in children and associated with abnormal vestibular function. Although attacks are usually self-limiting, they are very disturbing to the child and family.

Motion sickness can be very distressing in some children. Many over the counter remedies are available. Hyoscine hydrobromide appears the most effective medicine with antihistamines such as promethazine and cyclizine also useful. Although vertigo may be associated with middle ear disease, labyrinthitis or other inner ear problems in children, consideration should be given to other central causes for the symptom. Acute disturbances may be associated with vomiting and need anti-emetics.

THE NOSE

Acute rhinitis is likely to be virus-induced and therefore self-limiting. Persistence of symptoms, particularly if there is a purulent discharge, raises the possibility of secondary bacterial infection or possible underlying anatomical causes. The presence of a foreign body in the younger child should be considered. An appropriate antibiotic may become necessary at this stage. Chronic rhinitis is usually allergic in origin. Investigation for underlying allergic tendencies may be helpful in enabling preventative measures to be undertaken.

The distress of nasal obstruction from rhinitis may be eased by NaCI 0.9% nose drops or the short-term (<1 week) use of 0.5% ephedrine nose drops. Other topical sympathomimetic drugs, such as xylometazoline, can be useful but usage should be limited to no more than a few days because of the risk of rebound congestion on withdrawal. There are many over the counter treatments, containing drugs such as pseudoephedrine. Though less likely to cause rhinitis medicamentosa, most oral preparations should not be used for more than a few days. Simple suction may clear nasal obstruction in infants. Humidification of inspired air may help. Antihistamines may thicken the secretions of infective rhinitis, thus worsening symptoms unlike the dramatic improvement they often give when treating allergic rhinitis.

In allergic rhinitis second generation antihistamines such as loratadine and cetirizine are well-tolerated.

Allergic rhinitis may also be treated topically, with nasal sprays or drops. Sodium cromoglicate (sodium cromoglycate) has a low side-effect profile, although it is less effective than topical steroids. Preparations of beclometasone dipropionate (beclomethasone diproprionate), flunisolide and fluticasone propionate are all effective. There continue to be concerns about possible systemic effects for nasally administered steroids and of long-term local side-effects.

Idiopathic rhinitis is less commonly recognised in children and may have a neurogenic origin. It appears to respond to ipratropium bromide.

Sinus disease is uncommon in children and can be difficult to diagnose with subtle symptoms. It is common in a variety of syndromes such as cystic fibrosis and immotile cilia syndrome, where it should be actively looked for. Sinusitis will commonly complicate upper respiratory tract infections, particularly when there is allergic rhinitis. Clear-cut infective sinus disease responds well to antibiotics covering common upper respiratory pathogens. Generally a 10-14 day course is prescribed although there is no clear evidence for or against this. Subacute or chronic sinusitis seems to require more prolonged treatment for a number of weeks. Other ancillary treatments are similar to that for rhinitis, although there is no clear-cut evidence from controlled studies of the overall effectiveness of these treatments for sinusitis.

Peri-orbital cellulitis is a complication of sinusitis. The area around the eye becomes red and swollen. Orbital cellulitis, where the extra-ocular muscles are involved, (patient may have diplopia) is an ophthalmological emergency because of the risk of blindness. Referral to an ophthalmologist or ENT surgeon is essential.

Epistaxis may complicate infection or occur with allergic disease, vascular anomalies, and (rarely) clotting deficiencies. It usually settles with simple first aid measures involving local pressure and calming the child. Persistent bleeding may respond to a topical sympathomimetic spray, but local cautery or (rarely) packing may be needed. If infection is suspected, local application of chlorhexidine and neomycin (Naseptin®) cream helps.

Endocrine

DIABETES

TYPE 1 DIABETES

Diabetes presenting without ketoacidosis. If the child is well with a high blood glucose, glycosuria and few ketones, and is tolerating oral fluids, start with subcutaneous insulin. Starting insulin type and dose is not evidence-based and depends on personal preference. Each department should have clear written guidelines. Options are either isophane insulin alone, or a mixture of soluble and isophane such as Human Mixtard® 20 (or equivalent). Usual dose is 0.5 units/kg/day, given as three-fifths to two-thirds of the total dose in the morning and two-fifths to one-third of the total dose in the evening. A greater dose (up to 0.7 units/kg/day) may be needed if the child is in puberty or has heavy ketonuria. Blood glucose should be measured before meals and before bed and also if symptoms of hypoglycaemia occur. If glycosuria but no ketonuria consider maturity-onset diabetes of the young (MODY) and if obese Type 2 diabetes. If the child has been started on oral fluids and subcutaneous insulin but deteriorates, start treatment for diabetic ketoacidosis (DKA) as below.

Diabetes presenting with ketoacidosis (DKA). The diagnosis from the history, signs and biochemical findings is usually clear, the key features being hyperglycaemia, dehydration, acidosis and heavy ketonuria, usually with associated vomiting and/or hyperventilation. The following is based on the *British Society for Paediatric Endocrinology and Diabetes Guidelines*, 2001. http://www.bsped.org.uk

Management of diabetic ketoacidosis

Initial management

☐ **Resuscitate the child (Airway, Breathing, Circulation).** If vomiting or semiconscious, insert a nasogastric tube. If the child is severely dehydrated correct shock with 10mL/kg NaCl 0.9% or colloid solution as quickly as possible, and repeat as necessary (maximum x 3). Then commence IV therapy as below.

☐ **IV therapy.** If the child is dehydrated >3% and clinically acidotic, correct dehydration over 24 hours. To avoid excessive fluid replacement, which may be a risk factor for cerebral oedema, calculate the deficit as if the patient is no more than 10% (usually work on 7.5%) dehydrated. Add deficit to maintenance and give at a constant rate over 24 hours. If the blood glucose is very high or the child very young, it may be prudent to rehydrate over 48 hours. Use NaCl 0.9%. Carefully document all administered fluids, including those given in Accident and Emergency.

☐ **Potassium.** Potassium should be started immediately unless anuria is suspected or if there are peaked T waves on the ECG. Add 20mmol potassium chloride to 500mL IV fluid. Blood levels of potassium will fall once insulin is commenced, regardless of the initial level. Use a cardiac monitor and check frequently for T wave changes.

□ **Insulin.** Start 0.1 units/kg/hour soluble insulin (made up as 50 units in 50mL NaCl 0.9% given via a syringe pump) once fluids are running. Continuous low-dose IV infusion is the preferred method. There is no need for an initial bolus. Do not add insulin directly to the fluid bag. If the rate of blood glucose fall exceeds 5mmol/L/hour, reduce the insulin infusion rate to 0.05 units/kg/hour. Do not reduce the insulin infusion further than this as insulin is required to switch off ketone production. Consider adding extra glucose (50mL glucose 50% added to 500mL glucose 5% will increase the glucose concentration to approximately 10%) rather than reducing/stopping the insulin.

□ **Bicarbonate.** There is no experimental evidence to support the use of bicarbonate in the treatment of metabolic acidosis in DKA unless myocardial function is impaired. If acidosis persists, consider giving further colloid, increasing the dose of insulin, and excluding sepsis.

Observations

□ Measure hourly blood glucose, test every urine sample for glucose and ketones, measure weight twice daily, evaluate neurological status at least hourly, measure electrolytes after 2 hours and then at least 4 hourly during IV therapy, monitor ECG for T wave changes

□ Accurate documentation of fluid balance is very important. All fluid input and output must be recorded, including oral fluids. Only replace losses if urine output is excessive.

Continuing management

□ Once blood glucose is <12mmol/L, change IV therapy to NaCl 0.45% and glucose 5% and consider reducing insulin to 0.05 units/kg/hour, but no further. Plan to maintain a gradually increasing plasma sodium, as a falling level has been implicated in the development of cerebral oedema. If necessary (e.g. blood glucose falls below 7mmol/L) add extra glucose to the infusion.

Response to treatment

□ If no improvement – re-evaluate IV therapy, acidosis and consider sepsis. If acidosis is not correcting, resuscitation may have been inadequate; therefore consider giving more NaCl 0.9%/colloid.

□ If neurological deterioration and/or severe headache – exclude hypoglycaemia, consider cerebral oedema (which requires urgent intervention – see below).

□ Continue with IV fluids until the child is drinking well and able to tolerate food. Do not expect ketones to have disappeared completely before changing to SC insulin. Discontinue the insulin infusion 60 minutes after the SC injection to allow SC insulin to start working.

Coma and cerebral oedema. Suspect cerebral oedema if there is any deterioration in conscious level, severe headache or signs of raised intracranial pressure. It requires urgent intervention. Inform senior staff immediately and give mannitol 500mg/kg stat (2.5mL/kg mannitol 20% over 15 minutes). It should be given within 5-10 minutes of the initial deterioration. Restrict IV fluids to two-thirds maintenance and replace the deficit over 72 rather than 24 or 48 hours. Move the child to the intensive care unit. If necessary intubate and hyperventilate to reduce blood pCO_2. Exclude other diagnoses by computed tomography (CT) brain scan once child is stable – other intracerebral events such as thrombosis, haemorrhage or infarction may present in the same way. Inform neurosurgeons. Intracerebral pressure monitoring may be required. A further dose of mannitol may be necessary.

Insulin Regimens in Type 1 Diabetes
Suggested regimens

□ Twice daily isophane insulin: often the initial regimen; soluble insulin added in when necessary for blood glucose control.

□ Twice daily mixtures of soluble and isophane: either free mixed or as fixed combinations e.g. 20/80 or 30/70 of soluble/isophane.

□ Three times daily: combination of soluble/isophane in the morning, soluble only before evening meal, isophane only before bed; suitable for children who have at least 2 hours between teatime and bedtime injections.

□ Multiple injection regimen: isophane before bed, then either soluble or rapid-acting insulin before meals; most suitable for those who need flexibility. New long-acting insulin (glargine) may be useful for this regimen.

□ Continuous subcutaneous insulin infusion pump: using either soluble or rapid-acting insulin. Only used in a few centres at present.

Insulin should be given half an hour before meals except for rapid-acting, which should be given immediately before meals.

Endocrine

Doses

☐ Most prepubertal children require around 0.7-1 units/kg/day once they are beyond the honeymoon period. Therefore increase the dose at most clinic visits.

☐ During puberty, boys may need up to 1.5-2 units/kg/day, especially during the growth spurt. Girls generally require slightly less (up to 1.5 units/kg/day).

☐ Around one year after menarche in girls or after the growth spurt in boys, the dose needs to be reduced to avoid excessive weight gain.

Treatment of Hypoglycaemia.

Symptoms vary between individuals. If the child is conscious, there may be enough time to check blood glucose level. Give sugar or food containing sugar immediately: e.g. glucose tablets (<5 years 2 tablets, >5 years 3 tablets), or Lucozade® 60mL (30mL = 10g carbohydrate) or any sweet drink such as lemonade (not 'diet'), orange juice or one heaped tablespoon of sugar in water. This must be followed by a longer-acting carbohydrate: e.g. biscuits, toast or sandwiches, which are absorbed more slowly.

Hypostop®. If the child is unable to co-operate but can swallow, use Hypostop®. Hypostop® may be safely smeared on to the buccal mucosa of semi-conscious patients in whom the swallowing reflex is preserved. An initial dose of half a tube is recommended. The dose should be repeated if there is no clinical response within 10 minutes. Do not use in unconscious patients.

Glucagon. If the child is unconscious or fitting, or does not respond after 10 minutes, administer glucagon. It acts by mobilising liver glycogen stores and may not therefore be effective after repeated use, or after alcohol. The recommended dose is 500 microgram if under 10 years of age and 1mg if over 10 years by SC or IM injection. Nausea and vomiting are frequent side-effects following use.

Glucose 10%. In hospital, give 2-5mL/kg of glucose 10% (200-500mg/kg glucose) IV followed by an infusion of glucose 5-10% until the child is awake. Do not give glucose 50% solution, as it is very hypertonic and carries a risk of fatal haemolysis.

SURGERY FOR A CHILD WITH DIABETES.

Admit the child to hospital, continue insulin, and remember that starvation before a general anaesthetic will increase the risk of hypoglycaemia. The following is one suggested guideline. Other protocols are used. It is important that each hospital has in place a protocol agreed by the anaesthetic service.

Elective surgery. Ideally the child should be first on the morning list. Admit in the afternoon of the day before (or before 8am if minor surgery) and inform the anaesthetist and the diabetic team so that they can oversee the blood glucose control.

☐ Evening prior to surgery. Check pre-mealtime, and pre-bedtime blood glucose levels. Look for ketones and sugar in the urine and treat ketoacidosis if present. Give the usual evening insulin with a bedtime snack.

☐ Morning operations. No solids from midnight, give clear fluids up to 4 hours before the operation but also check with anaesthetist. Omit the morning dose of insulin (or give only half long-acting insulin and omit fast-acting component if a minor procedure expected) and set up fluids and insulin (see below). If a very short procedure is expected, IV fluids and insulin may not be necessary. Measure capillary glucose every hour before surgery, every half-hour during surgery and until recovery from anaesthetic, then hourly for 4 hours and then 2 hourly until the usual insulin regimen is recommenced. Adjust the insulin infusion to maintain the blood glucose between 7-13mmol/L. Continue the infusions until the child is taking oral fluids and snacks, and then at the next mealtime give the usual dose of insulin subcutaneously and stop the insulin infusion 1 hour later.

☐ Afternoon operations. Give one-third of the usual dose of insulin in the morning. Offer a light breakfast at 8am and then fast for solids. Give clear fluids up to 4 hours before the operation, but also check with the anaesthetist. Start IV fluids and insulin (see below) at 12:00 hours at the latest and proceed as above.

Maintenance fluid. Use glucose 10%, NaCl 0.18% with 10mmol added potassium chloride per 500mL bag.

Insulin infusion. 50 units of soluble human insulin in 50mL NaCl 0.9% (1 unit in 1mL). Infuse by syringe pump at 0.025mL/kg/hour. Adjust hourly using a sliding scale to keep blood glucose level between 7-13mmol/L. If the child is unwell, the infusion may need to be started at 0.05mL/kg/hour.

Emergency surgery. Ketoacidosis can present as an 'acute abdomen', and acute illness may provoke ketoacidosis. Do not feed, check body weight, and check blood for electrolytes, glucose, venous pH/bicarbonate, and urine for ketones. If ketoacidosis is present, delay operation until circulation is restored and acidosis under control; if not, proceed as for elective surgery.

TYPE 2 DIABETES

Rare in children but becoming more common as obesity increases, particularly in some ethnic groups. Suspect if no ketones at diagnosis, family history of type 2 diabetes, obesity or very low insulin requirements (if insulin commenced). Confirm with oral glucose tolerance test (including measurement of insulin levels). Start treatment with diet, then move to an oral hypoglycaemic agent (most experience with metformin). Treat with insulin if control remains poor.

HYPOGLYCAEMIA FROM CAUSES OTHER THAN DIABETES

Prompt treatment of hypoglycaemia from any cause is essential to prevent subsequent neurological damage. If the aetiology is unknown, a blood sample should be obtained prior to treatment for measurement of serum concentrations of glucose, insulin, C-peptide, growth hormone, cortisol, non-esterified fatty acids, lactate and ketone bodies, and the next available urine sample should be collected for analysis (ketones and organic acids).

Glucose 10% (10g/100mL). 200-400mg of glucose/kg body weight of glucose 10% (i.e. 2-4mL/kg) should be infused intravenously over 4-6 minutes followed by a continuous infusion of glucose sufficient to maintain euglycaemia. The usual requirement is 4-6mg/kg/minute, and the requirement for infusions in excess of this indicates hyperinsulinism. Stronger concentrations of glucose should be avoided to prevent the risk of cerebral oedema and haemolysis.

Hypostop®. As a holding measure Hypostop® may be used. See above for further information.

Glucagon may be used as an alternative to parenteral glucose for the treatment of hypoglycaemia when the patient has adequate glycogen stores as may occur in hyperinsulinism, but not in glycogen storage disease. It is therefore not a first line treatment for undiagnosed hypoglycaemia. See above for further information.

HYPERINSULINISM

Diagnostic criteria are:

☐ Laboratory blood glucose below 2.6 mmol/L

☐ Glucose requirement above 6-8mg/kg/minute to maintain blood glucose above 2.6-3 mmol/L

☐ Detectable plasma insulin (with raised C-peptide) at time of hypoglycaemia.

☐ Inappropriately low blood free fatty acid and ketone body levels.

☐ Absent ketonuria.

☐ Glycaemic response to glucagon when hypoglycaemic.

Persistent susceptibility to severe hypoglycaemia is an urgent indication for carefully supervised transfer to a specialist centre. Trial drug management must not be allowed to delay definitive treatment unless promptly effective.

Glucagon is particularly useful as an interim measure when intravenous access is problematic. However, it may not be effective after repeated use due to exhaustion of glycogen stores.

Diazoxide may be given orally. When successful in suppressing the need for excessive intravenous glucose, this may be used long-term but may cause hypertrichosis.

Chlorothiazide. The effect of diazoxide is potentiated by the use of thiazide diuretics such as chlorothiazide, which should be given concurrently.

Octreotide. If diazoxide and chlorothiazide fail to suppress excessive glucose requirements then octreotide may be added. Tachyphylaxis and gastrointestinal disturbances are common. Although octreotide may suppress growth hormone secretion, there is little evidence that this has any long-term adverse effects on growth.

Alternative treatments for hyperinsulinaemic states are being evaluated, including calcium-channel blocking agents such as nifedipine. The evidence for their clinical efficacy is awaited.

THYROID DISORDERS

Congenital hypothyroidism. Neonatal capillary blood screening for elevated thyroid stimulating hormone (TSH) detects congenital hypothyroidism in approximately 1 in 3,500 infants. Screening programmes need to be linked to an efficient process for fast-track referral, confirmation, and counselling. The recommended starting dose of levothyroxine (thyroxine) is 10-15 microgram/kg/day, recognising that normal neonates have relative hyperthyroxinaemia. Levothyroxine dosage is then titrated to sustain free thyroxine in the upper normal adult range and TSH in the normal adult range. A useful guide is that children have a levothyroxine requirement approximating to 100 microgram/m^2/day.

Acquired (Hashimoto) autoimmune hypothyroidism is commoner in girls and there is often a family history of thyroid disease. Young persons tolerate a relatively rapid increase in levothyroxine (thyroxine) dosage, aiming for free thyroxine in the upper normal adult range and TSH in the normal adult range. Recognised but infrequent problems linked to diagnosis and treatment include benign intracranial hypertension and slipped upper femoral epiphysis.

Permanent levothyroxine replacement is necessary for confirmed autoimmune hypothyroidism. The differential diagnosis includes subacute thyroiditis, a self-limiting disorder presenting with tender goitre and variable thyroid dysfunction.

Juvenile hyperthyroidism is rare in the first decade and has a marked female preponderance. Elevated plasma thyroxine and/or tri-iodothyronine with suppressed TSH provide biochemical confirmation. The main cause is Graves' disease, usually presenting with goitre, eye involvement, and detectable TSH receptor stimulating antibodies. Low titres of antithyroid microsomal antibodies also occur. The early 'toxic' phase of Hashimoto autoimmune thyroiditis may also present as hyperthyroidism, however, eye involvement is less common and there are usually higher titres of thyroid autoantibodies.

Prolonged medical management is the preferred approach in young patients and it should be under the direction of specialists. High dosage carbimazole is administered until euthyroid. There are then two approaches: either to adjust the carbimazole dose to the minimum that sustains normal thyroid function, or to continue high dosage and give levothyroxine (thyroxine) replacement. The 'block and replace' approach is indicated when dosage adjustment is uncertain, or early relapse a problem. It is difficult to anticipate the likelihood of remission but it is reasonable to attempt carbimazole withdrawal after 1 to 2 years. Relapse warrants a further prolonged course of carbimazole.

Agranulocytosis, though rare, is the most serious side-effect of carbimazole treatment. Families should be given written advice to stop treatment and seek an urgent blood count if patients develop an unusual sore throat or other infection. Agranulocytosis is most likely to occur in the first 3 months of treatment. Hyperthyroidism itself is a cause of mild neutropenia. Serious or recurrent side-effects justify changing to propylthiouracil, although this drug is also a potential cause of agranulocytosis.

Active disease for more than 4 to 5 years, inability to tolerate anti thyroid drugs or major compliance problems are indications for either partial thyroidectomy or radio-iodine. The prejudice against the latter in young patients needs to be balanced against increasing evidence of efficacy and safety.

Fetal and neonatal hyperthyroidism occurs in an estimated one in 70 pregnancies in mothers with past or present Graves' disease. High maternal titre of TSH receptor antibody signals risks to the fetus, with tachycardia potentially emerging from 24 weeks gestation. The neonatal presentation is delayed if mothers have been treated with carbimazole or propylthiouracil. Affected infants are treated with carbimazole until resolution, usually within 8-12 weeks. Severe symptomatic disease merits initial iodine as Lugol's solution to block the thyroid, and propranolol for its peripheral action.

CALCIUM DISORDERS

These disorders are at the interface between nutrition, metabolism, nephrology and endocrinology. It is important that all appropriate samples have been collected prior to the initiation of any treatment otherwise the clinical picture becomes hard to interpret in retrospect.

Hypocalcaemia. The differential diagnosis broadly divides into vitamin D deficiency, or a failure of secretion (hypoparathyroidism), or resistance to parathyroid hormone (PTH) (pseudohypoparathyroidism). Hypoparathyroidism and pseudohypoparathyroidism are characterised by a low plasma calcium and elevated plasma phosphate but this combination may also be rarely seen in severe vitamin D deficiency. Measurements of 25-hydroxyvitamin D and serum PTH are therefore critical to the correct diagnosis. Vitamin D status is normal in hypoparathyroidism and pseudohypoparathyroidism, with inappropriately low or elevated PTH levels respectively. Hypocalcaemia due to vitamin D deficiency also produces an elevated PTH. Individuals with pseudohypoparathyroidism may or may not have physical features of Albright hereditary osteodystrophy. Individuals with acquired hypoparathyroidism should be regularly checked for the development of adrenal insufficiency.

Mild asymptomatic hypocalcaemia may be managed with oral calcium supplements. Severe symptomatic hypocalcaemia requires an intravenous infusion of calcium gluconate 10% (0.3mL/kg) over 5 to 10 minutes repeating the dose if symptoms persist. In exceptional cases it may be necessary to maintain a continuous calcium infusion over a day or more. Persistent hypocalcaemia requires an oral regimen based on calcium supplements and either a vitamin D analogue (alfacalcidol or calcitriol) for hypoparathyroidism and pseudohypoparathyroidism or native vitamin D (calciferol) if due to vitamin D deficiency. It is important to monitor plasma and urinary calcium on long-term maintenance therapy.

Hypercalcaemia. This has a broad differential diagnosis and is less commonly seen than hypocalcaemia. The key investigation is serum PTH which should be suppressed below normal but is elevated in primary and tertiary hyperparathyroidism and within or just above the normal range in benign familial hypercalcaemia. Assessment of vitamin D metabolites, urinary calcium excretion and evidence of familial hypercalcaemia will help clarify the diagnosis. Acute symptomatic hypercalcaemia should be treated with furosemide (frusemide) and volume expansion with NaCl 0.9%. Subsequent treatment depends on the aetiology.

☐ Primary and tertiary hyperparathyroidism – surgery
☐ Vitamin D toxicity – withdraw vitamin D
☐ Benign familial hypercalcaemia – no treatment
☐ Williams syndrome/granulomatous disorders – low calcium and vitamin D diet and/or steroids
☐ Malignancy or immobilisation – consider intravenous disodium pamidronate.

Rickets. This can be divided according to aetiology into calcipenic (due to calcium/vitamin D problems) or phosphopenic (due to phosphate deficiency). The key investigation to distinguish these is serum PTH, which is elevated in calcipenic rickets and normal in untreated phosphopenic rickets. Measurements of vitamin D metabolites, renal function and renal tubular reabsorption of phosphate (%TRP) will also help clarify the diagnosis. Treatment depends on the cause:

☐ Vitamin D deficiency – calciferol for 6 weeks to 4 months
☐ Vitamin D-dependent rickets type 1 – alfacalcidol or calcitriol long-term
☐ Vitamin D-dependent rickets type 2 – high-dose alfacalcidol or calcitriol long-term. High-dose oral or intravenous calcium may be required to heal rickets
☐ Hypophosphataemic rickets – phosphate supplements with alfacalcidol or calcitriol
☐ Rickets due to distal renal tubular acidosis will heal with correction of the acidosis and does not require vitamin D.

In vitamin D-deficiency rickets treatment should be discontinued once biochemistry returns to normal rather than prolonging it until deformity of legs improves which may take up to 2 years.

Osteoporosis. This is uncommon in children and may be primary (osteogenesis imperfecta or idiopathic juvenile osteoporosis) or secondary e.g. steroids, immobilisation, inflammatory disorders. Careful investigation and management requires the input of a clinician familiar with osteoporosis in children. There is increasing experience with the use of bisphosphonates especially disodium pamidronate in children with a good short-term safety profile although concerns about potential long-term adverse effects remain.

PITUITARY FUNCTION TESTS
Stimulation tests may focus on either one hormone pathway, frequently growth hormone (GH), or be combined to examine two or more of GH, luteinising hormone (LH), follicle stimulating hormone (FSH), thyroid stimulating hormone (TSH), adrenocorticotrophic hormone (ACTH) and prolactin (PRL).

Growth hormone axis. GH levels are regulated by interplay between growth hormone releasing hormone and somatostatin, the former governing the magnitude of secretory pulses and the latter their timing. Pharmacological agents that act through the hypothalamic-pituitary axis to stimulate GH release include glucagon, clonidine, arginine, and levodopa. The use of insulin-induced hypoglycaemia as a stimulus to GH secretion carries considerable risks and should only be performed in centres able to provide intensive supervision.

Indications for GH tests include:

☐ Growth failure not explained by environmental restraint or non-endocrine organic disease
☐ Congenital and acquired structural hypothalamic-pituitary disorders (confirmed by magnetic resonance imaging). This includes congenital multiple pituitary hormone deficiency
☐ Growth failure following cranial irradiation.

Low plasma levels of insulin-like growth factor-1 (IGF-1) and its binding protein (IGFBP3) support but do not prove GH deficiency. It is essential that GH assays be performed within external quality assurance schemes.

Endocrine

Commonly used GH tests (contact specialist centres for detailed guidelines)
☐ Glucagon: intramuscular 100 microgram/kg to a maximum 1mg.
    Sampling at baseline, 30, 60, 90, 120, 150, 180 minutes.
    Caution: risk of delayed hypoglycaemia.
☐ Clonidine: oral 150 microgram/m².
    Sampling at baseline, 30, 60, 90, 120, 150 minutes.
    Caution: risk of hypotension.

Gonadorelin (gonadotrophin–releasing hormone; LH–RH) test. Sensitive assays of basal gonadotrophin samples and ovarian ultrasound imaging have reduced the indications for this test.

Protirelin (thyrotrophin–releasing hormone; TRH) test. Sensitive assay of basal TSH samples has reduced the indications for this test. It is used to confirm hypothalamic-pituitary disorders when basal TSH may be in the low normal range with a low free thyroxine.

Tetracosactide (tetracosactrin; Synacthen®) tests. These are used to investigate the ACTH-cortisol axis. A basal 09:00 hours plasma cortisol level at or above 500nmol/L suggests an intact ACTH-cortisol axis; a level below 100nmol/L, especially in a stressed or hypoglycaemic patient, indicates an impaired axis. Levels in between may require further clarification as guided by the clinical picture. Glucagon stimulation (and the restricted insulin-induced hypoglycaemia test) may be used to test the hypothalamic-pituitary-adrenal axis directly. However, paired baseline ACTH and cortisol samples followed by tetracosactide stimulation are more widely used in clinical practice. The low-dose tetracosactide stimulation test is considered to be more sensitive than the conventional dosage test for confirming partial, established adrenal insufficiency, such as that caused by high-dose inhaled corticosteroid.

Corticotrophin releasing factor (CRF). Used for detailed assessment of pituitary ACTH release under specialist guidance.

Antidiuretic hormone (ADH) assessment. The combination of an established hypothalamic-pituitary abnormality or multiple pituitary hormone deficiency with excessive thirst, polyuria, hypernatraemia and inappropriately hypo-osmolar urine is indicative of ADH deficiency. It is important to recognise that cortisol deficiency masks ADH deficiency, and that ADH therapy in the absence of adequate cortisol replacement can cause hazardous water retention and hyponatraemia.

Isolated partial diabetes insipidus (DI) is more difficult to diagnose, especially in older children who maintain fluid balance with increased thirst. Confirmation and differentiation from behavioural over-drinking may require a water deprivation test. A normal response to deprivation is a plasma osmolality in the normal range (282-295 mOsm/kg) and a maximum urine osmolality of greater than 750 mOsm/kg. Plasma osmolality above 295 mOsm/kg with urine osmolality less than 300 mOsm/kg confirms severe DI. A test dose of desmopressin resulting in an increase in urine osmolality by 20% or more confirms central diabetes insipidus; a deficient response suggests nephrogenic DI. Careful fluid balance measurement must be ensured before and after a test dose of desmopressin to prevent over-hydration and hyponatraemia.

GROWTH HORMONE THERAPY
Synthetic human GH (somatropin) is currently licensed for use in children with:
☐ GH insufficiency usually defined as a persistently low height velocity together with two or more biochemical
    confirmatory tests
    Dose 25-35 microgram/kg/day or 0.7-1mg/m²/day
☐ Turner syndrome
    Dose 50 microgram/kg/day or 1.4mg/m²/day
☐ Prepubertal chronic renal disease
    Dose 50 microgram/kg/day or 1.4mg/m²/day
☐ Prader-Willi syndrome for which the benefit is based on metabolic criteria as well as improved growth
    Dose 35 microgram/kg/day or 1mg/m²/day.

GH is administered as a daily SC injection or needle-free delivery. Monitoring includes 3-6 monthly growth review and serial plasma IGF-1 measurement. Failure of the predicted growth response requires review of diagnosis and compliance.

GH therapy may be stopped at the end of effective height growth without graded dose reduction. Patients with permanent severe GH deficiency, especially when associated with multiple pituitary hormone deficiency, are candidates for lower dose GH replacement as adults.

ADRENAL STEROID REPLACEMENT

The main indications for adrenal steroid replacement are:

☐ Hypopituitarism – usually panhypopituitarism; rarely isolated ACTH deficiency.

☐ Primary adrenal insufficiency.

☐ Congenital adrenal hyperplasia (the aim being suppression of the ACTH drive to androgen production).

Hypopituitarism (see also: thyroxine, GH, sex hormone and ADH replacement).
Disorders of the hypothalamic-pituitary axis result in glucocorticoid deficiency (secondary adrenal failure); aldosterone secretion remains intact. The typical plasma biochemical profile comprises hypoglycaemia, hyponatraemia without hyperkalaemia, low cortisol levels with impaired response to tetracosactide (tetracosactrin) tests, and low ACTH levels.

Primary adrenal insufficiency. The majority of patients require both glucocorticoid and mineralocorticoid replacement. The biochemical confirmation of dual deficiency is provided by hyponatraemia with hyperkalaemia, an impaired cortisol response with elevated ACTH levels, reduced aldosterone and a compensatory increase in plasma renin activity.

Glucocorticoid replacement in childhood is conventionally provided as hydrocortisone, 12-$15mg/m^2$/**day** divided in three doses. Freedom from symptoms, an active lifestyle, and normal growth while using this regimen avoids the need for frequent biochemical monitoring.

Mineralocorticoid replacement is provided with fludrocortisone in the dose range 50-200 microgram/**day** aiming for electrolyte balance confirmed by normal plasma renin activity and blood pressure.

Congenital adrenal hyperplasia. The conventional approach to suppression of the ACTH-adrenal androgen axis in childhood is to use hydrocortisone. A dose of 12-$15mg/m^2$/**day** divided into three doses is usually adequate but may need to be increased to 15-$20mg/m^2$/**day** to fully suppress androgen levels. Plasma or salivary profiles of 17-hydroxyprogesterone may be used to refine the dose regimen. Adolescents may be better managed with prednisolone or dexamethasone. The dosage of the more potent corticosteroids requires careful titration because of uncertain bio-equivalence. Mineralocorticoid replacement as listed above is required for patients with salt losing forms of congenital adrenal hyperplasia.

SEX STEROID REPLACEMENT

Sex hormone replacement is indicated for:

☐ Gonadotrophin deficiency

☐ Gonadal disorders

☐ Delayed puberty that interferes with quality of life.

Male hormone replacement. For boys in whom gonadal failure is predicted testosterone replacement may be started at around age 12 years with gradually increasing dosage. For induction of puberty, a conventional strategy is based on monthly depot testosterone injections starting at 25mg/month and, escalating the dose in 6-12 monthly increments guided by response. An alternative oral regimen using testosterone undecanoate starts at 40mg on alternate days, increasing to 120mg per day. Replacement options for adult men include depot testosterone injections at 2 weekly intervals, or subcutaneous implant insertion at 4-6 monthly intervals guided by plasma testosterone levels. Topically active formulations of testosterone are established for adult replacement but are not yet approved for induction of puberty. In boys with gonadotrophin deficiency, testicular growth and potential fertility also require chorionic gonadotrophin (HCG) therapy under expert guidance. This is usually provided after induction of puberty unless small testicular size is an issue for the patient. Normal bone mineralisation is an important objective of replacement.

Options for temporarily assisting boys with delayed puberty, usually after age 14 years, include intramuscular testosterone depot 50mg/month, or oral testosterone undecanoate 40mg/day for 3-6 months. An alternative approach that promotes growth rather than sexual maturation uses oral oxandrolone 1.25-2.5mg/day for 3-6 months.

Female hormone replacement. Puberty induction from age 12 years is commenced with ethinylestradiol (ethinyloestradiol) 2 microgram/day, increasing at approximately 6-monthly steps to 5, 10 and then 20 microgram/day, guided by breast staging and uterine scans. Normal bone mineralisation is an important objective of replacement. Cyclical progestogen replacement is added after 12-18 months of oestrogen; potential progestogen regimens are levonorgestrel 30 microgram/day or norethisterone 5mg/day for the last 7 days of each 28 days. Once adult dosage of oestrogen has been reached, it is convenient to provide replacement either as a low dose oestrogen containing oral contraceptive formulation or as an oestrogen plus progestogen hormone replacement therapy preparation.

Turner syndrome. Ethinylestradiol 2 microgram/day is started after age 12 years. It may be preferable for final height gain to delay introduction until 14 years. Subsequent escalation follows the scheme above.

Puberty suppression

Gonadorelin agonists have a role in the control of central precocious puberty. Preliminary assessment should determine the:

☐ Underlying cause

☐ Pubertal stage, bone maturation and potential impact on final height

☐ Capacity of child and family to cope with early sexual maturity against the background of a secular trend towards earlier sexual maturation.

Injected formulations of gonadorelin analogues are more effective. Their safety profile justifies use if early puberty is likely to be disruptive to a child's well being. There is some uncertainty, however, as to whether they promote obesity and polycystic ovarian disease.

The management of precocious puberty driven by autonomous gonadal activity requires specialist guidance.

Eye

Administration of drugs to the eye

To administer drops, the lower lid should be gently pulled down and the drops instilled in the lower fornix. Instil only one drop at a time. Any excess drops should be wiped away. In an unco-operative child, stabilise the child's head whilst asking an assistant (preferably the mother), to hold the child's arms. For multiple therapy, a minimum of 3 minutes should be left between the administration of different substances to allow for absorption, and to prevent dilution and overflow. The order in which different drops are instilled is not particularly important, but drops which sting should be used last as they cause reflex tear secretion. Do not use topical agents to which there is known systemic sensitivity or risk of side-effects, such as beta-blockers (e.g. timolol) in asthma sufferers.

Eye ointments may be used instead of drops if a longer action is needed. When eye ointments and drops are used together, ointments are put in after drops. Drops and ointments containing preservatives should not be used in children wearing contact lenses without discussion with an ophthalmologist.

Reducing the risk of microbial contamination.

All preparations for the eye should be sterile prior to administration. Special caution should be taken in the use of multiple application formulations. One bottle is utilised per patient and if there is an infection in both eyes, the prescriber can opt to use different bottles for each eye. *In hospital wards,* eye drops for multiple application should be discarded 1 week after opening. If the drops do not contain a preservative they should be discarded after 1 day. *In operating theatres,* drops containing a preservative should not be kept for more than a month. Drops not containing a preservative should be refrigerated and not kept for more than a week.

Antibacterials

Most superficial eye infections are susceptible to topical treatments. Bacterial blepharitis is treated by lid hygiene together with application of an antibacterial eye ointment to the conjunctival sac; systemic treatment may occasionally be required. Conjunctivitis is treated with antibacterial eye drops. Gonococcal conjunctivitis is treated with both systemic and topical antibiotics. Corneal ulcers and keratitis require specialist advice and may need conjunctival/systemic treatment.

Endophthalmitis

Should be investigated with microscopy and culture of aqueous and vitreous biopsies before treatment. This is usually followed by administration of broad-spectrum intravitreal antibiotics e.g. vancomycin or cefazolin with amikacin or gentamicin. Chloramphenicol is the drug of choice in superficial eye infections; other broad-spectrum antibiotics include ofloxacin, ciprofloxacin, gentamicin, neomycin and framycetin. Gentamicin and tobramycin are active against *Pseudomonas aeruginosa.* Ciprofloxacin or erythromycin are used in the treatment of chlamydial infections. Fusidic acid is useful for staphylococcal infections. Propamidine isetionate is used for the treatment of *acanthamoeba keratitis*.

Antifungals

All suspected fungal infections should be investigated microbiologically by examination of smears and cultures of appropriate biopsies. There are no commercially available antifungal eye preparations but some (e.g. clotrimazole 1% eye drops) are available from Moorfields Eye Hospital.

Antivirals
Topical preparations of aciclovir (acyclovir) and ganciclovir or trifluorothymidine may be used to treat herpes simplex keratitis. Patients should be referred urgently to an ophthalmologist.

Corticosteroids and other anti-inflammatory agents
Although the relative potencies of steroids have been established from skin tests, there is little evidence to show that these figures can be used in treatment of the eye. The dose should be dependent on the severity of the condition. To prevent rebound inflammation it is important to wean the treatment gradually.

Topical side-effects of steroids include delay in healing rate, corneal ulceration or corneal oedema, and raised intra-ocular pressure. Clobetasone and fluorometholone are less likely than dexamethasone to cause raised intraocular pressure but may not penetrate the cornea so well. Do not use steroids in undiagnosed red eye, as inappropriate use could cause blindness. Steroids may mask or enhance the activity of eye infections.

Antihistamines can be used topically for short-term management of allergic conjunctivitis. Sodium cromoglicate (cromoglycate) and iodoxamide can be used in vernal catarrh, giant papillary conjunctivitis, and seasonal allergic conjunctivitis.

Antimuscarinics
These dilate the pupil and paralyse the ciliary muscle; they vary in potency and duration of action. Cyclopentolate and tropicamide are synthetic compounds with a lower risk than atropine of causing contact sensitivity. Both have a rapid onset of action and are short-acting, mydriasis occurring in about 15 minutes and cycloplegia taking a little longer. Tropicamide lasts for 4 to 6 hours and cyclopentolate for up to 24 hours. Atropine is the most potent of these compounds and lasts for about a week. It can cause significant systemic adverse effects particularly in very young children (in whom ointment should be used). Hyoscine is potent but should not be used in children due to the risk of hallucinations.

Sympathomimetics
These are used in ophthalmology to cause mydriasis (e.g. phenylephrine) or vasoconstriction and lowering of intraocular pressure (e.g. dipivefrine). The latter is thought to act principally by increasing aqueous humour outflow, although it is rarely used in children. Brimonidine, a newer sympathomimetic anti-glaucoma drug, should not be used in infants and only used with caution in children as it may cause cardiorespiratory depression.

Local anaesthetics
These cause stinging and irritation when first applied. They act by stabilising nerve cell membranes, preventing transmission of nerve impulses along the axons. Duration of action and depth of anaesthesia is dependent upon dose. Oxybuprocaine is used for tonometry, although proxymetocaine is better because it stings less.

GLAUCOMA
Glaucoma should always be managed by an ophthalmologist as it may result in blindness. Glaucoma is almost always due to reduced outflow of aqueous humour. Useful drugs include the beta-blockers, carbonic anhydrase inhibitors, cholinergics and prostaglandin analogues. In emergencies, intravenous hypertonic mannitol can be used to reduce intra-ocular pressure.

Beta–blockers cause a reduction in intraocular pressure with little, if any, effect on pupillary size. They vary with their specificity for beta-receptor sub-types. Betaxolol has a lower affinity than timolol for beta-2 receptors and may be of value in patients prone to asthma (though it should be used with extreme caution).

Carbonic anhydrase inhibitors may be topical or oral. Oral acetazolamide can halve aqueous humour production, but unpleasant side-effects are common. The carbonic anhydrase inhibitors are all sulphonamides, and must be avoided in children known to be sensitive to sulpha drugs.

Cholinergics (miotics) can cause brow ache and ciliary spasm, which reduces with time. They often cause some blurring of vision.

Topical prostaglandin analogues, latanoprost or travoprost, act by increasing aqueous outflow through uveoscleral pathways and are very effective pressure lowering agents. They have been associated with increased length and thickness of eyelashes, and with an increase in iris pigmentation. There are concerns that this colour change may predispose to iris melanoma, but no cases have so far occurred. Topical prostaglandin analogues also predispose to macular oedema, and should be used with caution in aphakic and inflamed eyes.

FEVER MANAGEMENT

Symptomatic drug treatment for fever in infancy and childhood can be justified on the basis of relief of discomfort to the child, reducing anxiety of parents and carers, and probably reducing the risk of febrile convulsion in those age groups at risk. Drugs may reduce the magnitude and duration of fever (irrespective of the underlying cause) but do not influence the underlying disease process. Symptomatic relief of fever must not distract attention from the need to establish an explanation for the cause of the fever. Physical intervention, such as tepid sponging and fanning, often cause disproportionate discomfort and are not recommended.

Paracetamol is the antipyretic drug of first choice and is widely used and well-tolerated by febrile children of all ages. It has mild analgesic but no anti-inflammatory effects. To avoid cumulative toxicity, especially if the drug is used for more than a few days, the dose must be correct for the age and weight of the child.

Ibuprofen is the second-line alternative. Its antipyretic properties are at least equal to those of paracetamol but (being a cyclo-oxygenase-inhibitor) it is also anti-inflammatory. Ibuprofen can be given in addition to paracetamol, as they do not interact.

Aspirin should not be given to children <12 years as an analgesic/antipyretic because of the risk of Reye syndrome unless medically indicated and should be avoided in children under 16 years if feverish. Aspirin still has a place in Kawasaki disease though.

Gastrointestinal

GASTRO-OESOPHAGEAL REFLUX (GOR)

Gastro-oesophageal reflux (GOR) in infancy is common. In most infants with repeated, effortless regurgitation who are otherwise well, the natural history is excellent and drug treatment is not justified. Some high-risk groups such as preterm infants and children with neurodevelopmental disorders, merit special consideration. This includes children with cerebral palsy and children with primary dysmorphic syndromes. Clinical assessment in this group is often difficult and special investigations should be considered early. In children with chronic respiratory disorders, which are difficult to control, or with unexplained exacerbations, reflux should be considered.

One approach to reflux management is based on the consensus statement of the European Society of Paediatric Gastroenterology and Nutrition – each level includes the previous one.

Level one	Parental reassurance, diet, alginate/antacid (e.g. Gaviscon®), thicken feeds, left lateral position
Level two	Domperidone or low-dose erythromycin
Level three	H₂ blockers (e.g. ranitidine), proton pump inhibitors (e.g. omeprazole), sucralfate, misoprostol
Level four	Fundoplication

Level one treatment may be prescribed after a clinical diagnosis of reflux. In children in whom symptoms persist or do not respond to the simple therapies, and in those with complications such as oesophagitis or recurrent respiratory problems, investigation is required. The principal investigations include prolonged oesophageal pH monitoring, endoscopy, and radiology. They are often undertaken by a paediatric gastroenterologist, in a special unit, in collaboration with a paediatric surgeon. Long-term use of acid suppression, the use of proton pump inhibitors, or any consideration of surgery should not be undertaken prior to full assessment.

Cisapride is currently suspended from routine use due to concerns about QT prolongation on the ECG (see cisapride monograph for further details). If cisapride is used an ECG must be obtained prior to therapy to exclude prolonged QT interval or other cardiac problems. Repeat 7 days after starting cisapride, after dose increase, before discharge, and every two months thereafter. Ensure serum potassium and magnesium are within the normal range before and during treatment.

Cisapride is still used in paediatric centres where clinical indications demand and is provided on a named patient basis from the manufacturer. A final international decision on cisapride is awaited. Alternative prokinetic agents include domperidone and low-dose erythromycin.

PEPTIC ULCER DISEASE

Duodenal and gastric ulcers are managed on the same principles as adult disease. In young children it is most important to consider other factors which may lead to secondary peptic ulceration and to deal with these (e.g. NSAIDs, stress-associated gastritis in the ill child).

In primary ulcer disease, *Helicobacter* eradication is most important (see below). Rapid symptom relief may be achieved with antacids. Ulcer healing requires suppression of acid secretion by proton pump inhibition or H_2 blockade for 6-12 weeks. Recurrence is well-recognised. Additional therapy, in resistant disease, includes misoprostol and sucralfate.

HELICOBACTER PYLORI

The role of *Helicobacter pylori* (HP) in gastrointestinal problems in children is not well defined. There is an association between HP and peptic ulceration. The relationship between HP infection and abdominal pain is still contentious. HP infection is frequently acquired in infancy. Faced with a child with upper gastrointestinal symptoms, epigastric pain or other symptoms of dyspepsia and in whom *Helicobacter* infection is present, it is reasonable to attempt to eradicate it. The optimal treatment regime for HP has not been established but a triple regime (two antibiotics and a proton pump inhibitor (PPI)) has a more superior eradication rate than a dual therapy regime (one antibiotic and a PPI) and the latter is not recommended. A two-week course offers higher eradication rates than a 1 week course but may be restricted by patient compliance and the incidence of adverse effects. These factors should be considered when determining length of treatment.

INFANTILE COLIC

Treatment of colic is problematic. Data are not available to provide useful guidelines. The choice of agent is dependent upon the child's age. It is mandatory to exclude any underlying pathology. Dimeticone is found in over the counter remedies such as Infacol®, and may help but evidence of benefit is uncertain. Artificially-fed infants could be tried on a hypoallergenic formula for a week.

ABDOMINAL PAIN

Children with recurrent abdominal pain should have underlying diseases excluded before being treated symptomatically or being labelled as having functional pain. Antispasmodic drugs consist of the antimuscarinics (dicyclomine, hyoscine butylbromide, and propantheline) and others such as mebeverine and peppermint. The antimuscarinics have an atropine-like action on smooth muscle, whereas mebeverine and peppermint are believed to have a more direct relaxant effect on intestinal smooth muscle.

ACUTE DIARRHOEA

Acute diarrhoeal disease in children leads to dehydration and is an important cause of morbidity and mortality worldwide. The mainstay of treatment is oral rehydration therapy; glucose-stimulated sodium and water absorption via mucosal cells is preserved even with extensive small bowel mucosal injury. Resistant vomiting and dehydration may require intravenous rehydration.

CHRONIC DIARRHOEA

There are many causes of chronic diarrhoea. The most common are chronic non-specific diarrhoea of childhood (often known as toddler diarrhoea) and the enteropathies, (e.g. cow's milk protein allergy and coeliac disease). Overflow causing soiling which can be misinterpreted as 'diarrhoea' can occur in chronic constipation. Chronic diarrhoea – when associated with blood or mucus in the stools, systemic upset or sub-optimal growth – merits full investigation before treatment.

Absorbents and bulk-forming drugs. These drugs are used mainly in children with excessive stool losses. It is important to monitor fluid, electrolyte, mineral, and vitamin balances. Ispaghula and methylcellulose are both bulk-forming drugs, which aid thickening.

Anti-motility drugs. Antidiarrhoeal agents should only be used in chronic diarrhoea of known cause after addressing the primary pathology, and in chronic non-specific diarrhoea of childhood once other pathologies are excluded. In general, symptomatic relief with anti-motility drugs should be used with caution and only for specific disorders in infants.

Chronic diarrhoea and excessive effluent losses, via colostomy and ileostomy, may be reduced by loperamide, codeine phosphate, and co-phenotrope. Caution is needed if there is hepatic dysfunction. The agents work by increasing transit time, thereby allowing fluid absorption. Loperamide also has an anti-secretory action.

Anion exchange resins. Colestyramine (cholestyramine) counteracts the irritant effect of non-resorbed bile acids, which may lead to diarrhoea in patients with a rapid transit time or short bowel syndrome. Because of the interference with the bile acid pool there is a danger of malabsorption of fat-soluble vitamins with chronic use. Hyperchloraemic acidosis has been described with colestyramine usage.

PROTEIN SENSITIVITY
Identifying a particular dietary component by exclusion is the treatment of choice for food sensitivity. Sodium cromoglicate (cromoglycate) may potentiate tolerance, although the evidence for this is scanty.

INFLAMMATORY BOWEL DISEASE
Crohn's disease. This may affect the patient anywhere from the mouth to the anus. Therapy is tailored towards the affected part of the bowel. Orofacial granulomatosis is more common in children than in adults and is difficult to treat. Topical steroid creams may be beneficial but oral steroids and occasionally azathioprine may be required for severe disease. Remission of small bowel disease can be achieved by using enteral feeding regimens, (usually of 4-6 weeks duration), or by oral steroids (in a tapering dose over 8-10 weeks). Remission of the colonic disease may be induced with prednisolone orally. Evidence is accumulating that enteral feeding regimens may also be useful in maintaining remission in colitis.

There are no good data supporting the use of maintenance steroid therapy in the long-term management of Crohn's disease in children. There is a risk of chronic steroid adverse effects, particularly growth suppression.

5-aminosalicylic acid (5-ASA) preparations such as sulfasalazine (sulphasalazine), olsalazine and mesalazine are beneficial in maintaining remission with ulcerative colitis and colonic Crohn's disease. The anti-inflammatory effects of the pH-dependent sustained-release preparation of mesalazine may benefit patients with distal small intestinal and right-sided colonic Crohn's disease.

Azathioprine and mercaptopurine act as steroid-sparing agents in extensive or recurrent inflammatory bowel disease. The effectiveness of azathioprine may not be apparent for up to three months and monitoring for rare but potentially serious marrow suppression is essential. The use of azathioprine for up to four years has not been shown to increase the risk of neoplastic disease.

Ulcerative colitis. Oral prednisolone is usually needed to achieve remission, and is tapered once symptoms have resolved. In left-sided colitis and mild disease, topical rectal preparations (of steroid and 5-ASA) may suffice. Maintenance treatment is with oral 5-ASA preparations.

Other treatments for inflammatory bowel disease. Should medical therapy fail then surgery is an option for both Crohn's disease and ulcerative colitis. Intravenous azathioprine and intravenous or oral ciclosporin (cyclosporin) have been tried in both diseases. Budesonide as an oral sustained-release steroid preparation has been used with reasonable effect in adults with terminal ileal and right colonic Crohn's disease. Its use is associated with less adrenopituitary suppression than systemic prednisolone. Trials of its use in children are under way. Metronidazole and (more recently), ciprofloxacin as well as topical tacrolimus may be beneficial in patients with perianal Crohn's disease.

Anti-tumour necrosis factor monoclonal antibodies (e.g. infliximab) are now being introduced for disease resistant to other strategies in adult patients. Experience in children is very limited and there are concerns regarding short and long-term side-effects. The treatment is very expensive.

CONSTIPATION
Dietary measures aimed at increasing the fibre and fluid content should be the first line of therapy. The result of prolonged constipation is megarectum and faecal overflow leading to soiling. Colonic inertia and lack of rectal sensation lead to faecal impaction.

Toilet training regimens based on daily attempts at faecal evacuation combined with laxative therapy lead to resolution of symptoms with time. It is essential to achieve colonic evacuation prior to initiating maintenance laxative therapy. Evacuation can be achieved by large doses of sodium picosulfate, or bowel cleansing solutions such as Klean-Prep®. Use softener first to aid evacuation, large doses of lactulose can be given.

Maintenance therapy can take the form of a faecal softener or (more usually), a combination of stimulant laxative and a softener. Oral laxative therapy is preferable to the use of regular suppositories and enemas, which are used only as a last resort.

Bowel preparation. For pre-operative and pre-colonoscopy bowel preparation, sodium picosulphate is a vigorous and effective stimulant laxative. Bowel cleansing solutions given rapidly in large volumes are an effective alternative. Phosphate enemas may be necessary but can lead to hyperphosphataemia and other electrolyte abnormalities (particularly in young children) so should be used with caution.

TOPICAL PREPARATIONS FOR PERIANAL CONDITIONS

Anal fissures are usually the result of chronic constipation. They are painful, and preparations containing local anaesthetic may give symptomatic relief. Laxatives (particularly stool softeners) should be given too.

Pruritus ani can be caused by threadworm infestation, and perianal erythema is frequently caused by local streptococcal skin infections. These conditions should be treated appropriately.

Infections

ANTIMICROBIAL THERAPY: PRINCIPLES OF USE

Resistance to antibiotics is increasing. Colonisation with resistant organisms can lead to spread between individuals in a community. The chances of infection caused by resistant organisms increases as a result. Resistance can develop by mutation during therapy and lead to treatment failure. Direct transfer of resistance genes can occur between bacteria of the same and different species. Resistance can be directed towards a single antibiotic, a group of closely related antibiotics or to an entire antibiotic class. Different resistance mechanisms (such as enzymes that hydrolyse the antibiotic, or changes that affect membrane bound antibiotic binding sites) can co-exist. Organisms resistant to one antibiotic are more likely to be resistant to unrelated agents. The clinical use of antibiotics inevitably drives the selection of resistant organisms. Antibiotics should therefore be used judiciously and not for trivial infections that resolve if left untreated. Parents are usually willing to accept thoughtful advice as to why antibiotics might not be necessary. Careful use of antibiotics also limits side-effects and costs.

Most antibiotic prescribing is started empirically but should be based on knowledge of the likely pathogens and their expected antibiotic sensitivities. Whenever possible, appropriate samples should be obtained for culture. When the results of culture and sensitivities are known, antibiotic treatment should be reviewed and rationalised, changing or stopping treatment if necessary. Local antibiotic prescribing policies should reflect prevailing antibiotic sensitivities of typical organisms (see table).

Likely distribution of antibiotic susceptibilities in the UK (guide only: always check local surveillance data)

	Strepto-coccus pyogenes	Strepto-coccus pneu-moniae	Staphy-lococcus aureus	Multiply-resistant S aureus (MRSA)	Entero-coccus	Neisseria menin-gitidis	Haemo-philus influenzae	Escherichia coli	Entero-bacter spp	Pseudo-monas spp
Penicillin										
Amoxicillin										
Co-amoxiclav										
Flucloxacillin										
Cefalexin										
Cefuroxime*										
Ceftazidime										
Meropenem										
Vancomycin										
Gentamicin										
Erythromycin										
Fusidic acid										
Rifampicin										
Trimethoprim										
Ciprofloxacin										

*cefotaxime and ceftriaxone show comparable sensitivity patterns to cefuroxime.

☐ Majority of strains resistant, or antibiotic not normally used in this situation
▨ 50–90% of strains sensitive
▨ >90% of strains sensitive, but resistance especially important
■ >90% of strains sensitive

Infections

COMBINATION THERAPY

A single agent is generally preferable to a combination. It reduces the risks of toxicity, and interactions, as well as cost. However, antibiotics are used appropriately in combinations for:

Empirical broad-spectrum treatment in severe sepsis. This applies to acute and potentially life-threatening infections in which the range of pathogens cannot be defined with certainty or covered by a single agent. For example, empirical treatment of meningitis in children under the age of 3 months is usually with cefotaxime and ampicillin.

Synergy. Two drugs occasionally have a greater effect in combination than when used alone. An example is the synergy between gentamicin and penicillin in group B streptococcal infection.

Anticipation of drug resistance. Formulations have been developed that combine a parent penicillin with a β-lactamase inhibitor (e.g. clavulanic acid, tazobactam) but infections that are sensitive to the parent penicillin should not be treated with the combined agent because the wider spectrum of activity of the combination is then unnecessary and side-effects, such as diarrhoea, may occur without any clinical gain.

Antibiotics such as rifampicin and fusidic acid should not normally be used as monotherapy, because of the high rate of emergence of resistant mutants during therapy leading to treatment failure.

Antituberculous regimens generally deploy three or more drugs, partly to prevent the development of a sub-population of resistant organisms.

ROUTES OF ADMINISTRATION

Oral drugs are absorbed mainly from the stomach and proximal small bowel. Although bioavailability is often best when taken on an empty stomach, this is rarely of clinical significance. It is generally more important to ensure that the antibiotic is taken reasonably regularly, in an appropriate dose, and for an adequate period of time. Liquid preparations are convenient and acceptable to the under 5s and these should be sucrose free so as not to contribute to dental caries and gingivitis.

Intravenous therapy is indicated for the seriously ill child when effective drug concentrations are required immediately at the site of infection. Otherwise it is restricted to situations in which oral administration is inappropriate, for example when there is vomiting and/or diarrhoea, or for agents (e.g. aminoglycosides) that are not absorbed from the gut.

Intramuscular treatment is painful. Drug absorption is unreliable, especially if the patient is poorly perfused. The main indication is for the prompt administration of benzylpenicillin for meningococcal meningitis or septicaemia if IV access is unavailable.

Topical agents are usually only active at the site of application but particular care is needed in newborn infants who are susceptible to systemic absorption through the skin. Their use is restricted to dermatomycoses, certain superficial skin and eye infections, mucosal candidiasis and eradication of carriage (e.g. nasal mupirocin).

Inhaled treatment is used predominantly to deliver maintenance antipseudomonal antibiotics, like colistmethate sodium (colistin), to the lungs in cystic fibrosis. Nebuliser equipment capable of generating an aerosol of appropriate particle size for effective pulmonary deposition and appropriate evacuation of exhaled antibiotic is essential.

DOSAGE REGIMENS

The clinical dose and frequency of administration depends on the pharmacokinetic properties of the drug (including the ability to penetrate different tissues); patient characteristics such as age and maturity, body weight, renal function; and the type and severity of infection.

The potential for toxicity is greater when the ratio between the therapeutic and toxic concentrations of a drug is low. For these agents, such as aminoglycosides and amphotericin, toxicity is monitored clinically and biochemically, and, for aminoglycosides, plasma antibiotic concentrations may require regular measurement.

With oral treatment, compliance declines with increasing frequency of administration or duration of therapy. In practice it is often unnecessary to prescribe oral antibiotics more than 3 times daily. An exception is oral aciclovir (acyclovir), which requires 5 doses in 24 hours. Conversely, once-daily administration is appropriate for antituberculous treatment and is a characteristic of some recently introduced agents, such as azithromycin.

Penetration of antibiotics to the site of infection

Antibiotics with good intracellular penetration	Antibiotics with good urinary penetration	Antibiotics with good biliary penetration
Ciprofloxacin	All β-lactams	Amoxicillin
Erythromycin	Trimethoprim	Most cephalosporins
Tetracyclines	Ciprofloxacin	Trimethoprim
Rifampicin	Aminoglycosides	Ciprofloxacin
Metronidazole	Glycopeptides (e.g. vancomycin)	

Antibiotics with good CSF penetration in the absence of meningeal inflammation	Antibiotics with adequate CSF penetration in the presence of meningeal irritation
Trimethoprim	Penicillin
Ciprofloxacin	Amoxicillin
Chloramphenicol	Cefotaxime
Rifampicin	Ceftriaxone
Metronidazole	Ceftazidime
	Imipenem/meropenem

LENGTH OF TREATMENT
The minimum duration of treatment will depend on the site of infection, type of organism and the clinical response. A reasonable (but not evidence based) guideline is to treat for 5 days beyond the last positive blood culture and for 48 hours beyond the last episode of fever, provided that there has been the expected clinical improvement. However, precise information is not available for most infections and longer courses are appropriate in deep-seated infection, in the immunocompromised, and in specific conditions such as neonatal meningitis (e.g. group B streptococcus 14 days, Gram-negative bacilli 21 days). Too short a course favours the survival of relatively resistant bacterial subpopulations and resurgence of infection. Too long a course increases the chances of resistance occurring within the commensal flora, and potential pathogenicity at a later date. When antibiotics are started for the possibility of infection but there is no subsequent evidence of bacterial sepsis, stop treatment as soon as possible.

SWITCHING FROM PARENTERAL TO ORAL TREATMENT
When the sensitivities of the causative organism have been defined, the choice of oral agent can be specific. There is no absolute requirement to use the same class of antibiotic as that given parenterally. When the organism has not been isolated but bacterial infection seems genuine, an agent is chosen with a similar spectrum of activity to that given parenterally. It is necessary to allow an overlap period so that the oral agent can achieve therapeutic levels before parenteral therapy is withdrawn. Early switch therapy is usually inappropriate in young children because of the relatively high incidence of bacteraemia in this age group.

MONITORING RESPONSE TO TREATMENT
It should not be assumed that antibiotics will necessarily cure the infection. If the child remains unwell, the clinical situation should be re-evaluated. Confirm that the antibiotic and dosage are appropriate; take further samples for culture; consider the possibility of focal or unexpected infection like an abscess, infected intravascular catheter, endocarditis, or opportunistic infection; consider the possibility of alternative or additional diagnoses such as immune deficiency or other systemic disorders. If a replacement antibiotic is needed it is wise to select one that is unlikely to show cross-resistance with the original agent. Bacteriostatic antibiotics should be avoided in the immunocompromised because host defences are required to eliminate non-replicating organisms.

PROPHYLAXIS
Preventative antibiotics should only be used when there is evidence of their efficacy in preventing infection in situations with a defined high risk of significant consequences (or with a lower risk but when the consequences of it are profound). In most situations the risk of infection is short-lived (such as in the treatment of close contacts of meningococcal disease) and the duration of prophylaxis should be correspondingly brief. There are few indications for longer-term prophyalxis. Here the microorganisms involved should have predictable sensitivities and the treatment should be well-tolerated, for example, the use of penicillin or erythromycin following splenectomy. Otherwise, the treatment of asymptomatic bacterial colonisation to prevent invasive disease carries an appreciable risk of selection of antibiotic-resistant microorganisms.

Infections

UNWANTED EFFECTS
The most frequent side-effect of antibiotics is a change to the host's normal flora. This occurs mainly with broad-spectrum agents. Overgrowth of *Candida* on mucocutaneous surfaces is a common problem and can lead to invasive disease in immunocompromised children. Poorly absorbed antibiotics, or those excreted into the gut after absorption, may predispose to antibiotic associated diarrhoea and to pseudomembranous colitis. The intestinal flora is also an important reservoir for the evolution of antimicrobial resistance.

COST
The costs of antibiotic treatment should not be put before the needs of the child but it is responsible to remember that there may be considerable differences in cost even between antibiotics with comparable activities and safety profiles. The temptation to prescribe newer and/or broad-spectrum antibiotics (both of which tend to be expensive) should be resisted unless there is good evidence to justify their use in preference to established treatments.

BACTERIAL INFECTIONS: COMMON ANTIBIOTICS
Comprehensive information about individual drugs is given in the monographs but they are outlined here to help in the selection of agents from the many available, and to emphasise important aspects of their use.

BETA-LACTAM ANTIBIOTICS (penicillins, cephalosporins, carbapenems)
This is the largest and most widely prescribed class of antibiotics. β-lactam antibiotics are widely distributed in tissues, and most are predominantly excreted in the urine. They do not cross the uninflamed blood-brain barrier but some penetrate the CSF in meningitis. ß-lactams should not be given directly into the CSF because of doubtful therapeutic benefit and the risk of serious encephalopathy.

β-lactam antibiotics are generally safe and well-tolerated. The most important side-effect is hypersensitivity, which is commonest with the penicillins. Much the most serious hypersensitivity reaction is anaphylaxis, which is estimated to occur in about 0.01% of all treatment courses. Non-anaphylactic, immediate, IgE mediated reactions occur in about 0.5% of courses and are manifest as urticaria or angioedema.

Non-allergic, maculopapular rashes are more frequent with ampicillin/amoxicillin (5%-10%) than natural penicillin (2%). There is 5%-10% cross-sensitivity between the penicillins and the cephalosporins and carbapenems. The latter two groups can usually be used with caution in patients who report hypersensitivity to penicillins but they should be avoided in children who have had an anaphylactic response. All injectable ß-lactams have potentially significant sodium contents.

Resistance to ß-lactam antibiotics may be due to ß-lactamase-mediated destruction, alteration of target binding proteins in the cell wall, or by decreased permeability through the outer membrane of Gram-negative bacteria. Different ß-lactam antibiotics are affected differently by these resistance mechanisms.

PENICILLINS
Benzylpenicillin (penicillin G) is for parenteral use and is effective in streptococcal, pneumococcal, gonococcal, meningococcal and some anaerobic infections. *However, it is no longer recommended for empirical treatment of possible pneumococcal meningitis or gonococcal infections because of increasing penicillin resistance in these bacteria.* Important indications include:

☐ Emergency treatment of suspected meningococcal disease in the community before urgent transfer of the child to hospital

☐ Combined with gentamicin in the empirical treatment of neonatal sepsis

☐ Pneumococcal infection. Because of the increasing incidence of penicillin resistance in pneumococci, penicillin is being increasingly replaced by other agents (such as the cephalosporins +/- vancomycin) for the empirical treatment of suspected pneumococcal infections. However, almost all penicillin-resistant pneumococci in the UK exhibit moderate resistance, and concentrations achieved at the site of infection (other than in meningitis) are usually adequate to treat infections with these strains

☐ When IV therapy is required for infections due to ß-haemolytic streptococci, e.g. *Streptococcus pyogenes*

☐ As part of the treatment regimen for specific conditions such as infective endocarditis, diphtheria, tetanus.

Phenoxymethylpenicillin (penicillin V) is given orally and has a similar range of activity to benzylpenicillin but is not used in serious generalised infections because of erratic absorption. The main indications are in the treatment of streptococcal tonsillitis and as prophylaxis against streptococcal infection following splenectomy, in sickle cell disease, and following acute rheumatic fever.

PENICILLINASE-RESISTANT PENICILLINS

Flucloxacillin is stable to staphylococcal penicillinases, and is the agent of choice for the oral and IV treatment of *Staphylococcus aureus* infections. However, flucloxacillin also has reasonable activity against streptococci and provides adequate cover in most mixed superficial infections (e.g. impetigo). It may be combined with fusidic acid in deep-seated infections, such as osteomyelitis. Resistance to flucloxacillin in staphylococci is mediated by alteration of the target penicillin binding protein. The majority of hospital-acquired coagulase-negative staphylococci are resistant to flucloxacillin, as are an increasing proportion of methicillin resistant staphylococcus aureus (MRSA). Flucloxacillin-resistant staphylococci are also resistant to other β-lactam antibiotics, and often to other classes of antibiotics. The glycopeptide antibiotics vancomycin and teicoplanin are the mainstay of treatment of infections with such strains.

EXTENDED-SPECTRUM PENICILLINS

Compared with benzylpenicillin and phenoxymethylpenicillin, ampicillin and amoxicillin have greater activity against enterococci, *Listeria* and Gram-negative bacteria, including *Haemophilus influenzae* and *Escherichia coli*. However, they are not β-lactamase-stable, and resistance due to altered penicillin-binding proteins also occurs. 90% of staphylococci and *Moraxella catarrhalis*, 15% of *H. influenzae* and 50% of *E. coli* are now resistant, limiting the value of these agents as empirical therapy. Maculopapular rashes are mediated by unknown mechanisms and do not indicate true penicillin allergy but occur commonly with both agents (5%-10%) and the incidence is much higher in children with concurrent infectious mononucleosis (Epstein-Barr virus or Cytomegalovirus).

Amoxicillin is significantly better absorbed than ampicillin and remains a good first choice for oral antibiotic treatment of otitis media and respiratory tract infections. It should not be used for treating uncomplicated sore throats because phenoxymethylpenicillin is adequate for streptococcal tonsillitis, and most other cases are viral. Amoxicillin can be combined with a β-lactamase inhibitor to overcome the resistance of many penicillinase-producing bacteria, but not penicillin binding protein-mediated resistance (see below).

Intravenous ampicillin or amoxicillin should only be used as empirical therapy in combination with another agent to ensure adequate cover. They may be combined with an aminoglycoside as an alternative to cephalosporin monotherapy in sepsis of gastrointestinal or urinary tract origin. They are also used to supplement cephalosporin therapy where cover against enterococci or *Listeria* is required.

PENICILLIN/β-LACTAMASE-INHIBITOR COMBINATIONS

β–lactamase inhibitors (e.g. clavulanic acid, tazobactam) are β-lactam compounds that have no useful antibacterial activity but which can inhibit β-lactamases by binding to them, so protecting the activity of the parent penicillin with which they are associated.

The β-lactamases of *Staph. aureus* and many Gram-negative bacteria including *Haemophilus* species, *M. catarrhalis*, many *E. coli* and *Klebsiella* species, and *Bacteroides* species are inhibited. However β-lactamase inhibitors are inactive against the β-lactamases of *Pseudomonas, Enterobacter, Serratia* and *Citrobacter* species. Enzymes similar to these are also increasingly being encountered in *E. coli* and other species that normally produce enzymes that can be inhibited. β-lactamase inhibitors penetrate CSF poorly.

<u>It is not appropriate to use a combined agent if the bacterium is sensitive to the parent penicillin alone.</u>

Co-amoxiclav combines amoxicillin and clavulanic acid, conferring activity against almost all *Staph. aureus* (except MRSA) and *M. catarrhalis,* over 90% of *H. influenzae* and *E. coli*; and many other Gram-negative bacteria, including anaerobes. This spectrum of activity is often unnecessarily broad, and probably accounts for the high incidence of associated gastrointestinal intolerance. Given orally, co-amoxiclav is the treatment of choice for human and animal bites, and other potentially mixed, soft tissue infections. Oral co-amoxiclav is otherwise a second-line agent, for example for recurrent otitis media, sinusitis, other respiratory tract infections, and urinary tract infections. Intravenous co-amoxiclav is an alternative to the combination of a cephalosporin and metronidazole as surgical prophylaxis.

Piperacillin plus tazobactam and ticarcillin plus clavulanic acid are combinations of an antipseudomonal penicillin and a β-lactamase inhibitor. These are very broad-spectrum antibiotics but lack of activity against *Enterobacter* and similar species is a significant disadvantage. They are used in some centres as empirical therapy for fever in neutropenic patients, usually combined with an aminoglycoside. Otherwise they should be reserved for serious infections resistant to other antibiotics.

CEPHALOSPORINS
These are useful and generally well tolerated broad-spectrum β-lactam agents. However, they are not active against enterococci, MRSA, *Listeria* species and anaerobes. Newer generation cephalosporins have greater activity against Gram-negative bacteria but sometimes at the expense of anti-Gram-positive activity.

First generation agents
Cefalexin is the most widely used in this category, and is given orally 3-4 times daily; **cefadroxil** has a longer half-life, allowing twice daily dosage. These agents are active against streptococci, *Staph. aureus*, and most community acquired *E.coli* and *Klebsiella*. None of them have reliable activity against *H. influenzae*. They do not cross the blood-brain barrier. Their main indication is in childhood urinary tract infections (especially because of increasing resistance to amoxicillin and trimethoprim) but they are also a suitable alternative to penicillins in mild skin and soft tissue infections. They are of limited value in respiratory infections because of the lack of activity against *H. influenzae*. They are not indicated in neonates.

Second generation agents
Compared to first generation cephalosporins, these agents provide similar Gram-positive cover, enhanced Gram-negative cover (including *H. influenzae*), and greater β-lactamase stability. **Cefuroxime** is the only widely used second generation agent for intravenous use. It is suitable for a wide range of serious infections, including infections of the urinary and respiratory tracts, skin and soft tissue, bones and joints. Combined with metronidazole it is also suitable for prophylaxis and treatment of intra-abdominal infections. Although it crosses the blood brain barrier, it sterilises CSF slowly *and should not be used for treating meningitis*. Cefuroxime in combination with metronidazole provides cover similar to co-amoxiclav, except that activity against enterococci and *Listeria* is lacking.

Orally-available second generation cephalosporins are not widely used because of doubts about their bioavailability and benefits over first generation agents.

Third generation agents
Although these agents have improved Gram-negative cover (sometimes encompassing *P. aeruginosa*) compared with second generation cephalosporins, these differences are not always clinically important. Nevertheless there are some clinical situations in which third generation parenteral cephalosporins have significant advantages over cefuroxime.

Parenteral
Cefotaxime and **ceftriaxone** are almost identical in activity. They have good activity against streptococci and *Staph. aureus* as well as Gram-negative bacteria. In particular, they are the most active cephalosporins against penicillin-resistant pneumococci and non- β-lactamase mediated amoxicillin-resistant *H. influenzae*. Ceftriaxone has a long half-life and once daily administration is effective. It is mainly cleared by the liver and can be associated with the formation of crystalline biliary sludge particularly in neonates. This is usually reversible when the drug is stopped. **Ceftazidime** has the broadest Gram-negative cover, which includes *Pseudomonas* species, but has much poorer activity against Gram-positive bacteria.

Parenteral cephalosporins – common indications in paediatrics

Cephalosporin (parenteral)	Common uses in paediatrics
Cefotaxime	Meningitis Meningococcal septicaemia Empirical treatment of severe sepsis Epiglottitis after securing the airway
Ceftriaxone	Similar indications to cefotaxime. Sometimes deployed as continuation therapy after initial control of infection has been achieved with cefotaxime
Ceftazidime	Broad anti-Gram-negative cover including *P. aeruginosa*
Cefuroxime	Lower respiratory tract infections in hospitalised children when penicillin or macrolide not appropriate Urinary tract infections requiring IV treatment Prophylaxis and treatment of intra-abdominal infections

Oral
Cefixime requires once daily oral administration and has good *in vitro* activity against *H. influenzae*, *M. catarrhalis*, and group A streptococci. It has Gram-negative cover similar to cefotaxime. It is not active against *Staph. aureus* and is less active than the second generation agents against *Streptococcus pneumoniae*. Cefpodoxime has less Gram-negative activity than cefixime but is active against *Staph. aureus* and has better activity against *Strep. pneumoniae*. It requires twice daily dosage. None of the oral third generation cephalosporins are currently first line agents in paediatrics.

Fourth generation agents
These agents have a very broad spectrum of activity. Cefpirome has comparable activity to first and second generation agents against Gram positive bacteria, and anti Gram negative activity similar to third generation cephalosporins (although it has poorer anti-pseudomonas activity than ceftazidime). It also has some activity against bacteria such as enterococci and *Enterobacter* species, which are normally resistant to cephalosporins. Cefpirome is not licensed for children under 12 years of age, and in any case a carbapenem antibiotic is usually a more reliable choice where very broad-spectrum cover is required.

CARBAPENEMS
These are exceptionally broad-spectrum ß-lactam agents for IV administration. They are active against most Gram-positive and Gram-negative bacteria, including anaerobes. They are stable against almost all ß-lactamases with penicillinase or cephalosporinase activity, and are therefore highly active against *Enterobacter* and other species that are commonly cephalosporin-resistant. However, they are inactive against MRSA, coagulase-negative staphylococci, *Stenotrophomonas maltophilia* and some enterococci. Therapeutic concentrations are established in the CSF. Their present role in paediatrics is generally restricted to serious hospital acquired infections unresponsive to standard therapy. There is limited experience with these agents in neonates.

Imipenem is combined with cilastatin, which inhibits the renal brush border inactivation of imipenem. This is essential to prevent the formation of nephrotoxic metabolites, and improves the urinary concentration of the active drug. There is a risk of seizures, mainly in patients with underlying CNS disease.

Meropenem is a more recent introduction that does not require stabilisation with cilastatin, and has a lower incidence of treatment induced seizures. It has a very similar spectrum of activity to imipenem, though infections with *Acinetobacter* species sometimes respond poorly even where the organism appears sensitive *in vitro*.

MACROLIDES (erythromycin, clarithromycin, azithromycin)
Erythromycin is the established macrolide used in paediatrics. Clarithromycin and azithromycin are newer macrolides whose main advantages are better tolerability, less frequent dosage, and in the case of azithromycin, shorter courses. All are active against streptococci, *Staph. aureus*, *Bordetella pertussis*, *Campylobacter* species and atypical pathogens including mycoplasmas, legionellae and *Chlamydia* species. Clarithromycin and azithromycin have greater activity against *H. influenzae* and *M. catarrhalis*. All have good tissue penetration and are concentrated intracellularly. Since low blood levels of azithromycin are achieved, it is not recommended in patients at risk of bacteraemia. The macrolides do not cross the blood-brain barrier, and excretion is mainly hepatic. Allergic reactions are uncommon.

Erythromycin is a good alternative to penicillin in penicillin allergy and is generally appropriate for mild to moderate infections if the organism is susceptible on culture. Other indications include atypical pneumonia and neonatal conjunctivitis due to *C. trachomatis*. Erythromycin eradicates *B. pertussis* from the nasopharynx and reduces the period of infectivity in children but does not alter the course of the disease; it is also used as prophylaxis for susceptible contacts of a case of pertussis. Erythromycin is less well absorbed than the newer macrolides and more likely to cause nausea, vomiting and abdominal discomfort. Orally, it is given 3-4 times daily. An IV formulation is available but this is very irritant to veins.

Clarithromycin requires twice daily oral administration and can also be administered IV. It is used in some eradication regimens for *Helicobacter pylori*.

Azithromycin is highly concentrated in the tissues, and slowly released. This allows once daily oral administration and a shortened duration of therapy (3 days for most infections).

The newer macrolides are alternatives to erythromycin where their better tolerability outweighs their greater cost. Their higher activity against *H. influenzae* means they are probably preferable to erythromycin in infections such as otitis media, sinusitis and pneumonia. They also have potent activity against many atypical mycobacteria.

Infections

AMINOGLYCOSIDES (amikacin, gentamicin, netilmicin, tobramycin)

These are rapidly bactericidal broad-spectrum antibiotics that are not absorbed from the gut. Penetration into the CSF is poor (but may be better in neonates). Excretion is mainly through the kidneys, and accumulation occurs in renal impairment. Aminoglycosides have excellent activity against Gram-negative bacteria (including *P. aeruginosa*) and staphylococci, but are inactive against anaerobes, streptococci and intracellular organisms. However, they may exhibit synergism with β-lactam antibiotics, especially against streptococci and enterococci.

The most important side-effects are ototoxicity (tinnitus, deafness, vestibular damage) and nephrotoxicity (usually reversible). Toxicity is directly related to duration of therapy, and is more common in patients receiving haemodialysis. The traditional view that high trough levels of the drugs contribute directly to toxicity has been challenged. It is now believed that it is the length of time for which serum levels exceed the threshold for binding to tissue receptors that is important. Once-daily administration shortens this period, and recent evidence suggests that it is associated with less toxicity and in most cases similar efficacy to conventional 8-12 hourly dosing. Evidence of efficacious once-daily gentamicin therapy for neonates is increasing and it is incorporated into treatment regimens in an increasing number of neonatal units. Plasma concentration monitoring is essential to avoid toxic levels on the one hand and ineffective ones on the other. For multiple daily dosing, concentrations should be measured 30-60 minutes after IV administration (peak) and again just before the next dose (trough). For once daily regimens it is essential to measure the trough level but there is no agreement as to if, or when, to measure peak levels.

Gentamicin and netilmicin are the most widely used aminoglycosides in paediatrics. They are indicated for serious infections, usually combined with a β-lactam antibiotic (and with metronidazole if anaerobic cover is important). Netilmicin may be less toxic than gentamicin, but is less active against *P. aeruginosa*. Tobramycin is slightly more active against *Pseudomonas aeruginosa* and slightly less active against other Gram-negative bacilli, although it is doubtful whether these differences are clinically important. It is predominantly used in combination with an antipseudomonal β-lactam in treating pseudomonas infections in cystic fibrosis.

Resistance to aminoglycosides is conferred by aminoglycoside converting enzymes. Different enzymes destroy different aminoglycosides, depending on their chemical structure. Amikacin is stable to many of these enzymes, and is reserved for serious infections where the organism is resistant to other aminoglycosides.

GLYCOPEPTIDES (vancomycin, teicoplanin)

These antibiotics are active against an extremely broad range of Gram-positive bacteria, but are inactive against Gram-negative bacteria. They are active against *Staph. aureus* (including MRSA) coagulase-negative staphylococci, streptococci, enterococci and *Clostridia*. Coagulase-negative staphylococci that are resistant to glycopeptides (especially teicoplanin) are occasionally seen, and MRSA that have reduced susceptibility to glycopeptides have recently been reported. Enterococci that are resistant to glycopeptides have emerged as important pathogens in some hospitals.

Glycopeptides are not absorbed after oral administration, and CSF penetration is poor. The glycopeptides are excreted unchanged in urine. Nephrotoxicity and ototoxicity are uncommon side-effects, but are more common with vancomycin. Vancomycin must be given by slow IV infusion over at least 60 minutes. Histamine release from non-allergic, direct mast cell degranulation occurs if the drug is given too quickly, causing flushing, urticaria, itching and sometimes, severe hypotension (red man syndrome). Red man syndrome is uncommon with teicoplanin, which can be given as a slow bolus or as an infusion over 30 minutes. Vancomycin is usually administered 2 or 3 times daily, whereas teicoplanin is once daily after initial loading. Monitoring of blood levels of vancomycin is currently recommended. Routine monitoring of teicoplanin levels to avoid toxicity is not necessary, but may help in children to optimise dosage.

Glycopeptides are important agents reserved for treatment of multiple antibiotic-resistant staphylococcal and other Gram-positive infections, and as prophylaxis against endocarditis. Oral vancomycin is a second-line agent for treating pseudomembranous colitis. Metronidazole is as effective, much cheaper, and does not risk promoting emergence of glycopeptide-resistant enterococci.

QUINOLONES (ciprofloxacin, moxifloxacin)

Most quinolones have a broad bactericidal Gram-negative spectrum, including *P. aeruginosa*, but are only moderately active against Gram-positive bacteria. Although more active against staphylococci than streptococci, resistance readily develops during treatment. They are well absorbed by mouth and achieve good tissue penetration. Intravenous administration offers no advantage over the oral route if the child can take oral medication. Excretion is mainly renal, but the gastrointestinal pathways become more important in patients with renal failure and dose adjustment is only necessary in severe renal failure. Quinolones are contra-indicated in G6PD deficiency.

Ciprofloxacin is the quinolone that is most used in children. It has only a limited paediatric licence because studies in juvenile animals indicated that quinolones damaged cartilage in weight-bearing joints, although there is no evidence of equivalent damage in children. Nevertheless, ciprofloxacin should only be used for serious infections and clear indications. Its main indications and uses at present are:

☐ Serious Gram-negative infections resistant to other agents

☐ Chronic *Pseudomonas aeruginosa* otitis media with perforation

☐ Children with cystic fibrosis who are colonised with *P. aeruginosa* and for whom oral therapy is considered necessary

☐ Resistant or complicated urinary tract infection unsuitable for treatment with other agents

☐ As an alternative in the treatment of invasive shigellosis or salmonellosis and in severe *Campylobacter* enteritis

☐ Enteric fever

☐ As an alternative to rifampicin in eradicating nasopharyngeal carriage of *Neisseria meningitidis*

☐ Anthrax.

Moxifloxacin is one of the first of a new generation of quinolones with enhanced activity against Gram-positive bacteria. Clinical experience with this agent is limited, and it is not licensed for use in paediatrics. However, it does have potential as an agent active against respiratory bacterial pathogens resistant to other oral agents.

LINCOSAMIDES & STREPTOGRAMINS (clindamycin, quinupristin with dalfopristin)

These agents are structurally unrelated to each other and to macrolides, but share a common mode of action. They have a predominantly anti-Gram-positive spectrum of activity, although clindamycin also has useful anti-anaerobic activity. They penetrate tissues well, but do not penetrate CSF. They are metabolised by the liver.

Clindamycin has good activity against staphylococci, streptococci and anaerobes. It is not usually used as a first-line antibiotic because of its association with pseudomembranous colitis. It is usually well tolerated in children, but treatment should cease immediately if the patient develops diarrhoea. It is well absorbed by mouth and is a suitable alternative to β-lactams in skin, soft tissue, and bone and joint infections, because of its excellent tissue penetration. It is also used in mixed infections with anaerobes, such as retropharyngeal abscesses, and as prophylaxis against infective endocarditis.

Quinupristin with dalfopristin is a recently introduced combination of two streptogramin antibiotics that act synergistically against staphylococci (including MRSA), streptococci and *Enterococcus faecium* (including strains that are glycopeptide-resistant). However *E. faecalis* is resistant. The product is not licensed for paediatric use but has been used successfully to treat infections with glycopeptide-resistant enterococci in children.

OTHER ANTIBIOTICS

Co-trimoxazole contains sulfamethoxazole and trimethoprim in a ratio of 5:1. The broad spectrum of activity is similar to either drug alone. The sulfamethoxazole component is responsible for most of the toxicity and, with the recognition that clinically useful synergism between the components is usually modest, co-trimoxazole is only recommended for specific indications such as prophylaxis and treatment of *Pneumocystis carinii* infection and treatment of brucellosis and nocardiosis.

Trimethoprim, a structural analogue of dihydrofolic acid, is bactericidal against *Strep. pyogenes, Strep. pneumoniae, H. influenzae*, and many strains of *E. coli*. Plasmid-encoded resistance is increasing. It is well absorbed, generally well tolerated, and mostly excreted unchanged in the urine. It is predominantly indicated in the prophylaxis and treatment of urinary tract infections in children.

Metronidazole is a nitroimidazole with a rapid bactericidal effect against obligate anaerobes such as *Bacteroides fragilis* and some parasites. It is metabolised in the liver and is generally well tolerated in children. It is generally combined with a β-lactam antibiotic to improve or provide anaerobic cover in the treatment of mixed infections. It is the treatment of choice for pseudomembranous colitis and is a component in some eradication regimens for *H. pylori*. It is the agent of choice in the treatment of *Giardia lamblia* infection.

Fusidic acid has potent bactericidal activity against staphylococci but when used systemically must always be combined with another agent to prevent the emergence of resistant escape mutants during therapy. It is indicated mainly for treatment of deep-seated infections, especially osteomyelitis, because of its excellent tissue penetration. It does not enter the CSF. Absorption after oral administration is high, and intravenous therapy is only indicated for patients unable to take or absorb oral medication; the bioavailability from the suspension (fusidic acid) is less than from the tablet formulation (sodium fusidate). Fusidic acid is metabolised and excreted by the liver.

Infections

Nitrofurantoin is rapidly excreted in the urine by filtration and tubular secretion, and is effective in uncomplicated urinary tract infections. It should not be used to treat pyelonephritis, because therapeutic blood and tissue levels of the agent are not achieved. _Proteus_ species are intrinsically resistant to nitrofurantoin, but acquired resistance in other species is uncommon. It is contra-indicated in G6PD deficiency and in infants under the age of 3 months but serious side-effects are rare in children.

Tetracyclines should not be given to children under the age of 12 years because they are deposited in immature teeth, which may become softened and permanently discoloured yellow-grey-brown. They are broad-spectrum and bacteriostatic. Widespread use of these agents in the past led to the rapid emergence of resistance, and they are now used infrequently as an alternative to macrolides in infections due to mycoplasma and chlamydia and for specific indications such as brucellosis and Lyme disease. Most tetracyclines are excreted in the urine: doxycycline is predominantly excreted by the liver, so may be used in renal failure. Oxytetracycline is still the first-line choice for the systemic treatment of acne.

Linezolid is the first of a new class of antimicrobials, the oxazolidinones, which inhibit protein synthesis. Linezolid is inhibitory against staphylcocci, enterococci and pneumococci, but has no bactericidal activity. It can be given orally or IV, but is not licensed for paediatric use. Given that there is currently more paediatric experience with quinupristin with dalfopristin, and that linezolid is not bactericidal, it is a second-line agent.

Antibiotics for specific bacteria

Outline of principal antibiotics for different organisms

Organism	Infection	First line treatment
Bacteroides species	Abscess, bacteraemia	Metronidazole
Bartonella henselae	Cat scratch fever	Usually none (macrolide)
Bordetella pertussis	Whooping cough	Macrolide (limits infectivity)
Borrelia burgdorferi	Lyme disease	Amoxicillin (macrolide)
		Ceftriaxone in CNS disease
Brucella species	Brucellosis	Co-trimoxazole +/- rifampicin
		(+ gentamicin in severe disease)
Campylobacter species	Enteritis	Erythromycin
Chlamydia pneumoniae	Atypical pneumonia	Macrolide
Chlamydia psittaci	Psittacosis	Macrolide
Chlamydia trachomatis	Eye infection	Oral macrolide + topical erythromycin
	Genital tract infection	Azithromycin (doxycycline)
	Pneumonia	Macrolide
Clostridium botulinum	Botulism	Seek advice
Clostridium difficile	Pseudomembranous colitis	Metronidazole
Clostridium tetani	Tetanus	Tetanus antitoxin + benzylpenicillin
Clostridium perfringens	Wound infection	Benzylpenicillin + metronidazole
Corynebacterium diphtheriae	Diphtheria	Benzylpenicillin + diphtheria antitoxin
Escherichia coli	Systemic infection	Cefotaxime/ceftriaxone + aminoglycoside
	Urinary tract infection	Cefuroxime
	Associated with diarrhoea	Usually none
Haemophilus influenzae	Invasive disease	Cefotaxime/ceftriaxone
	Otitis media	Amoxicillin or azithromycin (co-amoxiclav if fails to respond)
Helicobacter pylori	Gastritis, duodenal ulcer	Amoxicillin/clarithromycin/metronidazole in regimen with omeprazole
Klebsiella species	Pneumonia, systemic disease	Cefuroxime +/- gentamicin
Neisseria gonorrhoeae	Systemic disease	Benzylpenicillin or cefuroxime (check sensitivities)
Neisseria meningitidis	Meningitis / septicaemia	Urgent benzylpenicillin in community then cefotaxime in hospital
Legionella species	Legionnaires' disease	Macrolide (+ rifampicin in severe cases)
	Atypical pneumonia	Macrolide (ciprofloxacin if macrolide-allergic)

Organism	Infection	First line treatment
Leptospira species	Leptospirosis	Benzylpenicillin before 7th day
Listeria monocytogenes	Listeriosis	Ampicillin or amoxicillin + gentamicin
Moraxella catarrhalis	Otitis media, lower respiratory tract infection in children with chronic chest disease, or who are intubated	Oral: co-amoxiclav or macrolide IV: cefuroxime
Mycoplasma species	Atypical pneumonia Respiratory tract infection	Macrolide
Proteus species	Urinary tract infection	Cephalosporin
Pseudomonas aeruginosa	Cystic fibrosis	Ceftazidime + aminoglycoside
Salmonella species	Bacteraemia, gut infection	Ciprofloxacin (or trimethoprim)
Shigella species	Bacteraemia, gut infection	Amoxicillin (or ciprofloxacin)
Staphylococcus aureus	Cellulitis, abscess, osteomyelitis	Flucloxacillin +/- fusidic acid
Coagulase negative staphylococci	Bacteraemia	Vancomycin (or teicoplanin)
Streptococcus group A (*Streptococcus pyogenes*)	Tonsillitis, cellulitis	Penicillin (macrolide if allergic to penicillin)
Streptococcus group B (*Streptococcus agalactiae*)	Septicaemia, meningitis	Cefotaxime (or benzylpenicillin + gentamicin)
Enterococcus species	Urinary tract infection	Amoxicillin
Streptococcus pneumoniae (pneumococcus)	Pneumonia Meningitis Bacteraemia	Benzylpenicillin (+/- vancomycin) Cefotaxime (+/- vancomycin) Cefotaxime (+/- vancomycin)
Vibrio cholerae	Cholera	Ampicillin or amoxicillin (or trimethoprim or erythromycin)
Yersinia species	Yersinosis	Ciprofloxacin (or cefuroxime + gentamicin)

NEONATAL BACTERIAL INFECTIONS

Neonates are vulnerable to bacterial infection, and the lower the birth weight and the more preterm the baby, the greater the risk. Overwhelming sepsis may develop with little in the way of warning signs, and antibiotics are often given at the first suspicion of infection (after collecting all the necessary samples for culture).

Systemic infections

Bacteria acquired from the maternal genital tract predominate initially, giving way to organisms from the wider environment after 48-72 hours of age, and this affects the choice of antibiotics for empirical treatment. Individual neonatal units will have antibiotic policies, which take account of local circumstances, but the following tables outline a broad approach, which should be rationalised when culture results are available.

Summary of initial antibiotic choices for typical organisms in early and late neonatal sepsis

	Organism	First line treatment
Early onset sepsis	Group B streptococcus (*Strep. agalactiae*)	Penicillin + gentamicin
	E. coli	Cefotaxime
	Anaerobes	Metronidazole
	L.monocytogenes	Ampicillin + gentamicin
Late onset sepsis	Coagulase negative staphylococci	Vancomycin
	Staph. aureus	Flucloxacillin +/- gentamicin
	Enterococci	Ampicillin or amoxicillin + gentamicin
	Group B streptococcus (*Str. agalactiae*)	Penicillin + gentamicin
	Group A streptococcus (*Strep. pyogenes*)	Penicillin
	E. coli	Cefotaxime
	Klebsiella/Enterobacter species	Cefotaxime + gentamicin
	P. aeruginosa	Ceftazidime + gentamicin
	C. trachomatis or mycoplasmas	Erythromycin

Infections

Examples of initial neonatal antibiotic regimens in different clinical situations

Infection	Empirical treatment
Early-onset sepsis	Penicillin + gentamicin
Late-onset sepsis	Flucloxacillin + gentamicin
Meningitis on the NICU	Ceftazidime + ampicillin or amoxicillin +/- gentamicin
Meningitis outside the NICU	Cefotaxime + ampicillin or amoxicillin +/- gentamicin
Late-onset sepsis with resistant flora	Ceftazidime + gentamicin (or amikacin) OR: Vancomycin + ceftazidime
Necrotising enterocolitis	Penicillin + gentamicin + metronidazole
	OR: Ampicillin or amoxicillin + cefotaxime + metronidazole

Superficial infections
These should be taken seriously because of the risk of invasive disease. Relevant samples should always be taken for culture before starting antibiotics.

Outline of antibiotic treatment of common superficial infections in the newborn

Superficial infection	Initial treatment
Sticky umbilicus - moist but no flare	Local cleansing - send swab for culture
Umbilical sepsis - purulent discharge + erythema	Flucloxacillin +/- gentamicin
Paraonychia	Oral flucloxacillin (IV + gentamicin if ill)
'Septic spots'	Oral flucloxacillin (IV + gentamicin if ill)
Candidiasis	Nystatin or miconazole topically and orally
Conjunctivitis	Initially use topical neomycin
Conjunctivitis < 3 days old: ? gonococcal infection	IV penicillin or cefuroxime. Check antibiotic sensitivity If confirmed, counsel parents re: possible genital infection.
Conjunctivitis > 3 days old: ? C. trachomatis	Oral erythromycin + topical erythromycin. If Chlamydia confirmed, counsel parents re: possible genital infection.

CHILDHOOD BACTERIAL INFECTIONS
The following tables outline suggested initial treatment for common bacterial infections in children beyond the neonatal period. Treatment should be rationalised when culture and sensitivity results are available. Evidenced based recommendations continue to be developed and those endorsed by the Royal College of Paediatrics & Child Health are available on their website http://www.rcpch.ac.uk. Children with congenital or acquired immune deficiency are at risk of opportunistic infection. Recommendations for other infections are covered in the sections on individual systems.

Summary of initial treatment for upper respiratory tract infections

Upper respiratory tract infection	Organism	Initial treatment
Tonsillitis	Strep. pyogenes Viruses common C. diphtheriae rare	Penicillin (or erythromycin) for 10 days if swab confirms streptococcal infection otherwise, symptomatic treatment. In diphtheria, penicillin + diphtheria antitoxin (seek advice).
Peritonsillar abscess	Strep. pyogenes	Co-amoxiclav (clindamycin in β-lactam allergy)
Retropharyngeal abscess	Staph. aureus Anaerobes	Drainage of abscess
Otitis media	Strep. pneumoniae H. influenzae M. catarrhalis Anaerobes Viruses	Relieve pain Amoxicillin (co-amoxiclav if recurrent or not responding) Azithromycin (in penicillin allergy) Ciprofloxacin (if chronic with perforation)
Sinusitis	Strep. pneumoniae H. influenzae Strep. pyogenes Staph. aureus	Co-amoxiclav (azithromycin in penicillin allergy)
Acute epiglottitis	H. influenzae Strep. pneumoniae Staph. aureus	First, secure the airway. Then administer cefotaxime (use flucloxacillin for staphylococcal tracheitis)

Summary of initial therapy for community acquired pneumonia in previously healthy children requiring hospital admission.

Community acquired pneumonia	Organism	First-line treatment
Age 1- 3 months	Respiratory viruses Enteroviruses C. trachomatis (child may be afebrile) Streptococci (especially group B) Staph. aureus	Cefuroxime Macrolide if Chlamydia suspected
Age 3 months - 5 years	Strep. pneumoniae* Respiratory viruses Staph. aureus (mainly <1 year old) (H. influenzae)	Cefuroxime (or co-amoxiclav)
Age >5 years	Mycoplasma pneumoniae Strep. pneumoniae* Respiratory viruses	Benzylpenicillin if lobar Cefuroxime if bilateral signs, or fails to respond, or cause unclear. Macrolide if mycoplasma suspected

*In pneumococcal infection consider the addition of vancomycin to β-lactam therapy if there is a high local prevalence of penicillin resistance.

Summary of initial therapy for urinary tract infection

Urinary tract infection	Organism	First-line treatment
Acutely ill and/or < 3months of age	E. coli Proteus species Klebsiella species Other coliforms Enterococci	IV ampicillin or amoxicillin + gentamicin (or IV cefuroxime alone) Then oral therapy based on sensitivities Then trimethoprim prophylaxis until imaging complete
Mildly unwell and >3 months of age	E. coli Proteus species Klebsiella species Other coliforms Enterococci	Oral trimethoprim or cefalexin, guided by local sensitivity patterns Then trimethoprim or cefalexin prophylaxis until imaging complete

Commonest causes and initial treatment of bacterial meningitis by age

Bacterial meningitis	Organism	First-line treatment
Age 0-1 month	Group B streptococcus E. coli L. monocytogenes	Cefotaxime + ampicillin or amoxicillin
Age 1-3 months	N. meningitidis* Strep. pneumoniae Group B streptococcus H. influenzae* L. monocytogenes E. coli	Cefotaxime + ampicillin or amoxicillin†
Age 3 months - 5 years	N. meningitidis* Strep. pneumoniae H. influenzae*	Cefotaxime or ceftriaxone†
Over age 5 years	N. meningitidis* Strep. pneumoniae	Cefotaxime or ceftriaxone†

*For details of chemoprophylaxis for index case and contacts see prophylaxis section. †In pneumococcal infection consider the addition of vancomycin to β-lactam therapy if there is a high local prevalence of penicillin resistance.

Infections

Outline of initial treatment of acute bone and joint infections

Acute bone and joint infection	Organism	Initial treatment
Under age 6 years	Staph. aureus H. influenzae Strep. pneumoniae Strep. pyogenes	Cefuroxime +/- flucloxacillin for 3-6 weeks If Staph. aureus isolated, change cefuroxime to fusidic acid (clindamycin in β-lactam allergy)
Over age 6 years	Staph. aureus Strep. pneumoniae Strep. pyogenes	Flucloxacillin + ampicillin or amoxicillin for 3-6 weeks If Staph. aureus isolated, change to flucloxacillin + fusidic acid (clindamycin in β-lactam allergy)
Sickle-cell disease and in the immunocompromised	Salmonella species Other Gram-negative bacilli	Cefuroxime (or flucloxacillin + ciprofloxacin)

Summary of treatment of skin and soft tissue infections

Skin and soft tissue infection	Organism	Treatment
Otitis externa	Staph. aureus Strep. pyogenes	Flucloxacillin (or erythromycin)
Impetigo	Staph. aureus Strep. pyogenes	Flucloxacillin (or erythromycin)
Erysipelas	Strep. pyogenes	Penicillin or amoxicillin (or erythromycin)
Wound infection (including surgical wounds and burns)	Staph. aureus Streptococci Faecal flora (rare) P. aeruginosa (burns)	Flucloxacillin or co-amoxiclav (cefuroxime + metronidazole for post-laparaotomy wound infection). Superficial and localised infections may respond to topical mupirocin (Staph. aureus) or polymixins or silver sulfadiazine (Gram-negative bacteria). Isolation of faecal flora from superficial wounds is usually a result of colonisation rather than infection.
Bites (human or animal)	Staphyloccoci Streptococci Haemophilus species Anaerobes	Oral: co-amoxiclav or clindamycin IV: cefuroxime + metronidazole (consider need for tetanus toxoid)
Cellulitis	Staph. aureus Strep. pyogenes (H. influenzae)	Benzylpenicillin + flucloxacillin (change to cefuroxime if H. influenzae suspected)
Periorbital cellulitis (pre-septal)	Staph. aureus Strep. pyogenes (H. influenzae)	Cefuroxime Sinus disease may coexist
Orbital cellulitis (post-septal)	Staph. aureus Strep. pyogenes (H. influenzae) Anaerobes	Cefuroxime + metronidazole Urgent ophthalmological opinion Sinus disease likely to coexist
Necrotising fasciitis	Strep. pyogenes Anaerobes Coliforms	Benzylpenicillin + cefuroxime + metronidazole (or clindamycin + cefuroxime) Add gentamicin if neutropenia Emergency surgical debridement may be necessary

Summary of initial treatment of cardiovascular infections

Cardiovascular infection	Organism	Treatment
Intravascular device related	Coagulase-negative staphylococci *Staph. aureus* Coliforms	Cefuroxime. Add vancomycin if indicated on blood culture results.
Intravascular device related in haematology / oncology patients	Coagulase-negative staphylococci *Staph. aureus* Coliforms *P. aeruginosa*	Vancomycin + ceftazidime
Endocarditis (NO risk factors* for staphylococcal endocarditis)	*Streptococcus viridans* Enterococci	Amoxicillin + gentamicin Where possible, delay treatment until 3 sets of blood cultures have been obtained
Endocarditis (+ one or more risk factors* for staphylococcal endocarditis)	*Staph. aureus* Coagulase-negative staphylococci	Vancomycin + gentamicin Where possible, delay treatment until 3 sets of blood cultures have been obtained.

*Risk factors for staphylococcal endocarditis include: cardiac surgery in previous 12 months; central venous catheter present; haemodialysis; intravenous drug abuse

ANTITUBERCULOUS THERAPY
Treatment should always be given in collaboration with a paediatric or adult medicine physician experienced in tuberculosis therapy.

Mantoux test
The test is administered intradermally on the flexor aspect of the forearm. A control solution for Mantoux test is available and may be used at the same time but on the opposite forearm, to assess the response to the vehicle used in the active solution.

Mantoux test reagents and interpretation

Tuberculin PPD (Purified Protein Derivative)	Dosage	Response
100 units/mL (ampoules 1 in 1000)*	Intradermal: raise wheal **10 units** (0.1mL of 1 in 1,000)	Standard Mantoux test Read at 48-72 hours by measuring transverse diameter of **palpable induration**. Reaction ≥ 5mm is positive** If previous BCG, then ≥10mm suggestive and ≥15mm indicative, of infection.**
10 units/mL (ampoules 1 in 10,000)*	Intradermal: raise wheal **1 unit** (0.1mL of 1 in 10,000)	Special Mantoux test This is used only when very strong hypersensitivity to PPD is likely e.g. when erythema nodosum present. Read as above.

*Undiluted Tuberculin PPD (100,000 units/mL) is used only for the Heaf Multiple Puncture Test

** The Mantoux may be non-reactive initially in up to 50% of children with TB meningitis or miliary disease.

Antibiotic treatment
Prolonged therapy with more than one drug is required in order to prevent relapse and the emergence of drug resistance. In the initial phase of treatment (during which the bulk of the bacillary population is killed) isoniazid, pyrazinamide and rifampicin are given together for 2 months. Ethambutol should be included in the first 2 months, therapy when there is a risk of resistant infection. A continuation phase of at least 4 months follows, during which surviving bacteria are eliminated by isoniazid and rifampicin. Longer courses may be indicated for patients who are immunocompromised or have extra-pulmonary tuberculosis.

Summary of usual antituberculous therapy in children

Extent of tuberculosis	Recommended treatment (Single daily dose)	Duration
Pulmonary Glandular Genitourinary Pericarditis	Isoniazid Rifampicin Pyrazinamide	6 months 6 months First 2 months only
Bone and joint	Isoniazid Rifampicin Pyrazinamide	6-9 months 6-9 months First 2 months only
Meningitis	Isoniazid Rifampicin Pyrazinamide	12 months 12 months First 2 months only

Corticosteroid therapy
Adjunctive steroid therapy may be indicated to suppress hypersensitivity reactions, and in patients with extensive pulmonary disease, pleural effusion, pericarditis, tuberculosis affecting the ureter, and in meningitis once antibiotic therapy is established.

Compliance and toxicity
Compliance with therapy is a major determinant of its success. Treatment needs to be carefully supervised in families who cannot be relied upon to comply. An intermittent, supervised protocol is available for such situations. Seek advice. The incidence of clinically significant adverse reactions to the standard regime in children (most commonly gastrointestinal upset or skin rashes) is less than 2%.

Liver function should be checked before starting antituberculous therapy because all the standard drugs used are capable of causing hepatic toxicity. However, hepatotoxicity is less common in children than in adults. If pre-treatment liver function is normal (and there is no other reason to suspect liver disease) further measurements are only needed if the child develops fever, malaise, vomiting or jaundice or if unexplained deterioration occurs during treatment. This should be carefully explained to the child and carers so that any signs and symptoms can be recognised as soon as possible.

Drug resistance
Drug resistance in *Mycobacterium tuberculosis* is still uncommon in the UK. Isoniazid resistance is least uncommon, and is present in around 6% of isolates. Ethambutol, sometimes together with streptomycin, is used to replace isoniazid in the management of such cases. Treatment of multi-drug resistant *M. tuberculosis* has to be guided by antibiotic sensitivities but initial treatment should be with at least three drugs to which the bacterium is sensitive. Prolonged therapy with close monitoring is required for drug resistant tuberculosis. Treatment must be supervised by a paediatrician or adult physician experienced in managing such cases.

Chemoprophylaxis
Infants are highly susceptible to tuberculosis so chemoprophylaxis, followed by BCG if appropriate, is given to any infant who has close exposure to a case of smear-positive pulmonary tuberculosis. Chemoprophylaxis is also effective in preventing complications due to lymphohaematogenous and pulmonary spread in asymptomatic children of all ages who are tuberculin reactors.

Summary of chemoprophylaxis regimens against tuberculosis in children

Indication for chemoprophylaxis	Recommended treatment (Single daily dose)	Duration
Neonates of mothers with smear-positive pulmonary tuberculosis	Isoniazid 10mg/kg as a single daily dose	3 months, followed by BCG immunisation, provided that mother is no longer infectious
Children aged <2 years who are close contacts of a case of smear-positive pulmonary tuberculosis, and who have not received BCG	Isoniazid 10mg/kg as a single daily dose Or Isoniazid 10mg/kg as a single daily dose Rifampicin 10mg/kg as a single daily dose	6 months then perform Mantoux. If negative give BCG 3 months then perform Mantoux. If negative give BCG
Children aged <16 years with a strongly positive tuberculin test but no clinical evidence of disease	Isoniazid 10mg/kg as a single daily dose (max 300mg/**day**) Or Isoniazid 10mg/kg as a single daily dose (maximum 300mg/**day**) and rifampicin 10mg/kg as a single daily dose (maximum 600mg/**day**)	6 months 3 months

Outline of individual antituberculous agents

Comprehensive information about individual drugs is given in the monographs but they are outlined here to show the ways in which drugs are combined in therapy and to emphasise important aspects of their use.

Isoniazid is bactericidal and widely distributed, with good penetration into CSF. Peripheral neuropathy due to competitive inhibition of pyridoxine utilisation virtually never occurs in children in developed countries, but is a theoretical risk in patients with malnutrition or chronic renal failure. In these cases, prophylactic pyridoxine should be given for the duration of therapy. Isoniazid can inhibit the metabolism of anticonvulsants.

Rifampicin is widely distributed, but CSF penetration is less good than for isoniazid and it has less potent bactericidal activity. Rifampicin is excreted unchanged in the bile. Unlike the other commonly used antituberculous drugs, rifampicin has a broad spectrum of activity, including staphylococci, *N. meningitidis*, and *H. influenzae*. It is used in chemoprophylaxis after meningococcal or invasive *H. influenzae* type b disease (see prophylaxis section), and is occasionally used in conjunction with another agent for difficult staphylococcal infections. Otherwise it is reserved as much as possible for the treatment of tuberculosis. Urine, tears and saliva may be coloured orange-red during treatment, and soft contact lenses may be stained. Irregular treatment may be associated with flu-like symptoms that usually resolve when daily treatment is reinstituted. Rifampicin accelerates the metabolism of several drugs including phenytoin, corticosteroids, warfarin and oral contraceptives.

Pyrazinamide has an important function in the sterilisation of tuberculous lesions and is concentrated in macrophages. It achieves good CSF penetration and exerts its effects in the first 2-3 months of combined therapy. It is not active against *M. bovis* infections. Side-effects are rare in children.

Ethambutol is a less potent but useful antituberculous drug that is included in the treatment regime if isoniazid resistance is suspected or confirmed. Ethambutol is largely excreted in urine, and should be avoided in renal failure. Rarely it may cause optic neuritis. This is reversible if detected early and treatment stopped at once. Ophthalmological assessment should be made before and during treatment and is particularly important in children unable to report symptomatic visual changes.

Streptomycin is an aminoglycoside that is occasionally used when drug resistance is suspected or proven. It does not penetrate CSF. Plasma levels should be monitored particularly where there is the additional hazard of renal impairment.

Reserve drugs used in cases of multidrug resistance include thiacetazone, capreomycin, ethionamide, cycloserine, clarithromycin, amikacin and ciprofloxacin. Specialist advice in their use is essential.

Infections

COMMON VIRAL INFECTIONS

The range of antiviral agents currently available and suitable for children is limited, and treatment is mainly symptomatic and supportive.

Aciclovir (acyclovir) is active against herpes simplex and varicella-zoster viruses, by inhibiting new viral DNA synthesis. It is most effective when started early in the course of infection. Oral or intravenous therapy is substantially more effective than topical treatment. It can be life-saving in immunocompromised children, in whom it can also be used prophylactically. Resistance is beginning to be seen more widely.

Ganciclovir is related to aciclovir but is more active against cytomegalovirus (CMV). It is also significantly more toxic and should be used under specialist supervision. It may have a place in the prevention and treatment of CMV following organ transplantation and in CMV pneumonitis and organ disease.

Ribavirin (tribavirin) is a guanosine analogue and has activity against respiratory syncytial virus (and a range of other RNA and DNA viruses against which its role is not yet clear). In bronchiolitis it is inhaled after small particle aerosol generation into a head box or ventilator circuit. It may bring benefit to certain high risk and immunocompromised infants but it is not appropriate for routine use.

Antiretroviral therapy: see section on paediatric HIV infection.

Outline of common viral infections for which antiviral agents may be appropriate

Viral Infection	Treatment
Chickenpox - normal child	Symptomatic - avoid aspirin
Chickenpox - neonatal	IV aciclovir at first signs
Chickenpox - immunosuppressed	If cell-mediated defect: IV aciclovir at first signs
Chickenpox-contact - neonatal	Varicella-zoster immune globulin (VZIG) to baby if mother developed chickenpox or shingles ≤7 days before or after delivery. Give VZIG if baby born at <30 weeks or <1kg at birth but otherwise only if mother seronegative
Chickenpox-contact - immunosuppressed (including patients on steroids)	If seronegative, give VZIG. (Prednisolone 2mg/kg/24 hours for more than 7 days or 1mg/kg/24 hours for more than a month are considered to result in significant immunosuppression which may persist for 3 months after stopping treatment. If in doubt about an individual seronegative case, administer VZIG)
Cytomegalovirus (CMV)	Ganciclovir (+ human normal immunoglobulin if pneumonitis) Seek advice: treatment is potentially toxic
Hepatitis viruses	See Liver Disease section
Herpes simplex - neonatal	Suspected or established infection: IV aciclovir
Herpes simplex - immunocompromised	IV aciclovir. Seek advice
Herpes simplex - encephalitis	High dose IV aciclovir
Herpes simplex - gingivostomatitis	Aciclovir of benefit if started early
Herpes simplex - cold sores	Aciclovir usually not indicated. Topical use may contribute to viral resistance
Herpes simplex - keratoconjunctivitis	Seek ophthalmological advice. Topical aciclovir (+ IV aciclovir in neonatal cases)
Respiratory syncytial virus (RSV)	Supportive. Oxygen and nutritional care, respiratory support if necessary. Ribavirin (tribavirin) has a limited role in high risk groups - seek advice. Preventative treatment with monoclonal antibody given monthly through the RSV season may shorten length of clinical disease in very high risk groups, such as the baby with chronic lung disease requiring home oxygen therapy.

Paediatric Human Immunodeficiency Virus (HIV) infection
Antiretroviral therapy must be undertaken by a paediatric specialist familiar with the current treatment of children with HIV infection. Paediatricians in Europe, Canada and South America are co-operating in a series of studies coordinated by PENTA (Paediatric European Network for the Treatment of AIDS). Details of current trials are available in the UK from the Medical Research Council HIV Clinical Trials Centre (telephone 020 7380 9991). Recommendations continue to evolve.

Antiretroviral therapy is started in infected children meeting specific criteria, using triple therapy such as two nucleoside reverse transcriptase inhibitors and a protease inhibitor. Reduction in vertical transmission (mother to newborn) is achieved by avoidance of breast-feeding, and the use of antiretroviral therapy in pregnancy, at delivery, and for the newborn child. Caesarian section is no longer considered mandatory if the maternal viral load is undetectable prior to delivery.

Prophylaxis against *Pneumocystis carinii* with co-trimoxazole is recommended for all infants from the age of 6 weeks born to HIV-positive mothers. Prophylaxis can be discontinued once HIV infection of the infant has been excluded.

Further reading: Davies EG, Elliman DAC, Hart CA, Nicoll A, Rudd PT (Eds). The child with HIV infection. In: *Manual of Childhood Infections* (RCPCH), 2nd edition, 2001: W.B.Saunders Ltd; 125-136.

FUNGAL INFECTIONS (systemic therapy)
Individual agents are considered in detail in the drug monographs but are outlined here to show their comparative properties and uses.

Amphotericin B is the standard formulation for broad-spectrum systemic antifungal treatment. Liposomal amphotericin is associated with less nephrotoxicity even at much higher dosage. Experience with other lipid formulations is currently limited in children but they offer reduced toxicity compared with standard amphotericin and reduced cost compared to the liposomal product. Standard amphotericin remains first-line treatment for most situations but the lipid associated formulations should be considered if renal function is deteriorating or already impaired. Consult local prescribing policies.

Flucytosine should not be used as monotherapy because of the high incidence of resistant escape mutants during treatment. It is usually combined with amphotericin in systemic *Candida* or cryptococcal infections, especially when good CSF penetration is required. It is myelotoxic and blood levels should be monitored.

Fluconazole has a relatively prolonged half-life in neonates, but is not active against *Aspergillus* spp, and non-albicans *Candida* species may be resistant. It is effective against *Cryptococcus neoformans* and may be used prophylactically in AIDS. It has not been fully evaluated in dermatophyte infections in children. Generally well-tolerated.

Itraconazole is active against *Aspergillus* species and a wider spectrum of *Candida* species than fluconazole. It is also effective against dermatophytes but is not licensed for this purpose in children. Generally well-tolerated. It is recommended that levels be measured in long-term therapy.

Griseofulvin is well absorbed from the gut and is selectively concentrated in keratin where it is fungistatic for common dermatophytes. Side-effects are uncommon but relatively prolonged treatment courses are required. It is not indicated in neonates. The liquid formulation is no longer manufactured in the UK. Griseofulvin is still the recommended treatment for tinea capitis but may be superseded by terbinafine.

Terbinafine is an allylamine agent with a broad fungicidal spectrum, which was introduced for oral treatment of dermatophyte infections. It is not licensed for children for this purpose in the UK but has been successfully used to treat childhood tinea capitis and tinea unguium. It is generally well-tolerated in adults.

New antifungal agents. Limited clinical experience of these agents suggests that they are at least as effective, and better tolerated, than amphotericin B in children. They are currently only recommended for patients with progressive life-threatening fungal infections refractory to other treatments. **Voriconazole** is a triazole drug that is active against *Candida*, *Aspergillus* and *Cryptococcus* species. **Caspofungin** is the first member of a new class of antifungal drugs, the echinocandins, that inhibit fungal cell wall synthesis. It also has a broad spectrum of antifungal activity, but is inactive against *Cryptococcus* spp.

Systemic antifungal agents: outline comparison of principal characteristics

Anti fungal agent	Ampho- tericin (AMP)	Lipid associated amphotericin			Fluconazole	Itraconazole	Flucytosine
		Liposomal AMP (AmBisome®)	AMP colloidal dispersion (Amphocil®)	AMP Lipid complex (Abelcet®)			
Type	Polyene	AMP in liposomal vesicles	AMP in chemical particulate complex	AMP lipid complex	Triazole	Triazole	Fluorinated pyrimidine
Route	IV	IV	IV	IV	IV or oral	Oral	IV or oral
Anti- fungal spectrum	Candida species Aspergillus species Crypto- coccus Wide range of other fungi	Similar to AMP	Similar to AMP	Similar to AMP	Candida species Crypto- -coccus	Candida species Aspergillus species Sporothrix	Candida species Crypto- -coccus Resistance develops during mono- therapy
CSF levels	Low	Low	Low	Low	Good	Low	Good
Main toxicity	Fever, chills, renal toxicity, hypokalaemia	Similar to AMP but less renal toxicity	Similar to AMP but less renal toxicity	Similar to AMP but less renal toxicity Limited data in children	Low	Low	Myelo- suppression hepatic toxicty

THE IMMUNOCOMPROMISED CHILD

Infections in the immunocompromised child tend to be more severe and frequent, to show atypical features and be involved with opportunistic pathogens. More than one component of the immune system may be involved, and defects in cell-mediated immunity are often associated with defective antibody production as well. Each child has individual needs and risk factors depending upon the underlying disorder. Units caring for immunocompromised children will have specific protocols for the management of infection in different circumstances, but the following tables summarise the general ways in which antimicrobial agents are used.

Uses of antimicrobial agents

Immunological problem	Examples	Likely pathogens
Neutropenia	Congenital Autoimmune Post-chemotherapy Post-radiotherapy	Staph. aureus Coagulase-negative staphylococci Enteric Gram-negative bacteria Streptococcus species (Candida species) (Aspergillus species)
Neutrophil dysfunction	Chronic granulomatous disease Chemotactic defects Congenital disorders	Staph. aureus Enteric Gram-negative bacilli Candida species (Aspergillus species)

Uses of antimicrobial agents continued

Immunological problem	Examples	Likely pathogens
Antibody deficiency	Primary immunodeficiency Prolonged immunosuppression Post bone-marrow transplantation Absent or dysfunctional spleen Protein losing states	*Strep. pneumoniae* *H. influenzae* Enteric Gram-negative bacteria Enteroviruses *Giardia lamblia*

Defective cell-mediated immunity	Congenital
	Bone-marrow transplantation
	Solid organ transplantation
	Iatrogenic immunosuppression
	HIV infection
		Bacteria (intracellular)
		  Salmonella species
		  L monocytogenes
		  Mycobacterium species
		  Legionella species
		  Nocardia species
		Fungi
		  Pneumocystis carinii
		  Candida species
		  Aspergillus species
		  Cryptococcus species
		Viruses
		  Herpes group
		  Respiratory viruses
		  Enteroviruses
		Others
		  Toxoplasma gondii
		  Cryptosporidium

Outline examples of antibiotic combinations exhibited sequentially to the child with febrile neutropenia when cultures are unhelpful and there is no focus of infection.

Characteristics	Empirical treatment
Temperature >38°C Neutrophil count < 0.5 x 10^9/L Initial therapy	Piperacillin-tazobactam + gentamicin Or Imipenem/meropenem
Fever unremitting by 48-72 hours	Change to glycopeptide + ceftazidime or ciprofloxacin Consider adding amphotericin if neutrophils <0.1 x 10^9/L
Fever unremitting by 96 hours	Add amphotericin Consider imipenem/meropenem Add metronidazole if anaerobic enteric bacteria suspected

Infections

SCHEDULES OF PROPHYLAXIS

SUMMARY OF PREVENTION OF ENDOCARDITIS IN CHILDREN WITH HEART DISEASE.
Indications: – dental procedures involving the gingival margin (extractions, scaling, gingival surgery), ENT and genito-urinary procedures and surgery [additional information is available in the current British National Formulary (BNF)].

Procedures under local or no anaesthetic – no special risks:
Oral amoxicillin 1 hour before procedure

<5 years	750mg
5–10 years	1.5g
>10 years	3g

If penicillin-allergic or penicillin given in previous month:
Oral clindamycin 1 hour before procedure

<5 years	150mg
5–10 years	300mg
>10 years	600mg

or
Oral azithromycin 1 hour before procedure

<5 years	200mg
5-10 years	300mg
>10 years	500mg

Procedures under local or no anaesthetic – special risk group (history of endocarditis):
Treat as under general anaesthetic.

Procedures under general anaesthetic – no special risks:
No penicillin in previous month, no history of endocarditis:
IV + Oral amoxicillin

<5 years	250mg IV at induction then 125mg orally at 6 hours
5–10 years	500mg IV at induction then 250mg orally at 6 hours
>10 years	1g IV at induction then 500mg orally at 6 hours

If penicillin-allergic, or penicillin given in previous month, treat as in the next section:

Procedures under general anaesthetic – special risk group (prosthetic valve or history of endocarditis):
No penicillin in previous month:

<5 years	amoxicillin 250mg IV + gentamicin 2mg/kg (maximum 120mg) IV at induction then amoxicillin 125mg orally at 6 hours
5–10 years	amoxicillin 500mg IV + gentamicin 2mg/kg (maximum 120mg) IV at induction then amoxicillin 250mg orally at 6 hours
>10 years	amoxicillin 1g IV + gentamicin 2mg/kg (maximum 120mg) IV at induction then amoxicillin 500mg orally at 6 hours

Procedures under general anaesthetic – special risk group (prosthetic valve or history of endocarditis) continued:

If penicillin allergic, or penicillin given in previous month:

	all ages	Vancomycin 20mg/kg (maximum 1g) IV over 100 minutes; then gentamicin 2mg/kg (maximum 120mg) IV at induction
OR	all ages	Teicoplanin 6mg/kg (maximum 400mg) IV + gentamicin 2mg/kg (maximum 120mg) IV at induction
OR	<5 years	Clindamycin 75mg IV at induction then repeat orally or IV 37.5mg at 6 hours
	5–10 years	Clindamycin 150mg IV at induction then repeat orally or IV 75mg at 6 hours
	>10 years	Clindamycin 300mg IV at induction then repeat orally or IV 150mg at 6 hours

PROPHYLAXIS IN MENINGOCOCCAL AND *H. influenzae* TYPE B (Hib) INFECTION

MENINGOCOCCAL INFECTION

Indications for chemoprophylaxis

The index patient should receive prophylaxis as soon as oral medication can be taken, unless treated with ceftriaxone (which eliminates nasopharyngeal carriage).

Antibiotic prophylaxis for contacts is indicated as soon as possible, as follows:

☐ Contacts who have slept in the same house as the patient at any time during the 7 days before the <u>onset of symptoms</u>

☐ Boy/girl friends

☐ Health care workers or others who have administered mouth-to-mouth resuscitation or had some other prolonged, close, face-to-face contact with the patient.

Prophylaxis is sometimes indicated for other contacts (e.g. school mates where two or more linked cases have occurred). This will be instituted by the on-call Consultant in Communicable Disease Control (CCDC) or Public Health physician if appropriate.

Recommended prophylactic regimens for contacts of a case of meningococcal infection	
Children aged <1 year	Rifampicin 5mg/kg per dose, twice daily on two consecutive days
Children aged 1 - 12 years	Rifampicin 10mg/kg (maximum 600mg) per dose, twice daily for two consecutive days Or Age 5–12 years ciprofloxacin 250mg as a single oral dose
Children >12 years and adults	Ciprofloxacin 500mg as a single oral dose
Pregnant women	Ceftriaxone 250mg as a single IM dose

Hib INFECTION

Indications for chemoprophylaxis

The index patient should receive prophylaxis as soon as oral medication can be taken.

Antibiotic prophylaxis for contacts is indicated only where there is another child aged under 4 years, who has not been fully immunised, in the same household as the index case.

Hospital staff in contact with Hib infected patients do not require chemoprophylaxis.

Recommended prophylactic regimens for contacts of a case of invasive Hib disease	
Children aged 1-3 months	Rifampicin 10mg/kg per dose, once daily for 4 days
Children aged >3 months - 18 years	Rifampicin 20mg/kg (maximum 600mg) per dose, once daily for 4 days
Pregnant women	Seek advice from local CCDC or on-call public health physician
Adults	Rifampicin 600mg daily for 4 days

PROPHYLAXIS AGAINST *Pneumocystis carinii* INFECTION

Prophylaxis against *Pneumocystis carinii* infection
Co-trimoxazole, twice daily, for 2-3 days each week depending on treatment guidelines (see co-trimoxazole drug monograph)
Indicated for:
☐ HIV-positive children
☐ HIV-indeterminate children
☐ Children with congenital immunodeficiency
☐ Children undergoing prolonged continuous chemotherapy e.g. for leukaemia.
Co-trimoxazole contains trimethoprim and sulfamethoxazole in a ratio of 5:1.
Dosage is expressed as the combined amounts of each component e.g 480mg of co-trimoxazole contains 400mg of sulfamethoxazole and 80mg of trimethoprim.

PENICILLIN PROPHYLAXIS IN CHILDREN WITH AN ABSENT OR DYSFUNCTIONAL SPLEEN

Penicillin prophylaxis in children with an absent or dysfunctional spleen	
Age	Treatment
1 month-5 years	Phenoxymethylpenicillin 125mg twice daily
6 -12 years	Phenoxymethylpenicillin 250mg twice daily
>12 years	Phenoxymethylpenicillin 500mg twice daily

TUBERCULOSIS PROPHYLAXIS: SEE SECTION ON TUBERCULOSIS

TROPICAL DISEASES

Tropical diseases occur in the tropics because the warm humid climate is conducive to survival of the vectors (e.g. mosquitoes for malaria and filariasis, snails for schistosomiasis) or because eggs or larvae need warm moist soil for survival and development (e.g. *Ascaris lumbricoides* and hookworm). Other parasitic infections like tapeworms, amoebiasis, hydatid disease and toxocariasis, though often commoner in developing countries due to poor sanitation and hygiene, may also occur in industrialised countries. The prevalence of some parasitic diseases such as leishmaniasis (in Spain), toxoplasmosis and cryptosporidiosis have increased in industrialised countries due to immunosuppression associated with HIV infection. Some drugs developed many years ago for the management of parasitic diseases are still used in developing countries because of tradition or low cost.

Newer drugs considered to be more effective and with fewer side-effects have not been fully evaluated for some parasitic diseases; some older, and often toxic drugs, such as those used for trypanosomiasis (sleeping sickness), have not been replaced because of lack of commercial demand in industrialised countries. Drugs in this section are listed as (a) the drug of choice and (b) alternative drugs. The drug of choice is where possible the most effective, is easy to administer to children, and has the fewest side-effects.

Other drugs may be required in resistant cases. Expert advice on management should be obtained from schools of tropical medicine or infectious disease units for severe malaria, filariasis, trypanosomiasis, leishmaniasis, hydatid disease and the hyper infection syndrome of *Strongyloides stercoralis*.

Advice on specific problems available from:

PHLS Malaria Reference Laboratory (at London School of Hygiene and Tropical Medicine). Tel: 020 7636 3924

Birmingham Heartlands Hospital (Inf. Dis. Unit). Tel: 0121 424 0357

Glasgow, Scottish Centre for Infection and Environmental Health (registered users of Travax only).
Tel: 0141 300 1130 (weekdays 2–4 p.m. only)

Liverpool School of Tropical Medicine. Tel: 0151 708 9393

The Churchill Hospital, Headington, Oxford. Tel: 01865 225214

London:
PHLS Communicable Disease Surveillance Centre. Tel: 020 8200 6868

Hospital for Tropical Diseases
For treatment only ask for the medical officer on duty,
Patrick Manson Unit. Tel: 020 7387 9300
Travel prophylaxis. Tel: 020 7388 9600

MALARIA

Malaria is the commonest of imported diseases. There are approximately 2,000 cases each year in the UK of which about 15% are children. About half are caused by *Plasmodium falciparum*, a third by *P. vivax* and the remainder by *P. ovale*, *P. malariae* and mixed infections. Management depends on the degree of drug resistance in the area where infection was contracted and whether the condition is mild, severe or complicated. Prophylaxis depends on the extent of drug resistance in the area to be visited, and the age of the child. It must be emphasised that no drug can be relied on to prevent *P. falciparum* and travellers must be advised on measures to prevent mosquito bites (e.g. wearing protective clothing, using insecticides after dusk, and sleeping under mosquito nets impregnated with permethrin).

P. falciparum. The standard treatment is quinine for 7 days (or until the blood smear is negative). If quinine resistance is suspected this is followed by Fansidar® (single dose) or in children over 12 years and in whom Fansidar® resistance is suspected, doxycycline daily for 7 days. In children less than 12 years, clindamycin is an alternative to doxycycline. If the child is seriously ill or unable to take tablets, quinine should be given intravenously. For mild and uncomplicated cases Fansidar® (single dose), mefloquine (single or two divided doses) or Malarone® (proguanil with atovaquone) may be given. At present, mefloquine is not recommended for children under 5kg body weight or under 3 months of age. Alternative drugs may be required if *P. falciparum* is contracted in areas with multi-drug resistance such as South-East Asia. Artemesinin is a safe alternative and is given for 7 days. It may be combined with mefloquine to prevent recrudescence. Because of side-effects, especially on the heart, and interaction with other antimalarial drugs, halofantrine is reserved for multi-drug resistance when other drugs are unsuitable.

P. vivax **and** *P. ovale.* Oral chloroquine is given in a standard 3-day dose schedule. If the child cannot take it orally it may be given intravenously. A loading dose should not be given intravenously if the patient has recently received quinine or mefloquine. If chloroquine-resistant *P. vivax* is suspected, mefloquine or quinine may be given. Halofantrine should not be given if chloroquine has been administered recently. For eradication of the parasites in the liver and a radical cure, primaquine is given for 14 days, or 21 days for infections contracted in South-East Asia and Western Pacific. Before commencing primaquine, blood should be tested for G6PD activity since the drug may cause haemolysis in G6PD-deficient subjects. If G6PD deficiency is detected, primaquine is given weekly for 8 weeks.

P. malariae. Chloroquine should be given as for *P. vivax*. Primaquine is not required, as relapse is unlikely because *P. malariae* infection does not persist in the liver.

Protection against mosquito bites should be emphasised. Drugs used for prophylaxis are given according to the geographical area and should be commenced one week before departure and continued for 4 weeks after leaving the area. Weekly mefloquine should be commenced 2-3 weeks before departure to detect adverse reactions. Mefloquine is the drug of choice for most areas where infection with *P. falciparum* is a risk. However, because mefloquine is currently not recommended for children under 5kg body weight or under 3 months of age, they are given the combination of weekly chloroquine and daily proguanil. For children over 11kg daily Malarone® is an alternative. It is given 2 days before travel and stopped 1 week after leaving endemic area. Mefloquine is contra-indicated in children with a history of seizures, epilepsy in first-degree relatives or pre-existing psychiatric disorders. Chloroquine is also contra-indicated in children with seizures. For these children in areas without chloroquine resistance daily proguanil may be given. In areas with chloroquine resistance Malarone® may be used. Where there is a high risk of infection and mefloquine resistance exists (as in western provinces of Cambodia and borders of Thailand with Cambodia and Myanmar) dapsone combined with chloroquine may be used.

AMOEBIASIS

This is an infection of the colon caused by *Entamoeba histolytica*. The clinical spectrum ranges from asymptomatic colonisation, passage of cysts and colitis to extra intestinal disease such as amoebic liver abscess or pleuropulmonary disease. Management varies according to the site and severity of the condition.

Infections

Asymptomatic intestinal carriage. Diloxanide furoate is the treatment of choice. Other drugs include di-iodohydroxyquinoline (iodoquinol) and paromomycin.

Colitis. Treat with metronidazole; tinidazole is an alternative. Diloxanide furoate should also be given as a luminal amoebicide. *Balantidium coli* causes a colitis similar to *Entamoeba histolytica*. Metronidazole or tetracycline (children >12 years) is effective.

Liver abscess. Metronidazole and diloxanide furoate are given, as for colitis. Chloroquine, though less effective, may be added in difficult cases. Aspiration of a liver abscess may be required if rupture appears likely and if there is failure to respond to treatment within 3-5 days.

TRICHOMONAS VAGINALIS

This is an uncommon cause of vulvovaginitis in children. Metronidazole or tinidazole are given as a single dose and repeated if necessary.

GIARDIASIS

In symptomatic disease caused by *Giardia lamblia*, metronidazole or tinidazole are the treatments of choice. Furazolidone is less effective but well tolerated. It may cause haemolysis in G6PD-deficient children.

CRYPTOSPORIDIUM PARVUM

This causes a self-limiting disease in immunocompetent individuals. In immunodeficiency there may be prolonged, debilitating diarrhoea. A number of drugs have been tried with no clear benefit. The following drugs may be considered: paromomycin, spiramycin and azithromycin.

ISOSPORA BELLI

This is a protozoan similar to *Cryptosporidium*, and causes diarrhoea in immunodeficient patients. It responds to co-trimoxazole but relapse is common.

LEISHMANIASIS

This is caused by various *Leishmania* species and is transmitted by the sandfly. It has three main forms: cutaneous, mucocutaneous (Espundia, South American type), and systemic or visceral (Kala-azar). The different forms, and the response to treatment, vary geographically. The most likely forms to be seen in the UK are those contracted in Mediterranean and sub-Saharan Africa. Leishmaniasis is endemic in southern Spain and co-infection with HIV and leishmaniasis is not uncommon. Cutaneous leishmaniasis frequently heals spontaneously, but if it is extensive or unsightly, treatment is given as for visceral leishmaniasis.

Visceral leishmaniasis is treated with once daily sodium stibogluconate (pentavalent antimony) intravenously for 20-30 days depending on the resistance of the parasite. Antimony is rapidly excreted in urine (80% in a few hours) and 10 mg/kg twice daily may be a more effective regime, possibly enabling the duration of therapy to be reduced. The drug is cumulative and causes cardiac toxicity particularly in adults. ECG changes (T and ST and QT prolongation) are unlikely in treatment courses of up to 30 days. Recent studies have demonstrated the efficacy of liposomal amphotericin. Recovery is rapid with few or no side-effects. This is now the drug of choice. Other drugs for treatment of leishmaniasis include pentamidine isetionate and paromomycin in combination with sodium stibogluconate. For resistant cases, especially from India, expert advice should be sought.

Cutaneous leishmaniasis. If treatment is required, intravenous sodium stibogluconate is given as for visceral leishmaniasis. Topical ointment containing 15% paromomycin and 12% methylbenzethonium chloride may be effective. Oral itraconazole can be used. South American varieties should be treated as for visceral leishmaniasis.

TRYPANOSOMIASIS

This has African and South American (Chagas disease) forms. In the UK the African form is most likely to be seen, although it is very rare in travellers. It is transmitted by the tsetse fly. African trypanosomiasis produces initial systemic disease, which, if not treated, may progress to involvement of the CNS and typical sleeping sickness. In the rhodesiense type (East/Southern Africa) due to *Trypanosoma brucei rhodesiense* subjects may die in the acute phase (e.g. from myocarditis) before the disease of the central nervous system manifests itself. The type of disease transmitted by *T. b. gambiense* in West and Central Africa has a slower onset.

Systemic disease. Suramin is used for Rhodesian disease and pentamidine isetionate or suramin for Gambian disease. Suramin is given at intervals over a 4-week period and pentamidine isetionate for 7-10 days.

Central nervous disease. For involvement of the CNS, melarsoprol is given in increasing doses following initial doses of suramin. It is given at intervals over a 4 week period. Melarsoprol is a trivalent arsenical compound with severe side-effects. Eflornithine (given for 2 weeks) is an alternative for Gambian disease. Expert advice is required in the management of trypanosomiasis.

TOXOPLASMOSIS

Cats contract *Toxoplasma gondii* from infected prey such as mice. They pass infectious sporocysts in faeces, which may be ingested by a variety of animals (and humans). Infected animals develop tissue cysts (bradyzoites) in muscle, brain and other sites. Humans become infected by either ingesting sporocysts from cat faeces or by eating under-cooked meat or from transplacental infection. Toxoplasmosis is a common, usually self-limiting, infection. Major concerns include infection during pregnancy, eye involvement and infection in immunocompromised subjects such as HIV-infected children.

Toxoplasmosis in pregnancy and congenital infection. If *Toxoplasma* infection is suspected or confirmed during pregnancy, spiramycin is given throughout pregnancy if there is no evidence that the fetus is affected. If there is evidence of infection, from polymerase chain reaction (PCR) examination of the amniotic fluid or serology from fetal blood sampling, then spiramycin is replaced by pyrimethamine, sulfadiazine and calcium folinate (folinic acid).

At birth, if an infant has been exposed to infection *in utero*, but appears healthy, spiramycin is given pending laboratory investigation. If the infant appears not to be infected, spiramycin is continued for 6 months. If infection is confirmed, daily pyrimethamine plus twice daily sulfadiazine and thrice weekly calcium folinate (folinic acid) are given for a total of 12 months. At 6 months pyrimethamine is reduced to three times weekly and sulfadiazine is continued daily until completion of the course. At commencement a loading dose of pyrimethamine should be given. In addition, prednisolone 500 microgram/kg/dose twice daily is given until signs of CNS inflammation (high CSF protein >10g/L) or active chorioretinitis have settled, and then it is tailed off.

Ocular toxoplasmosis. Most cases of ocular toxoplasmosis have probably resulted from congenital infection. For acute exacerbation of disease a course of pyrimethamine plus sulfadiazine and calcium folinate (folinic acid) may be given until 1 to 2 weeks after inflammation has subsided. Clindamycin is an alternative to pyrimethamine/sulfadiazine combination. A short course of corticosteroids is usually given as well. Laser or cryotherapy may be of value.

HIV infection. For toxoplasmosis reactivation during HIV infection, a 6-week course of pyrimethamine plus sulfadiazine and calcium folinate (folinic acid) is given. To prevent relapse this is followed by maintenance of a quarter to half the dose of pyrimethamine and sulfadiazine plus calcium folinate (folinic acid) indefinitely. If reactions to sulphonamides occur, clindamycin, clarithromycin or azithromycin may be substituted. Dapsone is an alternative for maintenance.

Immunocompetent children. Specific therapy for infection in healthy children has not been shown to be effective. However, in protracted (>6 months) and incapacitating illness, the combination of pyrimethamine plus sulfadiazine and calcium folinate (folinic acid) may be tried.

HELMINTH INFECTIONS

Most of the parasites under this section are likely to have been contracted abroad apart from threadworms, toxocariasis, trichinosis and some tapeworms. Mebendazole is generally the treatment of choice; it is the least well absorbed but probably the safest. Albendazole is more useful in systemic disorders; it requires only a single dose but in high doses is associated with disorders of liver function and marrow depression. Tiabendazole (thiabendazole) is reserved for special situations because of side-effects. There is limited information on use of the above drugs in children less than 1 year of age, when helminth infections are rare. Soil-transmitted helminths are contracted by ingestion of eggs or larvae, or by larvae penetrating the skin (hookworm). Eosinophilia is common. Generally, they respond to a range of broad-spectrum anthelmintics with little difference in efficacy between them.

Ascaris lumbricoides. The eggs are ingested, hatch in the intestine and larvae migrate to the lungs. After development they pass back to the intestine via the trachea and oesophagus where they develop into adult worms. Most infections are small and asymptomatic. Complications include pulmonary symptoms, cough, wheeze, intestinal obstruction and blockage of the biliary or pancreatic ducts. In developing countries, large, recurrent infections are associated with malnutrition. Treatment is with mebendazole or albendazole. Other drugs include pyrantel embonate, piperazine and levamisole.

Toxocariasis is caused by the larvae of *Toxocara* species, usually *Toxocara canis*, occasionally *T. cati*. *T. canis* is a roundworm (nematode) infection of dogs, especially puppies. It is similar to *Ascaris lumbricoides* but it differs in that the life cycle is not completed in humans. Eggs from infected dogs are ingested, larvae are released in intestine and travel throughout the body. Larvae do not develop into worms in the intestine, so children are not infectious. There are two main clinical problems. One is visceral larva migrans (VLM) associated with migration of larvae. It consists of fever, hepatomegaly, wheezing and marked eosinophilia. Occasionally there may be seizures or myocarditis. Eye involvement is rare in VLM. The other clinical problem is isolated ocular disease. Larvae trapped in the retina may cause a local reaction and visual impairment. The diagnosis of ocular toxocariasis is difficult as serological tests (ELISA) are less sensitive than in VLM and the eosinophil count may not be raised. High antibody titres in the vitreous and aqueous humours are diagnostic. VLM is a self-limiting disease, however in severe cases drug therapy may alleviate symptoms. Albendazole is probably the drug of choice with the fewest side-effects. Other drugs include tiabendazole and diethylcarbamazine. Treatment of ocular *Toxocara* infection is difficult. Systemic or sometimes periocular corticosteroids are given to reduce local inflammation. Drugs as for VLM are given at the same time but are seldom effective. Visible larvae can be treated with laser. Surgery may be necessary.

HOOKWORMS

Hookworm disease (*ancylostomiasis*) is caused by *Ancylostoma duodenale* and *Necator americanus*. Eggs passed in the stool develop into larvae in warm moist soil. The larvae penetrate the skin of the host, migrate to the lungs and hence up the trachea and are swallowed. They attach themselves to the small intestine and suck blood. Heavy infections cause iron-deficient anaemia, particularly if the child's iron intake is low or loss is high. In malnourished subjects protein loss from the gut may lead to hypoalbuminaemia and oedema. Treatment is with mebendazole or albendazole. Other drugs include pyrantel embonate and levamisole. Mebendazole, albendazole, pyrantel embonate and levamisole will also treat *Ascaris lumbricoides* infection. Iron supplements may be required.

CUTANEOUS LARVA MIGRANS (CREEPING ERUPTION)

Cutaneous larva migrans is caused by the dog hookworm *Ancylostoma braziliense* or *A. caninum*. The hookworm penetrates the skin but does not develop further and 'wanders' in the subcutaneous tissue. In older children and adults the infection is usually in the feet but in infants who may be lying on infected soil, the infection can be on the buttocks or trunk. Local treatment with 10% tiabendazole may be used for single lesions. For multiple lesions add oral albendazole for 5 days. Oral tiabendazole is an alternative.

STRONGYLOIDES STERCORALIS

Infection with *Strongyloides stercoralis* is usually asymptomatic except in immunosuppressed individuals. Eggs passed in the stool usually develop into an early larval stage before excretion in faeces, thus diagnosis is by detection of larvae (rather than eggs) in faeces. Infection occurs when larvae penetrate the skin, following which they migrate to the lungs, proceed up the trachea and are swallowed and invade the small intestine. Autoinfection is an important complication, where larvae change into the infective form (filariform stage) before excretion and may penetrate the bowel wall or the skin. When infected larvae invade the bowel wall, they develop into adult forms and produce eggs from which larvae spread throughout the body. Cycles of autoinfection may result in persistent self-infection for many decades. Symptoms include periodic diarrhoea, and from migration of the larvae through the skin (larva currens) during autoinfection. The hyper infection syndrome occurs in immunosuppressed patients including those on corticosteroids. It results from repeated heavy autoinfection. Eosinophilia is not seen. Severe symptoms may occur affecting the gut, lungs and other organs. Albendazole is given for 3 days. An alternative is tiabendazole. Ivermectin (for 2 days) may be the most effective treatment. Hyper infection is difficult to eradicate and requires prolonged treatment (up to 2 weeks).

THREADWORMS

Enterobius vermicularis (thread or pinworm) The *Enterobius* worm lives in the caecum and upper colon and the gravid female migrates to the anus to deposit eggs. Irritation of the anus results in scratching and excoriation. Pinworms may enter the vulva and result in pruritus and discharge. Subjects are reinfected when ova contaminating the fingernails or clothing reach the mouth. If the person does not reinfect him or herself, the disease is usually self-limiting as the adult worms only survive 6-8 weeks. Management includes education in personal hygiene and drug treatment. Nails must be kept short, hands should be washed and nails scrubbed before meals and after defecation. Pants and if necessary, gloves should be worn at night. The perianal area should be washed before bedtime and after rising. Night attire and underclothes should be washed daily. All the family should be treated. Mebendazole is given as a single dose, and since reinfection is very common, repeated in 2–3 weeks time. An alternative is albendazole as a single dose. Other drugs include pyrantel embonate and piperazine. In intractable cases, the child, and if necessary, other family members may be given weekly doses of mebendazole for up to 3 months. Anthelminthics should be avoided in pregnancy especially during the first trimester. Although mebendazole is not recommended for children under 2 years it is probably safe in a **single** 100mg dose for infants over 6 months.

TRICHURIS TRICHURIA (WHIPWORM)
Trichuris worms usually inhabit the caecum where they are attached to the mucosa. When confined to the caecum they are usually asymptomatic. Heavy infection may extend to the rectum causing severe symptoms with chronic loss of blood and mucus, rectal prolapse, anaemia and failure to thrive. Mebendazole is given for 3 days. An alternative is albendazole in a single dose.

TRICHINOSIS
Trichinosis occurs when inadequately cooked pork infected by *Trichinella spiralis* cysts is consumed. Pigs may contract infection from eating infected offal or rats. Horses are occasionally infected. In humans larvae are released from the cysts in the intestine and penetrate the mucosa where they develop into adult worms. Female *T. spiralis* release larvae that migrate through the body causing an inflammatory reaction in organs including subcutaneous tissue, muscle, heart and brain before encysting in muscle. Infections are usually light and subclinical. Albendazole is given for 5 days and repeated if necessary. An alternative is tiabendazole (thiabendazole) for 7 days. In severe cases such as in myocarditis or central nervous system disease, corticosteroids may be beneficial.

TAPEWORMS (INTESTINAL CESTODES)
Taenia saginata (beef tapeworm). *T. saginata* is acquired by eating undercooked meat that contains the larvae of the parasite encysted in muscle (cysticerci). The worm attaches itself to the upper intestine. Gravid proglottides containing fertilised eggs are passed in the stool. Infected subjects are usually asymptomatic. Praziquantel is given after breakfast. An alternative is niclosamide. Following treatment, faeces are highly contaminated with eggs and safe disposal is advised.

Taenia solium (pork tapeworm) and cysticercosis. *T. solium* infection is usually contracted by eating undercooked pork, and intestinal infection is generally asymptomatic. More seriously however, ingestion of eggs passed by other humans or possibly by the patient him or herself can result in cysticercosis. Cysticercosis is caused by larvae released by the eggs in the intestine migrating throughout the body and encysting in organs such as subcutaneous tissue, muscle, CNS (neurocysticercosis), the myocardium and the eye. The commonest symptom of neurocysticercosis is epilepsy, followed by raised intracranial pressure and meningoencephalitis. With the availability of neuroimaging techniques, neurocysticercosis is found to be a commoner condition in developing countries than previously thought.

For intestinal infection, praziquantel is given in a single dose. An alternative is albendazole. Purgation is not necessary. Neurocysticercosis is a complex disease and expert advice is required in management. Anticonvulsants are used for seizures and shunts for hydrocephalus. As spontaneous resolution of intracranial lesions may occur, the efficacy of antiparasitic drugs is difficult to assess. However, albendazole or praziquantel with corticosteroids commenced before and continued throughout treatment, is accepted management of symptomatic disease in the presence of evidence of inflammation on neuroimaging. However, cysticidal drugs are not advised for cysticercotic encephalitis as they may exacerbate brain oedema. Dexamethasone and mannitol are administered to control intracranial hypertension. Surgery is the main treatment for ocular cysticercosis. There is a risk that antiparasitic drugs can induce an inflammatory response that can affect visual acuity. Drugs such as phenytoin, phenobarbital (phenobarbitone) and corticosteroids may lower blood levels of praziquantel and higher doses may be necessary. Conversely, corticosteroids may increase albendazole blood levels.

Hymenolepsis nana (dwarf tapeworm) and *Diphyllobothrium latum* (fish tapeworm) are treated with a single dose of praziquantel.

HYDATID DISEASE
This is caused by *Echinococcus granulosus* and much less commonly *E. multilocularis* that infect wild canines such as foxes and wolves. Dogs become infected with *E. granulosus* from eating the carcasses of sheep and less often cattle containing hydatid cysts. Humans contract the disease through contamination by eggs of the parasite in dogs' faeces. Larvae (oncospheres) penetrate the intestine and develop into hydatid cysts in the liver (50-70%) and less commonly

the lungs and peritoneum. Other organs including the brain and bone may be involved. Accessible large cysts are excised or less commonly they may be aspirated under computed tomography (CT) guidance. A scolicidal agent (e.g. 70-95% ethanol, 15-20% hypertonic saline or 0.5 % cetrimide) is injected into the cyst to sterilise it before removal. Albendazole is used pre and postoperatively, for inaccessible and multiple cysts. Pre-surgery 1-2 cycles should be given and 1-2 cycles post-surgery particularly if viable cysts persist. Praziquantel once a week in combination with albendazole may be more effective.

FLUKES

Schistosomiasis is caused by *Schistosoma haematobium*, *S. mansoni* and *S. japonicum*. *S. haematobium* worms live in the genito-urinary veins and usually present with haematuria and in advanced cases obstructive uropathy. *S.mansoni* and *S. japonicum* worms live in veins of the alimentary tract and present with diarrhoea, dysentery and in advanced cases, portal hypertension. Praziquantel 40mg/kg is given in two divided doses for *S. haematobium* and *S. mansoni*, and 60mg/kg in three divided doses for *S. japonicum* 4-6 hours apart. Follow-up parasitological examination of urine and stool should be undertaken at 2 months and 4-6 months to detect viable eggs and repeat treatment given if necessary. Praziquantel in appropriate dosage is also effective in infections by other flukes, *Clonorchis sinensis*, *Paragonimus* and *Fasciolopsis buski*. *Fasciola hepatica* does not respond to praziquantel. Triclabendazole taken after meals may be effective. Multiple courses may be required.

FILARIASIS

Filariasis is caused by mosquitoes and other biting flies which inject larvae of filaria worms into the skin. The larvae develop into adult worms and after mating the females produce microfilariae. *Wuchereria bancrofti* and *Brugia malayi* infections cause obstruction to lymphatics and elephantiasis. *Loa loa* is associated with inflammation of subcutaneous tissue (Calabar swelling) and *Onchocerca volvulus* with dermatitis, skin nodules and eye lesions, and is an important cause of blindness in endemic areas. Treatment of *W. bancrofti*, *B. malayi* and *Loa loa* is with diethylcarbamazine (DEC) or ivermectin. To minimise reactions DEC is commenced at 1mg/kg and increased gradually. In heavy infections there may be a febrile reaction and, in *Loa loa*, encephalopathy. Specialist advice should be sought. Addition of albendazole to DEC on ivermectin may enhance reduction of microfilaraemia. Ivermectin is the drug of choice for onchocerciasis.

DRACUNCULIASIS

Dracunliasis results from infection by the guinea worm *Dracunculus medinensis*. Guinea worm is contracted by swallowing water contaminated by the water flea cyclops that is infected by *Dracunculus* larvae. The larvae develop into adult worms and reside in subcutaneous tissue. When they mature, female worms extrude larvae through the skin causing a chronic skin condition usually in the legs. At present there is a strong drive worldwide for eradication of the worm. Traditional management is slow extraction of the worm by winding it around a small stick over a couple of weeks. Surgical removal may shorten the disability. Drug treatment has limited benefit. Metronidazole may shorten the time taken to extract the worm, perhaps by its anti-inflammatory action. Other drugs include tiabendazole (thiabendazole).

Life support

Life support must be given without delay to a child who is unconscious, pulseless or not breathing. Management focuses on Airway, Breathing, and Circulation (ABC). The aims are to ventilate, oxygenate, restore the circulation and tissue perfusion, and to diagnose and treat the underlying cause. This takes priority over giving drugs. Those involved with the emergency care of children should be familiar with the guidance given in *Advanced Paediatric Life Support* 3rd Edition BMJ Publishing Group (2000).

CARDIAC EMERGENCIES

Cardiac arrest, cardiac arrhythmias and cardiogenic shock are rare in childhood. Cardiac arrest is usually preceded by hypoxia or hypovolaemia, and recognition of this window of opportunity may prevent progression to cardiac arrest. The outlook following cardiac arrest is poor.

Protocol for asystole

Intubate and ventilate with high concentration of oxygen – establish intraosseous (IO) access, if no IV access available.

☐ **Adrenaline (epinephrine)** IV or IO (via endotracheal tube if no IV access)

☐ 3 minutes of basic life support and ventilation with oxygen

    External cardiac massage to ventilation ratio:

    5:1 – infants and small children

    15:2 – children over 8 years

☐ Repeat **adrenaline (epinephrine)** IV or IO

    In exceptional circumstances consider higher dose (e.g. presence of arterial monitoring, septicaemia, anaphylaxis)

☐ 3 minutes of basic life support and ventilation with oxygen

    Exclude treatable causes of cardiac arrest (e.g. hypoxia, tension pneumothorax, hypovolaemia, cardiac tamponade, electrolyte imbalance, hypothermia, and poisoning)

☐ Consider the use of sodium bicarbonate in prolonged cardiac arrest or documented severe metabolic acidosis.

The decision to discontinue resuscitation is extremely difficult, and demands discussion with senior colleagues. The management of supra-ventricular tachycardia, ventricular tachycardia, and bradycardia is given in the cardiac section.

RESPIRATORY EMERGENCIES

Respiratory emergencies are common in childhood and the initial aim of treatment is to ensure effective ventilation and oxygenation. Oxygen delivery should maintain a saturation of >95%. Treatment of upper airway obstruction and severe asthma are detailed in the respiratory section.

In the presence of upper airway obstruction with respiratory effort – the child's own attempts to clear the obstruction may be sufficient. In the absence of respiratory effort – ventilation with a bag and mask, or via an endotracheal tube is necessary.

SHOCK

The aetiology of shock determines the choice of fluid for volume replacement. Crystalloids or colloids may be appropriate. An initial bolus of 20mL/kg is repeated according to clinical response – see intravenous fluid therapy section.

ANAPHYLAXIS

Anaphylaxis describes a range of presentations from a rash to cardiovascular collapse and is potentially life-threatening. Anaphylactic shock requires effective airway management, treatment with **adrenaline (epinephrine)** and fluid resuscitation with boluses of 20mL/kg.

Administration of **adrenaline (epinephrine)** is by the IM route initially and should be repeated IM after 5 minutes if there is no clinical improvement. In the presence of airway obstruction with stridor, give nebulised adrenaline (epinephrine) in addition to the IM dose.

Chlorphenamine (chlorpheniramine) may be a useful additional treatment.

Hydrocortisone may also be beneficial.

HYPOGLYCAEMIA

The blood glucose must be checked urgently in any child presenting with an altered conscious level. Hypoglycaemia is treated with 5mL/kg of glucose 10% (more concentrated solutions offer no advantage and increase the likelihood of damage to the veins and of cerebral oedema). Management of hypoglycaemia in diabetic children is detailed in the endocrine section.

STATUS EPILEPTICUS

The initial management of status epilepticus is to maintain an adequate airway, ensure effective ventilation and oxygenation and to provide circulatory support. Coexisting hypoglycaemia or pyrexia must be recognised and treated.

The drug management of continuous fitting is given in the neurology section.

INTRAVENOUS FLUID THERAPY
Intravenous fluid and electrolytes are given to maintain or restore normal body composition when it is not possible or desirable to use the enteral route. Fluid and electrolytes are given as maintenance and/or replacement therapy. In each situation, it is necessary to be cautious as both hyper and hyponatraemia can occur.

Caution
Though uncommon, dilutional hyponatraemia is often an unheralded, but potentially fatal condition. It is due to complex neuro-endocrine mechanisms that can occur in children with a variety of conditions especially in the postoperative period. It is characterised by oliguria and a rapid fall in serum sodium concentration leading to cerebral oedema causing seizures and/or coning of the medulla oblongata. Slow correction and careful monitoring are required to prevent serious morbidity.

To prevent dilutional hyponatraemia and sodium overload, it is recommended that:
1 Body weight be accurately measured or estimated by a professional with substantial paediatric experience. The estimation of body weight can be made using the child's age; Body weight (kg) = (AGE+4) x 2. This weight should be plotted on a centile chart as a crosscheck. If the weight is beyond the 3rd or 97th centile range then the weight must be re-examined.

2 Fluid administration should reflect the composition of fluid lost or in deficit, especially as regards sodium content.

3 A baseline blood sample be sent for serum sodium, potassium, urea and blood sugar estimation. Regular and frequent serum sodium and blood sugar estimation is required and should be documented. This will usually mean at least one specimen per day in general maintenance situations, and at least two blood samples daily in the postoperative period and in deficit and significant ongoing loss situations. An indwelling heparinised cannula or capillary sample will avoid sampling difficulties in the anxious child or those with poor veins. Blood samples must not be taken from the same limb as the intravenous infusion.

4 An experienced doctor must assess fluid balance daily and take appropriate action to correct fluid loss or retention. Measurement of urinary sodium, potassium and urea should be helpful.

5 A child with acute hyponatraemia (<130 mmol/L) needs urgent referral to a hospital with paediatric high dependency facilities (asymptomatic hyponatraemia).

MAINTENANCE THERAPY
For this purpose fluid and electrolytes (chiefly sodium [Na⁺], chloride [Cl⁻] and potassium [K⁺]) are given together with glucose to replace the normal losses of water and electrolytes in quantities needed to maintain correct body composition. In infants and children, maintenance fluid and electrolyte requirements vary as a function of metabolic activity. The following normal requirements are derived from the relationship that exists between body weight and metabolic rate and may be used outside the neonatal period. The glucose requirement is that needed to minimise gluconeogenesis from amino acids obtained as substrate from muscle breakdown.

It is usual to meet these requirements by using a standard solution. For example, glucose 4% with NaCl 0.18% given in the volumes suggested below meets the fasting fluid, saline and glucose requirements for the purposes of most children under basal conditions. Solutions containing 20mmol/L of potassium chloride (KCl) also meet usual potassium requirements when given in the suggested volumes. Adjustments will need to be made if there is an inability to excrete fluids or electrolytes, excessive renal loss or continuing extra-renal losses. The exact requirements depend upon the nature of the clinical situation and types of losses incurred. See cautionary note about dilutional hyponatraemia above.

Fluid requirements/24 hours

Body weight <3kg	150mL/kg
	(start at 40–60mL/kg if newborn)
3–10kg	100mL/kg
For each kg between 10–20 kg	add 50mL/kg
For each kg over 20kg	add 20mL/kg to maximum of 2000mL in adult female and 2500mL in adult male
Sodium requirement	3mmol/kg
Potassium requirement	2mmol/kg
Glucose requirement	2.4–4.8g/kg

Intravenous fluid therapy

REPLACEMENT THERAPY

In general, initial intravenous replacement fluid is required if >10% dehydrated or if 5-10% dehydrated and oral and enteral rehydration is not tolerated or possible. Oral rehydration is adequate if tolerated in the majority of those <10% dehydrated. Subsequent fluid and electrolyte requirements are determined by clinical assessment of fluid balance, including measurement of ongoing excessive renal and extra renal losses, and measurement of plasma electrolytes, bicarbonate and glucose together with calcium, phosphate and magnesium where appropriate. In the United Kingdom oral rehydration is underused and severe dehydration overdiagnosed clinically.

Intravenous sodium is commonly given as a component of maintenance and replacement therapy. It may be given as NaCl 0.9% for initial fluid bolus in acute fluid loss and to replace ongoing gastrointestinal losses from the upper gastrointestinal tract. For maintenance and continuing replacement therapy it is usually given in combination with other electrolytes and glucose, the exact strength depending on the clinical situation. Other uses include promotion of saline diuresis in the management of some poisoning, as a vehicle for reconstitution and administration of intravenous medications and to maintain patency of arterial/venous catheters. It must be given with caution as sodium overload may be easily produced. Particular care is needed in those with renal insufficiency, cardiac failure, other cardio-respiratory disease, hepatic cirrhosis and those receiving glucocorticoids. Conversely, hyponatraemia with serious consequences can occur if maintenance and replacement fluids do not meet sodium requirements. See cautionary note about dilutional hyponatraemia above.

Solutions available
- ☐ Sodium chloride 0.45% – Na$^+$ 75mmol/L; Cl$^-$ 75mmol/L; osmolarity 154mOsm/L
- ☐ Sodium chloride 0.9% – Na$^+$ 150mmol/L; Cl$^-$ 150mmol/L; osmolarity 308mOsm/L
- ☐ Sodium chloride 1.8% – Na$^+$ 300mmol/L; Cl$^-$ 300mmol/L; osmolarity 616mOsm/L

Other infusion fluids containing sodium – see table.

Extreme care must be taken if giving sodium chloride in solutions stronger than 0.9% and there must be specific indications for their administration.

Intravenous potassium is commonly given as a component of maintenance and replacement intravenous therapy and in the correction of severe hypokalaemia where oral potassium is insufficient or not possible. For maintenance and continuing replacement therapy it is most usually given in combination with glucose and other electrolytes. Whilst it is often added to glucose/saline solutions, ready-prepared infusion fluid containing these together with potassium may be adequate in many cases and their use may decrease the number of errors in its administration. The quantity required is calculated according to usual maintenance requirements with adjustment for any deficit and ongoing loss. As always, the situation must be monitored by clinical assessment and measurement of plasma potassium concentration. Potassium should not be given in established hyperkalaemia and should only be given with extreme caution and close monitoring where there is renal impairment or coincidental administration of drugs which may cause hyperkalaemia. Potassium should only be given as a slow infusion and it is recommended that the concentration of the solution should not exceed 40mmol of potassium per litre. ECG monitoring should be used where there is concern regarding hypo or hyperkalaemia, together with frequent measurement of plasma potassium.

Solutions available
- ☐ Strong potassium chloride (15%)® – K$^+$ 2mmol/mL; Cl$^-$ 2mmol/mL
- ☐ Strong KCl should be diluted with not less than 50 times its volume of compatible intravenous fluid, mixed well and given as a slow infusion. Where possible, compounding should be performed in a pharmacy. For other infusion fluids containing potassium – see table.

Intravenous glucose is given in maintenance and replacement therapy to minimise gluconeogenesis and is also used specifically in the treatment of hypoglycaemia. For maintenance and continuing replacement therapy it is most usually given in combination with other electrolytes. In hypoglycaemia an initial bolus of 200mg/kg of glucose given as 2mL/kg of 10% glucose over 2-3 minutes is recommended.

Solutions available
- ☐ Glucose 5 % – osmolarity 278mOsm/L
- ☐ Glucose 10 % – osmolarity 555mOsm/L
- ☐ Glucose 20 % – osmolarity 1110mOsm/L

☐ Glucose 40 % – osmolarity 2220mOsm/L
☐ Glucose 50 % – osmolarity 2775mOsm/L

For other infusion fluids containing glucose – see below. Solutions stronger than 10% glucose should NOT be used except in exceptional circumstances because of the dangers of hyperosmolarity.

Intravenous bicarbonate is used in the management of metabolic acidosis. In most circumstances metabolic acidosis is secondary to hypoxia/hypovolaemia/hypoperfusion and treatment of any underlying condition with appropriate fluid replacement and cardiovascular support will improve or correct acidosis.

Bicarbonate may be given to correct the acid-base imbalance in severe metabolic acidosis or in specific circumstances, e.g. renal tubular acidosis. In the acute situation e.g. cardiac arrest, an initial bolus of 1mmol/kg may be given as a slow bolus if required (1mL/kg of 8.4% sodium bicarbonate or 2mL/kg of 4.2% sodium bicarbonate). The volume required of 8.4% sodium bicarbonate to correct a metabolic acidosis = base deficit x body weight (kg) x 0.3 for children other than newborns (x 0.5-0.6 in premature neonate; x 0.4 in term neonates). Half this volume is usually given initially by slow infusion and progress monitored by clinical assessment and measurement of plasma pH or H^+ concentration before giving the remaining half. The standard sodium bicarbonate solutions available are hypertonic. Venous damage or thrombophlebitis may occur at the site of infusion, and extravasation can cause severe tissue injury. Continued administration can lead to hypernatraemia and overdosage of sodium bicarbonate may cause diarrhoea, nausea and vomiting, hyperpnoea and convulsions.

Solutions available
☐ Sodium bicarbonate 1.26% – Na^+ 150mmol/L; $HCO3^-$ 150mmol/L; – osmolarity 300mOsm/L
☐ Sodium bicarbonate 4.2% – Na^+ 500mmol/L; $HCO3^-$ 500mmol/L; – osmolarity 1000mOsm/L
☐ Sodium bicarbonate 8.4% – Na^+ 1000mmol/L; $HCO3^-$ 1000mmol/L; – osmolarity 2000mOsm/L

THAM (tris-hydroxymethyl aminomethane trometamol) is an organic buffer used for correction of metabolic acidosis. It is an alternative to sodium bicarbonate when there is concern about carbon dioxide retention, hypernatraemia or renal impairment. THAM is available as 3.6% or 7.2% solution, and should be used as 3.6% solution when given intravenously. 1mL of 7.2% solution (2mL of 3.6% solution) is equivalent to 1mmol of bicarbonate ion.

Lactate was previously used in the management of metabolic acidosis but is now not recommended because of the risk of producing lactic acidosis, especially in those with hepatic impairment or poor tissue perfusion. Any solutions containing lactate should not be given to those with impairment of hepatic function.

Solutions available
☐ Sodium lactate M/6 – Na^+ 167 mmol/L; lactate 167 mmol/L

For other infusion fluids, which contain lactate – see table.

Combined intravenous fluids

	Na^+ (mmol/L)	Cl^- (mmol/L)	K^+ (mmol/L)	Other (mmol/L)	Osmolarity †(mOsm/L)	Energy (kcal/L)
Glucose 2.5%/NaCl 0.45%	75	75	–	–	293	100
Glucose 4%/NaCl 0.18%	30	30	–	–	263	160
Glucose 5%/NaCl 0.45%	75	75	–	–	432	200
Glucose 5%/NaCl 0.9%	150	150	–	–	586	200
Glucose 10%/NaCl 0.18%	30	30	–	–	567	400
Glucose 10%/NaCl 0.45%	75	75	–	–	660	400
Glucose 5%/KCl 0.15%	–	20	20	–	318	200
Glucose 5%/KCl 0.2%	–	27	27	–	332	200
Glucose 5%/KCl 0.3%	–	40	40	–	358	200
Glucose 4%/NaCl 0.18% with KCl 0.15%	30	50	20	–	322	160
Glucose 4%/NaCl 0.18% with KCl 0.2%	30	57	27	–	336	160

Combined intravenous fluids continued

	Na⁺ (mmol/L)	Cl⁻ (mmol/L)	K⁺ (mmol/L)	Other (mmol/L)	Osmolarity †(mOsm/L)	Energy (kcal/L)
Glucose 4%/NaCl 0.18% with KCl 0.3%	30	70	40	–	362	160
Glucose 5%/NaCl 0.45% with KCl 0.15% (Alder Hey Special K)	75	95	20	–	426	200
NaCl 0.9%/KCl 0.15%	150	170	20	–	340	0
NaCl 0.9%/KCl 0.2%	150	177	27	–	354	0
NaCl 0.9%/KCl 0.3%	150	190	40	–	380	0
Ringer's – compound sodium chloride	147.5	156	4	Calcium – 2	310	0
Hartmann's – compound sodium lactate	131	111	5	Lactate – 29 Calcium – 2	278	0
Half Hartmann's with glucose 5%	66	56	3	Lactate – 14 Calcium – 1	418	200
Darrow's – lactated potassic saline	121	103	35	Lactate – 53	312	0

†Osmolarity may differ slightly depending on brand. The figures quoted are mainly for Baxter products.

COLLOIDS

These are used for plasma replacement or expansion. They may be natural products like human albumin solution (HAS) and fresh frozen plasma (FFP), or synthetic: based on gelatin like Gelofusine® (succinylated gelatin) and Haemaccel® (urea-linked gelatin); or hydroxyethyl starches (HES) like Pentastarch®; or dextrans. HAS and gelatins are essentially plasma substitutes, whereas hydroxyethyl starches and dextrans are true plasma expanders – they produce an increase in plasma volume greater than the volume of colloid infused. A meta-analysis of clinical trials has suggested that use of HAS may be associated with increased mortality across all age ranges; a more recent review of studies in newborns could not confirm this finding. NaCl 0.9% is often an effective crystalloid alternative for rapid volume expansion in resuscitation, sepsis and dehydration. There is no justification for use of FFP as a plasma substitute unless there is also a coagulopathy.

4.5% HAS has been the standard fluid used in neonates and infants, but it is expensive and there is a small risk of anaphylaxis or infection. More recently, there has been concern about possible variant CJD (vCJD) transmission from UK sources of HAS. A synthetic gelatin is a cheap and safe alternative to 4.5% HAS. A succinylated gelatin is preferable to a urea-linked gelatin as the reported anaphylactoid reaction rate is lower (0.05% and 0.1% respectively). Dextrans are not routinely indicated because of increased side-effects compared to gelatins and hydroxyethyl starches.

Hydroxyethyl starches (HES) have anaphylactoid reaction rates similar to gelatins but as HES are true plasma expanders the risk of fluid overload is greater. For this reason, HES are probably best restricted to an intensive care setting.

Liver

Acute hepatitis. This is often due to hepatitis A virus infection but it may be the first presentation of serious liver disease. Serology, liver function tests and coagulation studies should be undertaken in all cases. No specific treatment is necessary in the vast majority of cases. All cases not due to hepatitis A virus or where coagulation studies are abnormal should be referred for further investigation.

Hepatitis B. Hepatitis B infection rarely causes acute hepatitis in childhood but may result in chronic carriage. Chronic infection and carriage is more likely to occur the younger the age at which the infection is acquired. It is usually asymptomatic in childhood but, if untreated, carries a high lifetime risk of progression to cirrhosis and hepatocellular carcinoma.

All pregnant women in the UK are screened for hepatitis B. Perinatal vaccination, plus immunoprophylaxis where indicated, provides 97% protection against perinatal infection. Universal vaccination against hepatitis B has decreased the incidence of hepatocellular carcinoma in endemic areas but has not been implemented in the UK.

The aim of drug treatment is to induce immune responsiveness to the virus with subsequent viral clearance. Interferon alfa treatment for 16 weeks appears to be successful in about 40% of cases but the response may be significantly less in those with perinatal infection. Lamivudine treatment appears to be safe and induces a rapid fall in circulating virus but relatively few patients seroconvert. The long-term role of this agent is still unclear and currently children should only be treated in the context of a clinical trial (therefore no drug monograph).

Hepatitis C. With the introduction of effective blood product screening, perinatal transmission has become the major route of infection in childhood. The risk of the latter is approximately 7%. Acute symptoms are rare with chronic infection and carriage being the rule, with similar lifetime sequelae to hepatitis B infection. The goal of treatment is to abolish viraemia and prevent ongoing liver damage. Experience in adults suggests that the combination of ribavirin (tribavirin) and interferon alfa offer the best chance of sustained response. Studies of this combination in children more than 3 years old are planned. At present children with hepatitis C should only be treated in the setting of a clinical trial.

Autoimmune hepatitis. This is the commonest cause of chronic liver disease in later childhood. It may present as acute hepatitis, with complications of chronic liver disease or as liver failure. It is characterised by specific autoantibodies and histological appearance. Treatment is with immunosuppression. Prednisolone is the mainstay and is started at 2mg/kg/day (maximum 40mg/day). With biochemical control prednisolone is rapidly decreased to the minimum effective dose. Azathioprine is used either as a steroid-sparing agent from the start, or as an add on if relapse occurs on prednisolone. Liver function, prothrombin time and full blood count should be checked weekly in the first month of treatment, monthly while steroids are being decreased, and subsequently 3 monthly. An attempt may be made to withdraw steroids where there has been at least one year of complete biochemical remission and in the absence of histological activity. A significant proportion will relapse and require long-term immunosuppression. Second-line treatment – ciclosporin (cyclosporin) or tacrolimus – should be reserved for non-responsiveness or severe side-effects on first- line treatment.

Acute liver failure. This syndrome is characterised by severe liver dysfunction in a child without recognised underlying chronic liver disease. The severity of liver dysfunction is best judged by the degree of coagulopathy, which is invariably present. In view of the high mortality of this condition all cases should be discussed with a unit skilled in the management of acute liver failure and with facilities for emergency liver transplantation, so that a management and transfer protocol can be agreed.

Prior to transfer, supportive treatment should be commenced:
☐ Glucose 10–20% infusion at two-thirds of normal fluid requirements
      Intravenous ranitidine
      Oral lactulose (if conscious)
☐ Mannitol 20% if evidence of worsening encephalopathy or development of cerebral oedema.

If the cause of liver failure is, or could be, paracetamol poisoning, acetylcysteine treatment should be commenced irrespective of the time of ingestion.

Variceal bleeding. The principle of treatment is resuscitation and maintenance of haemodynamic stability, followed by timely therapeutic endoscopy. The first choice drug treatment is octreotide. Blood glucose and electrolytes should be monitored daily during treatment. An alternative is terlipressin by intermittent bolus injection. The use of vasopressin (see argipressin monograph) is limited by side-effects in up to 33% of cases and should rarely be necessary. If used, it should be combined with glyceryl trinitrate to limit its side-effects. In children with cirrhosis, broad-spectrum antibiotics should be commenced and the use of lactulose considered. The use of beta-blockers is not recommended for primary or secondary prophylaxis in children.

Pruritus. In addition to drug treatment, attention should be paid to physical measures like keeping nails short, and moisturising the skin.

First line: Ursodeoxycholic acid

Second line: Rifampicin

Third line: Colestyramine (cholestyramine), phenobarbital (phenobarbitone), or sedative antihistamines

Fourth line: Ondansetron.

In general, a single drug should be used with a stepwise increase until effective or maximum dose reached. First and second line drugs are effective in 40-60%. Colestyramine is rarely feasible in younger children but can be disguised in food and drink.

Nutritional support. Children with liver disease, especially cholestatic liver disease, often have severe fat and fat-soluble vitamin malabsorption. Treatment relies on providing sufficient net calorie intake to allow normal growth, which usually implies a gross energy intake of at least 120% of average requirements for age. Similarly, fat-soluble vitamin supplementation is usually required, often in a high-dose.

Cholestatic liver disease. Commence standard doses of vitamins A, K, E and alfacalcidol, and monitor 3 monthly vitamin A and E levels, prothrombin time, calcium, phosphate and alkaline phosphatase. Adjust individual vitamin dosages as necessary. Occasionally, parenteral supplementation is necessary if there is no response to high-dose oral treatment.

Ascites and fluid retention. Sodium should be restricted to the minimum necessary for growth. Spironolactone should be increased slowly. If this is not effective, only then should furosemide (frusemide) be added. Furosemide is more likely to contribute to metabolic and renal complications and should be started and increased in small increments. Depending on the clinical state of the patient, weight, electrolytes and renal function may need to be checked daily on introduction and following dose increases. Subsequent monitoring frequency should be weekly and then at least monthly.

Wilson disease. Penicillamine is still the drug of first choice. The dose should be increased over 2-3 weeks if tolerated. It should be combined with pyridoxine. Full blood count and urinalysis should be undertaken after 1 week and fortnightly for the first 2 months and subsequently 2 monthly. If serious side-effects develop, penicillamine should be withdrawn and either slowly reintroduced or alternatives used. Efficacy is shown by improvements in liver function, which should occur within weeks, and is monitored by measuring 24 hour urinary copper excretion every 6 months. Trientine has a similar mode of action and side-effect profile to penicillamine, but paediatric experience is limited.

Zinc, which is safe and well tolerated, is recommended in addition to penicillamine where there is acute liver dysfunction. There is increasing evidence that zinc monotherapy is effective in patients who have been successfully decoppered by chelation, or in presymptomatic patients with normal liver function. It may become the treatment of choice for this patient group.

Where the initial presentation is neurological, neurological deterioration may occur whatever therapy is used. Low-dose penicillamine is usually used but close clinical supervison is imperative.

Tyrosinaemia type 1. The management of this condition has been transformed by the introduction of NTBC (2-(2-nitro-trifluoromethylbenzoyl)-1,3-cyclohexanedione). Absolute indications for this treatment in tyrosinaemia include liver failure and porphyria-like neurological crises but its use is associated with clinical improvement in almost all treated patients. Treatment once started is probably lifelong, or until liver transplantation.

Metabolism

LIPID DISORDERS

The process of atherosclerosis begins in childhood. Elevated blood levels of cholesterol have been positively linked with coronary heart disease (CHD) in adulthood. Lowering the cholesterol to a safe level without hindering growth and development in children and adolescents at risk for CHD should reduce the morbidity and mortality from CHD in later life. Treatment might be considered if children have a total cholesterol of >5.2mmol/L (200mg/dL) with a family history of hypercholesterolaemia and premature CHD. When the parents or grandparents have hypercholesterolaemia but no evidence of CHD, screening of children and adolescents should include a complete lipid profile. If total cholesterol is >5.2mmol/L (>200mg/dL) or low-density lipoprotein-C (LDL-C) >3.4mmol/L (>130mg/dL) the lipid profile needs to be repeated. Total cholesterol of >7mmol/L (>270mg/dL) or LDL-C is >4.9mmol/L (>189mg/dL) strongly suggests familial hypercholesterolaemia, and screening for LDL-receptor mutations should be done if possible. Secondary causes of hypercholesterolaemia include diabetes mellitus, hypothyroidism, nephrotic syndrome, obstructive biliary disease, glycogen storage disease and drugs such as corticosteroids. These secondary causes can be excluded by clinical assessment and simple investigations.

Metabolism

The classification of risk category for children and adolescents with familial hypercholesterolaemia is as follows.

Low risk:
☐ Total serum cholesterol 5.3–6.9mmol/L and either no family history of early CHD, or a female, with CHD only in male family members
☐ Total serum cholesterol 7–9.9mmol/L female and no family history of early CHD.

Moderate risk:
☐ Cholesterol 5.3–6.9mmol/L male, with family history of early CHD or female, with family history of early CHD in females
☐ Cholesterol 7-9.9mmol/L male, no family history of early CHD
☐ Cholesterol ≥10mmol/L female, no family history of early CHD.

High risk:
☐ Cholesterol ≥10mmol/L male, no family history of early CHD
☐ Cholesterol ≥10mmol/L female, with family history of early CHD
☐ Cholesterol ≥7mmol/L male, with family history of early CHD.

Early CHD defined as CHD in first or second degree relatives: <40 years in males and <50 years in females.

Diet. Dietary intervention remains the mainstay of treatment in children. The general aim of dietary therapy is to lower the cholesterol levels enough to reduce the risk of atherogenesis while ensuring adequate growth. This may be achieved by limiting saturated fatty acids to 10% of total calorie intake and total fat to less that 30% of the total daily calories.

Drug therapy is indicated in children >5 years and adolescents in the 'high-risk' group if their LDL-C remains >4.9mmol/L or their total cholesterol remains >7mmol/L during an adequate (6-12 month) trial of dietary intervention. It should also be strongly considered in those with moderate risk. Dietary therapy should continue even if lipid-lowering drugs have been introduced.

Lipid-lowering drugs. The bile acid sequestrants (colestyramine (cholestyramine) and colestipol) should be considered if diet therapy fails to achieve cholesterol concentrations in the mild risk band. However, compliance with these agents is generally poor. The 3-hydroxy-3-methylglutaryl coenzyme A (HMG CoA) reductase inhibitors (statins) - atorvastatin, simvastatin, pravastatin and fluvastatin - should be considered in moderate-risk children and are generally indicated in high-risk children if dietary therapy and resins prove unsuccessful. If diet, resins and statins together are not successful, then nicotinic acid or the fibric acid derivatives (bezafibrate, ciprofibrate, fenofibrate, and gemfibrozil) may be beneficial.

INHERITED METABOLIC DISORDERS

In patients with acute metabolic decompensation, the load on affected pathways can be reduced by preventing catabolism and stimulating anabolism. Stop all exogenous protein and give glucose intravenously (5-10mg/kg/minute). Aim to maintain the blood glucose at 7-10mmol/L, if necessary giving insulin at 0.05 units/kg/hour. Dialysis may be required to remove toxic metabolites. Other measures include maintaining urinary output and giving carnitine intravenously (100mg/kg/day, or 200mg/kg/day if already on 100mg/kg/day) either as a continuous infusion or in 3 or 4 divided doses. Treat hyperammonaemia when ammonia >150 micromol/L with sodium benzoate, sodium phenylbutyrate and arginine hydrochloride 10%. Although dietary treatment may be the most effective therapy for certain disorders (e.g. phenylketonuria) drug treatment is indicated in a number of others (see table). Because of the rarity of individual inborn errors of metabolism, evidence of efficacy of the therapies is rarely based on clinical trials. Clinicians need to be aware of the lack of proof of efficacy and weigh the potential for benefit against the possible risks of the treatment. Physicians without experience in the use of particular medications are advised to contact specialist centres involved in the care of patients with inborn errors of metabolism.

Drugs used in inherited metabolic disorders

General advice on the use of medicines in metabolic disorders can be sought from:
Dr Andrew Morris   Tel: 0161 727 2137/2138
                     Email: andrew.morris@cmmc.nhs.uk
Dr George Rylance   Tel: 0191 202 3033 or 0191 232 5131
                     Email: george.rylance@ncl.ac.uk

Metabolism

Disorder	Drug and diet therapy	Disorder	Drug and diet therapy
Urea cycle disorders		Tetrahydrobiopterin	
Carbamylphosphate	arginine	metabolism disorders	
synthase deficiency	citrulline	Tetrahydrobiopterin	tetrahydrobiopterin
	carbamylglutamate	synthesis defects	5-hydroxytryptophan
	sodium benzoate		co–careldopa
	sodium phenylbutyrate	Dihydrobiopterin	tetrahydrobiopterin
Ornithine carbamyl	arginine	reductase deficiency	5-hydroxytryptophan
transferase deficiency	citrulline		co–careldopa
	sodium benzoate		folinic acid
	sodium phenylbutyrate	Mitochondrial disorders	
Arginosuccinic aciduria	arginine	Isolated carboxylase defects	biotin
	sodium benzoate	Defects of biotin metabolism	biotin
	sodium phenylbutyrate	Mitochondrial myopathies	ubiquinone
Citrullinaemia	arginine	Lactic acidosis due to	dichloroacetate
	sodium benzoate	pyruvate dehydrogenase	
	sodium phenylbutyrate	complex defects	
Arginase deficiency	sodium benzoate	Congenital lactic acidosis	riboflavin
	sodium phenylbutyrate		thiamine
N-acetylglutamate	carbamylglutamate	Mitochondrial respiratory	thiamine
synthase deficiency		chain defects	
Amino acid disorders		Others	
Non-ketotic	L-tryptophan	Menke disease	copper histidine
hyperglycinaemia	ketamine	Gaucher disease	alglucerase
	dextromethorphan		imiglucerase
	Sodium benzoate	Homocystinuria (classic and	betaine
Tyrosinaemia type I	NTBC	remethylation)	pyridoxine
Maple syrup urine disease	thiamine		hydroxocobalamin
(MSUD)			folinic acid
Tyrosinaemia type III	vitamin C	Wilson disease	ammonium
Transient tyrosinaemia of	vitamin C		penicillamine
the newborn			tetrathiomolybdate
Hawkinsuria	vitamin C		trientine
Organic acidaemias		Acrodermatitis enteropathica	zinc sulphate
Isovaleric acidaemia	glycine	Pyridoxine dependent seizures	pyridoxine
	carnitine	Smith-Lemli-Opitz syndrome	cholesterol
Methylmalonic acidaemia	hydroxocobalamin		ursodeoxycholic acid
	carnitine		chenodeoxycholic acid
Propionic acidaemia	carnitine	Cystathioniuria	pyridoxine
Glutaric aciduria type I	carnitine		
Glutaric acidaemia type I & II	riboflavin		

Pain in musculoskeletal conditions. The techniques used for management of pain in musculoskeletal conditions are similar whatever the aetiology. Treatment must be tailored to the individual child and must consider the psychological, emotional and social aspects as well as the sensory component. Simple analgesics such as paracetamol in addition to physical treatments such as the application of heat or cold, transcutaneous electrical nerve stimulation (TENS) and cognitive behavioural techniques are often helpful.

Musculoskeletal pain syndromes. Arthralgia in the absence of evidence of inflammation occurs in joint hypermobility syndromes and the nocturnal idiopathic pain syndrome (growing pains) and is usually best managed with local massage, physiotherapy and simple analgesics such as paracetamol or ibuprofen. Patellofemoral pain syndromes, common in adolescence, are best treated with strengthening of the muscles around the knee. Arthralgia also occurs in chronic fatigue syndrome which is best managed using a graded exercise regime, supportive psychotherapy, and simple analgesics as required. Reflex sympathetic dystrophy and the idiopathic musculoskeletal pain syndromes often respond to a similar approach. Occasionally, tricyclic antidepressants or selective serotonin re-uptake inhibitors may be helpful.

Acute musculoskeletal inflammatory conditions. Soft tissue injuries and sprains can often be managed with rest, the local application of heat or cold, analgesia and non-steroidal anti-inflammatory drugs (NSAIDs). Viral or reactive arthritis may be treated in a similar way, although higher dose NSAIDs will be required (as for juvenile idiopathic arthritis). Prophylaxis with oral penicillin is recommended following recurrent post-streptococcal reactive arthritis and is mandatory in the presence of carditis. Aspiration or drainage of the affected joint may also be required as well as adequate analgesia. Tenosynovitis may respond to rest with splinting if necessary. A local corticosteroid injection may be helpful in persistent cases.

JUVENILE IDIOPATHIC ARTHRITIS (JIA)

The management of children with JIA requires a multidisciplinary approach. The aim of treatment is to induce remission, but until this is achieved physiotherapy and splinting are important to maintain joint position and function.

NSAIDs are used for the relief of symptoms in JIA. Different drugs may suit different children in terms of their efficacy, side-effect profile, dosage regimen and formulation. The mean time course of response to NSAIDs is 4 weeks and may be as long as 12 weeks. Slow-release formulations given with the evening meal are especially useful in treating early morning stiffness. Although they are sometimes used, there are no data in children showing that NSAID combinations are additive or synergistic but they appear to be more toxic than single drugs. NSAIDs appear generally to be better tolerated in children than in adults. The majority of children with asthma tolerate NSAIDs well, although parents and children should be advised about the potential effect on lung function. Gastrointestinal bleeding is a rare complication of using NSAIDs in children, therefore the routine use of gastroprotective agents is not necessary. Ranitidine may be helpful in children who develop NSAID-related abdominal pain. If this is ineffective, the use of omeprazole may be considered. Indometacin (indomethacin) appears to be less well tolerated than some other NSAIDs and should only be tried when others have failed. In adolescents with NSAID intolerance it is reasonable to consider the use of the preferential cyclo-oxygenase-2 (COX-2) inhibitor meloxicam. Salicylates are not recommended for JIA because of the concern about Reye syndrome.

CORTICOSTEROIDS

Systemic corticosteroids have a limited role in the management of JIA because of their deleterious effects on bone metabolism and growth. The relative inability of children with JIA to exercise causes osteopenia, which is compounded by the addition of long-term corticosteroid therapy. Indications for systemic corticosteroids are life-threatening systemic diseases such as pericarditis, pleuritis, severe anaemia, or polyarticular joint disease unresponsive to other therapies. The lowest dose that controls the disease should be used and that dose subsequently weaned as soon as possible according to the clinical status of the child. In some cases, alternate day administration (or alternate high-dose, low-dose) may be possible, thus reducing pituitary-adrenal suppression. An additional dose of NSAID may be helpful on the low/no dose evening.

Intermittent pulsed intravenous methylprednisolone is effective at controlling severe systemic symptoms and may have fewer long-term adverse effects. The use of pulses of oral steroids is an alternative approach.

Intra-articular corticosteroid injections are effective in controlling synovitis and may be used alone as therapy for oligoarticular disease. Triamcinolone hexacetonide gives the longest lasting effect. The shorter acting hydrocortisone acetate is often preferred for injecting tendon sheaths. Localised soft tissue atrophy may occur due to steroid leak from the site of injection.

Slow-acting anti-rheumatic drugs (SAARDs). Joint damage occurs early in JIA and may be modified by the earlier use of disease-modifying drugs. Extra caution should be exercised in the use of SAARDs in systemic JIA as adverse effects are more frequent and severe.

Methotrexate has been shown in randomised controlled trials to be more efficacious than placebo and to produce radiological improvement in children with JIA and is therefore the first-line SAARD for polyarticular and extended pauciarticular JIA. It is usually given once a week, although this dosage schedule has never been shown to be optimal. Response may take up to 3 months. Absorption after a single oral dose is highly variable. The absorption of oral methotrexate at doses greater than $20mg/m^2$ is particularly unpredictable. If higher doses are required parenteral administration is advised. Home administration by patient or parents is made practicable by the availability of long-life pre-filled syringes. Full blood count and liver function tests should be monitored regularly. Common adverse effects such as nausea may be limited by evening administration, the addition of oral folic acid or folinic acid, splitting the methotrexate dosage over 24 hours, or parenteral administration. Elevation of transaminases may respond to a temporary reduction in dosage. Omission of a dose should be considered if the transaminase level is greater than three times the upper limit of normal. NSAIDs can alter methotrexate pharmacokinetics and vice versa, resulting in the potential for increased toxicity in patients receiving the combination. Gradual reduction in dosage is recommended after control of disease for a period of 12 months. Abrupt discontinuation of methotrexate may lead to a disease flare.

Sulfasalazine (sulphasalazine) is a useful drug in JIA, particularly in the enthesitis-related and rheumatoid factor positive arthropathies. Side-effects appear to be more frequent and serious in systemic onset JIA. Gradual introduction of the drug with graduated increases in dose lessens the incidence of adverse effects.

Hydroxychloroquine is useful in some cases of JIA. It has a low incidence of adverse effects and routine blood tests to monitor for toxicity and monitoring of visual fields are not required.

Tumour necrosis factor–α inhibitors (TNF). Etanercept is licensed for the treatment of polyarticular JIA refractory to methotrexate. Children commencing this biological therapy must be notified to the British Paediatric Rheumatology Group Registry.

Other treatments. Ciclosporin (cyclosporin) has been studied in JIA only in uncontrolled trials and its use remains experimental except in uveitis. Immunosuppressive agents such as azathioprine, cyclophosphamide, mycophenolate mofetil, and chlorambucil are occasionally also used in treating severe disease unresponsive to other agents. Chlorambucil is used for systemic amyloidosis. The value of combinations of slow-acting anti-rheumatic drugs is as yet unknown. A randomised placebo-controlled trial failed to demonstrate benefit from high dose IV immunoglobulin in systemic onset JIA.

Close collaboration with an ophthalmologist is essential when managing JIA. All children with JIA should be screened for uveitis.

OTHER DISORDERS
Connective tissue diseases and vasculitis. There are no definitive trials to guide the management of this spectrum of diseases in childhood. Therapy should be tailored to the individual child according to the pattern of organ involvement, pathology, and severity of the disease. NSAIDs should be used for arthritis and arthralgia as in JIA. If there is photosensitivity, topical sunblocks should be applied to all exposed skin. Hydroxychloroquine may be used for mucocutaneous disease, fatigue and joint symptoms. When anticardiolipin antibodies and lupus anticoagulant are present, antiplatelet treatment should be considered. In the presence of thrombosis, anticoagulant therapy may be necessary. Low-dose oral prednisolone therapy (<500 microgram/kg/day) is used for the treatment of fever and serositis. High-dose oral prednisolone is used for control of CNS disease, more severe forms of nephritis, and acute haemolytic anaemia in systemic lupus erythematosus and systemic vasculitis. The use of initial IV pulsed methylprednisolone therapy provides a more rapid response in severe disease with major organ involvement. Gut vasculitis may limit absorption of oral treatment. Following control of the acute manifestations of the disease, the prednisolone dosage should be tapered gradually to the lowest possible dose that will maintain the child's health. Pulsed cyclophosphamide with corticosteroids is the current treatment of choice for systemic vasculitis. Immunoregulatory drugs (including azathioprine, methotrexate, ciclosporin and chlorambucil) may be used in any of these diseases.

Raynaud phenomenon. Treatment involves warm clothing and, if necessary, the use of vasodilators or calcium-channel blockers such as nifedipine. In very severe cases, where digital infarction is imminent, IV infusions of the synthetic prostacyclin analogue iloprost may be helpful.

Henoch–Schönlein purpura. Treatment is supportive in most cases, with prednisolone being reserved for the management of severe gastrointestinal disease or haemorrhage.

Kawasaki disease. IV immunoglobulin should be administered on diagnosis. A subsequent dose is recommended for children who remain symptomatic, or in whom symptoms recur after the first infusion. Anti-inflammatory doses of aspirin should be given in the acute phase of the disease and then antiplatelet doses during the convalescent phase. Aspirin therapy should be continued at this antiplatelet dose until the ESR and platelet count return to normal, or indefinitely if aneurysms are present.

Polyarteritis. This may be related to a preceding streptococcal infection, and recurrences may be prevented by the use of prophylactic penicillin.

Wegener granulomatosis. Low dose methotrexate may be an alternative to cyclophosphamide, and co-trimoxazole may be valuable as prophylaxis against recurrences/relapses.

Juvenile dermatomyositis (JDM). The mainstay of therapy is prednisolone but the dose and route of administration remain controversial. Steroid-sparing agents used in JDM include ciclosporin (cyclosporin), azathioprine, methotrexate and IV immunoglobulin, with cyclophosphamide being reserved for life-threatening vasculitis. There is no proven treatment for calcinosis. Physiotherapy and splinting are essential ingredients in the treatment schedule.

Scleroderma. The need for drug therapy is dependent on the disease pattern. Treatment of localised morphoea is often unnecessary. Linear scleroderma or scleroderma *en coup de sabre* may respond to oral or IV corticosteroids during periods of extension when there is active inflammation. Maintenance therapy with penicillamine or methotrexate may be employed, but these drugs have not been studied in placebo-controlled trials in children.

Musculoskeletal symptoms occur frequently in other systemic inflammatory diseases and NSAIDs are often required.

Familial Mediterranean fever (FMF). Prophylactic colchicine reduces the severity and duration of attacks and prevents the development of amyloidosis.

Behçet disease. Corticosteroids and immunosuppressive therapy are often required. Colchicine has also been used.

Neurology

Not all seizures or even convulsions are epileptic and epilepsy is often misdiagnosed. Always consider the possibility that the seizures may be syncopal, emotional, or due to raised intracranial pressure. When epilepsy is diagnosed always think about an underlying cause and investigate appropriately.

EPILEPSY
The decision when to start treatment with an antiepileptic drug (AED) and with which medication depends on the child, frequency of seizures, neurological findings, the identification of an epilepsy syndrome, and the wishes of the parents/carers. Treatment is probably not recommended after a single, brief, generalised, tonic-clonic seizure, or after a few with long intervals in between, or automatically required in a child with severe physical and learning disabilities who develops infrequent myoclonic or atypical absence seizures. In contrast, most clinicians would prescribe an AED after a cluster of seizures or frequent seizures of any kind. The objective of treatment is to achieve seizure control without unacceptable adverse effects using a single drug in the lowest effective dose and in the most appropriate formulation.

Selecting a drug. Approximately 70-75% of children with epilepsy can be controlled with a single AED. The currently 'recommended' first-line drugs are sodium valproate for generalised seizures and carbamazepine for partial seizures.

Drug treatment of epilepsy

Seizure type/ Epilepsy syndrome	First choice	Alternatives
Generalised tonic-clonic (tonic and/or clonic)	Sodium valproate Carbamazepine	Gabapentin, lamotrigine, levetiracetam, phenobarbital (phenobarbitone), phenytoin, topiramate
Atonic (astatic)	Sodium valproate	Clobazam, lamotrigine, phenytoin, topiramate
Myoclonic	Sodium valproate	Clonazepam, lamotrigine, levetiracetam

Drug treatment of epilepsy continued

Seizure type/ Epilepsy syndrome	First choice	Alternatives
Absence	Sodium valproate	Clonazepam, ethosuximide, lamotrigine
Partial simple/complex	Carbamazepine	Gabapentin, lamotrigine, levetiracetam, sodium valproate, topiramate, vigabatrin
Infantile spasms (West syndrome)	Vigabatrin	Nitrazepam, prednisolone hydrocortisone or tetracosactride (tetracosactrin), sodium valproate
Lennox-Gastaut	Sodium valproate	Carbamazepine, clobazam, lamotrigine topiramate
Landau-Kleffner	Prednisolone	Clobazam, lamotrigine, sodium valproate, vigabatrin

The treatment of infantile spasms varies. In European centres vigabatrin or sodium valproate are most commonly prescribed, whereas in the United States the preferred drug is corticotropin (corticotrophin) which is only available on a named patient basis in the UK where the synthetic polypeptide tetracosactide (tetracosactrin) in depot formulation is more commonly used. In the UK a more commonly prescribed alternative to tetracosactide is prednisolone.

There is no evidence that regular anticonvulsant medication prevents febrile seizures or the development of late epilepsy and prophylactic treatment is not recommended. Rectal diazepam at the time of fever can be helpful in children with repeated febrile seizures, but the timing of administration and induced drowsiness are practical difficulties.

Using drugs. Higher per kg doses of AEDs are usually required for children under 3 years of age because of a higher rate of metabolism and increased clearance. Selected drugs should be used alone and in sequence. Adverse effects are more common with larger starting doses than when using a more gradual escalation. Should unacceptable adverse effects occur before optimal control is achieved, an additional drug will be required. If complete seizure control is achieved with the combination, the first drug could be gradually withdrawn after a seizure-free period of around 2-3 months. In the event of the initial drug being wholly ineffective, it would be appropriate simultaneously to replace the first drug with the second and maintain monotherapy.

Combination therapy. Treatment with two AEDs can significantly improve seizure control in 5-10% of children but potentially at the expense of difficulties in interpreting the effects of each drug and an increase in drug interactions. The choice of a second AED will depend on seizure type/epilepsy syndrome, safety profile and whether or not it acts synergistically or antagonistically with the other drug. The use of three AEDs is generally only acceptable when one drug is being introduced as another is withdrawn.

Stopping therapy. This can usually be tried after a 1 or, more commonly, 2-year seizure free period dependent on the seizure syndrome and therefore recognised prognosis. Drug therapy should be gradually withdrawn, e.g. over 2-3 months by reducing the usual daily dose by 10-25% at 1-2 weekly intervals, using convenient dose sizes i.e. using knowledge of liquid concentrations and tablet doses. There is usually no need to withdraw a drug over longer than 3 months.

Blood monitoring in AED treatment. In most situations the dose of AED is appropriate when the patient is seizure-free and experiencing no, or mild and acceptable, adverse effects. Routine measurement of AED blood levels is not justified, as the target ranges are arbitrary and often vary between individuals. However, AED concentrations should be measured in children presenting with worsening seizures, status epilepticus, major non-compliance, or when there are problems identifying adverse effects in children with learning difficulties (especially if receiving phenytoin). Similarly, haematological and biochemical monitoring should only be undertaken if clinically indicated, or possibly before initiating therapy to identify specific, pre-existing dysfunction e.g. liver function tests (phenytoin, sodium valproate, lamotrigine), blood counts (carbamazepine, sodium valproate, phenytoin, ethosuximide) and electrolytes (carbamazepine). However, routine testing may not be sufficiently sensitive to identify those at most risk and is not generally undertaken in the UK. Hepatotoxicity with sodium valproate appears to be greatest in children under 3 years with severe cryptogenic epilepsy featuring myoclonic seizures, additional learning difficulties and receiving at least one other AED.

Neurology

Continuing epileptic seizures, convulsive status epilepticus. The aims of treatment are to secure the airway, maintain cerebral blood flow and stop the seizures. Exclude and, if necessary, treat hypoglycaemia. If seizures last more than 15 minutes, consider taking blood for urea and electrolytes, blood gases, glucose, calcium, AED concentration, toxicology and culture. Start an intravenous infusion and give drug therapy as outlined in the table opposite.

Conventionally, diazepam is given rectally by parents, carers, or nurses at special schools to terminate a tonic-clonic seizure that lasts over 5 or 6 minutes or repeated, serial seizures. Midazolam, either given into the buccal cavity (i.e. between the cheeks and gums) or into the nostril, may be an effective and more acceptable drug (and route) for children.

CEREBRAL PALSY

Drugs for spasticity – oral. Benzodiazepines, particularly nitrazepam and diazepam, reduce tone in muscles. Their undoubted efficacy in some children may be accompanied by side-effects, mainly drowsiness and excessive drooling. Skin patches containing hyoscine hydrobromide will counteract drooling. The use of benzodiazepines over months can induce tolerance and thus may reduce efficacy. They are particularly effective in the young infant with severe spasticity or dystonia. Baclofen by mouth also reduces tone in some children, but again its use is limited by the side-effects of drowsiness. Dantrolene may be used in resistant cases. Tone may be increased in children with cerebral palsy who are in pain, particularly from gastro-oesophageal reflux or dislocating hips. Tizanidine is a newer antispasticity drug that may be less sedating than baclofen; paediatric experience is very limited and the drug should not be used without specialist advice.

Drugs for spasticity – injection. Phenol or alcohol injections into muscle have been used to reduce tone. They work by irreversibly destroying the motor nerves. These are used less since the introduction of botulinum toxin injection. The manufacturers of the two commercially available botulinum A toxin preparations give guidelines on the maximum dose per kilogram body weight per injection or set of injections. The two preparations are both measured in units but the units are of differing potencies and the two are not interchangeable.

Drugs for spasticity – intrathecal. Baclofen may be given as a continuous infusion into the lumbar intrathecal space via an indwelling catheter and subcutaneous pump. The rate of infusion may be altered according to the clinical needs of the child at different times of the day. This is a therapy currently available only at a very few specialised centres.

Drugs used in dystonia. Severe dystonia as part of cerebral palsy may partially respond to levodopa. Children should be started on the smallest possible dose of combined levodopa/carbidopa (co-careldopa) - such as Sinemet-110® half a tablet once daily - with a gradual increase while monitoring for clinical improvement. Children may experience some nausea within 2 hours of taking co-careldopa. Improvement will be apparent within 2 weeks of starting treatment. Video recordings of a child before and after treatment are useful to decide on functional improvement and control of dystonic movements. Most children with dopa-sensitive dystonia (Segawa syndrome – an enzyme defect in the production of dopamine) are exquisitely sensitive to small doses of levodopa and may be completely symptom free on this drug. Occasionally, children with this condition present with symptoms suggestive of a slowly progressive dystonic disease, not dissimilar from dystonic cerebral palsy. A response to levodopa is usually seen within a few days, but occasionally, improvement is delayed and slow over a period of a year. In dystonic cerebral palsy, treatment with co-careldopa at higher doses can induce some of the 'on-off' treatment effects seen in adults with Parkinson's disease. Benzodiazepines have some role in the management of dystonia, limited by their side-effects. Botulinum toxin injections are effective in the management of focal dystonia. Intrathecal baclofen is effective in controlling generalised dystonia, either as part of cerebral palsy, or following head injury. Doses needed are higher than used to control spasticity.

MIGRAINE

Treatment of the acute attack. Ibuprofen is the most effective medication used to control the acute pain of migraine. Other NSAIDs may be used. Analgesics given very early in the acute attack are more likely to provide relief than those given later. In migraine where there is persistent vomiting, metoclopramide may be used as an anti-emetic either by mouth or by injection. In these circumstances, oral analgesics may not be tolerated and a suppository preparation of drugs such as paracetamol or diclofenac may be used.

Sumatriptan is effective in treating the acute migraine attack in children. Onset of relief of pain is quicker with nasal spray than with tablets. The commonest reported side-effect is an alteration in taste. Side-effects are slightly dose-related. Some children do relapse within 24 hours and a second dose within that 24 hours is not always effective. One should ensure that children and parents understand the circumstances in which a second dose within 24 hours can be taken. As sumatriptan is a vasoconstrictor, there have been concerns that it may exacerbate associated symptoms of migraine where vasoconstriction is thought to be the cause (e.g. visual field defects, mild hemiparesis). These concerns

Treatment guideline for an acute tonic-clonic convulsion including established convulsive status epilepticus.

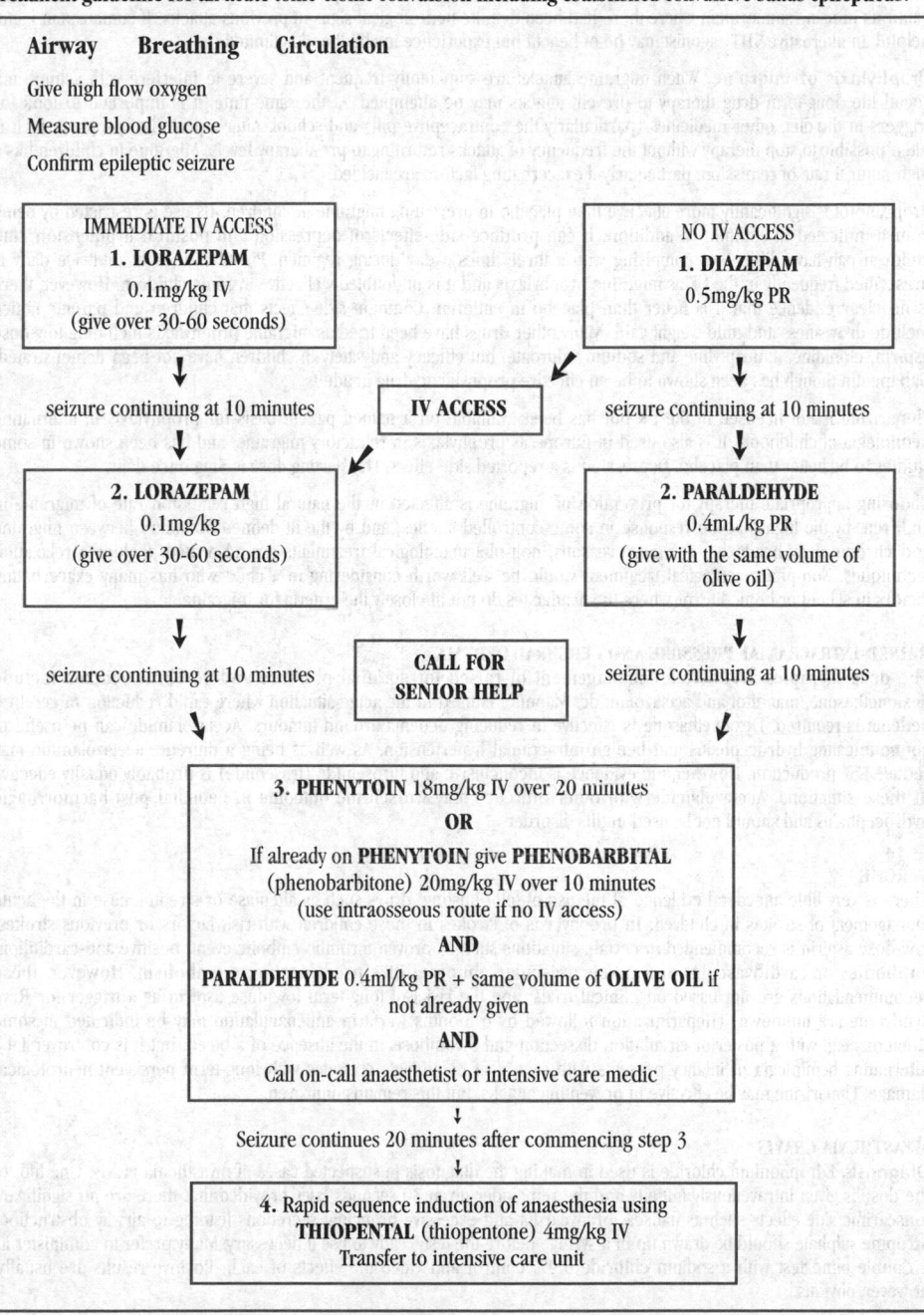

Airway   Breathing   Circulation

Give high flow oxygen

Measure blood glucose

Confirm epileptic seizure

IMMEDIATE IV ACCESS
1. LORAZEPAM
0.1mg/kg IV
(give over 30-60 seconds)

NO IV ACCESS
1. DIAZEPAM
0.5mg/kg PR

seizure continuing at 10 minutes

IV ACCESS

seizure continuing at 10 minutes

2. LORAZEPAM
0.1mg/kg
(give over 30-60 seconds)

2. PARALDEHYDE
0.4mL/kg PR
(give with the same volume of olive oil)

seizure continuing at 10 minutes

CALL FOR SENIOR HELP

seizure continuing at 10 minutes

3. PHENYTOIN 18mg/kg IV over 20 minutes

OR

If already on **PHENYTOIN** give **PHENOBARBITAL**
(phenobarbitone) 20mg/kg IV over 10 minutes
(use intraosseous route if no IV access)

AND

PARALDEHYDE 0.4ml/kg PR + same volume of **OLIVE OIL** if
not already given

AND

Call on-call anaesthetist or intensive care medic

Seizure continues 20 minutes after commencing step 3

4. Rapid sequence induction of anaesthesia using
THIOPENTAL (thiopentone) 4mg/kg IV
Transfer to intensive care unit

Neurology

have not been borne out in studies, although there is the occasional report of an ischaemic event. One would be cautious in using sumatriptan where there had been definite neurological signs in previous attacks. If sumatriptan is not helpful an alternative $5HT_1$ agonist may be of benefit but experience in childhood is limited.

Prophylaxis of migraine. When migraine attacks are sufficiently frequent and severe to interfere with school and social life, long-term drug therapy to prevent attacks may be attempted. At the same time, it is important to look for triggers in the diet, other medicines (particularly the contraceptive pill) and school. After a period of prophylaxis, it is often possible to stop therapy without the frequency of attacks returning to pre-therapy levels. Migraine in children has a high natural rate of remission, particularly if exacerbating factors are tackled.

Propranolol is significantly more effective than placebo in preventing migraine in children. Its use is restricted by being contra-indicated in asthma. In addition, it can produce side-effects of depression and postural hypotension, and children can have difficulties complying with a three times a day dosing regimen. Pizotifen at night or twice daily is prescribed frequently in the UK as migraine prophylaxis and it is undoubtedly effective in some children. However, there is no clear evidence that it is better than placebo in children. Common side-effects that children and parents notice include drowsiness and mild weight gain. Many other drugs have been tried as migraine prophylaxis including low-dose aspirin, clonidine, amitriptyline and sodium valproate, but efficacy and safety in children have not been demonstrated. Gabapentin though has been shown to be an effective prophylactic drug in adults.

Flunarizine is not licensed in the UK but has been available on a named patient basis for prophylaxis in alternating hemiplegia of childhood. It is also used in Europe as prophylaxis in refractory migraine, and has been shown in some studies to be better than placebo. Depression is a reported side-effect. The starting dose is 5mg once daily.

Choosing appropriate therapy for prevention of migraine is affected by the natural high remission rate of migraine in children, by the high placebo response in some controlled studies, and by the ill-defined boundary between migraine and chronic daily headache. For these reasons, non-pharmacological treatments are advocated, including relaxation techniques. Non-pharmacological treatment would be well worth considering in a child who has many exacerbating factors in school or home life, or where the headaches do not fit closely the criteria for migraine.

RAISED INTRACRANIAL PRESSURE AND CEREBRAL OEDEMA.
The drug therapies available for management of raised intracranial pressure and cerebral oedema include dexamethasone, mannitol and acetazolamide. Mannitol is used in the acute situation where rapid reduction of cerebral oedema is required. Dexamethasone is effective in reducing oedema around tumours. Acetazolamide can be useful in communicating hydrocephalus and benign intracranial hypertension. As well as being a diuretic, acetazolamide may reduce CSF production. However, the evidence is inconclusive and furosemide (frusemide) is probably equally effective in these situations. Acetazolamide with other diuretics may worsen the outcome in neonatal post-haemorrhagic hydrocephalus and should not be used in this disorder.

STROKE
There is very little anecdotal evidence of the use of 'clot-busting' drugs such as alteplase or streptokinase in the acute management of strokes in children. In prophylaxis of strokes in those children with risk factors or previous strokes, low-dose aspirin is recommended in certain situations such as proven thrombo-embolic event, positive anti-cardiolipin antibodies or cardiovascular and cerebrovascular abnormalities predisposing to embolism. However, these recommendations are not based on clinical trials, and the risks of long-term low-dose aspirin as a trigger for Reye Syndrome are unknown. (Heparinization followed by 6 months warfarin anticoagulation may be indicated in some situations e.g. with a posterior circulation dissection and thrombosis in the absence of a bleed, but it is controversial.) Alternating hemiplegia of infancy presents with recurrent hemiplegic episodes with long-term persistent neurological damage. Flunarizine may be effective in preventing attacks, but this remains unproven.

MYASTHENIA GRAVIS
Diagnosis. Edrophonium chloride is used in making the diagnosis in suspected cases of myasthenia gravis. One fifth of the dose is given intravenously initially and the remainder given 30 seconds later provided that there are no significant muscarinic side-effects such as nausea, bradycardia and excessive bronchial secretions leading to airway obstruction. Atropine sulphate should be drawn up in a syringe before the test, ready to use if necessary. Many prefer to administer as a double blind test with a sodium chloride 0.9% control and video the effects of each. Positive results are usually, however, obvious.

Treatment. Once the diagnosis has been established, the child should be started on maintenance anticholinesterase drugs. The drug of choice is pyridostigmine, given every 4-5 hours during waking hours. The dose and frequency of doses should be titrated against clinical symptoms. Neostigmine is used less frequently due to the shorter half-life of 4 hours, and greater risk of muscarinic side-effects. It may be given by injection, and has a role in infants so weak as to be unable to feed. In severe cases, a child may require a course of steroid therapy, particularly when antibodies to the acetylcholine receptor are present in high titre. Pulsed methylprednisolone therapy followed by maintenance therapy may be used. Alternatively, the methylprednisolone may be followed by a course of intravenous immunoglobulin. Intractable cases have required plasma exchange therapy before anticholinesterase therapy has been effective and some respond well to thymectomy.

There are rare familial forms of myasthenia not related to antibodies to acetyl-choline receptors, but caused by defects elsewhere in transmission between nerve and muscle at the neuro-muscular junction. Anticholinesterase drugs may be ineffective, and in rare cases may exacerbate the condition. 3,4-Diaminopyridine has been used in some of these disorders within regional neuromuscular centres.

GUILLAIN-BARRÉ SYNDROME (GBS)
Treatment of the acute attack of GBS is focused on good supportive care, management and prevention of complications, and symptomatic therapy. Immunoglobulin therapy is the treatment of choice with evidence of increased speed of recovery. Plasmapheresis has a similar efficacy but is more difficult in the young child.

ACUTE PAROXYSMAL AND CHRONIC MOVEMENT DISORDERS
The idiopathic acute paroxysmal choreoathetoses and dystonias are differentiated by time, frequency, and triggers of attacks. Some may be difficult to differentiate from epilepsy, particularly when occurring during sleep. Paroxysmal kinesigenic choreoathetosis (triggered by movement) responds well to phenytoin or carbamazepine. Paroxysmal dystonic choreoathetosis may be improved by clonazepam, acetazolamide, or haloperidol.

Choreoathetosis as a symptom of an underlying metabolic, inflammatory or degenerative disorder is difficult to treat. Levodopa or benzatropine may be effective. Chorea associated with systemic lupus erythematosus usually responds to corticosteroid therapy. The chorea of rheumatic fever may be helped by carbamazepine, haloperidol or pimozide.

Focal dystonia may respond to levodopa, clonazepam or benzatropine (benztropine). Botulinum toxin is licensed in adults for treatment of blepharospasm and orofacial dystonias. Levodopa is less effective in generalised genetic dystonia or dystonia secondary to encephalopathy, traumatic brain injury or strokes.

The movement disorder of Tourette Syndrome responds equally well to haloperidol and pimozide. Symptomatic relief of severe drug induced movement disorders can be gained with trihexyphenidyl (benzhexol), benzatropine (benztropine), or diazepam. Initial treatment may have to be given intravenously, and should be continued orally for 2-3 days. Essential tremor can be successfully relieved by propranolol.

MUSCULAR DYSTROPHIES
There is no treatment that will reverse the symptoms of muscular dystrophy. Rarely, steroid therapy may temporarily increase muscle strength in Duchenne muscular dystrophy in boys who are rapidly losing strength, but this must be weighed against the potential side-effects of steroids - in particular, weight gain, oedema, and steroid-induced myopathy and osteopenia. Maintaining ambulation, spinal surgery and nocturnal minimally invasive ventilation prolong and improve quality of life.

MYOTONIA
The myotonic and paramyotonic disorders are slowly being separated into distinct clinical and genetic entities, some of which are related to sodium and other ion channel defects. Acetazolamide is used to prevent attacks of cramps. Carbamazepine or phenytoin may also be effective both as treatment for the acute attack and as prophylaxis.

DEMYELINATING DISORDERS
Demyelination is an integral part of the pathologies of optic neuritis, acute disseminated encephalomyelitis, multiple sclerosis and its variants. The treatment of the acute attack is based on steroid therapy. Various regimens have been used. Currently, the preferred treatment is high dose methylprednisolone (500mg in children under 12 years and 1g for

Neurology

children 12 years and over) given daily intravenously for 3 days, followed by prednisolone reducing over 14 days. This hastens recovery from the acute attack, but whether it has any effect on frequency of relapse of multiple sclerosis or on the progression of optic neuritis to multiple sclerosis is uncertain. The role of interferon beta in preventing progression of childhood multiple sclerosis is not yet known.

HYPOKALAEMIC PERIODIC PARALYSIS
Oral potassium chloride can be given as a regular prophylaxis and in an acute attack, but the dose is limited by the unpleasant taste. Acetazolamide, spironolactone, and oral contraceptives have all been used for long-term prophylaxis. The initial benefit obtained from acetazolamide therapy may wear off. The benefit may reappear when the acetazolamide is reintroduced after a period without treatment.

FACIAL PARALYSIS
This can sometimes complicate acute or chronic otitis media, Lyme disease, or hypertension, but is most often idiopathic (Bell palsy). The latter is believed to be a post-infectious, allergic or immune demyelinating facial neuritis which may follow Epstein-Barr virus, herpes virus or mumps virus infections. There is no good evidence that steroids are helpful, but in cases of total paralysis they are often used. Ideally, steroids should be used within the first 24 hours. Doxycycline is the antibiotic of choice for Lyme disease.

Neurally medicated syncope
In young children Reflex Asystolic Syncope typically manifests as Reflex Anoxic Seizures. Attacks are easily mistaken for epileptic seizures, 'breath-holding' or 'temper tantrums'. Specific treatment is reserved for rare cases where attacks are so severe or frequent as to cause significant handicap to the child and family. Atropine sulphate or even cardiac pacing may be indicated but, if considered, ictal recording of an attack is recommended to exclude other mechanisms. In older children and teenagers there is usually an associated drop in peripheral vascular resistance. If causing significant handicap then fludrocortisone, ephedrine, disopyramide or a beta-blocker has been used. Other causes of recurrent syncope should be investigated, including cardiac arrhythmias e.g. prolonged QT syndromes.

Nutrition

COMPLETE ENTERAL FEEDS
Infant (0-12 months). Term infants with normal gastrointestinal function are fed either breast milk or normal infant formula during the first year of life. The average intake is between 150mL and 200mL/kg/day. Formulas are based on whey or casein dominant protein, lactose, +/- maltodextrin and amylose, vegetable oil and milk fat. The composition of all normal and soya infant formulas in the UK have to meet The Infant Formula and Follow-on Formula Regulations 1995, which enact the European Community Regulations 91/321/EC. The composition of other enteral and specialist infant formulas has to meet the Commission Directive (1999/21/EC) on Dietary Foods for Special Medical Purposes.

An infant who is failing to thrive may be given one of two high energy feeds, each of which contains a percentage energy from protein between 9 and 11%. Alternatively, energy supplements may be added to normal infant formula to achieve a higher energy content, but this will reduce the protein/energy ratio, or normal infant formula concentration may be slightly increased from the norm of around 13% up to 17%. Care should be taken not to present an osmotic load of >500mOsmol/kg water to the normal functioning gut, otherwise an osmotic diarrhoea will result. Concentrating or supplementing feeds should not be attempted without the advice of a paediatric dietitian.

Children 1-6 years (8-20kg). A number of nutritionally-complete 1.0kcal/mL ready to use feeds designed for the 1-6 year age group are available. They are all based on caseinates, maltodextrin and vegetable oils ± added medium chain triglyceride (MCT) oil and contain residual lactose only. They are well-tolerated and effective in improving nutritional status in this age group. They should be administered at a rate of 85-110mL/kg/day depending on age, weight, condition and nutritional requirements. There are also 1.5kcal/mL ready-to-use nutrient dense formulas produced for young children with high energy requirements or for those who require small feed volumes.

Children over 6 years – 1kcal/mL feeds. There are no standard nutritionally complete polymeric 1kcaL/mL feeds specifically produced for children over 6 years. There is little choice but to use adult 1kcaL/mL feeds for this group, although the nutritional profile is not ideal. Protein, electrolyte, vitamin and trace mineral intake should be assessed to ensure this is not excessive. They should be given at a rate of 50-70mL/kg/day depending on age, weight, clinical condition and nutritional requirements.

Children over 6 years – 1.5kcal/mL feeds. There are no standard nutritionally-complete polymeric 1.5kcal/mL feeds produced for children over 6 years. Adult feeds containing 1.5kcal/mL are used but all those containing over 6g protein/100mL have been excluded from the tables as they are considered to be too high in protein (daily protein requirements of 7-14 year old children vary from 19.7g to 42g daily). If 1.5kcal/mL feeds are used, the intake of protein, electrolytes, vitamins and trace minerals should be carefully assessed and monitored.

FIBRE-ENRICHED FEEDS

Fibre-enriched formula feeds are specifically formulated for the 1-6 year old age group. These paediatric feeds (1kcal/mL and 1.5kcal/mL) contain fibre between 0.5g-0.75g/100kcal. There is little data on the long-term efficacy of fibre-containing feeds in young children but fibre-enriched feeds may be helpful for children with chronic constipation and/or diarrhoea. All adult fibre-enriched feeds containing fibre over 2g/100mL have been excluded.

SPECIALISED FORMULA

It is essential that any infant or child who is intolerant of breast milk or normal infant formula, or whose condition requires nutrient specific adaptation, is prescribed a nutritionally-complete replacement formula in adequate volume. In the first 4 months of life, a volume of 150-200mL/kg/day is recommended. After 6 months, should the formula still be required, a volume of 600mL/day should be maintained in addition to solids.

Products for cow's milk protein allergy and/or lactose intolerance. There are a number of infant formulas designed for cow's milk protein allergy and/or lactose intolerance. If a low intake of these formulas is consumed, it may be necessary to supplement with calcium, and possibly a vitamin and mineral supplement.

Liquid soya milks purchased from supermarkets and health food stores are nutritionally incomplete and should never be used for infants <1 year of age. Low lactose formulas based on whole cow's milk protein are unsuitable for infants with cow's milk protein allergy.

Protein hydrolysate formulas based on casein, whey, meat and soya, are suitable for infants with disaccharide and/or whole protein intolerance. Some of the formulas contain a significant proportion of their fat source in the form of medium chain triglyceride (MCT) oil and are prescribable for indications where amino acids or peptides are necessary in conjunction with MCT oil. There is only one peptide-based feed which has been specifically produced for children over 1 year of age (Pepdite 1+). All the other peptide-based formulas are designed for adults and when used for children, the intake of electrolyte, vitamins and minerals should be carefully assessed and modified to meet the nutritional requirements of the child. They have a high osmolality when given at recommended dilution and need careful introduction.

Elemental (amino acid–based formula). There is only one elemental nutritionally-complete formula designed for infants (Neocate®). There is some evidence to demonstrate that tolerance of and growth on this formula is satisfactory. In addition, there is only one elemental formula based on L-amino acids specifically produced for young children (Neocate® Advance). Adult elemental formulas may be used for children over the age of 6 years. The intake of electrolytes, vitamins and minerals should be carefully assessed and modified to meet the nutritional requirements of children. They have a high osmolality when given at recommended dilution and need careful introduction.

Modular feeds. A modular feed is one which is based on individual protein, fat, carbohydrate, vitamin and mineral components/modules so that these components and their concentrations can be adapted to meet the specific needs of an infant or child. Modular feeds are used when nutritionally-complete specialised formulas are not tolerated or if the fluid and nutrient requirements are changed with a varying clinical state, e.g. in gastrointestinal, renal or liver disease. The chief advantage of modular feeds is their flexibility; disadvantages include their complexity and preparation difficulties. Modular feeds should not be used without the supervision of a paediatric dietician.

Miscellaneous formulae. A number of highly specialised formulas are available in which nutrients have been modified to meet the specific requirements of various clinical conditions such as in renal and liver diseases. When using these formulas, careful monitoring of growth and biochemistry should be undertaken.

Nutrition

FEED THICKENERS

Carob-based thickeners. These may be used to thicken feeds for infants <1 year of age. Breast-fed infants can be offered the thickener as a paste from a spoon prior to feeds.

Starched based thickeners. These can be used to thicken liquids and feeds for children >1 year of age.

Pre-thickened formula. This is casein-based infant formula, which contains small quantities of pre-gelatinized starch. Pre-thickened formula is prepared in the same way as normal infant formula. The feeds do not thicken on standing but thicken in the stomach when exposed to its acid pH. The feeds flow through a standard teat. The pre-thickened formula is designed primarily for infants with mild reflux.

DIETARY SUPPLEMENTS FOR ORAL USE

Three types of prescribable fortified dietary supplements are available – fortified milk shakes providing 1kcal/mL and 1.5 kcal/mL fortified non-milk tasting supplements and fortified desserts. The daily quantity recommended is age dependant and the following is a useful guide, 1-2 years, 200kcal (840kJ); 3-5 years, 400kcal (1680kJ); 6-11 years, 600kcal (2520kJ); and over 12 years, 800kcal (3360kJ). Adult designed supplements, containing 1.5 kcal/mL should not be used for children 1-3 years of age as these are too high in protein. All supplements containing greater than 6g protein/100mL have been excluded. Ideally, supplements should be administered after meals or at bedtime so as not to impair appetite. Many supplements are high in sugar or maltodextrin. Care should be taken to prevent prolonged contact with teeth.

OTHER DIETARY SUPPLEMENTS

A number of dietary supplements based on carbohydrates, fat and/or protein are available to enhance the nutrient density of feeds or diet or used as the components of modular feeds. Details are shown in the tables. For infants and children receiving carbohydrate-based supplements, careful attention to dental hygiene is necessary.

PRODUCTS FOR METABOLIC DISEASE

There is a large range of disease-specific infant formulas and amino acid supplements for metabolic diseases. Unfortunately many of the product names are so similar that care should be taken that the correct supplement is being prescribed to avoid potential metabolic derangement. Also, some are nutritionally incomplete and require vitamin and/or other nutrient supplementation.

Intravenous nutrition

INTRAVENOUS NUTRITION

Parenteral nutrition (PN; intravenous feeding) should be considered whenever an adequate supply of nutrients cannot be provided using the enteral route. A functional small bowel should be used whenever feasible, although this sometimes requires access by feeding tube (e.g. nasogastric, nasojejunal, gastrostomy, gastro-jejunal or jejunostomy). The need for severe fluid restriction or difficulty maintaining enteral access may mean PN is preferable to enteral feeding even in the presence of normal gut function; complete enteral starvation, however, should usually be avoided. Nutritional support can be optimised through a multidisciplinary team approach.

PN solutions are complex and must be prepared in the pharmacy under strict aseptic conditions. Their osmolality will generally be high and this will determine whether they can be safely infused into a peripheral vein or if central venous access is required. For long-term PN (e.g. in a patient with short bowel syndrome) a tunneled Broviac®-type central venous catheter is preferred. To reduce the risk of catheter-related bloodstream infection there must be strict adherence to protocols for aseptic technique during the setting up and discontinuing of parenteral feed administration.

Biochemical and anthropometric monitoring are used to ensure homeostasis and the effectiveness of nutritional support. Quantities of nutrients will vary with patient age and underlying condition but age-related IV nutritional targets can be used as a guide and in some cases will allow the use of standardised mixtures of nutrients.

In neonatal paediatric practice pharmaceutical considerations (e.g. high calcium concentration destabilises the lipid emulsion) make it unusual to be able to deliver all nutrients from a single feed container. Such an 'all in one' feed can

Characteristics of proprietary infusion solutions commonly used in neonatal and paediatric PN

PRODUCT	Nitrogen g/litre	Energy (non-protein kcal/litre)	Electrolytes						Comments
			Na	K	Ca	Mg	acetate	Cl	
Amino acid solutions									
Dipeptiven®									Additive containing glutamine dipeptide providing 135mg glutamine/mL
Glamin®	22.4						62		Contains glutamine dipeptide; for older children (unlicensed <2 years)
Nephramine®	6.4		5				44	<3	Essential amino acids, histidine, used in renal failure
Primene®	15							16	Cord blood profile, contains taurine and neonatal essential amino acids
Vaminolact®	9.3								Breast milk profile, contains taurine and neonatal essential amino acids
Vamin 9 Glucose®	9.4	400	50	20	2.5	1.5		50	Egg protein profile; glucose energy source; for older children
Vamin 18®	18						110		For older children who are fluid restricted
Fat emulsions									
Intralipid® 20%		2000							Soya oil, glycerol, phosphate 15mmol/L
Intralipid® 30%		3000							Soya oil, glycerol, phosphate 15mmol/L
Lipofundin® MCT/LCT 20%		1900							Soya oil, glycerol, phosphate 15mmol/L
Clinoleic®		2000							Olive oil 80%, soya oil 20%, phosphate 15mmol/L
Glucose solutions									
Glucose 5%		200							
Glucose 10%		400							
Glucose 50%		2000							

Other preparations used in neonatal and paediatric PN.

Trace element solutions
Additrace® contains multiple trace elements and is suitable for children >40kg. Dose 10mL daily.
Peditrace® contains multiple trace elements and is suitable for infants and children.
Dose 1mL/kg daily to a maximum of 15mL.
Individual trace elements may be available as 'specials' from NHS and commercial specials manufacturers.
Check the compatibility of trace elements with other PN components before use.

Intravenous nutrition

Intravenous nutrition

VITAMIN CONTENT of PARENTERAL MULTIVITAMIN PRODUCTS
with reference dietary requirements

VITAMIN	DoH recommended intake/day	Other recommended intakes/day	MVI paediatric (in 5mL)	Cernevit® (in 5mL)	Multibionta® (in 10mL)	Solivito N®+ Vitlipid N® infant/adult (in 10mL)
A (retinol as palmitate)	<6 years 400 microgram >6 years 700 microgram	Infants 450 microgram Older children 700 microgram	700 microgram	1.064mg	3.043mg	<11years 690 microgram >11years 1.004mg
D (cholecalciferol/ ergocalciferol)	1–3 years 1 microgram	<3 years 10 microgram	10 microgram	5.5 microgram (220 units)	Nil	<11years 10 microgram >11years 5 microgram
E (alpha tocopheryl acetate)	–	3–12mg	7mg	10.2mg	5mg	<11years 6.4mg >11years 9.1 microgram
K$_1$ (phytomenadione)	–	infants 2 microgram/kg	200 microgram	Nil	Nil	<11years 200mg >11years 150microgram
C (ascorbic acid)	30mg	20–60mg	80mg	125mg	500mg	113mg
B$_1$ (thiamine)	1–3 years 500 microgram 4–6 years 700microgram	20–40 microgram/ 100 kcal diet	1.2mg	3.51mg	50mg	3.1mg
B$_2$ (riboflavin)	1–3 years 500 microgram 4–6 years 700 microgram	1.1–1.7mg	1.4mg	4.14mg	10mg	4.9mg
B$_6$ (pyridoxine)	1–3 years 500 microgram 4–6 years 700 microgram	400 microgram at 1 year increasing to 2mg in adults	1mg	4.53mg	15mg	4.9mg
Niacin (nicotinic acid)	1–3 years 500 microgram 4–6 years 700 microgram	15–20mg Nil	17mg	Nicotinamide 46mg	Nil	Nicotinamide 40mg
Pantothenate	–	3–7mg	5mg	17.25mg	25mg (as dexpanthenol)	16.5mg
Biotin	–	10–200 microgram	20 microgram	70 microgram	Nil	60 microgram
Folate	1–3 years 70 microgram 4–6 years 100 microgram	Infants 50 microgram increasing to 400 microgram in adults	140 microgram	414 microgram	Nil	400 microgram
B$_{12}$ (hydroxocobalamin/ cyanocobalamin)	1–3 years 500 nanogram 4–6 years 800 nanogram	1–2 microgram	1 microgram	6 microgram	Nil	5 microgram

be used for older children, particularly if receiving home PN. Most infants and children will receive water-soluble nutrients (e.g. amino acids, glucose, electrolytes, trace minerals) from one container and lipid and vitamins from another. The two solutions are infused simultaneously and mixed as close to the catheter as possible via a Y-connector. The inclusion of heparin in PN solution is unnecessary and leads to lipid droplet formation after mixing has taken place in the catheter lumen. Use of sodium glycerophosphate allows the incorporation of adequate amounts of calcium and phosphate even for preterm babies. Acetates used in place of some chloride salts help avoid hyperchloraemic acidosis. Glutamine is important for immune function and maintaining gastrointestinal mucosal integrity, and may become essential under conditions of stress. However, the role of glutamine is still being assessed in children and as yet it is not routinely incorporated into PN solutions.

The main problems associated with PN are mechanical complications related to central venous catheter insertion and maintenance, catheter-related bloodstream infection, and metabolic imbalance from over or under provision of nutrients (unexpected serious disturbance is rare). They can be avoided by ensuring recognised procedures for prescribing, handling, administration and monitoring are adopted, preferably under the supervision of a nutritional care team. Cholestatic jaundice is particularly associated with long-term PN and enteral 'starvation' (with prematurity and sepsis being additional major risk factors) and may respond to an increase in enteral feeding, cyclic PN and/or decrease in intake of lipid emulsion.

Weaning from short-term PN can be achieved over a few days as enteral feeds are introduced and tolerated. Patients with major gastrointestinal abnormalities often require a prolonged period of combined parenteral and enteral nutrition until the small bowel adapts to absorb sufficient nutrients. In such cases (beyond the newborn period) PN is usually given as an overnight infusion; this may protect against hepatic complications as well as freeing the patient from infusion pumps in the day.

Vitamins and minerals

The Department of Health has produced tables, which can be used as a guide to prescribing appropriate doses although they are based on data from populations. Except for iron-deficiency anaemia, a primary vitamin and/or mineral deficiency due to simple dietary inadequacy is rare in the developed world.

Children at risk of developing deficiencies because of an inadequate intake:
☐ Preterm infants (who have inadequate stores at birth)
☐ Infants born of mothers who are vegans or of women who are themselves deficient in minerals and vitamins. Maternal vitamin B12 deficiency can cause developmental delay or encephalopathy in the first 6 months of life
☐ Neglected children or children fed on foods of poor nutrient quality due to poor parenting
☐ Adolescents who do not eat enough calcium and iron to support their rapid growth spurt
☐ Children fed on restrictive diets for religious or cultural reasons (e.g. vegans, Rastafarians, and Seventh Day Adventists)
☐ Children with metabolic and other disorders requiring restrictive diets.

Diseases which may lead to deficiencies:
☐ Malabsorption syndromes – cystic fibrosis, short bowel syndrome, coeliac disease, Crohn disease
☐ Kidney disease and liver disease; leading to impaired vitamin synthesis.

Other causes of deficiency:
☐ Certain drugs which impair absorption or metabolism of vitamins – warfarin and vitamin K
☐ Excessive intakes of specific nutrients which are vitamin dependent for their metabolism – polyunsaturated fatty acids and vitamin E, tryptophan and niacin
☐ Excessive intake of one mineral absorbed in preference to another – e.g. excessive zinc impairs copper absorption
☐ Excessive dietary phytate (which impairs the absorption of certain minerals).

Many vitamin supplements are described as 'multivitamin' but few contain the whole range of essential vitamins and many contain very high amounts of vitamins A and D. Care should be taken to ensure the correct dose is not exceeded.

Vitamins and minerals

Reference Nutrient Intakes for Vitamins.

Department of Health report on Health and Social Subjects 41.
Dietary reference values for food energy and nutrients for the UK. 1991 HMSO.

Age	Thiamine mg/day	Riboflavin mg/day	Niacin *mg/day	Vit B_6 micro-gram/day	Vit B_{12} micro-gram/day	Folate micro-gram/day	Vit C mg/day	Vit A micro-gram/day	Vit D micro-gram/day
0–3 mth	0.2	0.4	3	0.2	0.3	50	25	350	8.5
4–6 mth	0.2	0.4	3	0.2	0.3	50	25	350	8.5
7–9 mth	0.2	0.4	4	0.3	0.4	50	25	350	7
10–12 mth	0.3	0.4	5	0.4	0.4	50	25	350	7
1–3 yrs	0.5	0.6	8	0.7	0.5	70	30	400	7
4–6 yrs	0.7	0.8	11	0.9	0.8	100	30	500	-
7–10 yrs	0.7	1	12	1	1	150	30	500	-
Male									
11–14 yrs	0.9	1.2	15	1.2	1.2	200	35	600	-
15–18 yrs	1.1	1.3	18	1.5	1.5	200	40	700	-
Female									
11–14 yrs	0.7	1.1	12	1	1.2	200	35	600	-
15–18 yrs	0.8	1.1	14	1.2	1.5	200	40	600	-

* Based on protein providing 14.7% of the energy. Niacin–nicotinic acid equivalent.

Reference Nutrient Intakes for Minerals (SI Unit).

Department of Health report on Health and Social Subjects 41.
Dietary reference values for food energy and nutrients for the UK. 1991 HMSO.

Age	Ca mmol/day	P[1] mmol/day	Mg mmol/day	Na[2] mmol/day	K[3] mmol/day	Cl[4] mmol/day	Iron micro-mol/day	Zn micro-mol/day	Cu micro-mol/day	Se micro-mol/day	I micro-mol/day
0–3 mths	13.1	13.1	2.2	9	20	9	30	60	5	0.1	0.4
4–6 mths	13.1	13.1	2.5	12	22	12	80	60	5	0.2	0.5
7–9 mths	13.1	13.1	3.2	14	18	14	140	75	5	0.1	0.5
10–12mths	13.1	13.1	3.3	15	18	15	140	75	5	0.1	0.5
1–3 yrs	8.8	8.8	3.5	22	20	22	120	75	6	0.2	0.6
4–6 yrs	11.3	11.3	4.8	30	28	30	110	100	9	0.3	0.8
7–10 yrs	13.8	13.8	8	50	50	50	160	110	11	0.4	0.9
Male											
11–14 yrs	25	25	11.5	70	80	70	200	140	13	0.6	1
15–18 yrs	25	25	12.3	70	90	70	200	145	16	0.9	1
Female											
11–14 yrs	20	20	11.5	70	80	70	260[5]	140	13	0.6	1
15–18 yrs	20	20	12.3	70	90	70	260[5]	110	16	0.8	1.1

1 Phosphorus RNI is set equal to calcium in molar terms.
2 1 mmol sodium = 23mg.
3 1 mmol potassium = 39mg.
4 Corresponds to sodium 1 mmol = 35.5mg.
5 Insufficient for adolescents and young women with high menstrual losses where the most practical way of meeting iron requirements is to take iron supplements.

In infants and children as in adults, pain, anxiety and fear are often associated. All concerned with the care of children have a duty to anticipate and avoid, as well as relieve pain and the psychological and emotional threats of illness and injury. For further guidance and references to primary sources see *Prevention and Control of Pain in Children: a Manual for Health Care Professionals*, Royal College of Paediatrics and Child Health, BMJ Publications, London, 1997.

Assessment, measurement and awareness of pain. All children should have regular assessment for the presence or absence of pain and, if present, enquiry made about its severity, exacerbating factors and relieving factors. Pain assessment should be undertaken and documented as regularly as the measurement of vital signs. Behavioural and physiological indicators can be used in infants and young children, while self-reporting by the child from age 3 years is possible using appropriate pain assessment tools (see Morton NS. Pain assessment in children. *Paediatric Anaesthesia* 1997;7:(4) 267-272 and Royal College of Nursing guidelines on the recognition and assessment of acute pain in children. (www.rcn.org.uk)). Covert suffering is often identified in children in hospital settings by this proactive approach and making pain visible in this way allows more effective treatment. Intervention to reduce pain should be undertaken early on the basis of assessments. Intervention to prevent pain whenever it can reasonably be anticipated should be the standard of care. Pain prevention and treatment should be given a high priority when managing children of all ages (including the preterm) as all age groups can feel pain.

Managing the emotional and physical components of pain in children. Pain management can be difficult and is sometimes inadequate. The reasons for this include: a failure to recognise or anticipate pain and the distress it causes; an undue fear of masking clinical signs and symptoms (e.g. of an acute abdomen); an apprehension of side-effects (e.g. of opioids); a concern about inducing dependency; the child's fear of the treatment (children fear injections and may rather suffer pain in silence than receive an injection).

All staff concerned should have training in pain management in children. They should know how to recognise and assess fear and pain. Young children cannot describe their experience, although they can show their feelings. Older children may mask or deny their feelings or suffering. Staff must decide when to tell a child about a forthcoming procedure, why it is to be done, whether it will be painful or not, and how any pain will be eased. When decisions on care are made, the child should participate as far as understanding allows. It may not be possible to remove all pain or anxiety, and children and their parents should not be misled. Having parents close by, providing they understand what is happening and know how to help, is important to a child. The environment should be friendly and as peaceful as other necessary activities allow. Many clinical procedures (e.g. venepuncture and cannulation of an artery) are threatening to the child and should be done by someone with appropriate skill, not the least experienced member of the clinical team. The procedure may need to be repeated, and a bad experience can have a lasting effect. Simple measures such as sucrose by mouth in newborn infants and topical anaesthesia benefit many children.

Particular circumstances. There are circumstances when the needs of children call for additional specialised skills and knowledge. These circumstances include:
☐ Care in the emergency department
☐ Care before and after operations
☐ Care of sick newborn infants
☐ Management of children in intensive care
☐ Management of children with long-term pain, and pain during terminal care
☐ Management of children with pain due to sickle cell disease
☐ Sedation and analgesia for painful diagnostic or therapeutic procedures.

Pain management teams. Many hospitals now have a multidisciplinary pain management team (specialist nurses, anaesthetists, pharmacists, physiotherapists and psychologists) who can share in the management of acute, chronic and palliative pain and associated symptoms. In some specialist centres these teams are also involved in providing a service for children undergoing diagnostic or therapeutic procedures.

PRINCIPLES OF DRUG THERAPY FOR PAIN PREVENTION AND PAIN CONTROL
A pre-emptive approach to the use of analgesic drugs complements the management of the emotional component of pain most effectively. The child who recovers after surgery free of pain requires lower total doses of analgesics to continue good pain control and needs potent analgesia for a shorter time than the child who has severe pain during the early recovery phase. Poor management of pain in early life lowers the threshold for pain for a long time afterwards as sensitization to pain can occur. Experience has shown that multimodal analgesia (the concurrent use of analgesics with

different modes of action) is highly effective and very safe in children. The foundation of multimodal analgesia is local or regional anaesthesia then (in various proportions) opioids, NSAIDs and paracetamol. Local anaesthesia should be used as part of the pain management plan for every child unless there is a specific contra-indication.

LOCAL ANAESTHETICS

Local anaesthetics can be used topically, or infiltrated or infused, to produce nerve block. Systemic toxicity can occur with excessive dosage, inadvertent IV injection, or transcutaneous absorption. Whenever local anaesthetics are used, a means of resuscitation should be at hand.

Lidocaine (lignocaine) is effective for 30 minutes to 1 hour or up to 2-4 hours if mixed with adrenaline (epinephrine).

Bupivacaine has a slower onset but is effective for up to 3-7 hours.

Levobupivacaine is the pure L-isomer of bupivacaine, and has less cardiotoxicity and less CNS toxicity than the racemic mixture.

Ropivacaine is an S-enantiomer, which is somewhat less potent than bupivacaine and has less propensity to produce cardiac or CNS toxic effects.

Prilocaine is shorter acting than either and is the least toxic (except in preterm neonates in whom absorption might cause methaemoglobinaemia). It is most often used as Emla® which is a eutectic mixture of lidocaine (lignocaine) and prilocaine.

Tetracaine (amethocaine) does not carry the risk of methaemoglobinaemia in neonates. It has a more rapid onset of action than Emla®.

Gels and creams are applied to intact skin, but not mucous membranes (except for lidocaine (lignocaine) gel – see below) or inflamed skin. Emla® or tetracaine (amethocaine) gel are applied before venepuncture or venous cannulation. Lidocaine (lignocaine) gel is used before urethral catheterisation. Tetracaine (amethocaine) or oxybuprocaine eye drops are used for local anaesthesia in eye surgery.

Lidocaine (lignocaine) or bupivacaine can be infiltrated around wounds for local analgesia, and bupivacaine can also be instilled into dressings. Nerve block should only be performed by those trained and experienced in giving regional anaesthesia. Intravenous block and central neural blockade should only be undertaken by trained and experienced anaesthetists with facilities for resuscitation to hand.

NON-OPIOID ANALGESICS

Paracetamol is a widely used analgesic and antipyretic, and is well tolerated by children of all ages. It acts on the CNS but not other tissues. It does not cause respiratory depression. It is now recognized that a higher loading dose is needed at least 90 minutes to 2 hours in advance to achieve therapeutic concentrations in the CNS, particularly when the rectal route of administration is used. To avoid cumulative toxicity, the correct dose must be given at an appropriate dosing interval with a maximum daily dose for a specified duration, especially if the drug is to be used for more than a few days. An overdose of paracetamol can result in liver damage and failure. Particular care is required in the child who has a viral illness and is not eating or drinking adequately.

Aspirin is analgesic, anti-inflammatory and antipyretic. It is a gastric irritant. Because of its association with Reye syndrome, aspirin should not be given to children <12 years as an analgesic/antipyretic unless medically indicated and avoid in children under 16 years if feverish. Aspirin still has a place in Kawasaki disease.

Non-steroidal anti-inflammatory drugs (NSAIDs) are anti-inflammatory, antipyretic and analgesic. Children are less prone than adults to side-effects, but long-term treatment increases the risk of gastric irritation and platelet disorders. NSAIDs should not be given in renal impairment. NSAIDs potentiate the analgesia from local and regional blocks. NSAIDs can be combined with paracetamol. When combined with opioids they allow a lower dose of opioid to achieve the same level of analgesia (opioid-sparing effect). NSAIDs can relieve mild to moderate musculo-skeletal pain, the pain of inflamed soft tissues and joints, pain from bony metastases, dental pain, post-operative pain, and ureteric colic. Ibuprofen is an alternative to paracetamol, though a second-line choice. It has similar antipyretic properties but is also anti-inflammatory. It is less likely than other NSAIDs to cause gastro-intestinal side-effects. Diclofenac is available as an enteric-coated preparation, but this takes an hour to work and is not, therefore, suitable for relief of acute pain. There is a dispersible form, which is quicker to act. Suppositories for rectal administration are effective within an hour. The rectal route does not remove the risk of gastric bleeding. Naproxen is recommended in children with chronic pain. Piroxicam sublingual melts are useful and can be given once a day. Some parenteral NSAIDs are available.

OPIOID ANALGESICS
Most act on both the central and peripheral nervous systems. Their analgesic effects are specific and not part of the general depression of brain function that occurs with general anaesthetics. Opioids are invaluable drugs in the control of severe pain in children, but those who prescribe or administer them must be experienced in the recognition and assessment of pain and distress in children and on the safe and effective use of the drugs and their side-effects. Children who are given opioids must be observed closely and monitored. The important side-effects of opioids are respiratory depression, excessive sedation, nausea and vomiting, pruritus, constipation, urinary retention and muscle spasms. Opioids must not be used in airway obstruction. Tolerance occurs, but dependence is rarely a problem when opioids are used for the control of pain.

Weak opioids
Codeine phosphate is a weak opiate. The analgesic effect does not increase beyond a certain dose, but side-effects, including respiratory depression, do. Respiratory depression is reversed with naloxone. Codeine phosphate should not be given intravenously. Constipation is usual so prophylactic lactulose should be started at the same time. Codeine phosphate can be used alone, with NSAIDs or paracetamol, or with both. There is no evidence that the effects of dihydrocodeine differ from those of codeine.

Strong opioids
The strong opioids do not show the analgesic limit of codeine. The degree of monitoring required depends on whether they are given for acute or chronic pain. When strong opioids are given for acute pain the level of sedation, respiratory effectiveness and airway control must be monitored, with professionals skilled in airway management and respiratory support immediately available. There must be frequent monitoring and observation if a child is unstable and pain control is poor. Continuous opioid infusions may be used safely and effectively in children of all ages provided the correct dosing schedule is used and appropriate monitoring is maintained. Children from age 5 years may be taught to use patient-controlled analgesia devices very effectively.

Morphine is extremely valuable in the control of both acute and chronic pain. It is well absorbed, and oral preparations are suitable for the control of chronic pain. The taste is usually accepted. In children from 6 months to 5 years of age, morphine is metabolised more rapidly than in adults, and in newborn infants less rapidly.

Diamorphine is metabolised to morphine. It is more water-soluble and may be more convenient for subcutaneous or intravenous injection.

Fentanyl has a shorter duration of action than morphine, is less sedative and hypnotic, but is a powerful respiratory depressant. It can cause muscle rigidity of the chest wall and/or jaw. Fentanyl injection should only be used in an operating theatre or intensive care unit by experienced anaesthetists or intensivists.

MANAGEMENT OF THE SIDE-EFFECTS OF OPIOIDS
Anticipation, prompt recognition, and effective management of side-effects are essential when administering opioids.

Respiratory depression. The priority is to maintain the airway, breathing and circulation, using paediatric life support measures. If a child needs high levels of analgesia, ventilatory support may be needed. If powerful analgesia is no longer required, naloxone may be given in addition to life support measures. Naloxone reverses all the effects of opioids with the return of pain. It is not a substitute for life support. Doxapram is a respiratory stimulant, which does not reverse the other effects of opioids but may cause excitation.

Nausea and vomiting. Cyclizine is useful for opioid-induced nausea. Prochlorperazine may also be effective. Ondansetron may be effective when these fail and has the significant advantage of not producing sedation.

Pruritus. Chlorphenamine (chlorpheniramine) is used, but not in infants. It is sedative. Low dose naloxone is useful for pruritus due to epidural opioids.

Constipation. Constipation can cause severe pain, and should be anticipated and treated early by agents such as lactulose, sodium docusate, bisacodyl suppositories, or Micralax® micro-enemas.

Pain management

Pain management

NEUROPATHIC PAIN
Opioids give only partial relief of pain arising from invasion or compression of nerves. Tricyclic antidepressants and anticonvulsants are useful. Amitriptyline may relieve the burning pain of nerve compression or tumour invasion, or neuropathic pain caused by vincristine. Carbamazepine may give relief to neuropathic pain, which has a shooting or stabbing quality. Gabapentin may also be effective. These agents should only be used by experts in chronic pain management as part of a multidisciplinary evaluation and management of pain and associated symptoms.

PAIN DUE TO MUSCLE SPASM
Such pain can be severe in disease of the CNS and might be aggravated by pain elsewhere. Diazepam, ibuprofen, or baclofen may give relief. When any agent used alone fails, the combination of diazepam and baclofen may be effective. For post-operative lower limb muscle spasm, epidural analgesia is highly effective. Low-dose midazolam infusion with appropriate monitoring is also used in specialist centres.

INHALATIONAL ANALGESIA WITH NITROUS OXIDE
Entonox (oxygen 50% and nitrous oxide 50%) provides inhalational patient-controlled analgesia if the facemask or mouthpiece is held by the child. It takes 3-5 minutes to achieve peak effect, which wears off over several minutes. Entonox should not be used after injuries to the head or chest that might introduce air into a closed compartment, nor in cases of bowel obstruction. The sedative and respiratory depressant effects of all sedatives are potentiated by nitrous oxide.

In dental practice, analgesia and conscious sedation ('relative analgesia') with titrated inspired concentrations of nitrous oxide are used very safely via a nasal hood system.

PREMEDICATION
The main objective of premedication is to allay fear and anxiety before clinical procedures or operations, while avoiding over-sedation (which may make the child disorientated and difficult to manage). Use of sedative premedication can be reduced by providing a child-friendly environment, full parental involvement in the child's care, and managing the emotional and the physical components of the child's fear, anxiety and pain. If the child is in pain, adequate analgesia should be provided first, as non-analgesic sedatives cause the child to be more distressed in such circumstances. Sedative premedicants should be avoided when there is a compromised airway, CNS depression, or a history of sleep apnoea.

The ideal premedicant for children is pleasant to take, with rapid anxiolysis, but with no hangover or side-effects.

Midazolam. Oral midazolam has a bitter acidic taste which can be disguised with a sweet liquid. Unlike other benzodiazepines, its quick onset and short duration make it suitable for day cases. Recent evidence suggests that benzodiazepines are effective in reducing late post-operative behavioural disturbance. However, midazolam can cause severe disinhibition and restlessness in some children shortly after administration and in the recovery period.

Temazepam or diazepam are alternatives to midazolam in older children.

Alimemazine (trimeprazine) has sedative, antiemetic and neuroleptic properties but is a poor anxiolytic. Recent studies have shown it to cause increased crying and struggling. Moreover, neuroleptic drugs such as alimemazine (trimeprazine) may induce a cataleptic state in which the child appears tranquil and dissociated from the surroundings but is actually in a state of masked restlessness. In low dose it produces a useful anti-emetic effect for ear, nose and throat surgery.

Atropine or glycopyrronium. These anticholinergic drugs are given orally by some anaesthetists to prevent bradycardia during induction of anaesthesia. This is most common in neonates and infants but may occur in any child. Anticholinergics are also used to reduce salivation or give dry conditions when the airway or intubation would be difficult or where ketamine anaesthesia is to be used. Anticholinergics should not be so used in children with cystic fibrosis.

SEDATION FOR DIAGNOSTIC AND THERAPEUTIC PROCEDURES
Clinical procedures in children often call for immobility or sleep, and relief of pain and anxiety. The need for pharmacological intervention can be reduced considerably by careful preparation of the child and parents. A range of behavioural techniques including play therapy, distraction and guided imagery have very useful sedative-sparing effects. Parental involvement is also very helpful in reducing the need for sedative agents.

Where procedures are known to be painful, distressing to an individual child, or prolonged, or in a young or sick child, serious consideration should be given as to whether general anaesthesia would be safer and more effective.

The state of sedation is difficult to achieve in children. There is such variability in the pharmacokinetics and pharmacodynamics of sedative drugs in children that responses to sedation may vary from slight depression of the conscious level to complete anaesthesia. Sedation is a continuum, and it is not always possible to predict how an individual patient receiving sedation will respond. Sedation is defined as 'a technique in which the use of a drug or drugs produces a state of depression of the CNS enabling treatment to be carried out but during which verbal contact is maintained throughout the period of sedation. The drugs and techniques used should carry a margin of safety wide enough to render unintended loss of consciousness unlikely. Loss of consciousness is a state of anaesthesia with all its attendant risks'.

Where drugs are to be used to induce sedation, it should be carried out in the right environment by experienced staff. The standards of care before, during, and after the procedure should be the same as those for a general anaesthetic. The child must be carefully screened for contra-indications to sedation. The sedative chosen should be right for the procedure and for the child, taking into account the time to take effect and its duration, the route, the child's response to other drugs, and the child's medical condition. Psychological upset can be minimised by anxiolysis and brief amnesia, for which benzodiazepines are a common choice. For painful procedures, a local anaesthetic or systemic analgesic (which might include an opioid) are needed and should be given first when possible to prevent and control pain. All sedatives potentiate the CNS depressant effects of each other, and extreme caution must be exercised when combinations of drugs with sedative properties are given.

A sedated child must be closely observed and monitored, with the means of resuscitation to hand. Only appropriately trained and experienced staff should sedate children. There must be at least two trained and experienced staff present so that one can give their full attention and effort to monitoring the child.

Sedation for painless procedures, lasting less than 20 minutes.
Oral midazolam can be given 15-30 minutes in advance of the procedure. Monitoring must commence immediately and continue until full recovery. Oral temazepam is an alternative.

Sedation for painless procedures lasting 20–60 minutes.
Oral chloral hydrate usually gives effective sedation, particularly in pre-school children. Secobarbital (quinalbarbitone) can be used in older children. The recovery time for both is several hours.

Sedation for painful procedures.
The above techniques may be supplemented with local anaesthesia for the painful sites (topical, infiltration or nerve block as appropriate) and NSAIDs/ paracetamol. Supplementation of the above techniques with opioids produces an unacceptable incidence of adverse effects and should only be conducted by a trained and experienced anaesthetist or intensivist. Consideration should be given to a formal general anaesthetic. General anaesthetic agents such as propofol or ketamine, or potent opioids such as fentanyl, should only be used by trained and experienced anaesthetists or intensivists.

Nitrous oxide inhalation (titrated up to 70% inspired concentration or as premixed 50% (Entonox)) in oxygen is highly effective for brief painful procedures in cooperative children. It can also be given for longer periods in dental practice. It is often supplemented by local anaesthesia. Supplementation with other sedatives or with opioids should only be carried out by a trained and experienced anaesthetist or intensivist.

The child who has been sedated must not be discharged until fully recovered, and then only after medical examination.

Palliative care and symptom control

INTRODUCTION
The aim of this section is to provide a guide to how medications have been used to treat distressing symptoms in children. In some cases there is an evidence base (often only in adults); in other cases it simply describes an approach that those working largely or entirely with dying children have found helpful.

PAIN
The main principle of the management of pain in children is that appropriate analgesia should not be withheld from a child simply because of a fear of the medications involved. It is quite common for children to require a combination of opioid and adjuvant.

Palliative care

Opioid. Codeine and dihydrocodeine are more or less equivalent and it is worth remembering that a large dose of a minor opioid may have the same effect as a small dose of a major opioid. There is, however, a limit to the analgesic effect of codeine. Codeine and dihydrocodeine are both powerfully constipating, probably more so than morphine in relation to their analgesic potency. Buprenorphine can be given sublingually and is helpful when swallowing is a problem but should be used with caution when combined with other major opioids as it is a partial agonist.

Morphine, diamorphine and fentanyl are the mainstays of major opioid therapy in children. Diamorphine has the advantage of being more soluble than morphine and is therefore the usual parenteral choice. It can be combined with a variety of other medications in the same syringe driver. The conversion from oral morphine to parenteral diamorphine is three to one (i.e. the dose of parenteral diamorphine is one third that of morphine orally). Fentanyl has some advantages in the child unable to tolerate first-line opiods for moderate to severe pain. It is available as a transcutaneous patch, and causes less constipation and sedation than morphine. Although the conversion from morphine to fentanyl often requires quite a large dosage increase, children seem to be resilient to this and fentanyl is a useful second -line major opioid.

Methadone has been used only rarely in children. It may have a particular role in managing neuropathic pain.

Adjuvants. Very few types of pain are wholly resistant to opioids, and opioids are usually the most effective form of analgesic medication irrespective of the cause of the pain. However, appropriate adjuvants can significantly enhance their effect. An adjuvant medication is one that may not have analgesic effectiveness in its own right, but may relieve pain nevertheless when used in certain specific situations. There are four common situations in which an adjuvant may be helpful:

BONE PAIN
Bone pain from metastatic cancer is caused by deformation of the microarchitecture of the bone, and mediated through a complex series of inflammatory cytokines. The most effective adjuvant therapy is often radiotherapy. Pharmacologically, NSAIDs such as diclofenac may be effective. The incidence of serious adverse effects is relatively low but can be further reduced using prophylactic omeprazole or misoprostol, a gastric mucosal protectant. An alternative approach is to use a cyclo-oxygenase-2 selective NSAID.

Bone pain may be due to osteopenia. There is much evidence to suggest that malignant or non-malignant bone pain can be moderated by use of bisphosphonates (such as disodium pamidronate) in adults. Bisphosphonates have been used in children.

NEUROPATHIC PAIN
Antidepressants and anticonvulsants have both been shown to be effective in neuropathic pain models. Amitriptyline and carbamazepine are both frequently used in children and are therefore good starting choices. The decision about which to start first depends on the situation; for example, a child in whom depression is likely may obtain more benefit from amitriptyline whereas carbamazepine would be more appropriate in a child with a seizure disorder. If one is not tolerated, or is ineffective after 3-4 weeks, it is worth changing to the other. Amitriptyline is usually well-tolerated by children but imipramine or nortriptyline may be better alternatives for some.

Ketamine is widely used in adult palliative care for neuropathic pain and has also been used in children. Although it is effective, it is not always well-tolerated so should be used with caution. There are wide variations in the doses that have been used in children.

Dexamethasone has a role when neuropathic pain is caused by pressure on a nerve (for example by tumour). Its mechanism is believed to be the reduction of oedema around the tumour. The longer there has been pressure the less likely it is that any damage will be reversible by these means. To be effective, dexamethasone should probably be prescribed within 24 hours of the onset of neuropathic pain. Because of their side-effect profile in long-term use, steroids should be used with caution in palliative care (see below).

ABDOMINAL COLIC
Colicky abdominal pain can be relatively resistant to opioids. Because the pain is intermittent but severe, there is a risk of alternating between over- and undertreatment. A dose which is effective for the worst of the pain may be toxic at other times. More commonly, the child has the worst of both worlds; inadequate pain relief when it is at its worst and toxicity at other times. If possible, it is better to reduce the number of spasms of colic. This can sometimes be achieved with hyoscine butylbromide.

MUSCLE SPASM

Pain in children with non-malignant life-limiting conditions is often caused by muscle spasm. There is an extensive literature on the use of orthopaedic interventions and botulinum toxin to relieve this. Diazepam and baclofen (orally, parenterally or even intrathecally) are effective in reducing muscle spasm.

GASTROINTESTINAL SYMPTOMS

Nausea, vomiting and constipation are the commonest gastrointestinal symptoms children experience. The mechanisms are complex and perhaps for this reason there is often a temptation to use a 'one size fits all' approach characterised, for example, by the prescription of lactulose for constipation irrespective of the mechanism. In fact, gastrointestinal symptoms lend themselves well to a rational and systematic approach based on an understanding of the pathophysiology.

CONSTIPATION

The commonest causes of constipation in children needing palliative care are immobility, relative dehydration, and opioid therapy. Lactulose is a stool softener with little stimulant activity. Its breakdown products are stimulant enough to cause quite severe colic but probably not enough to have useful therapeutic action. Senna, bisacodyl, docusate and sodium picosulfate (picosulphate) are all good stimulant laxatives. Stimulants should usually be combined with softeners such as magnesium hydroxide.

Second-line alternatives include metoclopramide and domperidone. Domperidone is probably less effective than metoclopramide, but is also much less likely to cause dystonic reactions. Erythromycin (which acts directly on motilin receptors in the bowel) is used less commonly.

There is increasing evidence that oral naloxone can help relieve opioid-induced constipation. It is poorly absorbed systemically so there is little risk of reversing the therapeutic effects of opioids.

NAUSEA AND VOMITING

Nausea and vomiting have complex mechanisms which involve many different chemical messengers. Most anti-emetics block only one or two of these; phenothiazines block almost all of them. A logical approach is to select a first-line anti-emetic on the basis of the presumed pathophysiology and reserve phenothiazines for second-line treatment.

Cyclizine is an anticholinergic and antihistamine. It is thought to be particularly effective in centrally-mediated nausea and vomiting. It can be effective, but may cause drowsiness or even confusion. Domperidone, metoclopramide and haloperidol are all dopamine receptor blockers which act principally in the gut. Haloperidol and metoclopramide have additional central anti-emetic effects. Metoclopramide at high doses is also a $5HT_3$ antagonist similar to ondansetron. Of the dopamine receptor blockers, domperidone is probably the least effective but also carries the least risk of extrapyramidal side-effects. In adults, haloperidol has a particular role in opioid-induced nausea and vomiting. These adverse effects seem, however, to be rarer in children than in adults. Dexamethasone has been shown to improve the effectiveness of metoclopramide and ondansetron.

Hyoscine hydrobromide is an anticholinergic. The final common pathway of vomiting is through the vagus nerve and so anticholinergics have a role in controlling vomiting from most causes. Ondansetron is a pure $5HT_3$ blocker. It is most effective when the cause of vomiting can be traced to a damaged gut mucosa (e.g. post-chemotherapy and radiotherapy).

The most commonly used phenothiazines in paediatric palliative care are levomepromazine (methotrimeprazine) and chlorpromazine. Levomepromazine is to be preferred in children as it is less sedating and is a 'broad spectrum' anti-emetic which has additional beneficial effects such as analgesia.

Octreotide, a long-acting analogue of somatostatin, has been used to treat high-output vomiting in adults.

MOUTH CARE AND MUCOSAL BLEEDING

There are some simple, non-pharmacological approaches to maintaining a comfortable oral mucosa in the final stages of life even when adequate hydration is impossible to maintain. Ice chips or pineapple chunks keep the mouth moist; ascorbic acid dissolved on the tongue can help keep the mouth feeling fresh.

Mucosal bleeding from the mouth and nose are common problems in the terminal phase, particularly in the child suffering from haemopoeitic malignancy. Bleeding from the nose may be caused by a single bleeding point which can be arrested using cautery or dressing. Tranexamic acid, anti-fibrolytic agent, can be effective topically or systemically. Oral etamsylate (ethamsylate) increases platelet aggregation.

Palliative care

DIARRHOEA

If there is profuse diarrhoea, the integrity of the child's skin may be threatened. Bed sores and skin ulcers are extremely painful and difficult to manage once they occur. Avoiding them is therefore important. Loperamide can be useful for mild and moderate diarrhoea. Where there is a high volume of diarrhoea, octreotide may have a role.

SEIZURES

Intractable seizures are a relatively common symptom in children dying from non-malignant life-limiting conditions. They are frightening for child and family and merit treatment where possible.

Phenobarbital (phenobarbitone), orally or as a continuous subcutaneous infusion, is useful in gaining control of seizures. Continuous infusion of midazolam is an alternative. Both cause drowsiness, but this is rarely a concern in the context of terminal intractable seizures.

For breakthrough convulsions, a prescription of rectal diazepam, subcutaneous midazolam, or rectal paraldehyde may be appropriate.

With this approach, it is often possible to reduce the number of different anticonvulsants the child normally takes and sometimes to discontinue them altogether.

RESPIRATORY SYMPTOMS

Dyspnoea is a subjective sense that breathing has become unpleasant. It may not coincide exactly with how observers perceive it. For example, tachypnoea may not require treatment if it is not distressing the child. The mechanisms of dyspnoea are varied so it is important to have a systematic approach to the diagnosis. Where the cause is excessive secretions (such as the 'death rattle' which can complicate some children's final days) anticholinergics such as glycopyrronium and hyoscine hydrobromide are helpful. On the other hand, where the cause is secretions that are too thick, mucolytics such as acetylcysteine may be more appropriate. Many causes of dyspnoea are complicated by reactive bronchospasm, and a trial of bronchodilator therapy is often warranted.

There is no evidence that oxygen provides relief of dyspnoea unless the cause is hypoxaemia. Many hypoxic children have no dyspnoea and most children with dyspnoea are not hypoxic. A mask over the face is uncomfortable and unacceptable for some children who already feel they are suffocating. Where it is effective, oxygen therapy may be acting by providing a breeze on the face and an electric fan or open window may also provide this.

Dyspnoea and anxiety are closely linked. Anxiolytics have an important role in relieving dyspnoea. Ongoing anxiolysis can be provided with diazepam or a midazolam infusion. Breakthrough anxiolytics may be needed, particularly to break a cycle of panic and breathlessness. Sublingual lorazepam or subcutaneous midazolam are useful for this. Midazolam has been used intranasally.

Perhaps the most effective medications against dyspnoea are the opioids, which work at many different levels peripherally and centrally. Given systemically, the dose required for relief of dyspnoea is thought to be approximately half that required for analgesia. Nebulised opioids are probably no more effective than nebulised NaCl 0.9% but some patients seem to benefit, perhaps by providing the patient and family with a sense of control.

PSYCHOLOGICAL SYMPTOMS

Anxiety and depression in children present a diagnostic challenge. Children, particularly adolescents, who are in the palliative phase are almost always aware of the fact but often find it difficult to talk about. Paradoxically, this is usually due to reluctance on the part of adults who want to protect them.

Depression

Tricyclic antidepressants can be effective in children. They are generally well tolerated though the doses required to treat depression are somewhat higher than those required for neuropathic pain. Fluoxetine is an effective and safe alternative. As always, antidepressants should accompany rather than replace adequate psychological support.

Anxiety

Relief of anxiety can be provided by long-acting benzodiazepines such as diazepam, or by continuous infusion of the ultra short-acting benzodiazepine midazolam. Interventions for more acute episodes of anxiety (such as panic attacks) include short-acting benzodiazepines such as lorazepam sublingually or midazolam subcutaneously. Temazepam provides useful night-time sedation in some children.

Sedation
It is important to distinguish between anxiolysis and sedation. Benzodiazepines provide both, but chloral hydrate provides only sedation. On its own therefore, chloral hydrate simply masks anxiety rather than treating it. Haloperidol is often wrongly prescribed as a sedative. In fact, it is only poorly sedative though useful in delirium (see below).

Delirium
There is a syndrome of delirium in adults which has not been as clearly identified in children. It is characterised by disordered perception, such as hallucinations and confusion. Once underlying causes such as infection, dehydration or polypharmacy have been addressed, the mainstays of pharmacological intervention are haloperidol and benzodiazepines. Haloperidol has the advantage of being largely non-sedating.

Sleep disturbance
Children needing palliative care often have a disrupted sleep cycle. This is particularly true of children with non-malignant life-limiting conditions. It is often caused by a combination of central dysregulation and the chaotic lifestyle imposed by the condition. Before embarking on pharmacological therapy it is helpful to try to emphasise the difference between day and night by avoiding nocturnal interruptions, for example for administration of drugs. It is usually also possible to arrange prescribing times so that sedating medications are given in the evening rather than during daylight hours.

Melatonin is often helpful in managing sleep disorder. Night-time infusions of midazolam can further emphasise the difference between day and night.

Disturbed sleep is often a major factor influencing the quality of life for a child and their family and it is worth working hard to secure control if possible. Management is often easier in a children's hospice, where medical and nursing supervision can be combined with a home-like environment.

SKIN PROBLEMS
Pruritus
Pruritus is a relatively uncommon problem in children. Topical preparations such as calamine lotion, emollients (e.g. Eurax®), and antihistamines such as chlorphenamine (chlorpheniramine) are often helpful.

Less conventionally, ondansetron has been shown to be effective in some cases. Its good adverse effects profile combined with its extensive use in children make it a good choice. Oral naloxone has also been used. Where opioids are the cause, it may be appropriate to review the dose or to switch to an alternative opioid. Fentanyl is believed to cause less itching than naturally-occurring opioids.

Odour
In contrast with adults, fungating skin lesions are relatively uncommon. Where they occur, they can cause an unpleasant odour which is damaging for the dynamic of the child with carers and family. The odour may be caused by anaerobic organisms, so topical or systemic metronidazole may be helpful. Systemic metronidazole is associated with nausea and vomiting and therefore less desirable in a palliative context.

STEROIDS IN PALLIATIVE CARE
Steroids have a wide range of effects that are useful in relieving symptoms. Dexamethasone is the steroid conventionally preferred in palliative care. It has a number of different uses and the dose depends on the indication. It is helpful in reducing raised intracranial pressure due (for example) to tumour. It enhances the anti-emetic effect of metoclopramide and ondansetron and even acts as an appetite stimulant. It is also an adjuvant in the management of some forms of neuropathic pain.

With all its advantages, dexamethasone also carries the risk of effects on the appearance that can profoundly influence a child's self-image. It generally takes only a week or two before the benefits of the steroid are outweighed by these adverse effects. One way to try to minimise the problems while capitalising on its strengths is to prescribe dexamethasone in short courses of 5 days. These can be repeated as often as indicated by the symptomatology. While this approach does not eliminate the risk of adverse effects, it does ensure that the balance of burden and benefit to the child is constantly under review.

Palliative care

DEALING WITH ANALGESIC SIDE-EFFECTS

Children are fairly resistant to opioids and often need a higher dose per kilogram body weight than adults do. However, anecdotal evidence suggests that children are more prone to certain adverse effects such as urinary retention (which can be eased by carbachol or bethanechol). Opioid-induced pruritus is less common – see above.

NSAIDs are generally safe in children. Gastrointestinal side-effects can be minimised by antacids such as Gaviscon® and proton pump inhibitors such as omeprazole. There is little evidence supporting the use of H_2 blockers in this context. Misoprostol, a gastric protectant, is combined with diclofenac in some preparations. Co-prescription of a NSAID with steroids should be avoided when possible, but if it is unavoidable it is particularly important to ensure adequate prophylaxis. Cyclo-oxygenase-2 selective non-steroidals may be equally effective with fewer adverse effects though this is yet to be proven.

Poisoning

Acute poisoning in children is responsible for approximately 40,000 hospital attendances at Emergency Departments each year in England and Wales. Most children have taken a trivial ingestion of a non-poisonous substance. If the overdose is deemed as being of low toxicity then no treatment is required.

A proportion will require a short period of observation whilst only a few will require treatment and admission.

The management of most acute poisoned patients is supportive.

Death from poisoning in childhood is exceptionally rare. In 1978-1998 there were 1868 deaths in England and Wales related to poisons in children under the age of 15 years. The most common causes were as follows:

- ☐ Carbon monoxide – 782
- ☐ Polyester fumes and smoke – 721
- ☐ Antidepressants – 55
- ☐ Opiates – 27
- ☐ Co-proxamol – 21
- ☐ Paracetamol – 19
- ☐ Butane, propane – 15
- ☐ Hydrogen cyanide and cyanide gas – 8
- ☐ Iron – 8.

Most childhood poisoning is accidental. Other causes include intentional overdose, drug abuse, iatrogenic and deliberate poisoning (Munchausen by proxy and child abuse). Any child taking an intentional overdose should be referred to a child or adolescent psychiatrist prior to discharge.

Information about the management of poisoning can initially be obtained on the internet from Toxbase at http://www.spib.axl.co.uk. New users of Toxbase will need to register with the Edinburgh branch of the National Poisons Information Service (NPIS) first (Tel: 0131 228 6907). Poisons advice can also be provided through the central number of NPIS (0870 600 6266).

Tictac is a tablet and capsule identification system available on CD ROM and held by all NPIS centres and many Medical Information Centres.

MANAGEMENT

A child who presents with acute poisoning should initially be triaged. The Manchester Triage Group produced the following flow chart:

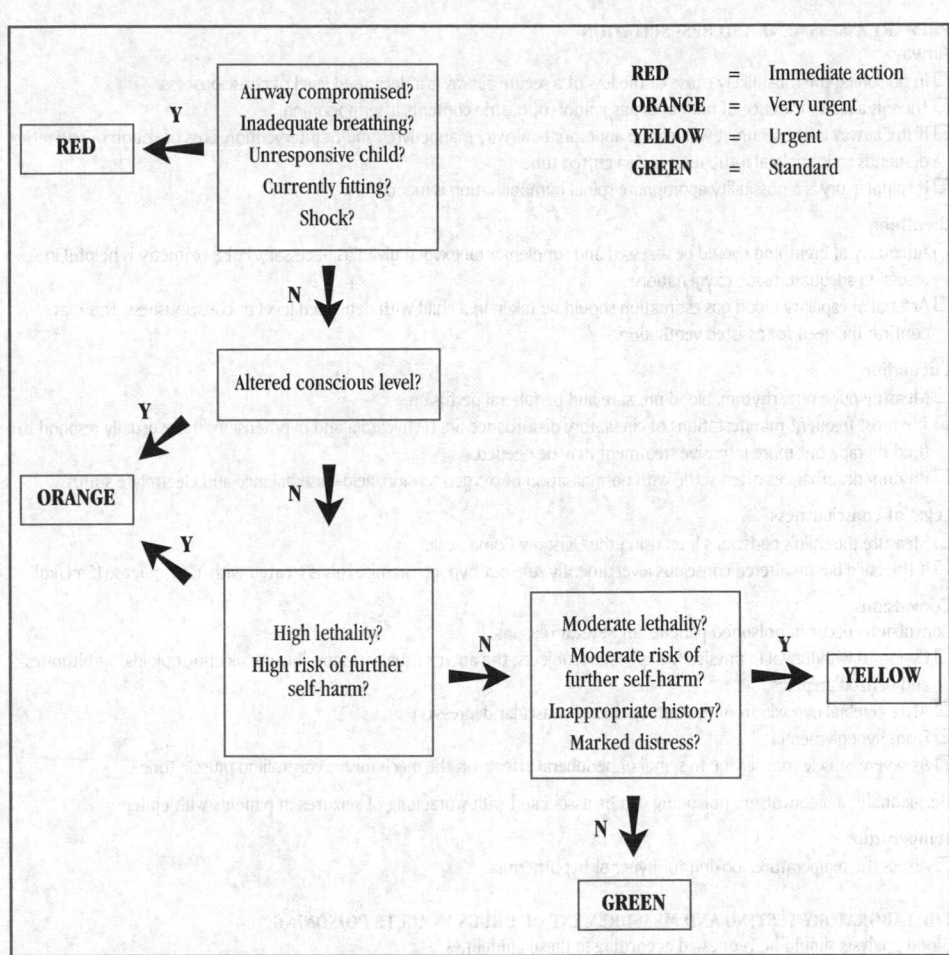

Poisoning

SPECIFIC DISCRIMINATORS

Lethality – the potential of the substance taken to cause harm. Advice from a poisons centre may be required to establish this. If in doubt assume a high risk.

Risk of further self-harm – the potential of the patient to actively attempt further self-harm. If in doubt assume a high risk.

Inappropriate history – if the alleged mechanism does not explain the apparent injury or illness, then the history is inappropriate.

Marked distress – patients who are mentally ill and/or markedly physically or emotionally upset fulfil this criterion.

Poisoning

PRIMARY ASSESSMENT AND RESUSCITATION
Airway
☐ In poisoning the most likely cause of the loss of a secure airway is a decreased level of consciousness.
☐ There is a high incidence of pulmonary aspiration of gastric contents after poisoning.
☐ If the airway is not secure it will require appropriate airway manoeuvres and/or intervention. Loss of cough or gag reflex demands endotracheal intubation with a cuffed tube.
☐ If spinal injury is a possibility appropriate spinal immobilisation is mandatory.

Breathing
☐ Adequacy of breathing should be assessed and supplemental oxygen given as necessary. Pulse oximetry is helpful in assessing adequate tissue oxygenation.
☐ Arterial or capillary blood gas estimation should be taken in a child with depressed level of consciousness. This may confirm the need for assisted ventilation.

Circulation
☐ Measure pulse rate, rhythm, blood pressure and peripheral perfusion.
☐ The most frequent manifestations of circulatory disturbance are tachycardia and hypotension. These usually respond to fluid therapy, but more intensive treatment may be needed.
☐ Rhythm disturbances often settle with normalisation of oxygen tension, acid-base balance and electrolyte status.

Level of consciousness
☐ Measure the child's conscious level using the Glasgow Coma Scale.
☐ If the child has an altered conscious level urgently rule out hypoglycaemia. This is treated with 10% glucose (5mL/kg).

Convulsions
Convulsions occur in poisoned patients for several reasons:
☐ Owing to withdrawal in physically dependent subjects; the agents usually responsible are alcohol, opioids, barbiturates, and benzodiazepines.
☐ After cerebral hypoxia from respiratory or cardiovascular depression.
☐ From hypoglycaemia.
☐ As severe muscle spasms due to spinal or peripheral effects on the mechanisms controlling muscle tone.

Occasionally, anticonvulsant poisoning can be associated with worsening of seizures in patients with epilepsy.

Temperature
☐ Assess the temperature, looking for hyper or hypothermia.

THE LABORATORY TESTING AND MEASUREMENT OF DRUGS IN ACUTE POISONING
Blood analysis should be requested according to these guidelines:
☐ If the patient is seriously ill (or deteriorating) then a drug screen may be performed immediately
☐ If a specific drug is suspected and when the knowledge of the actual concentration will affect the immediate therapy. In clinical practice measurement of paracetamol levels is the most commonly requested test in acute poisoning
☐ Alcohol measurement (breath, saliva, plasma, blood) again is commonly requested but only in patients whose breath smells of alcohol
☐ Salicylate measurement should not be routine but limited to cases of salicylate poisoning, unconscious patients, those with unexplained metabolic acidosis, or a toxidrome consistent with salicylate poisoning
☐ Other situations in which toxicology testing is useful include:
- carboxyhaemoglobin - digoxin
- iron - methaemoglobin
- theophylline - methanol
- lithium - ethylene glycol

Poisoning

Toxicity assessment

At the end of the primary assessment, assess the risk of death from the overdose. The following information is helpful:

☐ The substance
☐ Time taken
☐ Amount taken
☐ Description of the substance, bottle or label
☐ Age and weight of the patient
☐ Patient's condition.

GUT DECONTAMINATION

Position statements have been produced by the European Association of Poisons Centres and Clinical Toxicologists and American Academy of Clinical Toxicology regarding gastric lavage, ipecacuanha liquid mixture, single-dose activated charcoal, repeat-dose activated charcoal, cathartics and polyethylene glycol.

A common theme in these position statements is that the evidence regarding decontamination is lacking.

ACTIVATED CHARCOAL

The administration of a single-dose of activated charcoal may be considered if a patient has ingested a potentially toxic amount of a poison (which is known to be adsorbed to charcoal) up to one hour previously. There is no evidence that the administration of activated charcoal improves clinical outcome.

A second dose of charcoal may be warranted in patients whose blood level continues to rise, suggesting delayed gastric emptying, or who have taken enteric-coated preparations.

Contra-indications

☐ An unprotected airway
☐ A gastrointestinal tract not anatomically intact
☐ When activated charcoal therapy may increase the risk and severity of aspiration (e.g. hydrocarbons with a high aspiration potential).

Complications

Few serious adverse complications from single-dose activated charcoal have been reported. With inadequate airway management pulmonary aspiration has occurred and led occasionally to major respiratory problems.

MULTIPLE-DOSE ACTIVATED CHARCOAL

Many studies in animals and volunteers have demonstrated that multiple-dose activated charcoal increases drug elimination significantly. However, it has not been shown in a controlled study in poisoned patients to reduce morbidity and/or mortality. Based on experimental clinical studies multiple-dose activated charcoal should be considered only if a patient has ingested a life-threatening amount of the following:

☐ Carbamazepine
☐ Theophylline
☐ Quinine
☐ Phenobarbital (phenobarbitone)
☐ Dapsone.

The evidence for multiple-dose charcoal in salicylate poisoning is controversial, and advice should be obtained from NPIS.

GASTRIC LAVAGE

Gastric lavage is **seldom recommended** for children as benefit rarely outweighs risk. It should not be considered unless a patient has ingested a potentially life-threatening amount of poison and the procedure can be undertaken within 60 minutes of ingestion. Even then clinical benefit has not been confirmed in controlled studies. Unless a patient is intubated, gastric lavage is contra-indicated if airway protective reflexes are lost. It is also contra-indicated if a hydrocarbon with high aspiration potential or corrosive substance has been ingested.

Poisoning *(side tab)*

Complications

☐ Aspiration pneumonia
☐ Laryngospasm
☐ Hypoxia and hypercapnia
☐ Mechanical injury to the throat, oesophagus and stomach
☐ Fluid and electrolyte imbalance
☐ Combative patients may be at greater risk of complications.

Technique for performing gastric lavage

The patient should be placed in the left lateral/head down position (20° tilt on the table). A 24-28 French gauge tube should be used in children. The tube should be lubricated before being passed. Lavage fluid of 10mL/kg body weight of preferably warm (38°C) NaCl 0.9% should be used. Lavage should be continued until the lavage fluid has cleared of particulate matter.

IPECACUANHA

Historically, ipecacuanha syrup has played a principal role in the management of children's poisoning. However, there is no evidence from clinical studies that ipecacuanha improves the outcome of poisoned patients and its routine administration in the Emergency Department should be abandoned. A number of toxicologists have discouraged against its use in any circumstances.

CATHARTICS

The administration of cathartics alone has no role in the management of the poisoned patient and is not a recommended method of gut decontamination. The routine use of a cathartic in combination with activated charcoal is not endorsed.

Cathartics should not be administered to young children because of the likelihood of laxatives causing fluid and electrolyte imbalance.

ANTIDOTES

Modern resuscitation techniques and supportive care are the mainstay of management of a seriously poisoned patient. However, in certain circumstances, antidotes may be lifesaving or may shorten the duration of toxicity or diminish its severity, increasing the chances of recovery and reducing side-effects.

The International Programme On Chemical Safety has recommended that the following antidotes are available, as their effectiveness is well documented.

Indications	Antidotes
Alpha-adrenergic agonists	Phentolamine
Beta-adrenergic agonists	Beta-blockers (ß-1 and ß-2, preferably short-acting)
Beta-blockers	Isoprenaline (isoproterenol) and glucagon
Carbon monoxide	Oxygen
Central anticholinergic syndrome from atropine and derivatives	Physostigmine
Cyanide	Oxygen, sodium thiosulfate, dicobalt edetate, sodium nitrite and/or hydroxocobalamin
Digoxin/digitoxin, other digitalis glycosides	Digoxin-specific antibody fragments [F(ab)]
Ergotism	Sodium nitroprusside
Ethylene glycol	Fomepizole (4-methylpyrazole)
Heparin	Protamine sulfate
Hydrofluoric acid, fluorides, oxalates	Calcium gluconate or other soluble calcium salts
Hydrogen sulphide	Oxygen
Insulin	Glucose
Methanol, ethylene glycol	Ethanol
Methaemoglobinaemia	Methylthioninium chloride (methylene blue)
Opiates	Naloxone
Organophosphorus compounds and carbamates	Atropine

EMERGENCY TREATMENT OF SPECIFIC POISONING
PARACETAMOL

Only a small number of children will have ingested a toxic amount. Young children seem to be at less risk of liver damage than adults. However, treat according to the guidelines agreed by the National Poisons Information Service (NPIS) in 1999 in collaboration with the British Association for Accident & Emergency Medicine and the Royal College of Paediatrics and Child Health.

Hepatocellular necrosis is the major toxic effect of paracetamol poisoning. Acute renal tubular damage and necrosis may occur usually in association with hepatocellular necrosis.

For further advice, on staggered overdose, severe liver damage, abnormalities of liver function, adverse reactions to acetylcysteine, or any concerns regarding management, contact the NPIS.

Management of children (<12 years)

Consider activated charcoal if more than 150mg/kg paracetamol has been taken within the previous hour. If more than 150mg/kg (more than 75mg/kg in those with enhanced risk of toxicity) take a sample for plasma paracetamol levels at four hours. Plasma concentrations taken within four hours should not be requested as they cannot reliably be interpreted because of the possibility of continuing absorption and distribution of the drug.

If there is absolute certainty that the levels as stated above have not been exceeded then it can be considered reasonable to not perform a blood level.

After measuring a four-hour level, refer to the treatment line (see paracetamol monograph) to determine whether antidotal therapy with acetylcysteine is required.

Enhanced risk

Patients at enhanced risk include the following groups:

☐ Patients on enzyme-inducing drugs (carbamazepine, phenobarbital, phenytoin, primidone, rifampicin, St John's Wort)

☐ Underweight children with 'failure to thrive' whatever the cause

☐ Anorexia nervosa

☐ Cystic fibrosis

☐ Patients who regularly consume alcohol in excess of currently recommended limits (particularly those who are malnourished)

☐ HIV infection.

Staggered Overdose

In patients who have taken several overdoses of paracetamol over a short period of time, the plasma paracetamol concentration will be meaningless in relation to the treatment graph. Such patients should be considered at a serious risk and treated with acetylcysteine.

Acetylcysteine

Acetylcysteine (NAC) is best commenced within eight hours. Adverse reactions occur in 5% of patients and are anaphylactoid in nature. They usually respond to stopping the infusion, treating with either antihistamines, or in severe cases corticosteroids. Once the reaction has settled recommence acetylcysteine infusion at the lower infusion rate of 50mg/kg over four hours.

After treatment with NAC blood should be taken for creatinine, LFTs and clotting – including INR.

TRICYCLIC ANTIDEPRESSANTS

Tricyclic overdoses must be treated seriously. Observe for six hours if asymptomatic. Patients who remain asymptomatic and with a normal ECG after six hours are unlikely to develop late complications.

Clinical features

☐ Anticholinergic effects - dry mouth, blurred vision, dilated pupils, urinary retention, absent bowel sounds, pyrexia, myoclonic twitching.

☐ Cardiovascular effects – sinus tachycardia, QRS prolongation, QT prolongation, arrhythmias, hypotension.

☐ CNS effects – drowsiness, coma, convulsions, hyperreflexia, ophthalmoplegia.

☐ Metabolic effects – metabolic acidosis, hypokalaemia.

Poisoning

Poisoning

Treatment

Consider gastric lavage only if within one hour of a potentially fatal overdose. Give activated charcoal by mouth or naso-gastric tube if a toxic amount has been ingested within one hour, provided the airway can be protected. Consider a second dose of charcoal after two hours in patients with features of toxicity.

Protect airway, ventilate if necessary.

Treat delirium and agitation with intravenous benzodiazepine.

Seizures – treat with benzodiazepines and correct acidosis if prolonged.

QRS prolongation – if QRS is >0.16 seconds, or accompanied by hypotension, correct acidosis.

Hypotension – correct hypotension by raising the foot of the bed or in severe cases by expanding intravascular volume. Treat with fluid challenge. If this fails consider inotropes and intensive care. Consider mechanical support (aortic balloon pump, cardiac bypass) for refractory hypotension/cardiac arrest.

Ventricular tachycardia – treat by correction of acidosis and lidocaine (lignocaine). Consider overdrive pacing.

Alkalinisation has been shown to reduce the toxic effects on the heart.

OPIODS (including methadone)

Opioid overdose results in respiratory depression, pinpoint pupils and coma. The effects of overdose will be potentiated by co-ingestion of alcohol and other central depressant drugs.

Management of unconscious patients

Give naloxone, preferably intravenously if coma or respiratory depression are present. Repeat the dose if no response after two minutes.

Plasma half-life of naloxone is shorter than most opioids and repeated dosages of naloxone may be required. This can be achieved by an intravenous infusion of naloxone (dose is two thirds of the initial dose per hour). All patients must be observed for at least six hours after the last dose of naloxone.

IRON

Clinical as well as laboratory assessment of severity of poisoning must be performed.

The dose of elemental iron ingested may give some guide to the severity of poisoning. More than 20mg/kg body weight of ingested elemental iron is likely to result in features of toxicity. Measurement of serum iron taken at four hours after ingestion is the best laboratory measure of severity.

A plain abdominal x-ray is of value, as a screening for iron ingestion, if less than two hours have elapsed since ingestion. After two hours the tablets may have disintegrated and therefore not show up on the film.

Clinical signs and symptoms in the first six hours include nausea, vomiting, abdominal pain and diarrhoea. Leucocytosis and hypoglycaemia suggest toxicity. Less common features in severe poisoning include haematemesis, rectal bleeding, drowsiness, convulsions and metabolic acidosis. Coma and shock indicate severe poisoning. After twelve hours in serious cases hepatocellular necrosis occurs with or without hypotension.

Treatment

Consider gastric lavage in children who have ingested more than 60mg/kg elemental iron in the previous hour. Activated charcoal does not adsorb iron. Measure serum iron concentration. In severe cases replace fluid loss and correct acidosis. Give desferrioxamine intravenously. Check all serious cases with the NPIS.

SALICYLATES

Salicylate poisoning is potentially fatal. Contact NPIS in serious cases.
Features of poisoning include:
☐ Vomiting
☐ Tinnitus
☐ Sweating
☐ Hyperventilation.

In younger children a metabolic acidosis is common. In older children a mixed respiratory alkalosis and metabolic acidosis is more common.

Assess the severity of poisoning by measuring plasma salicylate concentration.

Clinical features that suggest severe poisoning include:
☐ Confusion
☐ Impaired consciousness
☐ Metabolic acidosis.

Treatment

Give oral activated charcoal to children who have ingested more than 250mg/kg body weight salicylate within one hour.

Measure the plasma salicylate concentration. A repeat sample should be taken after a further two hours in patients with suspected severe toxicity because of the possibility of continuing absorption. Repeat levels until concentrations are falling.

Assess acid-base balance. Venous or capillary blood gases are acceptable.

Check the serum potassium, clotting (including INR) and blood glucose.

Alkalinisation will improve excretion of salicylate. If the salicylate level in a child is greater than 350mg/L (2.5mmol/L) give 1mmol/kg sodium bicarbonate. Correct serum potassium if low before giving sodium bicarbonate. Toxbase suggests the following dose of bicarbonate – 1mL/kg 8.4% bicarbonate diluted in 500mL in 5% glucose or NaCl 0.9% at 2-3mL/kg/hour.

Attempt to maintain the urinary pH at a level of 7.5-8.5. Alkalinisation of the urine may be complicated by hypokalaemia so re-check the plasma potassium. Forced diuresis is no longer used.

Haemodialysis is the treatment of choice with severe poisoning and should be considered in patients with:
☐ Plasma concentration > 700mg/L (5.1mmol/L)
☐ Renal failure
☐ Pulmonary oedema
☐ Convulsions
☐ CNS effects not resolved by correction of acidosis
☐ Persistently high salicylate concentration unresponsive to urinary alkalinisation
☐ Severe metabolic acidosis.

Children who require haemodialysis should be discussed with the NPIS, a paediatric intensivist and a paediatric nephrologist.

CARBON MONOXIDE

Carbon monoxide poisoning is a common cause of death in house fires and from faulty heating appliances. It is important to maintain a high index of suspicion. Acute symptoms include headache, nausea, vomiting, dizziness, weakness, and depressed conscious level.

Undertake a neurological assessment including tests of co-ordination, a mini mental state examination, serial 7s and short-term memory testing.

Measurement of blood carboxyhaemoglobin may be confirmatory but does not rule out exposure, particularly if there is delay in measurement or in chronic cases.

All suspected cases require the highest possible concentration of oxygen on admission, ideally with a tight fitting face masking and non-rebreathing reservoir bag. Consider treatment for six hours. If symptoms persist oxygen therapy should be continued.

Hyperbaric therapy is an option, where readily available, although the evidence base is limited, particularly for children.

Discuss severe cases with neurological features or high levels of carbon monoxide with the NPIS.

Poisoning

Poisoning (side tab)

ALCOHOL

Alcohol is frequently ingested by children. Severe cases of poisoning are uncommon but severe features include:

☐ Coma
☐ Convulsions
☐ Respiratory depression
☐ Hypotension
☐ Risk of aspiration of stomach contents
☐ Hypothermia.

Children are particularly prone to the complication of hypoglycaemia.

Alcohol potentiates the effects of other CNS depressants.

Management

Includes maintenance of the airway and ventilation. Symptomatic treatment, particularly look for and treat hypoglycaemia. Observe for at least four hours. Gastric decontamination is not warranted.

ECSTASY

Ecstasy, or MDMA (3-4 Methylenedioxymethamfetamine) is an amphetamine derivative. In general, most cases of MDMA toxicity result only in mild symptoms. However, severe toxicity may develop after typical recreational doses.

Most cases of MDMA toxicity result in mild symptoms but severe and sometimes fatal reactions may occur such as:

☐ Fulminant hyperthermia (over 39°C)
☐ Convulsions
☐ Disseminated intravascular coagulopathy
☐ Rhabdomyolysis with myoglobinaemia and acute renal failure
☐ Cardiovascular collapse
☐ Hepatocellular necrosis
☐ Adult respiratory distress syndrome (ARDS)
☐ Hyponatraemia.

Treatment

Initial treatment is supportive. Patients with severe toxicity will require intervention such as intubation and ventilation and intensive care management. Activated charcoal may be given if the patient is seen within one hour of MDMA ingestion.

Hyperthermia

In severe cases management should be aggressive. Patients should be treated with a combination of sedation and cooling measures. If this is ineffective the patient should be paralysed, ventilated and transferred to an Intensive Care Unit. Dantrolene is controversial but can be considered.

Hyponatraemia

Fluid restriction should help to correct hyponatraemia. The syndrome of inappropriate antidiuretic hormone secretion may be present (confirm by measuring serum and urine osmolarity and urinary sodium). In severe cases of hyponatraemia, consider infusion of NaC1 0.9% or hypertonic saline.

FUNGI

Mushrooms and toadstools are fungi. Toxic effects are extremely uncommon. Most childhood cases involve undistinguished small brown fungi. It is vital to exclude serious poisonous fungi. Identification can be helped by using the CD ROM titled *Poisonous Plants and Fungi in Britain and Ireland* produced by Nightshade – a joint initiative by the Royal Botanic Gardens, Kew and the Medical Toxicology Unit, Guy's and St Thomas's Hospitals NHS Trust.

Mushrooms that cause features within six hours of ingestion are likely to be toxic.

Mushrooms found in gardens or on lawns are highly unlikely to be seriously toxic but may cause gastrointestinal upset, or be hallucinogenic.

Amanita phalloides (death cap mushroom) is the most toxic species in the UK but symptoms do not usually start until six hours or more after ingestion. Clinical presentation is of intractable vomiting and watery diarrhoea. Hypoglycaemia may occur. Delayed presentation includes hepatotoxicity and fulminant hepatic failure. Multiple-dose activated charcoal may be effective. During the acute gastroenteritis phase fluid should be replaced and hypoglycaemia promptly treated.

Management
The benefit of gastric decontamination is uncertain. Consider activated charcoal if the patient presents within one hour of ingestion. Observe for six hours to exclude gastrointestinal symptoms and CNS effects. Treat symptomatically. Consult NPIS for further help with identification of fungi, and more specific advice about the treatment of poisoning.

Psychiatry

Psychiatric disorders in children and adolescents are usually managed by psychological means and only a few of the children affected by them will need medication. Nevertheless, pharmacological treatments are an essential part of a comprehensive approach. They will nearly always be combined with psychological or psychosocial interventions and follow a full assessment. Most drug dosages are increased in a stepwise manner until either an adequate effect or the limit of tolerance is achieved. A dose per kilogram approach can give an indication of initial doses to be used but should not be used rigidly and is not employed in this section. With the exception of hypnotics, psychotropic drugs are rarely given to pre-school age children.

Many psychoactive drugs are metabolised through the cytochrome P450 system and a small proportion of the population are slow metabolisers through this route. They will only need small doses of medication and have a high rate of dose-related adverse effects.

There may be an indicative family history.

AFFECTIVE DISORDER
A meta-analysis of group studies concluded that tricyclic antidepressants have not been shown to be effective for depression in childhood. Nevertheless, many clinicians believe that a few depressed children, particularly older and more severely affected ones, do respond to tricyclics. Current evidence favours selective serotonin re-uptake inhibitors (SSRIs) as the drugs of first choice. These should only be used after assessment by experienced clinicians. Assessment includes a diagnostic interview including a mental state examination, a baseline record of symptoms/signs reported by both child and parents and usually a self-completed questionnaire. A low starting dose with gradual increase over 3 weeks or so helps minimise adverse effects which otherwise are a common reason for poor adherence. In children and adolescents the final dose sometimes needs to be higher than conventionally recommended for adult practice because of loss on first pass metabolism. Once a working dose level is reached, 8 weeks, treatment should be given before deciding that there has been no effect. A successful response means at least 6 months' treatment followed by gradual withdrawal over a further 3 months and reinstating full doses for a further 3 months if there is a relapse. In the prophylaxis of recurrent depressive or bipolar (manic-depressive) disorder, lithium or a mood-stabilising anticonvulsant such as sodium valproate or carbamazepine is analogous with psychiatric practice in adult patients. Similarly, mania can be treated directly with lithium or sodium valproate, though the response time is relatively slow compared with symptomatic control obtained by antipsychotics.

ATTENTION DEFICIT HYPERACTIVITY DISORDER (ADHD)
Methylphenidate is the drug of first choice because of the greater volume of research on it. A trial will be needed for all severe combined ADHD cases, for milder cases that do not respond to educational or psychological measures and other children where attentional or hyperactive/impulsive problems cause substantial impairment. Sustained-release preparations are appearing which reduce the stigma of having to take tablets at school. Dexamfetamine (dexamphetamine) is used as a second-line drug for non-responders to methylphenidate or where there is intolerance. Medication should always be part of a comprehensive treatment package including advice on management to parents and educational measures to support academic deficits. Gains will often be more evident in the classroom than at home and should be measured using frequent reports such as Conners' questionnaires and by monitoring academic progress. Personal review including measuring weight and height should be regular. The impact of stimulants on hyperactivity in children with autistic spectrum disorder and/or severe mental retardation (severe general learning disability/difficulty) can be very beneficial although unpredictable and should be undertaken cautiously. Misery is more likely as an adverse effect in such children.

Psychiatry

Imipramine is less powerful and does little to improve attention but may be given once daily. It does not show the adverse effects on sleep or appetite but can be cardiotoxic. Low doses of imipramine (25-75mg/day) are normally safe but with higher doses it is wise to obtain a baseline ECG, and repeat this on treatment. Consult a cardiologist if there are any ECG abnormalities. It is unwise to combine tricyclic antidepressants and CNS stimulants because of possible cardiac toxicity. Bupropion is a third-line agent.

Clonidine (50-150 micrograms daily in divided doses) is sometimes used with younger children (4-8 years) and children with co-morbid tic disorders or aggressive behaviour (who may require a higher dose). It has a beneficial effect on impulsive restlessness but less so on attention. Some clinicians use it in combination with a CNS stimulant, prescribing it as an evening dose to take advantage of the drowsiness which is a common side-effect. The child's blood pressure will need to be monitored to avoid unwanted hypotension. Withdrawal should be gradual to avoid rebound hypertension and parents should be warned accordingly. A baseline ECG recording should be obtained, and regular ECG monitoring is recommended if clonidine is combined with a CNS stimulant.

AGGRESSIVE BEHAVIOUR
Apart from aggressive behaviour associated with hyperactivity disorders, which often responds to stimulants and/or clonidine, most aggressive behaviour requires psychological management. Medication is an intervention of last resort. Sedation should be avoided.

Chlorpromazine and haloperidol have traditionally been used but there is dubious value in their use except for very short periods of time. Risperidone is increasingly popular but the evidence base is slim and its advantages have frequently offset by weight gain. Carbamazepine has been shown to reduce aggressive behaviour in some children without epilepsy, as has lithium, but these are best reserved for specialist practice.

Benzodiazepines can have unpredictable effects when used to manage aggressive behaviour and need close monitoring. Levomepromazine (methotrimeprazine)can be used for rapid tranquillisation.

SLEEP DISORDERS
Problems settling a young child at night are best managed psychologically, though as part of an overall management programme it is occasionally humane to give a sedative or hypnotic to the child for a few nights to help exhausted parents catch up on lost sleep. Promethazine or alimemazine (trimeprazine) are traditionally used but habituation is a common problem with prolonged use. They may have to be given an hour or two before the desired sleep time. Melatonin is gaining in popularity but the evidence base and safety information are both limited. So-called night waking is usually a problem of failing to settle after normal waking during the night. It is not logical to treat it by sedation except for a very few nights to ease the burden for parents before implementing psychological management. Very high doses are required to sedate a child who cries in the night and there are usually hangover effects the next day.

Parasomnias (sleep walking, night terrors etc.) usually respond to psychological techniques such as anticipatory waking but, as a last resort, can be abolished by a sleep stage 4 blocker such as diazepam or zopiclone. Either of these can be tried empirically for approximately one month with subsequent gradual withdrawal.

ANXIETY DISORDERS
The pharmacological management of anxiety in childhood is not well understood. Sedative antihistamines are ineffective. Benzodiazepines are best avoided because of their unpredictable effects on mood and the remote possibility of dependence. Nevertheless, alprazolam and lorazepam are sometimes used for panic disorder in adolescents. SSRIs are increasingly popular and the ultimate dose may be higher than required in depression. Some clinicians use buspirone for general anxiety but there is a substantial therapeutic delay (3-6 weeks). Simple phobias are normally managed with behaviour therapy.

OBSESSIVE-COMPULSIVE DISORDER (OCD)
SSRIs, often in higher doses than conventionally recommended for depression, are now the drugs of first choice for children and adolescents with OCD. Those resistant to them will improve with adequate doses of clomipramine (up to about 250mg/day). It is sensible to use ECG monitoring and review blood pressure with high doses (>75mg/day). Because of the high relapse rate on discontinuation, cognitive behaviour therapy is employed alongside pharmacological management.

TIC DISORDERS

Transient (simple) tics do not need medication. Chronic (usually multiple) tics may do and Tourette syndrome usually does. The purpose of medication is to help the child achieve near normal life and development, not necessarily the complete abolition of all tics. The characteristic waxing and waning of tic intensity needs to be taken into account when evaluating drug effects so trials of an agent need to be several weeks in duration. Clonidine, titrated upwards from 50-100 microgram a day until enduring drowsiness, fatigue or hypotension supervene is the drug of first choice but is not always effective. Dopamine receptor blockers such as risperidone, sulpiride, haloperidol or pimozide are more widely effective but have a high rate of adverse effects. ECG screening for QTc prolongation (>450 milliseconds) is necessary before starting pimozide.

SCHIZOPHRENIA

The principles of treatment in children are essentially the same as in adults, though quite often there is less symptomatic improvement than with older age groups. Because of the likelihood of protracted treatment, the newer (atypical) antipsychotics are preferred since they are less likely to produce extrapyramidal effects in the long term. Nevertheless these may have other adverse effects such as weight gain and hyperglycaemia and need close monitoring. They are also expensive. Clozapine is a second-line agent, reserved for those cases that do not respond to first-line medications.

Renal and urological

Primary nocturnal enuresis. Do not treat until at least 5 years of age. Behavioural therapies with star charts and enuresis alarms should be used in the first instance. Desmopressin is useful for short periods, for example on holidays, when the need to be dry is greater. However, there seems to be no problem with prescribing desmopressin for longer periods, although patients tend to relapse on stopping treatment. There is some evidence that a gradual reduction of the desmopressin dose may reduce the likelihood of relapse. Studies have suggested that use of desmopressin with enuresis alarms can improve efficacy.

Urge incontinence/Unstable bladder. Children presenting with symptoms suggestive of an unstable bladder should firstly have possible provoking factors excluded, particularly urinary tract infection. Relief can then be obtained using oxybutynin. Side-effects are relatively common and oxybutynin should be started at the lower dose. They usually wane after 7-14 days if benefits from treatment are thought to warrant perseverance. They can be reduced by administering the drug intravesically in patients on intermittent catheterisation regimens. A newer anti-muscarinic drug, tolterodine, may have fewer side-effects and is increasingly being used in children.

URINARY TRACT INFECTION (UTI)

UTI should be considered in all febrile or sick infants and toddlers. UTI identified by dipsticks for nitrite and leucocyte esterase should be confirmed by microscopy and culture. It is important to initiate treatment promptly, as delays in treatment have been implicated in the development of renal scar formation.

Antibiotic therapy. Oral trimethoprim is a reasonable blind first-line therapy. Intravenous ampicillin and gentamicin should be used for UTI if the child is under two months, or if there is evidence of shock, septicaemia, vomiting, dehydration or acute pyelonephritis. Failure to respond or persistence of fever beyond 48 hours is an indication to review antibiotic sensitivity and to investigate the urinary tract for obstruction and other complicating anatomical factors. 24-48 hours after resolution of fever, it is reasonable to change the treatment from IV to oral therapy, except in neonates when it is customary to give IV therapy for 5 days. The duration of treatment after the neonatal period depends on the clinical situation. Ten days is recommended for children with systemic illness but children with mild illness can be given a 5 day course.

Prophylaxis. Long-term low-dose prophylaxis with trimethoprim or nitrofurantoin has been shown to be effective in reducing the risk of recurrence in children with frequent re-infections. There is little published evidence of benefit from other antibiotics.

Single-dose treatment. Single-dose and very short-course treatment is not recommended in young children or those with underlying anomalies. However, this form of therapy may be acceptable for the management of girls over 8 years old with recurrent symptomatic infection and normal urinary tracts.

Asymptomatic bacteriuria. Asymptomatic bacteriuria is common at all ages, particularly in girls. Extensive studies in infants and schoolgirls have demonstrated no benefit from treatment in the complete absence of symptoms. It has been demonstrated that courses of antibiotic can alter the perineal flora and increase the risk of a new ascending infection.

NEPHRITIS

Treat any underlying sepsis and manage fluid balance, electrolyte disturbances, acute renal failure and hypertension. In some immunological disorders, such as systemic lupus erythematosus and Wegener granulomatosis, immunosuppression is indicated. Antiplatelet agents and anticoagulants may have a limited role, but this has not yet been established in controlled trials in children. Angiotensin-converting enzyme (ACE) inhibitors are effective in the management of hypertension and proteinuria and are thought to have a beneficial effect on the progression of renal failure by reducing intra-glomerular hypertension and protecting the glomerular capillaries and basement membrane.

NEPHROTIC SYNDROME

This is defined as proteinuria >200mg/mmol of creatinine or Albustix® +++ for three days, accompanied by low serum albumin (<25g/L) and oedema. Management of the nephrotic state requires careful control of fluid and sodium intake, weight, blood pressure, nutrition and sepsis and cautious use of diuretics. Albumin 20% with furosemide (frusemide) may be used to promote a diuresis in children with gross oedema if diuretics alone have failed. However, use of albumin can result in life-threatening pulmonary oedema, so respiratory rate and oxygen saturations should be monitored. Because of the relapsing and remitting nature of this condition, prescription of suitable sticks for urine monitoring at home is essential. Parents should be taught to test the urine, keep a record of urinalysis and drugs given, and told who to contact in the event of sepsis or relapse.

Acute hypovolaemia is a serious and potentially life threatening complication of nephrotic syndrome which requires urgent treatment with NaCl 0.9% or albumin 4.5%, monitoring for hypertension and pulmonary oedema in a children's high dependency unit.

Immunomodulation. Over 90% of children presenting have steroid sensitive nephrotic syndrome and achieve remission, i.e. reduction of proteinuria to less than 20mg/mmol creatinine or Albustix® negative or trace, following treatment with prednisolone for 4 weeks. A small proportion remit after a further period of up to 4 weeks. Once remission has been achieved (Albustix® trace or negative, or protein to creatinine ratio of <20mg/mmol) it is customary to reduce steroids to alternate days for a further 4 week period and then stop. Time to relapse is longer in children treated with longer courses of prednisolone at full dosage, but this benefit should be balanced against the increase in steroid side-effects.

Frequent relapsers. Two-thirds of children relapse and need further courses of prednisolone to induce remission. Frequent relapsers – more than four per year or two in 6 months – may be maintained in remission with a small dose of alternate day steroids, however, the use of long-term alternate day prednisolone is likely to result in reduced growth velocity and delayed puberty. The dose of alternate day steroids that prevents relapse can be carefully titrated. Second-line therapy should be considered in children with frequent relapses requiring >500 microgram/kg alternate days or if growth failure or delayed puberty.

Second- and third-line therapy. Levamisole is relatively safe. Third-line treatment is with cyclophosphamide for 8 weeks. Chlorambucil and ciclosporin (cyclosporin) are alternatives.

Prevention of infection. Consider pneumococcal vaccine and ensure immunisations are up to date when the child is in remission and has been off steroids for 3 months.

ACUTE RENAL FAILURE

Acute renal failure is characterised by a rising urea and creatinine usually accompanied by oliguria (<1mL/kg/hour). Renal failure may develop due to pre-renal, intrinsic renal or post-renal problems. Preliminary management is aimed at establishing the extent of fluid and electrolyte disturbances and looking for the underlying cause.

All fluid losses including a calculated insensible loss should be recorded and all intake measured. The bladder should be catheterised or nappies weighed if the child cannot co-operate. If there is any possibility that the child is shocked or hypovolaemic, NaCl 0.9% or albumin 4.5% (10-20mL/kg) should be given over 30-60 minutes and furosemide (frusemide) 2mg/kg, increasing to 5mg/kg, administered once hypovolaemia has been corrected. Fluids must be stopped if there is any sign of fluid overload because of the risk of pulmonary oedema or hypertensive encephalopathy.

Fluid overload should be managed by water restriction, augmented by diuretics and dialysis. Polyuria often accompanies partial obstruction, and follows relief of obstruction or recovery from acute renal failure. All measured fluid and electrolyte losses should be replaced on an hourly basis after correction of initial imbalances.

Acidosis and electrolyte disturbances should be corrected as soon as possible. Potassium, sodium and protein intake may need restricting while calorie intake should be supplemented, if possible. The dose of water-soluble drugs should be reduced according to the level of renal function, and the dosage interval lengthened. Hypertension, sepsis and urinary infection should be sought, and if present, treated. Nephrotoxic drugs and drugs prone to cause interstitial nephritis should be stopped or reduced. Specific immunological therapy may be required in rapidly progressing nephritis. Dialysis should be introduced well before life-threatening situations – hyperkalaemia, pulmonary oedema and hypertensive encephalopathy – develop.

CHRONIC RENAL FAILURE

Chronic renal failure causes complex metabolic changes due to the loss of homeostasis of fluids and electrolytes, accumulation of waste products and loss of its hormonal activities (erythropoeitin, renin, vitamin D, parathyroid hormone (PTH), aldosterone). This leads to loss of appetite, failure to thrive, poor growth, anaemia, metabolic bone disease (rickets and hyperparathyroidism) and hypertension. Monitoring and treatment need to be rigorously structured.

Fluids. It is important that fluid input is adequate, particularly if oral fluids are being withheld (e.g. surgery or gastroenteritis) when IV fluids may be needed.

Nutrition. Supplementation of water-soluble vitamins with Ketovite® tablets is important. Calorie supplementation is often required because of anorexia associated with uraemia. Electrolyte supplementation may be necessary, particularly with sodium.

Anaemia. Before starting erythropoietin, check for haematinic deficiency (ferritin, folate and vitamin B12) and measure serum aluminium levels. Ensure good control of metabolic bone disease. Exclude chronic blood loss and infection. Maintain serum ferritin concentration at upper limit of normal using appropriate iron supplements. Erythropoietin should be used to help achieve a haemoglobin of at least 9.5g/dL in children under 6 months of age, 10g/dL in children aged 6 months to 2 years and 10.5g/dL in children over 2 years.

Renal bone disease. Control serum phosphate levels by a low phosphate diet and use of calcium carbonate as a phosphate binder. Calcium acetate and magnesium carbonate may also be used. Sevelamer, a new phosphate binding polymer, free of aluminium and calcium, has recently been licensed in the UK for use in adults and has been available for much longer in the United States. It has the additional benefit of lowering cholesterol and low density lipoproteins and is therefore a welcome addition to the treatment of hypophosphataemia. Remember to compare serum phosphate measurements with age-matched controls. Maintain the serum calcium levels at the upper end of the normal range by use of alfacalcidol and calcium supplements. Serum PTH levels should be kept as near to the normal range as possible. PTH levels slightly above the normal range may be optimal. If control of PTH levels is hampered by hypercalcaemia, use of low calcium dialysate fluids should be considered. Alternatively, pulse alfacalcidol or calcitriol 2-3 times per week, either orally or IV, has been shown to be effective in adults.

HYPERTENSION

Accurate measurement of blood pressure requires the correct cuff size. A simple rule is to use the largest cuff possible and the bladder must encircle at least 80% of the arm circumference. Assess diastolic pressure at point of muffling (4th Korotkov sound) and use the appropriate centile chart to establish if blood pressure is abnormally high.

Mild hypertension. Modify the diet and where relevant, the life-style. Make modest reductions in sodium intake and give potassium supplements. Encourage weight loss and regular exercise. If drug treatment is required, use nifedipine or beta-blocker + thiazide diuretic. If considering a calcium antagonist in younger children who are unable to swallow one of the sustained-release nifedipine preparations, amlodipine can be given once or twice a day. It is available in a tablet form, which can be dispersed and administered as a liquid.

Atenolol is usually the first-choice beta-blocker. It has the advantage of a long duration of action requiring only once-a-day dosing, availability as a syrup, relative cardio-selectivity and being water-soluble is less likely to enter the brain so cause less sleep disturbance and nightmares. However, some patients do not tolerate atenolol, with headaches being a particular problem. Switching to metoprolol (a more lipid-soluble drug) can help in this situation.

Renal and urological

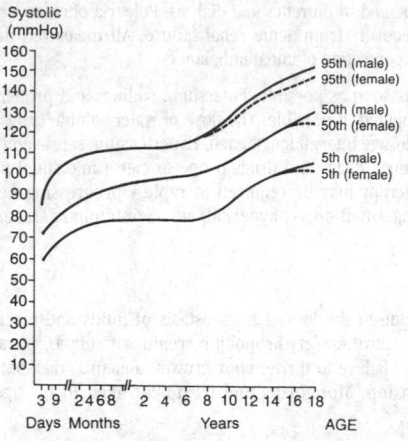

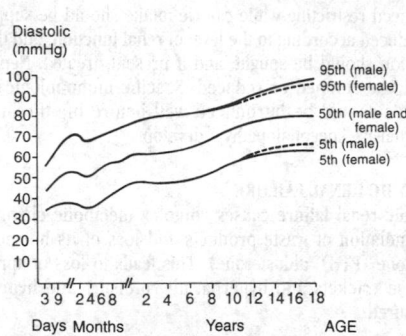

Moderate/severe hypertension. 80-90% is secondary to renal disease. Investigate the cause and treat accordingly. If it is secondary to parenchymal renal disease (particularly with proteinuria) the first-line therapy should include an ACE inhibitor. Renal function should be monitored because of the risk of renal hypoperfusion in renovascular disease. Add a calcium antagonist, a beta-blocker, a diuretic and a vasodilator as required. Refractory hypertension may require additional treatment with agents such as minoxidil or clonidine.

Hypertensive emergencies. Controlled reduction in blood pressure over 72-96 hours is essential to avoid cerebral ischaemia, particularly optic nerve damage. Controlled reduction is achieved by infusions of labetalol or sodium nitroprusside, particularly in encephalopathic patients, or those who are vomiting or uncooperative. The intravenous calcium antagonist nicardipine is also becoming increasingly popular in the United States, administered as a continuous infusion, although it is not licensed in the UK. In less severe cases, oral nifedipine capsules can be used. Either drug has the advantage of potentially increasing cerebral blood flow, thereby reducing the risk of cerebral ischaemia. Diazoxide can be used in resistant cases, although it may cause sudden hypotension. Other antihypertensive drugs which can be given intravenously by bolus or infusion include hydralazine, clonidine and methyldopa. Intravenous access is essential, particularly during the first 12 hours, to allow expansion of plasma volume should the blood pressure drop too rapidly. Hypertension in acute nephritis is secondary to salt and water retention. This should be treated with salt and fluid restriction and furosemide (frusemide) as well as other antihypertensive agents. Once blood pressure control is achieved oral therapy should be instigated.

Phaeochromocytoma requires special consideration. Surgery should not take place until there is adequate pharmacological blockade of both alpha and beta-sympathetic receptors (alpha-blockers – phenoxybenzamine and prazosin, beta-blocker – propranolol). Nifedipine can also be used to control blood pressure. If accelerated hypertension develops, IV labetalol can be used. At surgery, the blood pressure is controlled using short-acting antihypertensive agents - phentolamine, labetalol, sodium nitroprusside. If necessary, supplies of plasma and blood are given to fill the vascular space. Ensure good intravascular filling, as ligation of the vascular supply to the tumour can cause vasodilatation and hypotension. Avoid anaesthetic agents which stimulate sympathetic activity. Surgery should only be carried out at a specialist centre.

Management of hypertension

	1st line	2nd line	3rd line
Mild	Dietary modification ↓Na⁺, ↑K⁺, ↓Weight	Calcium-channel blocker	Atenolol Thiazide diuretic
Moderate/Severe	ACE inhibitor Calcium-channel blocker	Atenolol Diuretic Hydralazine	Minoxidil Prazosin Clonidine
Emergency	Nifedipine Labetalol	Sodium nitroprusside Hydralazine	Clonidine Methyldopa Diazoxide

HYPERKALAEMIA

Emergency management

☐ Stop the intake of potassium-containing food and fluids, stop drugs which promote hyperkalaemia, and monitor the ECG. If there is significant widening of the QRS complex or arrhythmia, the myocardium can be stabilised with IV calcium.

☐ Rapid reduction of plasma potassium can be achieved with salbutamol, either IV or nebulised.

☐ Reduction of total potassium can be achieved with ion exchange resins. Calcium Resonium® can be administered orally or rectally. If given orally, repeated doses can cause constipation which should be treated with lactulose.

☐ Insulin with glucose will also move potassium intracellularly. It requires careful monitoring of blood glucose.

☐ If hyperkalaemia is associated with acidosis, correction of the acidosis with bicarbonate will again move potassium intracellularly. Bicarbonate is of little benefit in the absence of acidosis.

☐ Persistent hyperkalaemia requires dialysis to remove potassium.

PERITONEAL DIALYSIS

The main complication is peritonitis; the clinical diagnosis is based on finding two out of three from: cloudy dialysis fluid (WBC >100/mm^3 of which >50% are polymorphonuclear neutrophils); sudden onset of abdominal pain and rebound tenderness; and isolation of organisms from dialysis effluent.

Each paediatric renal unit has its own protocol for treating peritonitis in children on peritoneal dialysis and there is wide variation in the drugs and dosages used. The rate of methicillin-resistant organisms causing peritonitis has increased significantly and this favours the use of a glycopeptide. There is, however, concern about the spread of vancomycin resistance. Ototoxicity and nephrotoxicity are strong arguments against the use of aminoglycosides. Based on these considerations, the paediatric peritonitis guidelines recently generated by an International Expert Committee recommend combining a glycopeptide with ceftazidime for children at risk for a severe clinical course (as indicated by age less than 2 years, severe abdominal pain or signs of systemic infection) and/or a previous or current infection with a methicillin-resistant *Staphylococcus aureus*. Asymptomatic patients with cloudy fluid, without such risk factors, should receive a first generation cephalosporin combined with ceftazidime. These antibiotics should be administered intraperitoneally (IP).

Antibiotic	Loading dose	Maintenance dose
Vancomycin	20mg/kg	25mg/L
Cefazolin	250mg/L	125mg/L
Cefuroxime	1000mg/L	250mg/L
Ceftazidime	250mg/L	125mg/l

It is recommended that Gram-positive infection be treated for 2 weeks, except *S. aureus* which should be treated for 3 weeks. Infections caused by a single Gram-negative organism should also be treated for 2 weeks, but 3 weeks if *Pseudomonas* or *Stenotrophomonas* species are implicated or multiple organisms or anaerobes are involved. Relapsing Gram-positive infections may respond to a 3 week course of vancomycin IP and rifampicin orally. Heparin is also added to the peritoneal dialysis fluid at a dose of 500–1000 units per litre if necessary. Consideration should also be given to the use of oral antifungal prophylaxis during the course of antibiotics.

Fungal peritonitis is treated with fluconazole which may be given orally or IV; it can also be given IP (6mg/kg in 250-350mL dialysis fluid, left for 6 hours and then 3mg/L IP in each bag) PLUS flucytosine which can also be given orally, IV and IP (to a concentration of 50mg/L). Treat for 2 weeks if the catheter is removed and 6 weeks if it is left in place. Intravenous liposomal amphotericin may be used in resistant cases, although peritoneal penetration is poor. Amphotericin should not be given intraperitoneally.

RENAL TRANSPLANTATION

Immunosuppression. Renal transplantation is an emergency procedure (except for live donors) and effective immunosuppression must be provided from the time of the operation. This is achieved using methylprednisolone given intravenously (600mg/m^2) over 4 hours during the pre- and peri-operative period. Protocols for immunosuppression vary but a typical example will be triple therapy with azathioprine, ciclosporin (cyclosporin) microemulsion and prednisolone. There continues to be a rapid development of new agents, with enhanced immunosuppressive effects and the promise of reduced side-effects, in particular nephrotoxicity. Tacrolimus, another calcineurin inhibitor, and mycophenolate mofetil, which inhibits lymphocyte proliferation by blocking the *de novo* synthesis of purine nucleotides, have been used in paediatric practice for a number of years. Newer agents include basiliximab, a monoclonal antibody that prevents T cell proliferation and is used for prophylaxis against acute rejection. Sirolimus is a new potent non-calcineurin inhibiting immunosuppressant which has the advantage of not being nephrotoxic. Trials of these agents in paediatric patients continue and while they may have enhanced immunosuppressive action, this must be balanced against the possible increased risks of sepsis and cancer.

Acute rejection is treated with methylprednisolone 400mg/m^2 for 3-5 doses on consecutive days. Failure to respond to this treatment is an indication for renal biopsy. Further acute rejection is normally treated with Anti-Thymocyte Globulin (ATG) or muromonab-CD3 (OKT3).

Immunisations. Pre-transplantation immunisation with live vaccines for measles, chickenpox and mumps will reduce the risk of death due to these common infections. The chickenpox vaccine is an attenuated virus and may be given after transplantation.

CYSTINOSIS
Fanconi syndrome develops in infancy and requires replacement of electrolytes (sodium, potassium, bicarbonate and phosphate) not reabsorbed in the proximal tubule. Vitamin D analogues are required to prevent hypophosphataemic rickets. Later, the biochemical and haematological problems of chronic renal failure predominate, followed by hypothyroidism and diabetes mellitus. Renal replacement therapy and prevention of cystine accumulation with phosphocysteamine or cysteamine bitartrate has dramatically improved the prognosis. These compounds and their metabolites have a distinctive and unpleasant odour which can limit their tolerability. Pre-dose white cell cystine levels should be monitored and levels maintained in the heterozygote range (<1mg/g protein). There is a register for patients in the UK.

Respiratory

RESPIRATORY FAILURE IN THE NEWBORN
Prevention. Pulmonary immaturity due to lack of surfactant is the commonest reason for respiratory failure in the early neonatal period and affects most babies born more than 10 weeks early. Betamethasone or dexamethasone given to the mother at least 12 hours before delivery (preferably 48 hours before), substantially enhances the chemical maturity of the lung at birth. Surfactant production also increases rapidly, even in the preterm baby, within three days of delivery so the primary objective of good neonatal care is to tide the baby over this vulnerable period without further iatrogenic problems. Try to avoid hypoxia, atelectasis, acidosis and cold stress, all of which interfere with surfactant production. Optimising early lung expansion by establishing an adequate functional residual capacity is the first need in any preterm baby who remains cyanosed after birth. Avoid overdistension of the lung which will cause local injury and damaging inflammatory responses.

Surfactant. Oxygen dependent babies of less than 30 weeks gestation requiring intubation at birth benefit from having surfactant instilled prophylactically down the endotracheal tube into the lung. The tube can then be removed or retained depending on the clinical state of the baby. More mature babies needing ventilation with >40% oxygen in the first 48 hours may also benefit from surfactant administration. Trials have established that surfactant treatment is also of benefit to some term infants with meconium aspiration syndrome and there is some evidence to suggest that the same may be true of the baby with intrapartum streptococcal infection.

Other strategies. Warmth, rest, minimal handling and selective pain relief are all part of good basic care. Neuromuscular blockade should be considered in babies requiring high-pressure ventilation, especially if they fail to breathe in phase with the ventilator. Look first for evidence of pain, correctable hypoxia, respiratory acidosis, inadequate respiratory support or inappropriate respiratory rate. Infants with neuromuscular blockade should not be left without pain relief. Morphine is the analgesic about which most is known. The dose needed to control visceral pain in the neonatal period is probably considerably higher than the usual sedative dose. Benzodiazepine anxiolytics do not prevent pain, and problems have been reported with their sustained use.

CONTINUED CENTRAL CYANOSIS
Once structural heart disease has been excluded, the management of cyanosis in the ventilated baby consists of optimising lung expansion and cardiac output, and reducing pulmonary vascular resistance. Sequential ventilator adjustments will help to establish the mean airway pressure that provides the best balance between optimal alveolar

blood flow and optimal alveolar aeration. Low systemic vascular resistance can be as potent a cause of right-to-left shunting as raised pulmonary vascular resistance. A dobutamine infusion should be started if left ventricular function and cardiac output are poor. Blood is the logical fluid to give if there is clinical evidence to suggest that hypovolaemia has been caused by concealed bleeding or feto-maternal blood loss. High dose dopamine, adrenaline (epinephrine) or noradrenaline (norepinephrine) may help if poor peripheral vascular tone is contributing to systemic hypotension (e.g. septic shock). Indometacin (indomethacin) or ibuprofen may help to reduce ductal shunting while a prostaglandin infusion can be used to maintain ductus patency in suspected duct-dependent congenital heart disease.

Pulmonary vasodilators. These should be tried if cyanosis persists after systemic circulatory output and lung expansion have been optimised. Tolazoline will have an immediate effect if it is going to work at all, as will epoprostenol. Magnesium sulphate can be of value but works more slowly. All these agents lower systemic as well as pulmonary blood pressure. Inhaled nitric oxide (NO) has such a short half-life that it only affects pulmonary vascular tone. If NO is available then its use would be logical at this stage. However, if it is only partially effective, extra-corporeal membrane oxygenation (ECMO) may be the only option. Once NO has been started withdrawal may lead to deterioration even if introduction of NO produced little improvement. Transfer to an ECMO centre would then have to be accomplished with continued administration of NO in transit.

Respiratory stimulants. Apnoea in babies of less than 34 weeks postconceptional age (gestational plus postnatal age) is best managed with caffeine citrate. The addition of doxapram may be of benefit when problems persist despite high dose caffeine. Caffeine can also be used to help wean the preterm baby from ventilator support.

INFECTIONS

Cough is a frequent symptom in children and is usually due to a viral upper respiratory tract infection. Often the cough itself does not need treatment. When it is distressing or interferes with sleep or causes vomiting, parents may seek help. Enquiry into possible underlying causes such as asthma and cystic fibrosis should be made before offering symptomatic relief. A cough linctus such as Simple Linctus may offer benefit. Compound cough mixtures are best avoided. Decongestants administered systemically or locally may provide symptomatic relief but should be used sparingly. A systematic review of 'over the counter' medications for acute cough in children and adults concluded that there was no good evidence for or against their effectiveness.

Croup (laryngotracheobronchitis) presents with inspiratory stridor, a barking cough, hoarseness and variable degrees of respiratory distress. Randomised controlled trials have shown nebulised budesonide and oral dexamethasone to be of benefit in children with mild to moderately severe croup. Nebulised adrenaline (epinephrine) is of value although the initial improvement in the child's condition is often not sustained. Because of this it should only be administered to children who require admission to hospital. Mist is not helpful in the management of croup. Croupettes may be dangerous.

Systemic corticosteroids are used in children who are intubated for croup. They reduce the duration of intubation and the need for reintubation.

Stridor. Any child at risk of significant obstruction to airflow should be sent to hospital. Attempts should be made to calm the child. In hospital, oxygen is given and oxygen saturation is monitored. If necessary, seek the assistance of an anaesthetist experienced in controlling a child's airway. Procedures such as examining the pharynx, obtaining x-rays of the neck, attempting IV access, sedating or lying the child flat, are usually unhelpful and may be dangerous if undertaken before the child is intubated.

Acute epiglottitis. Since the introduction of the *Haemophilus influenzae* type b (Hib) vaccine, this is rare. The main consideration is control of the airway. Intubation is usually required but generally not for long. Intravenous antibiotics – third generation cephalosporins – are generally continued until after extubation. The usual course of treatment is 5 days. There is no evidence that nebulised adrenaline (epinephrine) or steroids are beneficial.

Bacterial tracheitis is a rare life-threatening condition due to *Staphylococcus aureus*, Streptococci, *Moraxella catarrhalis* or *Haemophilus influenzae*. Children usually require intubation for many days. Treatment is with ampicillin and flucloxacillin or a third generation cephalosporin and reviewed once the results of cultures are known.

Retropharyngeal abscess. Early assessment by an ear, nose and throat (ENT) surgeon is essential, as the abscess may require drainage. Intravenous antibiotics are required whether or not the lesion is drained. Benzylpenicillin and flucloxacillin or a third generation cephalosporin, are used. Metronidazole is often added to cover anaerobes.

Pneumonia. If a bacterial cause is suspected, treat with benzylpenicillin or erythromycin. Amoxicillin (amoxycillin) or third generation cephalosporins may also be used; under 3 months of age, cefuroxime or co-amoxiclav is generally the first-line treatment (or erythromycin if Chlamydia is suspected). If the child is not seriously ill antibiotics may be given orally. Oxygen saturations should be monitored and humidified oxygen administered if appropriate. Atypical pneumonias, when suspected, should be treated with a macrolide antibiotic. Erythromycin should be given for a period of 2 weeks. Newer macrolide antibiotics have not been shown to be superior to erythromycin but may have fewer side-effects and, because of the need for less frequent administration, aid compliance.

Bronchiolitis is usually due to respiratory syncytial virus (RSV). Many infants with RSV infection are cared for at home but a few become distressed and require admission. As a minority of infants require assisted ventilation, all infants should be monitored closely for evidence of exhaustion. Oxygen is given to maintain oxygen saturations as measured by continuous pulse oximetry at a minimum of 92%. To avoid dehydration oro/nasogastric feeds should be given to infants unable to take adequate fluids orally. Infants with severe distress may need IV fluids. Antibiotics are only indicated if there is evidence of a secondary bacterial infection. Ribavirin (tribavirin) is licensed for use in the treatment of bronchiolitis due to the respiratory syncytial virus (RSV). Evidence for benefit in infants with RSV bronchiolitis is equivocal and therefore it is not indicated for routine use. It may be considered in infants with RSV bronchiolitis if they have underlying cardiac disease, chronic lung disease, or an immunosuppressive illness – but the evidence of benefit is no better in these groups. Babies with chronic lung disease and those born extremely prematurely and under 6 months of age at the beginning of the bronchiolitis season can be given passive immunisation with the monoclonal antibody palivizumab.

Pertussis is a prolonged, distressing illness causing a spasmodic cough often accompanied by an inspiratory whoop. In severely affected infants pulse oximetry should be used to monitor arterial oxygen saturation at all times. Humidified oxygen should be administered when the child is hypoxic, particularly during coughing spasms and continuously if the child is hypoxic between coughing spasms. Adequate hydration is ensured with nasogastric or IV fluids. Erythromycin may be of benefit in the catarrhal stage of the illness (a suspected contact) and may reduce transmission. There is no evidence that it is of benefit during the paroxysmal stage of the disease although it is frequently administered. Erythromycin may be given for prophylaxis to siblings and immunocompromised contacts.

OPPORTUNISTIC PNEUMONIAS
Children who are immunocompromised frequently present with acute respiratory distress due to an opportunistic pneumonia; it is important to try to identify the causative organism. Without such identification the only safe course of action is to administer treatment for likely causative organisms.

Pneumocystis carinii pneumonia is diagnosed by broncho-alveolar lavage or transbronchial lung biopsy. Treatment is with high dose intravenous co-trimoxazole for 10–21 days depending on the clinical response, with the addition of steroids if necessary. An alternative treatment is intravenous pentamidine. Prophylaxis with either oral co-trimoxazole or nebulised pentamidine should be considered in all children who are known to be immunocompromised and particularly in those children who have already experienced an episode of *Pneumocystis carinii* pneumonia.

Cytomegalovirus (CMV) pneumonia should be treated promptly with intravenous ganciclovir for 2 weeks. CMV immunoglobulin may also be used in addition to a specific antiviral agent. Prophylaxis with oral aciclovir (acyclovir) or CMV immunoglobulin IV may be considered in the high-risk patient.

Aspergillus infection can occur in the lungs as in many other parts of the body. Medical treatment may be used in addition to, or instead of, surgery. Amphotericin in combination with flucytosine is most commonly prescribed. Ketaconazole liquid is also used.

Varicella zoster pneumonia. A primary infection with chickenpox in an immunocompromised patient is frequently associated with chickenpox pneumonia. This should be treated with high-dose IV aciclovir for a period of 2 weeks.

Herpes simplex pneumonia may present with superficial lesions on the lips and these then progress into the mouth and oropharynx and from there, down the trachea into the lungs. Mortality from herpes simplex pneumonia is very high. Treatment should be with high dose IV aciclovir.

ASTHMA
Emergency management of acute childhood asthma
It is essential to assess the severity of the child's symptoms accurately. The following signs should be recorded:
☐ Pulse rate: increasing tachycardia generally denotes worsening asthma

☐ Respiratory rate and degree of breathlessness: i.e. too breathless to complete sentences in one breath or to feed
☐ Use of accessory muscles for respiration
☐ Amount of wheezing. May become biphasic or less apparent with increasing airway obstruction
☐ Degree of agitation and conscious level
☐ Oxygen saturation.

Note: Clinical signs may correlate poorly with severity of airways obstruction. Some children with acute severe asthma do not appear distressed.

Acute asthma treatment in children aged under 2 years in hospital
Assess asthma severity; signs of moderate and severe cases are described below. If a patient has signs and symptoms across the categories, always treat according to their most severe features.

Moderate: $SpO_2 \geq 92\%$; audible wheezing; using accessory muscles; still feeding.
Severe: $SpO_2 < 92\%$; cyanosis; marked respiratory distress; too breathless to feed.

Most infants are audibly wheezy with intercostal and subcostal recession but may not appear distressed. Life-threatening features include apnoea, bradycardia and poor respiratory effort.

Immediate management: oxygen via close-fitting facemask or nasal prongs to achieve normal saturations. Give trial of ß₂ agonist: salbutamol or terbutaline up to 10 puffs via spacer and facemask, or nebulised salbutamol 2.5mg, or nebulised terbutaline 5mg. Give 1-4 hourly if responding in moderately severe patients.

If poor response: add nebulised ipratropium bromide 250 microgram (up to 4 hourly only). Consider soluble prednisolone 10mg daily for up to 3 days.

Assess response to treatment: heart rate, pulse rate, pulse oximetry; supportive, calm nursing care; consider need for chest x-ray.

If not responding or any life-threatening features: discuss immediately with senior paediatrician or Paediatric Intensive Care Unit (PICU) team.

Note: Infants often respond poorly to bronchodilators. Nebulised ß₂ agonists have been associated with mild paradoxical bronchoconstriction and transient worsening of oxygen saturation. Response to prednisolone may also be poor in this age group.

Acute asthma treatment in children aged 2–5 years in hospital
Assess asthma severity; signs of moderate, severe and life-threatening exacerbations are described below. If a patient has signs and symptoms across the categories, always treat according to the most severe features.

Moderate exacerbation: $SpO_2 \geq 92\%$: no clinical features of severe asthma.

Severe exacerbation: $SpO_2 < 92\%$: too breathless to talk or eat; heart rate >130/minute; respiratory rate >50/minute; use of accessory neck muscles.

Life-threatening exacerbation: $SpO_2 < 92\%$; silent chest; poor respiratory effort; agitation/altered consciousness; cyanosis.

Treatment: oxygen via facemask/nasal prongs should be given to achieve normal oxygen saturation. Nebulisers should always be driven with oxygen.

Moderate exacerbation: ß₂ agonist 2-4 puffs via a spacer device plus facemask; increase agonist dose by up to 2 puffs every 2 minutes up to 10 puffs according to response; give soluble, oral prednisolone 20mg and reassess within 1 hour.

Severe exacerbation: ß₂ agonist 10 puffs via spacer device plus facemask or nebulised salbutamol 2.5mg or nebulised terbutaline 5mg; give soluble prednisolone 20mg or IV hydrocortisone 4mg/kg. Repeat ß₂ agonists up to every 20-30 minutes according to response. In severe exacerbations a Cochrane Review suggests frequent doses (every 30 minutes) of ipratropium bromide (250microgram/dose) over the first 2 hours may be of benefit. Then reduce ipratropium bromide to 4-6 hourly. It may be mixed with ß₂ agonist solutions.

Life-threatening exacerbation: Give nebulised ß₂ agonists: salbutamol 2.5mg or terbutaline 5mg plus ipratropium bromide 250 microgram. In severe exacerbations a Cochrane Review suggests frequent doses (every 30 minutes) of ipratropium bromide (250microgram/dose) over the first 2 hours may be of benefit. Then reduce ipratropium bromide to 4-6 hourly. Give IV hydrocortisone 4mg/kg. Discuss with a senior paediatrician or anaesthetist or the PICU team. Repeat ß₂ agonist bronchodilators every 20-30 minutes.

Respiratory

Assess response to treatment: measure respiratory rate, heart rate and oxygen saturation. If a patient with a severe exacerbation or life-threatening exacerbation is not responding arrange high dependency/paediatric intensive care unit transfer. Consider:

☐ Chest x-ray and blood gases

☐ IV salbutamol 15 microgram/kg bolus over 10 minutes following by continuous infusion 1-5 microgram/kg/minute (dilute to 200 microgram/mL) or

☐ IV aminophylline 5mg/kg loading dose over 20 minutes (omit in those receiving oral theophyllines) followed by continuous infusion 1mg/kg/hour.

Patients responding to treatment: continue on bronchodilators 1-4 hourly as required; discharge when stable on 4 hourly treatment; continue oral prednisolone 20mg/day for up to 3 days.

At discharge: ensure patient is stable on 4 hourly treatment; review need for regular treatment and use of inhaled corticosteroids; review inhaler technique; provide a written management plan for treatment of future attacks; arrange follow up according to local policy.

Acute asthma treatment of children over 5 years in hospital
Assess asthma severity; signs of moderate, severe or life threatening exacerbations are described below. If a patient has signs and symptoms across the categories described below, always treat according to their most severe features.

Moderate exacerbation: SpO_2 ≥92%, PEF≥50% best or predicted, no clinical features of severe asthma.

Severe exacerbation: SpO_2<92%, PEF≤50% best or predicted, heart rate >120/minute, respiratory rate >30 minute, use of accessory neck muscles.

Life threatening exacerbation: SpO_2<92%, PEF<33% best or predicted, silent chest, poor respiratory effort, altered consciousness, cyanosis.

Treatment: oxygen should be given by facemask/nasal prongs to achieve normal oxygen saturation. Nebulisers should always be driven with oxygen.

Moderate exacerbation: ß₂ agonist 2-4 puffs via a spacer; increase ß₂ agonist dose by 2 puffs every 2 minutes up to 10 puffs according to response; give soluble oral prednisolone 30-40mg and re-assess within 1 hour.

Severe exacerbation: ß₂ agonist 10 puffs via a spacer or nebulised salbutamol 2.5-5mg or nebulised terbutaline 5-10mg. Give oral prednisolone 30-40mg or IV hydrocortisone 4mg/kg if vomiting. In severe exacerbations a Cochrane Review suggests frequent doses (every 30 minutes) of ipratropium bromide (250microgram/dose) over the first 2 hours may be of benefit. Then reduce ipratropium bromide to 4-6 hourly. Repeat ß₂ agonist bronchodilators up to every 20-30 minutes according to response.

Life-threatening exacerbation: give nebulised ß₂ agonist; salbutamol 5mg or terbutaline 10mg plus ipratropium bromide 250 micrograms. Repeat ß₂ agonists every 20-30 minutes as required. In severe exacerbations a Cochrane Review suggests frequent doses (every 30 minutes) of ipratropium bromide (250microgram/dose) over the first 2 hours may be of benefit. Then reduce ipratropium bromide to 4-6 hourly only. Give IV hydrocortisone 4mg/kg. Discuss with a senior paediatrician or anaesthetist or the PICU team.

Assess response to treatment: measure respiratory rate, heart rate, oxygen saturation and PEF/FEV_1 every 1-4 hours.

If responding poorly to treatment: with severe, life-threatening exacerbations, continue 20-30 minute nebulisers and arrange HDU/PICU transfer. Consider:

☐ Chest x-ray and blood gases

☐ IV salbutamol 15 microgram/kg bolus if not already given. Continuous IV infusion of salbutamol 1-5 microgram/kg/minute (200 microgram/mL solution)

☐ IV aminophylline 5mg/kg loading dose over 20 minutes followed by continuous infusion 1mg/kg/hour (omit loading dose in those receiving oral theophyllines).

Discuss with consultant in PICU the possibility of a bolus infusion of magnesium sulphate (40mg/kg (maximum dose 2g)) over 20 minutes although studies of efficacy, however, have been inconsistent in proving benefit.

Patient responding to treatment: continue bronchodilators 1-4 hourly when required; discharge when stable on 4 hourly treatments. Continue oral prednisolone 30-40mg for up to 3 days.

At discharge: ensure stability on 4 hourly inhaled treatment; review the need for regular treatment and the use of inhaled corticosteroids; review inhaler technique; provide a written management plan for treating future attacks; arrange follow up according to local policy.

Maintenance therapy in childhood asthma

Outlined below is a stepwise approach to asthma management. Before changing any treatments, ensure the patient is adhering to his/her treatment and has a good inhaler technique.

Maintenance asthma therapy of children under 5 years

Step 1. Occasional use of relief bronchodilators: an inhaled short-acting $ß_2$ agonist is the bronchodilator of choice as a short-term reliever therapy. Use inhaled medication whenever possible. Oral $ß_2$ agonists are much less effective and have more systemic side-effects.

Step 2. Regular inhaled preventive therapy: give inhaled short-acting $ß_2$ agonists as required. Add inhaled steroids up to a dose of 200-400 microgram/day of beclometasone (beclomethasone) or budesonide and 100-200 microgram/day of fluticasone propionate. Administer via a spacer device +/- a facemask. Children who have only virus-associated wheeze with no interval symptoms do not usually benefit from regular inhaled steroids. Always titrate down to the lowest dose of inhaled steroid required.

Step 3. Add on therapy: give inhaled short-acting $ß_2$ agonists as required. Give inhaled steroids at a dose of 400 microgram/day of beclometasone (beclomethasone) or budesonide and at 200 microgram/day for fluticasone propionate. Leukotriene receptor antagonists are licensed from 2 years upwards. No studies have been performed using long-acting $ß_2$ agonists in children under 4 years of age.

Step 4. Refer to specialist in paediatric respiratory care.

Stepping down: regularly review the possibility of stepping therapy down.

General comments: always consider the differential diagnosis in a young child with wheeze and cough. This is particularly important in children under the age of 2 years. Response to bronchodilators may be poor in this age group.

Maintenance asthma therapy of children 5–12 years

Step 1. Inhaled short-acting $ß_2$ agonists: inhaled short-acting $ß_2$ agonists, as short-term reliever therapy, should be used for all patients with symptomatic asthma. If needed more than once a day, move to Step 2.

Step 2. Introduction of regular preventive therapy: give inhaled short acting $ß_2$ agonists 'as required'. Inhaled steroids are the recommended preventive medicine for children, for achieving overall treatment goals. The threshold for introduction of inhaled steroids is not firmly established. Patients requiring short-acting $ß_2$ agonists more than 2-3 times per day should be treated with inhaled steroids, but patients with lower inhaler requirements may benefit. Consideration should also be given for frequent exacerbations; nocturnal asthma, or impaired lung function. Give 200-400 microgram/day of beclometasone (beclomethasone) or budesonide or fluticasone at 100-200 microgram/day. The child should be started on a dose of inhaled steroids appropriate to the severity of their disease and the dose titrated to the lowest dose at which effective control of asthma is maintained. Antihistamines and ketotifen are ineffective.

Step 3. Inhaled steroid plus long-acting $ß_2$ agonist: patients are already on as required $ß_2$ agonists plus inhaled steroid. At this step it is recommended that a trial of other treatments starting with a long-acting $ß_2$ agonist, is given prior to increasing the dose of the inhaled steroid. If there is no benefit, stop the long-acting $ß_2$ agonist and consider sequential trials of: a leukotriene receptor antagonist; a slow-release theophylline. If there is benefit but control is still inadequate, go to Step 4.

Step 4. Poor control on moderate dose of inhaled steroid plus add-on therapy: continue inhaled short-acting $ß_2$ agonists as required: continue add-on therapy from Step 3. Inhaled steroids may be increased to 800 microgram per day i.e. inhaled beclometasone or budesonide 800 microgram per day, or fluticasone 400 microgram per day via a spacer device. If control is incomplete, consider referring patient for specialist paediatric respiratory care. Go to Step 5.

Step 5. Addition of regular steroid tablets: refer to specialist in paediatric respiratory care if this is considered necessary. Prescribe daily oral steroid (usual practice is to give on alternate days if possible – e.g. prednisolone 10mg alternate days). Use in lowest dose that provides adequate control.

Give an inhaled short-acting ß₂ agonist as required with inhaled beclometasone or budesonide 800 microgram per day, or fluticasone 400 microgram per day via a spacer device. Patients may be tried on long-acting ß₂ agonists or leukotriene receptor antagonists or theophyllines. Some patients may benefit from higher doses of inhaled corticosteroids but such decisions should be made by specialist respiratory paediatricians.

Stepping down: stepping down therapy once asthma is controlled is recommended but not often implemented. Regular review of patients is important as they step down. The decision on which drug to step down first and at what rate needs to take into account the severity of the asthma, the side-effects of the treatment and the benefit achieved. Patients should be maintained at the lowest possible dose of inhaled steroid. Reduction in inhaled steroid dose should be slow as patients deteriorate at different rates. Previous guidelines have suggested that reduction should take place every 1-3 months by decreasing the dose by approximately 25-50% at each step.

Exercise–induced asthma
Immediately prior to exercise, an inhaled short-acting ß₂ agonist is the drug of choice.

In most patients, exercise-induced asthma is an expression of poorly controlled asthma and regular inhaled steroids are therefore recommended. If persistent exercise-induced symptoms occur in patients taking inhaled steroids, the following drugs may be considered:
☐ Long acting ß₂ agonists
☐ Leukotriene receptor antagonists
☐ Theophyllines.

Choice of inhaler devices for children under 5 years of age:

Device	1–3 years	3–5 years
MDI plus spacer and facemask	First	First
MDI plus spacer	Second	Second
Nebuliser	Third	Third
Breath-activated MDI	Avoid	Avoid
Dry powder inhalers –		
ß₂ agonists	Avoid	Not recommended
Corticosteroids	Avoid	Not recommended

Facemasks attached to spacers are usually required for children of 3 years and under but may also be needed in older children. Apply the mask firmly to the face to ensure there is no air leak. Giving medication to a young child who is crying will result in a lower dose of drug being inhaled.

When using a nebuliser, the mask should be held as close to the face as possible. Any gap will dramatically reduce the dose received.

Inhaled steroids should be administered via a spacer device. There are several spacer devices with masks available. The dose received varies between devices and age groups. Spacers are as effective, cheaper and less time-consuming than nebulisers for preventer and reliever therapy.

Adrenal suppression
Recent case reports have highlighted that adrenal suppression leading to adrenal crisis may occur in children receiving inhaled steroids. Symptoms and signs associated with adrenal suppression and crises may be under-recognised, particularly in children receiving higher than licensed doses of corticosteroids. NB: presenting symptoms of adrenal suppression and crisis are non-specific and include anorexia, abdominal pain, weight loss, tiredness, headache, nausea, vomiting, decreased levels of consciousness, hypoglycaemia and seizures. Situations that may potentially trigger acute adrenal crisis include infection, trauma, surgery or any rapid reduction in dosage.

CYSTIC FIBROSIS
Antibiotics
Patients with cystic fibrosis (CF) may develop repeated infections with *Staphylococcus aureus* and *Haemophilus influenzae* in the first few years of life. Ultimately more than 80% of patients become chronically infected (colonised) with *Pseudomonas aeruginosa*. Antibiotic therapy is aimed at treating these bacteria, but may need to be changed if less usual organisms (e.g. *Burkholderia cepacia*, *Stenotrophomonas maltophilia*) are isolated.

Oral antibiotics are given at higher doses and for longer periods to children with CF. Broad spectrum antibiotics, such as amoxicillin (amoxycillin), are used in children without Pseudomonas infection. A course of ciprofloxacin is prescribed at the first isolation of *Pseudomonas aeruginosa* (along with nebulised colistin), and further courses may be given at times of deterioration in chronically infected children. There is evidence that prophylactic flucloxacillin is beneficial in the first 2 years of life but there is currently no consensus as to how long to continue with it.

Nebulised. Three months, treatment of first isolates of *Pseudomonas aeruginosa* with oral ciprofloxacin, together with nebulised colistin has been shown to postpone, or reduce, the rate of chronic infection (colonisation). Nebulised colistin is used regularly in those with Pseudomonas. Other antibiotics, which may be nebulised, are tobramycin, gentamicin, ceftazidime and temocillin (particularly for *Burkholderia cepacia*). High-dose tobramycin (Tobi®) has been shown to increase lung function significantly when used on alternate months compared with placebo. All antibiotics are nebulised twice daily following physiotherapy. The first dose should be given under supervision and if there is bronchoconstriction, beta agonists should be given prior to nebulised antibiotics. There is no study to lead the clinician to prefer one nebulised antibiotic over another.

Intravenous. Infective exacerbations are usually treated with at least a 2 week course of intravenous antibiotics usually on an 'as required' basis but some patients benefit from regular 2 to 3 monthly intravenous courses. Some advocate routine 3 monthly intravenous antibiotics for all CF patients but this is not the policy in the UK. Two different classes of antibiotics are used to prevent resistance. The choice depends on bacteriological sensitivities but one is frequently an aminoglycoside. There is a trend towards using once daily aminoglycosides in CF but the results of clinical studies are awaited. Aminoglycoside levels are measured before and after the third dose. If colistin is used intravenously, renal function should be measured weekly.

ANTI-INFLAMMATORY THERAPY
Although it is debatable whether inflammation may be present without infection in CF, it is known that there is an overwhelming inflammatory process present in the lungs of even very young infants. Various treatment strategies have been considered to modify this process.

Corticosteroids
Inhaled steroids: the evidence is conflicting and a randomised study of inhaled steroid withdrawal in the UK has commenced. A clinical trial of inhaled steroids may be considered, especially in the atopic wheezy child with CF, but should be discontinued if there is no benefit.

Oral steroids: long-term alternate day steroids improve lung function but their benefits are outweighed by their side-effects. Short courses are indicated for acute wheeze and allergic bronchopulmonary aspergillosis. Intermediate courses are used for chronic steroid sensitive airflow obstruction. Oral steroids may also provide useful palliation in terminal care.

Ibuprofen. One randomised controlled trial showed this may be useful in CF. Side-effects are not uncommon, in particular, acute renal failure if the child is also given intravenous aminoglycosides.

Macrolides. There is growing interest in the anti-inflammatory properties of these antibiotics. They may be used for treatment of acute infective exacerbation. Some centres are using them as prophylaxis but their effects on antibiotic resistance and acquisition of *Pseudomonas aeruginosa* infection need to be determined. Their long-term safety has also to be established in CF patients.

Mucolytics
Neutrophil degradation results in large amounts of deoxyribonucleic acid (DNA) in CF sputum, which therefore becomes very viscous.

Dornase alfa (rhDNase/Pulmozyme®) lyses the DNA in sputum and is nebulised once a day at least one hour before physiotherapy. A trial for 1 to 3 months should be considered in any child older than 5 years who is chronically productive of sputum, compliant with conventional therapy and has forced expiratory volume in 1 second (FEV_1) of <70% predicted. An improvement in lung function of >10% is considered clinically beneficial. Alternate day therapy may be just as effective as daily treatment.

Hypertonic saline. This may be of benefit if dornase alfa therapy fails but it does require twice daily dosing.

Acetylcysteine (Parvolex®) and mesna (Mistabron®). Some centres use these drugs if treatment with the above mucolytics fails but evidence for benefit is lacking.

Bronchodilator therapy

Patients with CF often have episodes of bronchoconstriction necessitating the use of short-acting ß agonists. These partially reverse the bronchoconstriction and if beneficial should be used before physiotherapy to help mobilise secretions. They may however cause paradoxical worsening of lung function and so their effects need to be monitored. Occasionally, oral theophyllines or long-acting ß agonists are helpful. There is no evidence of long-term benefit for any bronchodilator. There is anecdotal evidence that subcutaneous terbutaline infusions may be useful if severe bronchoconstriction complicates an infective exacerbation.

ALLERGIC BRONCHOPULMONARY ASPERGILLOSIS (ABPA)

This is characterised by increasing breathlessness and wheeze, with pleuritic chest pain, and with no response to antibiotics. Aspergillus is often present in sputum, and blood tests show a high total immunoglobulin E (IgE), Aspergillus-specific IgE, and *Aspergillus precipitins*. There may be large wedge-shaped infiltrates on chest x-ray and skin prick tests are positive. ABPA is treated with oral steroids. A randomised controlled trial of ABPA in asthmatic adults showed benefit by adding itraconazole to oral steroids. But there are limited data in CF patients. Recent evidence suggests that itraconazole may increase systemic steroid side-effects by reducing clearance. Some have used nebulised amphotericin and long-term intravenous liposomal amphotericin in patients who are chronically infected with Aspergillus and not responding to standard ABPA treatment.

PANCREATIC ENZYME REPLACEMENT

More than 85% of patients with CF have pancreatic insufficiency. Proper dietary assessment is essential. There are many pancreatin preparations available. Capsules of enteric-coated pancreatin microspheres are commonly used, approximately one capsule per 3-4g of fat. For babies, the capsules can be opened and the microspheres mixed with apple sauce; start with half a capsule per feed and increase in half capsule increments (1/2 capsule of Creon 10,000®, Pancrease®, Nutrizym 10®, Nutrizym GR®). Pancreatin powder is rarely needed. Pancreatin is inactivated by stomach acid, so ranitidine or omeprazole may enable lower doses to be used. Due to concerns about the development of fibrosing colonopathy in patients on high-dose pancreatin, the Committee on Safety of Medicines recommends using no more than 10,000 lipase units/kg/day. It is important to optimise fat absorption and to avoid the possibility of distal intestinal obstruction syndrome or fibrosing colonopathy. Other diagnoses (e.g. coeliac disease) need to be considered if malabsorption continues.

FAT SOLUBLE VITAMINS

Absorption of the fat-soluble vitamins A, D, E and K is reduced. Patients are started on vitamin E and multivitamins at diagnosis. Vitamin K is used in patients with evidence of liver disease.

GASTRO-OESPHAGEAL REFLUX

This can occur in CF. Domperidone is used together with ranitidine. The use of the latter may reduce the number of pancreatic enzymes required. Alternative treatments include Gaviscon® Infant and low-dose erythromycin.

LIVER DISEASE

As children grow older their chance of liver disease increases. Most centres check liver function tests annually. If liver enzymes remain elevated after 6 months (+/- liver ultrasound changes) ursodeoxycholic acid, a bile acid, is commenced in an attempt to improve bile flow. There is little evidence-based information relating to the improvement in the natural history of CF related liver disease but the liver enzymes invariably fall within the normal range after commencement of urso. As with other causes of liver disease, vitamin K is given if there is any evidence of abnormal blood clotting.

DISTAL INTESTINAL OBSTRUCTION SYNDROME (DIOS)

If children with CF develop constipation they should be started on lactulose, and an adequate fluid intake given. If an intestinal obstructive picture develops, the use of oral Gastrografin® with or without rectal Gastrografin® can be helpful. Klean-Prep® is an alternative. Because these preparations are osmotic in action it is essential to ensure adequate hydration, particularly in babies who are prone to develop hypernatraemic dehydration. Oral acetylcysteine (Parvolex®) is used in some centres. The evidence base for all these therapies is poor. Once the acute episode is treated, it is important to institute a thorough review of the patient's diet and pancreatic enzyme intake.

CF-RELATED DIABETES MELLITUS

This is uncommon in young children but the prevalence increases with age. Some centres, at the annual clinical review, perform a glucose tolerance test from 10 years of age. Early abnormalities (blood glucose >9mmol/L at one hour but normal at 2hours) define 'glucose alert' highlighting that patient to be at high risk of developing CF-related diabetes. An abnormal blood glucose at 2hours probably warrants the commencement of insulin. Oral hypoglycaemic agents are rarely used.

SALT REPLACEMENT

In hot weather it is essential that dehydration and salt depletion are prevented in patients with CF. Patients who can swallow them are given sodium chloride tablets. Parents of younger children are advised to give salty snacks and a high fluid intake. Fluoride should be given if the local drinking water contains <300 microgram/L of fluorine.

BONE DISEASE

Low bone mineral density is found in some patients with CF. It is essential that patients have good nutritional support, normal vitamin D levels, and at least the normal dietary intake of calcium. Exercise may increase bone mineral density. There is some evidence that bisphosphonates such as disodium etidronate and disodium pamidronate may be beneficial in increasing bone mineral density although these medications have been reported to produce very severe bone pain during their treatment.

PUBERTY

This is often delayed. Testosterone and oxandrolone may be used to induce puberty and promote growth in males. Hormone replacement with oestrogen may be used in girls but in both sexes the delay in puberty is usually related to severe CF disease, poor nutrition and chronic chest infections.

ARTHROPATHY

Pain from CF arthropathy occurs in some children with cystic fibrosis and is often best controlled with NSAIDs. Other causes of arthropathy need to be excluded if pain persists.

UPPER AIRWAYS DISEASE

Nasal polyps occur in some patients. If symptomatic, treatment is with intra-nasal steroids but polypectomy is often required. Chronic sinusitis may occur. Long-term (4 weeks) antibiotics may be of benefit. Surgery is rarely required.

IMMUNISATIONS

In line with Department of Health guidelines an annual influenza immunisation (which confers 70-80% protection) is recommended from 6 months of age. As protective antibody levels may take up to 10-14 days to develop it is best given in October to early November. Those with anaphylaxis to egg products can be safely immunised in hospital. Routine immunisation against *Streptococcus pneumoniae* is not necessary because pneumococcus is not a common pathogen in the CF lung. If the vaccine is given, the protective effect lasts approximately 5 years. As with any child, it is important that children with CF have their routine immunisations.

Skin

UMBILICAL CORD

Most umbilical cords do not need any specific treatment other than keeping the area clean and dry with normal bathing. If the cord becomes sticky, as it usually does prior to separation, it is usually sufficient to clean the area with cotton wool moistened in cooled boiled water.

If the cord is very smelly, or the skin around it becomes red, then a swab should be taken for culture and consideration given to starting parenteral antibiotics. Antibiotics should be started if the redness is extending or there is induration of the skin.

Umbilical granulomas can be treated with topical silver nitrate. The surrounding skin should be protected from staining by application of Vaseline®.

CRADLE CAP

This occurs mainly in babies under 3 months of age and appears as thick yellow/orange scales on the scalp, particularly around the anterior fontanelle. It may spread and cover much of the body (seborrhoeic eczema). Often no treatment is required. It is self-limiting and causes no discomfort but a bland emollient (e.g. olive oil or aqueous cream) can be used. With increased parental anxiety or for children more severely affected, thick scaling can be removed by massaging coconut oil, emulsifying ointment, or a mixture of emulsifying ointment 25% in coconut oil into the scalp once or twice daily. Arachis (peanut) oil is probably best avoided in children under 5 years because of potential sensitisation leading to peanut allergy. Frequent shampooing and harsh brushing should be avoided.

HEAD LICE

If nits are seen, head lice infestation (pediculosis) should be confirmed by finding live lice before starting treatment with an insecticide. Automatic treatment of family members is unnecessary but contacts should have detection combing for live lice and then be treated if positive. Either alcoholic lotions or aqueous liquids of carbaryl or malathion can be used, but shampoos may not kill lice so are not recommended. Alcohol lotions can sting and give off fumes which may irritate very young children and those with asthma. Although one treatment application should suffice, a second application 7 days after the first is recommended because some eggs may survive. At least 50mL (100mL for thick hair) should be applied to the whole scalp and left on for at least 12 hours. Alternatively, permethrin is available as a cream rinse which can be washed off after 10 minutes. Resistance to insecticides can occur, but is rare with carbaryl. If one insecticide fails or reinfection occurs, a different one should be used.

Mechanical methods such as combing of hair soaked in conditioner, for about 30 minutes every fourth day, with a special 'nit comb' have the attraction of not using an insecticide but reports of benefit are anecdotal. They remain reasonable approaches when insecticides continue to fail or when families refuse insecticide treatment.

ACNE

Topical agents are sufficient for mild acne with superficial inflammation but may cause irritation. They work by removing sebum, bacteria and squames from the skin. Washing with soap and water is helpful. Benzoyl peroxide is very effective, but the patient must be warned that it may bleach coloured clothing. Excessive redness and peeling can be avoided by selecting a suitable concentration (2.5% increasing to 5% or 10%), frequency of application (alternate days to twice daily), and area of application (single spots to whole affected area). The topical retinoids, tretinoin 0.01% or 0.025% and isotretinoin 0.05% gel, are useful when comedones predominate (azaleic acid and the newer retinoid adapalene may be less irritant). Topical antibiotics (erythromycin, tetracycline and clindamycin) are probably no more effective than benzoyl peroxide, and may promote the emergence of resistant organisms.

Systemic treatment is required for widespread acne with substantial inflammation. Oxytetracycline or tetracycline taken in a single daily dose on an empty stomach for a minimum of 3 months and for as long as required (years if necessary) is commonly used and effective in many cases. They are contra-indicated in children under 12 years as they stain teeth. Erythromycin is similarly effective if oxytetracycline is contra-indicated or ineffective. Minocycline is better absorbed, but may cause irreversible pigmentation and a lupus-like syndrome with hepatitis. Cyproterone acetate given as the oral contraceptive Dianette® may be used for adolescent girls. Adolescents with severe or chronic acne unresponsive to the above, especially when deep inflammatory nodules and scarring are present, should be referred to a dermatologist for consideration of oral treatment with the vitamin A derivative isotretinoin orally.

Infantile acne requires treatment with oral erythromycin because topical agents are not well tolerated and oxytetracycline is contra-indicated in this age group.

PSORIASIS

Topical treatment of psoriasis is messy and time-consuming, and must not be made more burdensome than the condition itself. The aim should be relief of symptoms and embarrassment rather than complete clearance of all lesions at all times.

Chronic plaque psoriasis. Emollients relieve dryness, scaling, cracking and itching. They must be used liberally and often. Salicylic acid 2% added to an emollient facilitates the removal of scale. Tar preparations are moderately antipsoriatic but some children object to the smell. Calcipotriol, a vitamin D derivative, is an effective and cosmetically acceptable alternative to tar. It is irritant in some individuals, and absorption might theoretically lead to hypercalcaemia. Tacalcitol, a related substance, is downgraded by ultraviolet (UV) light so can only be applied at bedtime and topical calcitriol has no published data supporting its use in children under 12years. Dithranol, the most effective topical antipsoriatic agent, stains and is irritant, and is best used under skilled supervision. Adverse effects are minimised by using the 'short contact technique' (washing the cream off 20 minutes after application) and by starting at a lower concentration (0.1%) which may be increased cautiously every few days. Topical steroids should be avoided because of the risk of skin atrophy with long term use, and because they merely suppress rather than clear psoriasis. However, hydrocortisone 1% is sometimes used intermittently for short periods for facial or flexural psoriasis not responding to emollients alone, or where other antipsoriatic agents are too irritant. For intertriginous areas, hydrocortisone should be combined with an antibacterial and anti-candidal agent.

Guttate psoriasis is easily irritated and should be treated with emollients moving on to tar 5% if necessary. Sometimes hydrocortisone 1% (which can be combined with tar) is required to control itching or soreness.

Scalp psoriasis. Thick scaling must first be removed with oils (e.g. olive or coconut oil), salicylic acid, or combinations such as compound coconut ointment left in at least overnight to exert maximum effect. Tar, calcipotriol, dithranol and steroids are all available as scalp applications. Many are in an alcoholic base which improves cosmetic acceptability but can sting; for children, an aqueous base is therefore preferable.

Systemic therapy is used for severe psoriasis which is resistant to or intolerant of topical treatment, and should be initiated and supervised by a dermatologist. Treatments include phototherapy with UVB light, photochemotherapy with psoralen and UVA light (PUVA), acitretin, methotrexate and ciclosporin (cyclosporin).

ICHTHYOSIS

Topical treatment of ichthyosis is unrewarding. The application of emollients is messy and laborious and the benefit short-lived. Emollients must be applied liberally and frequently to have any effect. Greasier preparations are more effective, but less cosmetically acceptable. Penetration is enhanced by occlusion under tubular bandages. Some patients opt to apply a thick layer of ointment under bandages at night and a light cream or lotion during the day. There is a vast array of emollients available (see monograph on emollients) and the main determinant of efficacy is probably the quantity used.

Bathing emollients. Emulsifying ointment applied liberally to the skin before bathing or showering is probably more effective than oils added to the bath water. Detergents (bubble baths) must be avoided. Salicylic acid as a keratolytic improves the efficacy of emollients in ichthyosis, but may lead to toxicity through absorption. Urea is a hydrating agent.

Systemic treatment. Acitretin is very effective in some ichthyoses, but the condition relapses as soon as the drug is stopped. It is toxic (teratogenic, and affects serum lipids) and can only be prescribed by dermatologists.

Neonates with ichthyosis presenting as collodion membrane or harlequin ichthyosis should be coated liberally with liquid paraffin 50% with white soft paraffin 50%, to minimise loss of heat and fluid while awaiting a dermatological opinion.

EPIDERMOLYSIS BULLOSA

Neonates with blisters should be coated liberally with liquid paraffin 50% with white soft paraffin 50% to reduce friction and fluid loss while awaiting a dermatological opinion.

WARTS AND VERRUCAS

Warts are common, benign, self-limiting and usually asymptomatic, and treatments are not very effective. Wart applications work by (1) destroying warty tissue and (2) inflaming the lesions and breaking down infected cells, thereby exposing the immune system to the antigen. Treatments available include salicylic acid, glutaraldehyde, formaldehyde and podophyllum. These are all available as wart paints, which are applied daily to warts after rubbing off any superficial debris. Even duct tape has been used successfully. Children allergic to Elastoplast® will react to paints containing collodion. Formaldehyde lotion is used to soak large mosaic plantar warts. In addition to its direct action on the wart, it reduces sweating in the surrounding skin, discouraging further spread of the verrucas. Sensitisation can occur. Cryotherapy with dry ice or liquid nitrogen is a more aggressive and painful method of inflaming and destroying warts. A single treatment is rarely enough. More often, repeated fortnightly treatments are required, and patients often default before the warts have gone. Genital warts are treated with podophyllin paint, applied weekly by a trained nurse. It is an irritant and should only be applied to the warts, not to the surrounding skin, and should be washed off after 4 hours. It is fetotoxic and should not be handled during pregnancy. The management of genital warts includes considering the possibility of sexual abuse. Warts in immunosuppressed individuals will respond only to aggressive destructive measures. Adequate cryotherapy is very painful and should, if possible, be timed to coincide with another procedure requiring general anaesthesia.

Skin

SCABIES

Topical malathion and permethrin are both effective. Aqueous preparations are preferable to alcoholic lotions which sting excoriated skin. Persistence of symptoms after treatment is usually due to inadequate treatment or reinfection. Drug resistance has not been reported. When using malathion, the following rules must be explained to the patient:

☐ Apply the lotion to the whole body, from the neck down in adults and children, and including the head in infants

☐ Allow it to dry on the skin

☐ Leave the lotion on for 24 hours (if the hands are washed then more must be applied)

☐ Treat all contacts even if they are ill, pregnant, eczematous, very young, very old, or asymptomatic

☐ Treat everybody on the same day to avoid reinfection of the first-treated.

Norwegian (heavily crusted) scabies occurs in children who are immunosuppressed or immobile due to illness or disability. The antiscabetic agent should be applied daily for 3 days. Post-scabies itch can persist for several weeks after eradication of the mites. It may be relieved by topical crotamiton with or without hydrocortisone, and antihistamines.

IMPETIGO

This is usually due to penicillin-resistant *Staphylococcus aureus*. Minor infections can be treated with mupirocin ointment 3 times daily. Fusidic acid ointment should not be used for more than a few days because *Staphylococcus aureus* rapidly becomes resistant. More extensive infections require an oral anti-staphylococcal antibiotic such as flucloxacillin or erythromycin. Infections not responding to either of these should be swabbed for antibiotic-resistant *Staphylococcus aureus* or streptococci, and treated accordingly. Family contacts should be advised to add chlorhexidine to the bath and use their own towels.

TINEA (ringworm)

Specimens of scale, nail or hair should be sent for mycological examination before starting treatment, unless the diagnosis is certain.

Tinea corporis (body) and tinea pedis (athletes foot) respond to topical imidazoles (clotrimazole, econazole, miconazole, sulconazole, or terbinafine applied 2-3 times daily and continued for two weeks after the condition has cleared. Nystatin is less effective against tinea.

Tinea unguium (nails) may respond to topical amorolfine or tioconazole applied as a lacquer. Affected nails should be kept short. If it is resistant to topical treatments, symptomatic, and confirmed on mycological examination of nail clippings, systemic treatment can be considered. Griseofulvin is not very effective and treatment must be continued until the affected nail has grown out completely (up to 6 months for toenails). Terbinafine is more effective but not yet licensed in children. Previous marketing surveillance has not shown any evidence of greater problems in children than adults, but data are limited.

Tinea capitis (scalp) requires systemic treatment. Griseofulvin is usually effective. Mild infections may clear in 6 weeks, but most children require 3 months treatment. Children intolerant of griseofulvin can be treated with oral terbinafine or itraconazole (neither of which are licensed for use in children). All children in the family should use an antifungal shampoo (ketoconazole or selenium sulphide).

URTICARIA

Oral antihistamines. Histamine is not the only vasoactive mediator causing urticaria, so it is not surprising that treatment with antihistamines is not always effective. Different antihistamines act by different mechanisms, so it is worthwhile trying others if the first does not work. For an acute attack, chlorphenamine (chlorpheniramine) 6 hourly remains a good first choice. If sleep is disturbed by itching, it is logical to give a non-sedating antihistamine during the day (for example cetirizine or loratadine) and a sedating antihistamine at bedtime (such as hydroxyzine, promethazine or alimemazine (trimeprazine).

Topical agents. Topical antihistamines and local anaesthetics are ineffective and can cause sensitisation. Calamine lotion is soothing and safe. Calamine cream, oily calamine lotion or aqueous cream are preferable in children with eczema.

NAPKIN DERMATITIS

Occlusion must be minimised by frequent changes of napkin and avoiding waterproof pants. Leaving the napkin off for prolonged periods is ideal but rarely practical. At each napkin change the bottom should be washed with warm water and liberally coated with a barrier containing dimethicone, titanium dioxide, paraffins or zinc. The choice of ointment is less important than the frequency of changing. A napkin liner prevents the barrier cream from blocking the absorbency of disposable napkins. If thrush is suspected, a topical anticandidal such as nystatin or clotrimazole should be applied 4 times daily. If there is considerable inflammation and erosion, topical hydrocortisone may help. It should be applied sparingly twice daily for not more than a week, and should be combined with an anti-candidal and antibacterial agent (e.g. Nystaform-HC® cream or ointment, or Terra-Cortril Nystatin® cream). The barrier preparation must still be applied on top of the hydrocortisone.

PHOTOSENSITIVE DISORDERS

Topical agents. The Sun Protection Factor (SPF) indicates how much longer a sunscreen allows a person to stay in the sun before the skin begins to burn and becomes red. For example, SPF8 means that it takes 8 hours in the sun to develop erythema with the sunscreen compared with 1 hour without. Physical (i.e. reflective) sunscreens containing titanium dioxide or zinc provide excellent protection against all wavelengths of UV, but they are opaque, and therefore cosmetically unacceptable. All prescribable sunscreens now contain a proportion of titanium dioxide but it is in a micronised form that is much more cosmetically acceptable. Chemical (absorptive) sunscreens differ according to which wavelength of UV light they absorb most. Fair skinned individuals and those with vitiligo require protection against sunburn caused by the shorter (UVB) wavelengths, which are absorbed by aminobenzoates and cinnamates. Photosensitive dermatoses are often provoked by longer (UVA) wavelengths which are absorbed by dibenzoylmethanes. The benzophenones absorb both UVB and UVA, and most sunscreens contain a mixture of constituents. The SPF refers only to the burning (UVB) rays. Other factors to consider in selecting a sunscreen include the base (alcohol is less messy but may sting) and additives such as fragrance and parabens which may sensitise.

Oral agents. Beta carotene, mepacrine, and the antimalarials chloroquine and hydroxychloroquine are used in some photosensitive disorders.

ANTIPERSPIRANTS

Topical agents. aluminium chloride hexahydrate 20% in alcohol is available as a roll-on application suitable for axillae, palms or soles. It should be applied twice daily to washed and dried skin, but irritation often limits its use. Daily iontophoresis of tap water using a commercially available electrical device ('Drionic®') can be used to treat hyperhidrosis.

Oral agents. The anticholinergic agent propantheline reduces sweating, but causes unpleasant side-effects.

ATOPIC ECZEMA

Atopic eczema is common, affecting more than 10% of all children. Scratching is a constant feature which damages the skin and disrupts sleep. The dry, ichthyotic skin and the erythematous, lichenified patches look unpleasant. Assessment of treatment is complicated by the marked fluctuation in severity, which may vary from hour to hour. To doctors it is a skin disease, but to severely affected children it can be a disabling handicap. Children often dislike topical treatment. If the parent can do it, the best approach is a combination of firmness and the use of play techniques, such as painting a face on the child's skin with the cream or ointment before gently rubbing it in.

Damage from scratching. Distraction and a cool environment are the best remedies. Damage from scratching can be reduced by daily filing of the nails and by the use of cotton sleep suits which enclose the hands, or the use of cotton tubular bandage mittens at night. There is no drug that will control scratching in eczema. Sometimes the application of a simple emollient gives relief, although emollients have no specific antipruritic properties.

Sedative antihistamines such as alimemazine (trimeprazine), promethazine, or chlorphenamine (chlorpheniramine) have no known direct effect on the eczematous process and no effect on itching, but act by helping the child to fall asleep. Large doses are needed (see drug monographs for details). Morning drowsiness, which limits the use of bedtime sedatives in schoolchildren, can be minimised by giving the drug early in the evening (e.g. 5-6pm).

Emollients. Some degree of dryness of the skin is found in most cases. Emollients improve hydration of the skin by reducing evaporation, and emollient ointments may act as a barrier, protecting the skin from water at bathtime. Emollient ointments such as emulsifying ointment or white soft paraffin are more effective than emollient creams, and the absence of preservatives or stabilisers reduces the risk of irritation or contact sensitisation. However, some patients and parents prefer emollient creams such as aqueous cream. Patient preference is important; people are unlikely to use topical preparations which they strongly dislike. There is no evidence from controlled trials that expensive proprietary emollients are better than more cost effective generic emollients. Some children are helped by a regular bath once or twice a day, whereas others are better off avoiding baths and having an occasional shower. There is no evidence from controlled trials of benefit from bath oils. However, an application of emollient to the skin prior to a bath is sometimes helpful.

Skin

Topical steroids. The basic principles are to use ointment rather than cream preparations, and to use the least potent preparation as sparingly as possible. The first choice is hydrocortisone 1% ointment; it is uncommon for more potent preparations to be needed for children. When other steroid preparations are used, the potency must be checked. The different potencies of topical steroids cause confusion among doctors and parents alike. Many parents believe that topical steroids are dangerous, and any prescription must be accompanied by an explanation of the different potencies.

The major hazard of topical steroids is skin atrophy. This results from regular use of the more potent preparations, especially on the face. Severe and heavily lichenified patches of eczema (e.g. on hands, front of knees, ankles) may occur, particularly in older children. Such lesions may not respond well to mildly potent steroids, and the benefits of moderately potent preparations usually outweigh the risk of skin atrophy.

The larger the area of skin affected, and the more inflamed it is, the greater the risk of systemic absorption of a topical steroid. Thus there is a theoretical risk of iatrogenic Cushing syndrome with widespread application of topical steroids. However, the dearth of reported cases suggests that this is exceedingly rare. While atopic eczema is not a fatal condition, the resulting handicap and psychological damage can be severe. To withhold mild or moderately potent steroids in such patients for fear of side-effects is unreasonable. Growth impairment occurs in up to 10% of children with atopic eczema, but there is no evidence that use of mild or moderately potent topical steroids contributes to this, although the long-term use of potent or very potent preparations over large areas of skin can inhibit growth.

Tacrolimus, an immunosuppressive agent formulated as an ointment (0.03% for children aged 2-12 years and 0.1% for children over 12 years), is licensed for the treatment of moderate to severe atopic eczema in children who failed to respond adequately to conventional therapies. It is recommended that tacrolimus ointment should only be prescribed by dermatologists and physicians with extensive experience in the treatment of atopic eczema. Tacrolimus ointment 0.03% should be applied as a thin layer to the affected areas of skin, and may be used on any part of the skin (including the face, neck and flexures) until clearance occurs, when treatment should be discontinued. Tacrolimus ointment should be started at twice a day, and thereafter the frequency reduced until clearance is achieved. Occlusion should not be used. Tacrolimus ointment should not be applied to infected skin and users should be aware of the risk of spreading bacterial, herpes simplex, varicella-zoster and wart infections. Emollients should not be applied up to 2 hours before or after the use of tacrolimus. Exposure of the treated skin to sunlight should be avoided. Burning and stinging are very common side-effects, seen in about 40% of cases. The main advantage of tacrolimus ointment over topical steroids is that its use is not associated with skin atrophy. The disadvantage is that there is a dearth of information about the long-term use of this agent in children.

Complications
Bacterial infection.
The features suggesting secondary bacterial infection are pustules, crusting, a weeping discharge, or a sudden flare-up of eczema. Secondary bacterial infection is common. In mild cases the causative organism is *Staphylococcus aureus*, but in more severe cases, beta haemolytic streptococci are often also present. In infected eczema there are usually multiple scattered infected lesions, and treatment with an oral anti-staphylococcal antibiotic is essential. Because of the increasing incidence of antibiotic resistance in staphylococci, obtaining a skin swab for bacteriology is mandatory before starting antibiotic treatment. Oral flucloxacillin is the drug of choice, or a cephalosporin such as cefadroxil in cases of penicillin allergy. Erythromycin is less useful because of the increasing prevalence of resistant staphylococci. Strains of *staphylococcus* resistant to erythromycin, fusidic acid and flucloxacillin are increasing common in both the community and hospitals, and the antibiotic treatment of these strains must be discussed with a microbiologist. In some situations clindamycin may be appropriate, but in others a combination of two second-line anti-staphylococcal agents may be required.

A trial of oral anti-staphylococcal antibiotics should be considered for any child with a flare-up of atopic eczema. Topical antibiotics are avoided because of the widespread nature of the skin lesions, and the risks of sensitisation and resistance. Topical steroids should be continued. The role of antiseptic-corticosteroid combinations (e.g. clioquinol with hydrocortisone) is uncertain and parents must be warned that clioquinol causes permanent yellow-brown staining to white clothing. Recurrence of infection is common and difficult to prevent. Long-term anti-staphylococcal antibiotics are contra-indicated because of the inevitable rapid emergence of antibiotic-resistant staphylococci. Antiseptics in the bath water and the use of antiseptic hair shampoos are logical, but unproven strategies.

The increasing prevalence of methicillin-resistant *Staphylococcus aureus* (MRSA) often makes antibiotic treatment, particularly of recurrent infections, especially difficult. In children with recurrent relapses of eczema due to bacterial infection it is worth considering increasing the topical steroid therapy, because better control of the eczema in this way is likely to reduce the number of infective relapses.

Viral skin infection. Infection with the herpes simplex virus (HSV) causes vesicles in children with atopic eczema (eczema herpeticum). This is usually a self-limiting, if unpleasant problem, but occasionally secondary bacterial infection causes severe illness.

Treatment is aimed primarily at preventing secondary bacterial infection. For recurrences of HSV, this is all that is required. In severe cases of initial infection, when there is a high fever and general malaise, admission to hospital and intravenous treatment with the antiviral agent aciclovir are required. The need for oral aciclovir in less severe initial infections is unproven.

Vaccines and immunoglobulins

Vaccines and immunoglobulin preparations are used to prevent the development of certain infectious diseases. Occasionally, immunoglobulin preparations are used to modify the course of disease. For most preparations, official recommendations are based on advice received from the Joint Committee on Vaccination and Immunisation (JCVI). These recommendations are aggregated and published at intervals in book form and sent to all doctors and relevant nurses[1]. Urgent alterations and major changes are notified to professionals by way of CMO letters or Updates. Guidance is also given specifically on overseas travel by the World Health Organisation[2] and Department of Health[3]. Before giving a specific vaccine, the manufacturers data sheet should be consulted, but it must be borne in mind that the advice contained in them is often somewhat conservative and may have been overtaken by more recent research. Where the two conflict, advice from the JCVI should be followed.

Many vaccines are given routinely to all children unless there are specific contra-indications. Others are only given to children who are at significantly greater than average risk. The table sets out the routine schedule in operation in the United Kingdom from November 2001.

Current UK Immunisation Schedule – November 2001

AGE	VACCINE
8 weeks	Diphtheria/pertussis/tetanus/Hib (DTPHib)
	Meningococcal C
	Oral polio (OPV)
12 weeks	DTPHib, meningococcal C and OPV
16 weeks	DTPHib, meningococcal C and OPV
12–18 months	Measles/mumps/rubella (MMR)
Preschool	Diphtheria/tetanus/acellular pertussis (DTaP) and OPV
	MMR second dose, if not already given
10–14 years	BCG if Heaf test negative*
13–18 years	Low dose diphtheria/tetanus (Td) and OPV

*Not given in a few exceptional areas.

As millions of doses of vaccine are given each year, often to children of an age when fits are relatively common and neurodevelopmental anomalies are becoming apparent, it is no surprise that various adverse events have been recorded in association with vaccination. Studies and systematic reviews have shown that such events are either coincidental or only rarely caused by the vaccines. Parents, understandably, may be anxious about the advice given on immunisations. Time should be spent advising them of the risks and benefits of immunisation and addressing specific concerns.

CONTRA-INDICATIONS
Unless there are overriding clinical indications, all vaccinations are contra-indicated if the potential recipient is suffering from an acute illness, apart from a minor illness without fever or systemic upset, or has had a severe reaction to the vaccine or a constituent of it when administered previously. Other lesser reactions are not contra-indications. An existing stable neurological disorder such as cerebral palsy or Down syndrome is not a contra-indication for vaccination.

Live vaccines may be contra-indicated in individuals who are immunosuppressed. Any one of the following circumstances could fall into this category (For details see the RCPCH document *Immunisation of the*

Skin

Immunocompromised Child. http://www.rcpch.ac.uk/publications/recent_publications/Immunocomp.pdf).

☐ All patients currently receiving or recently completing courses of immunosuppressive therapy whether radiotherapy or chemotherapy.

☐ Children receiving prednisolone, orally or rectally, at a daily dose (or its equivalent) of 2mg/kg/day for at least 1 week, or 1mg/kg/day for 1 month.

☐ Anyone taking more than 40mg prednisolone per day for more than 1 week should be considered immunosuppressed. Lower doses of corticosteroids given in combination with cytotoxic drugs should also be considered immunosuppressive.

☐ Children who have had a bone marrow transplant.

☐ Patients with impaired cell mediated immunity.

☐ HIV -positive individuals (but see individual vaccines).

☐ Patients with minor deficiencies of antibodies are not at risk and those with major antibody deficiencies will be receiving antibodies to polio, measles, mumps and rubella as part of their immunoglobulin treatment.

Inactivated vaccines are not contra-indicated in individuals who are immunosuppressed, but the immunological response may be reduced and in some cases it may be appropriate to give further doses of vaccine depending on antibody measurements. However, interpretation of the results may be difficult.

These contra-indications will only apply to a small number of children. Advice should be sought from the consultant managing their underlying condition.

Vaccine supply

At the time of writing (October 2002), the supply of many vaccines and some immunoglobulin preparations is in a state of flux. It is important that prescribers make themselves aware of the current situation and note any variations in product characteristics.

Prematurity

There is little evidence for the efficacy of the routine vaccines in very premature babies when given according to the UK schedule of 2, 3 and 4 months. Most premature babies can be fully immunised using the routine schedule. The date of immunisation should be calculated from the child's actual date of birth, not from expected date of delivery. This may mean that some babies are immunised while they are still in special care or neonatal units. As the evidence is not yet conclusive, it has been suggested that in babies born at 28 weeks gestation or earlier, a blood test should be done after completing their immunisations to check that they do have adequate protection against Hib, Meningococcal C and hepatitis B.

1. Department of Health. *Immunisation against infectious disease.* London: HMSO, 1996.

2. *International Travel and Health.* Geneva: World Health Organisation, 2001.

3. *Department of Health. Health Information for Overseas Travellers.* London: The Stationery Office, 2001.

3,4–Diaminopyridine

Enhances neuromuscular transmission and is particularly useful in presynaptic disorders of neuromuscular transmission.

USES
Lambert-Eaton myasthenic syndrome, congenital myasthenia, myasthenia gravis and botulism.

PRESENTATION
Tablet: 20mg (scored) – named patient.

DOSAGE
Use of 3,4-diaminopyridine is largely experimental and experience is limited; a consultant paediatric neurologist should be consulted. Used in combination with pyridostigmine.

Route	Age		Frequency	Notes
	2–12 years	**12–18 years**	**(times daily)**	
Oral	≥ 6 years		3-4	Starting dose.
	5mg	5mg		Doses up to 100mg daily have been
	(maximum 10mg)	(maximum 20mg)		used in adults but are associated with
				a higher incidence of side-effects.
				Experience of use in children
				< 6 years is extremely limited.

ADMINISTRATION
Oral: taking the tablets with food can help prevent epigastric distress. Taking the last dose at least 2 hours before bedtime can prevent insomnia.

CONTRA-INDICATIONS & WARNINGS
There have been isolated reports of seizures in adult patients receiving 3,4-diaminopyridine. There is a theoretical risk of QT-interval prolongation.

INTERACTIONS, PREGNANCY, BREAST-FEEDING, POISONING/TOXICITY
No data available.

SIDE-EFFECTS
These would appear to be dose-related and have included light-headedness or heavy-headedness and fatigue. Many patients experience perioral and digital paraesthesia shortly after administration, lasting for 5-10 minutes. Perioral paraesthesia is made worse by taking on an empty stomach or concurrently with pyridostigmine. Some patients experience abdominal cramps and diarrhoea which are prevented by taking the dose with food or antacid. Difficulty with sleeping after the evening dose, rhinorrhoea, increased tear production and frequent micturition have also been reported. There have been a few reports of seizures in adult patients who had received 100mg per day. The patients had no further seizures when restarted on lower doses of 3,4-diaminopyridine.

PHARMACOKINETIC PROPERTIES
The onset of beneficial effects is usually noticed within 20-30 minutes of the dose. Duration of action is approximately 5 hours with peak activity between 90-120 minutes. Pyridostigmine potentiates the effect and prolongs the duration. Optimal response is reported 3-4 days after a dose change.

LICENSED STATUS
Not licensed for use in the UK.

FURTHER INFORMATION
Available from IDIS World Medicines.

5–Hydroxytryptophan

Provides exogenous source of amines.

USES
Treatment of amine deficiency in defects of tetrahydrobiopterin synthesis and dihydrobiopterin reductase (DHPR) deficiency.

A

PRESENTATION
Capsule: 20mg and 50mg – manufactured 'special'.

DOSAGE

Route	Age				Frequency (times daily)	Notes
	birth-1 month	1 month-2 years	2-12 years	12-18 years		
Oral	← 250-500 microgram/kg →				4	Starting dose. Dose then increased every 4–5 days to the maintenance dose.
	← 2-2.5mg/kg →				4	Maintenance dose.

Dose adjusted according to individual response.
Dose needs to be regularly reviewed and updated according to weight and CSF amine metabolic concentrations.

ADMINISTRATION
Oral: give at the same time as L-dopa (as co-careldopa). Give 30 minutes before main meals and at night. Adjustments in the timing of administration may need to be made according to individual response.

CONTRA-INDICATIONS & WARNINGS, INTERACTIONS, PREGNANCY, BREAST-FEEDING
No information available.

SIDE-EFFECTS
Side-effects are infrequent but nausea, fidgetiness and/or abnormal movements may be seen due to excess dopamine.

PHARMACOKINETIC PROPERTIES
Need to monitor CSF levels of amine metabolites.

EXCIPIENTS
Contact manufacturer for further details.

LICENSED STATUS
Available as 'specials' and as such are unlicensed.

FURTHER INFORMATION
20mg capsules available from Martindale Pharmaceuticals.
50mg capsules available from Special Products Limited.

Acetazolamide

Carbonic anhydrase inhibitor.

USES
Epilepsy (third choice treatment for partial seizures and refractory absence seizures), glaucoma, diuresis and raised intracranial pressure.

PRESENTATION
Capsule: (modified release) 250mg – Diamox® SR.
Injection: (as sodium salt) 500mg vial – Diamox®.
Oral liquid: may be extemporaneously prepared.
Tablet: 250mg – Diamox®.

DOSAGE

Indication	Route	Age				Frequency (times daily)	Notes
		birth-1 month	1 month-2 years	2-12 years	12-18 years		
Epilepsy	Oral/ IV bolus	← 2.5mg/kg →			250mg	2-3	Starting dose.
		← 5-7mg/kg →				2-3	Maintenance dose.
					250mg	2-4	Maximum dose: <12 years 750mg/day ≥12 years 1g/day.

DOSAGE continued

Indication	Route	Age				Frequency (times daily)	Notes
		birth–1 month	1 month–2 years	2–12 years	12–18 years		
Diuresis	Oral/IV bolus	←	5mg/kg	→	250–375mg	1	
Raised intracranial pressure	Oral/IV bolus	-	← 8mg/kg →		-	3	Initial dose. A gradual increase in dose may be required; doses of up to 100mg/kg/day have been used.
Glaucoma	Oral/IV bolus	←	5mg/kg	→	250mg	2-4	Maximum dose: <12 years 750mg/day ≥12 years 1g/day.
	Oral			-	250mg	1-2	Sustained release preparation.

Renal failure
No dose adjustment is required in patients with a creatinine clearance >20mL/minute/1.73m^2. If creatinine clearance 10-20mL/minute/1.73m^2 then reduce the frequency to twice daily, less than 10ml/minute/1.73m^2 avoid (as ineffective).

ADMINISTRATION
Oral: injection solution is alkaline but can be given orally.
IV: reconstitute each vial with 5mL Water for Injections, and administer as a bolus.

CONTRA-INDICATIONS & WARNINGS
Contra-indicated in situations in which sodium and/or potassium plasma levels are depressed, in cases of marked liver and kidney disease or dysfunction, suprarenal gland failure, and hyperchloraemic acidosis. Long-term use is contra-indicated in patients with chronic non-congestive closed-angle glaucoma. Avoid in patients with known sulphonamide hypersensitivity. Increasing the dose does not increase the diuresis and may cause increased incidence of paraesthesia and/or drowsiness. Patients on long-term therapy should be counselled to report any unusual skin rashes; blood cell counts and electrolytes may be monitored and if necessary, the drug discontinued.

INTERACTIONS
Carbamazepine and acetazolamide may be synergistic in partial (simple and complex) seizures. Possible increased risk of osteomalacia with *phenytoin*. Acetazolamide reduces excretion of *quinidine*.

PREGNANCY
Acetazolamide has been reported to be teratogenic and embryotoxic in animal studies. Although there is no evidence of these effects in humans, there are no adequate and well controlled studies in pregnant women and use in pregnancy should be avoided, especially during the first trimester.

BREAST-FEEDING
Acetazolamide has been detected in low levels in breast milk although it is unlikely that this will lead to any harmful effects in the infant.

SIDE-EFFECTS
Adverse effects during short-term therapy are usually non-serious and can include nausea, paraesthesia, thirst, polyuria, headache, fatigue, irritability and depression. Chronic adverse effects include metabolic acidosis, renal calculi and low white blood cell count.

POISONING/TOXICITY
There is no specific antidote. Treatment is supportive with correction of electrolyte and fluid balance.

PHARMACOKINETIC PROPERTIES
Absorption is complete after oral administration. Plasma half-life is 4-8 hours. Excreted unchanged in the urine. Plasma protein binding 70-90%.

EXCIPIENTS
Contact manufacturers for further details.

LICENSED STATUS
Glaucoma and diuresis are not licensed indications in children; raised intracranial pressure and epilepsy are not licensed indications.

Derivative of the naturally occurring amino acid L-cysteine. It is used to detoxify an intermediate paracetamol metabolite that is present in paracetamol overdosage. Also acts as a mucolytic.

A

USES
Treatment of paracetamol overdosage. Use in post-liver transplantation if lactate >2mmol/L at 4 hours or if concerns about graft function. Acute liver failure.
Mucolytic in the treatment of cystic fibrosis used occasionally when other mucolytics fail (use is controversial). Treatment of abdominal complications associated with cystic fibrosis (distal intestinal obstructive syndrome [DIOS]). Treatment of meconium ileus in newborn infants.

PRESENTATION
Injection: 20% (200mg in 1mL), 10mL ampoule – Parvolex®.
Granules: 100mg and 200mg sachets – named patient.

DOSAGE

Paracetamol Overdose
Newborn infants (birth to 1 month)
Acetylcysteine is unlikely to be required for use in newborn infants, but the dose would be based on body weight, as for patients in other age groups.

WARNING
1. Calculate the dose for each patient carefully and note that:
    Each millilitre of Parvolex® contains 200mg of acetylcysteine
    Each ampoule of Parvolex® contains 2g acetylcysteine.
2. Get your arithmetic checked before starting the infusion.

Child

Indication	Route	Age/Weight			Frequency	Notes
		under 12 years		12–18 years		
		<20 kg	>20 kg			
Treatment of paracetamol overdosage	IV infusion over 15 minutes	150mg/kg in 3mL/kg	150mg/kg in 100mL	150mg/kg in 200mL	single dose	May be used up to 24 hours after paracetamol overdose. After 24 hours seek guidance from a National Poisons Information Centre.
	then	then	then	then		
	IV infusion over 4 hours	50mg/kg in 7mL/kg	50mg/kg in 250mL	50mg/kg in 500mL	single dose	
	then	then	then	then		
	IV infusion over 16 hours	100mg/kg in 14mL/kg	100mg/kg in 500mL	100mg/kg in 1 litre	single dose	

See paracetamol monograph for graph showing treatment lines.
High risk treatment line to be used if patient is on liver enzyme inducing drugs (e.g. carbamazepine, phenytoin, phenobarbital (phenobarbitone), primidone, St John's Wort and rifampicin), chronic alcohol abuser or those with conditions causing glutathione depletion (e.g. malnutrition and HIV infection).

Other Indications
Newborn infants (birth to 1 month)

Indication	Route	Age	Frequency	Notes
		birth–1 month	(times daily)	
Meconium ileus	Oral (injection orally)	1–2mL	2–3	Of the 20% injection solution and dilute 1 in 4 to 50mg in 1mL – see administration.

Child

Indication	Route	Age			Frequency (times daily)	Notes
		1 month–2 years	2–12 years	12–18 years		
Mucolytic in cystic fibrosis patients	Oral (granules)	100–200mg	200mg	200–400mg	3	Use is controversial.
	Nebulised	←	3–5mL	→	2–4	Of the 20% injection solution and then dilute 1 in 2 to 100mg in 1mL
Treatment of distal intestinal obstructive syndrome	Oral (injection orally)	2–15mL	<7 years 10–15mL >7 years 20–30mL	20–30mL	single dose single dose	Of the 20% injection solution and then dilute 1 in 4 to 50mg in 1mL – see administration.
Post liver transplantation	IV infusion	←	100–150mg/kg/day	→	continuous over 24 hours	Use if lactate >2mmol/L at 4 hours post liver transplant or if concerns about graft function.
Acute liver failure	IV infusion	←	100mg/kg/day	→	continuous over 24 hours	See administration – higher concentration of glucose can be used as a diluent if patient is hypoglycaemic. Concentration maybe increased up to 50mg in 1mL if fluid restricted.

ADMINISTRATION

IV infusion: infuse in glucose 5%, if for any reason glucose is unsuitable, NaCl 0.9% may be substituted. A change in colour of solution to light purple has sometimes been noted and is not thought to indicate significant impairment of safety or efficacy. Monitoring of plasma potassium concentration recommended as hypokalaemia may occur. Acetylcysteine can be added to potassium-containing infusion fluids.

Oral: the granules should be dissolved in a glass of water before administration. The injection solution diluted to 50mg in 1mL (1 in 4 dilution) can be given orally but it is very bitter. Orange or blackcurrant syrup, or coca-cola, can be used to dilute the injection solution.

Inhaled: the injection solution diluted to 100mg in 1mL (1 in 2 dilution) with NaCl 0.9% can be nebulised.

CONTRA-INDICATIONS & WARNINGS

Contra-indicated if previous hypersensitivity to any of the ingredients. Use with caution in patients with asthma or a history of bronchospasm.

PREGNANCY

The limited data available on the use of acetylcysteine in pregnancy does not indicate that it is associated with an increased risk of fetal toxicity. It is important for the well-being of both the mother and the fetus that the mother should be detoxified as soon as possible after the overdose. If the blood levels of paracetamol indicate that acetylcysteine is required, withholding the antidote increases the risk of toxicity both for the mother and the fetus.

BREAST-FEEDING

No information available on the excretion of the drug into breast milk.

SIDE-EFFECTS

Anaphylactoid or 'hypersensitivity-like' reactions occur in up to 15% of patients. These include nausea, vomiting, flushing, urticarial rash, angioedema, tachycardia, hypotension, bronchospasm and rarely tachycardia or hypertension. These have usually occurred between 15-60 minutes after the start of the infusion and have usually been relieved by stopping the infusion. Occasionally antihistamines or corticosteroids are required. Once an anaphylactoid reaction is under control, the infusion can normally be restarted at the lowest infusion rate. Hypokalaemia and ECG changes have been noted in patients with paracetamol poisoning irrespective of the treatment given and monitoring of plasma potassium 12 hourly is therefore recommended.

PHARMACOKINETIC PROPERTIES

Following IV administration at the high rate of infusion, initial concentrations of the drug are reported to be very high (300-900mg/L have been reported). Concentrations fall rapidly and a mean steady state of 35mg/L is maintained after 12 hours. The plasma half-life on discontinuing infusion is 2-6 hours.

EXCIPIENTS

Contact manufacturers for further details. pH of Parvolex® is 6.5-7.5.

A

LICENSED STATUS
Licensed for use in children and adults for paracetamol overdosage.
Other indications are not licensed.

FURTHER INFORMATION
For information on treating late presentation (>24 hours) of paracetamol overdose contact local National Poisons Information Centre. Acetylcysteine granules are available from IDIS World Medicines.

Aciclovir (acyclovir)

A synthetic purine nucleoside analogue with *in vitro* activity against herpes viruses.

USES
Aciclovir is an antiviral indicated for the treatment of herpes simplex and varicella-zoster viruses and prophylaxis of herpes simplex in immunocompromised patients.

PRESENTATION
Cream: 5% – Zovirax® and non-proprietary.
Eye ointment: 3% – Zovirax®.
IV infusion: 250mg and 500mg – Zovirax® and non-proprietary; 1g – non-proprietary.
Suspension: 200mg in 5mL and 400mg in 5mL – Zovirax®.
Tablet (dispersible): 200mg, 400mg and 800mg – Zovirax® and non-proprietary.
Tablet: 200mg, 400mg and 800mg – non-proprietary.

DOSAGE
The cream and ophthalmic ointment may be used 5 times daily for herpes simplex infection and herpes simplex keratitis respectively of the skin. Continue the eye ointment for 3 days after healing.

Newborn infant (birth to 1 month)

Route	Age		Frequency (times daily)	Notes
	Up to 7 days	Over 7 days		
IV infusion	← 10mg/kg →		3	Usually for 10 days.

Child – Herpes simplex virus treatment

Route	Age			Frequency (times daily)	Notes
	1 month–2 years	2–12 years	12–18 years		
Oral	100mg	← 200mg →		5	Normal immune states.
	200mg	← 400mg →		5	Severely immunocompromised or with reduced absorption.
IV infusion	<3 months 10mg/kg	250mg/m²	5mg/kg	3	Normal immune status.
	3 months–2 years 250mg/m²			3	
	<3 months 10mg/kg	500mg/m²	10mg/kg	3	Immunocompromised.
	3 months–2 years 500mg/m²			3	

Herpes simplex prophylaxis

Route	Age			Frequency (times daily)	Notes
	1 month–2 years	2–12 years	12–18 years		
Oral	100mg	← 200mg →		4	Herpes simplex prophylaxis.
	200mg	← 400mg →		4	Severely immunocompromised.

Chickenpox and shingles treatment

Route	Age			Frequency	Notes
	1 month–2 years	2–12 years	12–18 years	(times daily)	
Oral	←	DOSE BY WEIGHT	→		Use IV route in immunocompromised
		20mg/kg		4	children for at least 5 days first.
	DOSE BY AGE	DOSE BY AGE	DOSE BY AGE		
		2–5 years			
	200mg	400mg		4	
		6–12 years			
		800mg		4	
			800mg	5	
IV Infusion	≤3 months	250mg/m²	5mg/kg	3	Normal immune status.
	10mg/kg				
	3 months–2 years				
	250mg/m²			3	
	≤3 months	500mg/m²	10mg/kg	3	Immunocompromised.
	10mg/kg				
	3 months–2 years				
	500mg/m²			3	

Dose adjustment in renal or liver failure

In mild renal impairment give a dose every 12 hours. In moderate impairment (creatinine clearance 10-50mL/minute/1.73m²) give one dose once daily and in severe impairment (creatinine clearance <10mL/minute/1.73m²) give 50% of dose once daily. Monitor urea and creatinine.

ADMINISTRATION

IV: reconstitute to 25mg/mL or may be diluted further to 5mg/mL with NaCl 0.9% or glucose 5%. Peripheral administration – use 5mg/mL only and infuse over at least 1 hour. Central line administration – 25mg/mL may be given if fluid restricted, administer via a syringe pump over a minimum of 1 hour. Displacement volume negligible. Not given by IV bolus to avoid crystallisation in the renal tubules and a rapid increase in blood urea and creatinine levels.

CONTRA-INDICATIONS & WARNINGS
Contra-indicated in patients hypersensitive to aciclovir. Polyuric renal failure has occurred with high doses therefore ensure adequate hydration and avoid dehydration.

INTERACTIONS
May produce extreme lethargy with *zidovudine*. Increased levels and risk of toxicity with *probenecid* and *cimetidine*. Risk of renal damage is increased with the concurrent use of other *nephrotoxic drugs*.

PREGNANCY
Limited data – use must outweigh risk to fetus. Contact local Medicines Information Centre for advice.

BREAST-FEEDING
Excreted in breast milk therefore use with caution in nursing mothers.

SIDE-EFFECTS
Severe local inflammatory reactions and phlebitis have occurred at the site of injection. Reversible neurological reactions have been reported.

POISONING/TOXICITY
Adequate hydration is essential to reduce the risk of crystal formation in the urine. Aciclovir can be removed by haemodialysis.

PHARMACOKINETIC PROPERTIES
Most of the drug is excreted unchanged in the urine. Tubular secretions contribute to the renal excretion of the drug. Plasma protein binding is low. Plasma half-life is about 2-9 hours.

EXCIPIENTS
Each 250mg of powder contains 1.1mmol of sodium. Aciclovir liquid is sucrose free.

LICENSED STATUS
Oral treatment and prophylaxis of varicella-zoster and treatment of herpes simplex in immunocompromised children are unlicensed uses.

FURTHER INFORMATION
The use of the oral route in neonates is based on anecdotal evidence and the pharmacokinetics are uncertain.

Synthetic derivative of vitamin A that reverses hyperkeratotic and metaplastic skin changes in psoriasis and ichthyosis.

USES
Severe psoriasis resistant to other forms of therapy and ichthyosis.

PRESENTATION
Capsule: 10mg, 25mg – Neotigason®.
Oral suspension: can be extemporaneously prepared.

Use only under the supervision of a consultant dermatologist.
Not recommended for children except in exceptional circumstances; sometimes used in Harlequin ichthyosis in neonates which is a very specialised use and a consultant dermatologist should be consulted.

Maximum duration of continuous treatment is 6 months.

DOSAGE

Route	Age	Frequency	Notes
	12–18 years	(times daily)	
Oral	500 microgram/kg	1	Occasionally doses up to 1mg/kg daily are needed up to a maximum of 35mg daily for limited periods.

ADMINISTRATION
Oral: to be taken once daily with meals or milk.
The capsules should not be opened by women who are or may become pregnant, when a suspension is prepared. A suspension should only be prepared if strictly necessary e.g. when acitretin is to be used to treat a neonate with Harlequin ichthyosis.

CONTRA-INDICATIONS & WARNINGS
Do not use in hepatic or renal impairment.
A bone scan is recommended before treatment is started; monitor for any abnormalities of musculoskeletal development. Liver function and fasting blood lipids to be monitored initially and thereafter at 3 monthly intervals.

INTERACTIONS
Tetracyclines: possible increased risk of benign intracranial hypertension.
Methotrexate: plasma concentration increased with acitretin.
Vitamin A preparations: risk of hypervitaminosis A.

PREGNANCY/BREAST-FEEDING
Contra-indicated: acitretin is a known human teratogen. Pregnancy must be first excluded and then prevented throughout treatment and then avoided for 2 years after cessation of treatment.

SIDE-EFFECTS
Dryness of mucous membranes, skin, conjunctiva, reversible hair thinning and alopecia, myalgia and arthritis, photosensitivity, hyperlipidaemia. See manufacturers SPC for further details.

POISONING/TOXICITY
Acute vitamin A toxicity symptoms, e.g. severe headache, nausea, vomiting, drowsiness, irritability and pruritus. Symptoms will subside without treatment. Gastric lavage recommended.

PHARMACOKINETIC PROPERTIES
Peak plasma levels achieved within 1–4 hours. Elimination half-life 2 days. May metabolise to etretinate which has elimination half-life of 120 days due to deposition in adipose tissue.

EXCIPIENTS
See manufacturers SPC for further details..

LICENSED STATUS
Only for use in children in exceptional circumstances.

FURTHER INFORMATION
Specialist dermatological supervision only. Available to hospital pharmacies and specified retail pharmacies only.

A powerful adsorbent and is used to prevent absorption of poisons or to interrupt their enterohepatic circulation.

USES
The oral administration of activated charcoal can both reduce absorption and enhance elimination of toxins. Single doses and (less commonly) multiple doses are given to reduce absorption of toxins from the gut. Multiple oral doses enhance the elimination of some toxins from the blood.

PRESENTATION
Powder: 25g, 50g – Carbomix®.
Granules: 5g sachet – Medicoal®.
Oral suspension: 50g – Actidose-Aqua® Advance; 50g – Charcodote®.

DOSAGE
The dose of activated charcoal in children is related more to the dose of poison than to the age or weight of the child. When the weight (amount) of poison is known, 10 times that amount of activated charcoal can be given. If amount unknown give dose as in table. If in any doubt contact a National Poisons Information Centre.

Route	Age			Frequency	Notes
	1 month–2 years	2–12 years	12–18 years	(times daily)	
Oral	DOSE BY WEIGHT				Single dose treatment (see USES).
	←	1g/kg	→	single dose	In most cases, charcoal should be given
	DOSE BY AGE				within one hour of ingestion.
	-	25–50g	50g	single dose	
	DOSE BY WEIGHT				Multiple dose treatment (see USES).
	←	500mg - 1g/kg	→	4 hourly	Ideally continue until features of toxicity have
	DOSE BY AGE				resolved or until adverse effects of the charcoal
	-	25–50g	50g	4 hourly	make continued administration impracticable.

ADMINISTRATION
None of the preparations are readily accepted by patients. Palatability may be improved by adding blackcurrant cordial or flat cola immediately prior to administration. Compliance may also be improved by placing the activated charcoal in a covered cup and drinking through a straw.

CONTRA-INDICATIONS & WARNINGS
Because of the risk of aspiration, charcoal should never be given to a child with an absent gag reflex or impaired consciousness unless the airway is first protected by an endotracheal tube. Aspiration of charcoal has been reported to cause airway obstruction.

INTERACTIONS
Charcoal will adsorb most drugs – concurrently administered drugs should be given via the parenteral route.

PREGNANCY/BREAST-FEEDING
Insufficient data, but it is pharmacologically inert and is not absorbed from the gastrointestinal tract. No hazard is therefore anticipated.

SIDE-EFFECTS
Unpalatable, black stools, some patients may experience constipation or diarrhoea. Aspiration of activated charcoal may cause airway obstruction.

PHARMACOKINETIC PROPERTIES
Not absorbed from the gut and is eliminated in the faeces or by vomiting. Pharmacologically inert – a powerful adsorbent.

EXCIPIENTS
Actidose-Aqua® includes sucrose. See manufacturers SPC for further details.

LICENSED STATUS
Licensed for use in children and adults.

FURTHER INFORMATION
Povidone in Medicoal® may cause aspiration pneumonitis.

Retinoid-like drug possibly less irritant than other topical retinoids.

USES
Mild to moderate acne where comedones, papules and pustules predominate.

PRESENTATION
Cream: 0.1% – Differin®.
Gel: 0.1% – Differin®.

DOSAGE/ADMINISTRATION
Topical: wash and dry affected area and apply a thin film before bedtime.
Physician should assess if there is continued improvement after 3 months treatment.

CONTRA-INDICATIONS & WARNINGS
Hypersensitivity to any ingredient of the product. Avoid eyes, lips, angles of nose and mucous membranes. Best suited for use on dry and fair skin. Exposure to ultraviolet irradiation or excessive sunlight should be avoided.

INTERACTIONS
None known but other retinoids or drugs with similar mode of action should not be used concurrently.

PREGNANCY
Should not be used in women of childbearing age unless on effective contraception.

BREAST-FEEDING
Avoid contact exposure of the infant when feeding. Application to the chest should be avoided.

SIDE-EFFECTS
Skin irritation and stinging.

EXCIPIENTS
See manufacturers SPC for further details.

LICENSED STATUS
Licensed for ≥12 years of age.

Additrace®

USES
As part of a complete IV nutrition regimen providing a source of trace elements for children >40kg.

PRESENTATION
Solution: trace elements (traces of Fe^{3+}, Zn^{2+}, Mn^{2+}, Cu^{2+}, Cr^{3+}, Se^{4+}, Mo^{6+}, F^- and I^-), 10mL ampoule – Additrace® (see manufacturers SPC for further details).

DOSAGE
0.2mL/kg up to a total dose of 10mL. Where higher doses are considered necessary, up to 20mL may be administered daily in at least 1L of fluid. Where not administered as part of an IV feed give in a compatible IV fluid, e.g. glucose 5%, over not less than 2 hours to minimise renal losses. Maximum administration time 24 hours.

ADMINISTRATION
As part of a PN regimen.

CONTRA-INDICATIONS AND WARNINGS
Injection should not be given undiluted. *Caution*: impaired liver function especially cholestasis (monitor manganese levels), impaired renal function and fructose intolerance.

PHARMACOKINETIC PROPERTIES
Excreted both by biliary route (manganese) and renally.

LICENSED STATUS
Licensed for use in adults and children >40kg body weight.

Slows conduction through the AV node.

USES
Antiarrhythmic to terminate supraventricular tachycardia (SVT) and to elucidate mechanism of tachycardia.

PRESENTATION
Injection: 3mg in 1mL, 2mL vial – Adenocor® and 10mL vial for infusion – Adenoscan®.

DOSAGE

Route	Age				Frequency	Notes
	birth–1 month	1 month–2 years	2–12 years	12–18 years		
IV bolus	← 50 microgram/kg →			3mg	single dose	Initial dose.
	increase after 2 minutes			increase after		
	if necessary to			2 minutes if		Subsequent doses if required,
	← 100 microgram/kg →			necessary to 6mg		as shown.
						Increments should not be
	Increase further in 50 microgram/kg			Increase after a		given if high level AV block
	increments at 2 minute intervals until			further 2 minutes		develops at any particular
	tachycardia terminated or to a maximum dose of:			if necessary		dose.
	300 microgram/kg <1 month			to 12mg		
	or 500 microgram/kg >1 month.					

ADMINISTRATION
IV injection: give into central or large peripheral vein over 2 seconds, with cardiac monitoring, followed by rapid IV flush with NaCl 0.9%.

CONTRA-INDICATIONS & WARNINGS
Second or third degree heart block, AV block, sick sinus syndrome and asthma. Beware of torsades de pointes in child with prolonged QT interval.

INTERACTIONS
Effect enhanced with *dipyridamole*, if need to use adenosine, reduce the dose of adenosine by factor of 4. Effect antagonised by *theophylline/xanthines*.

PREGNANCY/BREAST-FEEDING
No data available. However, no effect on the fetus would be expected. Contact local Medicines Information Centre for advice.

SIDE-EFFECTS
Transient facial flushing, chest pain, dyspnoea, bronchospasm, choking, nausea and light-headedness occur commonly. Severe bradycardia has been reported.

POISONING/TOXICITY
The half-life in blood is very short, hence duration of toxic effects likely to be limited.

PHARMACOKINETIC PROPERTIES
Very short half-life (less than 10 seconds).

EXCIPIENTS
See manufacturers SPC for further details.

LICENSED STATUS
Not licensed for use in children.

Adrenaline (epinephrine)

Direct-acting sympathomimetic agent exerting its effect on both alpha and beta adrenoreceptors.

USES
CPR, acute anaphylaxis, croup and low cardiac output.

A

PRESENTATION

Injection: 1 in 10,000 (100 microgram in 1mL), 10mL ampoule – non-proprietary; 1mL and 10mL prefilled syringe – non-proprietary; 3mL and 10mL disposable syringe – Min-I-Jet® Adrenaline.

Injection: 1 in 1000 (1mg in 1mL) 0.5mL, 1mL, 2mL, 5mL and 10mL ampoule – non-proprietary; 1mL prefilled syringe (for IM or SC) – non-proprietary; 1mL disposable syringe (for IM) – Min-I-Jet® Adrenaline; 1mL disposable syringe (for SC) – Min-I-Jet® Adrenaline.

IM injection for self-administration: 300 microgram, single dose pen — Anapen® 0.3mg, EpiPen® Auto-injector 0.3mg. 150 microgram, single dose pen – Anapen® Junior 0.15mg, Epipen® Jr Auto-injector 0.15mg.

SC or IM injection for self-administration: 300 microgram, prefilled syringe delivers 2 doses of 300 microgram or can be adjusted to administer smaller doses for children – named patient, Ana-Guard®.

DOSAGE

Newborn infant (birth - 1 month)

Indication	Route	Age	Frequency	Notes
		birth–1 month		
Cardio-pulmonary resuscitation (CPR)	IV/ endotracheal tube (ETT)	10 microgram/kg (0.1mL/kg of 1 in 10,000)	initial dose	Endotracheal route is accepted but has unproven effectiveness in resuscitation at birth.
		10-30 microgram/kg (0.1-0.3mL/kg of 1 in 10,000)	subsequent doses	

Child

Indication	Route	Age				Frequency	Notes
		birth–1 month	1 month–2 years	2–12 years	12–18 years		
Cardio-pulmonary resuscitation (CPR)	IV rapid bolus/ intraosseous	-	10 microgram/kg (0.1mL/kg of 1 in 10,000)		1mg (10mL of 1 in 10,000)	initial and usual subsequent dose	If given by intraosseous route, flush with NaCl 0.9%.
		-	100 microgram/kg (0.1mL/kg of 1 in 1000 or 1mL/kg of 1 in 10,000)		5mg (5mL of 1 in 1000)		Maximum dose is 5mL of 1 in 1000. Subsequent doses in exceptional circumstances e.g. arterial monitoring, septicaemia, anaphylaxis.
	Endotracheal tube (ETT)	-	100 microgram/kg (0.1mL/kg of 1 in 1000 or 1mL/kg of 1 in 10,000)		5mg (5mL of 1 in 1000)	initial dose	
Acute anaphylaxis	Deep IM	← 10 microgram/kg (0.01mL/kg of 1 in 1000) →			0.5–1mg (0.5–1mL of 1 in 1000)	single dose	Repeat at 5 minute intervals if necessary according to clinical response.
Low cardiac output	IV infusion	← 10 nanogram – 1 microgram/kg/minute →				continuous	Start at lower doses.
Croup	Nebulised	← 1-5mL of 1 in 1000 →			-	single dose	Produces a transient improvement, rarely alters the long-term course of the illness. Observe closely with ECG and oxygen saturation monitoring.

A

ADMINISTRATION
ETT: inject quickly down a narrow-bore suction catheter beyond the tracheal end of the endotracheal tube and then flush with 1-2mL NaCl 0.9%.
IV: do not use if injection is discoloured or has a precipitate. For IV infusion can dilute with NaCl 0.9% or glucose 5%. Inactivated by sodium bicarbonate.
Nebulised: larger volumes of 3-5mL used undiluted and smaller volumes can be diluted to 2-3mL with NaCl 0.9%.

CONTRA-INDICATIONS & WARNINGS
More susceptible to arrhythmia if taking tricyclic antidepressants. May lose blood sugar control in diabetic patients.

INTERACTIONS
Risk of arrhythmia with *volatile anaesthetics*. Severe hypertension with *beta-blockers* and *doxapram*.

PREGNANCY/BREAST-FEEDING
Not applicable in a life support situation. However, there is some evidence of a slightly increased risk of fetal abnormalities and it will have fetal cardiac effects.

SIDE-EFFECTS
Tremor, tachycardia, arrhythmia and cold extremities. Headache, dizziness, nausea and vomiting.

POISONING/TOXICITY
Overdose may cause cardiac arrhythmia, cerebral haemorrhage and pulmonary oedema. Treatment is symptomatic and supportive.

PHARMACOKINETIC PROPERTIES
Rapidly metabolised and then excreted in the urine.

EXCIPIENTS
Contact manufacturers for further details.

LICENSED STATUS
1:10,000 injection ampoule (Martindale Pharmaceuticals) is licensed for the treatment of children and adults with acute anaphylaxis when the IM route has been ineffective. 1mL prefilled syringe (CPR) licensed for CPR for <12 years of age. 10mL prefilled syringe is licensed for the treatment of >12 years of age for CPR and all ages with acute anaphylaxis when the IM route has been ineffective. Min-I-Jet® 1:10,000 is licensed for CPR in children and adults.
1:1000 injection ampoule (Martindale Pharmaceuticals) is licensed for the treatment of anaphylactic reactions, as a vasopressor in anaphylactic shock, as a cardiac stimulant and as a bronchodilator for ≥1 year of age. 1mL prefilled syringe (IM or SC) is licensed for treatment of anaphylaxis or acute allergy in all ages. Min-I-Jet® 1:1000 is licensed for emergency treatment of anaphylaxis or acute angioneurotic oedema with airway obstruction, or acute allergic reactions for >12 years of age.
Anapen® 0.3mg and EpiPen® Auto-injector 0.3mg are licensed for use in >30kg as an IM injection for self-administration. Anapen® Junior 0.15mg and Epipen® Jr Auto-injector 0.15mg are similarly licensed for use in children 15-30kg.
Ana-Guard® is not licensed in UK.

FURTHER INFORMATION
Ana-Guard® is available from IDIS World Medicines.

Albendazole

Anthelmintic.

USES
Treatment of hydatid cysts caused by *Echinococcus granulosus* or *E. multilocularis*. First-line medical therapy or as adjunct to surgery either pre- or post-operatively.
Treatment for large roundworm, hookworm, *Strongyloides stercoralis*, threadworm, whipworm, trichinosis, tapeworm cysticercosis, cutaneous larva migrans and toxocariasis.

PRESENTATION
Tablet: 200mg, 400mg – Zentel® (imported).
Tablet: 400mg (chewable) – Zentel® (imported).
Suspension: 200mg in 5mL – Zentel® (imported).

A

DOSAGE

Indication	Route	Age		Frequency	Notes
		2-12 years	12-18 years	(times daily)	
Whipworm, threadworm, hookworm, large roundworm	Oral	← 400mg →		single dose	Treatment may be repeated in 2-3 weeks for threadworms.
Strongyloides stercoralis	Oral	← 400mg →		1 for 3 days	Treatment may be repeated after 3 weeks if necessary
Trichinosis	Oral	← 400mg →		1 for 5 days	Repeat if necessary.
Tapeworm	Oral	← 400mg →		1 for 3 days	
Neurocysticercosis	Oral	← 7.5mg/kg (maximum 400mg) →		2 for 14-28 days	Take with food. Repeat as necessary. Treatment should be initiated under steroid cover. Use prednisolone 1.5mg/kg daily (maximum 60mg per day). Anticonvulsant cover may be required. In young children raised intracranial pressure may be a problem and a shunt may be needed. Maximum dose in adults should not exceed 400mg twice daily.
Hydatid disease (echinococcosis)	Oral	← 7.5mg/kg (maximum 400mg) →		2 for 28 days	Take with food. Treatment should be followed by 14 drug-free days and then repeated for up to 2-3 cycles.
Cutaneous larva migrans	Oral	← 400mg (see notes for children <2 years) →		daily for 5 days	For children <2 years give 10mg/kg twice daily for 5 days.
Toxocariasis	Oral	10mg/kg (maximum 400mg)	400mg	2 for 5 days	Steroid cover for symptomatic cases, especially if ocular involvements (see above for doses).

ADMINISTRATION

Oral: absorption increased when administered with fatty foods. For systemic infections, take with food. For intestinal parasites, take before food. Chewable tablets may be crushed, chewed or swallowed whole.

CONTRA-INDICATIONS & WARNINGS
Pregnancy or women of childbearing age not protected by non-hormonal contraception for duration of treatment and 1 month post-cessation. Can elevate liver enzymes and cause haematological changes. Baseline LFTs and blood counts recommended; repeat at least twice during treatment cycle.

INTERACTIONS
Induces cytochrome P450 system of liver, therefore theoretical risk of interaction with *theophylline, anticoagulants, anticonvulsants, oral contraceptives* (use non-hormonal contraception) and *oral hypoglycaemics*. Plasma concentrations of albendazole reported to be raised by concurrent administration of *dexamethasone, praziquantel* and *cimetidine*.

PREGNANCY
Shown to be teratogenic in some animal species. Contra-indicated in pregnancy or women of childbearing age not protected by non-hormonal contraception.

BREAST-FEEDING
Contact local Medicines Information Centre for advice.

SIDE-EFFECTS
Gastrointestinal upset, headache, dizziness, alopecia, haematological (leucopenia/pancytopenia) and elevation of liver enzymes (in up to 15% of cases).

POISONING/TOXICITY
No experience of overdosage. No specific antidote; treatment is symptomatic and supportive as required.

PHARMACOKINETIC PROPERTIES

Poorly absorbed from the gastrointestinal tract, but rapidly undergoes extensive first-pass metabolism. The principal metabolite, albendazole sulphoxide has anthelmintic activity and plasma half-life of about 8.5 hours. This and other metabolites appear to be primarily eliminated in bile.

EXCIPIENTS

Contact manufacturer for further details.

LICENSED STATUS

Not licensed for use in the UK.

FURTHER INFORMATION

Available from IDIS World Medicines.

Alendronic acid (sodium alendronate)

An aminobisphosphonate.

USES

Alendronic acid may be of use in the following conditions: steroid-induced osteoporosis, immobilisation osteoporosis e.g. high-spinal injury and cerebral palsy, idiopathic juvenile osteoporosis, juvenile idiopathic arthritis, osteogenesis imperfecta.

PRESENTATION

Tablet: (as alendronate sodium) 5mg and 10mg – Fosamax®.

DOSAGE

Experience in the use of bisphosphonates in children is limited; expert advice should be sought and the drug should be used only in specialist centres experienced in its use.

ADMINISTRATION

Oral: tablets should be taken in the morning, at least 30 minutes before the first food or drink of the day, with a full glass of plain water only. Patients should be advised not to lie down for 30 minutes after taking the tablet. Tablets should not be chewed, crushed or sucked.

CONTRA-INDICATIONS & WARNINGS

Hypersensitivity to alendronic acid, or any excipient in the formulation. Abnormality of the oesophagus or any factor which may delay oesophageal emptying. Inability to stand for less than 30 minutes. Hypocalcaemia. Not recommended in patients with creatinine clearance <35mL/minute/1.73m². Alendronic acid may cause irritation of the upper gastrointestinal mucosa. Caution is therefore necessary when upper gastrointestinal disease or abnormality including dysphagia, oesophageal disease, gastritis, duodenitis or peptic ulcers, is present. Oesophageal reactions may occur and be sufficiently severe to require hospitalisation. They include oesophagitis, oesophageal ulcers and erosions. Patients should be advised to seek medical advice if they experience symptoms of oesophageal irritation such as dysphagia, pain on swallowing, retrosternal pain or new or worsening heartburn.

INTERACTIONS

Concurrent use of other *bisphosphonate drugs* is contra-indicated. Concurrent use of *NSAIDs* or *aspirin* may increase the frequency of upper gastrointestinal adverse events. Bisphosphonate drugs form complexes with *divalent metal ions* and oral absorption may be impaired if they are given at the same time as *food, antacids* and *mineral supplements.*

PREGNANCY

Avoid during pregnancy due to risk of adverse effects on bone formation in the fetus.

BREAST-FEEDING

As a consequence of animal experiments which indicate that other bisphosphonate drugs are excreted in breast milk it is advised that mothers should not breast-feed whilst receiving this treatment.

SIDE-EFFECTS

Abdominal pain, dyspepsia, oesophagitis, oesophageal erosions and ulceration, dysphagia and abdominal distension. Rash and erythema are reported rarely. Musculoskeletal pain, constipation, diarrhoea, flatulence, and headache are also reported.

POISONING/TOXICITY
Theoretical risk of hypocalcaemia, hypophosphataemia and upper gastrointestinal adverse events may be anticipated. Serum calcium should be monitored and calcium supplements administered orally or parenterally as appropriate. Due to the risk of oesophageal ulceration patients should not be permitted to lie down and vomiting should not be induced. Calcium salts and/or antacids may be used to bind alendronic acid after oral ingestion.

PHARMACOKINETIC PROPERTIES
Oral absorption is approximately 45% when administered 1 hour before breakfast. Bioavailability is reduced by 60% if taken with coffee or orange juice and oral absorption is virtually abolished if given with, or up to 2 hours after, food. Transient distribution into soft tissue occurs after administration, after which redistribution into bone occurs rapidly. Volume of distribution, excluding bone is greater than 28 litres in adult humans. Concentrations in blood are too low for analytical detection. Protein binding is approximately 80%. Alendronic acid is not metabolised and is excreted in the urine. 50% of the administered dose is recovered in 72 hours with the terminal half-life in humans estimated to exceed 10 years, reflecting uptake into, and release from, the skeleton.

EXCIPIENTS.
See manufacturers SPC for further details.

LICENSED STATUS
Not licensed for use in children.

Alfacalcidol (1α-hydroxycholecalciferol)

Vitamin D derivative.

USES
Prevention and treatment of renal bone disease.
Vitamin D dependent and hypophosphataemic rickets.
Hypoparathyroidism and neonatal hypocalcaemia.
Pseudohyproparathyroidism.

PREPARATIONS
Capsule: 250 nanogram and 1 microgram – AlfaD®, One-Alpha®; 500 nanogram – One-Alpha®.
Injection: 2 microgram in 1mL, 0.5mL and 1mL ampoules – One-Alpha®.
Oral drops: 2 microgram in 1mL (100 nanograms per drop) – One-Alpha Drops®.

DOSAGE

Indication	Route	Age				Frequency	Notes
		birth–1 month	1 month–2 years	2–12 years	12–18 years	(times daily)	
Hypo-phosphataemic rickets	Oral/IV			DOSE BY WEIGHT PER KG <20kg			Initial dose. Adjust the dose according to response to avoid hypercalcaemia.
		←—— 25–50 ——→ nanogram/kg		25–50 nanogram/kg	-	1	
				DOSE BY WEIGHT RANGE/AGE >20kg			
		-		1 microgram	1 microgram	1	
Neonatal hypocalcaemia	Oral/IV	50–100 nanogram/kg	-	-	-	1	Up to 2 microgram/kg may be needed in severe cases. 100 nanogram/kg/**day** has proven effective as prophylaxis against early neonatal hypocalcaemia in premature infants.

DOSAGE continued

Indication	Route	Age				Frequency (times daily)	Notes
		birth–1 month	1 month–2 years	2–12 years	12–18 years		
Prophylaxis of vitamin D deficiency in renal patients	Oral/IV			DOSE BY WEIGHT PER KG			
		← 15–30 → nanogram/kg		<20kg 15–30 nanogram/kg	–	1	
				DOSE BY WEIGHT RANGE/AGE			
		–		>20kg 250–500 nanogram	250–500 nanogram	1	

Indices of response include plasma levels of calcium (ideally corrected for protein binding), alkaline phosphatase, parathyroid hormone, as well as radiological and histological investigations. Monitor carefully for hypercalcaemia.

In the management of renal bone disease the aim is to maintain parathyroid hormone level at or slightly above the normal range. Oversuppression can result in adynamic bone disease.

ADMINISTRATION

Oral: measure oral drops using the dropper provided by the manufacturer. The solution may be diluted with milk immediately prior to administration for doses under 100 nanogram; discard any remaining drug/milk solution.

IV: administer by IV bolus over approximately 30 seconds. May be given via the return line at the end of haemodialysis.

CONTRA-INDICATIONS & WARNINGS

Ensure adequate control of serum phosphate levels to reduce risk of metastatic calcification.

The injection should be avoided in those with known hypersensitivity to propylene glycol and used with caution in premature infants.

INTERACTIONS

Patients taking *barbiturates* or *anticonvulsants* may require larger doses of alfacalcidol to produce the desired effect.

PREGNANCY

Has been used in pregnancy for many years without apparent ill consequence, and may be used if there is no alternative.

BREAST-FEEDING

It is excreted into breast milk and high doses may cause hypercalcaemia in the infant. Avoid use in breast-feeding. Contact local Medicines Information Centre for advice.

SIDE-EFFECTS

Hypercalcaemia and associated symptoms.

POISONING/TOXICITY

Hypercalcaemia is treated by stopping alfacalcidol.

Severe hypercalcaemia may be additionally treated with a loop diuretic and with IV fluids or with corticosteroids.

May need peritoneal dialysis with low calcium or calcium-free dialysis fluid.

EXCIPIENTS

AlfaD® capsules include arachis (peanut) oil. One-Alpha® capsules include sesame oil. Oral drops include ethanol and sorbitol. Injection includes polyethylene glycol. See manufacturers SPC for further details.

LICENSED STATUS

One-Alpha® is licensed for use in all ages; AlfaD® is licensed for use in patients ≥20kg body weight.

Alfentanil (controlled drug)

Short-acting synthetic opioid analgesic related to fentanyl with actions similar to morphine.

USES

Adjunct to anaesthesia (particularly in short procedures and day case surgery). Analgesic for patients in intensive care on assisted ventilation.

PRESENTATION

Injection: (as hydrochloride) 500 microgram in 1mL; 2mL and 10mL ampoule – Rapifen®.

Intensive care injection: (as hydrochloride) 5mg in 1mL, 1mL ampoule – Rapifen®.

A

DOSAGE

Route	Age				Frequency	Notes
	birth–1 month	1 month–2 years	2–12 years	12–18 years		
IV bolus over 30 seconds	← 20–50 microgram/kg →				single dose	Initial dose. Assisted ventilation required.
	← 15 microgram/kg →				single dose	Supplemental doses. Assisted ventilation required.

Route	Age				Frequency	Notes
	birth–1 month	1 month–2 years	2–12 years	12–18 years		
IV bolus over 10 minutes	← 50–100 microgram/kg →				single loading dose	Assisted ventilation required.
then IV infusion	← then 500 nanogram/kg/minute – 1 microgram/kg/minute →				continuous	Assisted ventilation required.

Should only be prescribed/administered by a trained anaesthetist or intensivist.

ADMINISTRATION

IV: compatible infusion fluids are NaCl 0.9%, glucose 5% or compound sodium lactate infusion BP. The resultant solutions should be used within 24 hours. Administer last bolus dose 10 minutes before end of procedure or discontinue infusion 30 minutes before end of procedure to avoid prolonged respiratory depression after completion.

CONTRA-INDICATIONS & WARNINGS

Contra-indications: obstructive airways disease, respiratory depression (non-ventilated patients), in labour or before the clamping of the cord during caesarian section.
Cautions: hypothyroidism, liver or renal impairment, epilepsy.
Warnings: following administration, a transient fall in blood pressure may occur.

INTERACTIONS

Plasma concentration increased with *erythromycin, fluconazole, ketoconazole* and *cimetidine*, increased risk of respiratory depression, increased sedative effects with *anxiolytics* and *hypnotics*, antagonism of the gastrointestinal effects of *cisapride, metoclopramide* and *domperidone*, CNS excitation or depression with *MAOIs*, possible bradycardia and/or hypotension with *beta-blockers* and *anaesthetic agents*, bradycardia and possibly asystole with *non-vagolytic muscle relaxants*.

PREGNANCY

Alfentanil rapidly crosses the placenta to the fetus. Severe respiratory depression has occurred in neonates whose mothers were given alfentanil during caesarian section.

BREAST-FEEDING

Alfentanil is excreted into breast milk but this is not likely to be of clinical significance.

SIDE-EFFECTS

Respiratory depression, bradycardia and hypotension, muscle rigidity during induction (prevented by slow IV injection, lower doses, premedication with benzodiazepines or administration of muscle relaxant just prior to alfentanil), nausea and vomiting.

POISONING/TOXICITY

Symptoms of toxicity include bradycardia (treat with anticholinergic such as atropine or glycopyrrolate), respiratory depression (the opioid antagonist naloxone may be required if not controlled by oxygen and assisted or controlled respiration), muscle rigidity (treat with an IV neuromuscular blocking agent).

PHARMACOKINETIC PROPERTIES

Alfentanil has a rapid onset and short duration of action. Peak effect may be seen within 1.5-2 minutes of IV bolus injection with analgesia lasting for up to 10 minutes. It is metabolised to inactive metabolites in the liver and these are excreted in the urine. Its terminal elimination half-life is 1-2 hours. It can cross the blood-brain barrier.

EXCIPIENTS

See manufacturers SPC for further details.

LICENSED STATUS

Rapifen® is licensed for use in children and adults; Rapifen® intensive care is licensed for use in adults only. The use of alfentanil to treat children in intensive care is an unlicensed indication.

Phenothiazine derivative with a central sedative effect. It has H_1-receptor antagonist properties, and some antimuscarinic actions.

A

USES
Night sedation, premedication, urticaria and pruritus (antihistamine).

PRESENTATION
Tablet: 10mg – Vallergan®.
Syrup: 7.5mg in 5mL – Vallergan®.
Syrup forte: 30mg in 5mL – Vallergan Forte®.

DOSAGE

Indication	Route	Age			Frequency	Notes
		1 month–2 years	2–12 years	12–18 years	(times daily)	
Sedation	Oral	← 1.5–3mg/kg →		up to 90mg	single dose	Two hours before bedtime for night sedation or two hours prior to a procedure.
Antihistamine dose	Oral	DOSE BY WEIGHT				
		6 months –1 year	2–4 years	–		
		250 microgram/kg	2.5mg		3-4	
		DOSE BY AGE				
		>1 year	5–12 years	–		
		2.5mg	5mg		3-4	
		–	–	10mg	2-3	Up to a maximum of 100mg per day.

ADMINISTRATION
Oral: tablets – the blue film coating can be washed off the tablets to enable them to be more easily crushed if this is required. Syrups may be diluted, if required, using simple syrup (without preservative).

CONTRA-INDICATIONS & WARNINGS
Avoid in patients with hepatic or renal dysfunction, epilepsy, hypothyroidism. Caution in use <6 months because of a possible association with sudden infant death syndrome.

INTERACTIONS
Enhanced CNS depression with other *sedatives.* Respiratory depression may occur. Increased hypotensive effect with *most antihypertensives.* Enhanced anticholinergic effect with other *anticholinergic agents.* Decreased absorption of alimemazine with *antacids.*

PREGNANCY
Inadequate evidence of safety in pregnancy, but has been widely used for many years without apparent ill consequence.

BREAST-FEEDING
Alimemazine is excreted in breast milk, in levels too low to affect the infant.

SIDE EFFECTS
Minor side-effects include nasal stuffiness and dry mouth. Can cause restless irritability next day and morning drowsiness.

POISONING/TOXICITY
Symptoms of overdose include drowsiness or loss of consciousness, hypotension, tachycardia, ECG changes, ventricular arrhythmias and hypothermia. Severe extra-pyramidal dyskinesia may occur.
Up to 6 hours after ingestion activated charcoal can be given. There is no specific antidote.

PHARMACOKINETIC PROPERTIES
Well absorbed following oral administration. Usually needs to be given 2 hours before desired onset of effect.

EXCIPIENTS
Syrups include sugars and ethanol.

LICENSED STATUS
Licensed for use ≥2 years. Manufacturers maximum recommended dose for premedication is 2mg/kg/dose.

FURTHER INFORMATION
Usually need to give 2 hours before desired onset of effect.

A

USES

Prevention of urate nephropathy in tumour lysis syndrome associated with haemopioetic malignancy. Prevention of gout in glycogen storage disease type I (GSD) and methylmalonic acidaemia (MMA), and prevention of urolithiasis in phosphoribosyl pyrophosphate (PRPP) synthetase superactivity, Lesch-Nyhan syndrome and adenine phosphoribosyltransferase (APRT) deficiency.

PRESENTATION

Injection: 200mg powder for reconstitution – named patient.
Suspension: may be extemporaneously prepared.
Tablet: 100mg and 300mg – Zyloric® and non-proprietary.

DOSAGE

Indication	Route	Age			Frequency (times daily)	Notes
		1 month–2 years	2–12 years	12–18 years		
Hyperuricaemia due to tumour lysis syndrome	IV/oral	←	100mg/m²	→	3	Commence 24 hours before giving cytotoxic drugs.
GSD and MMA	Oral	←	10-15mg/kg (maximum dose 400mg <15 years)	→	1	Start if serum urate > 0.36mM. (>0.36 mmol/L).
PRPP synthetase superactivity and Lesch-Nyhan syndrome	Oral	←	10-20mg/kg (maximum dose 400mg <15 years)	→	1	Starting dose, adjust to minimum needed to maintain normal serum urate.
APRT deficiency	Oral	←	10mg/kg (maximum dose 400mg <15 years)	→	1	

ADMINISTRATION

Oral: preferably after food.
IV: reconstitute with 5mL Water for Injections. Dilute to 50mL and infuse over 1 hour. Compatible with NaCl 0.9% or glucose 5%. IV solution is very alkaline (pH 10.8-11.8).

CONTRA-INDICATIONS & WARNINGS

Do not start during acute gout. Does not prevent neurological features of Lesch-Nyhan syndrome. Increased risk of toxicity (e.g. rashes) in hepatic and renal failure. Reduce dose in renal and hepatic failure. A high fluid intake and low purine diet are recommended in APRT deficiency, PRPP synthetase superactivity and Lesch-Nyhan syndrome, with urinary alkalinisation in the latter two.

INTERACTIONS

Risk of toxicity increased by *captopril*, especially if renal impairment. Increases toxicity of *azathioprine* or in *mercaptopurine*: reduce dose of these cytotoxics if given concurrently. May increase the level of *warfarin*, *acenocoumarol* and *ciclosporin (cyclosporin)*.

PREGNANCY

Toxicity not reported during pregnancy but manufacturer recommends that the drug is avoided if possible. Contact local Medicines Information Centre for advice.

BREAST-FEEDING

Allopurinol enters breast milk. Contact local Medicines Information Centre for advice.

SIDE-EFFECTS

Withdraw treatment if rash develops; if mild, reintroduce cautiously but discontinue immediately if recurrence. Hypersensitivity reactions (rare) include exfoliation, fever, lymphadenopathy, arthralgia, eosinophilia and vasculitis. Gastrointestinal disorders. Rarely headaches, drowsiness, visual or taste disturbance, neuropathy, alopecia, hepatotoxicity or blood disorders.

PHARMACODYNAMICS

Allopurinol and its main metabolite (oxipurinol) lower the level of uric acid by inhibition of xanthine-oxidase, the enzyme catalysing the oxidation of hypoxanthine to xanthine and xanthine to uric acid. In addition, *de novo* purine biosynthesis is depressed via feedback inhibition of hypoxanthine-guanine phosphoribosyltransferase.

PHARMACOKINETICS
Bioavailability varies from 67-90%. Peak plasma levels of allopurinol generally occur approximately 1.5 hours after oral administration. Allopurinol is negligibly bound by plasma proteins. Elimination of allopurinol is mainly by metabolic conversion to oxipurinol by xanthine oxidase and aldehyde oxidase, with less than 10% of the unchanged drug excreted in urine.

POISONING/TOXICITY
Massive inhibition of xanthine oxidase activity should have no untoward effect unless affecting concomitant medication, especially with azathioprine or mercaptopurine. Adequate hydration to maintain optimum diuresis facilitates excretion of allopurinol and its metabolites. If considered necessary haemodialysis may be used.

EXCIPIENTS
Contact manufacturer for further details.

LICENSED STATUS
Injection is supplied by GlaxoSmithKline on a named patient basis for tumour lysis syndrome. Suspension is an extemporaneous preparation and as such is unlicensed.
Tablets licensed for use in children for tumour lysis syndrome and enzyme disorders.

Alprazolam

Benzodiazepine.

USES
Anxiety and panic disorder.

PRESENTATION
Tablet: 250 microgram and 500 microgram (both scored) – Xanax®.

DOSAGE

Indication	Route	Age	Frequency	Notes
		12–18 years	(times daily)	
Anxiety	Oral	250–500 microgram	3	Can be increased if required to a maximum of 1mg 3 times daily. Use the lowest effective dose.
Panic disorder	Oral	500 microgram	3	Initial dose. Increase stepwise every 4 days, if required, to a maximum of 8mg per day in divided doses.

CONTRA-INDICATIONS & WARNINGS, INTERACTIONS, PREGNANCY/BREAST-FEEDING, SIDE-EFFECTS, POISONING/TOXICITY
See diazepam monograph.

PHARMACOKINETIC PROPERTIES
Following oral administration, alprazolam is rapidly and extensively absorbed from the gastrointestinal tract with negligible pre-systemic metabolism. Peak plasma levels occur 1-2 hours after administration. Half-life is 6-16 hours. Elimination is largely by oxidative metabolism in the liver followed by excretion of the metabolites in the urine.

EXCIPIENTS
See manufacturers SPC for further details.

LICENSED STATUS
Not licensed for use in children. Not prescribable under the NHS; private prescription required.

A

A glycoprotein that activates plasminogen directly to form plasmin.

USES
Fibrinolytic agent to dissolve intravascular thrombi. In the treatment of veno-oclusive disease (VOD).

PRESENTATION
Injection: powder for reconstitution (10mg ≡ 5.8 million international units); 10mg, 20mg, 50mg and 100mg vial – Actilyse®.

DOSAGE
Experience in children is limited; consult literature and expert advice before prescribing.

ADMINISTRATION
Injection: reconstitute with an appropriate volume of Water for Injections. Reconstituted solution may be further diluted with NaCl 0.9% (not Water for Injections or glucose), minimum concentration of 0.2mg/mL. The reconstituted solution is stable for 24 hours if refrigerated and up to 8 hours at room temperature.

CONTRA-INDICATIONS & WARNINGS
Should not be used in cases with a high risk of haemorrhage e.g. severe bleeding, history of stroke or CNS disease, haemorrhagic retinopathy, uncontrolled hypertension, bacterial endocarditis, peptic ulceration, pancreatitis, recent major surgery, severe liver disease. Experience in children is limited; consult literature and expert advice before prescribing.

INTERACTIONS
Risk of haemorrhage increases with the use of *anticoagulants* and *platelet aggregation inhibitors*.

PREGNANCY/BREAST-FEEDING
There is very limited experience. Benefit must be evaluated against the potential risk. Contact local Medicines Information Centre for advice.

SIDE-EFFECTS
Bleeding (either superficial or internal).

POISONING/TOXICITY
If severe bleeding results, infuse fresh frozen plasma or fresh blood. If necessary synthetic antifibrinolytics may be administered.

PHARMACOKINETIC PROPERTIES
When given IV, it remains relatively inactive in the circulation until it binds to fibrin, for which it has a high affinity. It is rapidly destroyed by the liver with a half-life of 5 minutes.

EXCIPIENTS
See manufacturers SPC for further details.

LICENSED STATUS
Not licensed for use in children.

FURTHER INFORMATION
It is not suspected to be antigenic.

Aluminium acetate

Astringent.

USES
Inflammation in otitis externa.

PRESENTATION
Ear drops 13%: aluminium sulphate 2.25g, calcium carbonate 1g, tartaric acid 450mg, acetic acid (33%) 2.5mL and purified water 7.5mL – manufactured 'special'.
Ear drops 8%: dilute 8 parts aluminium acetate ear drops 13% with 5 parts purified water. Must be freshly prepared.

DOSAGE/ADMINISTRATION
Ribbon gauze dressing can be soaked with aluminium acetate solution and used as a wet dressing for suppurating wounds and dermatitis. Local application in furunculosis.

POISONING/TOXICITY
Irritant and corrosive if ingested in large doses.

LICENSED STATUS
Available as 'specials' and as such are unlicensed.

Aluminium chloride hexahydrate

Potent antiperspirant.

USES
Topical treatment of hyperhidrosis specifically involving axillae, hands or feet.

PRESENTATION
Topical solution: 20% – Anhydrol Forte®, Driclor®.

ADMINISTRATION
Topical: apply to the affected sites at night, as required and allow to dry, wash off in the morning.

CONTRA-INDICATIONS & WARNINGS
History of hypersensitivity to any of the ingredients. Restrict application to the affected sites only. Keep away from the eyes and mucous membranes. Do not get into direct contact with clothing, polished surfaces, jewellery or metal. Do not bathe immediately before use, and if axillae are to be treated, do not shave or use depilatories on the area within 12 hours before or after use.

PREGNANCY/BREAST-FEEDING
No special precautions needed.

SIDE-EFFECTS
Irritation if applied too frequently (this may be treated with a mild hydrocortisone cream).

EXCIPIENTS
Anhydrol Forte® includes industrial methylated sprit BP.
Driclor® includes ethanol.

LICENSED STATUS
Licensed for use in children and adults.

Alverine citrate

Smooth muscle spasmolytic, effective on smooth muscle of the alimentary tract and uterus.

USES
Relief of smooth muscle spasm in conditions such as irritable bowel syndrome, painful diverticular disease of the colon and primary dysmenorrhoea.

PRESENTATION
Capsule: 60mg – Relaxyl®, Spasmonal®; 120mg – Spasmonal® Forte.

DOSAGE

Route	Age			Frequency (times daily)	Notes
	1 month–2 years	2–12 years	12–18 years		
Oral	–	–	60–120mg	1-3	

CONTRA-INDICATIONS & WARNINGS
Contra-indicated in paralytic ileus and known hypersensitivity to any of the ingredients.

PREGNANCY/BREAST-FEEDING
Not recommended. Contact local Medicines Information Centre for advice.

A

SIDE-EFFECTS
Nausea, headache, itching, rash, dizziness and allergic reaction.

POISONING/TOXICITY
Can produce hypotension and atropine-like toxic effects. Management is as for atropine poisoning with supportive therapy for hypotension.

EXCIPIENTS
See manufacturers SPC for further details.

LICENSED STATUS
Licensed for use ≥12 years of age.

Amikacin

Semi-synthetic aminoglycoside.

USES
Gram-negative infections resistant to gentamicin.
In cystic fibrosis patients – treatment of early *Pseudomonas aeruginosa* infections not cleared by oral ciprofloxacin plus nebulised colistin and treatment of moderate to severe exacerbations, in combination with other antibiotics (e.g. third generation cephalosporins, anti-pseudomonal penicillins, beta-lactam antibiotics and polymixins).

PRESENTATION
Injection: (as sulphate) 50mg in 1mL; 2mL vial – Amikin® paediatric; 250mg in 1mL; 2mL vial – Amikin® and non-proprietary.

DOSAGE
Many dose regimens exist for aminoglycosides depending on target concentrations aimed for and patient groups treated. The dose regimens below are generally accepted initial doses and dose adjustments should be made in the light of serum concentration measurement.

Divided daily dose regimen
Newborn infant (birth to 1 month)

Route	#Postconceptional age	Postnatal age	Dose	Frequency (times daily)	Notes
IV	<35 weeks	<14 days	10mg/kg	1	Aim for a 1 hour post dose (peak) level of 15-30mg/L
		>14 days	10mg/kg then 7.5mg/kg	loading dose 2	
	>35 weeks	<14 days	15mg/kg	1	
		>14 days	10mg/kg then 7.5mg/kg	loading dose 2	

#Postconceptional age = gestational plus postnatal age.

Prolongation of dosage interval is recommended in neonates presenting with patent ductus arteriosus (PDA), prolonged hypoxia or treated with indometacin (indomethacin).

Child

Route	Age			Frequency (times daily)	Notes
	1 month-2 years	2-12 years	12-18 years		
IV or IM	←	7.5mg/kg (maximum single dose of 500mg)	→	2	Aim for a 1 hour post dose (peak) level of 15-30mg/L ≥12 years – for life threatening infections up to 1.5g/day in 3 divided doses may be given for a maximum of 10 days.

Child continued

Route	Age			Frequency (times daily)	Notes
	1 month–2 years	2–12 years	12–18 years		
IV for cystic fibrosis patients	←	10mg/kg (maximum single dose of 500mg)	→	3	Starting dose; adjust according to drug levels. Aim for trough level of <10mg/L and 1 hour post dose (peak) level should not exceed 25-30mg/L

In patients with impaired renal function dosage and/or frequency of administration must be adjusted in response to serum drug concentrations and the extent of renal impairment. There are various methods to determine dosage and a wide variation in dosage recommendations. See manufacturers SPC for recommendations.

Single daily dose regimen
Newborn infant (birth to 1 month)

Route	#Postconceptional age/gestation		Frequency (times daily)	Notes
	32–35 weeks	>35 weeks		
IV	12mg/kg	15mg/kg	1	Aim for a 1 hour post dose (peak) level of 30mg/L; an 18 hour level of <3mg/L

#Postconceptional age = gestational plus postnatal age.

Use postconceptional age if >7 days postnatal age. There is little experience in neonates <32 weeks gestation.
Levels must be monitored and caution is required if impaired renal function is suspected.
Prolongation of dosage interval is recommended in neonates presenting with PDA, prolonged hypoxia or treated with indometacin (indomethacin).

Child

Route	Age			Frequency (times daily)	Notes
	1 month–2 years	2–12 years	12–18 years		
IV	←	15mg/kg	→	1	Aim for a 1 hour post dose (peak) level of 40–50mg/L; an 18 hour level of <3mg/L

Amikacin in a concentration of 2.5mg in 1mL may be used as an irrigation solution in abscess cavities, the pleural space, the peritoneum and the cerebral ventricles. See manufacturers SPC for full details.

ADMINISTRATION
IM or IV: give by IM injection, as a slow IV injection over 2-3 minutes or as an IV infusion over 20–30 minutes for once daily doses. Compatible with NaCl 0.9% and glucose 5%.
In general, amikacin injection should not be mixed with penicillins, cephalosporins, erythromycin, amphotericin, heparin or sodium bicarbonate. Adequate flushing between doses or administration at separate sites is suggested.

CONTRA-INDICATIONS & WARNINGS
Myasthenia gravis. As with other aminoglycosides patients should be well hydrated during amikacin therapy and renal function monitored. See manufacturers SPC for full details. Hearing tests are recommended for cystic fibrosis patients having repeated courses of aminoglycosides.

INTERACTIONS
Increased risk of ototoxicity and nephrotoxicity with *cephalosporins, vancomycin, ciclosporin (cyclosporin), cisplatin, diuretics* such as *furosemide (frusemide), amphotericin*. Enhances effects of *non-depolarising muscle relaxants* (calcium IV may reverse this effect). Antagonises effects of *neostigmine* and *pyridostigmine*.

PREGNANCY
Amikacin rapidly crosses the placenta appearing in the fetal circulation and amniotic fluid. Although no reports of congenital defects or fetal damage have occurred, fetal ototoxicity is well known following other aminoglycoside exposure and may occur with amikacin.

BREAST-FEEDING
Amikacin is excreted into breast milk in low concentration and since oral absorption is poor the potential for toxicity is low in the nursing infant.

A

SIDE-EFFECTS
As with all aminoglycosides, nephrotoxicity and ototoxicity can occur if optimum blood levels are exceeded.

POISONING/TOXICITY
In the event of overdose or toxic reaction, peritoneal or haemodialysis will aid in the removal of aminoglycosides from the blood.

PHARMACOKINETIC PROPERTIES
Amikacin distributes to achieve therapeutic concentrations in bone, heart, gallbladder and lung tissue. It is also well distributed into bile, sputum, bronchial secretions and interstitial, pleural and synovial fluids. CSF penetration is poor. The apparent volume of distribution is greater in neonates and young infants. This means greater doses on a mg/kg basis are required to produce serum concentrations comparable to those in adults. 94-98% of an amikacin dose is excreted unchanged by glomerular filtration. Plasma elimination half-lives are thus prolonged in neonates and in renal impairment. The manufacturers do not state target serum drug concentrations within the licence or manufacturers SPC. It is generally accepted with the **divided daily dose** regimen that to avoid toxicity a peak serum concentration measured one hour after injection of 30mg/L and a trough (taken immediately before the next dose) of between 2-5mg/L should not be exceeded. Serum levels should initially be measured around the third dose and then as required following dose adjustment. For **single daily dose** regimen: if 18 hour level is >3mg/L extend dosing interval.

EXCIPIENTS
See manufacturers SPC for further details.

LICENSED STATUS
Licensed in adults, children and neonates but some of the doses given in this monograph may be unlicensed e.g. dose for cystic fibrosis patients.

Amiloride

Potassium-sparing diuretic.

USES
Prophylaxis of diuretic (loop or thiazide) or amphotericin-induced hypokalaemia; nephrogenic diabetes insipidus (in conjunction with hydrochlorothiazide).

PREPARATIONS
Tablet: 5mg – non-proprietary.
Liquid: 5mg in 5mL – non-proprietary.

DOSAGE

Route	Age				Frequency (times daily)	Notes
	birth–1 month	1 month–2 years	2–12 years	12–18 years		
Oral	← 100–200 microgram/kg →			5–10mg	2	Prophylaxis of drug induced hypokalaemia.
	-	-	← 100 microgram/kg →		3	Nephrogenic diabetes insipidus.

CONTRA-INDICATIONS & WARNINGS
Risk of hyperkalaemia in renal impairment.
Do not use for nephrogenic diabetes insipidus in infants or young children (indometacin (indomethacin) is generally used instead).

INTERACTIONS
Risk of hyperkalaemia increased with *ACE inhibitors*. Increased risk of nephrotoxicity with *NSAIDs*.

PREGNANCY
Clinical experience is limited. Fetal and neonatal jaundice, fetal bone marrow depression and thrombocytopenia have been described.

BREAST-FEEDING
Contact local Medicines Information Centre for advice.

SIDE-EFFECTS
Gastrointestinal disturbances, dry mouth, rashes, hyperkalaemia, hyponatraemia.

Amiloride continued

POISONING/TOXICITY
The most likely signs and symptoms are dehydration and electrolyte imbalance, which should be treated by established methods.

PHARMACOKINETIC PROPERTIES
Plasma half-life is approximately 6 hours but prolonged in renal failure, hepatitis and cystic fibrosis patients.

EXCIPIENTS
Contact manufacturers for further details.

LICENSED STATUS
Not licensed for use in infants or children.

Aminophylline

A soluble salt of theophylline with ethylenediamine. It has a bronchodilating effect in asthma, acts as a respiratory stimulant in babies with apnoea, and produces diuresis.

USES
Idiopathic central or mixed apnoea. Diuretic, used before furosemide (frusemide) in intensive care. Bronchodilator in asthma and bronchodilator in anaphylaxis, if bronchospasm occurs.

PRESENTATION
Tablet (modified release): 100mg – Phyllocontin Continus® Paediatric; 225mg – Phyllocontin Continus® and non-proprietary; 350mg – Phyllocontin Continus® Forte.
Injection: 25mg in 1mL; 10mL ampoule – non-proprietary. 2mg in 1mL and 5mg in 1mL; 20mL ampoules – manufactured 'special'.

DOSAGE
Newborn infant (birth to 1 month)

Indication	Route	Age		Frequency	Notes
		birth–1 month		(times daily)	
Neonatal apnoea	IV (loading dose)	← 6mg/kg →		1	Give over at least 20 minutes either undiluted or diluted with NaCl 0.9% or glucose 5%. Start maintenance dose 24 hours after loading dose. Monitor theophylline plasma levels. Therapeutic range 8-12mg/L Due to the long half-life, a continuous infusion is not necessary.
	IV (maintenance dose)	← 2.5mg/kg →		2	

Child

Indication	Route	Age			Frequency	Notes
		1 month–2 years	2–12 years	12–18 years	(times daily)	
Diuresis in intensive care	IV infusion over 20–30 minutes	← 2–4mg/kg →		-	single dose	Synergistic effect if given 30 minutes before IV furosemide (frusemide). Doses of up to 6mg/kg have been used in critically ill children.
Bronchodilator in asthma or anaphylaxis	IV infusion over 20–30 minutes	← 5mg/kg (maximum 500mg) →			single loading dose over 20-30 minutes	Loading dose if no theophylline or aminophylline has been given in the last 24 hours.
	IV infusion	← 1mg/kg/hour →		500 microgram/kg/hour	continuous	Maintenance dose. Infusion can usually be stopped and not tapered down.

A

Child continued

Indication	Route	Age			Frequency (times daily)	Notes
		1 month– 2 years	2–12 years	12–18 years		
Bronchodilator in asthma or anaphylaxis	Oral	–	≥3 years 6mg/kg* for 1 week then 12mg/kg	100–225mg for 1 week then 200–450mg	2 2	*Round doses to nearest 100mg dose. Some children with chronic asthma may need 13-20mg/kg twice daily.

ADMINISTRATION

IV infusion: dilute infusion to 1mg in 1mL in NaCl 0.9% (preferred diluent), or glucose 5%. The infusion can usually be stopped and not tapered down. Give via a rate controlled infusion device. If patient is fluid-restricted, injection solution can be given undiluted.

Oral: swallow tablets whole; do not chew.

CONTRA-INDICATIONS & WARNINGS

Omit loading dose if patient has received oral aminophylline or theophylline in the last 24 hours. Clearance can decrease (blood levels increase) with reduced hepatic or cardiac function. Maintenance dose should be halved if reduced clearance is likely.

INTERACTIONS

Increased theophylline levels are seen with *cimetidine, erythromycin, ciprofloxacin, tiabendazole (thiabendazole), mexiletine, norfloxacin* and possibly *fluconazole, isoniazid, diltiazem and verapamil. Reduced levels with rifampicin, carbamazepine, phenobarbital (phenobarbitone), phenytoin, primidone* and *sulphinpyrazone.* Increased risk of hypokalaemia with high dose *salbutamol, salmeterol* and *terbutaline.* Increased risk of arrhythmias with *halothane.*

PREGNANCY

There have been no reports of congenital defects with the use of aminophylline in pregnancy. However, blood levels should be monitored to maintain non-toxic levels. Newborn infants may have therapeutic serum levels. Adverse effects in the newborn include transient ischaemia, irritability, feeding difficulties and vomiting.

BREAST-FEEDING

Theophylline is excreted in breast milk and has been shown to cause irritability in infants. Breast-feeding is not contra-indicated but it is recommended that a mother nurse her baby just prior to taking her next dose, when plasma theophylline levels are expected to be low.

SIDE-EFFECTS

Tachycardia, palpitations, hyperglycaemia, increased irritability, decreased gastric emptying with increased risk of vomiting and reflux, arrhythmias, headache and convulsions.

POISONING/TOXICITY

Symptoms characterised by nausea, vomiting, electrolyte imbalance and gastric irritation. Tachycardia, convulsions and hypotension may also occur. Correct metabolic abnormalities e.g. hypokalaemia. Monitor serum theophylline levels.

PHARMACOKINETIC PROPERTIES

Aminophylline readily liberates to theophylline in the body. Theophylline is metabolised in the liver to inactive metabolites. 10% is excreted unchanged in adults, however, in neonates this can be around 50%. Theophylline has a narrow therapeutic range, and the frequency of serious toxic effects increases progressively with plasma concentrations above 25mg/L; significant side-effects can occur when level exceeds 14mg/L in a neonate and 20mg/L in older children.

Sampling times

Prior to IV infusion if patient is already taking an aminophylline or theophylline preparation. 4-6 hours after beginning therapy. Modified release preparations sample prior to the next dose. *Asthma therapy*: therapeutic range is 10-20mg/L (55-110micromol/L). Apnoea therapy in neonates: therapeutic range is 8-12mg/L. *Loading doses*: a short infusion of 1mg/kg raises plasma theophylline levels by about 2mg/L.

EXCIPIENTS

Phyllocontin Continus® Paediatric 100mg includes saccharin sodium. Contact manufacturers for further details.

LICENSED STATUS

25mg in 1mL injection is licensed for use in asthma in children and adults. The 2mg in 1mL and 5mg in 1mL injection are available as 'specials' and as such are unlicensed. Neonatal apnoea and diuresis are unlicensed indications.

Phyllocontin Continus® Paediatric is licensed ≥3 years of age. Phyllocontin Continus ® tablets 225mg and 350mg licensed ≥12 years of age.

FURTHER INFORMATION
Special care calculating doses/administration volumes in neonates using 250mg in 10mL injection as frequently involved in medication errors. Aminophylline is compatible with hydrocortisone.

A

Amiodarone hydrochloride

An antiarrhythmic agent which prolongs the action potential duration in both the atrial and ventricular myocardium (Class III antiarrhythmic).

USES
Management of refractory supraventricular and ventricular arrhythmias and junctional ectopic tachycardia (JET), atrial fibrillation and flutter and tachyarrhthymias associated with Wolff-Parkinson-White syndrome. Shock resistant ventricular fibrillation and pulseless tachycardia in resuscitation.

PRESENTATION
Tablet: 100mg and 200mg – Cordarone X® (scored) and non-proprietary.
Injection: 30mg in 1mL, 10mL prefilled syringe – non-proprietary; 50mg in 1mL, 3mL ampoule – Cordarone X®.
Suspension: manufactured 'special'.

DOSAGE
Amiodarone must always be given under the direct supervision of a cardiologist. The minimum effective dose must be used at all times. The manufacturers do not recommend doses of amiodarone for paediatric patients. Doses vary but the following have been used.

Route	Age				Frequency	Notes
	birth-1 month	1 month-2 years	2-12 years	12-18 years	(times daily)	
Oral (loading dose)	← 5mg/kg → (maximum 200mg)				2-3	Give loading dose for 7-14 days (some neonatologists use
				200mg	3	a loading dose of 10mg/kg
Oral (mainten-ance dose)	← 5mg/kg → (maximum 200mg)				1	once daily), then reduce to minimum effective
				200mg	1	maintenance dose.
IV (loading dose)	← 5mg/kg →				single dose	Slow IV injection over 30 minutes. Loading doses up to 15mg/kg have been reported.
IV infusion	← 5-15 microgram/kg/minute → (maximum1.2g in 24 hours)				continuous	Give via a central line if possible. Adjust rate according to clinical response.
Rapid IV bolus	← 5mg/kg → (maximum 300mg)				single dose	In cardiopulmonary resuscitation (CPR) for shock resistant ventricular fibrillation and pulseless tachycardia.

ADMINISTRATION
Oral: it is possible to crush tablets and disperse in water. The IV formulation should not be given orally (contains Tween 80 – irritant).
IV: amiodarone IV should only be used when facilities exist for cardiac monitoring and defibrillation. When repeated or continuous infusion is anticipated, administration by a central venous catheter is recommended. IV amiodarone may be administered more rapidly in emergency situations, as a slow IV injection over at least 3 minutes. This should not be repeated for at least 15 minutes. The injection is compatible with glucose 5% only. Solutions containing less than 150mg of amiodarone in 250mL glucose 5% (600 microgram in 1mL, amiodarone) are unstable and should not be used.

A

CONTRA-INDICATIONS & WARNINGS

Evidence or history of thyroid dysfunction, sinus bradycardia and sino-atrial heart block.

IV amiodarone is contra-indicated in severe respiratory failure, circulatory collapse or severe arterial hypotension. Circulatory collapse may be precipitated by too rapid an administration or overdose. Congestive heart failure and cardiomyopathy are manufacturers contra-indications when using IV amiodarone as a bolus injection, but it is used in CPR. In small babies, the manufacturers warn that the IV preparation is potentially dangerous due to the benzyl alcohol content. Although the benzyl alcohol concentration is 20mg/mL, large quantities can cause a 'gasping syndrome' and may be fatal. Be aware of other products, used in neonates containing benzyl alcohol.

Hypersensitivity to amiodarone or iodine.

Precautions: due to the iodine content of the tablets and injection, caution is advised when administering to patients with known hypersensitivity to iodine. Too high a dose may lead to severe bradycardia and conduction disturbances. Caution should be exercised in patients with latent or manifest heart failure. Dosage adjustments should be considered in liver disease as the drug is extensively metabolised in the liver.

INTERACTIONS

Blood levels of *digoxin* approximately double with amiodarone, some individuals may show even greater increases; maintenance dose of *digoxin* should be halved. *Beta-blockers, certain calcium-channel blockers:* increase the risk of bradycardia, AV block and myocardial depression. Concomitant use of amiodarone and *phenytoin* can result in increased serum concentration of *phenytoin*, and decreased serum concentration of amiodarone. Monitor patients carefully. Amiodarone levels may be increased with concomitant use of *cimetidine. Ciclosporin (cyclosporin)* concentration can be increased with amiodarone. Monitor levels of *ciclosporin* and watch for evidence of toxicity.

Amiodarone may increase plasma levels of *oral anticoagulants*. Frequent monitoring of prothrombin time/INR is necessary during and for several months following concomitant amiodarone therapy. The risk of torsades de pointes may be increased when amiodarone is used in combination with other drugs which prolong the QT interval e.g. *certain antiarrhythmics,* or agents which may induce hypokalaemia and/or hypomagnesaemia.

Combination with other *antiarrhythmics* (especially Class I) needs careful consideration as increased myocardial depression can occur. Potentially severe complications have been reported in patients taking amiodarone undergoing *general anaesthesia*. The anaesthetist should be informed.

PREGNANCY

No teratogenic effects have been observed in animals. In view of the pharmacological properties of the drug on the fetus and its effect on the fetal thyroid gland, administration in pregnancy is not recommended.

BREAST-FEEDING

Amiodarone is present in breast milk in significant quantities and breast-feeding is generally not recommended.

SIDE-EFFECTS

Rapid administration of IV amiodarone has been associated with anaphylactic shock, hot flushes, sweating, nausea, a moderate and transient decrease in blood pressure. In cases of respiratory failure, notably in asthmatics, bronchospasm and/or apnoea may also occur.

Ophthalmological: patients on continuous therapy may develop microdeposits in the cornea. Slit lamp examination annually is recommended, unless blurred vision or decreased vision occurs.

Cardiac: bradycardia, sinus arrest or conduction disturbances.

Dermatological: photosensitivity (can be alleviated by use of total sun-block creams), skin rashes.

Thyroid: both hyper and hypothyroidism can occur. Clinical monitoring is recommended before starting treatment, after loading is complete and at 6 monthly intervals thereafter; continue monitoring for several months after stopping treatment.

Pulmonary: diffuse pulmonary alveolitis, pneumonitis and fibrosis have been reported. Chest X-ray before starting therapy should be considered.

Hepatic: monitor liver function particularly transaminases before starting treatment, when loading dose is complete and at 6 monthly intervals thereafter.

Neurological: peripheral neuropathy and/or myopathy have been reported. Nightmares, vertigo, headaches and sleeplessness may also occur.

Other: nausea, vomiting, metallic taste, fatigue, hypersensitivity reactions.

POISONING/TOXICITY

Nausea, vomiting, sweating, hypotension, cardiac arryhthmias, bradycardia and ECG changes may occur in overdose. Treatment should be supportive. Due to the long half-life of amiodarone, adequate and prolonged surveillance of the patient, particularly cardiac status is recommended.

PHARMACOKINETIC PROPERTIES

Absorption from the gastrointestinal tract is slow. Oral bioavailability is <50%. Pre-systemic metabolism is 13-39%. Mean plasma half-life in adults after chronic dosing is 50 days. Plasma protein binding is 96%. Amiodarone is extensively metabolised in the liver. Renal excretion appears to be negligible. Trough plasma levels are 0.5-2.5mg/L.

EXCIPIENTS
Contact manufacturers for further details.

LICENSED STATUS
Licensed for use ≥12 years of age.

Amitriptyline

Tricyclic antidepressant.

USES
Depression, nocturnal enuresis, neuralgic pain, idiopathic musculoskeletal pain syndromes.

PRESENTATION
Tablet: 10mg, 25mg and 50mg – non-proprietary.
Oral solution: (as hydrochloride) 10mg in 5mL - manufactured 'special'; 25mg in 5mL and 50mg in 5mL – non-proprietary.

DOSAGE

Indication	Route	Age		Frequency (times daily)	Notes
		2-12 years	12-18 years		
Nocturnal enuresis	Oral	≥ 6 years 10–25mg	25–50mg	1 (at night)	Unlikely to be indicated <6 years. Maximum period of treatment 3 months – review before further courses.
Depression	Oral	– –	25mg or 50mg	2–3 1 (at night)	Initial dose. Start at the lower dose and increase as tolerated if required. Usual maintenance dose 50–150mg daily.
Neuralgic pain	Oral	–	30mg	1 (at night)	Initial dose. May be increased, as tolerated, if required, up to 150mg daily.
Idiopathic musculoskeletal pain	Oral	> 8 years 10–50mg	10–50mg	1 (at night)	Start at the lower dose and increase as tolerated if required.

CONTRA-INDICATIONS & WARNINGS, INTERACTIONS, PREGNANCY, BREAST-FEEDING, POISONING/TOXICITY
See imipramine monograph. Rebound cholinergic symptoms such as sialorrhoea in the afternoon, can be minimised by dividing the dose.

SIDE-EFFECTS
As imipramine but more sedating.

PHARMACOKINETIC PROPERTIES
Rapidly absorbed from the gastrointestinal tract. Half-life range 9-25 hours (mean 15 hours). Onset of therapeutic effect 7-21 days.

EXCIPIENTS
Contact manufacturers for further details.

LICENSED STATUS
The 25mg in 5mL and 50mg in 5mL oral solutions are licensed for treatment of depression >16 years of age and enuresis >6 years of age. Neuralgic pain is not a licensed indication. The 10mg in 5mL oral solution is a 'special' and as such is not licensed.

FURTHER INFORMATION
Oral solutions available from Rosemont.

A

Calcium-channel blocker.

USES
Hypertension.

PREPARATIONS
Tablet: 5mg and 10mg – Istin®.
Suspension: may be extemporaneously prepared.

DOSAGE

Route	Age			Frequency	Notes
	1 month–2 years	2–12 years	12–18 years	(times daily)	
Oral	DOSE BY WEIGHT PER KG				Initial dose.
	← 100–200 micrograms/kg →			1	
	DOSE BY WEIGHT RANGE/AGE				Increase according to response.
	6–15kg 1.25mg	15–25kg 2.5mg	>25kg 5mg	5mg	1	Maximum 10mg daily.

ADMINISTRATION
Oral: the tablets disperse well in water.

CONTRA-INDICATIONS & WARNINGS
Dihydropyridine sensitivity, use in pregnancy and lactation contra-indicated. Caution in liver impairment.

INTERACTIONS
May increase *ciclosporin (cyclosporin)* levels. *Itraconazole* and *fluconazole* may possibly inhibit amlodipine metabolism, consider lower doses. *Rifampicin* may decrease amlodipine effects, higher doses may be required.

PREGNANCY/BREAST-FEEDING
Contra-indicated by manufacturers. Contact local Medicines Information Centre for advice.

SIDE-EFFECTS
Headache, oedema, rash, flushing, dizziness, nausea and fatigue.

POISONING/TOXICITY
Gastric lavage. Monitor urine output, cardiac and respiratory function, and elevate extremities. A vasoconstrictor may help restore vascular tone and blood pressure. Calcium gluconate may be of some benefit in reversing the effect of calcium-channel blockade.

PHARMACOKINETIC PROPERTIES
Oral bioavailability 64-80%. Half life 35-50 hours. Extensively bound to proteins.

EXCIPIENTS
See manufacturers SPC for further details.

LICENSED STATUS
Not licensed for use in children.

Ammonium tetrathiomolybdate

A chelating agent that aids the elimination of copper from the body.

USES
Treatment of Wilson's disease. Experimental drug that has had success in treating the initial disease. May be useful if patient has severe neurological symptoms.

PRESENTATION
Powder.

DOSAGE

Route	Age			Frequency	Notes
	1 month–2 years	2–12 years	12–18 years	(times daily)	
Oral	← 20mg →			3	With food
	and			and	and
	20–60mg			3	between meals.

CONTRA-INDICATIONS & WARNINGS, INTERACTIONS, PREGNANCY/BREAST-FEEDING, POISONING/ TOXICITY
No information available.

SIDE-EFFECTS
Bone marrow depression has been reported which has resolved on stopping treatment.

PHARMACODYNAMIC PROPERTIES
It forms unabsorbable complexes with copper in the intestinal lumen and also complexes free or loosely bound copper in plasma or tissues which are taken up into the reticuloendothelial cells and stored to be excreted in the urine. When it is given with food it blocks the intestinal absorption of copper and when taken between meals it combines with albumin and caeruloplasmin-bound copper.

LICENSED STATUS
Not licensed for use in the UK.

FURTHER INFORMATION
Powder available from Sigma Aldrich.
Ammonium tetrathiomolybdate undergoes oxidation, therefore may lose potency over time.

Amorolfine

Broad spectrum topical antimycotic.

USES
Treatment of fungal nail infections – nail lacquer.
Treatment of fungal skin infections – cream.

PRESENTATION
Cream: 0.25% – Loceryl®.
Nail lacquer: 5% – Loceryl®.

DOSAGE/ADMINISTRATION
Cream: apply once daily after cleansing in the evening for at least 2-3 weeks (up to 6 weeks for foot mycosis) continuing for 3-5 days after lesions have healed. There is, however, lack of clinical experience of the use of amorolfine in children.
Nail lacquer: apply to infected nails 1-2 times weekly after filing and cleaning; allow to dry (approx. 3 minutes). Treat finger nails for 6 months; toe nails for 9-12 months. Review 3 monthly.

CONTRA-INDICATIONS & WARNINGS
Avoid contact with eyes, ears and mucous membranes.

PREGNANCY/BREAST-FEEDING
Not recommended. Contact local Medicines Information Centre for advice.

SIDE-EFFECTS
Occasional transient burning sensation, erythema and pruritus.

POISONING/TOXICITY
Gastric emptying may be used following accidental oral ingestion.

EXCIPIENTS
See manufacturers SPC for further details.

LICENSED STATUS
Not licensed for use in children.

Amoxicillin (amoxycillin)

Broad-spectrum penicillin; a derivative of ampicillin.

USES
See ampicillin monograph. Oral pharmacokinetics make amoxicillin generally preferable to ampicillin as the oral aminopenicillin for general use. Prophylaxis of infective carditis (see infections guideline section – Summary of

prevention of endocarditis in children with heart disease). Adjunct in the eradication of *Helicobacter pylori* in patients with duodenal ulcers. In cystic fibrosis patients – treatment for asymptomatic *Haemophilus influenzae* carriage or minor exacerbations.

PRESENTATION
Capsule: 250mg and 500mg – Amoxil® and non-proprietary.
Injection: (sodium salt) 250mg, 500mg and 1g vials – Amoxil® and non-proprietary.
Oral suspension: 125mg in 1.25mL – Amoxil® paediatric; 125mg in 5mL and 250mg in 5mL – non-proprietary.
Sachet: 3g – Amoxil® and non-proprietary.
Syrup: 125mg in 5mL and 250mg in 5mL – Amoxil®.

DOSAGE
Neonate (birth to 1 month)

Route	Age	Dose	Frequency	Notes
Oral/IV/IM	<7 days	50mg/kg	12 hourly	Increase IV dose to 100mg/kg in suspected meningitis.
	7–21 days	50mg/kg	8 hourly	
	>21 days	50mg/kg	6 hourly	

Child

Route	Age			Frequency (times daily)	Notes
	1 month–2 years	2–12 years	12–18 years		
Oral	DOSE BY WEIGHT				Dose may be doubled in severe infection.
	8mg/kg		-	3	
	DOSE BY AGE				
	125mg	125–250mg	500mg	3	
IV/IM	30mg/kg			3	Dose may be doubled in severe infection, meningitis up to a maximum **daily** dose of 4g.
Oral for cystic fibrosis patients	DOSE BY WEIGHT				Treatment for asymptomatic *Haemophilus influenzae* carriage or mild exacerbations.
	16-33mg/kg			3	
	DOSE BY AGE				
	≤1 year	≤7 years			
	125mg	250mg	500mg	3	
	>1 year	>7 years			
	250mg	500mg		3	
Oral for *H. pylori*	>1 year	2-6 years			Treatment for 14 days with metronidazole and omeprazole.
	125mg	125mg	500mg	3	
		6-12 years			
		250mg		3	
	>1 year	2-6 years			Treatment for 14 days with clarithromycin and omeprazole.
	250mg	250mg	1g	2	
		6-12 years			
		500mg		2	

Reduce dose in renal impairment. If creatinine clearance is <50mL/minute/1.73m^2 increase dosage interval to 12 hourly. If <10mL/minute/1.73m^2 increase further to 18 hourly. Amoxicillin is removed by haemodialysis and peritoneal dialysis. In dialysis patients, a dose should be given after dialysis session.

ADMINISTRATION
Oral: administration little affected by food.
IV: each 250mg amoxicillin displaces 0.2mL. Reconstitute with Water for Injections: each 250mg vial with 4.8mL to give

50mg in 1mL; each 500mg vial with 9.6mL to give 50mg in 1mL; each 1g vial with 19.2mL to give 50mg in 1mL (some neonatal units reconstitute the 250mg vial with 2.4mL of water and the 500mg vial with 4.6mL to give 100mg in 1mL). Administer over 3-5 minutes. Higher doses may be given over 30 minutes. Compatible with glucose 5% and 10%, NaCl 0.9% and NaCl 0.45%.

CONTRA-INDICATIONS & WARNINGS, PREGNANCY, BREAST-FEEDING, SIDE-EFFECTS
See ampicillin monograph.

POISONING/TOXICITY
Treat symptomatically. Removed by haemodialysis and peritoneal dialysis.

PHARMACOKINETIC PROPERTIES
Oral: rapidly and almost completely absorbed following oral administration. Bioavailability reported as 75-92%. Peak levels occur 1-2 hours after oral dose. Linear relationship between dose and peak concentration or area under the serum concentration time curve (AUC). Peak levels 2-2.5 times ampicillin after oral dose. Presence of food may delay absorption but total drug absorbed is unaffected.
IM/IV: as ampicillin.

EXCIPIENTS
Amoxil® sachets include sorbitol; syrup includes sorbitol and saccharin sodium; paediatric oral suspension includes sucrose.
Injection: 1g amoxicillin sodium contains 3.3mmol sodium.
Contact manufacturers for further details.

LICENSED STATUS
Licensed for use in all ages.

Amphotericin

Polyene antifungal that is fungistatic rather than fungicidal in concentrations achieved in body fluids.

USES
Suspected or proven fungal infections. Active against a range of fungi and yeasts including *candida* species, *cryptococcus*, *blastomyces*, *histoplasma* and *aspergillus*, reducing the allergen load. May be of help in recurrent cases of allergic bronchopulmonary aspergillosis (ABPA) in cystic fibrosis.

PRESENTATION
IV infusion: 50mg vial – Fungizone®.
IV infusion: amphotericin 5mg in 1mL as a lipid complex (ABCL), 10mL and 20mL vial – Abelcet®.
IV infusion: amphotericin encapsulated in liposomes, 50mg vial – AmBisome®.
IV infusion: amphotericin as a complex with sodium cholesteryl sulphate (ABCS), 50mg and 100mg vial – Amphocil®.
Lozenge: 10mg – Fungilin®.
Tablet: 100mg (scored) – Fungilin®.

DOSAGE
Test doses
Manufacturers advise a test dose prior to each new course of treatment to exclude anaphylactic reactions which may occur. Test dose: 100 microgram/kg (maximum 1mg) infused over 30 minutes for conventional formulation or 10–15 minutes for ABCL, liposomal and ABCS formulations. Observe for 30 minutes and then continue treatment if no reaction.

Newborn infant (birth to 1 month)

Preparation	Route	Age	Frequency	Notes
		birth–1 month	(times daily)	
Conventional formulation	IV	250 microgram/kg	once daily	See test dose recommendations. Increase by 250 microgram/kg once daily (up to a maximum 1mg/kg/day in severe infections).

Newborn infant (birth to 1 month) continued

Preparation	Route	Age	Frequency	Notes
		birth–1 month	(times daily)	
Liposomal formulation	IV	1mg/kg increasing by 1mg/kg/day to	1	See test dose recommendations.
		3mg/kg or	1	Empirical treatment.
		5mg/kg	1	Proven systemic infection (unlicensed dose).

Child

Preparation	Route	Age			Frequency	Notes
		1 month–2 years	2–12 years	12–18 years	(times daily)	
Conventional formulation	IV	← 250 microgram/kg → increase by 250 microgram/kg/day to			once daily	See test dose recommendations. Adjust according to response and tolerance. If therapy interrupted for longer than 7 days, restart at low dose and increase as previously. Maximum dose is 1.5mg/kg/**day**.
		← 1mg/kg →			once daily	
Liposomal formulation	IV	← 1mg/kg → increase by 1mg/kg/day to			once daily	See test dose recommendations.
		← 3mg/kg → or			once daily	Empirical.
		← 5mg/kg →			once daily	Proven systemic infection.
		← 1–3mg/kg/day → for 10–21 days to a cumulative dose of 21–30mg/kg			once daily	Visceral leishmaniasis in immunocompetent patients.
		← 3mg/kg →			once daily on days 1–5, and days 14 and 21	Visceral leishmaniasis in immunocompetent patients. (USA guidance).
ABCS (Amphocil®) and ABCL (Abelcet®)	IV	← 1mg/kg → increase by 1mg/kg/day to			once daily	See test dose recommendations.
		← 3mg/kg → or			once daily	Empirical.
		← 5mg/kg →			once daily	Proven systemic infection.
Conventional formulation	Nebulised	<10 years 5mg ≥10 years 10mg		10mg	2 / 2	
	Bladder irrigation	← 50–100 microgram in 1mL solution →			2	Use appropriate volume.
Lozenges	Oral	← 10mg →			4	Treat for 10–15 days (continue for 48 hours after lesions have resolved). Increase to 8 times daily in severe infection.

Dose adjustment in renal impairment
No dose reduction is generally required in pre-existing renal failure. Dose reduction may be advisable if amphotericin is suspected of causing nephrotoxicity. Lipid complex formulations should also be considered in such situations. In renal dialysis patients, administration of amphotericin should commence only when dialysis is completed.

ADMINISTRATION
IV infusion: *conventional formulation* – reconstitute 50mg vial with 10mL Water for Injections to give a solution of 5mg in 1mL. The displacement volume is negligible. This solution must then be further diluted to a concentration of 100 microgram in 1mL with glucose 5% with a pH above 4.2. This may be ascertained by direct measurement of pH or ensured by adding a phosphate buffering solution to the glucose 5% before amphotericin addition. Concentrations up to 400 microgram in 1mL (unlicensed) may be used for fluid restricted patients providing administration is via a central line. Administer by slow IV infusion over 4-6 hours. May be reduced to a minimum of 2 hours if the 4-6 hour infusion is tolerated. Protect from direct sunlight.
Liposomal amphotericin – reconstitute 50mg vial with 12mL Water for Injections to give a solution of 4mg in 1mL. This solution must then be filtered, using the 5 micron filter provided, into the diluent solution of glucose 5% only. Dilute to a concentration between 200 microgram and 2mg in 1mL. Administer as a slow IV infusion over 1 hour. May be infused over 30 minutes if well tolerated or over more than 1 hour if acute infusion reactions occur.
ABCS – reconstitute the 50mg vial with 10mL Water for Injections and the 100mg vial with 20mL Water for Injections to provide a solution containing 5mg in 1mL. Dilute to a concentration of 625 microgram in 1mL with glucose 5% only.
ABCL – shake vial gently until any yellow sediment is removed. Withdraw the appropriate volume of solution and filter through the 5 micron filter needle in to the diluent solution (glucose 5% only) to provide a concentration of 1mg in 1mL.
Bladder irrigation: reconstitute a 50mg vial of conventional amphotericin with 10mL Water for Injections to give a 5mg in 1mL solution. Further dilute 2mL of this solution to 100mL with Water for Irrigation to produce a 100 microgram in 1mL solution, or 1mL to 100mL to produce a 50 microgram in 1mL solution for instillation into the bladder.
Lozenges: allow to dissolve slowly in the mouth.
Nebulised: add Water for Injections to a 50mg vial of amphotericin to achieve a concentration of 5mg in 1ml. Further dilute the required dose with Water for Injections to a volume of 3mL for nebulisation.

CONTRA-INDICATIONS & WARNINGS
Although lipid formulations, particularly liposomal amphotericin, may be less likely to cause severe side-effects it is still advisable to monitor all systemic formulations as conventional amphotericin. Hypersensitivity to amphotericin or any constituents of the formulations. Renal impairment may occur and discontinuation or reduction should be considered if urea or serum creatinine exceed twice the upper limit of normal. Monitor serum potassium, magnesium and phosphate as low serum levels may occur. Monitor LFTs and consider discontinuation if seriously deranged.
Avoid concurrent nephrotoxic drugs, antineoplastic agents if possible and also corticosteroids unless necessary to control drug reactions. Hyperkalaemia and arrhythmias can result if administered too rapidly.

INTERACTIONS
Conventional formulation
Increased nephrotoxicity with concurrent use of other *nephrotoxic drugs*.
Amphotericin-induced hypokalaemia may potentiate toxicity of *digitalis glycosides* and enhance effects of *skeletal muscle relaxants*. *Corticosteroids* may enhance potassium depletion. *Flucytosine* toxicity may be enhanced by increased cellular uptake and/or impaired renal function. *Zidovudine*: effects on bone

marrow and renal function may be enhanced. *Ciclosporin (cyclosporin)*: concomitant administration of Ambisome® and *ciclosporin* has reportedly resulted in increased *ciclosporin* levels.
Acute pulmonary reactions have occurred when amphotericin is given during or shortly after *leucocyte transfusions* Manufacturer advises separation of such infusions as far as possible and monitor pulmonary function. Manufacturers of Abelcet® report similar interactions. Manufacturers of Ambisome® and Amphocil® report that although no interactions with other drugs have been observed it is advisable to monitor closely.

PREGNANCY
Conventional amphotericin crosses the placenta. There are a few reports of use during pregnancy, including the first trimester, with no apparent adverse events. Caution is advised but the drug may be used in those patients who will clearly benefit from the drug.

BREAST-FEEDING
No data available of excretion into breast milk of any formulation. Contact local Medicines Information Centre for advice.

SIDE-EFFECTS
Conventional formulation
Acute infusion reactions are the most frequent adverse

A

reactions such as fever, shaking, chills, nausea, vomiting, headache, dyspnoea, tachypnoea, gastrointestinal effects, muscle and joint pains, pain at site of injection. These reactions are most severe and occur most frequently with initial doses and often lessen with subsequent doses. Febrile reactions may be managed by IV administration of hydrocortisone but keep dose and duration to a minimum. Other reactions may be decreased by use of antihistamines or paracetamol. Nephrotoxicity occurs to some degree in more than 85% of patients. Hypokalaemia, hypomagnesaemia, azotaemia, renal tubular acidosis, nephrocalcinosis and hyposthenuria can occur. Increased urea and serum creatinine, decreased creatinine clearance, GFR and decreased renal blood flow occur in many patients receiving conventional amphotericin. Renal function generally improves within a few months though some degree of permanent impairment may occur. Patients with higher serum low density lipoprotein (LDL) concentrations may be more susceptible to renal toxicity. Less common renal toxicity reactions are: anuria, oliguria, haematuria, urinary incontinence and acute renal failure.

Lipid complex formulations
While the lipid complex formulations (particularly liposomal and ABCL) appear to be associated with a lower risk (18-35%) of nephrotoxicity, or acute infusion reactions, and have been used in patients with pre-existing renal impairment (often due to conventional amphotericin B) with improvement or stabilisation of renal function, caution and monitoring is still advised as renal toxicity may occur.

Other rare adverse effects of amphotericin
Cardiovascular: arrhythmias, ventricular fibrillation, hypotension, hypertension. Bronchospasm, wheezing, angioedema and anaphylactic reactions have been reported with all formulations.
Haematological: coagulation defects, anaemia, agranulocytosis, leucopenia, thrombocytopenia, eosinophilia, leucocytosis.
Gastrointestinal: melaena, haemorrhagic gastroenteritis, anorexia, diarrhoea, epigastric pain, cramping, dyspepsia, weight loss, dry mouth, stomatitis.
Nervous system: malaise, depression, confusion, dizziness, vertigo, tinnitus, encephalopathy, peripheral neuropathy, convulsions, tremor, visual impairment.
Skin: maculopapular rash, pruritus, purpura, exfoliative dermatitis, alopecia, dry skin, skin discoloration.
Hepatic: increased LFTs, acute liver failure, hepatitis and jaundice have been reported but are rare.
Musculoskeletal: generalised pain, dystonia, muscle, bone and joint pain.

POISONING/TOXICITY
Overdose can result in cardio-respiratory arrest. Not removed by haemodialysis.

PHARMACOKINETIC PROPERTIES
Pharmacokinetics vary significantly depending on the formulation.
Usual doses of ABCS and ABCL result in lower serum concentrations and higher volume of distribution than conventional amphotericin. However, liposomal amphotericin produces a higher plasma concentration and lower volume of distribution.
The clinical importance of the differences in pharmacokinetics of the various formulations and effects on therapeutic efficacy are not clear. Amphotericin is poorly absorbed orally.

Conventional formulation
Distributed widely in body fluids and tissues including peritoneum, synovium and aqueous humour. Crosses the placenta. CNS penetration may be better in neonates. Plasma half-life is approximately 24 hours in adults but increases with length of treatment. Elimination half-life of up to 15 days has been reported. Highly protein bound (>90%) and not dialysable.
Eliminated slowly by kidneys, slow release from peripheral compartments may account for the long elimination half-life. Following discontinuation of amphotericin the drug can be detected in the blood for up to 4 weeks and in urine for 4-8 weeks. No information on tissue distribution or metabolic fate is currently available.

Liposomal Amphotericin (AmBisome®)
In animal studies higher levels are achieved in hepatic and splenic tissues and lower levels in renal tissue compared to conventional formulation. Concentrations in brain, CSF, thyroid, bone marrow, heart and muscle tissue are low. Detailed human tissue distribution and metabolic pathways have not been studied. Extensive uptake by reticulo-endothelial system occurs. Elimination half-life is 6-10 hours in adults.

ABCL (Abelcet®)
In animal studies high levels are achieved in hepatic, lung and splenic tissues and lower levels in renal tissue compared to conventional formulation. May achieve higher tissue concentrations although detailed studies have not been performed.

ABCS (Amphocil®)
In animal studies high levels are achieved in hepatic, lung and splenic tissues and lower levels in renal tissue compared to conventional formulation. May achieve higher tissue concentration although detailed studies have not been performed. May achieve higher levels in bone marrow than other formulations.

EXCIPIENTS
See manufacturers SPC for further details.

LICENSED STATUS
IV infusion preparations are not licensed for nebulisation. Conventional and lipid formulations of the IV infusion are licensed in children but unlicensed in neonates. Lozenges are not licensed for use in children.

Ampicillin

Broad-spectrum aminopenicillin.

USES
Treatment of susceptible Gram-negative and Gram-positive organisms.

PRESENTATION
Capsule: 250mg – Penbritin® and non-proprietary; 500mg – non-proprietary
Injection: (sodium salt) 500mg vial – Penbritin®.
Oral suspension: 125mg in 5mL and 250mg in 5mL – non-proprietary.

DOSAGE
Neonate (birth to 1 month)

Route	Age	Dose	Frequency	Notes
Oral/IV/IM	<7 days	50mg/kg	12 hourly	Increase IV dose to 100mg/kg/dose
	7–21 days	50mg/kg	8 hourly	in suspected meningitis or Group B
	>21 days	50mg/kg	6 hourly	streptococcal infection.

Child

Route	Age			Frequency (times daily)	Notes
	1 month–2 years	2–12 years	12–18 years		
Oral	12.5mg/kg	250mg	500mg	4	
IV/IM	←	25mg/kg	→	4	Maximum single dose 1g.
IV infusion	←	100mg/kg	→	4	Meningitis, septicaemia, CNS or severe infection. Maximum single dose 3g.

Patients with renal impairment
Severe impairment (creatinine clearance $<10mL/minute/1.73m^2$) reduce dose or frequency of administration.
Ampicillin is removed by haemodialysis. Patients undergoing haemodialysis should receive a supplemental dose of ampicillin after each dialysis period.

ADMINISTRATION
Oral: administer 30 minutes before food as food may affect absorption.
IV: each 250mg ampicillin displaces 0.2mL. Reconstitute with Water for Injections: 250mg vial with 4.8mL to give 50mg in 1mL; 500mg vial with 9.6mL to give 50mg in 1mL (some units reconstitute the 500mg vial with 4.6mL to give 100mg in 1mL). Administer as a slow IV injection over 3-5 minutes or inject into a flowing infusion. High dose therapy (100mg/kg/dose) may need to be infused over at least 10 minutes due to the volume administered.
IM: add 1.5mL Water for Injections to each 250mg vial to give 147mg in 1mL.

Compatible with NaCl 0.9%, use within 48 hours (central intravenous additive service [CIVAS] preparations only). Compatible with glucose 5% and 10%, and glucose/saline but must be used within 1 hour. Incompatible with dextrans, lipid emulsions and sodium bicarbonate. Do not mix with aminoglycosides: adequate flushing between doses or administration at separate sites is suggested.
As well as IV, IM and oral routes, ampicillin may be administered by the following routes in conjunction with systemic therapy; intraperitoneal, intrapleural, intra-articular and local use in abdominal surgery.

CONTRA-INDICATIONS & WARNINGS
Hypersensitivity to penicillins or cephalosporins. A high percentage of patients with infectious mononucleosis develop a rash with aminopenicillins and ampicillin should preferably not be used in these patients.
Monitor renal and hepatic function especially if prolonged therapy, high doses or pre-existing renal or hepatic insufficiency.

INTERACTIONS
With *allopurinol* increased frequency of skin rashes. *Chloroquine* reduces ampicillin absorption. *Probenecid* increases ampicillin levels. With *warfarin* prolongation of prothrombin time. Ampicillin decreases efficacy of *oestrogen containing oral contraceptives*.

PREGNANCY
Considered safe and appropriate to use if necessary during pregnancy.

BREAST-FEEDING
Trace quantities in breast milk but considered compatible. Usual precautions for antibiotics in breast-feeding should be considered.

SIDE-EFFECTS
Gastrointestinal upsets (nausea, diarrhoea), urticarial penicillin hypersensitivity rash; erythematous, maculopapular rash also reported in up to 10% of children in some studies. Incidence of rash may be higher in HIV patients.

POISONING/TOXICITY
Treat symptomatically.

PHARMACOKINETIC PROPERTIES
Oral: 30-60% absorbed from the gastrointestinal tract. Peak levels occur 1–2 hours after oral administration. Non-linear relationship between dose and peak serum concentration.
IM: peak levels occur within about 1 hour. Widely distributed in body fluids achieving therapeutic concentrations in ascitic, pleural and joint fluids. Distributed into bile and achieves concentrations 2 to 30 times higher than serum. Undergoes enterohepatic recycling. Some excreted in faeces. Little diffusion into CSF except when meninges inflamed. 20-40% of an oral dose and 60–80% of IV/IM dose excreted in urine within 6 hours of a dose. 20% bound to plasma proteins. Half-life of 1 to 1.5 hours is increased in neonates.

EXCIPIENTS
Contact manufacturers for further details.

LICENSED STATUS
Licensed in all ages.

Amsacrine

Intercalates DNA and inhibits topoisomerase II leading to DNA damage and cell death.

USES
Acute myeloid leukaemia.

PRESENTATION
Injection: 75mg ampoule and diluent vial, reconstituted solution contains 5mg in 1mL amsacrine (as lactate) – Amsidine®.

DOSAGE
** Always consult the current treatment protocol for details of dosage and scheduling. **

ADMINISTRATION
IV: infusion over 60-90 minutes in glucose 5%. Glass syringes are recommended for preparation, however, this is impractical. At The Royal Marsden Hospital, each ampoule of amsacrine is drawn up into standard individual syringes, without allowing the drug to come into contact with the rubber bung, then added to the diluent vials. One syringe is then used to draw up the total dose from the reconstituted solution which is added as quickly as possible to the infusion bag. Lines should be primed and flushed with glucose 5% prior to and after administration (sodium chloride solutions cause precipitation).

CONTRA-INDICATIONS & WARNINGS
Contra-indications: amsacrine should not be given to individuals who already have marked bone marrow suppression induced by other agents.

Cautions: the potential for cardiotoxicity may be increased by hypokalaemia, concurrent diuretics, aminoglycosides or other nephrotoxic drugs and previous exposure to anthracyclines.

Warnings: the terminal half-life is prolonged in patients with severe hepatic dysfunction.

INTERACTIONS
Incompatible with *sodium chloride solutions.*

PREGNANCY
Animal studies have indicated that amsacrine has fetotoxic and teratogenic properties. There is no information on use in human pregnancy, therefore the benefit verses risk considerations should be carefully weighed before administering amsacrine.

BREAST-FEEDING
Breast-feeding is not recommended.

SIDE-EFFECTS
Haematopoietic system: myelosuppression and pancytopenia are dose-limiting side-effects.

Gastrointestinal: nausea and vomiting, mucositis.

Central nervous system: a few cases of grand mal seizures have been reported.

Cardiac: ventricular tachycardia, congestive heart failure and cardiac arrest have been reported.

Hepatic: increased bilirubin and liver enzymes.

Renal: occasional haematuria, anuria and rarely acute renal failure.

Skin: local tissue irritation, necrosis and phlebitis have been reported. Alopecia occurs in 1 in 7 patients.

POISONING/TOXICITY
Supportive care only.

PHARMACOKINETIC PROPERTIES
Amsacrine distributes well in the body except to the brain and CSF. It undergoes extensive biotransformation in the liver and metabolites are excreted in bile by an active transport mechanism.

EXCIPIENTS
See manufacturers SPC for further details.

LICENSED STATUS
Licensed for use in adults.

FURTHER INFORMATION
Vesicant, therefore administration via a central line is preferable though not essential. Pain or phlebitis at the injection site may occur at doses >70mg/m^2.

Arachis (peanut) oil

Enemas containing arachis oil lubricate and soften impacted faeces.

USES
To soften impacted faeces promoting a bowel movement.

PRESENTATION
Enema: arachis oil retention enema containing 130mL arachis oil BP – Fletchers' Arachis Oil Retention Enema®.

DOSAGE

Route	Age			Frequency	Notes
	1 month–2 years	2–12 years	12–18 years	(times daily)	
Rectal	Not recommended	3-7 years $1/3 - 1/2$ enema 7-12 years $1/2 - 3/4$ enema	$3/4$ - 1 enema	when necessary	Use in children only under medical supervision.

ADMINISTRATION
Rectal: warm enema before use by placing in warm water.

A

CONTRA-INDICATIONS & WARNINGS
Contains peanut oil. Do not use if hypersensitive to arachis oil or peanuts. Inflammatory bowel disease except under medical supervision. Caution in children and in patients with intestinal obstruction.

PREGNANCY/BREAST-FEEDING
Only under medical supervision.

SIDE-EFFECTS
Local irritation.

LICENSED STATUS
Licensed for use in >3 years of age.

Arginine

USES
Carbamylphosphate synthetase (CPS) deficiency; ornithine carbamyltransferase (OCT) deficiency; citrullinaemia (argininosuccinic acid synthase deficiency [ASAS]); arginosuccinic aciduria (ASA) (argininosuccinic acid lyase deficiency [ASAL]); growth hormone secretion testing.

PRESENTATION
Injection: 10%, 200mL; 20%, 50mL, 100mL; 60%, 20mL – manufactured 'specials'.
Powder: as free base – manufactured 'special'.
Solution: 50mg in 1mL – may be extemporaneously prepared.
Tablet: 500mg – manufactured 'special'.

DOSAGE

Indication	Route	Age				Frequency (times daily)	Notes
		birth–1 month	1 month–2 years	2–12 years	12–18 years		
OCT and CPS deficiencies	Oral	←	25–35mg/kg		→	3–4	
	IV infusion	←	200mg/kg		→	single dose	Loading dose. Given over 90 minutes.
	IV infusion	←	200mg/kg/day		→	continuous	
Citrullinaemia and ASA	Oral	←	100–175mg/kg		→	3–4	Up to 700mg/kg/day.
	IV infusion	←	600mg/kg		→	single dose	Loading dose. Given over 90 minutes.
	IV infusion	←	600mg/kg/day (25mg/kg/hour)		→	continuous	
Growth hormone test	IV infusion	←	500 mg/kg		→	single dose	Over 30 minutes.

ADMINISTRATION
Oral: solution and powder may be mixed with milk, fruit juice or food to improve palatability. 10% and 20% injection solutions can be used orally.
IV: dilute to 20mg in 1mL with glucose 10% or 5%, maximum concentration is 100mg in 1mL. It can be infused at Y-site with carnitine, sodium benzoate and sodium phenylbutyrate (no data to support this but has been done in practice).

CONTRA-INDICATIONS & WARNINGS
Do not use in arginase deficiency.

INTERACTIONS/PREGNANCY/ BREAST-FEEDING
No information available.

SIDE-EFFECTS
No side-effects noted when arginine given orally. Nausea, vomiting, headache, flushing, numbness, local venous irritation and hypotension noted with IV infusion.

POISONING/TOXICITY
High concentrations of arginine seen in patients with arginase deficiency are thought to contribute to neurological damage therefore if give high doses of exogenous arginine it is possible that a similar effect will be seen. Monitor levels; target levels 50-200 micromol/L. The evidence for toxicity at 200 micromol/L is not strong.

PHARMACODYNAMIC PROPERTIES
Arginine administration catalyses the urea cycle allowing its continuation. It also reacts with nitrogen-containing substances earlier in the cycle to form less toxic compounds that are more readily excreted by the kidneys than ammonia itself (as citrulline in ASAS deficiency and argininosuccinic acid in ASAL deficiency).

PHARMACOKINETIC PROPERTIES
Well absorbed from the gastrointestinal tract.

LICENSED STATUS
Injections and tablet available as 'specials' and as such are unlicensed.
Powder is approved as a borderline substance for the treatment of patients with urea cycle disorders.

FURTHER INFORMATION
Powder available from Scientific Hospital Supplies and Special Products Ltd.
Oral solution formula is available from Pharmacy Department (not validated), Great Ormond Street Hospital, London.
Tablets available from Special Products Ltd.

Argipressin

Argipressin is 8-arginine vasopressin, a synthetic form of the naturally occurring antidiuretic hormone (ADH) in humans. It has both pressor and antidiuretic activity.

USES
Treatment of bleeding oesophageal varices.

PRESENTATION
Injection: 20 units in 1mL – Pitressin®.

DOSAGE

Route	Age			Frequency	Notes
	1 month–2 years	2–12 years	12–18 years		
IV infusion over 20–30 minutes	←	0.3 units/kg	→	single dose	Efficacy and tolerance may be improved by the simultaneous use of glyceryl trinitrate.
IV infusion	←	0.3 units/kg/hour	→	*continuous	Maximum rate of 1 unit/kg/ hour if bleed continues.

*A continuous infusion should only be administered when no alternative measures are available and should be discontinued at the earliest safe opportunity. Treatment should not normally continue for more than 72 hours. Patients should be monitored carefully.

ADMINISTRATION
IV: a loading dose is given as a short IV infusion over 20-30 minutes. Infuse in glucose 5% or NaCl 0.9% at a concentration of 0.2 unit/mL (maximum of 1 unit/mL). Extreme care should be taken to avoid fluid overload due to the risk of water intoxication with argipressin.

CONTRA-INDICATIONS & WARNINGS
Hypersensitivity to argipressin, or any component of the formulation. Chronic nephritis (until reasonable blood urea/creatinine concentrations attained). May induce water intoxication. Avoid or use with extreme caution in patients with systemic hypertension or vascular disease, particularly of the coronary arteries. Monitor closely for signs of anginal pain or skin ischaemia. Use with caution in patients with epilepsy, migraine, asthma, heart failure or any state in which a rapid addition to extracellular water may precipitate problems. Caution in acute/chronic renal failure. Monitor fluid intake and output, urine and serum sodium and osmolality.

INTERACTIONS
Carbamazepine, tricyclic antidepressants and *fludrocortisone* may decrease ADH activity. Large doses of *adrenaline (epinephrine)* and *heparin* may increase ADH activity.

A

PREGNANCY
Argipressin has been used for the treatment of diabetes insipidus in pregnancy with no reported adverse effect on the fetus. Possible oxytocic effects in the third trimester.

BREAST-FEEDING
Argipressin has been administered to breast-feeding mothers without apparent harm to the baby.

SIDE-EFFECTS
Local or systemic allergic reactions may occur in hypersensitive individuals. Myocardial ischaemia and infarction. Cardiac dysrhythmias, hypertension, venous thrombosis. Tremor, sweating, vertigo, circumoral pallor, 'pounding' in the head, abdominal cramps, diarrhoea, flatulence, nausea, vomiting, urticaria, wheezing, bronchial constriction, fluid retention, hyponatraemia. Peripheral and central ischaemia and gangrene have been reported rarely.

POISONING/TOXICITY
Water intoxication should be treated with fluid restriction, although in severe cases small amounts of hypertonic sodium chloride may be administered. Urea and/or mannitol may be helpful in the treatment of cerebral oedema. Glyceryl trinitrate should be given sublingually if the patient experiences anginal pain.

PHARMACOKINETIC PROPERTIES
Argipressin is rapidly inactivated by trypsin. No oral products are therefore available. Onset of action is 1 hour. Plasma half-life is approximately 7.5 minutes (range 5-15 minutes). Argipressin does not bind to plasma protein.

EXCIPIENTS
See manufacturers SPC for further details.

LICENSED STATUS
Not licensed for use in children.

Artemisinin and its derivatives

Dihydroartemisinin, artemether, sodium artesunate and arteether.

Potent antimalarials.

USES
Antimalarials for treatment of *P. falciparum* contracted in areas of multidrug resistance, such as south east Asia, Cambodia, Myanmar and Vietnam.

PRESENTATION
Several presentations of artemisinin and its derivatives including oral, parenteral and rectal formulations are available in some countries (artemisinin only as oral and rectal formulations), but none are licensed for use in the UK. Artemether is available as 50mg tablets and 40mg in 1mL, 80mg in 1mL and 100mg in 1mL IM injection which can be imported on a named patient basis.

DOSAGE/ ADMINISTRATION
Expert advice should be sought from one of the Schools of Tropical Medicine for optimum treatment including choice of preparation and dosage.

CONTRA-INDICATIONS & WARNINGS
First trimester of pregnancy.

INTERACTIONS
Caution with drugs that prolong the QT interval, such as *quinine* and *halofantrine*.

PREGNANCY
Use should be avoided during the first trimester of pregnancy, but in cases of severe malaria the risks have to be balanced against the benefits. Very limited documented data on use in pregnant women. No abnormalities were reported in 6-10 year follow-up of six children born to mothers who received IM artemisinin or artemether at 17-27 weeks gestation nor in a 3 month to 10 year follow-up of seventeen children born to mothers who received artemisinin at 16-38 weeks of pregnancy. At present no serious congenital defects have been reported passively.

BREAST-FEEDING
No information available. Contact local Medicines Information Centre for advice.

Artemisinin and its derivatives continued

SIDE-EFFECTS
Generally well tolerated at therapeutic doses; usually signs and symptoms cannot be differentiated from malaria-related effects. Neurotoxicity and cardiotoxicity have been demonstrated in high dose animal studies.

POISONING/TOXICITY
No information available.

PHARMACOKINETIC PROPERTIES
The pharmacokinetics of artemisinin and its derivatives are not yet known in detail. Studies have been hampered by lack of a suitable assay for measuring concentrations in biological fluids. In general, oral absorption seems to be rapid but incomplete. Following administration artemisinin and its derivatives are rapidly hydrolysed to the active metabolite dihydroartemisinin which is subsequently converted to inactive metabolites.

LICENSED STATUS
Not licensed for use in the UK.

FURTHER INFORMATION
Some presentations may be imported on a named patient basis via IDIS World Medicines or obtained through one of the Schools of Tropical Medicine.

Artificial salivas

These agents provide temporary relief for the symptoms of a dry mouth.

PRESENTATION
Aerosal spray: carmellose sodium 500mg/50g – Glandosone®.
Lozenges: mucin 65mg – AS Saliva Orthana®.
Mouthwash: lactoperoxidase, lactoferrin, lysozyme, glucose oxidase – Biotene®.
Oral spray: gastric mucin 3.5%, sodium fluoride 4.2mg/litre – AS Saliva Orthana®; carmellose sodium 390mg, sodium fluoride 258 microgram/60mL – Luborant®; carmellose sodium – Salivace®; carmellose sodium – Saliveze®.
Pastilles: Salivix®.
Saliva replacement gel: lactoperoxidase, glucose oxidase – Biotene Oralbalance®.
Tablets: SST®.
Toothpaste: lactoperoxidase, glucose oxidase, sodium monofluorophosphate 1000ppm – Biotene®.

DOSAGE/ADMINISTRATION
AS Saliva Orthana®: 2–3 sprays onto oral and pharyngeal mucosa when required; lozenges – suck as required.
Biotene®: mouthwash – gargle as often as necessary; toothpaste – put 1-1.5g on a toothbrush and brush for at least 30 seconds, twice daily.
Biotene Oralbalance®: apply as necessary to a dry mouth, coating the gums and tongue until they feel comfortable.
Glandosane®: spray onto oral and pharyngeal mucosa as required.
Luborant®: 2–3 sprays onto oral mucosa up to 4 times per day, or as directed.
Salivace®: 1–2 sprays onto oral mucosa as required.
Saliveze®: 1 spray onto oral mucosa as required.
Salivix®: suck 1 pastille as required.
SST®: allow 1 tablet to dissolve slowly in the mouth when required.

CONTRA-INDICATIONS & WARNINGS
Saliva Orthana® contains gastric mucin and thus may be unsuitable for those who have objections for religious or cultural reasons to ingestion of medicaments derived from a porcine source.
Do not use Biotene® products with toothpastes containing detergents or other tensioactive agents such as foaming agents. Close the tube of Biotene® toothpaste after each use to prevent contact with air which will in time deactivate the enzyme system contained in the paste. Biotene® toothpaste is unsuitable for children <6 years of age because of the 1000ppm fluoride content.

SIDE-EFFECTS/INTERACTIONS
None documented.

A

EXCIPIENTS
Contact manufacturers for further details.

LICENSED STATUS
AS Saliva Orthana®, Biotene Oralbalance®, Glandosone®, Salivace®, Saliveze® and Salivix® are ABCS listed for dry mouth associated only with radiotherapy or sicca syndrome.
Luborant® is licensed for any condition giving rise to dry mouth.

FURTHER INFORMATION
Only AS Saliva Orthana® oral spray, Biotene® toothpaste and Luborant® contain fluoride.

Asparaginase

Erwinase® Crisantaspase (asparaginase from *Erwinia chrysanthemi*).
Elspar® asparaginase aminohydralase derived from *Escherichia coli*.
Medac asparaginase derived from *Escherichia coli*.

See pegaspagase monograph for pegylated form of *E. coli* asparaginase.

Asparaginase inhibits protein synthesis in tumour cells dependent on exogenous asparagine, a non-essential amino acid in humans.

USES
Acute lymphoblastic leukaemia (ALL), acute myeloid leukaemia, non-Hodgkin lymphoma.

PRESENTATION
Injection: 5000 and 10,000 unit vial, powder for reconstitution – available from Medac; 10,000 unit vial, powder for reconstitution – Elspar® and Erwinase®.

DOSAGE
** Always consult the current treatment protocol for details of dosage and scheduling. **
Note: Elspar® brand of asparaginase and the Medac asparaginase are not equivalent and not interchangeable.

ADMINISTRATION
Erwinase®: IM is the recommended route of administration in all current 2002 UKCCSG protocols.
IM/SC/IV: reconstitute with 1-2mL of NaCl 0.9%. Must be administered within 15 minutes of reconstitution due to polymerisation of the enzyme. Avoid contact with rubber i.e. syringe plunger.
IV injection is rarely indicated but may be used (increased risk of anaphylaxis). Patients should be observed for signs of an anaphylactic type reaction for 30 minutes after asparaginase administration. Facilities for the management of anaphylaxis should be available. IV infusion is no longer recommended by the manufacturers of Erwinase®.
Elspar®: IM or IV administration. IM reconstitute with 2mL NaCl 0.9%. Use within 8 hours. IV reconstitute with 5mL and give directly or add to NaCl 0.9% or glucose 5% solutions for infusion. Use within 8 hours.
Medac Asparaginase: dissolve the powder in the 5000 unit vial with 2mL of Water for Injections and the 10,000 unit vial with 4mL of Water for Injections by squirting it carefully on the inner wall of the vial (not directly on the powder). For IM use no further dilution is needed. For IV continuous infusion, after reconstitution, further dilute in 250-500mL of NaCl 0.9% or glucose 5% and infuse over several hours.

CONTRA-INDICATIONS & WARNINGS
Contra-indications: previous allergic reaction to asparaginase.
Cautions: Erwinase® should preferably be given without interruption. If, however, an interruption cannot be avoided, treatment should be resumed with a low dose, 10 units/kg/day, and increased to the full dose over 5 days if tolerated.
Pretreatment with Elspar® also increases risk of hypersensitivity reactions at a later date. If skin testing indicates hypersensitivity, therapy should only be resumed after successful desensitisation.
Warnings: anaphylaxis is rare but facilities should be made available for management during administration.

INTERACTIONS
Asparaginase must not be mixed with any other drugs prior to administration.

PREGNANCY
There are no adequate and well-controlled studies with

Elspar®. Elspar® should only be used if the potential benefit outweighs the risk. Erwinase® should not be given to women who are, or who are likely to become pregnant. Medac asparaginase is contra-indicated in pregnancy.

BREAST-FEEDING

It is not known whether asparaginase is secreted into human milk and safety is not established. Therefore it is suggested that mothers receiving asparaginase should not breast-feed.

SIDE-EFFECTS

Undesirable effects are generally reversible and are less common with *Erwinia* L-asparaginase than with *E. coli* asparaginase. Patients receiving treatment with L-asparaginase from *E.coli* who develop hypersensitivity may be able to continue treatment with *Erwinia* L-asparaginase, and vice-versa, as the enzymes are immunologically distinct.

Neurological: neurotoxicity, CNS depression including somnolence, fatigue and coma, agitation, hallucinations.
Gastrointestinal: nausea and vomiting, acute pancreatitis.
Hepatic: elevation of bilirubin, serum glutamic oxaloacetic transaminase (SGOT), alkaline phosphatase (ALP) and cholesterol levels; decreases in fibrinogen and some clotting factors.

Renal: azotemia, acute renal failure.
Skin: rash, urticaria.
Other: life threatening sepsis and severe hypersensitivity have been described in patients treated with L-asparaginases. IM administration has a lower incidence of anaphylaxis than IV. Other effects reported with both enzymes include fever and various plasma biochemical changes. For these reasons, careful monitoring is therefore necessary and urine should be tested for glucose to exclude hyperglycaemia.

POISONING/TOXICITY

Undesirable effects are generally self-limiting. Facilities should be available to manage anaphylaxis. Monitoring of SGOT, ALP, bilirubin, clotting factors and glucose is recommended. No specific measures are recommended in overdose.

PHARMACOKINETIC PROPERTIES

Peak levels of Erwinase® are achieved in blood in 1-2 hours. The fall in enzyme levels follows first order kinetics with a half-life of 7-13 hours. Apparent volume of distribution is only slightly higher than plasma volume. L-asparaginase derived from different sources is not equivalent and substitution must take pharmacokinetic differences into account.

EXCIPIENTS
See manufacturers SPC for further details.

LICENSED STATUS
Medac asparaginase is not licensed for use in the UK.
Erwinase® is licensed for use in children and adults.
Elspar® is not licensed for use in the UK but is licensed for use in children and adults outside the UK.

FURTHER INFORMATION
The Elspar® *E.coli* derived asparaginase is currently recommended for the MRC UKALL trial. When the ALL 2003 trial opens, Medac asparaginase will be recommended. It is already in use for the Infant ALL trial.

Aspirin

A non-opioid analgesic with anti-inflammatory, antipyretic and antithrombotic actions.

PRESENTATION
Tablet: 75mg – Angettes 75®; 300mg – non-proprietary.
Tablet: (dispersible) 75mg and 300mg – non-proprietary.
Tablet: (enteric coated) 75mg and 300mg – Caprin®, Nu-Seals® Aspirin and non-proprietary.

USES
Kawasaki disease. Antiplatelet therapy e.g. management of post-operative patient with prosthetic heart valve, Fontan circulation or modified Blalock Taussig shunt.

A

DOSAGE

Indication	Route	Age			Frequency	Notes
		1 month–2 years	2–12 years	12–18 years	(times daily)	
Antiplatelet dose	Oral	← 10mg/kg →		75mg	1	
Kawasaki disease	Oral	← 25mg/kg → then		-	4	Give the higher dose until the 14th day of illness or until afebrile, followed by a single daily dose of 5mg/kg for 6-8 weeks for all patients. If no evidence of coronary lesions, discontinue after this period therwise seek cardiology opinion.
		← 5mg/kg →		-	1	

ADMINISTRATION

Oral: to give doses less than 75mg, dissolve one tablet in 10-15mL of water and use a proportion to obtain correct dose. Use immediately and discard remainder.

CONTRA-INDICATIONS & WARNINGS

Active peptic ulceration; haemophilia and other bleeding disorders. Do not give aspirin to children <12 years unless medically indicated and avoid in children aged up to and including 15 years if feverish. Use with caution in asthmatics, impaired renal or hepatic function, G6PD deficiency.

INTERACTIONS

Increased risk of bleeding with *anticoagulants*, increased side-effects with concomitant *NSAIDs*, decreased excretion of *methotrexate*, enhanced effect of *phenytoin* and *sodium valproate*.

PREGNANCY

There is clinical and epidemiological evidence of the safety of aspirin in pregnancy. However, it may prolong labour and contribute to maternal or neonatal bleeding. Hence is best avoided in the last trimester unless recommended by a doctor.

BREAST-FEEDING

Avoid – possible risk of Reye's syndrome. Regular use of high doses could impair platelet function and produce hypoprothrombinaemia in infants if neonatal vitamin K stores are low.

SIDE-EFFECTS

Bronchospasm, gastrointestinal irritation (including haemorrhage), and hypoglycaemia may occur with high doses.

POISONING/TOXICITY

Consider gastric lavage, forced alkaline diuresis and supportive therapy. Restoration of acid-base balance may be required. Major toxic signs include tinnitus, difficulty in hearing, sweating, dizziness, mental confusion; hyperventilation may lead to coma, cardiovascular collapse and respiratory depression.

PHARMACOKINETIC PROPERTIES

Oral absorption is >80%, is highly bound to plasma proteins and widely distributed.

EXCIPIENTS

Contact manufacturers for further details.

LICENSED STATUS

Not licensed for use <16 years of age.

Atenolol

Beta-blocker.

USES

Hypertension.

PREPARATIONS
Tablet: 25mg, 50mg and 100mg – Tenormin® and non-proprietary.
Syrup: 25mg in 5mL – Tenormin®.

DOSAGE

Route	Age				Frequency (times daily)	Notes
	birth–1 month	1 month–2 years	2–12 years	12–18 years		
Oral	←	1–2mg/kg	→	50mg	1	Adjust according to blood pressure and heart rate. May be given twice daily if necessary. Maximum of 100mg daily.

Renal failure
No dose adjustment is required in patients with a creatinine clearance >35mL/minute/1.73m². If creatinine clearance 10-35mL/minute/1.73m² give 50% dose, <10mL/minute/1.73m² give 30-50% dose and adjust according to response. In haemodialysis and CAPD give 30-50% of dose and adjust according to response. Also see propranolol monograph.

CONTRA-INDICATIONS & WARNINGS
Atenolol is relatively cardioselective but can still have an effect on airways resistance. Therefore it should be avoided in patients with a history of asthma. Atenolol may be used in patients with stable heart failure but initiation must be gradual.

INTERACTIONS, SIDE-EFFECTS, POISONING/TOXICITY
See propranolol monograph.

PREGNANCY
As propranolol monograph. Atenolol has been used under close supervision for the treatment of hypertension in the third trimester. Contact local Medicines Information Centre for advice.

BREAST-FEEDING
There is significant accumulation of atenolol in breast milk. Contact local Medicines Information Centre for advice.

EXCIPIENTS
Tenormin® syrup includes sorbitol. Contact manufacturers for further details.

LICENSED STATUS
Not licensed for use in children.

Atracurium besilate (besylate)

Atracurium is a short-acting non-depolarising neuromuscular blocking agent (competitive acetylcholine blocker).

USES
Neuromuscular blockade for ventilation and surgery.

PRESENTATION
Injection: 10mg in 1mL; 2.5mL, 5mL and 25mL ampoules – Tracrium® and non-proprietary.

DOSAGE

Route	Age				Frequency (times daily)	Notes
	birth–1 month	1 month–2 years	2–12 years	12–18 years		
IV bolus	*300–500 microgram/kg	←	300–600 microgram/kg	→	single dose	Initial dose. Supplemental doses of 100–200 microgram/kg can be given (up to 1mg/kg for rapid sequence induction).
IV infusion	*300–400 microgram/kg/hour	←	300-600 microgram/kg/hour (5-10 microgram/kg/minute)	→	continuous	

A

ADMINISTRATION
IV: infusion can be prepared using glucose 5% or NaCl 0.9% (both stable for 24 hours). Do not dilute to concentrations less than 500 microgram/mL. Requires no dose adjustment in renal or hepatic impairment.

CONTRA-INDICATIONS & WARNINGS
*Neonates may be more sensitive than children and adults (see dosage table). Little published information on its use in neonates.

INTERACTIONS
Blockade may be enhanced by *inhaled anaesthetics* such as *halothane, isoflurane* and *enflurane* and also by *aminoglycosides, lidocaine (lignocaine), furosemide(frusemide)* and *magnesium sulphate.*

PREGNANCY
In common with all neuromuscular blocking agents, atracurium should be used during pregnancy only if the potential benefit to the mother outweighs any potential risk to the fetus.

BREAST-FEEDING
Contact local Medicines Information Centre for advice.

SIDE-EFFECTS
Skin flushing and transient hypotension.

POISONING/TOXICITY
Reversed by atropine (20 microgram/kg) followed by neostigmine (80 microgram/kg).

PHARMACOKINETIC PROPERTIES
Elimination by non-enzymatic Hoffman degradation independently of liver or kidney function. It is non-cumulative, and only effective for 15-30 minutes.

EXCIPIENTS
Contact manufacturers for further advice.

LICENSED STATUS
Licensed for use >1 month of age.

FURTHER INFORMATION
Store at 2-8°C and protect from light.

Atropine sulphate

Antimuscarinic with central and peripheral actions.

USES
Premedication: to reduce salivation and dry airway secretions; to reduce bradycardia induced by anaesthetic agents, to counteract muscarinic effects of anticholinesterase agents during reversal of non-depolarising neuromuscular blockade.

PRESENTATION
Injection: 600 microgram in 1mL (other strengths also available) – non-proprietary.
Injection: prefilled disposable syringe 100 microgram in 1mL, 5mL, 10mL and 30mL – non-proprietary.
Injection: prefilled disposable syringe 200 microgram in 1mL, 5mL and 300 microgram in 1mL, 10mL – non-proprietary.
Oral solution: 500 microgram in 5mL – manufactured 'special'.
Tablet: 600 microgram – non-proprietary.

DOSAGE

Route	Age				Frequency (times daily)	Notes
	birth–1 month	1 month–2 years	2–12 years	12–18 years		
SC/IM	15 microgram/kg	← 10–30 microgram/kg → (minimum 100 microgram, maximum 600 microgram)		300–600 microgram	single dose	Not to be given IM in neonates. Administer 45 minutes before procedure.
IV bolus over 1 minute	15 microgram/kg	← 20 microgram/kg → (minimum 100 microgram, maximum 600 microgram)		300–600 microgram	single dose	Dose to be given at induction in the unpremedicated.
Oral	← 20–40 microgram/kg → (maximum 900 microgram)			900 microgram	single dose	Administer 1–2 hours pre-operatively.

A

ADMINISTRATION
Oral: injection can be given orally.

CONTRA-INDICATIONS & WARNINGS
Contra-indicated in urinary tract obstruction, thyrotoxicosis, fever, ileus, pyloric stenosis and glaucoma. Caution in conditions characterised by tachycardia, in obstructive disease of the gastro-intestinal tract, severe ulcerative colitis, hepatitis, asthma and myasthenia gravis.

INTERACTIONS
Many drugs have antimuscarinic effects; concomitant use of two or more such drugs can increase side-effects such as dry mouth, urine retention and constipation, e.g. *disopyramide, antihistamines, tricyclic antidepressants, phenothiazines.* Antagonism of *metoclopramide, domperidone.* Reduces gastric motility and may affect absorption of other drugs e.g. *ketoconazole.*

PREGNANCY
Possible association with limb reduction defects. Neonates may show a mild bradycardia after premedication of mothers with atropine.

BREAST-FEEDING
The passage of atropine into breast milk is controversial. No adequate data available, although no adverse effects have been reported in nursing infants whose mothers had been given atropine. Suggestions that atropine is secreted into breast milk in sufficient quantities to cause neonatal toxicity and that milk production is reduced have been challenged. The American Academy of Pediatrics considers atropine to be compatible with breast-feeding though it may be cautious to monitor the neonate.

SIDE-EFFECTS
Cardiovascular: tachycardia, cardiac arrhythmias.
CNS: confusion, tremor, drowsiness, restlessness, hallucinations.
GI: dry mouth, impaired gastrointestinal motility, constipation, oesophageal reflux.
Ophthalmic: blurred vision, pupilary dilation, raised intra-ocular pressure.
Other: urinary urgency plus retention, skin flushing, fever.

POISONING/TOXICITY
Symptoms: overdose produces exaggerated pharmacological effects, i.e. dry mouth and skin, blurred vision, constipation, urinary hesitancy, drowsiness, flushing, and tachycardia. Restlessness, confusion, ataxia, incoordination, hyperthermia, hypertension, tachypnoea, nausea, vomiting, rash, psychotic reactions, hallucinations, delirium and occasionally seizures can occur. In severe poisoning CNS depression may be seen with coma, circulatory and respiratory failure leading to death.
Treatment: neostigmine may be given to combat the peripheral anticholinergic effects.

PHARMACOKINETIC PROPERTIES
Well absorbed from the small bowel but not at all from the stomach. Intravenous administration should produce an effect within 30 seconds which lasts for at least 2 hours. Subcutaneous administration is maximally effective after 30–60 minutes. Crosses the blood-brain barrier. Incompletely metabolised in the liver, excreted as unchanged drug and metabolites.

EXCIPIENTS
Contact manufacturers for further details.

LICENSED STATUS
Injection is licensed for use in children. Oral administration of the injection is not licensed. Oral solutions available as 'specials' and as such are unlicensed.

FURTHER INFORMATION
Oral solution available from Rosemont.

Azathioprine

Immunosuppressant which inhibits the proliferation of B and T lymphocytes.

USES
To enhance survival/prevent rejection of organ transplants such as renal, cardiac and hepatic transplants.
As a steroid sparing agent in systemic lupus erythematosus; also used in other connective tissue and autoimmune diseases and vasculitis. Inflammatory bowel disease (ulcerative colitis and Crohn's disease).

PRESENTATION
Capsule: 10mg – manufactured 'special'.
Injection: (as sodium salt) 50mg – Imuran®.
Liquid: may be extemporaneously prepared.
Tablet: 25mg and 50mg – Imuran® and non-proprietary.

DOSAGE

Route	Age			Frequency (times daily)	Notes
	1 month–2 years	2–12 years	12–18 years		
Oral/IV	←	1.5–3mg/kg	→	1	The total daily oral dose may be given in 2 divided doses. Only use IV when the oral route is impractical.
Oral	←	2mg/kg	→	1	Inflammatory bowel disease. The total daily dose may be given in 2 divided doses.

During the first 4 weeks of therapy, full blood count (including platelets) should be performed at least weekly, and monthly thereafter. More frequent monitoring may be indicated if high dosage is used or in the presence of severe renal or hepatic impairment. Dosage should be reduced in renal failure. In transplantation, dose depends on the immunosuppressive regimen employed; always follow the protocol and seek expert advice before prescribing.

ADMINISTRATION
Oral: it is possible to split the tablets but this is not recommended due to the cytotoxic nature of the drug. Take with or after food.

IV: reconstitution and dilution should be carried out under full aseptic conditions. Any unused solution should be discarded as cytotoxic waste. Reconstitute vial with 5-15mL Water for Injections. Since azathioprine injection is alkaline (pH 10) and very irritant give slowly (over at least 1 minute) and flush through with 50mL of NaCl 0.9% or glucose 4%/NaCl 0.18%. Reconstituted solution can be diluted in NaCl 0.9% or glucose 5% and infused over 30–60 minutes.

The patient's eyes, skin and mucous membranes should be protected from the reconstituted or diluted solution. The patient's clothing, body and bedding should be protected by an absorbent disposable layer on top of a waterproof layer.

CONTRA-INDICATIONS & WARNINGS
Hypersensitivity to azathioprine or its metabolite, 6-mercaptopurine.

INTERACTIONS
Allopurinol inhibits the metabolism of an active metabolite of azathioprine. The azathioprine dose should be reduced to one quarter of the original dose when the two drugs are used together. Avoid concurrent use of other drugs which may cause bone marrow suppression. *Live vaccines* should not be given to patients on azathioprine therapy as atypical and potentially harmful reactions may be seen. In addition, a diminished response to killed vaccines is possible. *Trimethoprim* and *co-trimoxazole* may cause an increased risk of haematological toxicity when given with azathioprine in renal transplant patients.

PREGNANCY
Azathioprine crosses the placenta. It has been suggested that it may also affect sperm. Babies born to mothers receiving azathioprine may have an increased risk of myelosuppression and immunosuppression. Azathioprine is thought to exhibit borderline teratogenicity leading to a small increased risk of spontaneous abortion, congenital defects and a range of malformations. Intra-uterine growth retardation may also be associated with the drug. Although several studies found azathioprine to be relatively safe in pregnancy, there have been reports of anomalies and some references consider the drug to be potentially harmful. If azathioprine must be used in pregnancy, the lowest effective dose should be used. One report found that halving the dose in the third trimester, if the mother's leucocyte count is below normal, reduced the incidence of leucopenia and thrombocytopenia.

BREAST-FEEDING
Azathioprine or its metabolites are excreted in low amounts into breast milk. Contact local Medicines Information Centre for advice.

SIDE-EFFECTS
Bone marrow suppression (generally dose-related and reversible), nausea, vomiting, diarrhoea, malaise, dizziness, fever and rash. Pancreatitis and hepatitis.

POISONING/TOXICITY
Symptoms of overdosage include unexplained infection, ulceration of the throat, bruising and bleeding. However, these are likely to show with chronic overdosage rather than with a single acute overdose.

Treatment of acute overdosage – gastric lavage may be indicated. Subsequent monitoring, including haematological monitoring is essential in order to treat adverse effects as they occur.

PHARMACOKINETIC PROPERTIES
Blood levels of azathioprine are of no value in monitoring therapy with azathioprine.

EXCIPIENTS
Contact manufacturers for further details.

LICENSED STATUS
Licensed for use in children and adults but not for inflammatory bowel disease. Capsule is a 'special' and as such is unlicensed.

FURTHER INFORMATION
Capsule available from Nova Laboratories.

Azelaic acid

Antimicrobial and anticomedonal cream.

USES
Possible alternative to benzoyl peroxide or to a topical retinoid for treating mild to moderate comedonal acne, particularly of the face.

PRESENTATION
Cream: 20% – Skinoren® .

DOSAGE/ADMINISTRATION
Wash affected area with water alone, dry and apply cream sparingly. Rub in well. Use TWICE daily (morning and in the evening) but ONCE daily for the first week if sensitive skin. Reduce amount of cream per application if marked skin irritation. Distinct improvement apparent after 4 weeks. Should not be applied for more than 6 months.

CONTRA INDICATIONS/WARNINGS
Hypersensitivity to propylene glycol. Avoid contact with eyes. Rare reports of photosensitivity.

BREAST-FEEDING
The amount excreted in the breast milk is negligible. Avoid unless no suitable alternative.

PREGNANCY
Advisable to avoid but animal studies do not suggest any risk.

SIDE-EFFECTS
Local skin irritation.

EXCIPIENTS
See manufacturers SPC for further details.

LICENSED STATUS
No specific age limits stated in licence but use will be at discretion of prescriber and given appropriate indication. Safety and effectiveness not studied in infants and young children.

Azithromycin

A macrolide antibiotic active against a wide variety of Gram-positive and Gram-negative organisms.

USES
Lower and upper respiratory tract infections, skin and soft tissue infections, otitis media, uncomplicated genital infections due to *Chlamydia trachomatis, Cryptosporidiosis*. In cystic fibrosis patients – treatment of asymptomatic *Staphylococcus aureus* isolates or minor exacerbations, treatment for asymptomatic *Haemophilus influenzae* carriage

or minor exacerbations and treatment of atypical infection e.g. mycoplasma; some centres are using azithromycin for prophylaxis or treatment for longer than the licensed duration of 3 days, however long-term safety has yet to be established.

PRESENTATION
Capsule: 250mg – Zithromax®.
Oral suspension: 200mg in 5mL; 15mL, 22.5mL and 30mL pack – Zithromax®.
Tablet: 500mg – Zithromax®.

DOSAGE

Route	Age			Frequency (times daily)	Notes
	1 month–2 years	2–12 years	12–18 years		
Oral	← DOSE BY WEIGHT →				For 3 days. Continued treatment may be necessary to prevent relapse in cryptosporidiosis.
	>6 months 10mg/kg	10mg/kg	-	1	
		← DOSE BY AGE →			
		3–7 years 200mg	12–14 years 400mg	1	
		8–11 years 300mg	>14 years 500mg	1	
	-	-	1g	single dose	Sexually transmitted diseases caused by *Chlamydia trachomatis*.
Oral for cystic fibrosis patients	← 10mg/kg → (maximum dose 500mg)		500mg	1 for 3 days	Treatment of asymptomatic *S. aureus* isolates or minor exacerbations; asymtomatic *H. influenzae* carriage or mild exacerbation; atypical infection e.g. Mycoplasma. Repeat course 1 week later and then repeat as necessary.

ADMINISTRATION
Oral: administer 1 hour before or 2 hours after food.

CONTRA-INDICATIONS & WARNINGS
Avoid in patients with hepatic disease. Use with caution in severe renal failure. Observe for signs of bacterial/fungal superinfection.

INTERACTIONS
Antacids: administer azithromycin at least 1 hour before and 2 hours after *antacids.* May enhance effects and toxicity of *carbamazepine, ciclosporin (cyclosporin), digoxin* and *theophylline* – monitor levels. *Terfenadine* – possible risk of hazardous arrhythmias. Effect of *warfarin* may be enhanced – monitor INR.

PREGNANCY
Animal studies show azithromycin crosses placenta with no evidence of harm to fetus. No information in humans. Use only if no suitable alternative. Contact local Medicines Information Centre for advice.

BREAST-FEEDING
No data – use only if no suitable alternative. Contact local Medicines Information Centre for advice.

SIDE-EFFECTS
Nausea, abdominal discomfort (pain/cramps), vomiting, flatulence, diarrhoea, rash and photosensitivity, reversible elevation in liver transaminases, transient reduction in neutrophil count, reversible hearing impairment and cholestatic jaundice (rare). Serious allergic reactions e.g. angioneurotic oedema and anaphylaxis reported rarely.

POISONING/TOXICITY
Symptoms: hearing loss, severe nausea, vomiting and diarrhoea.
Treatment: general supportive measures.

PHARMACOKINETIC PROPERTIES
Following oral administration – widely distributed throughout the body. Time to peak plasma levels 2–3 hours. Elimination half-life is 2–4 days. Liver metabolism is the principal route of excretion.

EXCIPIENTS
Oral suspension contains sucrose. See manufacturers SPC for further details.

LICENSED STATUS
Licensed for >6 months of age.

FURTHER INFORMATION
Suspension is cherry/banana flavour.

Baclofen

Skeletal muscle relaxant derived from gamma-aminobutyric acid.

USES
Spasticity of voluntary muscle. Painful muscle spasticity following damage to the CNS e.g. palliative management of cerebral palsy, neurodegenerative conditions.

PRESENTATION
Tablet: 10mg (scored) – Lioresal® and non-proprietary.
Oral liquid: 5mg in 5mL – Lioresal®.
Intrathecal injection: 50 microgram in 1mL, 1mL ampoule; 500 microgram in 1mL, 20mL ampoule; 2mg in 1mL, 5mL ampoule – Lioresal®. 1mg in 1mL, 2mL ampoule, 12mL vial; 1.5mg in 1mL, 12mL vial; 2mg in 1mL, 12mL vial, 3mg in 1mL, 12mL vial and 6mg in 1mL, 12mL vial – manufactured 'special'.

DOSAGE

Route	Age			Frequency (times daily)	Notes
	1 month–2 years	2–12 years	12–18 years		
Oral	≥1 year 2.5mg	2.5mg	5mg	3	Initial dose. Increase gradually every 3 days.
			10–20mg	3	Maintenance dose. Maximum **daily** dose 100mg.
	≥1 year 5–10mg	2-6 years 10–15mg; 6-10 years 15–30mg; >10 years as 12–18 years	–	2; 2	Maintenance dose. Doses shown for a twice daily regimen; the total dose can be given as 2, 3 or 4 divided doses.
Intrathecal	–	≥ 4 years 25–50 microgram	25–50 microgram	single dose	Test dose.

Dosage adjustment in renal impairment
Reduce oral doses by at least 50% (maximum dose 5mg) in patients with impaired renal function and the frequency to three times daily (mild), twice daily (moderate) or daily (severe).

ADMINISTRATION
Oral: the liquid and tablet oral formulations are bioequivalent. If nausea is a problem despite dose reduction then baclofen may be ingested with food or milk.
Intrathecal: the 50 microgram in 1mL intrathecal injection is intended for administration as a test via a lumbar puncture or intrathecal catheter. The other preparations are intended to be given by implantable pumps in experienced centres and require careful dose titration – see manufacturers SPC for details.

CONTRA-INDICATIONS & WARNINGS
Oral baclofen is contra-indicated in peptic ulceration. *Cautions*: drowsiness and increased hypotonia may occur. Use with caution in patients suffering from cerebrovascular accidents, respiratory, hepatic or renal impairment and in epilepsy. Acute urinary retention can occur in patients with

pre-existing sphincter hypertonia. Monitor liver function tests and plasma glucose in patients with liver disease or diabetes mellitus. Drug withdrawal should be gradual over at least 1–2 weeks. Avoid abrupt withdrawal.

INTERACTIONS
Enhanced hypotensive effect with *antihypertensives*, enhanced sedative effect and possibly respiratory depression with *anxiolytics, opiates* and *hypnotics*. Muscular hypotonia with *tricyclic antidepressants*. Drugs producing renal insufficiency may lead to toxicity.

PREGNANCY
Crosses the placenta. Teratogenic effects demonstrated in rats only. Use with caution and in first 3 months of pregnancy and only if of vital necessity.

BREAST-FEEDING
Passes into breast milk but in such small quantities no undesirable effects on the infant are to be expected.

SIDE-EFFECTS
Mainly seen at start of treatment or if dose is escalated too quickly.
CNS: frequent effects include daytime sedation, drowsiness, nausea, headache, insomnia, occasional respiratory depression, hallucinations, tremor, ataxia, nystagmus, dry mouth and rarely lowering of the convulsion threshold.
Sense organs: occasional visual disturbances.
Gastrointestinal tract: frequent nausea, occasional diarrhoea or constipation.
Cardiovascular: occasional hypotension.
Urogenital: frequent reports of enuresis, dysuria and increased urinary frequency.

Skin: occasional hyperhydrosis, skin rash.

PHARMACOKINETIC PROPERTIES
Absorption from the gastrointestinal tract of liquid and tablet forms is rapid and almost complete. 30% plasma protein binding. Peak plasma concentration in 1-2 hours. Plasma half-life range 3–4 hours. CSF concentrations are 8.5 times lower than plasma levels after oral administration. Excreted largely unchanged in the urine. After a single intrathecal dose the onset is 30-60 minutes, peak 4 hours and duration 4-8 hours. CSF elimination half-life after a single intrathecal dose is 1-5 hours. After continuous intrathecal administration steady state concentrations are reached in 1-2 days. Very low plasma concentrations result. At steady state a mean concentration gradient of 4:1 from lumbar to cisternal CSF is achieved. Clinically this means spasticity in the lower extremities can be effectively treated with little effect on the upper limbs and fewer CNS side-effects.

POISONING/TOXICITY
Symptoms: prominent features are signs of central nervous depression, drowsiness, impairment of consciousness, respiratory depression and coma. Confusion, hallucinations, agitation, absent pupillary reflex, generalised muscle hypotonia, convulsions, hyporeflexia or areflexia, hypotension, bradycardia, hypothermia, nausea, vomiting, hypersalivation and diarrhoea are also liable to occur.
Treatment: no specific antidote. If oral ingestion, induction of vomiting, gastric lavage or activated charcoal may be given. Generous quantities of fluid should be given to encourage urinary excretion. Cardiac and respiratory supportive measures may be necessary and in the event of convulsions IV lorazepam or diazepam should be administered cautiously.

EXCIPIENTS
Lioresal® oral liquid includes sorbitol. See manufacturers SPC for further details.

LICENSED STATUS
Licensed for oral use in ≥1 year of age. Lioresal® intrathecal injection is not licensed for use <18 years of age in patients with spasticity of spinal origin but it is licensed in children and adults with spasticity of cerebral origin. The other intrathecal preparations are available as 'specials' and as such are unlicensed.

FURTHER INFORMATION
The intrathecal 'special' preparations are available from e.g. Victoria Pharmaceuticals, The Royal Hospitals, Belfast.

BCG vaccine (Bacillus Calmette–Guérin vaccine)

There have been repeated problems with supply of this vaccine and at the time of writing (May 2003) only one vaccine was available, i.e. BCG Vaccine SSI.

USES
To provide active protection against tuberculosis (TB). It is recommended in the following groups who have not previously been vaccinated (as evidenced by a characteristic scar, or definite documentation) and, except in the case of

infants under 3 months, those who are known to be tuberculin negative:-

☐ Contacts of cases of active pulmonary tuberculosis
☐ Immigrants from countries with a high prevalence of tuberculosis and their children (wherever born)
☐ Those intending to stay in countries with a high prevalence of TB for longer than 1 month
☐ Children between 10-14 years old
☐ Newborn babies, children or adults where immunisation is requested.

PRESENTATION
Injection: powder for suspension supplied in Diluted Sauton "SSI". Contains a living attenuated strain (Danish strain 1331) of bacteria derived from *Mycobacterium bovis*. Vaccine for intradermal use is available as 1ml or 2mL vials with between 2-8 million colony forming units per 1mL dose.

DOSAGE
For intradermal use the dose is 0.1mL (0.05mL for infants <12 months).

ADMINISTRATION
Intradermal: preferred site of injection is at the insertion of the deltoid muscle near the middle of the left upper arm. The upper and lateral surface of the thigh may be used for cosmetic reasons, if requested.

CONTRA-INDICATIONS & WARNINGS
As for vaccines generally and also the following:
The vaccination should always be preceded by a tuberculin test in people of ≥12 months old. BCG vaccine should not be given to individuals with a positive tuberculin test or a characteristic scar from previous BCG. Revaccination is not recommended routinely. Where BCG is indicated in individuals who have received it previously, it should be given only in those who have no scar and who have a negative tuberculin test. BCG vaccination is absolutely contra-indicated in anyone who is severely immunocompromised. Fatal disseminated BCG infection can occur in such individuals. It should not be given to the baby of an HIV positive woman until the baby is known to be HIV negative. The vaccine should only be given into healthy skin. No further injections should be given into the limb used for at least 3 months. The vaccine should not be given to individuals who are receiving anti-mycobacterial chemotherapy.

INTERACTIONS
An interval of at least 4 weeks should normally be left between the administration of BCG and *another live vaccine*, unless given at the same time. Oral polio vaccine can be given at any time in relation to BCG.
Viral infections, including infectious mononucleosis, and live viral vaccines may cause a tuberculin positive individual to become temporarily tuberculin negative. Before a tuberculin test is performed, 3 weeks should be allowed to elapse after a viral infection or receiving a live viral vaccine (4 weeks for MMR).
Three weeks should elapse after any injection, before giving BCG in the same limb. If BCG is given first, 3 months should elapse before giving another injection in the same limb.

PREGNANCY
There is no evidence available and it should be avoided in early pregnancy. Unless there is a clear indication, administration should be delayed until after delivery.

BREAST-FEEDING
Well documented experience is lacking, however, if it is necessary to give BCG to protect the mother, breast-feeding should not be terminated.

SIDE-EFFECTS
The incidence of adverse reactions depends in part on the origin of the vaccine as well as technique. Vaccine used in the UK rarely gives rise to major adverse effects. There is little reaction to BCG given percutaneously and a visible scar is unlikely to result. Most intradermal BCG injections result in a mild local reaction over the subsequent 1–2 months and sometimes a shallow ulcer up to 10mm across may develop. A small flat scar is the normal end result. Keloid formation is more likely to occur if the injection is given too high on the arm. Exaggerated local reactions such as large ulcers and abscess formation are usually, though not always, due to the injection being given too deeply. They may also occur in those individuals who were already tuberculin positive. The optimal treatment regimen for such reactions is not clear. Advice should be sought from a paediatric infectious diseases unit or chest clinic. Minor regional adenitis is common, but rarely may suppurate. Disseminated BCG infection is very rare, but less so in those who are immunocompromised. Anaphylactic reactions have been reported.

POISONING/TOXICITY
Overdose increases the risk of suppurative lymphadenitis and excessive scar formation.

PHARMACODYNAMIC PROPERTIES
Produces cell-mediated immunity approximately 2-3 months after immunisation.

B

EXCIPIENTS
Contains sodium glutamate, magnesium sulphate, dipotassium phosphate, citric acid monohydrate, L-asparagine monohydrate, ferric ammonium citrate, glycerol 85%.

LICENSED STATUS
Fully licensed for use as described.

FURTHER INFORMATION
The vaccine also protects against leprosy. Isoniazid resistant BCG is no longer recommended.
Store at 2-8°C and protect from light. Once reconstituted, it should be used within 4 hours.
BCG is produced in material, some of which is of animal origin, from sources known to be free of BSE. It is possible that there are trace amounts of these animal materials in the final product.

B

Beclometasone (beclomethasone) dipropionate

A corticosteroid which decreases tissue inflammation and bronchial hyper-reactivity within the respiratory tract.

USES
Prophylaxis of asthma. Prophylaxis and treatment of allergic rhinitis.

PRESENTATION
Aerosol inhalation: 50 and 100 microgram – Beclazone Easi-Breathe®, Becotide®, Qvar® and non-proprietary; 200 microgram – Becotide®; 250 microgram – Beclazone Easi-Breathe®, Becloforte® and non-proprietary.
Breath-actuated aerosal inhalation: 50 and 100 microgram – AeroBec Autohaler®, Qvar Autohaler®; 250 microgram – AeroBec Forte®
Dry powder for inhalation: 50 microgram – Asmabec Clickhaler®; 100 microgram – Asmabec Clickhaler®, Becodisks® and non-proprietary; 200 microgram – Becodisks® and non-proprietary; 250 microgram – Asmabec Clickhaler®; 400 microgram – Becloforte®, Becodisks® and non-proprietary.
Inhalation powder, hard capsule: 100, 200 and 400 micrograms per capsule – non-proprietary.
Nasal spray: 50 microgram per metered spray – Beconase® and non-proprietary.

DOSAGE

Route	Age			Frequency	Notes
	1 month-2 years	2-12 years	12-18 years	(times daily)	
Aerosol inhaler	>6 months			2	Asthma: preventor for regular use. **A smaller dose of Qvar® may be required.
	50–200 microgram	100–400 microgram			
Dry powder inhalation	–	>5 years		2	Asthma: preventor for regular use.
		100–400 microgram			
Intra-nasal	–	>6 years		2	Allergic rhinitis.
		100 microgram (2 sprays) into each nostril			

** A dose reduction may be needed when switching patients to Qvar® from a CFC-containing beclometasone preparation. This is because Qvar® is formulated as an 'extra-fine' aerosol which is said to deposit more drug in the lungs than conventional formulations. Patients with well-controlled asthma may require a smaller dose of Qvar® as compared with conventional formulations. Poorly controlled patients should be switched at the same microgram for microgram dose, up to 800 microgram daily. At present no definitive dosage recommendations can be made in children.

ADMINISTRATION
Inhaler: effect of medication may decrease when aerosol canister is cold. Volumatic® spacer and mask or Babyhaler® can be used for infants and younger children with aerosol inhaler. Rinse mouth with water after inhalation and wash face after use of mask.

B

CONTRA-INDICATIONS & WARNINGS
The propellant used with inhaled corticosteroids can occasionally cause paradoxical bronchospasm and therapy may need to be altered. If this is mild then use a dry powder inhaler or use a beta-2 agonist prior to use. Use with caution in respiratory infection.

INTERACTIONS
Very low plasma drug concentrations are achieved following inhaled doses, with low potential for drug interactions.

PREGNANCY
Administration of corticosteroids in pregnancy gives a very small risk of cleft palate and intra-uterine growth retardation. This risk is lower when corticosteroids are delivered directly to the lungs by the inhaled route. In practice, beclometasone has been used for many years without side-effects.

BREAST-FEEDING
It is reasonable to assume that beclometasone is excreted in milk. However, at inhaled or intra-nasal doses there is low potential for significant levels.

SIDE-EFFECTS
Candidiasis of the mouth and throat (increased incidence with doses >400 microgram/day). Hoarseness or throat irritation reduced by using a spacer device, or rinsing mouth with water after use. Paradoxical bronchospasm may occur, with an immediate increase in wheezing after dosing. Hypersensitivity reactions e.g. rashes, urticaria, pruritus and erythema, oedema of the eyes, face, lips and throat. Adrenal suppression may occur at high doses. Very rarely, nasal septum perforation with nasal spray.

POISONING/TOXICITY
Acute: inhalation of beclometasone in excess of the recommended doses may lead to temporary suppression of adrenal function. This is not an indication for emergency treatment. Beclometasone should be continued at a dose sufficient to control asthma. Adrenal function will recover in a few days.
Chronic: may lead to adrenal suppression. Treatment should be continued at a dose sufficient to control asthma.

EXCIPIENTS
See manufacturers SPC for further details.

LICENSED STATUS
All presentations are licensed for use in children except the 'high-dose' inhalers (>200 microgram per actuation), and Qvar® inhalers. Maximum licensed dose in children is 400 microgram/day.

Bendroflumethiazide (bendrofluazide)

Thiazide diuretic.

USES
Oedema, hypertension.

PREPARATIONS
Tablet: 2.5mg and 5mg – non-proprietary.
Liquid: may be extemporaneously prepared.

DOSAGE

Route	Age			Frequency (times daily)	Notes
	1 month–2 years	2–12 years	12–18 years		
Oral	◄— 50–100 microgram/kg —►		2.5-5mg	1	Maintenance dose. In children doses up to 400 microgram/kg may be needed initially, reducing to the maintenance dose.

ADMINISTRATION
Tablets disperse well in water.

CONTRA-INDICATIONS & WARNINGS, INTERACTIONS, PREGNANCY, BREAST-FEEDING, SIDE-EFFECTS, POISONING/TOXICITY, PHARMACOKINETIC PROPERTIES
See chlorothiazide monograph. Patients with renal failure are usually refractory to thiazides.

EXCIPIENTS
See manufacturers SPC for further details.

LICENSED STATUS
Aprinox® and Neo-NaClex® tablets are licensed for use in children.

Benzatropine (benztropine)

An antimuscarinic agent with actions similar to atropine.

USES
Treatment of drug induced dystonia.

PRESENTATION
Tablet: 2mg (quarter-scored) – Cogentin®.
Injection: 1mg in 1mL, 2mL ampoule – Cogentin®.

DOSAGE

Route	Age		Frequency	Notes
	2–12 years	12–18 years		
Oral	>3 years 20 microgram/kg	1–2mg	single dose	The dose can be given more than once a day, but frequency depends on the condition and response of the patient; benzatropine has a cumulative action and continued observation of the patient is necessary. Maximum 6mg/day.
IV or IM	>3 years 20–100 microgram/kg (maximum 2mg)	1–2mg	single dose	Followed, if necessary, by oral treatment.

ADMINISTRATION
IV bolus: given over 1–2 minutes.
Oral: give oral doses before food if patient experiences excessive dry mouth.

CONTRA-INDICATIONS & WARNINGS
Contra-indicated in children <3 years of age because of the atropine-like side-effects. Caution must be observed in patients with: tachycardia, hypertension, glaucoma, gastrointestinal or genito-urinary obstruction. In patients with abnormalities of sweating the possibility of hyperthermia should be considered. Not recommended in tardive dyskinesia.

INTERACTIONS
Drug interactions include increased antimuscarinic effects (blurred vision, dry mouth, constipation and urinary retention) with *nefopam, disopyramide, tricyclic antidepressants, antihistamines* and *phenothiazines*. Extra care if given concomitantly with *neuroleptics (e.g. phenothiazines, butyrophenones, thioxanthenes)* or *selective serotonin re-uptake inhibitors*. Patients should report gastro-intestinal complaints, confusion, hallucinations, fever or heat intolerance promptly.

PREGNANCY
There is a possible association with cardiovascular defects with first trimester exposure. Contact local Medicines Information Centre for advice.

BREAST-FEEDING
Contact local Medicines Information Centre for advice.

SIDE-EFFECTS
These are anticholinergic and particularly antimuscarinic.
Cardiovascular: tachycardia.
Digestive: constipation, paralytic ileus, dry mouth, nausea, vomiting.

Nervous system: confusion, psychosis, visual hallucinations, memory impairment, depression.
Special senses: blurred vision, dilated pupils.
Urogenital: urinary retention, dysuria.
Others: heat stroke, hyperthermia.

POISONING/TOXICITY

Physostigmine salicylate is reported to reverse the symptoms of anticholinergic intoxication but it is only used for diagnosis. After recent ingestion, induced emesis or gastric lavage are suggested. Supportive care for CNS depression, convulsions, respiratory depression, hyperpyrexia and circulatory collapse may be required.

PHARMACOKINETIC PROPERTIES

Pharmacokinetics are not well studied. Following IM injection the clinical effects are apparent within 10 minutes and maximal effects are seen within 30 minutes. Onset of action after oral dosing is 1-2 hours and duration 24 hours. After long-term therapy it may take up to 7 days to lose clinical effects. Thought to be hepatically metabolised. There is a non-linear relationship between daily dose and serum concentrations. Incremental dose increases result in several fold increases in serum anticholinergic activity.

EXCIPIENTS

See manufacturers SPC for further details.

LICENSED STATUS

Licensed for use in children ≥3 years of age.

FURTHER INFORMATION

Extemporaneous formulations using syrup are known of but are not research based. The injection can be used orally.

Benzoyl peroxide

Sebostatic and keratolytic agent with antibacterial activity against Propionibacterium acnes.

USES

Treatment of acne.

PRESENTATION

Aqueous gel: 2.5% – PanOxyl Aquagel®; 5% – Acnecide®, PanOxyl Aquagel®; 10% – Acnecide®, PanOxyl Aquagel®.
Aqueous alcoholic gel: 5%, 10% – PanOxyl®.
Cream (non-greasy): 5% – PanOxyl®.
Detergent based wash: 10% – PanOxyl®.
Lotion (non-greasy): 5%, 10% – PanOxyl®.

DOSAGE

Route	Age	Frequency	Notes
	12–18 years	(times daily)	
Topical	2.5% (see notes)	1–2	Start with 2.5% daily; decrease to alternate days, if excessive peeling and redness occur. Increase to 5% or 10% if necessary.

ADMINISTRATION

Topical: the affected area should be washed with soap and water and dried prior to application of the gel, lotion or cream to enhance efficacy. For the wash, wet the affected area, wash with the preparation, rinse first with warm water, then cold, and pat dry.

CONTRA-INDICATIONS & WARNINGS

Avoid in patients with known hypersensitivity to benzoyl peroxide. Avoid contact with eyes, mouth and other mucous membranes. Apply with care to neck and other sensitive areas. Benzoyl peroxide may bleach dyed fabrics.

PREGNANCY/BREAST-FEEDING

No restrictions on use during pregnancy and lactation.

SIDE-EFFECTS

Skin irritation. Temporary redness and skin peeling may occur.

POISONING/TOXICITY

If accidentally ingested, symptomatic and supportive treatment is advised.

EXCIPIENTS
See manufacturers SPC for further details.

LICENSED STATUS
PanOxyl aquagel®, cream, lotion and Acnecide® are licensed for use in children; PanOxyl® gel and wash are not.

Benzydamine hydrochloride

Analgesic, anti-inflammatory thought to work by stabilising the cellular membrane and inhibiting prostaglandin synthesis.

USES
Relief of painful inflammatory conditions of the oropharynx. To relieve the discomfort of oral ulceration and post-surgery. Gives some relief in post-irradiation mucositis.

PRESENTATION
Oral rinse: 0.15% – Difflam®.
Spray: 0.15% – Difflam®.

DOSAGE
Oral rinse: ≥12 years: 15mL every 1.5-3 hours as required.

Spray: <6 years: 1 puff per 4kg to a maximum of 4 puffs every 1.5-3 hours.
              6-12 years: 4 puffs every 1.5-3 hours.
              >12 years: 4-8 puffs every 1.5-3 hours.

ADMINISTRATION
Oral rinse: use as a rinse or gargle (diluted with water if stinging occurs), usually for not more than 7 days.
Spray: direct at the affected area.

CONTRA-INDICATIONS & WARNINGS
Oral rinse is not suitable for children <12 years.
Avoid contact with the eyes.

INTERACTIONS
None documented.

SIDE-EFFECTS
Slight numbness and stinging may be experienced. In the case of the latter dilute the oral rinse with equal volumes of water.

POISONING AND TOXICITY
Difflam® is unlikely to cause any systemic effects even if accidentally ingested. No special measures are advised.

EXCIPIENTS
Difflam® includes saccharin. See manufacturers SPC for further details.

LICENSED STATUS
Difflam® oral rinse is licensed for ≥12 years of age; the spray is licensed for use in children and adults.

FURTHER INFORMATION
Wipe the spray nozzle clean with a tissue after use to prevent clogging. Use and store the unit upright.

Benzylpenicillin (penicillin G)

A bactericidal antibiotic which acts by interfering with bacterial cell wall synthesis; useful against penicillin-sensitive bacteria but inactivated by beta-lactamases.

USES
A penicillin antibiotic used by injection to treat susceptible organisms. Not recommended for Pneumococcal meningitis (see Clinical Guidelines).

PRESENTATION
Injection: 600mg and 1.2g vial – Crystapen®.

DOSAGE
Newborn infant (birth to 1 month)

Route	Age		Frequency (times daily)	Notes
	Up to 7 days	Over 7 days		
IV	25mg/kg	-	2	Doses should be doubled when there is evidence of
IV	-	25mg/kg	3	meningitis (especially group B streptococcal meningitis).

Child

Route	Age			Frequency (times daily)	Notes
	1 month–2 years	2–12 years	12–18 years		
IV	←	25mg/kg	→	4	*In severe infection (including meningitis) doses of 50mg/kg may be given 6 times daily. Maximum single dose 2.4g. Maximum 14.4g/day.
	←	*50mg/kg	→	6	

Dose adjustment in renal failure
In moderate renal failure (creatinine clearance 10-50mL/minute/1.73m^2), dosage interval may be increased to 8-12 hours and in severe renal failure (<10mL/minute/1.73m^2) to every 12 hours.

ADMINISTRATION
IM, slow IV or IV infusion: on reconstitution 600mg powder displaces 0.4mL. For IM injection reconstitute 600mg in 1.6mL to give 300mg in 1mL. For IV injection dissolve 600mg in 4-10mL Water for Injections. For IV infusion dissolve 600mg in at least 10mL NaCl 0.9% or other transfusable solutions and administer over 10-30 minutes. Longer administration is advised when using doses of 50mg/kg to avoid CNS toxicity and convulsions. Reconstituted solutions may be stored for up to 24 hours at 2-8°C. Do not mix with aminoglycosides and do not administer down the same line without adequate flushing in-between.

CONTRA-INDICATIONS & WARNINGS
Allergy to penicillins. Very large dose may cause hypokalaemia and hypernatraemia.

INTERACTIONS
Increased levels of benzylpenicillin if given with *probenecid.*

PREGNANCY
There have been no reports of direct or indirect harmful effects on the fetus.

BREAST-FEEDING
As the drug is destroyed by gastric acid and poorly absorbed by the gut there is no contra-indication to its use by mothers during lactation unless the baby shows evidence of hypersensitivity (a very rare problem in the neonatal period).

SIDE-EFFECTS
Anaphylactic reactions, immediate and delayed hypersensitivity reactions. Rare reports of paraesthesia and haematological disorders in prolonged use.

POISONING/TOXICITY
Overdosage can be corrected by haemodialysis.

PHARMACOKINETIC PROPERTIES
Diffuses well into body fluids and tissues but only into inflamed meninges. Excretion is predominantly renal.

EXCIPIENTS
Each 600mg of powder contains 1.68mmol of sodium. See manufacturers SPC for further details.

LICENSED STATUS
Licensed for use in all ages.

FURTHER INFORMATION
Skin sensitisation may occur in persons handling the antibiotic.

B

Carotenoid precursor of vitamin A.

USES
Oral agent for reducing severity of photosensitivity reactions in patients with erythropoietic protoporphyria. Useful for longer wavelength light than that which causes sunburn (i.e. UVA rather than UVB).

PRESENTATION
Capsule: 15mg.

DOSAGE

Route	Age			Frequency	Notes
	1 month–2 years	2–12 years	12–18 years	(times daily)	
Oral	>1 year 60–90mg	2–4 years 60–90mg	12 years 120–150mg	1	All doses can be given in single or divided doses with meals. Protection is not total and generally 2–6 week, treatment resulting in a yellow colouration of the palms and soles is necessary before patients should attempt to increase their exposure to sunlight.
		5–8 years 90–120mg	13–15 years 150–180mg	1	
		9–12 years 120–150mg	>16 years 180–300mg	1	

SIDE-EFFECTS
Loose stools. Yellow discolouration of the skin. Bruising and arthralgia. High doses do **not** lead to abnormally high serum concentrations of vitamin A.

EXCIPIENTS
Contact manufacturers for further details.

LICENSED STATUS
Unlicensed.

FURTHER INFORMATION
Beta carotene capsules are available through IDIS World Medicines.

Betaine

USES
Treatment of homocystinuria; classical homocystinuria and remethylation defects: disorders of cobalamin metabolism, methylene tetrahydrofolate reductase deficiency.

PRESENTATION
Anhydrous powder: one level scoop (1.7mL) is equal to 1g of betaine anhydrous powder.
Oral solution: anhydrous betaine 5g in 10mL – 'special'.
Tablet: 500mg – manufactured 'special'.

DOSAGE

Route	Age				Frequency	Notes
	birth–1 month	1 month–2 years	2–12 years	12–18 years	(times daily)	
Oral	←	50mg/kg		→	2	Initial dose. Then adjusted according to homocysteine levels. Maximum dose 20g/day.

Dosage in renal impairment/liver failure: no information available.

ADMINISTRATION
Oral: powder may be mixed with a drink or feed. Solution 5g in 10mL can be prepared with distilled water: expiry 2 weeks.

CONTRA-INDICATIONS & WARNINGS, INTERACTIONS, PREGNANCY/ BREAST-FEEDING
No information available.

SIDE-EFFECTS
Serious side-effects are rare: gastrointestinal disturbances such as nausea and diarrhoea are the most commonly noted. Increases blood methionine. Not known to be toxic but reduce dose if levels exceed 800 micromol/L. On rare occasions, patients have developed cerebral oedema within a few months of starting the drug, which has resolved with prompt withdrawal of the drug.

POISONING/TOXICITY
In rats, death has occurred at 10g/kg.

PHARMACODYNAMIC PROPERTIES
Promotes conversion of homocysteine to methionine thus reducing homocysteine levels by using an alternative metabolic pathway.

PHARMACOKINETIC PROPERTIES
Need to monitor homocysteine and methionine levels. Onset of action is usually within 1 week. Has not been extensively studied.

EXCIPIENTS
Tablets are lactose-free. Contact manufacturers for further details.

LICENSED STATUS
Available as 'specials' and as such are unlicensed.

FURTHER INFORMATION
Anhydrous powder is available from Orphan Europe.
Oral solution available as an anhydrous betaine pack to prepare 100mL, from Special Products Ltd.
Tablets are available from IDIS World Medicines.

Betamethasone sodium phosphate

Corticosteroid.

USES
Inflammatory otitis externa. Inflammatory conditions of the nose.

PRESENTATION
Ear, eye or nose drops: 0.1% – 10mL Betnesol®; 5mL, 10mL Vista-Methasone®.

DOSAGE/ADMINISTRATION
Betnesol®
Ear: 2-3 drops into the affected ear(s) 2-3 hourly, reduce frequency when relief obtained.
Nose: 2-3 drops into each nostril 2–3 times daily.
Vista-Methasone®
Ear: 2-3 drops into the affected ear(s) 3-4 hourly, reduce frequency when relief obtained.
Nose: 2-3 drops into each nostril twice daily.

CONTRA-INDICATIONS & WARNINGS
Untreated infection. Perforated tympanic membrane.

PREGNANCY/BREAST-FEEDING
Contact local Medicines Information Centre for advice.

SIDE-EFFECTS
Local sensitivity. Excessive and prolonged use at doses above those recommended may introduce systemic side-effects.

POISONING/TOXICITY
Oral ingestion of the contents of one bottle of drops is unlikely to lead to any serious adverse effects.

B

Betamethasone sodium phosphate continued

EXCIPIENTS
Include disodium edetate and benzalkonium chloride.

LICENSED STATUS
Licensed for use in children and adults.

FURTHER INFORMATION
For reasons of hygiene do not use bottle for more than 28 days after first opening it.

Betamethasone and Neomycin

Corticosteroid with antibacterial.

USES
As for betamethasone drops with prophylaxis against secondary infection.

PRESENTATION
Ear, eye or nose drops: betamethasone 0.1% and neomycin 0.5% – 10mL Betnesol-N®; 5mL, 10mL Vista-Methasone N®.

DOSAGE
Ear: 2-3 drops into the affected ear(s) 3-4 times daily, reduce frequency when relief obtained.
Betnesol-N®
Nose: 2-3 drops into each nostril 2-3 times daily.
Vista-Methasone N®
Nose: 2-3 drops into each nostril twice daily.

CONTRA-INDICATIONS & WARNINGS	**SIDE-EFFECTS**
Otitis externa should not be treated when the eardrum is perforated because of the risk of toxicity. Potential for aminoglycoside toxicity (irreversible, partial or total deafness) if applied to broken skin and when high dose treatment is given to infants and small children.	Local irritation, stinging, burning or itching may occur.
	POISONING/TOXICITY
	Long-term intensive topical use may lead to systemic effects. Oral ingestion of the contents of one bottle is unlikely to lead to any serious adverse effects.
PREGNANCY/BREAST-FEEDING	
Contact local Medicines Information Centre for advice.	

EXCIPIENTS
Betnesol N® includes disodium edetate and benzalkonium chloride.
Vista-Methasone N® includes thiomersal.

LICENSED STATUS
Licensed for use in children and adults.

FURTHER INFORMATION
Treatment should not be continued for more than 7 days in the absence of clinical improvement. Prolonged use may lead to occult extension of infection due to the masking effect of the steroid. For reasons of hygiene do not use bottle for more than 28 days after first opening it.

Bezafibrate

Fibric acid derivative; lipid-modulating agent.

USES
Hyperlipidaemia, including familial hypercholesterolaemia in patients in whom diet therapy and resins have been unsuccessful.

PRESENTATION
Tablet: 200mg – Bezalip® and non-proprietary.
Tablet: (modified release) 400mg – Bezalip® Mono.

DOSAGE/ADMINISTRATION
Oral: 200mg/day has been used in adolescents, but experience in children is limited; refer to lipidologist.

CONTRA-INDICATIONS & WARNINGS
Severe hepatic and renal disease (reduce dose), gall bladder disease, nephrotic syndrome, pregnancy and breast-feeding.

INTERACTIONS
Warfarin: enhanced effect. *3-hydroxy-3-methylglutaryl coenzyme A (HMG-Co A) reductase inhibitors:* increased risk of rhabdomyolysis. *Bile acid sequestrants:* elevation in liver enzymes.

PREGNANCY
Animal studies have not shown any adverse effects on the fetus but manufacturers advise avoiding in pregnancy. Contact local Medicines Information Centre for advice.

BREAST-FEEDING
Manufacturers advise avoiding due to lack of information. Embryotoxicity in animal studies with some fibrates. Contact local Medicines Information Centre for advice.

SIDE-EFFECTS
Gastrointestinal: nausea, anorexia, gastric pain; headache, pruritus, urticaria, myopathy.

POISONING/TOXICITY
The effects of acute overdose are unknown although no serious biochemical or clinical effects are likely. Treatment, if necessary, should be symptomatic.

PHARMACODYNAMIC PROPERTIES
Lowers low density lipoprotein cholestrol (LDL-C) and triglycerides and increases high density lipoprotein cholestrol (HDL-C). Peripheral effects include decreased production of free fatty acids and increased secretion of cholesterol into biliary circulation.

EXCIPIENTS
See manufacturers SPC for further details.

LICENSED STATUS
Not licensed for use in children.

B

Biotin

An essential coenzyme in fat metabolism and in other carboxylation reactions.

USES
Isolated defects of carboxylases (most causes of isolated defects of carboxylases are not responsive to biotin); defects of biotin metabolism.

PRESENTATION
Tablet: 5mg – named patient.
Injection: 5mg in 1mL, 1mL ampoule – named patient.

DOSAGE

Route	Age				Frequency (times daily)	Notes
	birth–1 month	1 month–2 years	2–12 years	12–18 years		
Oral/ IV bolus	←	5–10mg		→	1	Initial dose.
	←	10–50mg		→	1	Maintenance dose, depending on condition: Isolated defects of carboxylases
	←	10mg		→	1	Holocarboxylase synthetase deficiency.
	←	5–20mg		→	1	Biotinidase deficiency.

ADMINISTRATION
Oral: tablets may be crushed and put into a drink.
IV: given as an IV bolus over 3-5 minutes.

CONTRA-INDICATIONS & WARNINGS, INTERACTIONS, PREGNANCY/BREAST-FEEDING, POISONING/TOXICITY
No information available.

PHARMACOKINETIC PROPERTIES
Biotin is rapidly absorbed following oral administration.

SIDE-EFFECTS
Few side-effects have been reported.

LICENSED STATUS
Not licensed for use in the UK.

FURTHER INFORMATION
Available, on a named patient basis, from John Bell and Croyden Ltd (Tel: 0207 935 5555). The Roche injection is licensed in France for IM use only but it was previously licensed for IV and IM use and the formulation has not changed.

Bisacodyl

Stimulant laxative.

USES
Constipation whenever a stimulant laxative is required.
Bowel clearance before surgery, labour or radiological investigation.

PRESENTATION
Tablet: 5mg (enteric coated) – Dulco-lax® and non-proprietary
Suppository: 5mg, 10mg – Dulco-lax® and non-proprietary.

DOSAGE

Indication	Route	Age			Frequency (times daily)	Notes
		1 month–2 years	2–12 years	12–18 years		
Constipation	Oral	5mg	<10 years 5mg >10 years 5-10mg	5-10mg	1 1	Give tablets at night. May be necessary to increase up to 15–20mg once daily.
	Rectal	5mg	<10 years 5mg >10 years 10mg	10mg	1 1	Give suppositories in the morning.
Preparation for radiological examination	Oral (and rectal if necessary see notes)	5mg	<10 years 5mg >10 years 10mg	10mg	1 1	Oral dose on each of the 2 nights before the investigation and rectal dose, if necessary, 1 hour before investigation.

May need doses up to twice the usual dose for age in opioid-induced constipation.

ADMINISTRATION
Oral: tablets are enteric coated for disintegration in the intestine; they should not be crushed or chewed and are therefore not suitable for infants and young children who cannot swallow them whole.

B

CONTRA-INDICATIONS & WARNINGS
Contra-indicated in intestinal obstruction and when any undiagnosed acute or persistent abdominal symptoms are present.

INTERACTIONS
Antacids should not be given within 1 hour of administering bisacodyl tablets.

PREGNANCY
No evidence of adverse consequences. Caution in first trimester unless expected benefit is thought to outweigh any possible harm to fetus.

BREAST-FEEDING
Contact local Medicines Information Centre for advice.

SIDE-EFFECTS
Griping has been reported. Prolonged use may result in the development of an atonic non-functioning colon and hyperkalaemia.

POISONING/TOXICITY
Colicky lower abdominal pain with possible signs of dehydration may be expected. Gastric lavage should be performed where appropriate. Maintain adequate hydration and monitor potassium levels. Antispasmodics may be of some value.

PHARMACOKINETIC PROPERTIES
Tablets taken after food act in 10-12 hours, suppositories produce a motion within 20 minutes to 1 hour of insertion.

LICENSED STATUS
Licensed for use in children and adults. The Dulco-lax® brand is NHS black-listed.

FURTHER INFORMATION
Reliable and predictable in its action, producing in most cases a soft formed stool without straining.

Bleomycin

Water soluble glycopeptide with cytotoxic activity – a cytotoxic antibiotic.

USES
Some germ-cell tumours, Hodgkin lymphoma, malignant effusions of serous cavities.
Specialist centre direction/use recommended.

PRESENTATION
Injection: powder for reconstitution (as sulphate), 15,000 units – non-proprietary.

DOSAGE
** Always consult the current treatment protocol for details of dosage and scheduling.**

ADMINISTRATION
IV: infusion in a suitable volume of NaCl 0.9% into established IV access.
For treatment of malignant effusions, the effusion is drained and the required dose of bleomycin is dissolved in a suitable volume of NaCl 0.9% and introduced into the cavity via the drainage needle or suitable cannula.

CONTRA-INDICATIONS & WARNINGS
Contra-indicated in patients with acute pulmonary infection or significantly reduced pulmonary function. In patients previously treated with bleomycin, exposure to high oxygen concentrations during general anaesthesia can result in fatal pulmonary toxicity.

INTERACTIONS
No specific drug interactions reported. Previous or intercurrent radiotherapy to the chest may exacerbate pulmonary fibrosis.

PREGNANCY & BREAST-FEEDING
Bleomycin should not normally be administered to patients who are pregnant or mothers who are breast-feeding.

SIDE-EFFECTS
Fever on day of injection, anorexia, tiredness and nausea. The most serious late effect is interstitial pneumonia, developing during or after the course of treatment. This may progress into fatal pulmonary fibrosis, particularly if high doses of bleomycin have been administered. Acute fulminant reactions with hyperpyrexia and cardiorespiratory collapse have been reported with high doses. Skin and/or oral lesions, induration, hyperkeratosis, reddening and tenderness of the fingertips, alopecia and stomatitis have also occurred. Late toxicity in particular appears to be dose related.

B

The acute reaction to an overdose would probably include hypotension, fever, rapid pulse, and general symptoms of shock. There is no specific antidote. Treatment consists of full symptomatic and supportive care. This may include antipyretics and parenteral chlorpromazine for treatment of hyperpyrexia. Parenteral or oral corticosteroids together with a broad-spectrum antibiotic are advised for treatment of respiratory complications.

PHARMACOKINETIC PROPERTIES

After IV bolus injection there is a biphasic plasma clearance with a terminal half-life of 3 hours. Total clearance approximately 41mL/minute/m^2, with renal clearance accounting for 65% of total drug clearance. In patients with creatinine clearance <50mL/minute/1.73m^2 dose reduction should be considered.

LICENSED STATUS

Licensed for use in children, under exceptional circumstances and in special centres.

FURTHER INFORMATION

Pulmonary function should be monitored during bleomycin therapy. Bleomycin has been found to be incompatible with a number of drugs, including aminophylline, ascorbic acid, dexamethasone, diazepam, hydrocortisone sodium succinate, benzylpenicillin, terbutaline and any agents containing sulphydryl groups.

Botulinum A toxin – haemagglutinin complex

USES

Predominant use in children is for dynamic equinus spasticity in cerebral palsy; also for spasticity of other muscle groups in cerebral palsy and after head injury; other uses are blepharospasm, hemifacial spasm, spasmodic torticollis.

PRESENTATION

Injection: powder for reconstitution, 100 unit vial – Botox®; 500 unit vial – Dysport®.
The 'unit' by which the potency of the preparations is measured is not the same for both preparations. Botox® and Dysport® are not interchangeable.

DOSAGE/ADMINISTRATION

Use of botulinum A toxin (dosage and administration) is highly specialised. It should only be prescribed and administered IM by a trained specialist experienced in its use.

Dynamic equinus spasticity in ambulant paediatric cerebral palsy
Botox®
Diluted Botox® is injected using a sterile 23-26 gauge needle. It is administered into each of two sites in the medial and lateral heads of the affected gastrocnemius muscle. The recommended total dose is 4 units/kg body weight. When both lower limbs are to be injected on the same occasion this dose should be divided between the two limbs.
Clinical improvement generally occurs within the first 2 weeks after injection. Repeat doses should be administered when the clinical effect of a previous injection diminishes but not more frequently than every 2 months.

Dysport®
Initial recommended dose is 20 units/kg body weight given as a divided dose between both calf muscles. If only one calf is affected, a dose of 10 units/kg bodyweight should be used. Consideration should be given to lowering this starting dose if there is evidence to suggest that this dose may result in excessive weakness of the target muscles, such as for patients whose target muscles are small or patients who require concomitant injections to other muscle groups. Following evaluation of response to the starting dose subsequent treatment may be titrated within the range 10 units/kg and 30 units/kg divided between both legs. The maximum dose administered must not exceed 1000 units/patient.
Administration should primarily be targeted to the gastrocnemius, although injections of the soleus and injection of the tibialis posterior should also be considered.
The use of electromyography (EMG) is not routine clinical practice but may assist in identifying the most active muscles. Clinical improvement may be expected within 2 weeks after injection. Injections may be repeated approximately every 16 weeks or as required to maintain response, but not more frequently than every 8 weeks.
To administer, the exposed central portion of the rubber stopper should be cleaned with alcohol immediately prior to piercing the septum. A sterile 23 or 25 gauge needle should be used. Dysport® is reconstituted with 1mL of NaCl 0.9% to yield a solution containing 500 units per ml of Dysport®. Dysport® is administered by IM injection into the calf muscles when treating spasticity.

B

CONTRA-INDICATIONS & WARNINGS
Generalised disorders of muscle activity (e.g. myasthenia gravis), pregnancy and lactation. Do not give with, or before, *aminoglycoside antibiotics or spectinomycin*. As it is a biological product there is a potential for anaphylaxis.

INTERACTIONS
The effect of botulinum A toxin may be potentiated by aminoglycoside antibiotics or other drugs that interfere with neuromuscular transmission e.g. *tubocurarine-type muscle relaxants. Polymixins, tetracyclines and lincomycin* should be used with caution.

PREGNANCY/ BREAST-FEEDING
Contra-indicated.

SIDE-EFFECTS
Pain at the injection site. Increased electrophysiologic jitters in some distant muscles; misplaced injections may paralyse nearby muscle groups and excessive doses may paralyse distant muscles; rash; transient burning after injection.
There have also been specific side-effects reported which are dependent on the condition being treated. For example: dysphagia and pooling of saliva can occur when treating torticollis. After treatment of dynamic equinus foot deformity, side-effects include falling, leg pain, weakness and urinary incontinence. Manufacturers SPC should be consulted for further details of reported side-effects. A small number of patients develop antibodies after one or more injections which can reduce efficacy of further treatments with botulinum A toxin.

POISONING/TOXICITY
Excessive doses may produce distant and profound neuromuscular paralysis. Respiratory support may be required where excessive doses cause paralysis of respiratory muscles. Should overdosage occur, the patient should be medically supervised for several days for signs or symptoms of systemic weakness or muscle paralysis. Specific antitoxin is only likely to be effective if given within 30 minutes of botulinum A toxin injection; it should generally not be expected to be beneficial; general supportive care is advised.

PHARMACODYNAMIC PROPERTIES
Botulinum A toxin blocks cholinergic transport at the neuromuscular junction by preventing the release of acetylcholine. The nerve endings of the neuromuscular junction no longer respond to nerve impulses and secretion of the chemotransmitter is prevented (chemical denervation). Peak effects seen 5-6 days after injection. Duration of action is 2 weeks – 8 months.

EXCIPIENTS
See manufacturers SPC for further details.

LICENSED STATUS
In children, Botox® and Dysport® are licensed for the treatment, in specialist centres with appropriately trained personnel, of dynamic equinus foot deformity due to spasticity in ambulant paediatric cerebral palsy patients of ≥2 years of age. Other paediatric indications are not licensed.

Bowel cleansing solutions

SPECIAL NOTE: Bowel cleansing solutions are not licensed as treatments for constipation.

Picolax® – sodium picosulfate (sodium picosulphate)

USES
Clearance of bowel prior to examination by radiography, endoscopy or surgery.

PRESENTATION
Oral powder: sodium picosulfate 10mg per sachet, with magnesium citrate formed in solution.
NB: see sodium picosulfate monograph for liquid preparation.

B

DOSAGE

Route	Age			Notes
	1 month–2 years	2–12 years	12–18 years	
Oral	1/4 sachet am and 1/4 sachet pm ≥1 year	1/2 sachet am and 1/2 sachet pm 2–4 years 1 sachet am and 1/2 sachet pm 4–9 years as for 12–18 years >9 years	1 sachet am and 1 sachet pm	Take on day prior to examination: first dose before 8am and second dose between 2pm to 4pm.

ADMINISTRATION

Oral: dissolve the contents of one sachet in about 25mL (1 fl oz) water (the solution becomes hot). After 5 minutes dilute to approximately 150mL (¼ pint) and swallow required amount. Low residue diet recommended for 2 days prior to endoscopic examination and liberal intake of clear fluids during treatment. Recommended diet/dosage sheet is supplied with the product. Expect frequent, loose bowel movements 3 hours after the first dose.

CONTRA-INDICATIONS & WARNINGS

General contra-indications to purgatives – avoid in any patient with undiagnosed abdominal pain or where intestinal obstruction is suspected.

INTERACTIONS

Sodium picosulfate increases rate of gastrointestinal transit. Absorption of other orally administered medications may be modified during the treatment period.

PREGNANCY

Caution during first trimester of pregnancy.

BREAST-FEEDING

Contact local Medicines Information Centre for advice.

SIDE-EFFECTS

Griping may occur.

POISONING/TOXICITY

Overdosage would lead to profuse diarrhoea. Treatment is with general supportive measures and maintenance of fluid intake.

EXCIPIENTS

Includes saccharin sodium; sugar-free.

LICENSED STATUS

Licensed for use >1 year of age.

Klean–prep®

USES

Bowel preparation before colonoscopy, colonic surgery, radiological examination and other related procedures. Used in cystic fibrosis patients, in the management of distal intestinal obstructive syndrome (DIOS), as an alternative to Gastrografin®.

PRESENTATION

Oral powder: polyethylene glycol 59g, anhydrous sodium sulphate 5.685g, sodium bicarbonate 1.685g, sodium chloride 1.465g, potassium chloride 743mg per sachet.

DOSAGE

Orally or via nasogastric tube or gastrostomy tube: 10mL/kg/hour for 30 minutes then 20mL/kg/hour for 30 minutes then increase to 25mL/kg/hour if well tolerated.

Maximum volume is 100mL/kg (or 4 litres whichever is smaller) over 4 hours. Patients must be reviewed at 4 hours when, if the output is not yet clean, a further 4 hours, treatment may be prescribed. Maximum total volume over 8 hours is 200mL/kg (or 8 litres whichever is the smaller amount) unless further treatment is approved by the consultant.

ADMINISTRATION
Oral: add the contents of 1 sachet to 1 litre of water. Older children/adults may sip/drink the required quantity every 10-15 minutes. If nasogastric administration is required, a pump may be used to provide accurate flow rates. Whenever possible this should be a special enteral pump which cannot be inadvertently connected to an IV cannula.

CONTRA-INDICATIONS & WARNINGS
Contra-indicated in gastrointestinal obstruction or perforation, ileus, gastric retention, acute intestinal or gastric ulceration, toxic colitis or megacolon and patients less than 20kg. Care in patients with impaired gag reflex, reflux oesophagitis and in ulcerative colitis. Patients who are semi-conscious should receive Klean-prep® via nasogastric route. Pulse, blood pressure, blood glucose, urine output and specific gravity should all be monitored. Should not be given to patients with phenylketonuria (PKU).

INTERACTIONS
Any oral medication given within 1 hour of administration of Klean-prep® may be flushed from the gastrointestinal tract and not absorbed.

PREGNANCY
Use in pregnancy only if essential.

BREAST-FEEDING
Contact local Medicines Information Centre for advice.

SIDE-EFFECTS
Nausea, abdominal fullness, bloating, abdominal cramps, vomiting and anal irritation. Fluid overload or dehydration; electrolyte disturbance, hypoglycaemia. Glucose and U&E levels should be monitored if any adverse effect is suspected and treatment is to continue beyond 4 hours. Urticaria and allergic reactions have been reported rarely.

POISONING/TOXICITY
If gross overdosage where diarrhoea is severe, conservative measures usually sufficient; generous amounts of fluid especially fruit juices should be given.

EXCIPIENTS
Contains aspartame. Contents of single sachet reconstituted with 1 litre of water contains:
Na^+ – 125mmol/L K^+ – 10mmol/L
SO_4^{2-} – 40mmol/L Cl^- – 35mmol/L
HCO_3^- – 20mmol/L.

LICENSED STATUS
Not licensed for use in children <20kg.

FURTHER INFORMATION
Metoclopramide or domperidone may be given 30 minutes before starting Klean-prep® to facilitate gastric emptying.

Citramag® – magnesium citrate

USES
Preparation of patient for all radiological examinations requiring a completely evacuated bowel; colorectal surgery.

PRESENTATION
Oral powder: effervescent, magnesium carbonate 11.57g, anhydrous citric acid 17.79g per sachet which produces 17.7g magnesium citrate in aqueous solution equivalent in alkalinity to 5mg magnesium oxide.

DOSAGE
Oral: before the examination or surgery.

5-9 years: one-third of a sachet
10-12 years: half a sachet
12-18 years: one sachet

ADMINISTRATION
Oral: hot water is needed to prepare the solution. Cool before drinking. Low residue or fluid only diet for 36 hours prior to the examination. Plenty of clear fluids should be drunk between taking Citramag® and the examination.

CONTRA-INDICATIONS & WARNINGS
No absolute contra-indications. Fruit juice should be avoided as routine fluid (due to its high potassium content) in conditions in which hyperkalaemia can occur. May be necessary to modify routine instructions regarding fluid intake in those patients with renal impairment. Risk of toxic hypermagnesaemia indicates need for caution in administration of magnesium citrate to patients in renal failure.

PREGNANCY/BREAST-FEEDING
Contact local Medicines Information Centre for advice.

EXCIPIENTS
Saccharin sodium.

LICENSED STATUS
Licensed for use $\geq$5 years of age.

B

Budesonide

A corticosteroid which decreases tissue inflammation and bronchial hyper-reactivity.

USES
Prophylaxis in the early management of babies at risk of bronchopulmonary dysplasia (BPD) and in the management of established BPD to reduce the need for systemic steroids; prophylaxis of asthma (especially if not fully controlled by bronchodilators); croup, Crohn's disease (affecting the ileum and/or ascending colon), ulcerative colitis.

PRESENTATION
Aerosol inhaler: 50 microgram and 200 microgram – Pulmicort®.
Dry powder for inhalation: 100 microgram, 200 microgram and 400 microgram - Pulmicort® Turbohaler®.
Nebuliser solution: 250 microgram in 1mL, 2mL unit and 500 microgram in 1mL, 2mL unit – Pulmicort® Respules®.
Capsule (enteric-coated): 3mg – Budenofalk®.
Capsule (enteric-coated, modified release): 3mg – Entocort® CR.
Enema: 2mg in 100mL when dispersible tablet is reconstituted in isotonic saline vehicle – Entocort®.
Nasal spray: 100 microgram per metered spray – Rhinocort Aqua® and non-proprietary.

DOSAGE
Birth to 4 months

Indication	Route	Age	Frequency	Notes
		birth–4 months	(times daily)	
Prophylaxis and management of BPD	Inhaled (spacer)	400 microgram/kg	2	For ventilated babies.
	Inhaled (nebuliser)	500 microgram	2	For non-ventilated babies. May be increased to 1mg twice daily in babies >2.5kg with severe symptoms.

Child

Indication	Route	Age			Frequency	Notes
		1 month–2 years	2–12 years	12–18 years	(times daily)	
Prophylaxis of asthma	Aerosol	50–400 micrograms		200–400 micrograms	2	Preventor for regular use. Can use up to 800 micrograms/day in periods of severe asthma.
	Turbohaler	-	100–400 micrograms		2	
	Nebuliser	> 3 months 250–500 micrograms		500 microgram –1mg	2	Higher doses have been used.
Croup	Nebuliser	← 2mg →			single dose	

Child continued

Indication	Route	Age			Frequency (times daily)	Notes
		1 month–2 years	2–12 years	12–18 years		
Crohn's disease	Oral modified release capsules	Not recommended		9mg	once in the morning	For up to 8 weeks, reducing the dose in the last 2-4 weeks. Induction of remission in mild to moderate disease affecting the ileum and/or the ascending colon.
	Oral	Not recommended		3mg	3	
Ulcerative colitis	Rectal	Not recommended		1 enema	once nightly	For 4 weeks. Recto and recto–sigmoid disease.

B

ADMINISTRATION
Inhaler: aerosol inhaler can be used via Nebuhaler® and mask for infants and young children.
Inhalation via spacer: in ventilated babies use a spacer of approximately 145mL (AeroChamber®) attached directly to the ET tube. Hand ventilate the baby using a bag system via the AeroChamber®. Once chest movement is established activate the metered dose device and then inflate the chest ten times for each dose.
Nebulisation: can be diluted to half strength with NaCl 0.9%. Compatible with terbutaline and ipratropium bromide nebuliser solutions. Rinse mouth with water and wash face after nebulisation.
Oral: capsules should be swallowed whole with water and not chewed. Take half to one hour before food. They can be opened and the granules taken in orange/apple juice without chewing.

CONTRA-INDICATIONS & WARNINGS
Hypersensitivity to budesonide. Local bacterial or viral infection is a contra-indication to use of the enema and the capsule should not be given in cases of bacterial, fungal or viral infection. In patients with compromised liver function, blood levels of glucocorticoid may increase. Use with caution in acute pulmonary tuberculosis.

INTERACTIONS
Very low plasma drug concentrations are achieved following inhaled doses. Therefore there is low potential for drug interactions. No information available on possible interactions with oral or rectal administration.

PREGNANCY
Avoid oral and rectal use in pregnancy unless there are compelling reasons. Contact local Medicines Information Centre for advice. Inhaled budesonide achieves very low plasma drug concentrations.

BREAST-FEEDING
No information available about the passage of budesonide into breast milk. Contact local Medicines Information Centre for advice.

SIDE-EFFECTS
Occasionally, mild irritation in the throat and hoarseness (reduced by use of a spacer device). Very occasionally inhaled drugs may provoke bronchoconstriction in hyper-reactive patients. Facial skin irritation has occurred occasionally if a nebuliser with a face-mask has been used (the face should be washed after use of a face-mask). With the oral preparation, side-effects characteristic of systemic corticosteroid therapy can occur although treatment with Entocort® results in lower systemic steroid levels than conventional oral steroid therapy. Adrenal suppression can occur with high-dose inhaled therapy.

POISONING/TOXICITY
Inhalation of large amounts of budesonide over a short period of time will suppress hypothalamic-pituitary-adrenal (HPA) function. No emergency treatment needs to be taken and treatment with budesonide at the recommended dose should be continued to control asthma. Overdosage of the rectal preparation is not thought to be a clinical problem. Acute overdosage of the oral preparation: supportive therapy as required.

PHARMACOKINETIC PROPERTIES
Very little of an inhaled dose of budesonide is absorbed systemically. Any corticosteroid that reaches the systemic circulation will be mainly metabolised in the liver but also in the kidney and is excreted in the urine. The maximal plasma concentration after inhalation of 1mg budesonide, delivered with a dry powder inhaler, is about 3.5nanomol/L and is reached after about 20 minutes.
Oral preparation; plasma protein binding 85-90%. Peak plasma concentration is 3-5 hours after a single oral dose. Maximal release occurs in the terminal ileum and caecum. The average elimination half-life is 3-4 hours and systemic availability is 9-13%.

EXCIPIENTS
Capsules include sucrose. See manufacturers SPC for further details.

LICENSED STATUS
Licensed inhaled dose in children is up to 800 microgram per day. Licensed nebulised dose in children is up to 2mg per day. The inhaled and nebulised routes are not licensed in children <3 months of age.
Capsules and enema are not licensed for use in children.
Nasal spray is licensed for ≥12 years of age.

FURTHER INFORMATION
Use individual respules within 12 hours of opening and respule pack within 3 months of opening foil envelope. Protect from light.

B

Bumetanide

Loop diuretic.

USES
Fluid overload, oedema.

PRESENTATION
Injection: 500 microgram in 1mL; 2mL, 4mL and 10mL ampoules – Burinex®.
Liquid: 1mg in 5mL – Burinex®.
Tablet: (scored) 1mg, 5mg – Burinex® and non-proprietary.

DOSAGE/ADMINISTRATION

Route	Age			Frequency	Notes
	1 month–2 years	2–12 years	12–18 years		
Oral	← 15–50 microgram/kg →		1–2mg	single dose	May be repeated up to 4 times daily.
IV infusion	← 25–50 microgram/kg →		1–2mg	single dose	Infuse in NaCl 0.9% or glucose 5% over 30 minutes.

CONTRA-INDICATIONS & WARNINGS, INTERACTIONS, PREGNANCY/BREAST-FEEDING, POISONING/TOXICITY
See furosemide (frusemide) monograph.

SIDE-EFFECTS
See furosemide monograph; also myalgia has been reported, especially with high doses in patients with renal failure.

PHARMACOKINETIC PROPERTIES
Oral bioavailability 80-95%. Elimination half-life (adults) 0.75-2.6 hours. Renal excretion accounts for about half the clearance with hepatic excretion responsible for the other half. There is an increase in half-life and a reduced plasma clearance in the presence of renal or hepatic disease.

EXCIPIENTS
Burinex® liquid includes sorbitol. Contact manufacturers for further details.

LICENSED STATUS
Not licensed for use in children.

FURTHER INFORMATION
An extemporaneous preparation can be made if a more concentrated liquid is required.

Bupivacaine hydrochloride

Local anaesthetic of the amide type.

USES
Infiltration and regional anaesthesia including peripheral nerve block, spinal and epidural block.

PRESENTATION
Injection: 0.25% and 0.5%, 10mL ampoule – Marcain® and non-proprietary.
Injection (epidural): several strengths and presentations – manufactured 'specials'.
Infusion (epidural): 0.1%, 100mL and 250mL bags; 0.125%, 250mL bag – non-proprietary.
Injection (spinal anaesthesia): 0.5% with glucose 8%, 4mL ampoule – Marcain Heavy®.
Injection: 0.25% with adrenaline (epinephrine) 1 in 200,000, 10mL ampoule and 0.5% with adrenaline (epinephrine) 1 in 200,000, 10mL ampoule – Marcain with Adrenaline®.

DOSAGE

Route	Age				Frequency (times daily)	Notes
	birth–1 month	1 month–2 years	2–12 years	12–18 years		
Local infiltration	← up to 0.8mL/kg of 0.25% → (up to 2mg/kg)			up to 60mL 0.25% (up to 150mg)	single dose	Do not administer more than every 8 hours.
Epidural block using plain solution	up to 0.8mL/kg of 0.25% (up to 2mg/kg)	≤8 years ← up to 1mL/kg of 0.25% → (up to 2.5mg/kg) ≥ 8 years ← 0.5mL/kg of 0.5% → (up to 2.5mg/kg)		15–30mL 0.5% (75–150mg/kg)	blocks all sensation for 2–8 hours	Given in fractionated doses.
Epidural infusion using plain solution	← ≤6 months → 0.1– 0.2mL/kg/hour of 0.125% (≡125–250 microgram/kg/hour) > 6 months 0.2–0.4mL/kg/hour of 0.125% (≡ 250–500 microgram/kg/hour) ← maximum dose per 4 hour period → ← (including top-up) 2mg/kg →			4–15mL/hour of 0.1% (≡ 4–15mg/hour) or 3.2–12mL/hour of 0.125% (≡ 4–15mg/hour)	continuous	Post-operative analgesia or acute pain relief. Use in ITU or high dependency care areas only. Infusion may require top-ups.
Epidural bolus (top-up) using plain solution	← ≤1 year → 0.1–0.3mL/kg of 0.25% (250–750 microgram/kg) ← >1 year → 0.1-0.2mL/kg of 0.375% (375–750 microgram/kg)			0.1–0.2mL/kg of 0.375% (375–750 microgram/kg)	4–12 hourly	Given in fractionated doses. May need less for thoracic epidural.

The dosage of bupivacaine will depend upon the site of injection and the procedure used. Expert advice should be obtained. Epidural administration should be carried out by, or under the supervision of, a consultant anaesthetist.

ADMINISTRATION
Injection: bupivacaine injection may be diluted with NaCl 0.9% injection.

CONTRA-INDICATIONS & WARNINGS
Contra-indications: IV regional anaesthesia (Biers block), complete heart block and hypovolaemia. The solution with adrenaline (epinephrine) should not be used for anaesthesia in digits or other appendages. *Cautions:* reduce dose in liver disease; impaired cardiovascular function.

INTERACTIONS
Possible increased myocardial depression in patients receiving *antiarrhythmics*, increased risk of bupivacaine toxicity with *propranolol*. Solutions with *adrenaline (epinephrine)* should be used with caution in patients receiving drugs known to produce blood pressure alterations.

PREGNANCY
There is no evidence of untoward effects in human pregnancy but use of large doses for paracervical or epidural block in labour may cause neonatal respiratory depression, hypotonia and bradycardia.

B

BREAST-FEEDING
Amount excreted in breast milk is too small to be harmful.

SIDE-EFFECTS
Hypersensitivity reactions may be provoked. Systemic adverse effects are likely to occur following accidental IV administration or following excessive dosage – see poisoning/toxicity.

POISONING/TOXICITY
Numbness of the tongue and perioral region may appear as an early sign of systemic toxicity. CNS excitation may occur leading to restlessness, nausea, vomiting and convulsions. This excitation may be followed by CNS depression leading to drowsiness, respiratory failure and coma. Effects on the cardiovascular system include myocardial depression, which may be severe and resistant to treatment, and peripheral vasodilatation leading to hypotension and bradycardia. Stimulates seizures and cardiovascular collapse may develop rapidly following inadvertent intravascular injection. Cardiac arrest may occur. This may be resistant to electrical defibrilation and resuscitation must be continued energetically for a prolonged period.

PHARMACOKINETIC PROPERTIES
Bupivacaine has a relatively slow onset taking up to 30 minutes for full effect and a long duration of action (2-8 hours). It is metabolised in the liver and the metabolites are excreted in the urine. Reported half-lives are from 1.5-5.5 hours in adults and about 8 hours in neonates. Bupivicaine is about 95% bound to plasma proteins.

EXCIPIENTS
Contact manufacturers for further details.

LICENSED STATUS
Licensed for use in all ages.

Bupropion

Atypical antidepressant, an aminoketone, related to phenylethylamines. Dopamine and noradrenaline (norepinephrine) agonist.

USES
Third-line treatment of attention-deficit hyperactivity disorder (ADHD).

PRESENTATION
Tablets: 150mg (modified-release) – Zyban®.

DOSAGE

Route	Age	Frequency	Notes
	12–18 years	(times daily)	
Oral	150–300mg	1 (morning)	Dose is usually 150mg in the morning.

ADMINISTRATION
Do not crush or chew tablets.

CONTRA-INDICATIONS & WARNINGS
Epilepsy or conditions (e.g. brain injury or tumour) that would predispose to seizures. Eating disorders, hepatic disease, bipolar disorder. Previous hypersensitivity to bupropion.

INTERACTIONS
Risk of seizures if patient is taking any ictogenic medication (*e.g. most antipsychotics, antidepressants, theophylline*) or likely to suddenly discontinue anticonvulsant or seizure-suppressing medicine. *Carbamazepine* and *valproate* alter balance of metabolites but significance unclear. Do not start bupropion until 14 days after stopping MAOI treatment.

PREGNANCY
Contra-indicated in pregnancy. No published data available about risk. Crosses placenta.

BREAST-FEEDING
Contra-indicated in breast-feeding. Excreted in breast milk.

SIDE-EFFECTS
Dry mouth, insomnia, anorexia, tinnitus, light-headedness, sweating, skin rash, seizures.

POISONING/TOXICITY
Seizures, tachycardia, hallucinations, nausea, coma. No antidote though activated charcoal recommended. Manage supportively. Treat seizures with intravenous benzodiazepine.

PHARMACOKINETIC PROPERTIES
Maximum concentration (in adults) at 2.5-3 hours. Steady state reached after 4-7 days. Metabolised extensively in liver to active metabolites through cytochrome P450 CYP2B6 pathway to threohydro-, erythrohydro- and hydroxybupropion. Elimination through urine, half-life approximately 20 hours.

EXCIPIENTS
See manufacturers SPC for further details.

LICENSED STATUS
Licensed for smoking cessation in adults only.

B

Buspirone hydrochloride

Azaspirodecanedione. It is an anxiolytic which lacks sedative, anticonvulsant and muscle relaxant properties.

USES
Anxiety. Hyperkinetic disorder (third-line).

PRESENTATION
Tablet: 5mg and 10mg – Buspar® and non-proprietary.

DOSAGE

Route	Age		Frequency (times daily)	Notes
	2–12 years	12–18 years		
Oral	5mg	5–10mg	2–3	Maximum dose in adults 45mg **daily** in divided doses.

CONTRA-INDICATIONS & WARNINGS
Hepatic and renal impairment, epilepsy, concurrent MAOI treatment.

INTERACTIONS
Can potentiate effects of *sedatives*.

PREGNANCY
No data on use in human pregnancy. Manufacturers state that use is contra-indicated during pregnancy. Contact local Medicines Information Centre for advice.

BREAST-FEEDING
Details of excretion not known. Manufacturers state that it is contra-indicated in breast-feeding. Contact local Medicines Information Centre for advice.

SIDE-EFFECTS
Nausea, light-headedness, dizziness, headache, vivid dreams and dry mouth.

POISONING/TOXICITY
Signs/symptoms: drowsiness and nausea.
Treatment: supportive measures only as no specific antidote.

PHARMACOKINETIC PROPERTIES
Rapidly absorbed following oral administration. It is then subject to considerable first-pass metabolism. Studies in adults have shown peak plasma levels to occur 60-90 minutes after dosing. Plasma concentration is linearly related to dose. Following multiple dosing, steady state plasma concentration is achieved within 2 days. Buspirone is 95% protein bound and eliminated primarily by liver metabolism. Half-life is 2-11 hours.

EXCIPIENTS
See manufacturers SPC for further details.

LICENSED STATUS
Not licensed for use in children.

FURTHER INFORMATION
May take several weeks to achieve effect.

Caffeine citrate

A xanthine derivative and thus a central nervous system stimulant.

USES
The drug of choice for idiopathic central or mixed apnoea in the neonatal period.
To speed extubation in the ventilator-dependent baby.

PRESENTATION
Oral liquid: 10mg in 1mL and 20mg in 1mL – manufactured 'specials'.
Injection: 5mg in 1mL, 2mL ampoule; 10mg in 1mL, 1mL, 2mL and 5mL ampoules; 25mg in 1mL, 2mL ampoule and 50mg in 1mL, 10mL ampoule – manufactured 'specials'.

DOSAGE
Newborn infant (birth to 3 months)

Route	Age	Frequency	Notes
	birth–3 months	(times daily)	
IV or oral loading dose	20mg/kg	single dose	
IV or oral maintenance	5mg/kg	1	Start maintenance dose 24 hours after loading dose. Some babies need a higher dose of 10mg/kg once daily. If more than 44 weeks post-conceptional age, some babies may need the 10mg/kg dose twice daily.

The doses are given here in terms of caffeine citrate. 2mg of caffeine citrate ≡ 1mg caffeine base. Always read labelling of products carefully.

ADMINISTRATION
IV: slow injection over 3-5 minutes, undiluted.
IV infusion: dilute with NaCl 0.9% or glucose 5% and administer over 20 minutes.

INTERACTIONS
Theoretical interaction with those drugs which interact with theophylline – no clinical data to support this theoretical risk.

SIDE-EFFECTS
Jitteriness, tachycardia and raised blood glucose.

POISONING/TOXICITY
Signs of toxicity do not occur until plasma levels exceed 50mg/L caffeine base (1mg/L = 5.14 micromol/L).

Tachycardia is the first sign of toxicity. Seizures, circulatory collapse and death can occur with ten times the recommended dose.

PHARMACOKINETIC PROPERTIES
Half-life more than 100 hours in neonates. The recommended dose aims to produce a therapeutic level of caffeine base of 10-20mg/L but levels of 25-35mg/L are occasionally needed. Routine monitoring is not necessary at standard dosage. Samples do not need to be collected at any set time.

EXCIPIENTS
Contact manufacturer for further details.

LICENSED STATUS
Available as 'specials' and as such are unlicensed.

Calamine lotion BP

Topical antipruritic.

USES
Relief of pruritus.

PRESENTATION
Lotion: calamine 15%, zinc oxide 5%, glycerol 5%, bentonite 3%, sodium citrate 0.5%, liquid phenol 0.5% in freshly boiled and cooled purified water in a homogenous suspension when shaken well.

DOSAGE/ADMINISTRATION
Topical: apply to the affected area as needed. For external use only.

LICENSED STATUS
Licensed for use in children and adults.

Calcipotriol

Vitamin D derivative that induces differentiation and suppresses proliferation of keratinocytes.

USES
Cream and ointment: topical treatment of mild to moderate plaque psoriasis affecting up to 40% of skin area.
Scalp solution: treatment of scalp psoriasis.

PRESENTATION
Cream: 50 microgram/g – Dovonex®.
Ointment: 50 microgram/g – Dovonex®.
Scalp solution: 50 microgram in 1mL – Dovonex®.

DOSAGE/ADMINISTRATION
All preparations: apply to affected area morning and evening. Do not apply to face. Wash hands after use to avoid inadvertent transfer to other body areas.
Cream/ointment: weekly maximum to be applied – 6-12 years, 50g; adolescents >12 years, 75g; adults, 100g.
Scalp solution: weekly maximum to be applied – adults, 60mL. When used with the cream/ointment, weekly maximum of total calcipotriol 5mg.

CONTRA-INDICATIONS & WARNINGS
Hypersensitivity. Do not use in patients with known disorders of calcium metabolism.

PREGNANCY
Avoid unless no safer suitable alternative.

BREAST-FEEDING
Not known if excreted in milk.

SIDE-EFFECTS
Transient local irritation. Dermatitis, pruritus, erythema, aggravation of psoriasis and photosensitivity.

POISONING/TOXICITY
Risk of hypercalcaemia if excessive amounts are applied. Greater risk at lower doses with generalised pustular or erythrodermic exfoliative psoriasis.

PHARMACOKINETIC PROPERTIES
Less than 1% of dose absorbed (single study with 5 patients).

EXCIPIENTS
See manufacturers SPC for further details.

LICENSED STATUS
Cream and ointment licensed for >6 years of age. Scalp solution not licensed in children.

USES
Calcitonin may have usefulness in the following conditions: steroid-induced osteoporosis, immobilisation osteoporosis e.g. high-spinal injury and cerebral palsy, idiopathic juvenile osteoporosis, hypercalcaemia in malignant disease, fibroplastic dysplasia of bone, juvenile idiopathic arthritis and osteogenesis imperfecta.

PRESENTATION
Injection: 50 units and 100 units in 1mL, 1mL ampoule; 200 units in 1mL, 2mL multidose vial – Miacalcic®; 100 units in 1mL, 1mL ampoule; 200 units in 1mL, 2mL multidose vial – Calsynar®.

DOSAGE
There is very limited experience of use in children; dose depends on the condition being treated; seek specialist advice.

ADMINISTRATION
IM/SC injection: for administration by IM or SC injection.
IV infusion: Miacalcic® may be diluted with NaCl 0.9% and given by IV infusion over at least 6 hours. There is a loss of potency of approximately 20% when diluted and this should be taken into account when calculating dosage.

CONTRA-INDICATIONS & WARNINGS
Long-term toxicity studies in the rat have shown a species and strain-specific increase in pituitary adenomas. For this reason long-term therapy is not recommended. In any patient with a history of allergy; a scratch or intradermal test challenge using a 1:100 dilution in NaCl 0.9% is recommended. Caution should be exercised in patients with renal or cardiac impairment. Careful surveillance of bone growth in children is recommended.

INTERACTIONS
Cardiac glycosides; calcitonin may cause serum calcium levels to fall transiently to below normal levels, particularly on initiating treatment; dose adjustment of *cardiac glycosides* may be necessary as their effect can be modified by changes in cellular electrolyte concentrations.

PREGNANCY/BREAST-FEEDING
No studies in human pregnancy are available. Animal studies suggest a risk of fetal growth retardation and inhibition of lactation. It is recommended that unless considered essential, calcitonin is not used in women of childbearing potential or nursing mothers. Contact local Medicines Information Centre for advice.

SIDE-EFFECTS
Severe hypersensitivity reactions have been reported, including bronchospasm, swelling of the tongue or throat and anaphylactic reactions. Allergic reactions should be distinguished from generalised flushing and hypotension. Nausea, vomiting, facial flushing, tingling in the hands and an unpleasant taste. Nausea and flushing are usually transient and rarely necessitate withdrawal of treatment. If difficulties persist, injections may be given at night with anti-emetic cover. Inflammatory reactions at injection sites. Calcitonin binding antibodies may develop after several months' treatment, particularly in patients receiving high doses. Titres are generally low and there is seldom a loss of clinical efficacy. Transient hypocalcaemia may occur, particularly at the time of commencing treatment and diminishing with time.

POISONING/TOXICITY
Facial flushing, and/or flushing of the extremities, and gastrointestinal disturbance may occur. Acute hypocalcaemia is unlikely to occur; should it do so appropriate supportive measures are recommended.

PHARMACODYNAMIC PROPERTIES
Calcitonin acts directly on bone osteoclasts to inhibit their activity and thus reduce bone resorption. It also has weak actions on the kidney enhancing the excretion of sodium, potassium, phosphate, calcium and magnesium, and renal production of 1,25-hydroxycholecalciferol. CNS effects include analgesic and anorectic effects.

PHARMACOKINETIC PROPERTIES
Following SC administration peak plasma levels occur after 15-45 minutes.

EXCIPIENTS
Miacalcic® multidose vial includes phenol. See manufacturers SPC for further details.

LICENSED STATUS
Calsynar® manufacturers recommend that in children it should not be used for periods of more than a few weeks, unless considered necessary on compelling medical grounds. Miacalcic® manufacturers give no recommendations for use in children due to limited experience.

FURTHER INFORMATION
The calcium lowering activity of calcitonin is measured in a rat bioassay. The relative amounts of calcitonin demonstrating 100 international units of activity are human calcitonin 1mg: salmon calcitonin 0.025mg (25 micrograms).

Calcitriol (1,25-dihydroxycholecalciferol)

Vitamin D derivative.

USES
Vitamin D-dependent rickets types 1 and 2. Hypophosphataemic rickets. Hypoparathyroidism and pseudohypoparathyroidism.

PRESENTATION
Capsule: 250 nanogram and 500 nanogram – Rolcaltrol®.

DOSAGE

Route	Age			Frequency (times daily)	Notes
	1 month–2 years	2–12 years	12–18 years		
Oral	15 nanogram/kg	15–25 nanogram/kg	250 nanogram	1	Starting dose. Titrate according to response in increments of 5 nanogram/kg/day (child) or 250 nanogram/day (adult), every 2–4 weeks until maintenance achieved.

ADMINISTRATION
Oral: capsules should be swallowed with a little water.

CONTRA-INDICATIONS AND WARNINGS
Hypersensitivity to calcitriol or any excipient of the formulation; hypercalcaemia, metastatic calcification. Concurrent administration of other compounds, including foods and food supplements, should be undertaken with caution. Continued control of serum phosphate remains essential.

INTERACTIONS
Use with caution when given concurrently with other agents which may cause a rise in serum calcium levels.

PREGNANCY
Administration during pregnancy is not advised. Contact local Medicines Information Centre for advice.

BREAST-FEEDING
It is likely that calcitriol is excreted into breast milk. Caution with high systemic doses; may cause hypercalcaemia in the infant. Contact local Medicines Information Centre for advice.

SIDE-EFFECTS
Hypercalcaemia and hypercalciuria may occur and indicate excessive dosage. As such, the following which are signs and symptoms of hypercalcaemia may be seen: anorexia, nausea, vomiting, headache, weakness, apathy, somnolence, thirst, dehydration, polyuria, nocturia, abdominal pain, paralytic ileus, cardiac arrhythmias, overt psychosis, metastatic calcification. Mild, non-progressive and reversible elevations of LFTs occur occasionally.

POISONING/TOXICITY
If hypercalcaemia should occur, supportive measures, including adequate hydration, should be initiated. After oral overdosage gastric lavage may be helpful if performed within 6-8 hours of ingestion.

PHARMACOKINETIC PROPERTIES
Calcitriol is well absorbed following oral administration, with peak plasma levels occurring 4-6 hours after dosing. Plasma half-life is 3-6 hours, but the duration of pharmacological activity is 3-5 days. Approximately 10% of the administered dose appears in the urine in 24 hours with biliary excretion and enterohepatic recirculation also occurring.

EXCIPIENTS
See manufacturers SPC for further details.

LICENSED STATUS
Not licensed for use in children.

Calcium carbonate

USES
Phosphate binding agent. Hyperphosphataemia.

PRESENTATION
Tablet: calcium carbonate 1.25g (calcium 500mg or Ca^{2+} 12.6mmol) – Calcichew® (chewable); Cacit® (effervescent); Calcium-500.
Tablet: (chewable) calcium carbonate 1.5g, (calcium 600mg or Ca^{2+} 15mmol) – Adcal®.
Tablet: (chewable, scored) calcium carbonate 2.5g, (calcium 1g or Ca^{2+} 25mmol) – Calcichew Forte®.
Tablet: calcium carbonate 300mg – manufactured 'special'.
Tablet: calcium carbonate 420mg (calcium 168mg or Ca^{2+} 4.2mmol) and glycine 180mg – Titralac®.
Liquid: 600mg in 5mL – manufactured 'special'; other strengths available.

DOSAGE

Route	Age			Frequency (times daily)	Notes
	1 month–2 years	2–12 years	12–18 years		
Oral	≤1 year 120mg	2-6 years 300mg		3–4	Initial dose. Subsequently adjusted according to plasma phosphate levels.
	>1 year 300mg	6-12 years 600mg	1.25g	3–4	

Note: dose is dependent on serum phosphate levels and should be adjusted until serum phosphate is in the normal range.

ADMINISTRATION
Oral: take immediately prior to food to bind phosphate in the food. Cacit® tablets must be dissolved in a glass of water and the solution should then be drunk immediately after complete dissolution of the tablet. Titralac® may be chewed, allowed to dissolve in the mouth or swallowed whole as desired. Calcium-500 tablets should be swallowed whole.

CONTRA-INDICATIONS & WARNINGS
Severe hypercalcaemia, hypercalciuria and osteoporosis due to immobilisation. Patients treated with high doses of vitamin D or who are receiving prolonged calcium treatment, should undergo regulatory measurements of plasma calcium levels which should be interpreted in conjunction with measurements of plasma protein levels. Serum phosphate levels should be measured in all patients receiving phosphate binders, to prevent the development of a phosphate depletion syndrome.

SIDE-EFFECTS
Hypercalcaemia and hypophosphataemia are possible complications of vigorous therapy.

EXCIPIENTS
Calcichew® tablets contain aspartame and are unsuitable for phenylketonuria patients. Contact manufacturers for further details.

LICENSED STATUS
Calcichew®, Calcichew® Forte, Calcium-500 and Titralac® are licensed for phosphate binding in children and adults; this is not a licensed indication for Cacit®. 300mg tablets are available as a 'special' and as such are unlicensed.

FURTHER INFORMATION
300mg tablets are available as a 'special' from Guy's and St. Thomas' Hospital manufacturing unit, London.

Calcium chloride

USES
Hypocalcaemia or electrolyte disturbances.

PRESENTATION
Injection: 10% (100mg in 1mL) disposable syringe (6.8mmol calcium in 10mL) – Min-I-Jet® Calcium Chloride 10% and non-proprietary; 1mmol in 1mL, 5mL, 10mL ampoules and 0.5mmol in 1mL, 5mL, 10mL ampoules.

DOSAGE

Route	Age			Frequency	Notes
	1 month–2 years	2–12 years	12–18 years		
IV	← 0.2mL/kg → of the 10% injection		5–10mL	single dose	Cardiopulmonary resuscitation - ONLY when there is electrolyte disturbance.

CONTRA-INDICATIONS & WARNINGS
Can cause severe tissue necrosis on extravasation. In cardiac resuscitation, calcium is contra-indicated in the prescence of ventricular fibrillation.

INTERACTIONS, SIDE-EFFECTS, PREGNANCY/BREAST-FEEDING, POISONING/TOXICITY
See calcium gluconate monograph.

EXCIPIENTS
Contact manufacturers for further details.

LICENSED STATUS
Min-I-Jet® Calcium Chloride 10% is licensed for use in children and adults for CPR and hypocalcaemic disturbances. The 10% disposable syringe from Aurum is not licensed for use in children.
Ampoules are licensed in children and adults for treatment of hypocalcaemia or electrolyte disturbance.

FURTHER INFORMATION
Calcium chloride is no longer recommended for routine use in CPR. Should only be used in CPR when there is an electrolyte disturbance.

Calcium folinate (folinic acid)

An essential coenzyme for nucleic acid synthesis.

USES
Dihydrobiopterin reductase (DHPR) deficiency. Uridine monophosphate synthase (UMPS) deficiency (hereditary orotic aciduria). Methylene synthase deficiency. Hereditary folate malabsorption. Methylene tetrahydrofolate reductase deficiency. Some disorders of cobalamin metabolism. Folate rescue after methotrexate therapy.

PRESENTATION
Tablet: 15mg (scored) – non-proprietary.
Injection: 3mg in 1mL, 1mL and 10mL ampoules; 7.5mg in 1mL, 2mL ampoule; 10mg in 1mL, 5mL, 10mL, 30mL and 35mL vials – non-proprietary.
Injection: powder for reconstitution 15mg and 30mg vials – non-proprietary.

DOSAGE

Route	Age				Frequency (times daily)	Notes
	birth–1 month	1 month–2 years	2–12 years	12–18 years		
Oral/IV	←		15mg	→	1	Metabolic indications. Larger doses may be required in older children.

Folate rescue after methotrexate therapy: see methotrexate monograph for full details.

ADMINISTRATION
Oral: injection solution can be given orally.
IV: for IV injection, give over 2 minutes; for slow IV infusion, dilute with NaCl 0.9% or glucose 5% and give over a period of 30 minutes.

CONTRA-INDICATIONS & WARNINGS
Treatment of pernicious anaemia or other megaloblastic anaemias where vitamin B12 is deficient. Should not be administered simultaneously with a folic acid antagonist.

INTERACTIONS
Large amounts may antagonise the anti-epileptic effect of *phenobarbital (phenobarbitone), phenytoin* and *primidone* and increase the frequency of seizures in susceptible patients.

PREGNANCY
No adequate well controlled studies in pregnant women; reproduction studies in rats and rabbits have revealed no evidence of teratogenicity. Contact local Medicines Information Centre for advice.

BREAST-FEEDING
No data available.

SIDE-EFFECTS
Adverse effects are rare; occasional reports of pyrexia following parenteral administration.

POISONING/TOXICITY
No reported sequelae in patients who received significantly more than the recommended dose. No specific antidote; treatment, if necessary, is supportive.

PHARMACOKINETIC PROPERTIES
Rapidly and extensively converted to other tetrahydrofolic acid derivatives including 5-methyl tetrahydrofolate, which is the major transport and storage form of folate in the body.

LICENSED STATUS
Licensed for folate rescue following methotrexate therapy in children and adults. Not licensed for the various metabolic indications stated.

Calcium gluconate

USES
Hypocalcaemia, cardiac arrest and as part of a PN regimen.

PRESENTATION
Injection: 10% (calcium 8.9mg or Ca^{2+} 220 micromol in 1mL), 10mL ampoule – non-proprietary.

DOSAGE

Route	Age				Frequency (times daily)	Notes
	birth–1 month	1 month–2 years	2–12 years	12–18 years		
IV bolus over 5–10 minutes	← 0.07mmol/kg (0.3 mL/kg of 10% injection) →				single dose	**Hypocalcaemia urgent correction:** some neonatologists advocate the use of 0.46mmol/kg (2mL/kg of 10% solution) which is a higher dose than that recommended in most UK texts but conforms to practice in the USA.
IV infusion	0.5mmol/kg (0.1mL/kg/hour of 10% injection)	1mmol/kg (0.2mL/kg/hour of the 10% injection)	← 8.8mmol total (40mL of the 10% injection) →		continuous over 24 hours	**Hypocalcaemia maintenance treatment:** IV infusion maintenance may be necessary for a few days but the danger of extravasation usually makes oral maintenance preferable. Dilute to at least 0.045mmol/mL with glucose 5% or NaCl 0.9%.
IV bolus	← 0.3mL/kg of 10% solution →				single dose	**Cardiopulmonary resuscitation:** only when there is electrolyte disturbance.
IV	1mmol/kg	0.2–1mmol/kg	0.2mmol/kg	5–10mmol total	continuous over 12–24 hours	**As part of a PN regimen:** quantities are approximate. It depends on individual requirements to maintain normal serum calcium levels.

CONTRA-INDICATIONS & WARNINGS
Hypercalcaemia. Parenteral administration may cause local reactions at injection site – soft tissue calcification. Do not administer via scalp veins. Not recommended by SC or IM route. Caution in impaired renal function. Monitor plasma calcium closely.

INTERACTIONS
Digoxin with large IV doses of calcium can precipitate arrhythmias.

SIDE-EFFECTS
Associated with hypercalcaemia. Local irritation on injection.

POISONING/TOXICITY
Hypercalcaemia: treat by rehydration followed by furosemide (frusemide) or another loop diuretic to enhance calcium excretion; consider calcitonin and bisphosphonates.

PHARMACOKINETIC PROPERTIES
Excreted in urine (also faeces, sweat, hair, skin and nails).

EXCIPIENTS
Contact manufacturers for further details.

LICENSED STATUS
Not licensed for use in children for the indications listed.

Calcium (oral supplements)

C

USES
Correction of dietary calcium deficiency or when normal requirements are high.

PRESENTATION
Tablet: (effervescent) calcium lactate gluconate 930mg, calcium carbonate 700mg and anhydrous citric acid 1.189g (calcium 400mg or Ca^{2+} 10mmol) – Sandocal®-400.
Tablet: (effervescent) calcium lactate gluconate 2.327g, calcium carbonate 1.75g and anhydrous citric acid 2.973g (calcium 1g or Ca^{2+} 25mmol) – Sandocal®-1000.
Tablet: (effervescent) calcium gluconate tablets 1g (calcium 89mg or Ca^{2+} 2.25mmol) – non-proprietary.
Syrup: calcium glubionate 1.09g and calcium lactobionate 727mg (calcium 108.3mg or Ca^{2+} 2.7mmol) per 5mL – Calcium-Sandoz®.

DOSAGE

Route	Age				Frequency (times daily)	Notes
	birth–1 month	1 month–2 years	2–12 years	12–18 years		
Oral	← 0.25mmol/kg →		2–4 years 0.25mmol/kg	10mmol	4	
			5–12 years 0.2mmol/kg		4	

ADMINISTRATION
Tablets: effervescent tablets must be dissolved in one third to half a tumbler full of water.
Syrup: in neonates doses may be mixed with the first (small) part of milk feeds.

CONTRA-INDICATIONS & WARNINGS
Contra-indicated in hypercalcaemia, severe hypercalciuria and renal calculi. Precautions in mild hypercalciuria, or renal failure, or where there is evidence of stone formation in the urinary tract; adequate checks must be kept on urinary calcium excretion. The likelihood of hypercalcaemia is increased in pregnant women in whom calcium and vitamin D are co-administered. Calcium glubionate is converted to galactose so Calcium-Sandoz® syrup should not be given to patients with galactosaemia.

INTERACTIONS
Oral calcium administration may reduce the absorption of oral *tetracycline* or *fluoride* preparations. An interval of 3 hours should be observed if the two are to be given.

PREGNANCY
Epidemiological studies have shown no evidence of harm to the fetus if used in the doses recommended.

BREAST-FEEDING
Although supplemented calcium may be excreted in

breast milk the concentration is unlikely to be sufficient to produce any adverse effects in the baby.

SIDE-EFFECTS
Mild gastrointestinal disturbances (e.g. constipation, diarrhoea) have occurred rarely. Although hypercalcaemia would not be expected in patients unless their renal function was impaired, the following symptoms could indicate the possibility of hypercalcaemia: nausea, vomiting, anorexia, constipation, abdominal pain, bone pain, thirst, polyuria, muscle weakness, drowsiness or confusion.

EXCIPIENTS
Calcichew Forte® tablets include aspartame. Contact manufacturers for further details.

LICENSED STATUS
Calcium-Sandoz® liquid is licensed for use in all ages including neonates. Sandocal® tablets are licensed for use in adults and children (although the oral syrup is used in children <1 year of age).

Calcium polystyrene sulphonate

Ion exchange resin.

USES
To remove excess potassium in mild or moderate hyperkalaemia.

PRESENTATION
Powder: Calcium Resonium®.
Enema: may be extemporaneously prepared (see below).

DOSAGE

Route	Age				Frequency (times daily)	Notes
	birth–1 month	1 month–2 years	2–12 years	12–18 years		
Rectal	125–250mg/kg	←	125–250mg/kg	→	4	
Oral	–	←	125–250mg/kg	→	4	Do not give orally to neonates.

Monitor plasma electrolytes.

ADMINISTRATION
Oral: mixed with water or as a paste. Avoid using squashes/ fruit juices because of the high potassium content.
Rectally: mix 1g with 5-10mL methylcellulose 1%. Retain in rectum for at least 9 hours if possible, then irrigate to remove resin.

CONTRA-INDICATIONS & WARNINGS
Contra-indicated in bowel obstruction, oral administration or reduced gut motility in neonates, hyperparathyroidism. Caution in patients with high calcium. Inadequate dilution or excessive dosages may cause impaction in children. Stop if plasma potassium lower than 5mmol/L.

PREGNANCY
Use with caution. Contact local Medicines Information Centre for advice.

BREAST-FEEDING
Contact local Medicines Information Centre for advice.

SIDE-EFFECTS
Rectal ulceration following rectal administration, colonic necrosis when enemas containing sorbitol used for irrigation. Gastric irritation, nausea, vomiting, anorexia and constipation. Faecal impaction following rectal administration in children. Bleeding and hypercalcaemia.

PHARMACOKINETIC PROPERTIES
Not absorbed.

LICENSED STATUS
Licensed for use orally and rectally in children.

EXCIPIENTS
See manufacturers SPC for further details.

Angiotensin-converting enzyme (ACE) inhibitor.

USES
Hypertension (particularly secondary to hyperreninaemia) and heart failure.

PRESENTATION
Tablet: 2mg – named patient; 12.5mg, 25mg and 50mg – Capoten® (12.5mg and 50mg are scored) and non-proprietary.
Solution: 5mg in 1mL (imported).
Suspension: may be extemporaneously prepared.

DOSAGE

Route	Age				Frequency (times daily)	Notes
	birth–1 month	1 month–2 years	2–12 years	12–18 years		
Oral	10–50 microgram/kg	◄— 100 microgram/kg —►		6.25mg	single dose	Test dose with patient supine. Monitor blood pressure every 15 minutes for 1–2 hours.
	10–50 microgram/kg	◄— 100 microgram–2mg/kg —►		–	3	Start at the low dose and titrate up to the maximum
	–	–	–	12.5–50mg	2–3	if necessary. Use the lowest effective dose. Maximum daily doses: <1 month 2mg/kg/day 1 month–1 year 4mg/kg/day 1 year–12 years 6mg/kg/day.

C

ADMINISTRATION
Oral: tablets can be halved and will disperse in water.

CONTRA-INDICATIONS & WARNINGS
Avoid where possible in neonates (particularly preterm) due to the risk of renal failure, anuria and hypotension. Risk of marked hypotension if volume depleted. Renal impairment if renovascular disease. Patients with renal impairment may respond to smaller or less frequent dosage – titrate dose to response. Removed by dialysis, give 25% dose after dialysis. Should not be used in patients with bilateral renal artery stenosis or outflow tract obstruction. In patients with evidence of prior renal disease, urine should be tested for protein monthly for first 9 months of treatment. Anaphylactoid reaction can occur during dialysis with high-flux polyacrylonitrile membranes.

INTERACTIONS
Diuretics – potentiate the anti hypertensive effect of ACE inhibitors and hyperkalaemia with *potassium-sparing diuretics*.
NSAIDs – reduced hypotensive effect of ACE inhibitors. Enhanced hypotensive effect with *anaesthetics*, *antihypertensives*, *anxiolytics* and *hypnotics*.

PREGNANCY
Use is contra-indicated in pregnancy and women of childbearing potential unless protected by adequate contraception. Exposure of the mother in the second and third trimesters of pregnancy has been associated with oligohydramnios and neonatal hypotension and/or anuria.

BREAST-FEEDING
Excreted in breast milk in amounts which are probably too small to be harmful, but manufacturers advise avoidance. Contact local Medicines Information Centre for advice.

SIDE-EFFECTS
Hypotension, gastrointestinal upset, hyperkalaemia, angioedema, blood disorders (increased incidence in renal failure) and cough.

POISONING/TOXICITY
In the event of overdose, blood pressure should be monitored and if hypotension develops volume expansion is the treatment of choice. Removable by dialysis.

PHARMACOKINETIC PROPERTIES
Maximal decrease in blood pressure 1-1.5 hours after oral administration. It may take several weeks of therapy before full hypotensive effect is seen. The half-life is dependent upon renal and cardiac function, range in children 0.98-2.3 hours (mean 1.5 hours). In infants with congestive heart failure half-life range 1.2-12.4 hours. Renal elimination; titrate dose against response.

EXCIPIENTS
Contact manufacturers for further details.

LICENSED STATUS
12.5mg, 25mg and 50mg tablets are licensed for use in all ages for congestive heart failure and severe hypertension, although experience in neonates is limited. Not licensed for the treatment of mild to moderate hypertension in children. 2mg tablets and 5mg in 1mL solution are not licensed for use in the UK.

FURTHER INFORMATION
Solution available via IDIS World Medicines.

Carbamazepine

Antiepileptic.

USES
Epilepsy; neuropathic pain (dose in the therapeutic range for seizure control can be used); some movement disorders (eg: paroxysmal kinesigenic choreoathetosis); mood stabilisation; attention deficit hyperactivity disorders (ADHD).

PRESENTATION
Liquid: 100mg in 5mL – Tegretol®.
Suppository: 125mg and 250mg – Tegretol®.
Tablet: (scored) 100mg, 200mg and 400mg – Tegretol® and non-proprietary.
Tablet: (modified release) 200mg and 400mg – Tegretol® Retard (both scored), Teril® CR and Timonil® Retard.
Tablet: (chewable) 100mg and 200mg – Tegretol® Chewtabs.

DOSAGE

Route	Age				Frequency (times daily)	Notes
	*birth–1 month	1 month–2 years	2–12 years	12–18 years		
Oral	← 5mg/kg → or			-	1 (at night)	Starting dose. Increase by 2.5–5mg/kg every 3–7 days until maintenance dose achieved, to reduce incidence of ataxia and drowsiness.
	← 2.5mg/kg →			-	2	
	-			100–200mg	1–2	
	← 5mg/kg →			400–600mg	2–3	Usual target maintenance dose. Doses of up to 20mg/kg/day may be needed.
Oral 'M/R' tablets	-	← 5–10mg/kg →		400–600mg	2	Usual target maintenance dose (see also non-modified release tablets).
Rectal	-	use approximately 25% more than oral dose (maximum 250mg)			Maximum of 4	Use usually limited to short-term replacement of oral therapy.

* Experience with use of carbamazepine in the neonatal period is very limited.

ADMINISTRATION
Oral: bioavailability unaffected by food. Tegretol® Retard tablets can be halved but should not be chewed. Oral liquid rapidly absorbed and may cause drowsiness.
Rectal: oral liquid has been given rectally, may have a laxative effect and should be retained for at least 2 hours.

CONTRA-INDICATIONS & WARNINGS
A-V conduction abnormalities, history of bone marrow depression, intermittent porphyria, MAOIs within last 2 weeks, sensitivity to tricyclic antidepressants. Do not

use carbamazepine for myoclonic or absence seizures, which are both exacerbated. Counsel on recognition of haematological, skin and liver adverse effects. Warn of drowsiness particularly at start of treatment and not to cease therapy without advice. Extensively metabolised by oxidation in the liver so dose reduction may be required in advanced liver disease.

INTERACTIONS

Synergy with *acetazolamide* in partial (simple and complex) seizures. *Sodium valproate* often raises plasma concentration of an active metabolite of carbamazepine. Increased toxicity with *lamotrigine*. Numerous potentially serious interactions mainly with drugs that inhibit carbamazepine metabolism and by acceleration of metabolism of other drugs by carbamazepine. Consult appropriate references when changing dose of carbamazepine or interacting drugs or when changing drug therapy. Reduces the effectiveness of the standard dose *oral contraceptive pill*. A higher oestrogen dose-containing *oral contraceptive* will be required.

PREGNANCY

Increased risk of neural tube defects and other malformations, especially if more than one antiepileptic used. Specialist counselling, management and screening required. Administer folate supplements before and during pregnancy. Blood levels may be altered. Administer vitamin K during last weeks of pregnancy and to newborn to prevent bleeding disorders in the newborn. Neonates may have withdrawal symptoms if the mother has taken carbamazepine during pregnancy. Contact local Medicines Information Centre for advice.

BREAST-FEEDING

Passes into breast milk such that infants receive about 10% of a therapeutic dose but not considered a significant hazard. Breast-feeding is appropriate if maternal dose is normal.

SIDE-EFFECTS

Dose dependent adverse effects include nystagmus, diplopia, nausea and/or vomiting, ataxia and drowsiness. Chronic adverse effects include mental slowing, hyponatraemia and low white blood cell count. Monitor pre-treatment electrolytes and blood count and thereafter if clinically indicated.

POISONING/TOXICITY

Signs and symptoms involve CNS, CVS and respiratory systems. Contact UK National Poisons Information Service. Measure blood levels.

PHARMACOKINETIC PROPERTIES

Peak plasma levels 12, 6 and 2 hours after standard tablets, chewable tablets and oral liquid respectively with steady state plasma levels in 1-2 weeks. Initial elimination half-life 36 hours falling to 16-24 hours as auto-induction of carbamazepine metabolism occurs; maximal after 4 weeks; dose may require increasing. Bioavailability of suppositories approximately 75% of oral dose forms. Metabolised by CYP 3A4, co-administration of inhibitors and inducers will affect carbamazepine levels. Monitor blood levels if clinically indicated (see therapeutic section). Target range is a trough concentration of 6-12mg/L measured after 1-2 weeks.

EXCIPIENTS

Tegretol® Retard tablets and liquid include polyethoxylated castor oil. Tegretol® Chewtabs and liquid include sorbitol. See manufacturers SPC for further details.

LICENSED STATUS

Licensed for use in adults, children and infants, although some formulations e.g. Tegretol® Chewtabs are not recommended for young children or infants.

FURTHER INFORMATION

Different preparations may vary in bioavailability; to avoid reduced effect or excessive side-effects, it may be prudent to avoid changing the formulation. Prescriptions should include brand name to ensure consistency of drug delivery. Problems unlikely if Tegretol® Chewtabs sucked or swallowed whole.

Carbamylglutamate

USES

N-acetyl glutamate synthase (NAGS) deficiency.
Carbamylphosphate synthase deficiency.

PRESENTATION

Tablet: 200mg (dispersible/scored) – named patient.

DOSAGE

Route	Age				Frequency (times daily)	Notes
	birth–1 month	1 month–2 years	2–12 years	12–18 years		
Oral	←	12.5–25mg/kg		→	4	Use only with specialist advice.

ADMINISTRATION

Oral: tablet should be dispersed in 5-10mL water, administered orally or via a nasogastric tube. Store in the refrigerator until opened. After first opening of the tablet container, store at room temperature, do not refrigerate – it is stable for up to 1 month. Tablets are scored to give dosage portions of 50mg.

CONTRA-INDICATIONS & WARNINGS, INTERACTIONS, PREGNANCY/BREAST-FEEDING, SIDE-EFFECTS, POISONING/TOXICITY
No information available.

PHARMACODYNAMIC PROPERTIES
N-carbamyl glutamate is an analogue of N-acetyl glutamate, which is the naturally occurring activator of carbamylphosphate synthetase of the urea cycle.

EXCIPIENTS
Contact manufacturers for further details.

LICENSED STATUS
Not licensed for use in the UK.

FURTHER INFORMATION
Tablet available from Orphan Europe on a named patient basis.

Carbaryl

Parasiticidal agent.

USES
Eradication of head louse infestation.

PRESENTATION
Liquid: 1% in an aqueous basis – Carylderm®.
Lotion: 0.5% in an alcoholic basis – Carylderm®.

DOSAGE/ADMINISTRATION
Topical: rub gently into dry hair and scalp until all the hair is thoroughly moistened. Comb and allow to dry naturally, away from heat or sunshine, in a well ventilated room. A contact time of 12 hours or overnight is recommended. Then, wash in ordinary shampoo and remove the dead lice and eggs with a fine toothed comb whilst the hair is still wet. Repeat after 7 days only if live lice are found again.

CONTRA-INDICATIONS & WARNINGS
Avoid contact with eyes. Do not use on broken or secondarily infected skin. Do not use more than once a week for 3 weeks at a time. Alcoholic lotion is not recommended for head lice treatment in asthmatics or small children.

PREGNANCY/BREAST-FEEDING
Can be used with caution.

SIDE-EFFECTS
Skin irritation may occur.

POISONING/TOXICITY
Treat by gastric lavage, assisted respiration, and in the case of massive ingestion, administration of atropine. May be necessary to counteract cholinesterase inhibition.

EXCIPIENTS
See manufacturers SPC for further details.

LICENSED STATUS
Licensed for use in children and adults, but children <6 months should only be treated under medical supervision.

FURTHER INFORMATION
In the light of conclusions (based on experimental data in animals) it would be prudent to consider carbaryl as a potential human carcinogen, therefore it has been restricted to prescription use only. Treat all affected members of the family/household on the same day.

Carbimazole

Antithyroid drug.

USES
Hyperthyroidism, including diffuse toxic goitre (Grave's disease), and neonatal thyrotoxicosis.

PRESENTATION
Tablet: 5mg, 20mg – Neo-Mercazole®.
Oral suspension: manufactured 'special'.

DOSAGE

Route	Age				Frequency (times daily)	Notes
	birth–1 month	1 month–2 years	2–12 years	12–18 years		
Oral	← 250 micrograms/kg →			10mg	3	Initial dose. Maximum **total daily dose** 40mg. Administer until euthyroid and then gradually reduce the dose to the minimum (usually given once daily) that sustains normal thyroid function. Alternatively, once euthyroid, continue high dose carbimazole and add levothyroxine (thyroxine) 100 microgram/m²/**day** for replacement. Monitor thyroid function.

CONTRA-INDICATIONS & WARNINGS
Hyperthyroidism due to nodular goitre. Use with caution in liver disease.

INTERACTIONS
Increased sensitivity to *warfarin* has been observed in hyperthyroidism and careful control of dosage is required as the patient is rendered euthyroid.

PREGNANCY
Carbimazole crosses the placenta and may cause neonatal goitre and hypothyroidism – the lowest dose that will control the hyperthyroid state should be used (requirements in Grave disease tend to fall during pregnancy). Rarely, carbimazole has been associated with aplasia cutis of the neonate.

BREAST-FEEDING
Carbimazole, as methimazole, is excreted into breast milk but this does not preclude breast-feeding as long as neonatal development is closely monitored and the lowest effective dose is used (if possible <15mg daily).

SIDE-EFFECTS
Nausea, headache, rashes, pruritus and arthralgia; rarely alopecia and jaundice. If jaundice develops withdraw carbimazole and consider an alternative treatment. Agranulocytosis: patients should be asked to report symptoms and signs suggestive of infection, especially sore throat or mouth ulcers. A white cell count should be performed if there is clinical evidence of infection and carbimazole should be stopped if there is evidence of neutropenia.

POISONING/TOXICITY
Acute overdosage may be associated with minor and transient changes in thyroid hormone levels, no specific treatment is indicated.

PHARMACOKINETIC PROPERTIES
Absorption of oral carbimazole is rapid and virtually complete and it is rapidly converted to the active metabolite methimazole. Plasma half-life is approximately 5 hours and is unaffected by thyroid status but is prolonged in both hepatic and renal disease. Methimazole is actively concentrated by the thyroid and it is thought to stay in the thyroid for approximately 20 hours. Over 90% of orally administered carbimazole is excreted in the urine as either methimazole or its metabolites, the remainder appearing in faeces.

EXCIPIENTS
Tablets include sucrose. See manufacturers SPC for further details.

LICENSED STATUS
Tablets licensed for use in children and adults. Oral suspension is a 'special' and as such is unlicensed.

FURTHER INFORMATION
Oral suspension is available as a 'special' from Martindale Pharmaceuticals.
Propylthiouracil may be substituted for carbimazole, where 1mg of carbimazole ≡ 10mg propylthiouracil.

Carboplatin

Platinum-containing complex; a derivative of cisplatin.

USES
Current UK protocols for treatment of: Stage 4 neuroblastoma; germ-cell tumours (including intracranial); low-grade gliomas (including astrocytomas); neuroectodermal tumours (including medulloblastoma); rhabdomyosarcoma (metastatic and non-metastatic disease) and soft-tissue sarcomas. Other applications include treatment of retinoblastoma, Wilms tumour and some liver tumours.

PRESENTATION
Injection: 10mg in 1mL; 5mL, 15mL, 45mL and 60mL vials – Paraplatin® and non-proprietary.

DOSAGE
** Always consult the current treatment protocol for details of dosage and scheduling. **
Total cumulative doses vary with protocol. An increasing number of protocols employ doses based on glomerular filtration rate (GFR) (e.g. UKCCSG GC2, MMT 98) or EDTA half-life (e.g. UKCCSG CNS 2000 01).

Paediatric dosing equations:

$$\text{Dose (mg)} = \text{Target AUC (mg/mL/minute)} \times (\text{GFR (mL/minute)} + [0.36 \times \text{weight (kg)}])$$

$$\text{Dose (mg)} = \text{AUC} \times \{[0.693 /^{51}\text{Cr EDTA } t_{1/2} \text{ (min)}] \times [0.52 \times (843 \times \text{BW}^{0.891})] + 0.36 \times \text{BW}\}$$

Where BW = body weight.

GFR is uncorrected and paediatric treatment regimens aim to deliver a target carboplatin AUC of 6-10mg/mL/minute.

ADMINISTRATION
IV: infusion over 1 hour, or greater if dictated by fluid volume. May be diluted with glucose 5% or NaCl 0.9% to concentrations as low as 500 microgram in 1mL.

Carboplatin continued

CONTRA-INDICATIONS & WARNINGS
Severe, pre-existing renal impairment; prior myelosuppressive therapy.

INTERACTIONS
Co-administration with potentially *nephrotoxic agents* should be avoided due to the risk of acute reduction in GFR and hence decreased carboplatin clearance.

PREGNANCY
Safe use in pregnancy has not been established.

BREAST-FEEDING
It is not known if carboplatin is excreted in human milk. Breast-feeding is not advised.

SIDE-EFFECTS
Common side-effects include nausea and vomiting, myelosuppression and persisting thrombocytopenia (nadir often delayed until 3 weeks). Occasional side-effects include ototoxicity, raised hepatic alkaline phosphatase and mild nephrotoxicity with little or no reduction in GFR. Occasional hyponatraemia and/or hypomagnesaemia due to renal tubular loss. Rare side-effects of neurotoxicity, rashes, anaphylaxis, and alopecia have also been reported.

POISONING/TOXICITY
Full supportive measures including the use of growth factors should be considered. Carboplatin is removed by haemodialysis and the use of this technique in the case of carboplatin overdosage would be a reasonable management option.

PHARMACOKINETIC PROPERTIES
Carboplatin is eliminated primarily by renal excretion. Dosing of carboplatin on the basis of GFR produces more consistent drug exposure than surface-area based dosing.
Median (range) pharmacokinetic parameters:
Clearance: 75 (42–130) mL/minute/m^2.
Half-life: 82 (45–258) minutes.

EXCIPIENTS
Contact manufacturer for further details.

LICENSED STATUS
Not licensed for use in children.

Carmellose sodium

USES
Mechanical protection of oral and circumoral lesions.

PRESENTATION
Protective paste: 16.7% – Orabase®.
Powder: Orahesive®.

DOSAGE/ADMINISTRATION
The paste or powder needs to be applied to dry oral mucosa if it is to be retained over the lesion(s). Gauze can be used to dry the mucosa before application.
Protective paste: a thin layer should be smeared over the affected area.
Powder: sprinkle on the affected area.

CONTRA-INDICATIONS & WARNINGS
The paste or powder are difficult to apply especially in more inaccessible areas of the mouth.

INTERACTIONS/SIDE-EFFECTS
None documented.

POISONING/TOXICITY
No incidents reported.

PHARMACODYNAMIC/PHARMACOKINETIC PROPERTIES
The paste/powder are inert and act only as a mechanical barrier.

EXCIPIENTS
Both the paste and powder contain the three hydrocolloids carmellose sodium, pectin and gelatin, which act in combination to stick to wet surfaces to provide the protective barrier. The paste also contains Plastibase®.

LICENSED STATUS
These products are classed as medical devices. They are promoted for use as a skin barrier for people with stomas and are not recommended by the manufacturers for application to oral lesions (although it can be noted that there is published data to support the use of both the paste and powder for oral lesions).

Carnitine

USES
Primary and secondary carnitine deficiency, organic acidaemias and fatty acid oxidation defects.

PRESENTATION
Oral liquid: L-carnitine 1g in 10mL (as single dose bottles); L-carnitine paediatric 30% solution, 20mL – both Carnitor® Injection: L-carnitine 200mg in 1mL; 5mL ampoule – Carnitor®.

DOSAGE

Route	Age				Frequency (times daily)	Notes
	birth–1 month	1 month–2 years	2–12 years	12–18 years		
Oral	←	25–50mg/kg		→	2	May be increased to 175mg/kg/**day** or 3g/**day**.
IV infusion	←	100mg/kg		→	single dose	Loading dose. Give over 30 minutes.
IV infusion (continuous)	←	100mg/kg/day		→	continuous infusion	Start immediately after loading dose.
IV bolus	←	25–50mg/kg		→	2–4	Give over 5–10 minutes. Usually given as an infusion.

ADMINISTRATION
Oral: solution can be mixed with flavoured drinks.
IV: can be diluted in glucose 5%, glucose 10%, NaCl 0.9% and Ringers solution.
IV compatibilities: can be infused at Y-site with arginine, sodium benzoate and sodium phenylbutyrate (no data to support this but has been done in practice).

CONTRA-INDICATIONS & WARNINGS
Do not use racemic mixture, only L-carnitine. Caution in renal impairment.

INTERACTIONS
No information available.

PREGNANCY
There is no documented experience of use in pregnant patients with primary systemic carnitine deficiency.

BREAST-FEEDING
L-carnitine is a normal component of human milk. Supplementation in nursing mothers has not been studied.

SIDE-EFFECTS
Nausea, vomiting, abdominal pain, diarrhoea, body odour; more commonly seen at higher doses.

PHARMACODYNAMIC PROPERTIES
Repletion of carnitine stores. Removal of toxic acyl-CoA intermediates in disorders of intermediary metabolism.

EXCIPIENTS
Paediatric solution contains sugar, but single oral dose vials contain saccharin.
Injection contains hydrochloride 10% to adjust the pH to 6-6.5.
Contact manufacturers for further details.

LICENSED STATUS
Paediatric solution 30% and injection licensed in newborn infants, children and adults.
Single dose vial only licensed >12 years of age.

A semi-synthetic second generation cephalosporin.

USES
Upper and lower respiratory tract infections; skin and soft tissue infections; otitis media, urinary tract infections including pyelonephritis and cystitis. Due to adverse effects not usually first-line treatment in paediatrics.
In cystic fibrosis patients – treatment for asymptomatic *Haemophilus influenzae* carriage or minor exacerbations.

PRESENTATION
Capsule: 250mg – non-proprietary; 500mg – Distaclor® and non-proprietary.
Tablet (modified release): 375mg – Distaclor MR®.
Suspension: 125mg in 5mL and 250mg in 5mL – Distaclor® and non-proprietary.

DOSAGE

Route	Age			Frequency	Notes
	1 month–2 years	2–12 years	12–18 years	(times daily)	
Oral	≤1 year 62.5mg	≤5 years 125mg	250mg	3	In severe infections, caused by less susceptible organisms doses may be doubled.
	>1 year 125mg	>5 years 250mg		3	
Oral modified release tablets	–	–	375mg	2	For the treatment of pneumonia the dose should be doubled.
Oral for cystic fibrosis patients	≤1 year 125mg	≤7 years 250mg	500mg	3	For treatment of asymptomatic *Haemophilus infuenzae* carriage or mild exacerbations.
	>1 year 250mg	>7 years 500mg		3	250mg three times daily can be given as 375mg twice daily. 500mg three times daily can be given as 750mg twice daily.

ADMINISTRATION
Oral: absorption of the modified release preparation is enhanced by administration with food therefore take with meals. Swallow whole, do not cut, crush or chew.

CONTRA-INDICATIONS & WARNINGS
Contra-indicated in patients with hypersensitivity to cephalosporins.
Caution in patients with hypersensitivity to penicillin, particularly type 1 reactions. Use with caution in renal impairment as the half-life is extended in moderate/severe impairment.

INTERACTIONS
Warfarin – increased prothrombin time; monitor INR and adjust dose as necessary. Renal excretion of cefaclor is inhibited by *probenecid*. False positive Coombs test. False-positive reaction for glucose in urine with Benedicts or Fehlings solution. Absorption of modified release tablets reduced by *aluminium* or *magnesium* containing *antacids*.

PREGNANCY
No evidence of teratogenicity.

BREAST-FEEDING
Cefaclor is excreted into breast milk in low concentrations but breast-feeding is not contra-indicated.

SIDE-EFFECTS
Gastrointestinal: diarrhoea, nausea, vomiting.
Skin: rash, urticaria, pruritus.
Haematological: eosinophilia. May cause serum sickness like reactions in susceptible individuals.

POISONING/TOXICITY
Toxicity expected to be low in acute overdose. Hypoprothombinaemia may follow prolonged or excessive use of some cephalosporins, especially in patients with renal impairment. Platelet dysfunction can occur up to 3 weeks after ingestion.

PHARMACOKINETIC PROPERTIES
Well absorbed from gastrointestinal tract. Half-life is between 30 minutes to 1 hour.

EXCIPIENTS
Distaclor® suspension includes sucrose. Contact manufacturers for further details.

LICENSED STATUS
Capsules and suspension licensed for >1 month of age. Modified release tablets not licensed for use in children.

Cefadroxil

First-generation cephalosporin with longer duration of action than other cephalosporins.

USES
Upper and lower respiratory tract infections, otitis media, osteomyelitis, septic arthritis, skin and soft tissue infections, genitourinary tract infections – cystitis, pyelonephritis, urethritis.

PRESENTATION
Capsule: 500mg – Baxan®.
Suspension: 125mg in 5mL, 250mg in 5mL and 500mg in 5mL – Baxan®.

DOSAGE

Route	Age				Frequency (times daily)	Notes
	birth–1 month	1 month–2 years	2–12 years	12–18 years		
Oral	DOSE BY WEIGHT		–	–	2	Limited experience of use in premature infants and neonates.
	12.5mg/kg	<1 year 12.5mg/kg				
		DOSE BY AGE 1–2 years 250mg	2–6 years 250mg	500mg–1g	2	
	–		6–12 years 500mg		2	

ADMINISTRATION
Oral: bioavailability and chemotherapeutic effects unaffected by food.

CONTRA-INDICATIONS & WARNINGS
Known hypersensitivity to cephalosporins. Caution in patients with a history of penicillin allergy.

INTERACTIONS
Probenecid raises serum levels of cefadroxil which might increase nephrotoxicity. Urine from patients receiving cefadroxil may give false-positive glycosuria reaction when tested with Benedicts or Fehlings solution – does not occur with enzyme-based tests. False positive Coombs' reaction may occur

PREGNANCY
Not shown to be teratogenic but safety in pregnancy not established. Contact local Medicines Information Centre for advice.

BREAST-FEEDING
Cefadroxil is excreted into breast milk in low concentrations, but breast-feeding is not contra-indicated.

SIDE-EFFECTS
Rash, pruritus, urticaria, angioneurotic oedema (rare). Nausea, vomiting, diarrhoea, dyspepsia, abdominal discomfort, dizziness, headache. Reversible neutropenia, minor elevation in transaminases and Stevens-Johnson Syndrome.

POISONING/TOXICITY
As for other cephalosporins (see cefaclor monograph).

PHARMACOKINETIC PROPERTIES
Well absorbed from gastrointestinal tract. Widely distributed to body tissues and fluids.

EXCIPIENTS
Suspension includes sucrose. See manufacturers SPC for further details.

LICENSED STATUS
Licensed for use in all ages.

Cefalexin (cephalexin)

First generation cephalosporin antibiotic.

USES
Infections due to sensitive Gram-positive and Gram-negative bacteria.

PRESENTATION
Capsule: 250mg and 500mg – Ceporex®, Keflex® and non-proprietary.
Oral suspension: 125mg in 5mL and 250mg in 5mL – Keflex® and non-proprietary.
Syrup: 125mg in 5mL, 250mg in 5mL and 500mg in 5mL – Ceporex®.
Tablet: 250mg and 500mg – Ceporex®, Keflex® and non-proprietary.

DOSAGE

Route	Age			Frequency	Notes
	1 month–2 years	2–12 years	12–18 years	(times daily)	
Oral	←	12.5–25mg/kg	→	2	Skin/soft tissue infections, pharyngitis; mild, uncomplicated urinary tract infections. Maximum single dose 1g.
	←	25mg/kg	→	4	Severe infection and otitis media. Maximum single dose 1g.
	62.5–125mg	-	-	2	Other infections.
	-	125–250mg	250–500mg	3	
	←	12.5mg/kg	→	1 at night	Urinary tract infection prophylaxis. Maximum dose 125mg.

Dosage adjustment in renal impairment
Reduce dose in severe renal impairment (creatinine clearance <10mL/minute/1.73m^2) by reducing dose frequency. Removed by dialysis thus an additional dose may be required after dialysis.

CONTRA-INDICATIONS & WARNINGS
Hypersensitivity to cephalosporins. Caution in those with hypersensitivity to penicillins.

INTERACTIONS
Urine from patients receiving cefalexin may give false-positive glycosuria reaction when tested with Benedicts or Fehlings solution – does not occur with enzyme-based tests. False-positive Coombs' reaction may occur.

PREGNANCY
No evidence of teratogenicity or fetotoxicity but use with caution.

BREAST-FEEDING
Excreted in low concentrations. Usual precautions apply.

SIDE-EFFECTS
Gastrointestinal: diarrhoea, dyspepsia, abdominal pain, rarely nausea and vomiting.
Hypersensitivity: allergic reactions in the form of rash, urticaria and angioedema have been reported. Other effects reported include headache, dizziness and fatigue.

POISONING/TOXICITY
Toxicity expected to be low in acute overdose. Symptoms may include nausea, vomiting, epigastric distress, diarrhoea and haematuria.

PHARMACOKINETIC PROPERTIES
Well absorbed from gastrointestinal tract. Bioavailability of 75-100% is only slightly reduced by food. Reduced absorption in young children and reduced to 50% in neonates. Peak levels appear 1 hour after dose in older children, within 2 hours in children 9-12 months of age, and 3 hours in infants <6 months old. Half-life: 1 hour in older children, 2.5 hours in infants aged 3-12 months, 5 hours in neonates. Widely distributed in body. Does not enter CSF. Not metabolised. Appears in bile in therapeutic concentration, 80% excreted in urine within 6 hours of a dose.

EXCIPIENTS
Contact manufacturers for further details.

LICENSED STATUS
Licensed for use in all ages.

A third-generation cephalosporin for oral administration. It has a long duration of action which allows once daily dosing.

USES
Upper and lower respiratory tract infections, otitis media, urinary tract infections. In cystic fibrosis patients – treatment for asymptomatic *Haemophilus influenzae* carriage or minor exacerbations but reserved for resistant cases.

PRESENTATION
Oral suspension: 100mg in 5mL, 37.5mL and 75mL – Suprax®.
Tablet: 200mg (scored) – Suprax®.

DOSAGE

Route	Age			Frequency	Notes
	1 month–2 years	2–12 years	12–18 years	(times daily)	
Oral	6 months–1 year	2–4 years			
	75mg	100mg	200–400mg	1	
	1–2 years	5–12 years			
	100mg	200mg		1	

ADMINISTRATION
Oral: food does not significantly affect serum levels but may increase time to maximum concentration.

CONTRA-INDICATIONS & WARNINGS
Known hypersensitivity to cephalosporins. Use with caution in patients with known hypersensitivity to penicillins and those with marked renal impairment.

INTERACTIONS
Urine from patients receiving cefixime may give false-positive glycosuria reaction when tested with Benedicts or Fehlings solution – does not occur with enzyme-based tests. False-positive Coombs' reaction may occur.

PREGNANCY
No evidence of teratogenicity in rats, but no studies in humans. Contact local Medicines Information centre for advice.

BREAST-FEEDING
No data available, but cephalosporins in general are not known to be harmful.

SIDE-EFFECTS
Pruritus and vaginitis. Mild transient changes in liver and renal function tests. Diarrhoea, abdominal pain, nausea, vomiting, rash and headache. Thrombocytopenia, leucopenia, eosinophilia, pseudomembranous colitis (rare) and hypersensitivity reactions.

POISONING/TOXICITY
As for other cephalosporins (see cefaclor monograph).

PHARMACOKINETIC PROPERTIES
Half-life is about 3-4 hours. Only 40-50% of an oral dose is absorbed from the gastrointestinal tract.

EXCIPIENTS
Oral suspension includes sucrose. See manufacturers SPC for further details.

LICENSED STATUS
Licensed for use ≥6 months of age.

Cefotaxime

Broad-spectrum bactericidal cephalosporin.

USES
Meningitis, respiratory tract, urinary tract, soft tissue, obstetric and gynaecological infections; prophylaxis for certain surgical procedures; epiglottitis. In cystic fibrosis patients – treatment of severe *Haemophilus influenzae* and *Staphylococcus aureus* infections.

PRESENTATION

Injection: (sodium salt) 500mg, 1g and 2g vials – Claforan® and non-proprietary; 1g and 2g vials with infusion connector – Claforan®.

DOSAGE

Newborn infant (birth to 1 month)

Route	Age	Dose	Frequency (times daily)	Notes
IV	<7 days	50mg/kg	2	Severe neonatal infections, meningitis.
	7–21 days	50mg/kg	3	
	>21 days	50mg/kg	3–4	

Child

Route	Age			Frequency (times daily)	Notes
	1 month–2 years	2–12 years	12–18 years		
IV	← 50mg/kg →		1–3g	2	The frequency should be increased to four times daily in meningitis and other severe infections.
IV for cystic fibrosis patients	← 50mg/kg →			3–4	Treatment of severe exacerbations of *Haemophilus influenzae* infection.

Dosage adjustment in renal impairment

Due to extra-renal elimination it is only necessary to reduce dose in severe renal impairment (creatinine clearance <10mL/minute/1.73m^2). A normal single dose should be given as a loading dose then the daily dose should be halved without a change in frequency.

ADMINISTRATION

For Claforan®, reconstitute with Water for Injections by adding 1.8mL to 500mg vial to give 500mg in 2mL; 3.5mL to 1g vial to give 1g in 4mL; 8.8mL to 2g vial to give 2g in 10mL to account for the displacement volume. For non-proprietary products see the manufacturers SPC for details.

IV bolus: reconstitute as shown and give over 3–5 minutes.

IV infusion: dilute 4-10 times in glucose 5% or NaCl 0.9% and infuse over 20–60 minutes.

CONTRA-INDICATIONS & WARNINGS

Known or suspected allergy to cephalosporins/ penicillins (particularly type 1 penicillin hypersensitivity).

INTERACTIONS

High doses should be given with caution to patients receiving *aminoglycosides* or *potent diuretics* due to the combination having an adverse effect on renal function. A positive Coombs' test may be seen.

PREGNANCY

Animal studies have shown no adverse effect on developing fetus – safety in humans not established. Contact local Medicines Information Centre for advice.

BREAST-FEEDING

Cefotaxime is excreted in breast milk in low concentrations; breast-feeding is not contra-indicated but there is the possibility of modification of the infant's bowel flora.

SIDE-EFFECTS

Generally infrequent, mild and transient. Effects reported include; candidiasis, rashes, fever, transient rises in liver transaminase and/or alkaline phosphatase and diarrhoea. Pseudomembranous colitis may occur rarely – stop drug. Changes in renal function have been observed rarely with high doses. Hypersensitivity reactions include skin rashes, drug fever and very rarely anaphylaxis.

Granulocytopenia and more rarely agranulocytosis may occur. Eosinophilia, neutropenia, thrombocytopenia and haemolytic anaemia have been reported – if treatment for longer than 10 days monitor full blood count. Transient pain may be experienced at the site of injection.

PHARMACOKINETIC PROPERTIES

Following IV administration cefotaxime is widely distributed into body tissues and fluids. It is partially metabolised in the liver to active metabolite and is excreted principally in urine. In term and preterm neonates the half-life is extended.

EXCIPIENTS
1g vial contains 2.09mmol sodium. Contact manufacturers for further details.

LICENSED STATUS
Licensed for use in all ages.

Cefpodoxime

Third-generation cephalosporin.

USES
Upper and lower respiratory tract infections.

PRESENTATION
Tablet: (proxetil salt) 100mg – Orelox®.
Oral suspension: (proxetil salt) 40mg in 5mL, 100mL – Orelox®.

DOSAGE

Route	Age			Frequency (times daily)	Notes
	1 month–2 years	2–12 years	12–18 years		
Oral	←	4mg/kg	→	2	Maximum single dose 200mg.

Dosage adjustment in renal impairment
The dose frequency should be reduced in renal impairment.

Creatinine clearance (mL/minute/1.73m²)	Dose frequency
10–40	24 hourly
<10	48 hourly

Patients on haemodialysis should receive the usual dose 3 times weekly, or following dialysis.

ADMINISTRATION
Oral: administer orally with food to maximise absorption. Suspension is not very palatable.

CONTRA-INDICATIONS & WARNINGS
Hypersensitivity to cephalosporin antibiotics or type I hypersensitivity to penicillins.
Suspension contains aspartame thus contra-indicated in patients with phenylketonuria.

INTERACTIONS
Absorption decreased by *antacids* or *histamine H$_2$ antagonists*.

PREGNANCY
No evidence of teratogenicity or fetotoxicity in animal studies.

BREAST-FEEDING
Excreted in breast milk. Cephalosporins in general are not known to be harmful.

SIDE-EFFECTS
Diarrhoea, nausea, vomiting and abdominal pain can occur. Occasional reports of headache, allergic reactions.

POISONING/TOXICITY
Treatment is symptomatic and supportive.
Encephalopathy may occur particularly in patients with renal insufficiency. Usually reversible once cefpodoxime plasma levels have fallen.

PHARMACOKINETIC PROPERTIES
Cefpodoxime proxetil is inactive and metabolised in intestinal epithelium to release active cefpodoxime into the blood stream. Bioavailability is 50% on empty stomach but increases in presence of food. Absorption reduced in conditions of low gastric acidity. 30%-40% bound to plasma proteins. Half-life of 2 to 3 hours. Excreted unchanged in urine. Reaches therapeutic concentrations in respiratory and genito-urinary tracts and bile.

EXCIPIENTS
Oral suspension includes aspartame and sucrose. See manufacturers SPC for further details.

LICENSED STATUS
Licensed for >14 days of age.

Cefradine (cephradine)

A first generation cephalosporin.

USES
Upper and lower respiratory tract infections; skin and soft tissue infections; otitis media, urinary tract infections including pyelonephritis and cystitis. In cystic fibrosis patients – continuous anti-staphylococcal therapy.

PRESENTATION
Capsule: 250mg and 500mg – Velosef® and non-proprietary.
Injection: 500mg and 1g vials – Velosef®.
Syrup: 250mg in 5mL – Velosef®.

DOSAGE

Route	Age			Frequency	Notes
	1 month–2 years	2–12 years	12–18 years	(times daily)	
Oral	← 12.5mg/kg → or 25mg/kg		250–500mg or 500mg–1g	4 2	Doses may be doubled in severe infection. Maximum of 4g/**day**.
	← 3mg/kg →		–	1 (at night)	Prophylaxis for urinary tract infections (if no symptoms present).
IV/IM	← 12.5–25mg/kg →		500mg –1g	4	Doses may be doubled in severe infection. Maximum of 8g/**day**.
Oral for cystic fibrosis patients	**DOSE BY WEIGHT** ← 12.5–25mg/kg →		–	2	Continuous anti-staphylococcal therapy. Daily dose can be given in four divided doses if necessary. Maximum of 4g/**day**.
	DOSE BY AGE <1 year 500mg >1 year 1g	<7 years 1g >7 years 2g	2g	2 2	

Renal impairment
Reduce dose in moderate renal impairment to 50% of a dose every 6 hours or in severe impairment to 25% of a dose every 6 hours.

ADMINISTRATION
Oral: after food.
IM: add 2mL to a 500mg vial, or 4mL to a 1g vial, of Water for Injections or NaCl 0.9%.
IV: reconstitute with Water for Injections. To account for displacement volume add 4.6mL to the 500mg vial and 9.2mL to the 1g vial to give 100mg in 1mL. Inject slowly over 3-5 minutes.
IV infusion: reconstitute as for the IV injection then dilute with Water for Injections (50mg in 1mL cefradine solutions are approximately isotonic), NaCl 0.9% or glucose 5% and infuse over 30 minutes.

CONTRA-INDICATIONS & WARNINGS
Contra-indicated in patients with hypersensitivity to cephalosporins. Caution in patients with hypersensitivity to penicillin, particularly type 1 reactions. Use with caution in renal impairment.

INTERACTIONS
False-positive reaction for glucose in urine with Benedicts or Fehlings solution. False-positive Coombs' reaction may occur.

PREGNANCY
No evidence of teratogenicity.

BREAST-FEEDING
Cefradine is excreted into breast milk and should be used with caution in lactating mothers.

SIDE-EFFECTS
Gastrointestinal: diarrhoea, nausea, vomiting. *Skin:* rash, urticaria.
Haematological: eosinophilia.

PHARMACOKINETIC PROPERTIES
Well absorbed from gastrointestinal tract.

EXCIPIENTS
Contact manufacturers for further details.

LICENSED STATUS
Capsules, injection and syrup licensed for use in children, except for prophylactic use in cystic fibrosis patients. Not licensed for use in neonates.

Ceftazidime

C

A third-generation cephalosporin antibiotic which is resistant to most beta-lactamases and is active against a wide range of Gram-positive and Gram-negative bacteria.

USES
Infections due to sensitive Gram-positive and Gram-negative bacteria. In cystic fibrosis patients – treatment of early *Pseudomonas aeruginosa* infections not cleared by ciprofloxacin plus colistin and treatment of moderate to severe exacerbations in combination with an aminoglycoside; for the treatment of more severe *Burkholderia cepacia* infection, discuss with local microbiology department; nebulised for chronic *Burkholderia cepacia* infection.

PRESENTATION
Injection: 250mg – Fortum®; 500mg, 1g and 2g – Fortum®, Kefadim®; 3g vials – Fortum®.

DOSAGE
Newborn infant (birth to 1 month)

Route	Age	Frequency	Notes
	birth–1 month	(times daily)	
IV	30mg/kg	2	
IV	50mg/kg	2	Dose for treatment of suspected or proven meningitis.

Child

Route	Age			Frequency	Notes
	1 month–2 years	2–12 years	12–18 years	(times daily)	
IV or IM	←	30mg/kg	→	2–3	Doses of up to 50mg/kg given 3 times daily may be used in severe infection to a maximum of 6g **per day**. Single dose >1g by IV route only.
IV for cystic fibrosis patients	←	50mg/kg	→	3	Daily dose can be given in two divided doses if necessary. Maximum of 9g **per day**.
Nebulised for cystic fibrosis patients	←	1g	→	2	Treatment of chronic *Burkholderia cepacia* infection. Dissolve in 3mL of Water for Injections.

Dosage adjustment in renal failure
In mild impairment give a dose every 12 hours, in moderate impairment (creatinine clearance 10-50mL/minute/1.73m^2) give a dose once daily and in severe impairment (creatine clearance <10mL/minute/1.73m^2) give 50% of dose once daily. Levels may be monitored if clinically indicated.
In haemodialysis: the appropriate maintenance dose should be repeated after dialysis.
In peritoneal dialysis: 125–250mg may be added to 2L of dialysis fluid, and given in addition to the IV dose.

ADMINISTRATION
IV, IV infusion & IM: displacement values - Fortum® displaces 0.2mL per 250mg and Kefadim® displaces 0.6mL per 1g. For IM injection the powder may be reconstituted with 0.5% or 1% lidocaine (lignocaine) hydrochloride injection to a concentration of 250mg in 1mL. IV injection should be diluted to 100mg in 1mL. IV infusions should be given over 30 minutes. Ceftazidime and aminoglycosides should not be mixed in the same giving sets or syringe. Precipitation has been reported with vancomycin therefore giving sets and lines should be flushed between administration of these two agents.
Nebulisation: dissolve in 3mL of Water for Injections.

CONTRA-INDICATIONS & WARNINGS
Contra-indicated in patients with a known sensitivity to cephalosporins. Special caution in patients with type I or immediate hypersensitivity to penicillin.

INTERACTIONS
Possible antagonism of effect of ceftazidime if given with *chloramphenicol*. Caution when given with *nephrotoxic drugs*.

PREGNANCY
No evidence of teratogenic effects.

BREAST-FEEDING
Excreted in breast milk – caution exercised when given to nursing mothers.

SIDE-EFFECTS
Infusion related phlebitis, thrombophlebitis and pain on injection. Via nebulisation – sensitivity reactions and local effects.

POISONING/TOXICITY
Overdose can lead to neurological sequelae including encephalopathy, convulsions and coma. Serum levels can be reduced by haemodialysis.

PHARMACOKINETIC PROPERTIES
80-90% excretion unchanged by the kidneys.

C

EXCIPIENTS
See manufacturers SPC for further details.

LICENSED STATUS
Licensed for use in all ages.

Ceftriaxone

Third-generation cephalosporin.

USES
Infections due to sensitive Gram-positive and Gram-negative bacteria (see cefotaxime).

PRESENTATION
Injection: (sodium salt) 250mg, 1g and 2g vials – Rocephin®; 1g and 2g – non-proprietary.

DOSAGE
Newborn infant (birth to 1 month)

Route	Age	Frequency	Notes
	birth–1 month	(times daily)	
IV	20–50mg/kg	1	Do not exceed 50mg/kg. Infuse over 10-30 minutes (doses of 50mg/kg over at least 60 minutes). Avoid in premature, acidotic or hyperbilirubinaemic neonates.

Child

Route	Age			Frequency (times daily)	Notes
	1 month–2 years	2–12 years	12–18 years		
IV or IM	←	20–50mg/kg	→	1	Maximum single dose 4g.
IV	←	80mg/kg	→	1	Severe infections, meningitis. Infuse over at least 30 minutes.

Dose adjustment in renal or liver failure
In severe renal failure reduce dose to a maximum of 2g or 50mg/kg.
No dose adjustment required in hepatic impairment.

If both hepatic and severe renal impairment monitor serum concentrations. In patients undergoing dialysis no supplemental dose required but serum concentration monitoring advisable.

ADMINISTRATION

May be given by deep IM or IV injection.
IV: doses below 50mg/kg may be given by slow IV injection over 3-5 minutes. Higher doses should be infused over at least 30 minutes. Compatible with glucose 5% or 10%, NaCl 0.9% or 0.45%, and glucose 4%/NaCl 0.18%. Displacement value is 0.194mL for each 250mg.
IM: injection may be reconstituted with 1% lidocaine (lignocaine) hydrochloride. Manufacturer recommends a concentration of 250mg in 1mL but higher concentrations have been studied and may be more practical, e.g. adding 2.1mL to a 1g vial gives a concentration of 350mg in 1mL. Doses greater than 1mg should be divided and injected at more than one site.
Incompatible with calcium containing solutions, amsacrine, aminoglycosides, fluconazole, vancomycin, filgrastim and labetolol.

CONTRA-INDICATIONS & WARNINGS

As for cefotaxime. Use with caution in pre-existing disease of biliary tract, gallbladder, liver or pancreas. Ceftriaxone may displace bilirubin from albumin binding site and should not be used in jaundiced, hypoalbuminaemic or acidotic newborn infants. Should probably not be used in premature infants for this reason.

INTERACTIONS

As for cefotaxime. Interferes with cupric sulphate method for urinary glucose determination. Glucose oxidase method unaffected. May displace *phenytoin* from albumin binding site.

PREGNANCY

No evidence of teratogenicity or fetotoxicity in animal studies. Safety in human pregnancy not established. Contact local Medicines Information Centre for advice.

BREAST-FEEDING

Minimal amounts excreted in breast milk. Apply normal precautions.

SIDE-EFFECTS

As for cefotaxime.
Urinary precipitates of calcium ceftriaxone have occurred rarely; immobile, dehydrated and young patients are most at risk. A similar precipitate has been reported in the gallbladder and may be seen on ultrasound as shadows. If biliary symptoms develop, ceftriaxone should be discontinued and ultrasound performed. Biliary precipitates generally disappear on discontinuation and non-surgical management is recommended. Those most at risk are patients with pre-existing renal or hepatic disease, dehydration or receiving concurrent parenteral nutrition.

POISONING/TOXICITY

No specific antidote; treatment should be symptomatic. Not removed by haemodialysis or peritoneal dialysis.

PHARMACOKINETIC PROPERTIES

IM bioavailability 100% but produces lower serum concentrations. Widely distributed in body tissues and fluids of gallbladder, lungs, bone, bile, sputum, tears, pleural, peritoneal, synovial cavities. Concentration-dependent binding to plasma albumin. The plasma free (unbound) fraction is approximately 5% over most of the therapeutic concentration range, increasing to 15% at concentrations of 300mg/L. 50-60% of a dose renally excreted by glomerular filtration, remainder via biliary and intestinal excretion. Elimination half-life approximately 8 hours; prolonged in neonates and in renal impairment.

EXCIPIENTS

Each gram of ceftriaxone (sodium salt) contains 3.6mmol of sodium. Contact manufacturers for further details.

LICENSED STATUS

Licensed for use in all ages.

A second-generation cephalosporin antibiotic which is resistant to most beta-lactamases and is active against a wide range of Gram-positive and Gram-negative organisms.

USES
Infections due to sensitive Gram-positive and Gram-negative bacteria. In cystic fibrosis patients – treatment of severe *Haemophilus influenzae* infections, not routinely used orally.

PRESENTATION
Injection: (sodium salt) 250mg, 750mg and 1.5g – Zinacef®.
Sachet: 125mg – Zinnat®.
Suspension: 125mg in 5mL – Zinnat®.
Tablet: 125mg and 250mg – Zinnat®.

DOSAGE
Newborn infant (birth to 1 month)

Route	Age	Dose	Frequency (times daily)	Notes
IV	<7 days	30mg/kg	2	Treatment of infection.
	>7 days	30mg/kg	3	
	birth–1 month	50mg/kg	2	Severe infection.

Child

Route	Age			Frequency (times daily)	Notes
	1 month-2 years	2-12 years	12-18 years		
IV or IM	←	10–30mg/kg	→	3	20mg/kg/dose is appropriate for most infections. Maximum single dose is 750mg.
	←	50–60mg/kg	→	3-4	Severe infection – reduce the dose after 3 days or when clinical improvement occurs to 100mg/kg/**day**. Maximum single dose is 1.5g.
IV for cystic fibrosis patients	←	50mg/kg	→	3-4	Severe exacerbations of *Haemophilus influenzae* infection. Maximum single dose is 1.5g.
Oral	>3 months 125mg	250mg	*250mg	2	*May be doubled in severe infection.

Dose adjustment in renal or liver failure
Reduce dose in moderate renal failure. When the creatinine clearance is >20mL/minute/1.73m^2 dosage interval should be not less than 8 hours; 10-20mL/minute/1.73m^2 give 12 hourly and <10mL/minute/1.73m^2 give 24 hourly. Cefuroxime is significantly removed by haemodialysis. During continuous peritoneal dialysis increase the dose interval to 12 hourly.

ADMINISTRATION
IV, IV infusion or IM: on reconstitution 250mg powder displaces 0.2mL and 750mg displaces 0.5mL. IM injection – reconstitute with Water for Injections to a final concentration of 250mg in 1mL. Shake gently to produce a suspension. IV infusion – dilute reconstituted dose with NaCl 0.9% or glucose 5%, and give over 30 minutes.

CONTRA-INDICATIONS AND WARNINGS
Known hypersensitivity to cephalosporins. Cross sensitivity to penicillin has been reported, particularly in type 1 or intermediate hypersensitivity to penicillin.

INTERACTIONS
High doses should be given with caution with other nephrotoxic drugs e.g. *diuretics/aminoglycosides*.

PREGNANCY
No evidence of teratogenicity but give with caution in early months of pregnancy.

BREAST-FEEDING
Excreted in breast milk – caution should be exercised when given to nursing mothers.

SIDE-EFFECTS
Hypersensitivity reactions including rashes and fever. Gastrointestinal disturbances and rarely transient rises in liver function tests.

POISONING/TOXICITY
Overdose can cause cerebral irritation leading to convulsions; serum levels can be reduced by haemodialysis or peritoneal dialysis.

PHARMACOKINETIC PROPERTIES
Peak levels reached 35-40 minutes after IM injection and the drug is excreted unchanged in the urine. Oral absorption is poor and requires presence of food to maximise absorption.

EXCIPIENTS
Each 1g of powder contains 2.4mmol of sodium. See manufacturers SPC for further details.

LICENSED STATUS
Licensed for use in all ages.

C

Cernevit®

Multivitamin preparation.

USES
Multivitamin supplement for patients receiving PN.

PRESENTATION
Solution: powder for reconstitution – Cernevit®.
Each vial contains:

Alpha tocopheryl	11.2 international units
Cholecalciferol	220 international units
Retinol	3500 international units
Ascorbic acid	125mg
Biotin	69 micrograms
Folate	414 micrograms
Glycine	250mg
Niacin	46mg
Pantothenate	17.25mg
Pyridoxine	5.5mg
Riboflavin	4.14mg
Thiamine	3.51mg
Vitamin B12	6 micrograms

DOSAGE
Child: >11 years of age 1 vial per day.

ADMINISTRATION
IV: dissolve initially in 5mL Water for Injections, NaCl 0.9% or glucose 5%; then administer in infusion fluid as intermittent infusion or nutritional parenteral mixtures. Use within 24 hours of reconstitution.

CONTRA-INDICATIONS & WARNINGS
Contra-indicated in patients who are hypersensitive to any ingredient, especially thiamine. May require supplementation with vitamin D and vitamin K. Vitamin A dose is relatively high.

INTERACTIONS
Do not administer with other preparations containing *vitamin A*. ALT has been seen to rise in patients with inflammatory enterocolitis. Drugs affected by folate levels should be monitored, e.g. *phenytoin*. Pyridoxine may reduce the effects of *levodopa*.

PREGNANCY
Untested. Contact local Medicines Information Centre for advice.

BREAST-FEEDING
Untested; not recommended as it is known that some vitamins are excreted in maternal milk. Contact local Medicines Information Centre for advice.

POISONING/TOXICITY
Overdosage of vitamin A and D leading to symptoms of hypercalcaemia may occur with prolonged overdosage.

EXCIPIENTS
See manufacturers SPC for further details.

LICENSED STATUS
Licensed for use in patients >11 years of age.

FURTHER INFORMATION
pH 5.9 when reconstituted with Water for Injections.

Cetirizine

Non-sedative antihistamine.

USES
Symptomatic relief of allergy such as hay fever, urticaria; also used in perennial rhinitis.

PRESENTATION
Tablet: 10mg (scored) – Zirtek®, 10mg – non-proprietary.
Oral solution: 5mg in 5mL – Zirtek® and non-proprietary.

DOSAGE

Route	Age		Frequency (times daily)	Notes
	2–12 years	12–18 years		
Oral	2-6 years 5mg	10mg	1	The total daily dose can be given in 2 divided doses.
	6-12 years 10mg		1	

Renal impairment
It is recommended to administer 50% of above doses daily.

PREGNANCY
Studies have not shown any adverse effects in animals, but there is little information regarding its use in human pregnancies, therefore use of cetirizine should, if possible, be avoided during pregnancy.

BREAST-FEEDING
Contact local Medicines Information Centre for advice.

SIDE-EFFECTS
Mild and transient side-effects such as headaches, dizziness, drowsiness, agitation, dry mouth and gastrointestinal discomfort occasionally reported. Such effects are minimised by splitting daily dose into two and taking every 12 hours.

POISONING/TOXICITY
Drowsiness can occur in adults, agitation can occur in children; in cases of massive overdose, gastric lavage should be performed with the usual supportive measures. No specific antidote is available to date.

PHARMACOKINETIC PROPERTIES
Terminal half-life is approximately 10 hours in adults, 6 hours in children aged 6–12 years, and 5 hours in children aged 2-6 years, i.e. apparent plasma clearance is higher in children than in adults. Cetirizine is highly bound to plasma proteins.

EXCIPIENTS
Zirtek® oral solution includes sorbitol solution, saccharin sodium and is sugar-free. Contact manufacturers for further details.

LICENSED STATUS
Licensed for ≥2 years of age.

FURTHER INFORMATION
Tablets can be sold to the public for >12 years of age provided pack does not contain more than 10 days supply.

Chenodeoxycholic acid

A bile acid.

USES
Cerebrotendinous xanthomatosis and bile acid synthesis defects. Anecdotal use as additive therapy to cholesterol in Smith-Lemli-Opitz Syndrome, often in combination with ursodeoxycholic acid. For bile acid synthesis defects (e.g $3\text{ß-OH-}\Delta^5\text{-C}_{27}$ steroid dehydrogenase deficiency and Δ^4-3-oxosteroid 5ß reductase deficiency), chenodeoxycholic acid should, ideally, be given in combination with cholic acid but there are problems with the supply of the latter.

PRESENTATION
Capsule: 250mg – named patient.

DOSAGE

Indication	Route	Age				Frequency (times daily)	Notes
		birth–1 month	1 month–2 years	2–12 years	12–18 years		
Cerebro-tendinous xanthomatosis	Oral	←	5mg/kg		→	3	
Bile acid synthesis	Oral	←	Initially 5mg/kg then		→	3	
		←	2.5mg/kg		→	3	
Other indications	Oral	←	7mg/kg		→	1	Total daily dose may be given in divided doses.

ADMINISTRATION
To prepare a suspension of chenodeoxycholic acid, add the contents of a 250mg capsule to 25mL of sodium bicarbonate solution 1mmol/mL (8.4%w/v), to provide a suspension containing 10mg in 1mL. Administer a volume of suspension equivalent to dose required. This should be prepared immediately before administration and any remaining suspension discarded.

CONTRA-INDICATIONS & WARNINGS
Inflammatory disease of the small intestine and colon; peptic ulcer.

INTERACTIONS, PREGNANCY/BREAST-FEEDING, SIDE-EFFECTS, POISONING/TOXICITY
See ursodeoxycholic acid monograph.

PHARMACOKINETIC PROPERTIES
Rapidly and completely absorbed from the jejunum following oral administration.

EXCIPIENTS
Contact manufacturers for further details.

LICENSED STATUS
Not licensed for use in the UK.

FURTHER INFORMATION
Chenofalk® 250mg capsules may be imported via IDIS World Medicines.

Chloral hydrate

Short-term sedative and hypnotic.

USES
Sedation prior to procedures such as magnetic resonance imaging (MRI) and computerised tomography (CT) scans. Night sedation. Additional sedation for ventilated/intubated patients if IV therapy not sufficient. Chloral hydrate is sedative but not anxiolytic.

PRESENTATION
Elixir: 143mg in 5mL – Welldorm®, 200mg in 5mL – Chloral Elixir, Paediatric BP may be extemporaneously prepared.
Mixture: 500mg in 5mL – Chloral Mixture BP may be extemporaneously prepared.
Syrup: 500mg in 5mL – manufactured 'special'.
Suppository: 25mg, 50mg, 100mg, 250mg, 500mg and 750mg – manufactured 'specials'.
Tablet: chloral betaine 707mg (= chloral hydrate 414mg) – Welldorm®.

DOSAGE

Indication	Route	Age				Frequency (times daily)	Notes
		birth–1 month	1 month–2 years	2–12 years	12–18 years		
Sedation for painless procedures	Oral/rectal	←	25–50mg/kg	→	1–2g	single dose	Administer about 45–60 minutes prior to the procedure. Single doses up to 100mg/kg have been used prior to scans.
Long-term sedation	Oral/rectal	←	20–30mg/kg	→	-	4	Doses up to 50mg/kg administered 4 times daily have been used, but drug accumulation can occur.
Night sedation	Oral/rectal	←	30–50mg/kg	→	500mg–1g	single dose (at night)	

Chloral hydrate is sometimes used for sedation prior to painless procedures lasting more than 30 minutes such as scans. Preparation and management of the child should follow national and local guidelines. Chloral hydrate is used for sedation in intensive care. Other oral sedative agents such as alimemazine (trimeprazine) may be added.

Renal and hepatic impairment
No dosage adjustment is necessary in mild renal impairment. It should be avoided in patients with moderate to severe renal failure. Avoid in liver disease as it may precipitate coma.

ADMINISTRATION
Oral: mix with plenty of juice, water or milk to reduce gastric irritation and disguise the unpleasant taste. Care should be taken when administering to small babies to avoid gasping and aspiration.
Rectal: suppositories or the oral solution has been given rectally.

CONTRA-INDICATIONS & WARNINGS
Contra-indications: severe cardiac disease, porphyria, respiratory insufficiency, gastritis.
Cautions: caution in neonates, may accumulate and prolonged use can lead to hyperbilirubinaemia and metabolic acidosis.
Warnings: prolonged administration and abrupt withdrawal should be avoided to prevent the precipitation of withdrawal symptoms. Avoid contact with skin and mucous membranes as corrosive unless well diluted.

INTERACTIONS
Enhanced sedative effect with *anaesthetics, opioid analgesics, antidepressants, antipsychotics* and *nabilone.* If IV *furosemide (frusemide)* is to be given to patients who have recently received chloral then this should be done with caution as it can on occasion cause sweating, hot flushes, a variable blood pressure, tachycardia and uneasiness. This is thought to be due to the displacement of thyroid hormones from their binding proteins. May enhance the effects of *coumarin anticoagulants (e.g. warfarin).*

PREGNANCY
No reports have been found linking chloral hydrate with congenital defects. Contact local Medicines Information Centre for advice.

BREAST-FEEDING
Chloral hydrate and its active metabolite are excreted into breast milk at low levels. Although sedation of the infant may be possible from chloral in breast milk, the peak concentration is considerably lower than would be expected to be clinically important. Only trace amounts

are detectable after 10 hours. The American Academy of Pediatrics considers it to be compatible with breast-feeding but infants should be observed for signs of drowsiness.

SIDE-EFFECTS
Gastrointestinal: gastrointestinal irritation, abdominal distension, flatulence.
Skin: hypersensitivity reactions including skin rashes.
Respiratory: respiratory depression with large doses; airway patency may be compromised while patient is asleep.
CNS: drowsiness, light-headedness, ataxia, headache, hallucinations, nightmares, paradoxical excitement, confusion and a disinhibited state occur occasionally. Tolerance may develop and dependency can occur.
Haematological: leucopenia, eosinophilia and ketonuria may occur.

POISONING/TOXICITY
Symptoms: the irritant effect may cause vomiting and gastric necrosis leading to strictures. Toxic doses may cause drowsiness, sedation, ataxia, peripheral dilation, hypotension, ileus, myocardial suppression and arrhythmias. Significant overdosage can lead to hepatic and renal damage, coma, circulatory and respiratory depression and cardiac arrest.
Treatment: life support measures should be applied. Propranolol may be needed to control arrhythmias.

PHARMACOKINETIC PROPERTIES
Chloral is rapidly absorbed from the gastrointestinal tract following both oral and rectal administration and starts to act within 15-60 minutes. It is widely distributed throughout the body, metabolised in erythrocytes, liver and other tissues and excreted partly in urine and bile. Trichloroethanol is the active metabolite which has an elimination half-life of about 8 hours. Duration of action is from 60-120 minutes, but up to 8 hours has been reported. The half-life of trichloroethanol in babies is more than three times longer than in adults and may be further increased in preterm babies and those with hepatic or renal disease (up to 66 hours has been reported). This may result in drug accumulation which is a potential hazard with repeated administration. Metabolites may accumulate for several days even after the drug has been discontinued resulting in toxic reactions.

EXCIPIENTS
Welldorm® elixir includes glucose. Contact manufacturers for further details.

LICENSED STATUS
Welldorm® syrup not licensed for the indications given in the monograph. Welldorm® tablets not licensed in children <12 years or for this indication. Chloral hydrate 500mg in 5mL and suppositories are manufactured 'specials' and as such are unlicensed.

FURTHER INFORMATION
The quality and duration of sedation provided by chloral hydrate is variable, with higher doses producing more acceptable sedation at the expense of a prolonged recovery. Monitoring should be commenced from the time of administration until full recovery according to national and local guidelines. Chloral hydrate 500mg in 5mL is available from Rosemont Pharmaceuticals. The suppositories are available from Nova Laboratories.

Chlorambucil

Alkylating agent for oral administration.

USES
Hodgkin's disease and non-Hodgkin's lymphoma. Systemic amyloidosis and severe disease in juvenile idiopathic arthritis (JIA) unresponsive to other agents.

PRESENTATION
Tablet: 2mg – Leukeran®.

DOSAGE
Hodgkin's disease and non-Hodgkin's lymphoma
** Always consult the current treatment protocol for details of dosage and scheduling. **

Systemic amyloidosis and severe JIA
All ages: 100–120 microgram/kg orally once daily.

ADMINISTRATION
Oral: as a single daily dose.

CONTRA-INDICATIONS & WARNINGS
Contra-indication: previous hypersensitivity to chlorambucil.
Cautions: chlorambucil should not be given to patients who have recently undergone radiotherapy or received other cytotoxic agents. Careful monitoring should be performed in patients with impaired renal function and gross hepatic dysfunction.
Warnings: when lymphocytic infiltration of the bone marrow is present or the bone marrow is hypoplastic, the daily dose should not exceed 100 microgram/kg body weight.

INTERACTIONS
Possibility of enhanced chlorambucil toxicity with *phenylbutazone*.

PREGNANCY
Avoid wherever possible, especially during the first trimester. In any individual case, the potential hazard to the fetus must be balanced against the expected benefit to the mother. Contact local Medicines Information Centre for advice.

BREAST-FEEDING
Avoid if possible. Contact local Medicines Information Centre for advice.

SIDE-EFFECTS
Haematological: the most common side-effect is bone marrow suppression, which is usually reversible. However, irreversible bone marrow failure has been reported.
Gastrointestinal: nausea and vomiting, diarrhoea and oral ulceration are uncommon.
Hepatic: hepatotoxicity and jaundice have been reported after treatment.
Hypersensitivity: allergic reactions such as angioneurotic oedema and urticaria have been rarely reported following initial or subsequent dosing.
Skin: skin rashes are uncommon but have on rare occasions been reported to have progressed to serious conditions including Stevens-Johnson syndrome and toxic epidermal necrolysis.
Neurological: seizures have occurred in children with nephrotic syndrome. Movement disorders including tremor, twitching and myoclonia in the absence of convulsions have also been reported.
Fertility: chlorambucil may cause suppression of ovarian function and amenorrhoea has been reported following therapy. Azoospermia has been observed as a result of chlorambucil therapy in adult males. Chlorambucil administration to prepubertal and pubertal males has resulted in sterility.
Other: other reported adverse reactions include fever, peripheral neuropathy, interstitial pneumonia and sterile cystitis. Severe interstitial pulmonary fibrosis has been reported rarely in patients with chronic lymphocytic leukaemia on long-term therapy. However, this may be reversible on withdrawal.

POISONING/TOXICITY
Reversible pancytopenia following overdose. Neurological toxicity ranging from agitated behaviour and ataxia to grand mal seizures has also occurred. There is no known antidote. The blood picture should be closely monitored and general supportive measures instituted, together with appropriate haematological support.

PHARMACOKINETIC PROPERTIES
Peak levels occur at 40-70 minutes following oral administration. Absorption is rapid and almost complete. The parent drug has a terminal half-life in plasma of approximately 1.5 hours. Chlorambucil and the primary metabolites undergo some degree of spontaneous degradation in plasma and extensive hepatic metabolism. There is extensive protein binding of both drug and metabolites. Urinary excretion approaches 100%, almost entirely as metabolites.

EXCIPIENTS
See manufacturers SPC for further details.

LICENSED STATUS
Licensed for use in children for the treatment of Hodgkin's disease and non-Hodgkin's lymphoma. Not licensed for use in systemic amyloidosis or severe disease in JIA unresponsive to other agents.

Chloramphenicol

Broad-spectrum antibiotic.

USES
Orally or parenterally for serious infections.
In cystic fibrosis patients – for the treatment of chronic *Burkhoderia cepacia* infections.
Used topically in eye for bacterial conjunctivitis and in the ear for bacterial infection in otitis externa.

PRESENTATION
Capsule: 250mg – non-proprietary.
Injection: (as sodium succinate) 1g vial – Kemicetine®.
Ear drops: 5% and 10% – non-proprietary.

DOSAGE
Newborn infant (birth to 1 month)

Route	Age	Dose	Frequency (times daily)	Notes
IV bolus	<14 days	12.5mg/kg	2	Monitor levels and adjust dose accordingly.
	>14 days	12.5mg/kg	2–4	

Child

Route	Age			Frequency (times daily)	Notes
	1 month–2 years	2–12 years	12–18 years		
Oral or IV bolus	← 12.5mg/kg →		12.5mg/kg (maximum 1g)	4	Dose may be doubled for severe infection, meningitis, septicaemia, with blood level monitoring and high doses decreased as soon as clinically indicated.
Oral for cystic fibrosis patients	← 12.5mg/kg →			4	Treatment of chronic *Burkholderia cepacia* infections. Maximum single dose of 1g.
Ear drops	← 2–3 drops →			2–3	Eye ointment may be used in the ear.

ADMINISTRATION
IV: administer as bolus IV injection in NaCl 0.9% or glucose 5%.

CONTRA-INDICATIONS & WARNINGS
Can cause severe bone marrow depression; not to be used for trivial infection. Monitor plasma levels and full blood count. Grey baby syndrome (abdominal distension, cyanosis, circulatory collapse) may occur in babies with immature hepatic metabolism and/or with excessive doses.

INTERACTIONS
Increases plasma levels of *warfarin, phenytoin* and *sulphonylureas. Phenobarbital (phenobarbitone)* and *rifampicin* decrease chloramphenicol levels.

PREGNANCY
Risk of neonatal toxicity if used in third trimester. Manufacturer contra-indicates systemic use in pregnancy.

BREAST-FEEDING
Chloramphenicol and its metabolites are excreted in breast milk in concentrations approaching half the serum concentration and use is inadvisable in the lactating mother. Manufacturers contra-indicate use.

SIDE-EFFECTS
Blood disorders, peripheral or optic neuritis, headache, depression, dry mouth, nausea and vomiting, diarrhoea, urticaria. Superinfection with *Candida*. Sensitivity reactions to the ear drop vehicle may occur.

POISONING/TOXICITY
General supportive therapy. Seek advice from Poisons Centre.

PHARMACOKINETIC PROPERTIES
At fifth dose, trough blood level (immediately before dose) to be less than 10mg/L. Peak level (1 hour after IV and 2 hours after oral) 10-20mg/L.

EXCIPIENTS
Ear drops contain propylene glycol. Injection contains 3mmol sodium per gram. Contact manufacturers for further details.

LICENSED STATUS
All listed forms licensed for use in all ages. Using the eye ointment in the ear is unlicensed.

Antiseptic. Inhibits the formation of plaque on teeth.

USES
As an adjunct to oral hygiene measures; for the inhibition of dental plaque formation; for the prevention of gingivitis; as an aid in healing post surgery/trauma; useful in the management of aphthous ulceration, mucositis and other infections.

PRESENTATION
Dental gel: 1% – Corsodyl®.
Mouthwash: 0.12% Chlorohex 1200®; 0.2% – Corsodyl® and non-proprietary.
Oral spray: 0.2% – Corsodyl®.

DOSAGE
Dental gel: 1 inch of gel brushed around the teeth and gums once or twice daily for 1 minute. For gingivitis, apply for 1 month.
Mouthwash 0.12%: 15mL for 30 seconds twice daily.
Mouthwash 0.2%: 10mL for 1 minute twice daily.
Oral spray: up to 12 actuations to be used twice daily, morning and night. For the prevention of gingivitis, use for 1 month. In aphthous ulceration and oral infections use for 48 hours after the infection has cleared. Post oral surgery/trauma on the advice of the supervising clinician.

ADMINISTRATION
Dental gel: apply on a moistened toothbrush twice a day. For ulcerated areas the gel may be applied directly to the affected area once or twice daily for 1 minute.
Mouthwash: thoroughly rinse around the mouth twice a day before expectorating.
Oral spray: spray as directed onto the affected area and expectorate any excess.

C

CONTRA-INDICATIONS & WARNINGS
May discolour tongue and teeth with prolonged use.

INTERACTIONS
Chlorhexidine is inactivated by the *foaming agents in toothpastes* and therefore the mouth and toothbrush should be thoroughly rinsed after using toothpaste and before chlorhexidine is used (30 minute wait between using toothpaste and mouthwash is recommended).

SIDE-EFFECTS
Mucosal irritation (discontinue if desquamation); reversible brown staining of teeth, parotid gland swelling reported.

POISONING/TOXICITY
Ingestion of large quantities may cause nausea, vomiting and diarrhoea. Give liberal oral fluids.

EXCIPIENTS
Corsodyl® includes gel – polyoxyethylene hydrogenated castor oil; mouthwash – ethanol 96%, polyoxyethylene hydrogenated castor oil and sorbitol (in Corsodyl® mint); spray – ethanol 96 % and sorbitol.
Chlorohex® 1200 includes alcohol and saccharin.
Contact manufacturers for further details.

LICENSED STATUS
Licensed for use in children and adults.

FURTHER INFORMATION
Chlorhexidine is useful when the mouth is too sore for routine oral hygiene measures, for example in children with oral ulceration due to cytotoxic therapy. The carers of children with impairments may find chlorhexidine in gel form useful in controlling gingivitis when plaque removal is compromised.

Chlorhexidine and Neomycin

USES
Eradication of nasal carriage of Staphylococci.

PRESENTATION
Cream: chlorhexidine 0.1% and neomycin sulphate 3250 units/g, – Naseptin®.

DOSAGE/ADMINISTRATION
Topical eradication – apply to nostrils 4 times daily for 10 days.
Topical prophylaxis – apply to nostrils twice daily.

CONTRA-INDICATIONS AND WARNINGS	PREGNANCY/BREAST-FEEDING
Hypersensitivity to any ingredient. Existing hearing problems.	Unlikely to be of harm.

INTERACTIONS
None known.

SIDE-EFFECTS
Occasional allergic skin reactions. Rarely with long-term use there may be irritation, hearing difficulties or renal problems.

EXCIPIENTS
Include arachis (peanut) oil.

LICENSED STATUS
Licensed for use in all ages.

FURTHER INFORMATION
Do not use immediately after washing the face. For reasons of hygiene do not use tube for more than 28 days after first opening it.

Chloroquine

Antimalarial.

USES
Chemoprophylaxis and treatment of malaria.

PRESENTATION
Tablet: 150mg chloroquine base (as chloroquine sulphate 200mg) – Nivaquine®.
Tablet: 155mg chloroquine base (as chloroquine phosphate 250mg) – Avloclor®.
Syrup: 50mg chloroquine base in 5mL (as chloroquine sulphate 68mg in 5mL) – Nivaquine®.
Injection: chloroquine base 40mg in 1mL (as chloroquine sulphate 54.5mg in 1mL), 5mL ampoule – Nivaquine®.

DOSAGE
Doses expressed as chloroquine base.

Indication	Route	Age			Frequency	Notes
		1 month–2 years	2–12 years	12–18 years		
Malaria prophylaxis	Oral	← 5mg/kg → (maximum 300mg)		300mg	once weekly	Give for 1 week before entering and for 4 weeks after leaving an endemic area.
Malaria treatment	Oral/IV	← 10mg/kg → then		600mg then	initial dose	Maximum children's dose should not exceed the adult dose.
		5mg/kg then		300mg then	6–8 hours later	To eliminate liver forms of *P. vivax* or *P. ovale* follow with
		5mg/kg		300mg	daily for 2 days	primaquine.

ADMINISTRATION
Oral: tablets may be crushed if used immediately afterwards. Bioavailability is increased when given with food.
IV: can be given IV for treatment of malaria if oral therapy cannot be taken; give as an IV infusion over 8 hours, diluted in NaCl 0.9%.

CONTRA-INDICATIONS & WARNINGS

There are no absolute contra-indications.

Use with caution in renal or hepatic impairment. Dose may need to be reduced in renal failure. Full blood counts should be performed at regular intervals, as bone marrow suppression may rarely occur. Caution is advised in patients with G6PD deficiency. Use with caution in patients with a history of epilepsy as chloroquine may provoke seizures. Chloroquine may exacerbate psoriasis and myasthenia gravis.

Patients who are to receive chloroquine long-term (>12 months continuously or at weekly intervals for >3 years) should undergo ophthalmic examination before treatment and at 3 monthly intervals.

INTERACTIONS

Absorption of chloroquine may be reduced by *antacids* – administer at least 4 hours apart. Absorption of *ampicillin* may be reduced. *Chlorpromazine, ciclosporin (cyclosporin), digoxin* and *penicillamine* levels may be increased. *Cimetidine* may increase chloroquine levels – monitor for toxicity. Increased risk of ventricular arrhythmias with *amiodarone* and *halofantrine*. Antagonism of anticonvulsant effect with *antiepileptics*. Increased metabolism of *levothyroxine (thyroxine)*. Increased risk of convulsions with *mefloquine*.

PREGNANCY

Chloroquine crosses the placenta with fetal concentrations similar to those in the mother. The drug may accumulate in maternal and fetal eyes. Ocular or inner ear damage may occur in infants born to mothers who have received high doses of chloroquine throughout pregnancy.

There are reports of the safety of chloroquine as a weekly dose for malaria prophylaxis during pregnancy.

BREAST-FEEDING

Chloroquine is excreted into breast milk, but the amount ingested by the nursing infant is unlikely to pose a health risk.

SIDE-EFFECTS

Retinal damage may occur, particularly if treatment duration is greater than 1 year, but is unlikely with doses <4mg/kg/day. Short-term blurring of vision or difficulty in accommodation may occur at the start of therapy. Headache, gastrointestinal disturbances, pruritus and skin eruptions, depigmentation or loss of hair, ECG changes, dyskinesias, haematological effects: thrombocytopenia, agranulocytosis, aplastic anaemia.

POISONING/TOXICITY

Chloroquine is highly toxic in overdose, and children are particularly susceptible to its toxic effects. Symptoms of overdosage include circulatory collapse, cardiac dysrhythmia, respiratory arrest and coma. Gastric lavage should be carried out urgently, first protecting the airway and instituting artificial ventilation where necessary. In serious cases, there is a risk of cardiac arrest following aspiration of gastric contents. The administration of activated charcoal may reduce further absorption of the drug from the gut. Central venous pressure, respiration, plasma electrolytes and blood gases should be monitored, with correction of hypokalaemia and acidosis if indicated. If the patient has a cardiac arrhythmia, this should not be treated unless life threatening, and drugs with a quinidine-like effect in particular should be avoided.

Early administration of the following may be of benefit in serious poisoning to counteract cardiotoxicity before onset of cardiac arrhythmias:

☐ Adrenaline (epinephrine) infusion 250 nanogram/kg/minute initially with increments of 250 nanogram/kg/minute until adequate systolic blood pressure is restored.

☐ Diazepam infusion (2mg/kg over 30 minutes as a loading dose, followed by 1-2mg/kg/day for up to 2-4 days).

Due to the long half-life of chloroquine, the symptomatic patient should be observed for several days.

PHARMACOKINETIC PROPERTIES

Chloroquine is rapidly absorbed with peak concentrations achieved in 1-3 hours. It is excreted in the urine. Chloroquine has a long half-life of approximately 40 days in adults. This means it may take several months before steady state concentrations are reached.

EXCIPIENTS

Nivaquine® tablets include glucose.
Nivaquine® syrup includes sugars (including 65.73% sucrose).

LICENSED STATUS

Tablets licensed for treatment and prophylaxis of malaria in all age groups; injection licensed for malaria treatment in all age groups.

Thiazide diuretic.

USES
Oedema due to congestive cardiac failure (not first line treatment). Hypertension.
Hyperinsulinaemia (given with diazoxide).
Alternative to furosemide (frusemide) in babies with bronchopulmonary dysplasia requiring a diuretic.
Alternative to hydrochlorothiazide in nephrogenic diabetes insipidus in conjunction with amiloride or indometacin (indomethacin).

PRESENTATION
Tablet: 500mg – named patient.
Oral liquid: 250mg in 5mL – named patient.

DOSAGE

Indication	Route	Age				Frequency	Notes
		birth–1 month	1 month–2 years	2–12 years	12–18 years		
Diuresis	Oral	10–17.5 mg/kg	≤6 months 12.5–17.5 mg/kg >6 months 12.5mg/kg	12.5mg/kg	125–500mg	2 2	Doses up to 40mg/kg/**day** have been used in older children.
Nephrogenic diabetes insipidus	Oral	← 15–17.5mg/kg →			125–500mg	2	
Hyper-insulinism	Oral	← 3.5-5mg/kg →				2	

CONTRA-INDICATIONS & WARNINGS
Contra-indications: anuria, hypersensitivity to chlorothiazide or other sulphonamide-derived drugs, severe renal or hepatic failure, Addison disease, hypercalcaemia.
Warnings: fluid and electrolyte imbalance can occur. Hypokalaemia may develop which can sensitise the myocardium to digitalis glycosides. Sensitivity reactions may occur in patients with or without history of allergy or bronchial asthma. Thiazides may decrease urinary calcium excretion. Thiazides may impair glucose tolerance, latent diabetes may become manifest during thiazide therapy. In patients with renal disease, thiazides may precipitate uraemia. When creatinine clearance falls below 30mL/minute, thiazide diuretics become ineffective. Thiazides should be used with caution in patients with impaired hepatic function or progressive liver disease since minor alterations of fluid and electrolyte balance may precipitate hepatic coma.

INTERACTIONS
Increased risk of hypotension with *tricyclic antidepressant* and *antihypertensive drugs*. Antagonism of *antidiabetics*, which may therefore need adjustment of dose with concurrent use. Other *antihypertensive drugs* may have an additive effect. *Corticosteroids* or *corticotropin (corticotrophin, ACTH)* may intensify any electrolyte depletion. Hypokalaemia with *corticosteroids* and *other diuretics*. *NSAIDs* may attenuate the diuretic effects of chlorothiazide and increase risk of nephrotoxicity. Increased toxicity of *amiodarone, disopyramide, flecainide, quinidine, pimozide, sotalol, digoxin,* and *lithium* in hypokalaemia. Antagonism of *lidocaine (lignocaine)* and *mexilitine* in hypokalaemia. Reduced absorption with *colestyramine (cholestyramine)*.

PREGNANCY
Thiazides cross the placental barrier. Hazards include fetal or neonatal jaundice, thrombocytopenia and possibly other adverse reactions. Maternal effects could be hypovolaemia, increased blood viscosity and decreased placental perfusion.

BREAST-FEEDING
Thiazides appear in breast milk but not in amounts likely to be harmful. Large doses may suppress lactation.

SIDE-EFFECTS
Gastrointestinal: anorexia, gastric irritation, nausea, vomiting, diarrhoea, constipation, jaundice and pancreatitis.
CNS: dizziness, vertigo, paraesthesia, headache and yellow vision.
Haematological: leucopenia, agranulocytosis, thrombocytopenia, aplastic anaemia and haemolytic anaemia.

Cardiovascular: hypotension.
Hypersensitivity: purpura, photosensitivity, rash, urticaria and anaphylactic reactions.
Metabolic: hyperglycaemia, glycosuria, hyperuricaemia, electrolyte imbalance including hyponatraemia and hypokalaemia.
Renal: renal dysfunction, interstitial nephritis and renal failure.
Other: muscle spasm, weakness, restlessness and blurred vision.

POISONING/TOXICITY
The most common signs and symptoms of overdose are those caused by electrolyte depletion and dehydration. There is no known antidote. Treatment should be symptomatic and supportive.

PHARMACOKINETIC PROPERTIES
The bioavailability of oral doses of chlorothiazide is low. Plasma protein binding is approximately 70%. Chlorothiazide is not metabolised and is excreted almost completely as unchanged drug in the urine.
Plasma half-life in adults is 45-120 minutes though clinical effects of the oral preparation last approximately 12 hours.

EXCIPIENTS
Contact manufacturers for further details.

LICENSED STATUS
Liquid and tablets are not licensed in the UK.

FURTHER INFORMATION
Tablets are available via IDIS World Medicines. Oral liquid 250mg in 5mL is available via MSD.

C

Chlorphenamine (chlorpheniramine)

Antihistamine with sedative and antimuscarinic effects.

USES
Symptomatic relief of allergy. The injection is also used for anaphylactic reactions in emergency.

PRESENTATION
Injection: 10mg in 1mL, 1mL ampoule – non-proprietary.
Oral solution: 2mg in 5mL – non-proprietary.
Syrup: 2mg in 5mL – Piriton®.
Tablet: 4mg – Piriton® and non-proprietary.

DOSAGE

Route	Age			Frequency	Notes
	1 month–2 years	2–12 years	12–18 years	(times daily)	
Oral	1mg			2	Maximum **total daily doses** (oral):
	.	2–5 years			1 month–2 years: 2mg
		1–2mg		3	2–5 years: 6mg
		6–12 years			6–12 years: 12mg
		2–4mg		3–4	12–18 years: 24mg
			4mg	4–6	
IV, IM or SC	DOSE BY WEIGHT	2–5 years			Can be repeated up to 4 times in
	≤1 year	2.5–5mg	10–20mg	single	24 hours if necessary. Note adult
	250 microgram/kg			dose	maximum **daily dose** is 40mg. In
	DOSE BY AGE	6–12 years			anaphylaxis administer IV, as SC or IM
	>1 year	5–10mg			rarely acts quicker than oral dosing.
	2.5–5mg				

ADMINISTRATION
Injection: may be given by IM, IV, or SC routes. Give IV where a rapid response is required, e.g. treatment of anaphylaxis when it is injected slowly over 1 minute. For IV injection dilute in the syringe with 5–10mL of Water for Injections or NaCl 0.9%. It is not normally given as an infusion.

C

CONTRA-INDICATIONS & WARNINGS

Previous administration of MAOI within 14 days of treatment or concurrent MAOI treatment. Use with care in driving or operating heavy machinery due to potential to cause drowsiness. Use with caution in epilepsy, conditions with raised intra-ocular pressure (e.g. glaucoma), severe hypertension or cardiovascular disease, bronchitis, asthma, hepatic disease and thyrotoxicosis. Due to sugar content of the syrup, use with care in diabetes mellitus. Use with caution when taken with alcohol.

INTERACTIONS

Hypnotics, anxiolytics: increased sedative effect.
Phenytoin: chlorphenamine inhibits metabolism and can result in *phenytoin* toxicity.
MAOIs: intensification of anticholinergic effect.

PREGNANCY

Not recommended in pregnancy by manufacturers unless when clearly needed and potential benefits outweigh the potential unknown risks to the fetus. Use in the third trimester may result in reactions in neonates. Contact local Medicines Information Centre for advice.

BREAST-FEEDING

May be excreted in breast milk and inhibit lactation therefore use is not recommended during lactation unless therapeutic benefits of the drug outweigh the potential hazards to mother and baby. Contact local Medicines Information Centre for advice.

SIDE-EFFECTS

Sedation; varying from slight sedation to deep sleep. Inability to concentrate, lassitude, blurred vision, gastrointestinal disturbances, hepatitis (including jaundice), tachycardia, arrhythmias, hypotension, chest tightness, thickening of bronchial secretions, haemolytic anaemia and other blood dyscrasias. Allergic reactions e.g. exfoliative dermatitis, photosensitivity and urticaria. Twitching, muscular weakness and uncoordination, tinnitus, depression, irritability and nightmares. Paradoxical excitation can be seen in children.

POISONING/TOXICITY

Estimated lethal dose is 25-50mg/kg body weight. Signs and symptoms include sedation, paradoxical CNS stimulation, toxic psychosis, seizures, apnoea, convulsions, anticholinergic side-effects, dystonic reactions and cardiovascular collapse including arrhythmias. Symptomatic and supportive measures should be taken with special attention to cardiac, respiratory, renal and hepatic functions, and fluid and electrolyte balance. Treatment should include activated charcoal to minimise absorption. Treat hypotension and arrhythmias vigorously. CNS convulsions can be treated with IV diazepam or phenytoin. Haemoperfusion may be used in severe cases.

PHARMACOKINETIC PROPERTIES

Chlorphenamine is absorbed relatively slowly from the gastrointestinal tract and appears to undergo considerable first pass metabolism. It is largely protein bound in the plasma, widely distributed in the body and excreted in the urine. More rapid and extensive absorption, faster clearance and a shorter half-life have been reported in children.

EXCIPIENTS

Oral solution is sugar-free. Syrup includes sugar. Contact manufacturers for further details.

LICENSED STATUS

Licensed for use >1 year old by the oral route.
Other routes not licensed in children.

Chlorpromazine

Antipsychotic/neuroleptic (phenothiazine).

USES

Schizophrenia; mania or other causes of agitation, excitement or violent behaviour; intractable hiccup; nausea and vomiting of terminal illness; narcotic withdrawal symptoms in the baby of a drug abusing mother.

PRESENTATION

Injection: 25mg in 1mL, 1mL and 2mL ampoules – non-proprietary.
Oral solution: 25mg in 5mL and 100mg in 5mL – non-proprietary.
Syrup: 25mg in 5mL – Largactil®.
Suspension forte: 100mg in 5mL – Largactil®.
Tablet: 10mg, 25mg, 50mg and 100mg – Largactil® and non-proprietary.

DOSAGE
Newborn Infant (birth to 1 month)

Indication	Route	Age birth-1month	Frequency (times daily)	Notes
Withdrawal symptoms after birth in a baby of drug abusing mother	Oral or Oral/IV	1mg/kg or 550-750 microgram/kg	3 4	Dose can be doubled if withdrawal is severe. Maximum daily dose should not exceed 6mg/kg/day.

Child

Indication	Route	Age 2-12 years	Age 12-18 years	Frequency (times daily)	Notes
Schizophrenia, mania or other causes of agitation, excitement or violent behaviour	Oral	DOSE BY WEIGHT <6 years 500 microgram/kg DOSE BY AGE ≥6 years 10mg	25mg	4 3	Initial dose. Adjust according to response; 2-5 years – maximum 40mg/day. 6-12 years – maximum 75mg/day. 12-18 years – maximum 300mg/day.
Intractable hiccup	Oral	≥6 years 10mg	25–50mg	1–3 3–4	
Nausea and vomiting of terminal illness	Oral	500 microgram/kg	10–25mg	4	Maximum doses. <6 years – 40mg/day. 6-12 years – 75mg/day.

ADMINISTRATION
Oral: crushed tablets can cause skin contact hypersensitivity in those who crush them.

CONTRA-INDICATIONS & WARNINGS
Bone marrow depression; phaeochromocytoma.

INTERACTIONS
Plasma concentration increased by *propanolol*; enhances antimuscarinic effects of drugs; extrapyramidal effects increased by *lithium*.

PREGNANCY
Inadequate evidence of safety in human pregnancy but it has been widely used for many years without apparent ill consequence. It may occasionally prolong labour and at such a time should be withheld until the cervix is dilated 3-4cm. Possible adverse effects on the neonate include lethargy or paradoxical hyperexcitability, tremor and low Apgar score. Avoid unless considered essential.

BREAST-FEEDING
Excreted in breast milk: can cause drowsiness in baby. Breast-feeding should be suspended during treatment.

SIDE-EFFECTS
Drowsiness and sedation, antimuscarinic effects, hypotension, tachycardia, cardiac dysrhythmias, extrapyramidal symptoms and neuroleptic malignant syndrome, tardive dyskinesia after prolonged administration, hypothermia, gynaecomastia, galactorrhoea, impotence, menstrual disturbances, weight gain, lowered threshold for seizures, sensitivity reactions: bone marrow depression, leucocytosis, haemolytic anaemia, contact hypersensitivity, photosensitivity, rashes, cholestatic jaundice, corneal and lens opacities and skin pigmentation with prolonged use.

PHARMACOKINETIC PROPERTIES
Plasma levels unhelpful predictor of therapeutic response; rapidly absorbed and widely distributed in the body. Half-life is biphasic, initial 2 hours, terminal 30 hours; extensively metabolised in the liver to both active and inactive metabolites.

POISONING/TOXICITY
General sedation and depression of consciousness and respiration, hypothermia and tachycardia; consequent hypoxia and acidosis; seizures; dystonic reactions respond to antimuscarinic drugs, particularly benzatropine (benztropine) and procyclidine.

EXCIPIENTS
Largactil® syrup includes sucrose and the suspension forte includes sorbitol. Contact manufacturers for further details.

LICENSED STATUS
Licensed for use in children orally for childhood schizophrenia and autism (note that it is not actually an effective treatment for autism), and nausea and vomiting of terminal illness. Narcotic withdrawal symptoms in a neonate is not a licensed indication. Licensed for use in hiccup in adults only.

Cholera vaccine

The previously available cholera vaccine gave only limited personal protection, did not prevent spread of the disease and was not recommended for many years. Although alternative vaccines have been licensed in other countries, there is no cholera vaccine currently available in the UK.

Cholesterol

C

USES
Anecdotal evidence of use in Smith-Lemli-Opitz (SLO) syndrome (usually in conjunction with ursodeoxycholic acid and chenodeoxycholic acid).

PRESENTATION
Powder.

DOSAGE

Route	Age				Frequency (times daily)	Notes
	birth–1 month	1 month–2 years	2–12 years	12–18 years		
Oral	←	5–10mg/kg		→	3–4	Doses of up to 60mg/kg/day have been used.

ADMINISTRATION
The powder can be dissolved in vegetable oils.

CONTRA-INDICATIONS & WARNINGS, INTERACTIONS, PREGNANCY/BREAST-FEEDING
No information available.

SIDE-EFFECTS
None reported.

PHARMACODYNAMIC PROPERTIES
Smith-Lemli-Opitz syndrome is an autosomal recessive syndrome of multiple congenital anomalies. Defects in cholesterol biosynthesis in these patients has been reported resulting in low cholesterol levels. Exogenous cholesterol is given to try to correct this.

LICENSED STATUS
Not licensed for use in the UK.

FURTHER INFORMATION
Powder available from IDIS World Medicines.

Choline salicylate

USES
For the relief of pain and discomfort of mouth ulcers and teething.

PRESENTATION
Oral gel: 8.7% w/w choline salicylate – Bonjela®, Dinnefords Teegel®.

DOSAGE/ADMINISTRATION
Children ≥4 months: apply quarter of an inch of gel to the dried area of affected oral mucosa, no more frequently than once every 3 hours to a maximum of 6 applications in 24 hours.
>12 years: apply half an inch of gel with gentle massage not more often than every 3 hours.

CONTRA-INDICATIONS & WARNINGS
Preparations containing aspirin should not be given to children <16 years of age during treatment with choline salicylate. Not to be used in children <4 months.
The gel should not be used in children with active peptic ulceration or in those known to be allergic to salicylates.
Salicylates may precipitate bronchospasm and induce attacks of asthma in susceptible individuals.

INTERFERENCE WITH LABORATORY TESTS
Salicylates may produce falsely increased results for blood creatinine, urate (low dose aspirin) and urea. Falsely decreased results may be obtained for blood levothyroxine (thyroxine), urate and for urinary 5 hydroxyindole acetic acid (5-HIAA). Urinary vanillylmandelic acid (VMA) levels may be falsely increased or decreased depending on the method of analysis.

INTERACTIONS, PREGNANCY/BREAST-FEEDING, SIDE-EFFECTS, POISONING/TOXICITY,
As for salicylates. See aspirin monograph.

EXCIPIENTS
Bonjela® is sugar-free. See manufacturers SPC for further details.

LICENSED STATUS
Licensed for >4 months of age.

Chorionic gonadotrophin (human chorionic gonadotrophin; HCG)

USES
Investigation of testicular (Leydig cell) function in suspected primary hypogonadism and incomplete masculinisation. Stimulation of testicular development in hypogonadotrophic hypogonadism.

PRESENTATION
Injection: 1500 and 5000 unit ampoule – Pregnyl®.
Injection: 2000, 5000 and 10,000 unit ampoule – Profasi®.

DOSAGE

Indication	Route	Age			Frequency	Notes
		1 month– 2 years	2–12 years	12–18 years		
Short stimulation test	IM	←	1500-2000 units	→	Single dose	For 3 days. Testosterone (and androgen profile) at baseline and 4th day.
Prolonged stimulation test	IM	←	1500-2000 units	→	Twice weekly	For 3 weeks. Testosterone (and androgen profile) at baseline and 4-6 days after final dose.
Hypogonado-trophic hypogonadism	IM	←	1000-2000 units	→	Twice weekly	Seek expert advice. Used as an addition to testosterone replacement.

CONTRA-INDICATIONS & WARNINGS
Known or suspected androgen dependent tumours. Use with caution in prepubertal boys to avoid premature epiphyseal closure. Patients with cardiac failure, renal failure, hypertension, epilepsy or migraine should be monitored since sodium and fluid retention has been

observed with HCG. Prior to treatment, anatomical abnormalities of the genital organs or nongonadal endocrinopathies (e.g. thyroid or adrenal disorders) should be excluded.

PREGNANCY/BREAST-FEEDING
Not applicable.

EXCIPIENTS
See manufacturers SPC for further details.

LICENSED STATUS
Licensed for hypogonadotrophic hypogonadism.

SIDE-EFFECTS
Skin rashes, sodium and water retention is occasionally seen in males.

PHARMACOKINETIC PROPERTIES
HCG has a half-life of approximately 9 hours in its first phase and approximately 30 hours in its second.

Ciclosporin (cyclosporin)

Immunosuppressant which inhibits T-cell activation.

USES
Prevention of graft rejection following kidney, liver, heart, combined heart-lung, lung or pancreas transplant. Prevention of graft rejection following bone marrow transplantation and prophylaxis of graft-versus-host disease.
Psoriasis (severe psoriasis when conventional therapy is ineffective or inappropriate).
Short-term treatment (8 weeks) of severe atopic dermatitis.
Juvenile idiopathic arthritis (JIA), connective tissue diseases, vasculitis and uveitis. This use is largely experimental and should be reserved for specialist centres.
Severe, active ulcerative colitis and Crohn's disease (experience limited).

PRESENTATION
Capsule: 10mg, 25mg, 50mg and 100mg – Neoral®.
Injection: 50mg in 1mL, 1mL and 5mL ampoules – Sandimmun®.
Oral solution: 100mg in 1mL – Neoral®.
Note: Sandimmun® capsules and oral solution are available on a named patient basis for patients who are already established on this product. Doses are not equivalent between oral Sandimmun® and Neoral®. Both the Neoral® preparations are bioequivalent.

DOSAGE

Indication	Route	Age			Frequency	Notes
		1 month–2 years	2–12 years	12–18 years	(times daily)	
JIA, connective tissue disease, vasculitis and uveitis	Oral	←	1-2mg/kg	→	2	Initial dose. May be increased gradually if required but should not exceed 3mg/kg twice daily.
Organ transplantation	Oral	←	5-7.5mg/kg	→	2	Initial dose given 12 hours before transplantation and continued for 1–2 weeks post-operatively, gradually reducing to a maintenance dose as indicated.
		←	1-3mg/kg	→	2	Maintenance dose.
		←	1.5-4mg/kg	→	2	Low initial dose if ciclosporin given with other immunosuppressants as part of triple or quadruple therapy.

DOSAGE continued

Indication	Route	Age			Frequency (times daily)	Notes
		1 month–2 years	2–12 years	12–18 years		
Bone marrow transplantation (BMT)	Oral	←	6-7.5mg/kg	→	2	Initial dose. Started on the day before transplantation (this dose will vary depending on the type of BMT and protocol).
		←	6mg/kg	→	2	Maintenance dose.
Psoriasis, atopic dermatitis	Oral	←	1.25mg/kg	→	2	Initial dose. If no improvement after 2 weeks for dermatitis, or 1 month for psoriasis, the dose can be increased but should not exceed 2.5mg/kg twice daily. This dose can be used initially in severe cases requiring rapid control.
Severe ulcerative colitis	Oral	–	← 3-4mg/kg →		2	Experience is limited. Seek expert advice.
Crohn's disease	Oral	–	← 2.5-4.5mg/kg →		2	Experience is limited. Seek expert advice.

To convert a dose from oral to IV, divide the oral dose by three.

Doses used in organ transplantation can vary from those indicated depending on individual protocols. Sandimmun® concentrate for IV infusion is usually preferred for the initiation of therapy in bone marrow transplantation.

Monitor ciclosporin levels, according to local policy.
Hepatic or renal function may be impaired with ciclosporin, and close monitoring of serum creatinine, urea, electrolyte levels, bilirubin and liver enzymes is required. Dosage should be reduced if necessary. Regular monitoring of blood pressure is required during treatment as ciclosporin may cause hypertension (particularly in infants); antihypertensive therapy should be initiated if necessary.

ADMINISTRATION
Oral: oral solution should be mixed immediately before administration, preferably with apple juice, orange juice or squash, but not with grapefruit juice, as this may alter ciclosporin levels. Neoral® oral solution should not be mixed with chocolate or milk, as this will give a solution with a bad taste. The measuring device should not come into contact with the diluent and it should not be mixed with water, alcohol or other liquid.
IV: dilute the concentrated solution 1:20 to 1:100 with NaCl 0.9% or glucose 5% immediately before use, and give over 2-6 hours. The infusion time should not be prolonged beyond 6 hours, as ciclosporin can strip a component from PVC bags and tubing. A fresh solution should be prepared.

CONTRA-INDICATIONS & WARNINGS
Abnormal renal function, uncontrolled hypertension, uncontrolled infections, malignancy. Sandimmun® injection includes polyoxyl (polyethylated) castor oil – risk of anaphylaxis.

INTERACTIONS
Care should be exercised in patients who are being given other *nephrotoxic agents*. *Ketoconazole* (and to a lesser extent other *azole antifungals*), *erythromycin* and *clarithromyicn*, *oral contraceptives* and some *calcium-channel blockers* (in particular *diltiazem*, *nicardipine* and *verapamil*) have been found to increase ciclosporin levels. *Amiodarone, cisapride, doxorubicin, etoposide, colchicine* may increase ciclosporin levels. *Phenytoin, carbamazepine, barbiturates* and *rifampicin* may decrease ciclosporin levels. *Diclofenac* levels may be increased by ciclosporin (diclofenac dose should be halved).
Vaccination may be less effective during treatment with ciclosporin. The use of live vaccines should be avoided due to the risk of causing infection.
Nephrotoxicity may be increased when ciclosporin is given with *aminoglycosides* or *amphotericin (liposomal or conventional formulation)*.
St John's Wort (hypericum) markedly reduces ciclosproin levels – avoid concomitant use.

PREGNANCY
Ciclosporin crosses the placenta. There have been reports of various defects in infants born to women receiving ciclosporin (but most data comes from

mothers receiving multiple therapy rather than ciclosporin alone). No pattern of anomalies has emerged. Data is very limited, but the use of ciclosporin during pregnancy does not appear to pose a major risk to the developing fetus. Contact local Medicines Information Centre for advice.

BREAST-FEEDING

Ciclosporin is excreted in breast milk. Women treated with ciclosporin should not breast-feed due to the potential for adverse effects in the infant, including immunosuppression, neutropenia, growth effects and carcinogenesis.

SIDE-EFFECTS

Renal impairment, which may necessitate dosage reduction. Hypertension, which may necessitate withdrawal of ciclosporin, if unable to control with antihypertensives. Hypertrichosis, tremor, hepatic impairment, fatigue, gingival hypertrophy, abdominal pain, nausea, vomiting and diarrhoea, headache, rash and hyperkalaemia.

POISONING/TOXICITY

Signs of nephrotoxicity are generally reversible following withdrawal. Hypertension and convulsions may also occur in overdosage. Treatment is symptomatic.

PHARMACOKINETIC PROPERTIES

Neoral® is an improved pharmaceutical form of the active ingredient ciclosporin. It reduces the intra-patient variability of pharmacokinetic parameters, with a more consistent absorption profile affected less by concomitant food intake and the presence of bile.

EXCIPIENTS

Sandimmun® injection includes polyoxyl (polyethylated) castor oil. See manufacturers SPC for further details.

LICENSED STATUS

Not licensed for use in connective tissue disease, vasculitis, uveitis, ulcerative colitis or Crohn's disease in any age group, nor in rheumatoid arthritis and JIA in patients <18 years of age. Licensed for use in psoriasis >16 years of age and in prevention of graft rejection in children and adults.

FURTHER INFORMATION

Sandimmun® capsules and oral solution are available from Novartis.

Cimetidine

H_2-receptor antagonist.

USES

Oesophagitis, gastro-oesophageal reflux related respiratory disease, peptic ulcers, acid related dyspepsia, prevention of gastric bleeding in intensive care, reduction of degradation of pancreatic enzymes in cystic fibrosis, Zollinger-Ellison syndrome, prophylaxis against upper gastrointestinal bleeding/perforation in infants receiving high dose steroids for treatment for bronchopulmonary dysplasia. Persistant fat malabsorption despite optimal use of enzyme replacement in cystic fibrosis.

PRESENTATION

Tablet: 200mg, 400mg and 800mg – Tagamet® and non-proprietary.
Tablet: 400mg (effervescent) – Tagamet®.
Suspension: 200mg in 5mL – Dyspamet®.
Syrup: 200mg in 5mL – Tagamet®.
Injection: 100mg in 1mL, 2mL ampoule – Tagamet®.

DOSAGE

Route	Age				Frequency (times daily)	Notes
	birth–1 month	1 month–2 years	2–12 years	12–18 years		
Oral or IV infusion	5mg/kg	← 5–10mg/kg →			4	Total daily dose may be given in 2 divided doses.
				400mg	2–4	

ADMINISTRATION
IV: give over at least 10 minutes, continuous infusion may be preferred. Dilute in NaCl 0.9% to produce a solution not exceeding 10mg in 1mL.
Oral: in cystic fibrosis administer 1-2 hours before food.

CONTRA-INDICATIONS & WARNINGS
Rapid IV administration may lead to hypotension and arrhythmias. Reduce dose in hepatic impairment.
In mild to moderate renal impairment use 75% of the stated doses and in severe impairment use 50% of the dose, at the same time intervals.

INTERACTIONS
Cimetidine binds to cytochrome P450 very strongly, inhibiting the breakdown of those drugs metabolised by this enzyme in the liver, including *warfarin, opioid analgesics, ciclosporin (cyclosporin), theophylline, phenytoin, caffeine, intravenous lidocaine (lignocaine)*; monitor closely.

PREGNANCY
Crosses the placenta and should be used with caution in early pregnancy although teratogenicity has not been reported.

BREAST-FEEDING
Significant amounts in milk, but no known adverse effects.

SIDE-EFFECTS
Gastrointestinal side-effects include diarrhoea. Children may also report headache and tiredness.

POISONING
No significant ill effects with acute overdosage have been reported. Treatment is symptomatic and supportive.

PHARMACOKINETICS
Readily absorbed from the gastrointestinal tract. Bioavailability is 60-70%. Elimination half-life of about 2 hours. Partly metabolised but most excreted unchanged in the urine.

C

EXCIPIENTS
Tagamet® effervescent tablets include aspartame; sodium content 18mmol/tablet. Tagamet® syrup includes sucrose and saccharin. Dyspamet® suspension includes sorbitol (2.79g in 5mL) and is sugar-free.

LICENSED STATUS
Licensed for use in children and adults although use in children <1 year has not been fully evaluated.

Ciprofibrate

Fibric acid derivative; lipid-modulating agent.

USES
Hyperlipidaemia, including familial hypercholesterolaemia in patients in whom diet therapy and resins have been unsuccessful.

PRESENTATION
Tablet: (scored) 100mg – Modalim®.

DOSAGE/ADMINISTRATION
Oral: 2-4mg/kg (maximum 200mg) has been used in adolescents but experience in children is limited; refer to lipidologist.

CONTRA-INDICATIONS & WARNINGS, INTERACTIONS, PREGNANCY/BREAST-FEEDING, SIDE-EFFECTS, PHARMACODYNAMIC PROPERTIES, POISONING/TOXICITY
See bezafibrate monograph.

EXCIPIENTS
See manufacturers SPC for details.

LICENSED STATUS
Not licensed for use in children.

A synthetic 4-quinolone derivative.

USES
Treatment of infections due to sensitive Gram-negative or Gram-positive bacteria. In cystic fibrosis patients treatment of *Pseudomonas aeruginosa* infection – first isolates or in chronically infected patients who have a mild exacerbation.

PRESENTATION
IV infusion: (as lactate) 2mg in 1mL, in NaCl 0.9%, 50ml bottle – Ciproxin®; (as lactate) 2mg in 1mL, in Glucose 5%, 100mL and 200mL – Ciproxin® Flexibag.
Suspension: 250mg in 5mL – Ciproxin®.
Tablet: 100mg, 250mg, 500mg and 750mg – Ciproxin® and non-proprietary.

DOSAGE

Route	Age				Frequency (times daily)	Notes
	birth–1 month	1 month–2 years	2–12 years	12–18 years		
Oral	←	7.5mg/kg		→	2	Maximum single dose 750mg.
IV	←	5mg/kg		→	2	Maximum single dose 400mg.
Oral for cystic fibrosis patients	-	5–15mg/kg	≤5 years 5–15mg/kg >5 years 20mg/kg	20mg/kg	2 2	Treatment for *P. aeruginosa* infection – first isolates or in chronically infected patients with a mild exacerbation.
IV for cystic fibrosis patients	-	4–8mg/kg	≤5 years 4–8mg/kg >5 years 10mg/kg	- 10mg/kg	2 3	Maximum single oral dose is 750mg. Maximum single IV dose is 400mg.

Dose adjustment in renal or liver failure
In severe impairment (creatinine clearance <20mL/minute/1.73m^2) total daily dosage may be reduced by half, although monitoring serum levels provides the most reliable basis for dose adjustment. No adjustment in impaired hepatic function.

ADMINISTRATION
IV infusion: to be administered over 30-60 minutes. The 400mg dose should be administered over 60 minutes. The infusion should not be stored in the refrigerator.
Oral: well absorbed orally and achieves good tissue penetration. The IV route offers no advantage if the child can take oral medication.

CONTRA-INDICATIONS & WARNINGS
In children and growing adolescents ciprofloxacin is only recommended where the benefits outweigh the risk of arthropathy. Contra-indicated in patients with a known hypersensitivity to ciprofloxacin or other quinolones. Use with caution in epilepsy or CNS disorders – seizure threshold may be reduced by ciprofloxacin. Patients receiving ciprofloxacin should be well hydrated and excessive alkalinity of the urine avoided to prevent crystalluria. Patients with a familial history of G6PD activity may be prone to haemolysis.

INTERACTIONS
Ciprofloxacin tablets should not be administered within 4 hours of medication containing *magnesium, aluminium, calcium* or *iron salts. Theophylline* dose should be reduced when concomitant therapy given. Prolonged bleeding times have been reported on concomitant administration of *oral anticoagulants. Metoclopramide* may accelerate the absorption of ciprofloxacin. Increased risk of nephrotoxicity with *ciclosporin (cyclosporin)*.

PREGNANCY
No evidence of teratogenicity, however, ciprofloxacin causes arthropathy in immature animals and is not recommended in pregnancy.

BREAST-FEEDING
Excreted in breast milk – not recommended in nursing mothers.

SIDE-EFFECTS
Gastrointestinal disturbances: rarely pseudo-membranous colitis, CNS disturbances.
Hyper-sensitivity skin reactions: rarely erythema nodosum, Stevens-Johnson syndrome. Transient hepatic disturbances. Reversible arthralgia, joint swelling and myalgia. Reversible haematological disorders.

POISONING/TOXICITY
Reversible renal toxicity has been reported in overdose. In addition to routine supportive measures monitor renal function, including urinary pH and acidify, if required, to prevent crystalluria. Calcium or magnesium antacids may be administered soon after ingestion of ciprofloxacin tablets to prevent absorption. Serum levels are reduced by dialysis.

EXCIPIENTS
Contact manufacturers for further details.

LICENSED STATUS
Not licensed for use in children <1 year old. Not licensed for cystic fibrosis doses in children <5 years old.

Cisapride

Prokinetic agent without central antidopamine effects which directly stimulates myenteric plexus.

USES
The product licence was suspended in 2000 by the MCA, on advice from the CSM, due to continuing concern about rare cardiac arrhythmias and death.

Cisapride should only be prescribed to a patient after very careful consideration of all the known risks and potential benefits. The prescriber has to take personal responsibility for the child's safety and should be convinced that the child's condition, without cisapride, poses a greater threat to life than the potential cardiac side-effects of cisapride; which could result in sudden death. All the drugs and conditions which are contra-indicated or require special precautions MUST be taken into account.

Cisapride may be considered for use in patients with:
☐ proven gastro-oesophageal reflux disease, severe forms of other gastrointestinal motility disorders, gastroparesis (use restricted to motility disorders resistant to conventional measures and agents reducing gastric acid secretion)
☐ non-ulcer dyspepsia (patients not responding to antacids and gastric acid reducing agents)
☐ where alternative methods are inappropriate, the condition is life threatening, other therapies and risks having been considered.

PRESENTATION
Suspension: 1mg in 1mL – named patient Prepulsid®.
Tablet: 10mg (scored) – named patient Prepulsid®.
Suppository: 30mg – (imported).

DOSAGE

Route	Age				Frequency (times daily)	Notes
	birth–1 month	1 month–2 years	2–12 years	12–18 years		
Oral	←	200 microgram/kg	→	10mg	3-4	Do not exceed these recommended doses.
Rectal	←	400 microgram/kg	→	20mg	3	

ADMINISTRATION
Oral: tablets may be crushed. Administer 15-30 minutes before food.

CONTRA-INDICATIONS & WARNINGS
Do not use in patients in whom gastrointestinal stimulation might be dangerous e.g. gastrointestinal haemorrhage, obstruction or perforation.
Cisapride should not be used in patients with the following risk factors for cardiac arrhythmia: a personal or family history of QT-interval prolongation; a previous history of ventricular arrhythmia or torsades de pointes; combination with drugs known to prolong QT-interval (see interactions section). Cisapride should be avoided/used with caution in patients with other risk factors for arrhythmia such as those with clinically significant heart disease, uncorrected electrolyte disturbances, renal failure, significant chronic obstructive pulmonary disease or respiratory failure. Such patients should be carefully evaluated prior to

C

administration. An ECG should be part of this evaluation to exclude a prolonged QT-interval.

Cisapride should not be used in prematurely born infants (born at a gestational age <36 weeks) for up to 3 months after birth, due to the risk of QT-interval prolongation in this age group.

ECG must be monitored prior to therapy to exclude prolonged QT-interval or other cardiac problems. Repeat 7 days after starting cisapride, after dose increase, before discharge and every 2 months thereafter. Ensure serum potassium and magnesium are within the normal range before and during treatment.

INTERACTIONS

The main metabolic pathway of cisapride is through cytochrome P450 CYP3A4. The concurrent use of oral or parenteral drugs that significantly inhibit these enzymes may result in increased plasma levels of cisapride, and could increase the risk of QT-prolongation. Therefore the use of such drugs is contra-indicated. Examples include *azole antifungals*, *macrolide antibiotics* and *HIV-protease inhibitors*.

In patients receiving *anticoagulants* the prothrombin time may be increased. It is advisable to check the prothrombin time within the first few days of initiating or discontinuing cisapride treatment, and to adapt the dose of anticoagulant if necessary.

Drugs which prolong the QT-interval such as *amiodarone, quinine, sotalol, terfenadine, astemizole, thioridazine, chlorpromazine, lithium,* *pentamidine, haloperidol, pimozide, procainamide, bretylium,* are contra-indicated in patients receiving cisapride. Avoid *diuretics*.

PREGNANCY
Avoid use in pregnancy.

BREAST-FEEDING
Excretion into breast milk is minimal; however, the manufacturers suggest avoidance.

SIDE-EFFECTS
The most frequent side-effects reported are gastrointestinal. Increased gastrointestinal motility may be associated with colic/diarrhoea. In cases of severe cramps, it is recommended that the dose per administration is halved and the frequency of dosing doubled.

Rare cardiac toxicity: ventricular arrhythmias, cardiac arrest, sudden unexplained death and QT-prolongation. Most of these reactions have occurred in patients who were taking contra-indicated medication or who were suffering from underlying conditions known to increase the risk of ventricular arrhythmias or on a prescribed dose above the recommended dose.

POISONING/TOXICITY
Abdominal cramping and increased stool frequency. In infants mild sedation, apathy and atony, vomiting. Treat with activated charcoal and observe closely. Check for possible QT-interval prolongation and electrolyte disturbance.

EXCIPIENTS
Suspension includes sucrose. Contact manufacturer for further details.

LICENSED STATUS
Product licence suspended July 2000. Previously not licensed for use in children <12 years of age.

FURTHER INFORMATION
Suspension and tablets available from Janssen Cilag.
Suppositories available from IDIS World Medicines.

Cisplatin

Platinum-containing complex.

USES
Treatment of osteogenic sarcoma, Stage 4 neuroblastoma, some liver tumours, infant brain tumours and intracranial germ cell tumours.

PRESENTATION
Injection: 1mg in 1mL solution; 10mL, 50mL and 100mL vials – non-proprietary. Powder for reconstitution, 50mg vial (reconstituted solution 1mg in 1mL) – non-proprietary.

DOSAGE
** Always consult the current treatment protocol for details of dosage and scheduling. **

ADMINISTRATION
IV: 24 hour infusion, or 48 hour infusion in infant brain tumours. IV hydration is necessary to ameliorate renal damage and all protocols require hydration and an adequate urine output to be established at least 3 hours before, during and for at least 24 hours after completion of the cisplatin infusion or until the patient is able to tolerate oral fluids again. See protocol for details of IV hydration.

CONTRA-INDICATIONS & WARNINGS
Adequate hydration and diuresis must be established prior to, during and for at least 24 hours after cisplatin infusion.

INTERACTIONS
Co-administration of other potentially *nephrotoxic agents* should be avoided due to risk of acute reduction in glomerular filtration rate and hence reduction in cisplatin clearance. Also risk of additive renal toxicity. Concurrent administration of cisplatin and *etoposide* may reduce *etoposide* clearance.

PREGNANCY/BREAST-FEEDING
Safe use in pregnancy has not been established. Use should be avoided in pregnant and breast-feeding women, if possible.

SIDE-EFFECTS
Severe nausea and vomiting (may be delayed). Dose-limiting glomerular nephrotoxicity, hypomagnesaemia, hypokalaemia and hyperuricaemia. Ototoxicity, myelosuppression and alopecia. Occasional peripheral neuropathy and taste disturbance. Rarely, anaphylaxis may occur.

POISONING/TOXICITY
Full supportive measures. Plasmapheresis may be of value in cisplatin overdosage before established renal failure occurs.

PHARMACOKINETIC PROPERTIES
Median (range) pharmacokinetic parameters:
Clearance: 394 (213-931) mL/minute/1.73m^2.
Half-life: 48 (38-139) minutes.

EXCIPIENTS
Contact manufacturer for further details.

LICENSED STATUS
Licensed for use in children and adults.

Citalopram

Selective serotonin re-uptake inhibitor (SSRI).

USES
Depression, obsessive-compulsive disorder and anxiety.

PRESENTATION
Tablet: 10mg, 20mg and 40mg – Cipramil®.
Oral drops: 40mg in 1mL – Cipramil®.

DOSAGE

Route	Age	Frequency	Notes
	12–18 years	(times daily)	
Oral	20mg	1	Dose is usually given in the morning. Depending on the response, this can be increased to a maximum dose of 60mg.

CONTRA-INDICATIONS & WARNINGS, SIDE-EFFECTS, POISONING/TOXICITY
See fluoxetine monograph. Relatively more likely to cause weight gain than other SSRIs.

INTERACTIONS
Citalopram has a low potential for clinically significant drug interactions. *MAOIs* should not be used with SSRIs.

PREGNANCY
Animal studies have not shown evidence of teratogenic potential, but due to limited human data citalopram should only be used in pregnancy if considered necessary and under close supervision of a physician. Contact local Medicines Information Centre for advice.

BREAST-FEEDING
Citalopram appears in milk in very low concentrations, but it is not known what effect this may have on the infant.

EXCIPIENTS
See manufacturers SPC for further details.

LICENSED STATUS
Not licensed for use in children.

PHARMACOKINETIC PROPERTIES
Rapidly and completely absorbed following oral administration. The elimination is slow, with a terminal elimination half-life of 23-75 hours (mean 33 hours). During chronic administration, steady-state levels are attained within 1-2 weeks, consistent with the half-life. Citalopram is eliminated primarily by hepatic metabolism, with subsequent elimination of the metabolites in the urine and probably also in the faeces.

Citrulline

USES
Used in lysinuric protein intolerance (LPI) and as an alternative to arginine in severe carbamylphosphate synthase (CPS) and ornithine carbamyltransferase (OCT) deficiencies.

PRESENTATION
Powder.

DOSAGE

Route	Age				Frequency (times daily)	Notes
	birth–1 month	1 month–2 years	2–12 years	12–18 years		
Oral	←	42.5mg/kg		→	4	

CONTRA-INDICATIONS & WARNINGS, INTERACTIONS, PREGNANCY/BREAST-FEEDING
No information available.

SIDE-EFFECTS
None reported.

LICENSED STATUS
Not licensed for use in the UK.

FURTHER INFORMATION
Powder available from Scientific Hospital Supplies.

PHARMACODYNAMIC PROPERTIES
Citrulline is converted to arginine thus preventing arginine deficiency. Citrulline contributes one less nitrogen atom to the free amino acid pool than does arginine.

Clarithromycin

A macrolide antibiotic.

USES
Lower and upper respiratory tract infections, skin and skin structure infections, acute otitis media, adjunct in the eradication of *Helicobacter pylori* in patients with duodenal ulcers.
In cystic fibrosis patients – treatment of atypical infection e.g. mycoplasma; some centres using treatment courses of longer than the licensed 5-10 days.

PRESENTATION
Granules: 250mg – Klaricid®.
IV infusion: 500mg vial – Klaricid®.
Paediatric suspension: 125mg in 5mL, 70ml and 100ml – Klaricid®; 250mg in 5mL, 70mL – Klaricid®.
Tablet: 250mg and 500mg – Klaricid®.

DOSAGE

Route	Age				Frequency	Notes
	birth–1 month	1 month–2 years	2–12 years	12–18 years	(times daily)	
Oral	DOSE BY WEIGHT					For 5 10 days.
		<8kg or <1 year	–	–	2	Doses up to 500mg twice
	7.5mg/kg	7.5mg/kg				daily have been used to treat
		DOSE BY AGE				severe infection.
		1–2 years	3–6 years			
		62.5mg	125mg	250mg	2	
			7–9 years			
			187.5mg		2	
			10–12 years			
			250mg		2	
Oral for *H. pylori*		>1 year	2–6 years			Treatment for 14 days with
	–	62.5mg	125mg	500mg	2	amoxicillin and omeprazole,
			6–9 years			or metronidazole and
			187.5mg		2	omeprazole.
			9–12 years			
			250mg		2	
IV infusion	–	← 7.5mg/kg →		500mg	2	Do not give by IV bolus or IM injection.

ADMINISTRATION
Oral: food does not affect extent of bioavailability but may delay onset of absorption.
IV: reconstitute vial with 10mL of Water for Injections to give 50mg in 1mL concentration. Dilute reconstituted dose to 2mg in 1mL, with NaCl 0.9% or glucose 5%, and give over 1 hour via a large vein.

CONTRA-INDICATIONS & WARNINGS
Known hypersensitivity to macrolides or excipients. Monitor for signs of bacterial/fungal superinfection.

INTERACTIONS
Theophylline – increased serum levels and potential *theophylline* toxicity. *Digoxin, warfarin, carbamazepine* – reduced rate of excretion of these drugs, potentiation of effect, monitor levels; monitor prothrombin time for *warfarin. Terfenadine, astemizole* and *cisapride* – risk of cardiac arrhythmias – avoid concurrent use. *Ergot derivatives* and clarithromycin should not be co-administered; ergotism reported.

PREGNANCY
Safety not established. Some animal studies suggest embryotoxic effect. Contact local Medicines Information Centre for advice.

BREAST-FEEDING
Safety not established. Has been found in human breast milk. Contact local Medicines Information Centre for advice.

SIDE-EFFECTS
Nausea, vomiting, diarrhoea, abdominal pain, taste perversion, stomatitis and glossitis. Headache, allergic reactions – mild urticaria to Stevens-Johnson syndrome (rare). CNS effects including dizziness, anxiety, insomnia, bad dreams, pseudomembranous colitis (rare), altered LFTs.

POISONING/TOXICITY
Very little effect when taken in acute overdose. There may be gastrointestinal symptoms and skin rashes may occur if the patient is already allergic to clarithromycin. Gastric lavage is unnecessary. Symptomatic and supportive measures.

PHARMACOKINETIC PROPERTIES
Rapidly and well absorbed after oral administration.

EXCIPIENTS
Paediatric suspension contains sucrose. See manufacturers SPC for further details.

LICENSED STATUS
Oral route licensed for use in children (*H.pylori* eradication – children >12 years). IV route not licensed for use in children.

Clindamycin

A lincosamide antibiotic with a primarily bacteriostatic action.

USES
Staphylococcal bone and joint infections; peritonitis; endocarditis prophylaxis (see infections guideline section – *Summary of prevention of endocarditis in children with heart disease*). In cystic fibrosis patients – treatment of asymptomatic *Staphylococcus aureus* isolates or minor exacerbations; reserved for resistant isolates. Its use is limited because of serious side-effects. Consult with microbiology before use. Used topically for mild to moderately severe acne.

PRESENTATION
Capsule: 75mg and 150mg – Dalacin C®.
Gel: 1% – Zindaclin®.
Injection: (as phosphate) 150mg in 1mL, 2mL and 4mL ampoule – Dalacin C®.
Liquid: 75mg in 5mL – (import).
Lotion: 1% in aqueous basis – Dalacin T®.
Topical solution: 1% in an aqueous alcohol base – Dalacin T®.

DOSAGE

Route	Age				Frequency (times daily)	Notes
	birth–1 month	1 month–2 years	2–12 years	12–18 years		
Oral	<2 weeks 3–6mg/kg	–	–	–	3	
	≥2 weeks 3–6mg/kg	<1 year or <10kg 3–6mg/kg	–	–	3–4	In those <1 year or <10kg, the minimum recommended dose is 37.5mg three times a day.
	–	>1 year or >10kg 3–6mg/kg	3–6mg/kg	150–300mg (to a maximum of 450mg in severe infection)	4	
Oral for cystic fibrosis patients	–	← 5–7mg/kg →			4	Treatment of asymptomatic *S. aureus* isolates or minor exacerbations in cystic fibrosis patients. Maximum dose of 600mg four times daily.
IV/IM	5mg/kg	← 5–7mg/kg →		900mg	3	Up to 40mg/kg/day in severe infections or 4.8g/day.

Dental prophylaxis: see the infection therapeutic section.

Acne: topical treatment with lotion or solution ≥12 years – apply a thin film to the affected area, twice daily; with gel apply once daily.

Dose adjustment in hepatic impairment
Dose should be reduced in hepatic failure and liver function tests should be monitored. Not readily removed by dialysis or peritoneal dialysis.

ADMINISTRATION
IM: maximum 600mg (4mL) per dose.
IV: avoid rapid administration. Clindamycin must be diluted before IV administration to at least 6mg in 1mL, with NaCl 0.9% or glucose 5%, and infused over 10-60 minutes. Maximum rate 20mg/kg over 1 hour.

CONTRA-INDICATIONS & WARNINGS
Should only be used in the treatment of severe infections and contra-indicated in diarrhoeal states. Discontinue immediately if diarrhoea or colitis develops. Cases of diarrhoea have been reported during or even 2 or 3 weeks following treatment. When used topically avoid concurrent application of benzyl peroxide.

INTERACTIONS
Drug interactions include antagonism of *neostigmine* and *pyridostigmine* and enhancement of *non-depolarising muscle relaxants*.

PREGNANCY
Safety in pregnancy has not been established. Contact local Medicines Information Centre for advice.

BREAST-FEEDING
Small amounts of clindamycin may be present in breast milk in nursing mothers. Contact local Medicines Information Centre for advice.

SIDE-EFFECTS
Diarrhoea – discontinue treatment. Nausea and vomiting, antibiotic associated colitis, jaundice and altered LFTs, blood dyscrasias and erythema multiforme have been reported. With topical use skin dryness and irritation can occur.

POISONING/TOXICITY
In the case of overdose no specific treatment is indicated; treatment should be symptomatic and supportive. If the topical preparations come in contact with the eye, burning and irritation may occur; bathe with copious amounts of cool water.

EXCIPIENTS
Suspension includes sucrose. Injection includes benzyl alcohol which has been associated with fatal Gasping Syndrome in premature neonates. See manufacturers SPC for further details.

LICENSED STATUS
Oral use licensed in all ages. Injection licensed ≥ 1month. Topical use for acne ≥12 years.

FURTHER INFORMATION
Pseudomembranous colitis caused by growth of *Clostridium difficile* should be treated with metronidazole or oral vancomycin. Liquid is available via IDIS World Medicines.

Clobazam

Benzodiazepine antiepileptic.

USES
Third-line add-on treatment for absence (typical and atypical), tonic-clonic, atonic, myoclonic and partial seizures. May be used as monotherapy for catamenial (menstruation) seizures – either perimenstrually or continually. May be given over a short period for cluster seizures.

PRESENTATION
Tablet: 5mg – named patient, 10mg – Frisium®.
Liquid: may be extemporaneously prepared; 5mg in 5mL – manufactured 'special'.

DOSAGE

Route	Age				Frequency (times daily)	Notes
	birth–1 month	1 month–2 years	2–12 years	12–18 years		
Oral	–	◀— 125 microgram/kg —▶		10mg	2	Usual starting dose.
	–	◀— 250 microgram/kg —▶ (maximum 500 microgram/kg)		10–15mg (maximum 30mg)	2	Usual target maintenance dose. It takes 2–3 weeks to reach the maintenance dose, increasing every 5 days.

ADMINISTRATION
Oral: for catamenial seizures clobazam may only have to be given for 7-10 days each month, just before and during menstruation. Tablets should not be chewed.

CONTRA-INDICATIONS & WARNINGS
Contra-indications: acute severe respiratory insufficiency, alcohol or drug dependence, myasthenia gravis, sleep apnoea, hepatic insufficiency. Withdraw slowly if has been used daily for a week or more. Reduce dose in hepatic impairment. Dose may require adjustment in severe renal failure.

INTERACTIONS
May alter plasma levels of other *antiepileptics. Enzyme inhibitors (e.g. cimetidine)* may enhance the effects and *enzyme inducers (e.g. rifampicin)* may reduce the effects of clobazam.

PREGNANCY
Little data, but manufacturer advises not to be used in first trimester. May produce drowsiness, hypotonia and withdrawal symptoms in the neonate if used in third trimester. Contact local Medicines Information Centre for advice.

BREAST-FEEDING
Breast-feeding appropriate if maternal dose is normal.

SIDE-EFFECTS
Dose-dependent side-effects include sedation and irritability. Chronic adverse effects include tachyphylaxis, behaviour disturbance and cognitive dysfunction.

POISONING/TOXICITY
Hypotonia, ataxia, drowsiness, sedation and loss of consciousness may be seen. Flumazenil is a benzodiazepine antagonist but will also reduce anticonvulsant effect in patients with epilepsy.

PHARMACOKINETIC PROPERTIES
Blood reference range, up to 200 microgram/L.

EXCIPIENTS
Contact manufacturers for further details.

LICENSED STATUS
Licensed for use ≥3 years of age for epilepsy. Frisium® SPC state that it may be used between 6 months and 3 years of age for anticonvulsant treatment when there is a compelling indication. The 5mg tablets are unlicensed. The 5mg in 5mL liquid is a 'special' and as such is unlicensed.

FURTHER INFORMATION
Clobazam is NHS 'black-listed' for indications other than epilepsy. Endorse non-private prescriptions 'SLS' (Selected List Scheme). The 5mg in 5mL liquid is available as a 'special' from North Staffordshire Hospital manufacturing unit.

Clomethiazole (chlormethiazole)

Antiepileptic.

USES
Treatment of generalised tonic-clonic and focal seizures.

PRESENTATION
Capsule: 192mg – Heminevrin®.
Syrup: (as edisylate) 250mg in 5mL – Heminevrin®.

DOSAGE

Route	Age				Frequency (times daily)	Notes
	birth–1 month	1 month–2 years	2–12 years	12–18 years		
Oral	–	← 1.5–3mg/kg → (0.03–0.06mL/kg of syrup)			–	6	More frequent dosing may be required. Dose is equivalent to 10–20mg/kg/**day** of edisylate (syrup).

CONTRA-INDICATIONS & WARNINGS
Respiratory insufficiency and risk of respiratory depression. Tachyphylaxis can occur.

INTERACTIONS
Potentiates and may be potentiated by other *centrally acting depressant drugs*. Metabolism may be inhibited by *cimetidine* and other *enzyme inhibitors*.

PREGNANCY
Manufacturer recommends avoiding use in pregnancy, especially during first and last trimesters. Contact local Medicines Information Centre for advice.

BREAST-FEEDING
Excreted into breast milk, amount too small to be harmful.

SIDE-EFFECTS
Rapid infusion may produce apnoea, hypotension and tachycardia. Increased airway secretions, sedation and loss of consciousness. Fever and headache. Nasal and conjunctival irritation, and headache may occur with oral therapy. Paradoxical worsening of epilepsy may occur in the Lennox-Gastaut syndrome.

POISONING/TOXICITY
Unconsciousness, deep coma, respiratory and cardiovascular depression may be seen. Treatment is supportive.

PHARMACOKINETIC PROPERTIES
Rapid tissue redistribution, slower liver metabolism. Effects may be prolonged after ceasing therapy.

EXCIPIENTS
See manufacturers SPC for further details.

LICENSED STATUS
Not licensed for use in children. Epilepsy is an unlicensed indication.

FURTHER INFORMATION
One 192mg capsule is approximately therapeutically equivalent to 250mg in 5mL of syrup.

Clomipramine

Tricyclic antidepressant with marked serotonin re-uptake inhibition.

USES
Depression. Obsessive-compulsive disorder. Cataplexy in narcolepsy.

PRESENTATION
Tablet: 75mg (slow-release) – Anafranil SR®.
Capsule: 10mg, 25mg and 50mg – Anafranil® and non-proprietary.

DOSAGE

Route	Age		Frequency (times daily)	Notes
	2–12 years	12–18 years		
Oral	DOSE BY WEIGHT			The total daily dose may be given in divided doses or as a single dose at night. Start with low dose and titrate by gradual increases against clinical and side-effects. Obsessive compulsive disorder usually requires >100mg/**day**.
	>6 years 3mg/kg	3mg/kg	1 (see notes)	
	DOSE BY AGE			
	>6 years 10–120mg	25–250mg	1 (see notes)	

C

CONTRA-INDICATIONS & WARNINGS
As imipramine; particular care required in those with seizure disorders.

PREGNANCY, BREAST-FEEDING, SIDE-EFFECTS, POISONING/TOXICITY
See imipramine monograph.

INTERACTIONS
As imipramine, plus any *drug with serotonergic action*.

PHARMACOKINETIC PROPERTIES
Active substance completely absorbed following oral administration. Half-life range after oral administration is 12-36 hours (mean 21 hours).

EXCIPIENTS
Contact manufacturers for further details.

LICENSED STATUS
Not licensed for use in children.

Clonazepam

Benzodiazepine antiepileptic.

USES
Second or third-line treatment for myoclonic seizures (usually as add-on in patients with idiopathic generalised epilepsies) and third-line treatment of status epilepticus, particularly in neonates. May be useful in absence seizures with a myoclonic component.

PRESENTATION
Injection: 1mg in 1mL in solvent; for dilution with 1mL Water for Injections – Rivotril®.
Oral liquid: 500 microgram in 5mL and 2mg in 5mL – manufactured 'specials', 2.5mg in 1mL (100 microgram/drop) – named patient.
Tablet: (scored) 500 microgram and 2mg – Rivotril®.

DOSAGE

Route	Age				Frequency	Notes
	birth–1 month	1 month–2 years	2–12 years	12–18 years	(times daily)	
Oral	–	DOSE BY WEIGHT				Starting dose.
		◄— 25 microgram/kg —►		–	1	May be given at night.
		DOSE BY AGE				
		<5 years				Higher, divided doses have
		250 microgram		1mg	1	been used (up to
		5–12 years				100 microgram/kg/**day**).
		500 microgram			1	
	–	DOSE BY WEIGHT				Usual target maintenance
		◄— 80 microgram/kg —►		–	3	dose.
		DOSE BY AGE				The total daily dose may also
		<1 year				be divided into 2 or 4 doses.
		100–300 microgram		1–2.5mg	3	Increase dose from the
		1–5 years				starting dose every 4 days
		300 microgram – 1mg			3	over 2–4 weeks until satis-
		5–12 years				factory response, side-effects
		1–2mg			3	or maximum dose reached.
IV bolus over 30 seconds	–	◄— 50 microgram/kg —► (maximum 1mg)		1mg	single dose	Status epilepticus. Can be repeated.

DOSAGE continued

Route	Age				Frequency (times daily)	Notes
	birth–1 month	1 month–2 years	2–12 years	12–18 years		
IV short infusion	100 microgram/kg	–	–	–	single dose	Can be repeated every 24 hours.
IV infusion	–	10 microgram/kg/hour (up to 60 microgram/kg/hour has been given)		–	continuous	Bolus loading dose is usually administered first. Adjust to response.

ADMINISTRATION

Oral: initial oral dose may be administered at night to avoid drowsiness. Injection solution has been given orally (but see excipients).

IV: mix active substance with diluent before IV administration. IV bolus over at least 30 seconds. May be infused neat into suitably placed cannula, dilution preferred in glucose 5%, glucose 10%, NaCl 0.9% or glucose/saline, maximum concentration 12mg/L. Short infusion of 100 microgram in 1mL dilution preferred in neonates. Infusions should be changed every 12 hours.

Clonazepam can be adsorbed on PVC. The manufacturers therefore recommend that glass containers are used or, if PVC infusion bags are used, that the mixture is infused straight-away over a period of no longer than 2 hours. In practice problems do not seem to have been encountered with PVC-free syringes e.g. polypropylene plastic syringes or PVC-free infusion bags.

Rectal: injection (diluted) and oral solution have been given rectally.

CONTRA-INDICATIONS & WARNINGS

Porphyria, acute pulmonary insufficiency, respiratory depression, sleep apnoea, myasthenia gravis, renal and/or liver disease. Warn of drowsiness particularly at start of treatment and not to cease therapy without advice. Feeding may be difficult with hypersalivation.

INTERACTIONS

Enzyme inhibitors and other *drugs producing sedation or respiratory depression* may enhance the side-effects of clonazepam. *Enzyme inducers* may reduce clonazepam plasma levels.

PREGNANCY

Possible increased risk of neural tube defects especially if more than one antiepileptic used. Specialist counselling, management and screening required. Administer folate supplements before and during pregnancy. Blood levels may be altered. Fetal heart rate abnormality, hypotonia, poor sucking and hypothermia may be seen in the neonate when clonazepam is used in the third trimester or during labour. Contact local Medicines Information Centre for advice.

BREAST-FEEDING

Breast-feeding appropriate if maternal dose is normal.

SIDE-EFFECTS

Dose-dependent adverse effects include sedation, irritability, excess salivation and excess airways secretions. Chronic adverse effects include tachyphylaxis, behaviour disturbance and cognitive dysfunction. Hypotension, respiratory depression and apnoea may occur with IV injection.

POISONING/TOXICITY

Somnolence, muscle hypotonia and respiratory depression may be seen. Flumazenil is a benzodiazepine antagonist but will also reduce anticonvulsant effect in patients with epilepsy.

PHARMACOKINETIC PROPERTIES

Peak levels 1-4 hours after oral administration; long half-life of 1-2 days. Liver metabolism. Suggested therapeutic range of 25-85 microgram/L does not correlate well with efficacy or side-effects. Rapidly absorbed by rectal route.

EXCIPIENTS

Injection includes ethanol, glacial acetic acid, benzyl alcohol and propylene glycol. Contact manufacturers for further details.

LICENSED STATUS

Licensed for use in all ages except the liquid preparations which are unlicensed.

FURTHER INFORMATION

The 500 microgram in 5mL and 2mg in 5mL oral liquid are available as 'specials' from Rosemont.
The 2.5mg in 1mL oral liquid is available from IDIS World Medicines.

Alpha-2 adrenergic agonist.

USES
Hyperactivity, Tourette syndrome, hypertension (third-line therapy) and growth hormone secretion testing. Sedation, pain and opiate withdrawal.

PRESENTATION
Injection: 150 microgram in 1mL, 1mL ampoule – Catapres®.
Oral solution: may be extemporaneously prepared.
Tablet: 25 microgram – Dixarit®; 100 and 300 microgram – (both scored) Catapres®.

DOSAGE

Indication	Route	Age			Frequency (times daily)	Notes
		1 month–2 years	2–12 years	12–18 years		
Hyperactivity, Tourette syndrome	Oral	–	← >4 years → 25 microgram then increase by 25 microgram every 1-2 weeks, moving to divided doses (1-3 daily)		1	Usual maximum dose is 300 microgram. Titrate dose against symptoms and blood pressure. Monitor blood pressure and pulse on starting treatment and after each dose increase.
Hypertension	Oral	–	500 nanogram/kg – 1 microgram/kg		3	
	IV	–	← 2–6 microgram/kg →		single dose	
Growth hormone test	Oral	← 150 microgram/m² →			single dose	
Sedation, pain, opiate withdrawal	Oral	← 1 microgram/kg then escalate incrementally in steps of 1 to 3 to 5 micrograms/kg/dose if required →			single dose / 3	Test dose: monitor for hypotension. Maximum dose: 5 microgram/kg four times daily.
	IV infusion	← 250 nanograms/kg/hour →			continuous	Initial dose for sedation (PICU only). Then increase by 100 nanogram/kg/hour. Increase until adequate sedation is achieved. Most children require 1 microgram/kg/hour.

ADMINISTRATION
Oral: 100 microgram tablets can be crushed and dissolved in water.
IV: give by slow IV injection over 10-15 minutes. Compatible with NaCl 0.9% and glucose 5%.

CONTRA-INDICATIONS & WARNINGS
Porphyria; lowers blood pressure; can intensify depression; abrupt withdrawal can result in rebound hypertension; withdraw gradually.

INTERACTIONS
Caution with *tricyclic antidepressants* and *beta-blockers*, as clonidine withdrawal may cause rebound hypertension when these are also being taken.

PREGNANCY
No evidence of teratogenicity. Contact local Medicines Information Centre for advice.

BREAST-FEEDING
Passes into breast milk. No adverse effects in breast-fed

infants reported. Contact local Medicines Information Centre for advice.

SIDE-EFFECTS
Drowsiness, restlessness at night, dry mouth. Bradycardia, QT lengthening and hypotension. Subjectively cold extremities.

POISONING/TOXICITY
Symptoms include hypotension, bradycardia, sedation and coma. Treatment is symptomatic and supportive.

PHARMACOKINETIC PROPERTIES
Well absorbed after oral administration. Elimination half-life is 20-25 hours but this is increased to approximately 40 hours in severe renal impairment.

EXCIPIENTS
Contact manufacturers for further details.

LICENSED STATUS
Not licensed for use in hyperactivity, Tourette syndrome, growth hormone secretion testing or for hypertension in children.

Clotrimazole

Broad spectrum antifungal agent.

USES
Fungal skin infections.

PRESENTATION
Cream: 1% – Canesten® and non-proprietary.

DOSAGE/ADMINISTRATION
Apply 2-3 times daily continuing for 14 days after lesions have healed.

CONTRA-INDICATIONS & WARNINGS
Hypersensitivity to clotrimazole.

SIDE-EFFECTS
Occasional skin irritation or sensitivity.

PREGNANCY
Use only when necessary, although clotrimazole has been used in pregnant patients for ≥10 years without attributable adverse effects.

POISONING/TOXICITY
Oral ingestion – routine supportive measures should be performed as necessary.

EXCIPIENTS
Cream includes benzyl alcohol.

LICENSED STATUS
Licensed for use in children and adults.

Clozapine

Antipsychotic/neuroleptic.

USES
Treatment of resistant schizophrenia.

PRESENTATION
Tablet: 25mg (scored) and 100mg – Clozaril®.
Oral: liquid can be extemporaneously prepared.

DOSAGE

Route	Age	Frequency	Notes
	12–18 years	(times daily)	
Oral	12.5mg then	1 or 2	Initial dose (day1); only to in-patients.
	25mg	1 or 2	Second day, then increased gradually (if well tolerated) in steps of 25–50mg over 14–21 days to 300mg daily in divided doses (usual maintenance dose). May be increased to a maximum of 900mg **daily** if absolutely necessary. Must register the patient with Clozaril Patient Monitoring Service.

CONTRA-INDICATIONS & WARNINGS
Previous or current neutropenia, severe cardiac disease and poorly controlled epilepsy.

INTERACTIONS
Avoid drugs known to depress leucopoiesis *e.g. co-trimoxazole, carbamazepine* and many others.

PREGNANCY/BREAST-FEEDING
Contra-indicated.

SIDE-EFFECTS
Neutropenia/agranulocytosis (requires close monitoring in association with manufacturer). As chlorpromazine but more sedative and more antimuscarinic (though also associated with hypersalivation). Myocarditis, pericarditis and hypotension.

POISONING/TOXICITY
See chlorpromazine monograph.

PHARMACOKINETIC PROPERTIES
The absorption of orally administered clozapine is 90–95%; the rate or extent of absorption is not influenced by food. When steady-state conditions are reached, peak blood levels occur on average at 2.1 hours, with mean terminal half-life of 14.2 hours. Clozapine is almost completely metabolised prior to excretion.

EXCIPIENTS
See manufacturers SPC for further details.

LICENSED STATUS
Patient, prescriber and supplying pharmacist must be registered with Sandoz Clozaril® Patient Monitoring Service. Not licensed for use in children.

FURTHER INFORMATION
Initiation must be as hospital in-patient. Must monitor white count weekly initially (first 18 weeks) then fortnightly. Can monitor monthly if stable white count for 1 year. Withdraw if white cell count <3.5 x 10^9/L or if absolute neutrophil count <1.5 x 10^9/L.

Coal tar

Coal tar has anti-inflammatory and antiscaling properties.

USES
Treatment of psoriasis; shampoo is for the treatment of scalp disorders including psoriasis.

PRESENTATION
Cream: coal tar extract 1% – Clinitar®.
Cream: coal tar extract 5%, allantoin 2% – Alphosyl®.
Cream (in water-miscible basis): coal tar solution 10% – Carbo-Dome®.
Lotion: coal tar extract 5%, allantoin 2% – Alphosyl®.
Ointment: Coal Tar and Salicylic Acid Ointment BP – non-proprietary (may need to be extemporaneously prepared).

The above list is not exhaustive; there are several other preparations available including bath preparations, shampoos and other scalp preparations. Consult the current British National Formulary for details. Several preparations can also be extemporaneously prepared.

DOSAGE/ADMINISTRATION
Creams/lotions: apply 1-3 times daily.
Shampoos: wet hair, add sufficient of a preparation to produce lather, massage scalp, rinse hair thoroughly, then repeat if necessary. Use once or twice weekly. Consult individual product information for full details.

CONTRA-INDICATIONS & WARNINGS
Not for use in sore, acute or pustular psoriasis or in presence of infection. Avoid applying to eyes, mucosa and broken or inflamed skin.

PREGNANCY/BREAST-FEEDING
Although there is no direct evidence of the safety of coal tar used topically in pregnancy and lactation, it has been used over many years without known ill effect.

SIDE-EFFECTS
Skin irritation and acne-like eruptions, photosensitivity.

EXCIPIENTS
Contact manufacturers for further details.

LICENSED STATUS
Licensed for use in children and adults.

FURTHER INFORMATION
Some preparations stain skin, hair and fabric.

Co-amoxiclav (amoxicillin and clavulanic acid)

Amoxicillin is a broad-spectrum penicillin. Clavulanic acid itself has no significant antibacterial activity but, by inactivating penicillinases, it makes the combination active against penicillinase-producing bacteria that are resistant to amoxicillin.

USES
Infections due to penicillinase-producing strains (where amoxicillin alone is not appropriate) including respiratory tract, genito-urinary and abdominal infections, cellulitis, animal bites, severe dental infection with spreading cellulitis.

PRESENTATION
The proportions of amoxicillin and clavulanic acid in the following preparations are expressed in the form x/y where x and y are the strengths in milligrams of amoxicillin and clavulanic acid respectively.

Injection: 600mg vial (500/100) and 1.2g vial (1000/200) – Augmentin®.
Oral suspension: 125/31 in 5mL and 250/62 in 5mL – Augmentin® and non-proprietary; 400/57 in 5mL – Augmentin-Duo®.
Tablet: 375mg (250/125) and 625mg (500/125) – Augmentin® and non-proprietary.
Tablet: 375mg (250/125) (dispersible) – Augmentin®.

DOSAGE
Newborn Infant (birth to 1 month)

Route	Age		Frequency (times daily)	Notes
	<7 days	>7 days		
Oral	← 0.25mL/kg of the 125/31 suspension →		3	
IV	30mg/kg	–	2	Dosage is based on co-amoxiclav content.
	–	30mg/kg	3	

Child

Route	Age			Frequency (times daily)	Notes
	1 month–2 years	2–12 years	12–18 years		
Oral	≤1 year 0.25mL/kg of the 125/31 suspension	2–6 years 5mL of the 125/31 suspension	1 tablet (250/125)	3	Doses may be doubled in severe infections with the suspensions. In severe infections with the tablet give 1 tablet (500/125).
	≥1 year 5mL of the 125/31 suspension	7–12 years 5mL of the 250/62 suspension		3	
Oral Augmentin Duo®	2 months–2 years 0.15mL/kg	2–6 years 2.5mL	–	2	Doses may be doubled in severe infections with the suspension.
		7–12 years 5mL	–	2	
IV	← 30mg/kg →		1.2g	3	Dosage is based on co-amoxiclav content. Over 3 months of age the dose frequency can be increased to 4 times daily in severe infections.

Dose adjustment in renal impairment

Creatinine clearance (mL/minute/1.73m²)	Route	Dose/dose frequency (times daily)
10–30	Oral	Normal dose, twice daily.
	IV	Normal dose initially, then half dose twice daily.
<10	Oral	Half the normal dose twice daily.
	IV	Normal dose initially, then half dose once daily.

ADMINISTRATION

Oral: give at the start of a meal. Dispersible tablets should be stirred into a little water before taking.

IV: reconstitute a 600mg vial with 10mL Water for Injections (final volume 10.5mL) and a 1.2g vial with 20mL (final volume 20.9mL). Give by slow IV injection (over 3-4 minutes, within 20 minutes of reconstitution) or infuse over 30–40 minutes and complete infusion within 4 hours of reconstitution. For infusion the reconstituted injection can be diluted to 5 times its volume in NaCl 0.9%. Do not infuse in glucose solutions, as co-amoxiclav is less stable in infusions containing glucose.

CONTRA-INDICATIONS & WARNINGS

See ampicillin monograph. Caution in hepatic impairment (monitor hepatic function). Also see side-effects section of this monograph.

INTERACTIONS

See ampicillin monograph.

PREGNANCY

Animal studies have shown no teratogenic effects; limited data in human pregnancy. Contact local Medicines Information Centre for advice.

BREAST-FEEDING

Trace quantities excreted in breast milk but considered compatible with breast-feeding.

SIDE-EFFECTS

See ampicillin monograph. Also hepatitis, cholestatic jaundice; CSM has advised that cholestatic jaundice has been identified as an adverse reaction occurring during, or shortly after, the use of co-amoxiclav. An epidemiological study has shown that the risk of acute liver toxicity was about 6 times greater with co-amoxiclav than with amoxicillin; these reactions have only rarely been reported in children. Jaundice is usually self-limiting and very rarely fatal. The duration of treatment should be appropriate to the indication and not normally exceed 14 days. Erythema multiforme (including Stevens-Johnson syndrome), toxic epidermal necrolysis, exfoliative dermatitis, and vasculitis have been reported. Rarely, prolongation of bleeding time, headache, dizziness, convulsions, superficial staining of the teeth with the suspension and phlebitis at injection site.

POISONING/TOXICITY

Problems with overdosage of co-amoxiclav are unlikely to occur; if encountered, gastrointestinal symptoms and disturbance of the fluid and electrolyte balances may be evident. Treatment is symptomatic. Co-amoxiclav may be removed from the circulation by haemodialysis.

PHARMACOKINETIC PROPERTIES

The pharmacokinetics of the two components of co-amoxiclav are closely matched. Peak serum levels of both occur about one hour after oral administration. Absorption is optimised at the start of a meal. Both clavulanate and amoxicillin have low levels of serum binding; about 70% remains free in the serum. Doubling the dose of co-amoxiclav approximately doubles the serum levels achieved.

EXCIPIENTS

Dispersible tablets include saccharin sodium. Injection: sodium 1.6mmol and potassium 0.5mmol per 600mg vial. Suspension includes aspartame. Contact manufacturer for further details.

LICENSED STATUS

Licensed for use in all ages.

Co-careldopa

Provides exogenous source of amines.

USES

Treatment of defects in tetrahydrobiopterin synthesis and dihydrobiopterin reductase (DHPR) deficiency. Treatment of dopamine sensitive dystonia (Segawa syndrome) and dystonia as part of cerebral palsy.

PRESENTATION

Tablet: 110 (carbidopa 10mg & levodopa 100mg) (scored) – Sinemet-110®.
Tablet: 275 (carbidopa 25mg & levodopa 250mg) (scored) – Sinemet-275®.
Tablet: 62.5 (carbidopa 12.5mg & levodopa 50mg) (scored) – Sinemet-62.5®.
Tablet: 125 (carbidopa 25mg & levodopa 100mg) (scored) – Sinemet-Plus®.
Liquid: may be extemporaneously prepared.

DOSAGE

Indication	Route	Age				Frequency (times daily)	Notes
		birth–1 month	1 month–2 years	2–12 years	12–18 years		
Metabolic disorders	Oral	← 250–500 microgram/kg levodopa →				4	Starting dose. Increase stepwise every 4–5 days to maintenance dose below.
		← 2.5–3mg/kg levodopa →				4	Maintenance dose. Review dose regularly (every 3–6 months in early childhood); adjust if necessary according to weight and CSF amine metabolic concentration.
Dystonia	Oral	–	≥ 3 months – 18 years 250 microgram – 1mg/kg levodopa			2–3	Starting dose. Increase slowly every 2–3 days.

Treatment of dystonia on specialist advice. Published information is limited. Start with low dose and increase slowly until response established.

Dosage in renal impairment/liver failure – use with caution.

ADMINISTRATION

Oral: normally start at 1:4 mixture of carbidopa/levodopa, and only change if necessary for increased response. Give 30 minutes before main meals and at night. Adjustments in the timing and the balance of carbidopa/levodopa may need to be made according to individual response. Sinemet-62.5® tablets can be halved, but for infants, suspension needs to be made. In metabolic disorders give at the same time as 5-hydroxytryptophan.

CONTRA-INDICATIONS AND WARNINGS

Avoid in uncontrolled narrow angle glaucoma, psychosis or in patients with a history of melanoma or with a suspicious undiagnosed skin lesion. Avoid in endocrine, renal, hepatic and cardiac disorders when sympathomimetic amines are contra-indicated.

INTERACTIONS

Non-selective, irreversible MAOIs: hypertensive crisis.
Antihypertensives: enhanced hypotensive effect. *Iron*/high protein diet: absorption of co-careldopa may be reduced.
Antipsychotics/benzodiazepines: antagonism of effect of co-careldopa.
Phenytoin: increased metabolism of levodopa altering response.
Laboratory tests: false positives reported with Coombs test and urinary ketones. False negative urinary glucose using glucose oxidase methods.

PREGNANCY

Visceral and skeletal malformations have occurred in rabbits. No adverse outcomes have been noted in the few reports of human pregnancies.

BREAST-FEEDING

Levodopa inhibits prolactin release, however, it is not known whether carbidopa or levodopa is excreted in human milk. No published reports on levels in breast milk or effects on infant.

SIDE-EFFECTS

Side-effects due to excess dopamine include choreiform, dystonic and other involuntary movements. Muscle twitching and blepharospasm are early signs of the need to reduce dose. Mental changes include paranoid ideation, psychosis, depression and dementia. Nausea is common. Less commonly, palpitations, orthostatic hypotension, bradykinesia (on-off), anorexia, vomiting, dizziness and somnolence.

POISONING/ TOXICITY

General supportive measures with gastric lavage if the patient presents early. ECG monitoring for arrhythmias.

PHARMACOKINETIC PROPERTIES

Carbidopa doubles the bioavailability and half-life of levodopa and increases plasma levels five fold.

Levodopa is metabolised peripherally and centrally. Half-life of combination is 2 hours. Levodopa excreted in urine largely as metabolites. CSF levels of amine metabolites should be monitored for optimisation of dose in metabolic disorders. Measurement of plasma prolactin maybe useful in monitoring (prolactin is high if amine replacement is inadequate).

EXCIPIENTS
See manufacturers SPC for further details.

LICENSED STATUS
Not licensed in <18 years or for disorders of tetrahydrobiopterin synthesis.

FURTHER INFORMATION
Extemporaneous formulation e.g. Nova Laboratories using Suspension Diluent A (xanthan gum 1%) as a suspending agent has a shelf life of 8 days stored at room temperature.

Co-phenotrope

A mixture of diphenoxylate hydrochloride and atropine sulphate in the mass proportions 100 parts to 1 part respectively. Diphenoxylate is a pethidine analogue that inhibits gastrointestinal motility locally and centrally. In high doses it may produce an opiate effect. Atropine is added in subtherapeutic doses to prevent abuse by deliberate overdose.

USES
Adjunctive therapy to appropriate rehydration in diarrhoea. Control of stool formation after colostomy or ileostomy. Relief of symptoms in mild chronic ulcerative colitis.

PRESENTATION
Tablet: co-phenotrope 2.5/0.025 (diphenoxylate hydrochloride 2.5mg, atropine sulphate 25 microgram) – Lomotil®.

DOSAGE

Route	Age			Frequency (times daily)	Notes
	1 month–2 years	2–12 years	12–18 years		
Oral	–	2–4 years 1/2 tablet	13–16 years 2 tablets	3	Dose for >2 years has been stated as 300–400 microgram/kg/**day** in 2–4 divided doses (dose as diphenoxylate).
		4–8 years 1 tablet		3	
		9–12 years 1 tablet		4	
			≥16 years 4 tablets then 2 tablets	initial dose 4	

ADMINISTRATION
Oral: tablets may be crushed if necessary.

CONTRA-INDICATIONS & WARNINGS
Contra-indicated in patients with known hypersensitivity to ingredients, in patients with jaundice, intestinal obstruction, acute ulcerative colitis and diarrhoea associated with pseudomembranous colitis. Appropriate fluid and electrolyte therapy should be given. Use with extreme caution in patients with advanced hepatorenal disease and those with abnormal liver function as it may precipitate hepatic coma.

INTERACTIONS
Structure of diphenoxylate resembles pethidine, therefore concurrent use with *MAOIs* could precipitate hypertensive crisis. Diphenoxylate may potentiate the action of *CNS depressants* such as *barbiturates, tranquillisers* and *alcohol.*

PREGNANCY
Studies have demonstrated no adverse effects but safety in

pregnancy has not been established. Caution recommended when used in early pregnancy.

BREAST-FEEDING
Diphenoxylate and atropine may be excreted in human milk. Infant may exhibit some effects of the drugs. Contact local Medicines Information Centre for advice.

SIDE-EFFECTS
CNS: malaise, lethargy, sedation, somnolence, confusion, dizziness, restlessness, depression, euphoria, hallucinations and headaches.
Allergic: anaphylaxis, angioedema, urticaria and pruritus.
Gastrointestinal: paralytic ileus, toxic megacolon, gastrointestinal intolerance (e.g. nausea and vomiting), anorexia and abdominal discomfort.
Atropine effects: flushing, dryness of skin and mucous membranes, tachycardia and urinary retention.

POISONING/TOXICITY
Overdose may produce narcosis with respiratory depression or atropine poisoning or both, particularly in children. Symptoms include dryness of the skin and mucous membranes, flushing, hyperthermia and tachycardia, nystagmus, pinpoint pupils, hypotonic reflexes, lethargy, coma and severe respiratory depression. Onset of symptoms may be considerably delayed and respiratory depression may not become evident until as late as 12-30 hours after ingestion and may recur in spite of initial response to narcotic antagonists. Continuous observation should be maintained for at least 48 hours. Naloxone should be given if respiratory arrest occurs; repeated injections may be required. Activated charcoal may be indicated if the patient is not comatose.

PHARMACOKINETIC PROPERTIES
Duration of effect 3–4 hours. Peak plasma concentrations occur at approximately 2 hours. Metabolised in the liver; approximately 50% excreted unchanged in the faeces.

LICENSED STATUS
Licensed for ≥4 years of age.

Co-trimoxazole

A 5:1 mixture of two antibiotics, sulfamethaxazole (sulphamethoxazole) and trimethoprim.

USES
Use should be limited to drug of choice for *Pneumocystis carinii pneumonia* (PCP), toxoplasmosis and nocardiasis. Use for urinary tract infections where there is evidence of bacterial sensitivity and good reason to prefer co-trimoxazole to a single antibiotic. For use in otitis media there must also be good reason to prefer it to a single antibiotic. Prophylaxis of PCP e.g. oncology patients.
In cystic fibrosis patients – for the treatment of chronic *Burkholderia cepacia* and *Stenotrophomonas maltophilia* infections; discuss with local microbiology department.

PRESENTATION
240mg of co-trimoxazole consists of 200mg sulfamethoxazole and 40mg trimethoprim.
480mg of co-trimoxazole consists of 400mg sulfamethoxazole and 80mg trimethoprim.
960mg of co-trimoxazole consists of 800mg sulfamethoxazole and 160mg trimethoprim.

IV infusion: 480mg co-trimoxazole in 5mL ampoule – Septrin® and non-proprietary; 960mg co-trimoxazole in 10mL ampoule – non-proprietary.
Oral suspension: 240mg of co-trimoxazole in 5mL – Septrin® Paediatric and non-proprietary; 480mg co-trimoxazole in 5mL – Septrin® Adult and non-proprietary.
Tablet: 480mg co-trimoxazole – Septrin® and non-proprietary; 960mg co-trimoxazole – Septrin Forte® and non-proprietary.

DOSAGE
Newborn infant (birth to 1 month)
The use of co-trimoxazole is not generally recommended (and manufacturers contra-indicate use) under 6 weeks of age, but some neonatologists feel that there is no specific reason for this caution other than the risk of haemolytic anaemia in babies with G6PD deficiency and the risk of kernicterus because sulfamethoxazole competes for the protein binding sites usually available to bilirubin in babies with jaundice. If co-trimoxazole is used in newborn infants (an unlicensed use) it is given in the same dosage as for 6 weeks-5 months (see table below) but trimethoprim on its own is now usually preferred to co-trimoxazole.

Child

Indication	Route	Age			Frequency (times daily)	Notes
		1 month–2 years	2–12 years	12–18 years		
Systemic infection	Oral	**DOSE BY WEIGHT** 24mg/kg		–	2	Dose may be doubled in severe infection.
		DOSE BY AGE				
		6 weeks–5 months 120mg	2–5 years 240mg	960mg	2	
		6 months–2 years 240mg	6–12 years 480mg		2	
	IV	← 18–27mg/kg →			2	The higher dose stated is that used in severe infection. Maximum single dose 1.44g.
Prophylaxis of urinary tract infection	Oral	← 12mg/kg →		480mg	1 (at night)	Only if bacterial sensitivities indicate and there is good reason to prefer co-trimoxazole to a single antibiotic.
Pneumocystis carinii treatment	Oral/IV	← 60mg/kg or →			2	For 10–14 days. Oral route is preferred unless nausea is severe.
		← 30mg/kg →			4	
Pneumocystis carinii prophylaxis	Oral	body surface area 0.5–0.75m^2 240mg		960mg	2	Give on three days of the week eg. Mondays, Wednesdays and Fridays or on two consecutive days according to the appropriate protocol/guidelines.
		body surface area 0.76–1m^2 360mg			2	
		body surface area >1m^2 480mg			2	

Dosage is indicated in terms of the total amount of drug in milligrams or millilitres e.g. 24mg/kg is 20mg/kg sulfamethoxazole and 4mg/kg trimethoprim.

Dose adjustment in renal impairment

Creatinine clearance (mL/minute/1.73m^2)	Dosage/dose frequency adjustment
>30	Normal dose
15–30	Normal dose for 3 days then half the dose
<15	Avoid unless haemodialysis is available, and then give half the normal dose.

Co-trimoxazole is not removed by peritoneal dialysis

ADMINISTRATION

Oral: take with food or drink to minimise the possibility of gastrointestinal disturbances.
IV: IV infusion must be diluted before administration and dilution should be carried out immediately before use. Dilute 1 in 25 with NaCl 0.9% or glucose 5%. In severely fluid restricted patients dilute 1 in 10 with glucose 5%. Dilution to less than 1 in 10 is not possible as the propylene glycol precipitates out. After adding co-trimoxazole for infusion to the infusion solution shake thoroughly to ensure complete mixing. If visible turbidity or crystallisation appears at any time before or during an infusion, the mixture should be discarded. Infuse over 60–90 minutes. In severe fluid restriction, co-trimoxazole can be given undiluted via the central route.

CONTRA-INDICATIONS & WARNINGS

A history of hypersensitivity to sulphonamides, trimethoprim or co-trimoxazole; marked liver parenchyma damage; severe renal insufficiency where repeated measurements of the plasma concentration cannot be performed. Avoid in patients with serious haematological disorders except under specialist supervision; regular monthly blood counts are advisable when given for long periods; discontinue immediately if blood disorders or rash develops. A folate supplement should also be considered with prolonged high dosage. Infusion contains sulphite which may cause allergic-type reactions including anaphylaxis.

INTERACTIONS
Co-trimoxazole has been shown to potentiate the anticoagulant activity of *warfarin*. Co-trimoxazole prolongs the half-life of *phenytoin*. If co-trimoxazole is considered appropriate therapy in patients receiving other *anti-folate drugs* e.g. *methotrexate*, a folate supplement should be considered (see contra-indications & warnings section).

SIDE-EFFECTS
Of the reported adverse reactions most are mild and comprise nausea, with or without vomiting, and skin rashes. Fatalities, although rare, have occurred due to severe reactions including Stevens-Johnson syndrome, Lyell syndrome (toxic epidermal necrolysis), fulminant hepatic necrosis, agranulocytosis, aplastic anaemia. The majority of haematological changes are mild and reversible when treatment is stopped. The changes are mainly leucopenia, neutropenia, thrombocytopenia and, less commonly, agranulocytosis, megaloblastic anaemia and purpura. Co-trimoxazole may induce haemolysis in certain susceptible G6PD deficient patients. At the high dosages used for the therapy of PCP, rash, fever, neutropenia, thrombocytopenia and raised liver enzymes have been reported, necessitating cessation of therapy. Concomitant administration of IV chlorphenamine (chlorpheniramine) may permit continued infusion.

PREGNANCY
Since sulfamethoxazole and trimethoprim are both folate antagonists, the manufacturers contra-indicate use of co-trimoxazole in pregnancy. Teratogenicity has, however, been encountered only in folate deficient animals and the drug has been in widespread clinical use for more than 20 years. Sulphonamide-containing products should not be administered in late pregnancy because of the risk of kernicterus.

BREAST-FEEDING
Despite the excretion of sulfamethoxazole into breast milk, the administration of co-trimoxazole to lactating women represents a negligible risk to the suckling infant.

POISONING/TOXICITY
Nausea, vomiting, dizziness and confusion are likely symptoms of overdose. Bone marrow depression has been reported in acute trimethoprim overdosage. General supportive measures are recommended. Seek the advice of a Poisons Centre for specific measures which may be undertaken.

PHARMACOKINETIC PROPERTIES
Peak plasma levels of trimethoprim and sulfamethoxazole are higher and achieved more rapidly after 1 hour of intravenous infusion than after oral administration of an equivalent dose. Elimination half-life shows no significant differences following either the oral or intravenous route. Approximately 50% of trimethoprim in the plasma is protein bound. The half-life in adults is in the range 8.6-17 hours in the presence of normal renal function. It is increased by a factor of 1.5-3 when the creatinine clearance is less than 10mL/minute. The principal route of excretion of trimethoprim is renal and approximately 50% of the dose is excreted in the urine within 24 hours as unchanged drug. Approximately 66% of sulfamethoxazole in the plasma is protein bound. The half-life in man is approximately 9-11 hours in the presence of normal renal function. There is no change in the half-life of active sulphamethoxazole with a reduction in renal function. The principle route of excretion of sulphamethoxazole is renal; between 15%-30% of the dose recovered in the urine is in the active form.

EXCIPIENTS
Septrin® dispersible tablets include saccharin sodium, infusion includes ethanol and propylene glycol, paediatric suspension includes saccharin sodium and sorbitol, adult suspension contains syrup and sucrose. Contact manufacturers for further details.

LICENSED STATUS
Licensed for ≥6 weeks of age.

Coconut oil preparations

USES
Treatment of scaly scalp disorders.

PRESENTATION
Ointment: Emulsifying Ointment 25% in Coconut Oil – manufactured 'special'.
Scalp ointment: coal tar solution 12%, salicylic acid 2%, precipitated sulphur 4%, in coconut oil emollient basis – Cocois®.

ADMINISTRATION
Apply to scalp, leave on at least 1 hour. Emulsifying ointment 25% in Coconut oil may be left on overnight. Remove by washing hair with mild shampoo. Treatment can be daily.

CONTRA-INDICATIONS & WARNINGS	SIDE-EFFECTS
Sensitivity to any of ingredients. Cocois® may stain fabric and jewellery.	Cocois® contains coal tar that may cause skin irritation.

LICENSED STATUS
Emulsifying Ointment 25% in Coconut Oil is unlicensed but contains emollients that are suitable for use in young children. Cocois® is licensed for >6 years of age.

FURTHER INFORMATION
Emulsifying Ointment 25% in Coconut Oil is available from BCM Specials manufacturing.

Codeine phosphate

Opioid analgesic.

USES
Mild to moderate pain.

PRESENTATION
Injection: 60mg in 1mL – non-proprietary (controlled drug).
Linctus: 15mg in 5ml – Codeine Linctus BP, non-proprietary.
Suppository: 1mg, 2mg, 3mg and 6mg (other strengths on request) – manufactured 'specials'.
Syrup: 25mg in 5mL – non-proprietary.
Tablet: 15mg, 30mg and 60mg – non-proprietary.

DOSAGE

Route	Age				Frequency (times daily)	Notes
	birth–1 month	1 month–2 years	2–12 years	12–18 years		
Oral Rectal IM/SC	← 500 microgram – 1mg/kg →			30–60mg	4–6 (maximum daily dose 240mg)	Repeated doses increase the risk of respiratory depression. Avoid IM injections if possible. Use IM/SC cannula placed while under GA or topical LA. Codeine phosphate can cause severe constipation so prophylactic laxatives should always be prescribed.

Reduce dose in moderate/severe renal impairment if use cannot be avoided.

Although doses are given from birth in the above table, codeine is rarely recommended <3 months and is not licensed for use <1 year. There is little published experience of its use in the neonatal period and caution is necessary in neonates and children as they show an increased susceptibility to respiratory depression.

ADMINISTRATION
Must **not** be given intravenously as it causes histamine release, which may result in reduced cardiac output.

CONTRA-INDICATIONS & WARNINGS
Contra-indicated in paralytic ileus.
Warning: avoid in acute respiratory depression.
Caution: renal impairment; hepatic impairment may precipitate coma. High doses of codeine are pharmacologically very similar to small doses of morphine. If codeine provides inadequate analgesia, major opioids such as morphine should be the next step.

INTERACTIONS
Enhanced sedative effect with *anxiolytics* and *hypnotics*. Antagonism of gastrointestinal effects of *cisapride*, *metoclopramide* and *domperidone*. Possible increase of plasma concentration with *cimetidine*.

PREGNANCY
Use in the third trimester may depress neonatal respiration. Contact local Medicines Information Centre for advice.

BREAST-FEEDING
Amount in breast milk too small to be harmful.

SIDE-EFFECTS
May cause excessive sedation in children, constipation after long-term use, and respiratory depression with high doses.

POISONING/TOXICITY
Doses of 5mg/kg or more have resulted in respiratory failure. Naloxone may be used as an antidote.

PHARMACOKINETIC PROPERTIES
Codeine is metabolised by O- and N-demethylation in the liver. Codeine and its metabolites are excreted almost entirely by the kidney.

EXCIPIENTS
Contact manufacturers for further details.

LICENSED STATUS
Not licensed for use in children <1 year old. The rectal route is an unlicensed route of administration using an unlicensed product.

C

Colchicine

Thought to inhibit the motility of leucocytes, hindering their passage to the site of inflammation.

USES
Prophylaxis in Familial Mediterranean fever and other related periodic syndromes.

PRESENTATION
Tablet: 500 microgram – non-proprietary.

DOSAGE

Route	Age				Frequency (times daily)	Notes
	birth–1 month	1 month–2 years	2–12 years	12–18 years		
Oral	-	←	20-30 microgram/kg (maximum 2mg)	→	1	May be given in 2 divided doses.

CONTRA-INDICATIONS & WARNINGS
Should not be used in patients with blood dyscrasias of any nature. Colchicine should be used with caution in patients with decreased renal function as they are at increased risk of neuromuscular toxicity and bone marrow dysplasia. Use with caution in patients with gastrointestinal, hepatic or cardiac disease. Periodic blood counts should be performed in patients receiving long-term colchicine.

INTERACTIONS
Colchicine may increase *ciclosporin (cyclosporin)* levels. Absorption of *vitamin B_{12}* from the gastrointestinal tract may be reduced. *Erythromycin* may induce colchicine toxicity if the two drugs are used together.

PREGNANCY
It has been suggested that colchicine may affect sperm. Azoospermia has been reported. Colchicine crosses the placenta and has been shown to be teratogenic in animal studies. The limited human data available does not suggest a major teratogenic risk in humans. Caution must always be exercised in the use of colchicine in pregnancy, but in the treatment of Familial Mediterranean fever, the benefits may outweigh the risks. Contact local Medicines Information Centre for advice.

BREAST-FEEDING
Colchicine enters breast milk in high concentrations. In one case report, no adverse effects were seen in a nursing infant whose mother was receiving colchicine. Relevant information is limited, and caution is advised. Contact local Medicines Information Centre for advice.

SIDE-EFFECTS
Nausea, vomiting, diarrhoea, or abdominal pain may occur, and these symptoms are early signs of toxicity. Therapy with colchicine should be discontinued until

symptoms disappear. Bone marrow depression and blood dyscrasias including anaemia, leucopenia, neutropenia, pancytopenia and thrombocytopenia. Myopathy and neuropathy, especially after long-term therapy. Anuria and renal damage. Azoospermia.

POISONING/TOXICITY
Acute toxicity results in nausea, anorexia, pain, vomiting, ileus and diarrhoea which may be bloody. Also stomatitis, arthralgia, malaise, hypocalcaemia, fever and rashes may occur. Dehydration may lead to shock and cardiovascular collapse.
Acute renal failure and tender hepatomegaly have been seen. Other adverse effects include convulsions, delirium, muscle weakness, neuropathy and ascending paralysis of the CNS. Bone marrow depression with leucopenia may be followed by rebound leucocytosis.
There is no specific antidote. Treatment is symptomatic and supportive. Respiration, blood pressure and circulation should be controlled and fluid and electrolyte imbalances should be corrected.

PHARMACOKINETIC PROPERTIES
Colchicine is rapidly absorbed, and peak plasma concentrations are seen within 0.5-2 hours. The drug is partially metabolised in the liver.

EXCIPIENTS
Contact manufacturer for further details.

LICENSED STATUS
Licensed for gout. Not licensed for Familial Mediterranean fever.

Colecalciferol (cholecalciferol, vitamin D3)

USES
Rickets due to vitamin D deficiency.

PRESENTATION
Oral solution: 3000 units in 1mL; 10mL and 50mL vials – manufactured 'special'.
Tablets: see ergocalciferol monograph.

DOSAGE

Route	Age			Frequency (times daily)	Notes
	1 month–2 years	2–12 years	12–18 years		
Oral	< 6 months 3000 units	6000 units	10,000 units	1	
	> 6 months 6000 units			1	

Check biochemistry after 6 weeks of treatment which can be stopped once alkaline phosphatase and parathyroid hormone (PTH) are normal.

CONTRA-INDICATIONS & WARNINGS
Hypercalcaemia. No dose adjustment required in renal impairment, but effect may be reduced due to impaired metabolic activation.

INTERACTIONS
Concurrent administration of drugs which induce hepatic microsomal enzymes, such as barbiturates and anticonvulsants, is likely to reduce the half-life of colecalciferol and deplete stores in the liver.

PREGNANCY
Safety in pregnant women is not established. Contact local Medicines Information Centre for advice.

BREAST-FEEDING
Hypercalcaemia is likely to result if a nursing mother taking physiological doses of colecalciferol breast-feeds.

SIDE-EFFECTS
Infants and children are more susceptible to adverse effects. Hypercalcaemia and hypercalciuria may occur and indicate excessive dosage. Signs and symptoms of hypercalcaemia may be seen: anorexia, nausea, vomiting, headache, weakness, apathy, somnolence, thirst, dehydration, polyuria, nocturia, abdominal pain, paralytic ileus, cardiac arrhythmias, overt psychosis, metastatic calcification. Mild, non-progressive and reversible elevations of LFTs occur occasionally.

POISONING/TOXICITY
Gastric lavage may be helpful if performed within 6-8 hours of ingestion. If hypercalcaemia should occur, supportive measures, including adequate hydration, should be initiated.

PHARMACODYNAMIC PROPERTIES
Colecalciferol is the inactive precursor of 1,25-dihydroxycholecalciferol whose major therapeutic and physiological action is on the intestine where it acts to promote the absorption of calcium and phosphate. The active metabolite also acts on receptors on bone osteoblasts, and has a parathyroid hormone-like action on osteoclast bone resorption.

EXCIPIENTS
Contact manufacturers for further details.

LICENSED STATUS
The oral solution is a 'special' and as such is unlicensed.

FURTHER INFORMATION
Oral solution is available from Martindale Pharmaceuticals.

Colestipol hydrochloride

C

Ion-exchange resin which lowers plasma cholesterol levels through binding with bile acids in the intestinal lumen.

USES
Hyperlipidaemias including familial hypercholesterolaemia in patients who have not responded adequately to diet after 6 months-1 year.

PRESENTATION
Granules: 5g per sachet – Colestid® and Colestid® Orange.

DOSAGE/ADMINISTRATION
Oral: see colestyramine (cholestyramine) monograph; follow the same dosage recommendations.

CONTRA-INDICATIONS & WARNINGS
Complete biliary obstruction (unlikely to be of benefit).

INTERACTIONS, PREGNANCY/BREAST-FEEDING, SIDE-EFFECTS, POISONING/TOXICITY
See colestyramine monograph.

EXCIPIENTS
Colestid® Orange includes aspartame. See manufacturers SPC for further details.

LICENSED STATUS
Manufacturers SPC indicates that experience in children is limited but that it has been used in older children and young adults.

Colestyramine (cholestyramine)

Basic anion-exchange resin.

USES
Relief of pruritus associated with partial biliary obstruction; familial hypercholesterolaemia; relief of diarrhoea associated with ileal resection; Crohn's disease; vagotomy, diabetic vagal neuropathy; management of radiation-induced diarrhoea.

PRESENTATION
Powder: sachet, 4g colestyramine in 9g powder – Questran®; sachet, 4g colestyramine in 5g powder – Questran Light®.

DOSAGE

Indication	Route	Age		Frequency (times daily)	Notes
		2–12 years	12–18 years		
Cholesterol reduction	Oral	≥ 6 years $$dose = \frac{wt\ (kg) \times A\ (g)}{70}$$ where wt = child's weight and A = adult dose	1 sachet (4g) (see table 3 below for maintenance)	1	Starting dose: then adjust dose appropriate to symptom control and give as a single daily dose or in divided doses up to 4 times daily. Maximum dose of 9 sachets per day has been used in adults.
Cholestatic pruritis	Oral	< 6 years / Half a sachet (2g) ≥ 6 years / 1 sachet (4g)	1-2 sachets (4-8g)	1	
Diarrhoea	Oral	◄──── as cholesterol reduction above ────►		1	Initiate alternative therapy if no response within 3 days.

Colestyramine is not licensed for use in children <6 years, but the following doses have been used.

Age range	Dose	Frequency
Neonates	270mg Questran Light® (≡ 216mg colestyramine)	3 times daily
Infants <1 year	550mg Questran Light® (≡ 440mg colestyramine)	4 times daily
Children 1-6 years	As for children >6 years	

Children and adolescents with familial hypercholesterolaemia.

The following table is a guide to the number of 4g sachets of colestyramine required daily (depending on the total cholesterol and LDL-C levels after an adequate trial of dietary intervention of 6 months-1 year). Dietary intervention must continue in addition to colestyramine. Consider folic acid supplementation in familial hypercholesterolaemia.

Daily number of 4g colestyramine sachets	Total cholesterol		LDL–C levels	
	mmol/L	(mg/dL)	mmol/L	(mg/dL)
1	<6.3	(245)	<5.04	(195)
2	6.3–7.7	(245–300)	5.04–6.07	(195–235)
3	7.78–8.92	(310–345)	6.1–7.2	(236–280)
4	>8.92	(>345)		

ADMINISTRATION

The contents of the sachet should be mixed with water or other suitable liquid such as fruit juice, skimmed milk, thin soups and pulped fruits, such as apple sauce. The powder should not be taken dry.

CONTRA-INDICATIONS & WARNINGS
Unlikely to be of benefit in complete biliary obstruction. Consider folic acid supplementation in familial hypercholesterolaemia.

INTERACTIONS
Colestyramine may delay or reduce the absorption of *digoxin, tetracycline, chlorothiazide, warfarin, levothyroxine (thyroxine), fat-soluble vitamins (A, D, E and K)* and *mycophenolate mofetil*. Administration of these drugs, and others where normal bioavailability is critical, should be made 1 hour before, or 4-6 hours after, administration of colestyramine.

PREGNANCY/BREAST-FEEDING
Unlikely to be problematic. Consider possibility of interference of absorption of fat-soluble vitamins.

SIDE-EFFECTS
Impaired absorption of dietary and supplemental fat-soluble vitamins (A, D, E and K). Chronic treatment may result in an increased bleeding tendency and other effects of vitamin K deficiency. Hyperchloraemic acidosis is reported after prolonged treatment with anionic exchange resins. Constipation responds to usual treatments and often resolves with continuing treatment. Heartburn and flatulence, nausea and vomiting. Diarrhoea may occur with large doses.

POISONING/TOXICITY
Risk in overdosage should be minimal, with the most likely effect being obstruction of the gastrointestinal tract.

PHARMACODYNAMIC PROPERTIES
Colestyramine is not absorbed in the gut and its affinity for bile acids in the intestinal tract prevents their reabsorption. To compensate for the faecal loss of bile acids, their major precursor, cholesterol, is oxidised at an increased rate in the liver and plasma cholesterol levels are thus lowered.

EXCIPIENTS
Questran® includes sucrose. Questran Light® includes aspartame. See manufacturers SPC for further details.

LICENSED STATUS
Licensed for ≥6 years of age.

Colistin

A polymyxin antibiotic active against Gram-negative organisms, including *Pseudomonas aeruginosa*.

USES
In cystic fibrosis patients – nebulised treatment for first isolates of *Pseudomonas aeruginosa* (widely used as a long-term treatment for patients chronically infected) in combination with oral ciprofloxacin; IV treatment of early *Pseudomonas aeruginosa* infections not cleared by ciprofloxacin plus nebulised colistin, treatment of moderate to severe exacerbations in combination with an aminoglycoside and treatment of multiresistant organisms, in combination with an aminoglycoside, where there are no available alternatives.
Selective decontamination of the digestive tract (SDD).

PRESENTATION
Injection: 500,000 unit and 1 million unit vial (colistimethate sodium (colistin sulphomethate sodium)) – Colomycin®.
Solution: may be prepared extemporaneously.
Syrup: (as sulphate) 250,000 unit in 5mL – Colomycin®.
Tablet: (scored) 1.5 million unit – Colomycin®.

DOSAGE

Route	Age			Frequency	Notes
	1 month–2 years	2–12 years	12–18 years	(times daily)	
Nebulised	<1 year 500,000 units	<10 years 1 million units	2 million units	2	Cystic fibrosis.
	>1 year 1 million units	>10 years 2 million units		2	
IV infusion	16,666–25,000 units/kg	<60 kg 16,666–25,000 units/kg	>60kg 2 million units	3	Cystic fibrosis; multiresistant organisms.
Oral	–	<5 years 750,000 units	3 million units	4	Selective decontamination of digestive tract, given with tobramycin and amphotericin. Unlicensed and limited experience of use.
		5–12 years 1.5 million units		4	

ADMINISTRATION
Nebulised: reconstitute vial in 2-4mL Water for Injections or NaCl 0.9%. Administer after physiotherapy and bronchodilators. An active venturi nebuliser with outlet is recommended so that exhaled antibiotic can be discharged via a window otherwise an effective filter system should be used.
Colistin must not be mixed with tobramycin as they are chemically unstable. It may be mixed with gentamicin if time factor is crucial. Gentamicin dose may be added to colistin vial immediately before use and then made up to 3mL with NaCl 0.9%. Reconstituted vials for aerosol administration are stable for 1 week at room temperature or 1 month at 2-4°C.
IV: give over 30 minutes. Solutions for parenteral administration must be freshly prepared. Reduce IV dose in renal impairment.

CONTRA-INDICATIONS & WARNINGS

Contra-indicated in patients with known hypersensitivity to colistin or colistimethate sodium. Bronchospasm may occur when nebulised – treat with beta-agonist. Caution in acute porphyria.

INTERACTIONS

Enhanced muscle relaxant effect with *muscle relaxants*. Increased risk of ototoxicity and nephrotoxicity with *loop diuretics, aminoglycosides, ciclosporin (cyclosporin), amphotericin* and *cisplatin.*

PREGNANCY

Safety in pregnancy has not been established but colistin has been used in pregnant patients where benefits outweigh the risks. Contact local Medicines Information Centre for advice.

BREAST-FEEDING

Colistin is excreted in breast milk and is contra-indicated during breast-feeding. Contact local Medicines Information Centre for advice.

SIDE-EFFECTS

Bronchospasm if inhaled. Other side-effects are minimal with nebulisation but the following have been noted with IV administration: impaired renal function, muscle weakness, facial paraesthesia, slurred speech, visual disturbance and apnoea.

POISONING/TOXICITY

Unlikely with nebulisation. Following systemic administration, overdose can result in renal insufficiency, muscle weakness, and apnoea. There is no specific antidote; treatment should be supportive plus diuresis or dialysis to remove colistin or colistimethate sodium.

PHARMACOKINETIC PROPERTIES

Absorption from inhaled route negligible.

EXCIPIENTS

Syrup includes sucrose. See manufacturers SPC for further details.

LICENSED STATUS

Injection licensed for IV and nebulised use in children and adults, tablets and syrup licensed for use in children and adults; however the doses stated are higher than those recommended by the manufacturers e.g. IV doses over 16,666 units/kg per dose are unlicensed for <60kg. Although the syrup is licensed for bowel preparation, there is limited information on its use in SDD.

FURTHER INFORMATION

Various salts of colistin are not bioequivalent. 1mg colistimethate sodium ≡12,500 units; 1mg colistin sulphate ≡ 19,500 units; 1mg colistin base ≡ 30,000 units.

Copper histidine

USES

Menke's disease (anecdotal evidence of use).

PRESENTATION

Injection: 500 microgram elemental copper in 1mL – manufactured 'special'.

DOSAGE

It is important that the dosage be suited to the individual patient.

Route	Age				Frequency (times daily)	Notes
	birth–1 month	1 month–2 years	2–12 years	12–18 years		
SC	← 50–150 microgram elemental copper/kg →				1	
IM	← 200 microgram elemental copper →				1	Increase to 300 micrograms after 2 weeks then 400 micrograms after 7 weeks then 450 microgram after 9 weeks and then 1mg after 12 months if necessary.

CONTRA-INDICATIONS & WARNINGS
Hypersensitivity to any of the injection ingredients.

INTERACTIONS, PREGNANCY, BREAST-FEEDING
No information available.

SIDE-EFFECTS
Pain at the site of injection may be experienced. Copper supplementation in Menke's disease carries the risk of systemic copper overload especially in the kidney, heart, skeletal muscle, spleen and pancreas. Routine monitoring for side-effects of therapy include: FBC, measurement of creatinine, urea, liver enzymes, alkaline phosphatase, ammonia; serum protein electrophoresis, clotting tests (monthly); renal ultrasound (every 2 months); ECG and echocardiogram (every 4 months); fractional sodium excretion; tubular phosphate reabsorption; glucose, protein and amino acid excretion in the urine; 24 hour copper excretion tests.

POISONING/TOXICITY
Risk of copper overload (see side-effects).

PHARMACODYNAMIC PROPERTIES
Menke's disease is a disorder of copper handling, characterised by low serum, liver and brain copper levels. Copper histidine is given as replacement therapy as copper uptake by the liver and brain is thought to be mediated by histidine. The efficacy of early treatment may be the result of making copper available during the critical period of myelination and development of the CNS.

LICENSED STATUS
Available as a 'special' and as such is unlicensed.

FURTHER INFORMATION
The injection is available as a 'special' from Northwick Park Hospital, London.
It should be protected from light and stored in a refrigerator. Do not use if the solution is blue-black or black in colour; it should be a clear, bright, prussian blue coloured solution.

C

Corticosteroids (local oral use)

USES
Used as a local, topical application of steroid in the treatment of painful conditions of the oral and circumoral mucosa. The adherence of the paste to mucosa aims to prolong contact of the drug with the mucosa.

PRESENTATION
Inhaler: beclometasone (beclomethasone) dipropionate 50 microgram per metered dose inhaler – Becotide® 50 and non proprietary.
Oral paste: triamcinolone acetonide 0.1% in carmellose sodium – Adcortyl in Orabase®.
Pellets (lozenges): hydrocortisone 2.5mg (as sodium succinate) – Corlan®.
Tablet: (soluble) betamethasone 500 micrograms (as sodium phosphate) – Betnesol®.

DOSAGE/ADMINISTRATION
Inhaler: 1 puff directed onto the oral lesion 4 times daily.
Oral paste: apply a thin layer of paste 2–4 times daily to the affected area (do not rub in); use limited to 5 days in children.
Pellets: 2.5mg 4 times daily, allowed to dissolve slowly adjacent to the lesion.
Tablet: 500 micrograms dissolved in 15-20mLs of water and used as a mouthwash for 3 minutes, 4 times daily.
In severe cases the beclometasone inhaler and betametasone soluble tablets may be used in combination.

CONTRA-INDICATIONS & WARNINGS
Not advised in untreated oral infections. Not to be used in patients with a history of hypersensitivity to the product components, tuberculosis and most viral conditions, especially herpes and varicella. Only to be used in fungal or bacterial infections with simultaneous use of appropriate anti-infectives.

INTERACTIONS
As for other corticosteroids but unlikely in the dosages, and by the route administered. Limit to a 5 day course in children to avoid adrenal suppression.

SIDE-EFFECTS
May exacerbate existing local infection (which must be simultaneously treated). Any adverse effects reversed readily on stopping treatment.

POISONING/TOXICITY
As for corticosteroids but unlikely in dosages used. In suspected cases of overdosage, monitor and treat symptomatically.

EXCIPIENTS
Beclometasone inhalers – see beclometasone monograph for details. Betnesol® includes saccharin sodium.

LICENSED STATUS
Adcortyl in Orabase® and Corlan® are licensed for use in children and adults for the above indication but beclometasone inhalers are not. The use of Betnesol® tablets, as a mouthwash, is not a licensed indication.

Corticosteroids (topical)

Suppress various components of the inflammatory skin reaction.

USES
Treatment of inflammatory skin disorders such as eczema.

PRESENTATION

CORTICOSTEROID PRODUCTS

Drug Name	Proprietary Name	Presentation	Potency
Hydrocortisone	Several proprietary and non-proprietary preparations available	Cream 0.1%: 30g	Mild
		0.5%, 1%: 15g, 30g	
		Ointment 0.5%, 1%:15g,30g	Mild
Alclometasone dipropionate	Modrasone®	Cream 0.05%: 50g	Moderate
		Ointment 0.05%: 50g	Moderate
Clobetasone butyrate	Eumovate®	Cream 0.05%: 30g, 100g	Moderate
		Ointment 0.05%: 30g, 100g.	Moderate
Desoximetasone (desoxymethasone)	Stiedex®	Oily cream 0.05%: 30g,100g	Moderate
Fluocortolone	Ultralanum Plain®	Cream 0.25%: 50g	Moderate
		Ointment 0.25%: 50g	Moderate
Fludroxycortide/ Flurandrenolone	Haelan®	Cream 0.0125%: 60g	Moderate
		Ointment 0.0125%: 60g	Moderate
		Tape 4 microgram/cm² 7.5cm x 50cm, 7.5cm x 200cm	Potent
Betamethasone valerate	Betnovate RD®	Cream 0.025%: 100g	Moderate
		Ointment 0.025%: 100g	Moderate
	Betnovate®	Cream 0.1%: 30g, 100g	Potent
	non-proprietary also available for 0.1% cream and ointment	Ointment 0.1%: 30g, 100g	Potent
	Betnovate®, Betacap®	Scalp application 0.1%: 100mL	Potent
	Betnovate®	Lotion 0.1%: 100mL	Potent
	Bettamousse®	Foam (scalp application) 0.1%: 100g	Potent
Betamethasone dipropionate	Diprosone®	Cream 0.05%: 30g, 100g	Potent
		Ointment 0.05%: 30g,100g	Potent
		Lotion 0.05%: 30mL,100mL	Potent
Fluocinolone acetonide	Synalar 1 in 10 Dilution®	Cream 0.0025%: 50g	Mild
	Synalar 1 in 4 Dilution®	Cream, ointment 0.00625%: 50g	Moderate
	Synalar®	Cream, ointment, gel 0.025%: 30g	Potent

C

Drug Name	Proprietary Name	Presentation	Potency
Hydrocortisone butyrate	Locoid®	Cream 0.1%: 30g, 100g	Potent
		Lipocream 0.1%: 30g, 100g	Potent
	Locoid Crelo®	Ointment 0.1%: 30g, 100g	Potent
		Scalp lotion 0.1%: 100mL	Potent
		Topical lotion 0.1%: 100g	Potent
Fluocinonide	Metosyn®	Cream 0.05%: 25g, 100g	Potent
		Ointment 0.05%: 25g,100g	Potent
Fluticasone propionate	Cutivate®	Cream 0.05%: 15g, 50g	Potent
		Ointment 0.005%: 15g, 50g	Potent
Mometasone furoate	Elocon®	Cream, ointment 0.1%: 30g,100g	Potent
		Scalp lotion 0.1%: 30mL	Potent
Beclometasone (beclomethasone) dipropionate	Propaderm®	Cream 0.025%: 30g	Potent
		Ointment 0.025%: 30g	Potent
Diflucortolone valerate	Nerisone®	Cream 0.1%: 30g	Potent
		Oily cream 0.1%: 30g	Potent
		Ointment 0.1%: 30g	Potent
	Nerisone Forte®	Oily cream 0.3%: 15g	Very potent
		Ointment 0.3%: 15g	Very potent
Clobetasol propionate	Dermovate®	Cream 0.05%: 30g,100g	Very potent
		Ointment 0.05%: 30g,100g	Very potent
		Scalp application 0.05%: 30mL, 100mL	Very potent
Halcinonide	Halciderm Topical®	Cream 0.1%: 30g	Very potent

CORTICOSTEROID COMBINATION PRODUCTS

Corticosteroid	Other Active Ingredient	Proprietary Name	Presentation	Potency
Hydrocortisone 0.5% with	Nystatin 100,000 units/g, chlorhexidine 1%	Nystaform-HC®	Cream 30g	Mild
	Nystatin 100,000 units/g, benzalkonium chloride solution 0.2%, dimethicone '350' 10%	Timodine®	Cream 30g	Mild
Hydrocortisone 1% with	Clotrimazole 1%	Canestan HC®	Cream 30g	Mild
	Miconazole 2%	Daktacort®	Cream 30g	Mild
			Ointment 30g	Mild
	Fusidic Acid 2%	Fucidin H®	Cream 30g, 60g	Mild
			Ointment 30g, 60g	Mild
	Oxytetracycline 3%	Terra-Cortril®	Ointment 15g, 30g	Mild
	Clioquinol 3%	Vioform-Hydrocortisone®	Cream 30g	Mild
			Ointment 30g	Mild
	Nystatin 100,000 units/g chlorhexidine acetate 1%	Nystaform-HC®	Ointment 30g	Mild
	Nystatin 100,000 units/g oxytetracycline 3%	Terra-Cortril Nystatin®	Cream 30g	Mild
	Econazole nitrate 1%	Econacort®	Cream 30g	Mild
Hydrocortisone 1% with	Neomycin sulphate 0.4%, nystatin 100,000 units/g, polymixin B sulphate 7250 units/g	Gregoderm®	Ointment 15g	Mild
	Potassium hydroxyquinoline sulphate 0.5%	Quinocort®	Cream 30g	Mild

C

Corticosteroid	Other Active Ingredient	Proprietary Name	Presentation	Potency
Hydrocortisone butyrate 0.1% with	Chlorquinaldol 3%	Locoid C®	Cream 30g	Potent
			Ointment 30g	Potent
Betamethasone diproprionate 0.05% with	Salicylic Acid 3%	Diprosalic ®	Ointment 30g, 100g	Potent
	Salicylic acid 2%		Scalp application 100mL	Potent
	Clotrimazole 1%	Lotriderm®	Cream 15g	Potent
Betamethasone valerate 0.1% with	Clioquinol 3%	Betnovate C®	Cream 30g	Potent
			Ointment 30g	Potent
	Neomycin 0.5%	Betnovate N®	Cream 30g, 100g	Potent
			Ointment 30g, 100g	Potent
	Fusidic acid 2%	FuciBET®	Cream 30g, 60g	Potent
Clobetasol propionate 0.05% with	Neomycin 0.5%, nystatin 100,000 units/g	Dermovate NN®	Cream 30g	Very Potent
			Ointment 30g	Very Potent
Clobetasol butyrate 0.05 % with	Oxytetracycline 3%, nystatin 100,000 units/g	Trimovate®	Cream 30g	Moderate
Fluocinolone 0.025% with	Clioquinol 3%	Synalar C®	Cream 15g	Potent
			Ointment 15g	Potent
	Neomycin 0.5%	Synalar N®	Cream 30g	Potent
			Ointment 30g	Potent
Triamcinolone acetonide 0.1% with	Chlortetracycline hydrochloride 3%	Aureocort®	Ointment 15g	Potent

DOSAGE
Initial treatment, certainly in infants <12 months, should always be with the weakest topical steroid, hydrocortisone. Apply sparingly to the affected areas once or twice a day.

ADMINISTRATION
Topical: a small quantity of the preparation should be applied thinly to the inflamed areas of skin.

CONTRA-INDICATIONS & WARNINGS
Prolonged use of corticosteroids, especially preparations more potent than hydrocortisone, should be avoided on the face. Topical corticosteroids are contra-indicated in untreated fungal skin lesions, rosacea, perioral dermatitis and acne vulgaris.

PREGNANCY
There is inadequate evidence of safety in human pregnancy. Topical administration of corticosteroids to pregnant animals can cause abnormalities of fetal development including cleft palate and intra uterine growth retardation. There may therefore be a very small risk of such effects in the human fetus.

BREAST-FEEDING
Contact local Medicines Information Centre for advice.

SIDE-EFFECTS
Unlike the potent and very potent preparations, the moderate and mild corticosteroids are rarely associated with side-effects. The more potent the preparation, the larger the area to be treated and the younger the patient, the more care is required, as absorption through the skin can cause pituitary-adrenal-axis suppression and Cushing's syndrome.
Local: atrophic changes in the skin such as striae, thinning and dilation of the superficial blood vessels, especially with preparations more potent than hydrocortisone.

TOXICITY
Chronic overdose or misuse may cause the features of Cushing's syndrome.

EXCIPIENTS
The following additives may be associated with sensitisation of eczematous skin: wool fat (lanolin), chlorocresol, fragrances, ethylenediamine, benzylalcohol, butylated hydroxyanisole, butylated hydroxytoluene, hydroxybenzoates, polysorbates, propyl glycol and sorbic acid. Contact the manufacturers for further details.

LICENSED STATUS
All products are licensed for >1 year of age.

FURTHER INFORMATION
Dilution of these preparations is not recommended. However some preparations e.g. Betnovate® and Propaderm® are diluted 1 in 10 with aqueous cream or cetomacragol for wet wrap dressings with Tubifast® although this is not within the licensed applications.

Corticotropin (corticotrophin) (ACTH)

A naturally occurring hormone secreted by the anterior lobe of the pituitary gland.

USES
Drug of second or third choice for infantile spasms (particularly for the idiopathic type); rarely the drug of first choice. Rarely used in severe myoclonic epilepsy.

PRESENTATION
Injection: gelatin-containing depot preparation 40 units in 1mL – named patient.

DOSAGE

Route	Age				Frequency (times daily)	Notes
	birth–1 month	1 month–2 years	2–12 years	12–18 years		
IM/SC injection	-	←	20–80 units	→	1	Initial dose. Frequency of administration and duration of treatment are individually determined.

ADMINISTRATION
IM/SC: it must not be given by IV injection. Administer in the morning to minimise 'growth interference'. Rotate sites of administration.

CONTRA-INDICATIONS & WARNINGS
Hypersensitivity to corticotropin or any component of the injection, congestive heart failure, severe untreated bacterial and viral infections, peptic ulcer.

INTERACTIONS
As for corticosteroids (see prednisolone monograph).

PREGNANCY/BREAST-FEEDING
No data specific to corticotropin. See prednisolone monograph for information on corticosteroids in pregnancy.

SIDE-EFFECTS
Corticotropin stimulates the adrenals to produce cortisol (hydrocortisone) and mineralocorticoids; it therefore has the potential to produce similar adverse effects as those of the corticosteroids.
CNS: headache, mood swings, seizures, pseudotumour cerebri.
Dermatological: skin atrophy, bruising, hyperpigmentation, acne, hirsutism.

Endocrine and metabolic: amenorrhoea, Cushing syndrome, hyperglycaemia, bone growth suppression, sodium and water retention; considerable potassium loss may also occur.
Gastrointestinal: abdominal distension, ulcerative oesophagitis, pancreatitis.
Musculoskeletal: muscle wasting. Hypersensitivity reactions can also occur.

POISONING/TOXICITY
Overdosage may lead to fluid retention, hypokalaemia, hyperglycaemia and symptoms of Cushing syndrome. There is no known antidote; treatment should be symptomatic.

PHARMACOKINETIC PROPERTIES
Corticotropin is ineffective when given by mouth. The depot preparation formulated with gelatin is absorbed over a period of 8-16 hours and has a duration of action of 24 hours or more when administered SC or IM. It is excreted in the urine.

EXCIPIENTS
Contact manufacturer for further details.

LICENSED STATUS
Not licensed for use in the UK.

FURTHER INFORMATION
It may be imported via Farillon. If corticotropin gel is not available then tetracosactrin depot injection may be substituted. 40 units of corticotropin gel is approximately equivalent to 500 microgram tetracosactrin depot injection.

A polypeptide that stimulates the release of adrenocorticotrophic hormone from the anterior pituitary.

USES
Anterior pituitary testing for secretion of adrenocorticotrophic hormone.

PRESENTATION
Injection: 100 microgram vial, CRF (CRH) corticorelin (human) – named patient.

DOSAGE
1 microgram/kg to a maximum of 100 microgram by IV injection, as a single dose.

ADMINISTRATION
IV: the powder should be reconstituted with the diluent provided before administration by IV injection.

CONTRA-INDICATIONS & WARNINGS Hypersensitivity to CRF. **PREGNANCY/ BREAST-FEEDING** Contact local Medicines Information Centre for advice.	**SIDE-EFFECTS** Flushing of the face, neck and upper body, mild sensations of smell and taste. **POISONING/TOXICITY** Decreases in blood pressure with an accelerated cardiac action and an increased prolactin secretion may occur.

LICENSED STATUS
Not licensed for use in children.

FURTHER INFORMATION
CRH Ferring is available from Shire Pharmaceuticals.

Crotamiton

Antipruritic and weak acaricide.

USES
Treatment of itch, especially that associated with scabies.

PRESENTATION
Cream: 10% – Eurax®.
Lotion: 10% – Eurax®.

DOSAGE/ADMINISTRATION
Topical: after patient has had a warm bath and dried well, the preparation should be rubbed into the entire body surface excluding face and scalp. The application should be repeated once daily preferably in the evening for a total of 3-5 days. Children <3 years of age should not apply crotamiton more than once a day.

CONTRA-INDICATIONS & WARNINGS Avoid use near eyes and broken skin. Acute exudative dermatoses. **PREGNANCY** Not recommended during pregnancy, especially first trimester. Contact local Medicines Information Centre for advice. **BREAST-FEEDING** Not known if excreted in milk. Nursing mothers should	avoid applying crotamiton to nipple area. Contact local Medicines Information Centre for advice. **POISONING/TOXICITY** Symptoms of ingestion are nausea, vomiting and irritation of buccal and oesophageal and gastric mucosa. No specific antidote. General supportive measures and symptomatic treatment may be given. There is a risk of methaemoglobinaemia which may be treated with methylthioninium chloride (methylene blue).

EXCIPIENTS
See manufacturers SPC for further details.

LICENSED STATUS
Licensed for use in both children and adults.

Sedative antihistamine with antimuscarinic activity.

USES
Anti-emetic in the management of intractable vomiting of known causes including: drug-induced nausea and vomiting, post-operative nausea and vomiting, motion sickness, pharyngeal stimulation, mechanical bowel obstruction, raised intracranial pressure and irradiation sickness. Symptomatic management of vertigo caused by Meniere's disease and other vestibular disturbances.

PRESENTATION
Injection: (as lactate) 50mg in 1mL, 1mL ampoule – Valoid®.
Suppository: 12.5mg, 25mg, 50mg and 100mg – manufactured 'special'.
Suspension: may be extemporaneously prepared, manufactured 'special'.
Tablet: (scored) (as hydrochloride) 50mg – Valoid®.

DOSAGE

Route	Age			Frequency (times daily)	Notes
	1 month–2 years	2–12 years	12–18 years		
Oral/IV bolus	DOSE BY WEIGHT 500 micrograms – 1mg/kg ⟶			3	Maximum single dose: <6 years is 25mg. >6 years is 50mg.
Oral/rectal	DOSE BY AGE				
		2-5 years 12.5mg	12-18 years 50mg	3	
		6-12 years 25mg		3	
IV or SC infusion	3mg/kg	2-5 years 50mg	150mg	continuous infusion over 24 hours	Can be combined with other drugs. Check compatibility.
		6-12 years 75mg			

ADMINISTRATION
IV: by slow IV injection over 3-5 minutes. May be diluted if required to a maximum 1:1 dilution with Water for Injections only. Can be given as a continuous IV infusion.
Orally: tablets may be crushed and dispersed in water.
SC: occasionally associated with irritation at site of continuous SC infusion. If affected consider increasing the dilution of drug in the infusion or adding hyaluronidase or low dose hydrocortisone to the syringe. Do not mix with any solution containing chloride ions as this will lead to precipitate formation.

CONTRA-INDICATIONS & WARNINGS
Sedation. Cyclizine should be used with caution in patients with glaucoma, obstructive disease of the gastrointestinal tract and hepatic disease (may induce coma). Dose reduction may be necessary in renal impairment. Caution may be required in epilepsy and severe heart failure. Cyclizine injection may have a hypotensive effect.

INTERACTIONS
There may be additive effects with the co-administration of *CNS depressants*. May enhance the side-effects of other *anticholinergic drugs*. Increased antimuscarinic and sedative effects with *tricyclics, antimuscarinics, anxiolytics* and *hypnotics*.

PREGNANCY/BREAST-FEEDING
Contact local Medicines Information Centre for advice.

It is not known whether cyclizine or its metabolites are secreted in human milk.

SIDE-EFFECTS
Drowsiness, occasional dry mouth and blurred vision. Headache, psychomotor impairment and antimuscarinic effects such as urinary retention and gastrointestinal disturbance. Urticaria, drug rash, tachycardia, restlessness, nervousness, insomnia and hallucinations.

POISONING & TOXICITY
Symptoms of acute toxicity arise from peripheral anticholinergic effects and effects on the central nervous system including ataxia, hyperkinesia, extrapyramidal motor disturbance, convulsions and respiratory depression. The incidence of convulsions in children <5 years of age is about 60% when oral dose ingested exceeds 40mg/kg.

PHARMACOLOGY
Exerts its effect by acting upon the vomiting centre.

PHARMACOKINETIC PROPERTIES
Absorbed from the gastrointestinal tract and has an onset of action within 2 hours, with a duration of action lasting 4-6 hours. It is metabolised in the liver to the relatively inactive metabolite, norcyclizine. Both cyclizine and norcyclizine have plasma elimination half-lives of 20 hours.

LICENSED STATUS
Licensed ≥6 years of age, for all indications. Suppositories are 'specials' and as such are unlicensed.

FURTHER INFORMATION
Suspension and suppositories available from Martindale Pharmaceuticals and Aurum Pharmaceuticals Ltd.

Cyclophosphamide

Alkylating agent; oxazaphosphorine prodrug requiring hepatic activation to produce cytotoxic metabolites.

USES
Rhabdomyosarcoma; soft-tissue sarcomas; stage 4 neuroblastoma; Ewing tumour; non-Hodgkin's lymphoma (NHL); high-dose conditioning for bone marrow transplantation (BMT); neuroectodermal tumours (including medulloblastoma); infant brain tumours.
Nephrotic syndrome. Severe vasculitis, major renal involvement or CNS disease in systemic lupus erythematosus (SLE).

PRESENTATION
Injection: 200mg, 500mg and 1g vials – Endoxana® and non-proprietary.
Oral liquid: may be extemporaneously prepared.
Tablet: 50mg – Endoxana®.

DOSAGE
Treatment of malignant disease
Wide variation in dosage. Dose interval and cumulative dose vary depending on protocol.
** Always consult the current treatment protocol for details of dosage and scheduling. **

Other indications

Indication	Route	Age			Frequency	Notes
		1 month–2 years	2–12 years	12–18 years		
Nephrotic syndrome	Oral	←	2–3mg/kg	→	once daily in the morning	For up to 12 weeks.
Vasculitis' SLE	IV	←	500mg – 1g/m²	→	once monthly	More frequent administration may be necessary in severe disease.

ADMINISTRATION
IV: by slow IV bolus into established IV line; by IV infusion in glucose 5%, NaCl 0.9% or glucose/saline infusion. In order to prevent urothelial toxicity, hydration and mesna are required, particularly with higher daily doses of the drug. The manufacturers recommend concurrent mesna administration at daily doses of cyclophosphamide in excess of 10mg/kg (300mg/m²). In paediatric clinical practice, mesna is not required until higher daily or cumulative doses per course are exceeded, providing adequate hydration and micturition can be maintained, although in rheumatological practice, mesna is usually given whatever the dose.

Daily cyclophosphamide dose <10mg/kg (<300mg/m²)
No mesna. Maintain fluid intake; encourage micturition.

Daily, or total course cyclophosphamide dose 300mg/m² – 1g/m².
No mesna. IV hydration with glucose/saline at 3L/m²/24 hours commencing with first cyclophosphamide dose and continuing for at least 6 hours after last cyclophosphamide dose.

Daily, or total course cyclophosphamide dose >1g/m^2
IV hydration with glucose/saline containing mesna at 3L/m^2/24 hours. Mesna doses vary but in practice doses greater than 100% (mg:mg) of the prescribed daily cyclophosphamide dose are used. Start hydration 3 hours before first cyclophosphamide dose and continue for at least 12 hours after the last cyclophosphamide dose.

CONTRA-INDICATIONS & WARNINGS
Concurrent acute urinary tract infection or urothelial damage following previous cytotoxic chemotherapy or pelvic irradiation. Satisfactory full blood count and assessment of renal and hepatic function should be obtained prior to each course of therapy.

INTERACTIONS
Concurrent *dexamethasone* treatment may increase cyclophosphamide metabolism. Concurrent *allopurinol* administration may decrease cyclophosphamide metabolism. The clinical significance of these potential interactions has yet to be determined.

PREGNANCY
Should not be used in pregnancy, especially in the first trimester, unless the expected benefit is thought to outweigh the substantial risk to the fetus. Contact local Medicines Information Centre for advice.

BREAST-FEEDING
Mothers should not breast-feed while being treated with cyclophosphamide or for 36 hours after stopping treatment.

SIDE-EFFECTS
Dose-related nausea and vomiting. Alopecia, myelosuppression, mucositis/enteritis. Chemical or haemorrhagic cystitis if administered without mesna or with inadequate hydration and micturition. Occasional inappropriate antidiuretic hormone secretion. Rarely cardiotoxicity presenting as CCF, pericardial effusion and tamponade, possibly association with previous anthracycline therapy or mediastinal irradiation.

POISONING/TOXICITY
Full supportive measures. If recognised early, IV hydration plus mesna may ameliorate possible urothelial toxicity.

PHARMACOKINETIC PROPERTIES
The pharmacokinetic properties of cyclophosphamide are complex, and since the anti-tumour activity of the oxazaphosphorines rests with their metabolites, little information can be gained from the pharmacokinetics of the parent drug. No correlation between either total plasma alkylating activity or individual metabolite plasma AUCs and tumour response has been demonstrated. In children, the plasma half-life of cyclophosphamide ranges from 2.15-8.15 hours. Urinary excretion of cyclophosphamide and its metabolites is largely complete within 24 hours of administration. Plasma half-life, apparent volume of distribution and total body clearance increase with increasing dose. Daily administration of cyclophosphamide over 2-4 days results in auto-induction of metabolism but this cannot be demonstrated with repeated 3 weekly courses of the drug.

EXCIPIENTS
See manufacturers SPC for further details.

LICENSED STATUS
Not licensed for use in children. Nephrotic syndrome, vasculitis and SLE are unlicensed indications.

Cyproterone acetate

An anti-androgen.

USES
McCune-Albright syndrome (MAS); familial male precocious puberty (testotoxicosis).
Dianette$^{®}$ is indicated in women only, for the treatment of acne refractory to prolonged oral antibiotic therapy (and for moderately severe hirsutism). It also acts as an oral contraceptive.

PRESENTATION
Tablet: 50mg and 100mg – (scored) Androcur$^{®}$, Cyprostat$^{®}$ and non-proprietary.
Tablet: co-cyprindiol 2000/35 (cyproterone acetate 2mg, ethinyloestradiol 35 microgram) – Dianette$^{®}$.

DOSAGE/ADMINISTRATION
Seek expert advice on use in MAS or testotoxicosis.
Dianette$^{®}$: 1 tablet daily for 21 days starting on first day of menstrual cycle and repeated after a 7 day interval, usually for several months.

C

CONTRA-INDICATIONS & WARNINGS
Liver diseases, a history of, or existing, thrombosis or embolism, severe diabetes with vascular changes, sickle-cell anaemia. Dianette® is also contra-indicated in patients with disorders of lipid metabolism, undiagnosed abnormal vaginal bleeding or a history of herpes gestationis. The usual examination of the pelvic organs, breasts and blood pressure that should precede the prescribing of any combined oral contraceptive and which should be repeated regularly, should be carried out when prescribing Dianette®. All the usual reasons for stopping a combined oral contraceptive e.g. unusually frequent or severe headaches, signs of thromboembolism etc. also apply to Dianette®. The product literature for Dianette® should be consulted for full details of precautions/warnings.

INTERACTIONS
Hepatic enzyme inducers (e.g. phenobarbital (phenobarbitone), phenytoin, carbamazepine, rifampicin) and *antibiotics* can impair the contraceptive activity of Dianette®.

PREGNANCY/ BREAST-FEEDING
Contra-indicated.

SIDE-EFFECTS
Dianette®: in rare cases, headaches, gastric upset, nausea, vomiting, breast tenderness, changes in body weight and depressive moods can occur. Menstrual changes such as reduced menstrual flow, intermenstrual bleeding (especially in the first few cycles), can occur. Larger doses of cyproterone than are present in Dianette® can cause tiredness or breathlessness.

POISONING/TOXICITY
Overdose may cause nausea, vomiting and in females withdrawal bleeding. There are no specific antidotes and treatment should be symptomatic.

PHARMACOKINETIC PROPERTIES
Cyproterone is completely absorbed following oral administration. It is metabolised by various pathways including hydroxylations and conjugations. Some is excreted unchanged in the bile but most is excreted in the form of metabolites.

EXCIPIENTS
Dianette® includes sucrose. Contact manufacturers for further details.

LICENSED STATUS
Not licensed for use in children.

Cytarabine (cytosine arabinoside, ara-C, arabinosylcytosine)

Cell cycle phase specific antimetabolite. Metabolites of cytarabine competitively inhibit DNA polymerase after incorporation into the DNA chain.

USES
Acute lymphoblastic leukaemia, acute myeloid leukaemia, non-Hodgkin lymphoma.

PRESENTATION
IV/SC injection: 20mg in 1mL, 5mL and 25mL vial; 100mg in 1mL; 1mL, 5mL, 10mL and 20mL vial – non-proprietary.
IV/SC/intrathecal injection: 20mg in 1mL, 5mL vial – non-proprietary.

DOSAGE
** Always consult the current treatment protocols for details of dosage and scheduling. **
Maximum intrathecal dose is 30mg.
Consider dosage reduction when liver function is poor.

ADMINISTRATION
IV/SC/intrathecal: cytarabine can be given IV as a bolus or infusion. The high strength injection solution (100mg in 1mL) should not be given intrathecally due to the hypertonicity of the solution. May be diluted in Water for Injections, NaCl 0.9% or glucose 5%.

CONTRA-INDICATIONS & WARNINGS
Contra-indications: known hypersensitivity to the drug.
Cautions: prophylactic steroid eye drops (prednisolone

0.5%) must be given with high dose cytarabine i.e. ≥1g/m², to prevent conjunctivitis. Cytarabine is a potent bone marrow suppressant. Therapy should be started cautiously in patients with pre-existing drug-induced bone marrow suppression. Use the drug with caution and at reduced dose in patients whose liver function is poor. *Warnings:* severe and fatal CNS, gastrointestinal and pulmonary toxicity reactions have occurred with cytarabine at high doses. These reactions include reversible corneal toxicity; cerebral and cerebellar dysfunction, usually reversible; severe gastro-intestinal ulceration, including pneumatosis cystoides intestinalis, leading to peritonitis; sepsis and liver abscess; and pulmonary oedema. Cytarabine may induce hyperuricaemia secondary to rapid lysis of neoplastic cells.

INTERACTIONS
Absorption of oral *digoxin* may be substantially reduced as a result of temporary damage to the intestinal mucosa. Cytarabine may antagonise activity of *gentamicin* against *K. pneumoniae*, and of *flucytosine* against fungi.

PREGNANCY
Cytarabine is teratogenic in some animal species and should not be used in pregnant women, especially in the first trimester, or in those who may become pregnant, unless potential benefits outweigh the risks.

BREAST-FEEDING
Breast-feeding is not recommended.

SIDE-EFFECTS
Central nervous system: rarely, neurological effects such a quadriplegia and paralysis have been reported mostly with intrathecal administration. Isolated cases have also been reported with high IV doses.
Haematological effects: the major adverse effect of cytarabine is the haematological toxicity. Myelosuppression is manifested by megaloblastosis, reticulocytopenia, thrombocytopenia and anaemia.
Gastrointestinal: nausea and vomiting occur and are generally more frequent following rapid IV administration than with continuous IV infusion of the drug. Diarrhoea, anorexia, oral and anal inflammation or ulceration and less frequently abdominal pain, sore throat, oesphagitis, oesophageal ulceration and gastrointestinal haemorrhage may also occur.
Other: fever, rash, alopecia, skin ulceration, conjunctivitis, chest pain, urinary retention, dizziness, neuritis or neural toxicity and pain, cellulitis or thrombophlebitis at the site of injection. Cytarabine has also been associated with renal dysfunction, hepatic dysfunction and jaundice in some patients. It has also been associated with sepsis, irritation or sepsis at the injection site, neuritis or neurotoxicity rash, freckling, skin and mucosal bleeding, chest pain, joint pain and reduction in reticulocytes.
Cytarabine reaction: cytarabine syndrome/reaction is characterised by fever, myalgia, bone pain, occasionally chest pain, maculopapular rash, conjunctivitis and malaise. It usually occurs 6-12 hours after administration. Corticosteroids have been shown to be beneficial in treating or preventing this syndrome. If the symptoms of the syndrome are serious enough to warrant treatment, corticosteroids should be contemplated as well as continuation of cytarabine therapy.

POISONING/TOXICITY
The principal toxic effect is on the bone marrow. There is no antidote and bone marrow suppression must be managed with supportive measures including blood transfusions, antibiotics and growth factors. Corticosteroids can be used to treat/prevent 'cytarabine reaction'.

PHARMACOKINETIC PROPERTIES
Cytarabine is rapidly and widely distributed into tissues, crosses the blood brain barrier and also the placenta. CSF levels of 50% of plasma levels are achieved with IV infusion. Cytidine deaminase is concentrated in the liver and IV doses show biphasic elimination with half-lives of approximately 10 minutes and 1-3 hours.
After 24 hours 80% of a dose has been eliminated either as the inactive metabolite or as the unchanged cytarabine, mostly in urine but some in bile.
Intrathecal dosing results in slower elimination (half-life of 2-11 hours).

EXCIPIENTS
Contact manufacturer for further details.

LICENSED STATUS
Licensed for use in children and adults.

A cytotoxic drug thought to act as an alkylating agent in man.

USES
Hodgkin disease, as part of combination therapy (ABVD) with doxorubicin, vincristine and bleomycin.

PRESENTATION
Injection: powder for reconstitution (as citrate), 100mg, 200mg, 500mg, 600mg and 1g vials – non-proprietary; 200mg vial – DTIC-Dome®.

DOSAGE
** Always consult the current treatment protocol for details of dosage and scheduling. **

ADMINISTRATION
IV: reconstitute with Water for Injections (9.9mL, 100mg vial; 19.7mL, 200mg vial); the resulting solutions contain the equivalent of 10mg in 1mL. It can be given by slow IV injection over 2-3 minutes or diluted in 125-250mL glucose 5% or NaCl 0.9% and given as a short IV infusion over 15-30 minutes; consult the current protocol. The infusion set must be protected from light for the duration of the infusion.

CONTRA-INDICATIONS & WARNINGS
The injection solution is vesicant and extravasation should be avoided. In patients with hepatic and/or renal insufficiency, the elimination half-life may be significantly increased. Dose adjustment may be indicated together with close monitoring of hepatic and bone marrow function.

INTERACTIONS
Patients receiving dacarbazine should not be immunised with live vaccines as dacarbazine may impair the immunological response to the vaccine with the development of a generalised vaccinia.

PREGNANCY/ BREAST-FEEDING
Animal studies have shown dacarbazine to be carcinogenic and teratogenic. It should not be administered to women who are pregnant or may become pregnant or mothers who are breast-feeding unless the benefit clearly justifies the potential risk to the fetus.

SIDE-EFFECTS
Common reactions. Anorexia, vomiting and nausea are the most frequent side-effects; bone marrow depression, leucopenia, thrombocytopenia.

Less common reactions: *Dermatological:* transient rash, alopecia; general – a 'flu-like' syndrome of fever malaise and myalgia has been reported. *Gastrointestinal:* diarrhoea.
Hepatic: increases in transaminases, alkaline phosphatase, lactic dehydrogenase (levels usually return to normal within 2 weeks), hepatotoxicity accompanied by hepatic vein thrombosis and hepatocellular necrosis, resulting in death.
Nervous system: blurred vision, seizures, headache, facial paraesthesia, confusion, malaise and lethargy. Anaphylaxis has occurred very rarely.

POISONING/TOXICITY
Signs and symptoms: nausea, vomiting, diarrhoea and severe bone marrow depression.
Treatment: stop dacarbazine administration and institute supportive measures.

PHARMACOKINETIC PROPERTIES
Extensive hepatic metabolism and biliary excretion. Renal clearance can also account for up to 60% of total drug clearance. Terminal half-life is 5 hours which may be significantly increased in renal or hepatic impairment.

EXCIPIENTS
Contact manufacturer for further details.

LICENSED STATUS
Licensed for use in children and adults.

Dactinomycin (actinomycin D)

Cytotoxic, antineoplastic antibiotic with immunosuppressant properties.

USES
Ewing tumour, in combination chemotherapy with etoposide, vincristine, ifosfamide and doxorubicin.
Wilms tumour, in combination with vincristine +/- doxorubicin.
Rhabdomyosarcoma and other soft-tissue sarcomas, in combination with ifosfamide and vincristine.

PRESENTATION
Injection: powder for reconstitution, 500 microgram vial – Cosmegen Lyovac®.

DOSAGE
** Always consult the current treatment protocol for details of dosage and scheduling. **

ADMINISTRATION
IV: reconstitute with 1.1mL Water for Injections without preservative (other injection fluids may cause precipitation); reconstituted solution contains 500 microgram in 1mL of dactinomycin. Administer by slow IV injection over 2-3 minutes.

CONTRA-INDICATIONS & WARNINGS
The injection is vesicant and therefore extravasation should be avoided. Concurrent and recent radiotherapy may exaggerate toxicity. In cases of biliary obstruction (elevated serum bilirubin, jaundice) dose reduction should be considered.

INTERACTIONS
No specific drug interactions have been reported but caution with concurrent radiotherapy.

PREGNANCY
Shown to be teratogenic in animals and should not normally be given to pregnant women.

BREAST-FEEDING
Dactinomycin should not be administered to women who are breast-feeding.

SIDE-EFFECTS
General: malaise, fatigue, lethargy, fever, myalgia, proctitis, hypoglycaemia.
Oral: cheilitis, dysphagia, oesophagitis, ulcerative stomatitis, pharyngitis.
Gastrointestinal: anorexia, nausea, vomiting, abdominal pain, diarrhoea, gastrointestinal ulceration, hepatitis and liver function test abnormalities (rare with current dosing regimens), veno-occlusive disease.
Haematological: anaemia (even to the point of aplastic anaemia, agranulocytosis, leucopenia, thrombocytopenia, pancytopenia, reticulocytopenia). Platelet and white cell counts should be checked daily.
Dermatological: alopecia, acne, flare-up of erythema or increased pigmentation of previously irradiated skin.

POISONING/TOXICITY
In the event of overdosage, dactinomycin therapy should be withdrawn immediately. Limited information is available on overdosage in humans. Manifestations of overdosage have included nausea, vomiting, diarrhoea, stomatitis, gastrointestinal ulceration, severe haemopoietic depression, acute renal failure and death. There is no known antidote. Treatment should be symptomatic and supportive. It is advisable to check renal, hepatic and bone marrow functions frequently.

PHARMACOKINETIC PROPERTIES
Minimal hepatic metabolism. Renal excretion can account for up to 20% of total clearance, with biliary excretion accounting for between 50-90% of the total drug clearance.

EXCIPIENTS
See manufacturer's SPC for further details.

LICENSED STATUS
Licensed for use in children and adults.

Dalteparin sodium

A low molecular weight heparin (LMWH).

USES
Prophylaxis and treatment of thromboembolic disease.

PRESENTATION
Injection: 2500 units in 1mL; 4mL ampoule – Fragmin®.
Injection: 10,000 units in 1mL; 1mL graduated syringe and 1mL ampoule – Fragmin®.
Injection: 12,500 units in 1mL; 2500 units in 0.2mL syringe – Fragmin®.
Injection: 25,000 units in 1mL; 5000 units in 0.2mL, 7500 units in 0.3mL, 10,000 units in 0.4mL, 12,500 units in 0.5mL, 15,000 units in 0.6mL and 18,000 units in 0.72mL syringe, 4mL vial – Fragmin®.

DOSAGE

Indication	Route	Age				Frequency (times daily)	Notes
		birth–1 month	1 month–2 years	2–12 years	12–18 years		
Treatment dose	SC	← 100 units/kg →			–	2	
			–		200 units/kg	1	The single daily dose should not exceed 18,000 units.
Treatment dose if increased risk of bleeding	SC		–		100 units/kg	2	
Prophylaxis dose	SC	← 100 units/kg →			2500-5000 units	1	

Experience is very limited in children and even more limited in neonates.

Renal and hepatic impairment
Patients with severely disturbed hepatic function may need a reduction in dosage and should be monitored accordingly. The half-life is prolonged in uraemic patients as dalteparin sodium is eliminated primarily through the kidneys.

CONTRA-INDICATIONS & WARNINGS
Contra-indications include a history of confirmed or suspected immunologically mediated heparin induced thrombocytopenia, acute gastroduodenal ulcer; cerebral haemorrhage; known haemorrhagic diathesis; subacute endocarditis; injuries to and operations on the central nervous system, eyes and ears. When considered necessary, it is recommended that the antithrombotic effect be monitored by analysing anti-Factor Xa activity using a suitable assay. This is because dalteparin has only a moderate prolonging effect on clotting time assays such as APTT or thrombin time.

INTERACTIONS
The possibility of an enhancement of the anticoagulant effect by *anticoagulant/antiplatelet agents* should be considered.

PREGNANCY
This medicinal product has been assessed in pregnant women and no harmful effects are known with respect to the course of pregnancy and the health of the unborn and neonate.

BREAST-FEEDING
It is not known if dalteparin is excreted in breast milk. The oral absorption of dalteparin is unlikely. Contact local Medicines Information Centre for advice.

SIDE-EFFECTS
Commonly reported side-effects include subcutaneous haematomas at the injection site. Also rarely anaphylactoid reaction, thrombocytopenia, hyperkalaemia and allergic reactions (urticaria, pruritus, hair loss and skin necrosis).

POISONING/TOXICITY
The prolongation of the clotting time induced by dalteparin may be fully neutralised by protamine, but the anti-Factor Xa activity is only neutralised to about 25-50%. 1mg of protamine inhibits the effect of 100 international units (anti-Factor Xa) of dalteparin.

PHARMACOKINETIC PROPERTIES
The half-life following IV and SC administration is 2 hours and 3.5-4 hours respectively, twice that of unfractionated heparin. The bioavailability following SC injection is approximately 87% and the pharmacokinetics are not dose dependent.

LICENSED STATUS
Not licensed for use in children.

Dantrolene

A muscle relaxant acting directly on skeletal muscle.

USES
Chronic severe spasticity; painful muscle spasticity due to CNS damage e.g. palliative management of cerebral palsy, neurodegenerative conditions. Malignant hyperthermia.

PRESENTATION
Capsule: 25mg, 100mg – Dantrium®.
Oral liquid: may be extemporaneously prepared.
Injection: powder for reconstitution, 20mg vial – Dantrium Intravenous®.

DOSAGE

Indication	Route	Age			Frequency (times daily)	Notes
		1 month–2 years	2–12 years	12–18 years		
Spasticity	Oral	-	≥ 5 years 500 micrograms/kg	-	1	Initial dose for 7 days. Make dose changes every 7 days. Increase the frequency to 3 times
		-	-	25mg	1	daily, then increase the dose in increments of 500 microgram/kg/dose in children until satisfactory response is achieved.
			≥ 5 years 2mg/kg (maximum 100mg)	100mg	4	Maximum dose
Malignant hyperthermia	IV bolus	←	1mg/kg	→	single dose	Repeat as required, at 5-10 minute intervals to a maximum cumulative dose of 10mg/kg.

ADMINISTRATION
IV: the contents of 1 vial should be reconstituted with 60mL of Water for Injections. It is given as a bolus injection. The reconstituted solution should be protected from light and used within 6 hours; do not refrigerate or freeze and do not store above 30°C.

D

CONTRA-INDICATIONS & WARNINGS
Acute muscle spasm, hepatic impairment. Dantrolene has been associated with symptomatic hepatitis; liver function tests should be performed before starting treatment, 6 weeks after starting therapy and at regular intervals (at the physician's discretion) during treatment. Use with caution in patients with cardiovascular or respiratory disease.

INTERACTIONS
Use of dantrolene with other potentially *hepatotoxic drugs* should be avoided. Use of dantrolene IV with *calcium-channel blockers* is not recommended. *Metoclopramide* increases the oral bioavailability of dantrolene. Potential for interaction with *neuromuscular blockers*.

PREGNANCY
The safety in women who are or who may become pregnant has not been established. Potential benefits should be weighed against possible hazards to both fetus and mother. Dantrolene has been safely used shortly before delivery in mothers at risk of or who had previously suffered malignant hyperthermia during caesarian section.

BREAST-FEEDING
Use during lactation is not recommended as there are no case reports.

SIDE-EFFECTS
Oral therapy: the low starting dose and slow dose escalation is designed to reduce the transient side-effects of drowsiness, dizziness, weakness, malaise, fatigue and diarrhoea. The diarrhoea can be severe and necessitate withdrawal. Frequent side effects include anorexia, nausea, headache and rash. Less frequently constipation, dysphagia, speech and visual disturbances, confusion, nervousness, insomnia, depression, seizures, chills, fever and increased urinary frequency. Rarely tachycardia, erratic blood pressure, hyperkalaemia, dyspnoea, haematuria, possible crystalluria, urinary incontinence or retention, pleural effusion, pericarditis and dose-related hepatotoxicity.
IV: pulmonary oedema, thrombophlebitis and muscle weakness have been attributed to IV use in patients treated with short-term therapy for malignant hyperthermia.

POISONING/TOXICITY
After recent ingestion gastric lavage and general supportive measures are recommended. To prevent

crystalluria intravenous fluids should be administered in volumes, sufficient to induce diuresis.

PHARMACOKINETIC PROPERTIES
Absorption is reported as 80%. Mean half-life after single dose is 8.7 hours (oral) and 5 hours (IV) in adults. 80-90% bound to serum albumin. It is metabolised in the liver and has active metabolites. The main metabolite is as active as the parent drug and has a half-life ranging from 8-29 hours. 20% of a dose is excreted in the urine and 45-50% is excreted in the bile, mostly as metabolites.

EXCIPIENTS
See manufacturer's SPC for further details.

LICENSED STATUS
The capsules are not licensed for use in children. Injection is licensed for use in children and adults for treatment of malignant hyperthermia.

FURTHER INFORMATION
Extemporaneous formulation e.g. Nova Laboratories using Suspension Diluent A (xanthan gum 1%w/v). Further acidification of the suspension using 150mg citric acid per 100mL allows expiry to be extended to 1 month from 8 days. Store at room temperature.

Dapsone

Antibacterial; antileprotic.

USES
Immune blistering disorders (particularly dermatitis herpetiformis). Leprosy. Also used in some haematological disorders.

PRESENTATION
Tablet: 50mg and 100mg – non-proprietary.

DOSAGE

Route	Age			Frequency (times daily)	Notes
	1 month-2 years	2-12 years	12-18 years		
Oral	←	500 microgram/kg	→	1	Blistering skin conditions. Starting dose – titrate up or down as necessary in 12.5mg increments.
Oral	←	1-2mg/kg	→	1	Treatment of leprosy. In combination with rifampicin (see current *BNF* for details).

ADMINISTRATION
Oral: tablets may be crushed.

CONTRA-INDICATIONS & WARNINGS
Use with caution in cardiac or pulmonary disease, anaemia (treat severe anaemia first), G6PD deficiency.

INTERACTIONS
Plasma concentration reduced by *rifamycins*.
Probenecid reduces dapsone excretion – increased risk of side-effects.

PREGNANCY
Avoid if possible. Risk of neonatal haemolysis and megaloblastic anaemia in third trimester.

BREAST-FEEDING
Dapsone is excreted into breast milk and absorbed by the infant; risk of haemolytic anaemia. Breast-feeding of G6PD deficient children to be avoided.

SIDE-EFFECTS
Dose related.
CNS: peripheral neuropathy, insomnia, headache.
Dermatologic: exfoliative dermatitis.
Gastrointestinal: nausea, vomiting, cholestatic jaundice.

Haematological: haemolytic anaemia, methaemoglobinaemia, leucopenia, agranulocytosis.
Hepatic: hepatitis.
Ocular: blurred vision.
Otic: tinnitus.

PHARMACOKINETIC PROPERTIES
Well absorbed orally and distributed widely throughout the tissues. It is metabolised in the liver and is subject to enterohepatic recycling. About 10-20% of a dose is excreted in the urine unchanged with about 50% as conjugates of dapsone and 30% as N-oxidation products.

LICENSED STATUS
Licensed for use in children and adults.

Daunorubicin

Anthracycline glycoside antibiotic which inhibits synthesis of DNA and RNA primarily by intercalation of base pairs. It also interferes with DNA topoisomerase II and generates toxic free radicals.

USES
Acute lymphoblastic leukaemia. Acute myeloid leukaemia.

PRESENTATION
Injection: powder for reconstitution (as hydrochloride), 20mg – non-proprietary.

DOSAGE
** Always consult the current treatment protocol for details of dosage and scheduling. **

ADMINISTRATION
IV: reconstitute the contents of a 20mg vial with 4mL Water for Injections to produce a solution containing 5mg in 1mL. This solution should be further diluted with NaCl 0.9% to 1mg in 1mL. Daunorubicin should only be given IV. It should be given over a minimum of 20 minutes, although current guidelines for paediatric patients recommend infusion over 6 hours. The 1mg in 1mL solution may be given via a side arm of a free flowing infusion of NaCl 0.9% or the solution may be added to a minibag of NaCl 0.9% and this can be given via the side arm, as before. Always follow the guidelines in the protocol.

D

CONTRA-INDICATIONS & WARNINGS
Contra-indications: do not use in patients recently exposed to, or with existing, chickenpox or herpes zoster. Do not administer by the IM route. Do not use in patients with existing heart disease. Do not exceed a cumulative dose of 300mg/m^2 in children >2 years, or 10mg/kg in children <2 years.
Cautions: use with care in patients at risk of hyperuricaemia. Reduce dose in impaired renal and hepatic function.
Warnings: vesicant – avoid extravasation.

INTERACTIONS
Do not mix with *dexamethasone sodium phosphate* injection or *heparin sodium* injection – a precipitate will form. Protect solutions from sunlight.

PREGNANCY
Daunorubicin crosses the placenta and is mutagenic, carcinogenic and teratogenic. Treatment during pregnancy may cause delayed effects in the offspring.

BREAST-FEEDING
Breast-feeding should be discontinued during treatment owing to the potential for toxicity to the infant.

SIDE-EFFECTS
Haematological: bone marrow depression. Leucopenia is usually more significant than thrombocytopenia with the nadir occurring between 10-14 days.
Cardiac: cardiotoxicity if it occurs is likely to be heralded by either a persistent tachycardia, shortness of breath, swelling of feet and lower limbs or by minor changes in the ECG. For this reason an ECG examination should be made at regular intervals during the treatment. Cardiotoxicity usually appears within 1-6 months after initiation of therapy. It may develop suddenly and not be detected by routine ECG. It may be irreversible and fatal but responds to treatment if detected early. Routine echocardiogram measuring the fractional shortening is strongly recommended on a regular basis.
Gastrointestinal: stomatitis, diarrhoea, nausea and vomiting.
Other: alopecia, phlebitis, rash and red urine.

POISONING/TOXICITY
Overdosage may result in severe myelosuppression and severe cardiotoxicity with or without transient reversible ECG changes, leading to congestive heart failure. Treatment should be supportive and symptomatic.

PHARMACOKINETIC PROPERTIES
Daunorubicin is rapidly taken up by the tissues following infusion. It does not cross the blood-brain barrier. Release of drug and its metabolites is slow from the tissues (half-life is 55 hours). Daunorubicin is rapidly metabolised in the liver, and the major metabolite is also active. Daunorubicin is excreted slowly in the urine and by biliary excretion.

EXCIPIENTS
Contact manufacturer for further details.

LICENSED STATUS
Licensed for use in children and adults.

FURTHER INFORMATION
Vesicant. Extravasation may be treated with 5mL of sodium bicarbonate injection 8.4%w/v in the hope that the pH change will hydrolyse the drug. Change from red to blue-purple colour indicates decomposition of solution.
Tumour cell cross resistance has been seen between doxorubicin and daunorubicin. The brand name Cerubidin® was formerly used for daunorubicin injection.

Deferiprone

USES
Treatment of iron overload in patients with thalassemia major for whom desferrioxamine therapy is contra-indicated or not tolerated.

PRESENTATION
Tablet: (scored) 500mg – Ferriprox®.

DOSAGE

Route	Age			Frequency	Notes
	1 month–2 years	2–12 years	12–18 years	(times daily)	
Oral	–	> 6 years 25mg/kg (rounded to the nearest 250mg dose)	25mg/kg (rounded to the nearest 250mg dose)	3	Doses above 100mg/kg/**day** are not recommended because of the potential for an increased risk of adverse effects.

CONTRA-INDICATIONS & WARNINGS
Contra-indicated if history of agranulocytosis or recurrent episodes of neutropenia.
Deferiprone has been shown to cause neutropenia, including agranulocytosis. It is recommended that a patient's neutrophil count be monitored every week. There is limited data available on the use of deferiprone in children between 6-10 years of age.

INTERACTIONS
Due to the unknown mechanism of deferiprone-induced neutropenia, patients should not take medicinal products known to be associated with neutropenia or those that can cause agranulocytosis.
Interactions between deferiprone and other medicinal products have not been reported but the potential exists for interactions with *metallic ions* and *vitamin C*.

PREGNANCY/BREAST-FEEDING
Contra-indicated.

SIDE-EFFECTS
Commonly nausea, vomiting, abdominal pain and increased appetite. These effects are more frequent at the beginning of therapy with deferiprone and in most patients are resolved within a few weeks without the discontinuation of treatment. Also reddish/brown urine, agranulycocytosis, neutropenia and arthropathies.

POISONING/TOXICITY
There have been no reports of acute overdose with deferiprone.

PHARMACOKINETIC PROPERTIES
Is metabolised in the liver and excreted by the kidney. Deferiprone is rapidly absorbed from the upper part of the gastro-intestinal tract.
Peak serum concentration is reported to occur 45-60 minutes following a single dose in fasted patients. This may be extended to 2 hours in fed patients. The elimination half-life in most patients is 2-3 hours.

EXCIPIENTS
See manufacturer's SPC for further details.

LICENSED STATUS
Licensed for >6 years of age.

FURTHER INFORMATION
Patients should be advised to report immediately any symptoms indicative of infection such as: fever, sore throat and flu-like symptoms.

Deflazacort

Oxazoline derivative of prednisolone.

USES
Juvenile idiopathic arthritis (JIA); polyarticular disease unresponsive to other therapies, but not life-threatening.

PRESENTATION
Tablet: 1mg, 6mg and 30mg – Calcort®.

DOSAGE

Route	Age			Frequency (times daily)	Notes
	1 month-2 years	2-12 years	12-18 years		
Oral	← 250 microgram/kg-1.5mg/kg →		3-18mg	1	Doses up to 2.4mg/kg daily have been used in children. In adults up to 120mg has been used initially in acute disorders. The dose should normally be taken as a single dose in the morning. However, the total dose for two days can sometimes be taken as a single dose on alternate days in an attempt to reduce pituitary-adrenal suppression. The lowest effective dose should be used.

Dosage may need to be reduced in patients with hepatic impairment.

ADMINISTRATION
Oral: avoid *antacids* within 2 hours either side of administration of deflazacort as these will reduce absorption of the steroid.

CONTRA-INDICATIONS & WARNINGS, INTERACTIONS, SIDE-EFFECTS
See prednisolone monograph.

PREGNANCY
Deflazacort does cross the placenta. Administration of corticosteroids to pregnant animals can cause abnormalities of fetal development. There is no evidence that corticosteroids result in an increased incidence of congenital abnormalities in man. However, when administered for prolonged periods or repeatedly during pregnancy, corticosteroids may increase the risk of intra-uterine growth retardation. Hypoadrenalism may, in theory, occur in the neonate following prenatal exposure to corticosteroids but usually resolves spontaneously following birth and is rarely clinically important. As with all drugs, corticosteroids should only be prescribed when the benefits to the mother and child outweigh the risks. When corticosteroids are essential however, patients with normal pregnancies may be treated as though they were in the non-gravid state.

BREAST-FEEDING
Corticosteroids are excreted in breast milk, although no data are available for deflazacort. Doses of up to 50mg daily of deflazacort are unlikely to cause systemic effects in the infant. Infants of mothers taking higher doses than this may have a degree of adrenal suppression but the benefits of breast-feeding are likely to outweigh any theoretical risk.

POISONING/TOXICITY
There is no specific antidote, but it is unlikely that treatment would be required in case of acute overdosage. Serum electrolytes should be monitored.

PHARMACOKINETIC PROPERTIES
Deflazacort is rapidly absorbed and immediately hydrolysed to its active derivative.

EXCIPIENTS
See manufacturer's SPC for further details.

LICENSED STATUS
Licensed for use in children and adults.

FURTHER INFORMATION
Deflazacort may have a relatively bone-sparing effect compared with other corticosteroids at equivalent therapeutic dosages.

Desferrioxamine mesilate

A chelating agent for trivalent iron and aluminium ions; resulting chelates are stable and non-toxic.

USES
Iron overload; acute iron poisoning; primary and secondary haemochromatosis; aluminium overload in dialysis patients.

PRESENTATION
Injection: powder for reconstitution 500mg and 2g vials – Desferal®.

DOSAGE

Indication	Route	Age			Frequency	Notes
		1 month–2 years	2–12 years	12–18 years		
Acute iron poisoning	Oral	← 5g →		5–10g	single dose (in 50–100mL water)	The injection can be given orally. It may have to be given through a nasogastric tube, as the taste is very unpleasant.
	IM	← 1g →		2g	single dose (repeatable 8 hourly if necessary)	If there is any doubt about toxicity or if iron levels are unavailable, give IM dose and observe urine colour. A pink or port wine colour indicates free iron in the blood and therefore potential toxicity. If the iron level is toxic repeat at 8 hourly intervals until normal urine colour.
	IV infusion	← initially 15mg/kg/hour reducing after 4–6 hours as indicated →			continuous	If shocked, hypotensive or seriously ill, administer IV. Decrease rate of administration after 4–6 hours to ensure that total maximum dose does not exceed 80mg/kg/**day**. Continue until serum iron less than total iron binding capacity.
Pathological iron overload	IV infusion or SC infusion over 8–24 hrs	← 20mg/kg →		500mg	single dose	Seek specialist advice. Starting doses – give 4 to 5 nights per week. Increase and use lowest effective dose to give negative iron balance. Maintenance doses proportional to iron excretion rate. Do not exceed 50mg/kg/**dose**.
	IV infusion over 24 hours	up to ← 180mg/kg →		–	continuous	High dose therapy. Used in patients exhibiting cardiac damage due to iron overload.

DOSAGE continued

Indication	Route	Age			Frequency	Notes
		1 month–2 years	2–12 years	12–18 years		
Aluminium overload in dialysis patients	IV infusion	←	5mg/kg	→	once weekly	Haemodialysis or haemofiltration via fistula over the last hour of dialysis, for 3 months. Remeasure aluminium levels 4 to 8 weeks after completing course.
	IV, IM, SC or IP	←	5mg/kg	➤	once weekly	CAPD or CCPD. Give prior to the last exchange of the day.

ADMINISTRATION

Oral: injection is given orally in 50–100mL water. It has an unpleasant taste and may be given via the nasogastric tube following gastric lavage.

IV: administered as a 10% solution. Vial is reconstituted with 5mL Water for Injections and is diluted with glucose 5%, NaCl 0.9% or glucose-saline. Opaque, cloudy or discoloured solutions should be discarded. Infusion rate must not exceed 15mg/kg/hour to avoid hypotension. The iron-desferrioxamine complex is excreted in the urine, making it orange-red in colour. In acute iron poisoning administration of antidote should be stopped when the patient is clinically improved, free iron is no longer present in the plasma or the urinary screen for iron is negative.

Desferrioxamine can be administered through the infusion line (but not added to the blood bag), during blood transfusions (up to 2g per unit of blood).

The reconstituted solution should be used immediately or stored for a maximum of 24 hours at room temperature if reconstituted under validated aseptic conditions.

Intraperitoneal (IP): desferrioxamine can be added to dialysis fluid and given to patients on continuous ambulatory peritoneal dialysis (CAPD) or continuous cycling peritoneal dialysis (CCPD).

D

CONTRA-INDICATIONS & WARNINGS

Use with caution in patients with renal impairment since the metal complexes are excreted via the kidneys.

Disturbances of vision and hearing have been reported during prolonged therapy and therefore eye and ear examinations should also be carried out prior to the start of long-term therapy and at 3 monthly intervals during treatment.

INTERACTIONS

Avoid *prochlorperazine* (may lead to prolonged unconsciousness). Oral vitamin C 100mg (200mg in patients on high doses) may be given on treatment days to enhance urinary iron excretion.

PREGNANCY

Give desferrioxamine therapy with iron overdose in pregnancy if clinical evidence of moderate to severe iron intoxication. There is no evidence that desferrioxamine adversely affects the outcome of the pregnancy. If delivery occurs, the infant should be evaluated for iron overload or iron deficiency secondary to maternal desferrioxamine therapy.

BREAST-FEEDING

Not known whether it is excreted into breast milk or not, but no expected problems. Measure iron levels in the feeding baby.

SIDE-EFFECTS

Frequent: local reactions, pain, swelling, headache, urticaria.

Rare: gastrointestinal disturbance, hepatic and renal impairment, arrhythmia, rashes, anaphylactic reactions.

POISONING/TOXICITY

Toxicity: occasional tachycardia, hypotension and gastrointestinal symptoms.

Antidote: nothing specific; dialysable.

PHARMACOKINETIC PROPERTIES

Desferrioxamine is poorly absorbed from the gastrointestinal tract. Following parenteral administration, desferrioxamine chelates metal ions. It is metabolised, primarily in the plasma. Biphasic elimination: first phase half-life of 1 hour and second phase half-life of 6 hours. The iron desferrioxamine chelate is excreted in the urine and faeces.

EXCIPIENTS

See manufacturer's SPC for further details.

LICENSED STATUS

Licensed for use in children and adults.

Non-sedating antihistamine. Major active metabolite of the parent drug loratadine.

PRESENTATION
Syrup: 2.5mg in 5mL – Neoclarityn®.
Tablet: 5mg – Neoclarityn®.

USES
Non sedating relief of symptoms associated with seasonal allergic rhinitis and chronic idiopathic urticaria.

DOSAGE

Route	Age		Frequency	Notes
	2–12 years	12–18 years	(times daily)	
Oral	2-5 years 1.25mg	5mg	1	
	6-11 years 2.5mg		1	

CONTRA-INDICATIONS & WARNINGS
Known hypersensitivity to desloratadine, any of the excipients or to loratadine.
Use with caution in severe renal impairment.

INTERACTIONS
None with *erythromycin* or *ketoconazole* but metabolising enzyme not yet identified.

PREGNANCY/BREAST-FEEDING
Not advised unless benefit clearly outweighs risk. No teratogenic or mutagenic effects in animal trials.

SIDE-EFFECTS
Uncommon; fatigue, dry mouth, headache.

POISONING/TOXICITY
No clinically relevant effects observed in a multiple dose clinical trial.
Symptomatic and supportive if necessary.

PHARMACOKINETIC PROPERTIES
Well absorbed with maximum concentrations at 3 hours.

LICENSED STATUS
Licensed for ≥2 years of age.

EXCIPIENTS
See manufacturer's SPC for further details.

FURTHER INFORMATION
Manufacturer's claim for a decongestant effect cannot be fully evaluated.

Desmopressin

Vasopressin analogue.

USES
Nocturnal enuresis; central diabetes insipidus; mild to moderate haemophilia A and von Willebrand disease; pituitary function testing - assessment of anti diuretic hormone (ADH) secretion.

PRESENTATION
Injection: 4 microgram in 1mL – DDAVP®.
Intranasal solution: 100 microgram in 1mL, 2.5mL dropper bottle and catheter – DDAVP®.
Nasal spray: 2.5 microgram per metered dose spray – named patient, Low Dose Desmospray®; 10 microgram per metered dose spray – Desmospray®, Noctutil® and non-proprietary; 150 microgram per metered dose spray – named patient, Octim®.
Tablet: (scored, crushable) 100 microgram – DDAVP®, 200 microgram – DDAVP® and Desmotabs®.

DOSAGE

Indication	Route	Age				Frequency (times daily)	Notes
		birth–1 month	1 month–2 years	2–12 years	12–18 years		
Assessment of ADH secretion	Intranasal	–	← 1-5 microgram →			single dose	Infants with congenital ADH deficiency may be very sensitive to desmopressin and the dose should be reduced to one tenth of that stated.
Test dose for suspected diabetes insipidus	SC, IM or IV	–	400 nanogram	0.5-1 microgram	1 microgram	single dose	Restrict fluid input to maximum 1.5 times the urine volume from start of dehydration phase to the test. Monitor for HYPONATRAEMIA.
	Intranasal	–	5-10 microgram	10-20 microgram	20 microgram	single dose	
Established diabetes insipidus	Intranasal	1.25-5 microgram	2.5-5 microgram	5-20 microgram	10-20 microgram	1-2	Individual dose titration required. A trial of monitored treatment may be used as a diagnostic test.
	Oral	5 microgram	5-50 microgram	50-200 microgram	50-300 microgram	2-3	
Nocturnal enuresis	Intra-nasal	–		≥5 years 20 microgram		1 (at night)	Half the total dose is given into each nostril. Increase if necessary to a maximum of 40 microgram (20 microgram in each nostril) at night. Reassess after 3 months by stopping treatment for at least 1 week.
	Oral	–		≥5 years 200 microgram		1 (at night)	Increase if necessary to a maximum of 400 microgram at night. Reassess after 3 months by stopping treatment for at least 1 week.
Mild-moderate haemophilia A and von Willebrand disease	IV	–	>1 year ← 300 nanogram/kg →			single dose	Discuss with haematologist. Dilute in 30–50mL NaCl 0.9% and give over 20 minutes immediately before surgery. Can be repeated after 12 hours, only if no tachycardia.
	Intra-nasal	–	← 4 microgram/kg →			single dose	If used preoperatively, use 2 hours prior to procedures.

ADMINISTRATION

Intranasal: children requiring <10 microgram as a dose should receive the dropper bottle with catheter for nasal administration, or the named patient 2.5 microgram per spray product. If required, the intranasal solution may be diluted with NaCl 0.9% to a dilution of 10 micrograms in 1mL. It should be replaced into the original container, taking care to label with the appropriate strength, and stored in the fridge. It is stable for 28 days. This solution may be administered orally.

IV: it should not be diluted in patients with diabetes insipidus requiring dose of 4 microgram or less. When used for haemophilia A (Factor VIII deficiency) or von Willebrand disease doses are higher; dilute in 30-50mL NaCl 0.9%.

CONTRA-INDICATIONS & WARNINGS

Avoid water load. Stop drug if patient experiences concurrent episode of diarrhoea/vomiting. Exercise great caution with renal disease, cardiovascular disease and cystic fibrosis. Contra-indicated in cardiac insufficiency and other conditions requiring treatment with diuretic agents. The intranasal spray and solution are contra-indicated where hypersensitivity to the preservatives *benzalkonium chloride* or *chlorbutyl*, is known. The diagnosis of a psychogenic polydipsia should be excluded prior to treatment.

INTERACTIONS

Potentiated by *tricyclic antidepressants, carbamazepine, chlorpromazine* and *indometacin (indomethacin)*.

PREGNANCY
Available data suggest no increase in the rate of malformations in infants exposed to desmopressin throughout pregnancy.

BREAST-FEEDING
Concentration of desmopressin in breast milk is insufficient to influence diuresis.

SIDE-EFFECTS
Headache, stomach pain and nausea. Nasal administration may cause rhinitis and epistaxis. Treatment without concomitant reduction of fluid intake may lead to fluid retention, hyponatraemia and convulsions.

POISONING/TOXICITY
Overdose can lead to hyponatraemia and convulsions. If hyponatraemia occurs, stop desmopressin treatment and restrict fluid intake until serum sodium is normalised.

PHARMACOKINETIC PROPERTIES
The drug is well absorbed through the nasal mucosa, but because of degradation by gastric secretions, absorption from the gastrointestinal tract is poor (although sufficient is absorbed at the oral doses stated to produce therapeutic effects).

EXCIPIENTS
Intranasal solution contains chlorbutyl and the spray benzalkonium chloride as preservative. Contact manufacturer's for further details.

LICENSED STATUS
Licensed for use in all ages for diabetes insipidus and >5 years for nocturnal enuresis. Only the injection is licensed for haemophilia A and von Willebrand disease. ADH secretion testing is not a licensed indication.

FURTHER INFORMATION
The dose should be adjusted to allow a brief period of diuresis prior to the next dose. This helps to avoid overdosage. Tablets may be given when an upper respiratory infection makes intranasal administration unreliable.
Low Dose Desmospray® and Octim® are available from Ferring Pharmaceuticals UK.

Dexamethasone

Synthetic corticosteroid.

USES
To accelerate surfactant production in the fetal lung prior to preterm birth; to improve lung function in chronic lung damage ('bronchopulmonary dysplasia' or BPD); replacement therapy in adrenocortical disease; treatment of croup; as part of chemotherapy regimens for acute lymphoblastic leukaemia (ALL); as part of anti-emetic regimens following administration of moderately to highly emetogenic cytotoxic therapies; headache associated with raised intracranial pressure (ICP); to reduce tumour induced cerebral oedema prior to neurosurgery or palliative care of children with brain or other tumours.

PRESENTATION
Injection: dexamethasone sodium phosphate 5mg in 1mL (≡ dexamethasone phosphate 4.6mg in 1mL ≡ dexamethasone 3.8mg), 1mL ampoule and 2mL vial – non-proprietary (available from Organon); dexamethasone phosphate 4mg in 1mL (≡ dexamethasone 3.33mg in 1mL ≡ dexamethasone sodium phosphate 4.17mg in 1mL), 2mL vial – Decadron®, 1mL ampoule and 2mL vial – non-proprietary; 24mg in 1mL, 5mL vial – non-proprietary.
Oral solution: (as sodium phosphate) 500 microgram in 5mL – manufactured 'special'; 2mg in 5mL – non-proprietary; 10mg in 5mL – manufactured 'special'.
Tablet: 500 microgram – (scored) Decadron® and non-proprietary, 2mg – non-proprietary.

DOSAGE
3.8mg of dexamethasone base ≡ 4.6mg of dexamethasone phosphate ≡ 5mg of dexamethasone sodium phosphate. Prescribe in terms of **dexamethasone base**, with the exception of the treatment of cerebral oedema.

Indication	Route	Age			Frequency (times daily)	Notes
		1 month–2 years	2–12 years	12–18 years		
Croup	Oral	← 150 microgram/kg → OR 600 microgram/kg			2 or single dose	No definitive standard dose has been agreed in the UK. Suggested maximum single dose of 12mg.
Anti-emetic	IV/oral	<1 year 250 micrograms –1mg 1–2 years 1–2mg	2–5 years 1–2mg 6–12 years 2–4mg	4mg	3 3	Give IV doses with chemotherapy, then give IV or orally until 48 hours after chemotherapy.
Headache associated with raised intra-cranial pressure	IV/oral	← 250 microgram/kg →		–	2	For 5 days; then reduce the dose if possible to 62.5-125 micrograms/kg twice a day.
Short course to relieve symptoms of brain tumour	IV/oral	←125–500 microgram/kg→		–	2	Can also be used to reduce oedema around tumours compressing nerves.
Replacement	IV/oral	←250-500 microgram/m² →		–	2	

Fetal lung maturation: given to the mother
IM: 12mg **dexamethasone base**, repeated once after 24 hours if the risk of preterm delivery remains.
Oral: 6mg **dexamethasone base** orally twice daily for 4 doses.

Chronic lung damage ('bronchopulmonary dysplasia' or BPD)
The optimal regimen has not yet been finalised– see local policy. Regimens used have included:
250 microgram/kg **dexamethasone base** orally or IV twice daily for 3 days – regimen repeated once every 10 days until the baby is no longer oxygen dependent.
500 microgram/kg **dexamethasone base** orally or IV once daily for 3 days, then progressively reduced over a 6 week period to 100 microgram/kg on alternate days during the last week.

Post intubation laryngeal oedema
200 microgram/kg **dexamethasone base** orally or IV 8 hourly for a total of three doses, starting 4 hours before extubation.

Chemotherapy regimes
Always follow the dosage recommended in the chemotherapy protocol.

Cerebral oedema
High dose IV schedule (dose in terms of **dexamethasone phosphate**).

	Children <35kg	Children >35kg
Initial dose	20mg	24mg
1st–3rd day	4mg every 3 hours	4mg every 2 hours
4th day	4mg every 6 hours	4mg every 4 hours
5–8th day	2mg every 6 hours	4mg every 6 hours
Thereafter	decrease by daily reduction of 1mg	decrease by daily reduction of 2mg

ADMINISTRATION
Oral: the injection can be given orally (unlicensed route of administration). Tablets will disperse in water.
IV: can be given as a bolus over 3-5 minutes. The injection can be diluted in NaCl 0.9% or glucose 5%.

CONTRA-INDICATIONS & WARNINGS
There are concerns that postnatal use in preterm infants may be associated with an increased risk of cerebral palsy. May increase the risk of nephrocalcinosis if also on diuretics. Continuous treatment for over 10 days can produce adrenal suppression for 3-4 weeks. In palliative care, the adverse effects of long-term steroids often quickly begin to outweigh the beneficial ones so that it is often best to prescribe 5 day courses of steroids and repeat as indicated by symptoms.

INTERACTIONS

Reduced effect with *rifampicin, carbamazepine, phenobarbital (phenobarbitone), phenytoin* and *primidone.* Antagonises *antihypertensives* and *diuretics.* Increased risk of hypokalaemia with *acetazolamide, loop* and *thiazide diuretics.*

PREGNANCY

Intrauterine growth retardation has been observed. Contact local Medicines Information Centre for advice.

BREAST-FEEDING

No evidence that the baby will absorb/receive sufficient to produce adrenal suppression even if mother is taking doses equivalent to *prednisolone* 1mg/kg.

PHARMACOKINETIC PROPERTIES

Protein bound. Excretion mainly in urine.

EXCIPIENTS

Contact manufacturer's for further details.

LICENSED STATUS

Licensed for use in all ages; however BPD, fetal lung maturation, croup and anti-emetic use are not licensed indications. Oral solution 500 microgram in 5mL and 10mg in 5mL are 'specials', and as such are unlicensed.

FURTHER INFORMATION

Oral solution 500 microgram in 5mL available from Rosemont and 10mg in 5mL available from Nova Laboratories.

Dexamethasone with antibacterial

USES

Eczematous inflammation in otitis externa.

PRESENTATION

Ear or eye drops and ointment: dexamethasone 0.05%, framycetin 0.5% and gramicidin 0.005% – Sofradex® (drops 10mL and ointment 5g).
Ear spray: dexamethasone 0.1%, neomycin 3250 units/mL and glacial acetic acid 2%; 5mL pump-action aerosol – Otomize®.

DOSAGE/ADMINISTRATION

Ear drops: 2-3 drops 3-4 times daily.
Ear ointment: apply 1-2 times daily.
Ear spray: 1 metered dose spray 3 times daily.

CONTRA-INDICATIONS & WARNINGS

Otitis externa should not be treated when the eardrum is perforated because of the risk of ototoxicity. Hypersensitivity to any ingredient.

INTERACTIONS

None relevant to topical use.

PREGNANCY/BREAST-FEEDING

There is a risk of fetal ototoxicity if aminoglycosides are administered during pregnancy. Contact local Medicines Information Centre for advice.

POISONING/TOXICITY

Long-term intensive topical use may lead to systemic effects. Oral ingestion of the contents of one bottle is unlikely to lead to any serious adverse effects.

EXCIPIENTS

Otomize® includes hydroxybenzoates (parabens). Sofradex® drops include polysorbate 80.

LICENSED STATUS

Licensed for use in children and adults.

FURTHER INFORMATION

Treatment should not be continued for more than 7 days in the absence of clinical improvement. Prolonged use may lead to occult extension of infection due to the masking effect of the steroid. For reasons of hygiene do not use for more than 28 days after first opening it.

CNS stimulant.

USES
Hyperkinetic/attention-deficit disorders (often said to be the preferred drug in the presence of a poorly controlled seizure disorder). Narcolepsy.

PRESENTATION
Tablet: 5mg – Dexedrine®.

DOSAGE

Route	Age		Frequency	Notes
	2–12 years	12–18 years	(times daily)	
Oral	3–5 years 2.5mg 6–12 years 5–10mg	5–10mg	1–2 1–2	Initial dose shown in table. Then <6 years: increase if necessary by 2.5mg a day, at weekly intervals. Maximum 20mg per day. Then >6 years: increase if necessary by 5mg a day at weekly intervals. Maximum 40mg per day. Give maintenance dose as divided doses (usually 2–3 times daily).

ADMINISTRATION
Oral: tablets can be halved; unreliable dose if quartered.

CONTRA-INDICATIONS & WARNINGS, INTERACTIONS, SIDE-EFFECTS, POISONING, TOXICITY
See methylphenidate monograph. *Caution*: monitor growth in children, as growth rate retardation has been reported.

PREGNANCY
Dexamphetamine has been thought to produce embryotoxic effects in rodents, and retrospective evidence of uncertain significance in man has suggested a similar possibility. Avoid in pregnancy, especially during the first trimester.

BREAST-FEEDING
Passes into breast milk in significant amount; avoid in breast-feeding.

PHARMACOKINETIC PROPERTIES
Onset of action is 60-90 minutes. Peak serum concentration is reached within 3 hours of oral administration. Metabolised in the liver and excreted in the urine as unchanged drug and inactive metabolites.

EXCIPIENTS
Tablets include sucrose.

LICENSED STATUS
Licensed for use in children aged ≥3 years of age for treatment of hyperkinetic states.

Dextromethorphan

USES
Anecdotal evidence of use in non-ketotic hyperglycinaemia.

PRESENTATION
Oral liquid: 7.5mg in 5mL – Robitussin® Dry Cough; 3.75mg in 5mL – Robitussin® Junior Persistant Cough.
Oral suspension: 30mg in 5mL (long-acting) – Delsym® – named patient.

DOSAGE

Route	Age			Frequency (times daily)	Notes
	1 month–2 years	2–12 years	12–18 years		
Oral – liquid	←	1.25–2mg/kg	→	4	15 minutes before food.
Oral long-acting suspension	←	2.5mg/kg	→	2	Doses of up to 35mg/kg/**day** have been used.

CONTRA-INDICATIONS & WARNINGS
Respiratory failure.

INTERACTIONS
MAOIs may produce severe reactions, hyperpyrexia and fatalities have been reported.
Sodium valproate should be avoided if possible as it interferes with the activity of the glycine cleavage system to increase glycine levels in the blood and CSF.

PREGNANCY/BREAST-FEEDING
No information available.

SIDE-EFFECTS
At high doses somnolence, agitation and involuntary movements have been observed; if dose is decreased then side-effects are reduced. Dizziness and gastrointestinal disturbances occur rarely.

POISONING/TOXICITY
Lethargy, somnolence, ataxia, nystagmus and agitation. Overdose may be reversed by naloxone.

PHARMACODYNAMIC PROPERTIES
N-methyl-D-aspartate (NMDA) receptors are stimulated by glycine to cause seizures and irritability. Dextromethorphan is an antagonist of NMDA receptors and can help stop seizures.

PHARMACOKINETIC PROPERTIES
Rapidly absorbed from the gastrointestinal tract; metabolised in the liver and excreted in the urine as unchanged dextromethorphan and demethylated metabolites including dextrophan.

EXCIPIENTS
The long-acting preparation contains 1.7g of sugar in 5mL; it is alcohol-free.
Contact manufacturer's for further details.

LICENSED STATUS
Unlicensed for non-ketotic hyperglycinaemia.

FURTHER INFORMATION
The long-acting suspension is available on a named patient basis from IDIS World Medicines.

Di–iodohydroxyquinoline (iodoquinol)

A halogenated 8-hydroxyquinoline; a luminal or contact amoebicide.

USES
Amoebiasis; asymptomatic intestinal carriage (not the drug of choice).

PRESENTATION
Tablet: 210mg, 650mg – named patient (imported).

DOSAGE

Route	Age			Frequency (times daily)	Notes
	1 month–2 years	2–12 years	12–18 years		
Oral	← 10–13.3mg/kg →		630–650mg	3	For 20 days. Total daily dose should not exceed 1.95g.

ADMINISTRATION
Oral: take after meals. The tablets can be crushed and mixed with apple sauce or chocolate syrup.

CONTRA-INDICATIONS & WARNINGS
Known hypersensitivity to iodine or 8-hydroxyquinolines, impaired renal or hepatic function, pre-existing optic neuropathy. Use with caution in patients with thyroid disease. Discontinue the drug if hypersensitivity reactions occur. Its use is best avoided in patients with neurological disorders. Avoid long-term use.

INTERACTIONS
Protein-bound serum iodine levels may be increased during treatment with *iodoquinol* and therefore interfere with certain thyroid function tests. These effects may persist for as long as 6 months after discontinuation of therapy.

PREGNANCY/BREAST-FEEDING
Safe use during pregnancy or lactation has not been established.

SIDE-EFFECTS
The most serious adverse effect is neurotoxicity, which is related to dose and duration of therapy. Rarely the drug can cause optic neuritis, optic atrophy, and peripheral neuropathy, especially in children. Gastrointestinal effects are usually mild and include nausea, vomiting, abdominal cramps, diarrhoea, constipation and pruritus ani. Various forms of skin reactions have occurred including papular and pustular acneiform eruptions, bullae, and vegetating or tuberous iododerma. Other reported adverse effects include fever, chills, headache, vertigo, and slight enlargement of the thyroid.

POISONING/TOXICITY
Symptoms: see side-effects.
Treatment: no specific antidote; treatment is symptomatic and supportive.

PHARMACOKINETIC PROPERTIES
Partly and irregularly absorbed from the gastrointestinal tract. Excreted in the faeces.

LICENSED STATUS
Not licensed for use in the UK.

FURTHER INFORMATION
Available from IDIS World Medicines.

Diamorphine hydrochloride (controlled drug)

Opioid analgesic which is more potent than morphine.

USES
Control of severe pain. It has greater potency and water solubility than morphine and is preferred for parenteral administration in chronic pain or palliative care.

PRESENTATION
Injection: 5mg, 10mg, 30mg, 100mg and 500mg – non-proprietary.
Oral solution: may be extemporaneously prepared.
Tablet: 10mg – non-proprietary.

DOSAGE
Newborn infant

Route	Age		Frequency	Notes
	birth–1 month		(times daily)	
Slow IV bolus (over 30 minutes)	50 microgram/kg		single dose	Loading dose. Infant ventilated.
IV infusion	15 microgram/kg/hour		continuous	Maintenance dose. Infant ventilated.

The above doses have been used to provide analgesia and to improve synchrony during mechanical ventilation. Infusions of 2.5-7 microgram/kg/hour have been used in non-ventilated newborn infants.

Child

Prophylactic laxatives should always be prescribed when commencing major opioids.

Route	Age			Frequency	Notes
	1 month–2 years	2–12 years	12–18 years	(times daily)	
Oral	← 100–200 microgram/kg →		5–10mg	single dose	Repeat every 4 hours as necessary.
IV bolus	**1–3 months** 20 microgram/kg	-	-	single dose	Repeat every 6 hours as necessary.
	3–6 months 25–50 microgram/kg	-	-	single dose	Repeat every 6 hours as necessary.
	6–12 months 75 microgram/kg	-	-	single dose	Repeat every 4 hours as necessary.
	≥12 months ← 75–100 microgram/kg →		2.5–5mg	single dose	Repeat every 4 hours as necessary.
IV infusion	←12.5– 25 microgram/kg/hour→		-	continuous	
SC infusion	← 20–100 microgram/kg/hour →			continuous	
Extradural injection	← 25–50 microgram/kg/dose →			single dose	
SC/IM injection	-	-	5mg	single dose	Repeat every 4 hours as necessary. Use with caution if poor peripheral perfusion. Avoid IM injections if possible. Use SC/IM cannula placed while under GA or topical LA.

Renal impairment – in severe renal impairment give 50-75% of dose.
Liver disease – avoid or reduce dose as may precipitate coma.

ADMINISTRATION

IV infusion: glucose 5% is the preferred diluent but NaCl 0.9% may be used.
SC injection: reconstitute 5-100mg ampoules with 1mL Water for Injections and the 500mg ampoule with 2mL.
SC infusion: dilute reconstituted ampoules with Water for Injections or for doses up to 40mg in 1mL, NaCl 0.9% can be used but precipitation is more likely. Inspect solutions carefully for signs of precipitation after reconstituting and during administration.

The following drugs have been shown to be compatible with diamorphine in a syringe driver: haloperidol, hyoscine hydrobromide and butylbromide, levomepromazine (methotrimeprazine), midazolam, prochlorperazine.

The following drugs need to be used with caution: cyclizine – increased risk of precipitation above 10mg in 1mL of cyclizine; dexamethasone – care to avoid precipitation of dexamethasone when preparing; metoclopramide – if solutions become discoloured, they should be discarded.

CONTRA-INDICATIONS & WARNINGS

Contra-indications: paralytic ileus, phaeochromocytoma and raised intracranial pressure or head injury (may depress respiration and affect pupillary responses).
Cautions: acute respiratory failure and biliary colic in children <1 year (as they are more susceptible to respiratory depression – monitor oxygen saturation and respiratory rate).
Warnings: histamine release may provoke hypotension and tachycardia. In palliative care, there is no ceiling dose of major opioids.

INTERACTIONS

Enhanced sedative affect with *anxiolytics* and *hypnotics*, antagonism of gastrointestinal effects of *cisapride, metoclopramide* and *domperidone*.

Cimetidine inhibits metabolism of opioid analgesics leading to increased plasma level.

PREGNANCY

Use in the third trimester depresses neonatal respiration. Withdrawal effects are seen in neonates of dependant mothers.

BREAST-FEEDING

Therapeutic doses are unlikely to affect the breast-feeding infant but addicted mothers may often be discouraged from breast-feeding.

SIDE-EFFECTS

Sterile abscesses have been noted at subcutaneous sites. Nausea and vomiting, constipation and drowsiness. Larger doses may produce respiratory depression and hypotension. Nausea and hypotension may be less than seen with morphine. Histamine release with IV therapy may provoke hypotension and tachycardia.

POISONING/TOXICITY
The symptoms of serious overdose are respiratory depression, stupor or coma, muscle flaccidity, cold clammy skin, constricted pupils and occasionally bradycardia and hypotension. The specific antidote naloxone is indicated if coma or respiratory depression is present. In cases of fatal overdose, total morphine concentrations of 100-900 nanogram/mL have been detected in blood.

PHARMACOKINETIC PROPERTIES
Diamorphine is well absorbed from the gastrointestinal tract and following subcutaneous and intramuscular injection. Oral diamorphine is subject to extensive first pass metabolism to morphine. Parenteral doses are rapidly converted to morphine via an active metabolite. Up to 80% of a dose is recovered in the urine in 24 hours. Both diamorphine and its metabolite 6-acetylmorphine readily cross the blood-brain barrier.

EXCIPIENTS
Contact manufacturer's for details.

LICENSED STATUS
In children, diamorphine injection is only licensed for the treatment of those who are terminally ill.

Diazepam

Benzodiazepine.

USES
Short-term anxiety relief. Suppression of stage IV sleep in treatment of parasomnias. Relief of muscle spasm. Treatment of status epilepticus. Adjunct to anticonvulsants. Calming during alarming physical procedures, sedation for procedures. Pre-medication prior to surgery.

PRESENTATION
Injection: 5mg in 1mL – non-proprietary.
Injection: (emulsion) 5mg in 1mL – non-proprietary.
Oral solution: 2mg in 5mL – non-proprietary.
Strong oral solution: 5mg in 5mL – non-proprietary.
Rectal tube: 2mg in 1mL, 2.5mg and 5mg tube; 4mg in 1mL, 10mg tube – non-proprietary.
Suppository: 10mg – non-proprietary.
Tablet: (scored) 2mg, 5mg and 10mg – non-proprietary.

DOSAGE

Indication	Route	Age				Frequency	Notes
		birth–1 month	1 month–2 years	2–12 years	12–18 years	(times daily)	
Pre-medication	Oral	–	DOSE BY WEIGHT <u>≤1 year</u> 250 microgram/kg DOSE BY AGE <u>>1 year</u> 2.5mg	<u>≤5 years</u> 2.5mg <u>>5 years</u> 5mg	10mg	single dose single dose	
Sedation prior to procedures, calming during procedures	IV	–	← 100-200 microgram/kg →			single dose	IV only to be given by a trained anaesthetist or intensivist and very slow titration against symptoms or level of consciousness to a maximum of: 5mg <12 years 10-20mg >12 years. Orally give 45-60 minutes before procedure.
	Oral	–	← 200-300 microgram/kg →			single dose	
	Rectal	–	<u>>1 year</u> 5mg	<u>2-3 years</u> 5mg <u>>3 years</u> 5-10mg	10mg	single dose single dose	

D

DOSAGE continued

Indication	Route	Age				Frequency (times daily)	Notes
		birth– 1 month	1 month– 2 years	2–12 years	12–18 years		
Status epilepticus	IV bolus	← 300–400 microgram/kg →			10–20mg	single dose	Lorazepam is first choice benzo-diazepine IV (see guidance section).
	IV infusion	50 microgram /kg/hour (maximum 300 microgram /kg/hour)	100 microgram/kg/hour (maximum usually 125 micrograms/kg/hour but doses of up to a maximum of 400 microgram/kg/hour have been used in PICU)		125 microgram/ kg/hour	continuous	Diazepam IV is an alternative. Repeat diazepam IV bolus after 10 minutes if necessary. IV infusion: start at the lower dose, increasing if necessary to the maximum as indicated.
	Rectal	1.25–2.5mg	5mg	5–10mg	10mg	single dose	If needed, repeat after 5 minutes.
Short-term anxiety relief	Oral	–	–	2–3mg	2–10mg	3	Unlikely to be effective <12 years. Keep daily dose below 10mg in this category.
Suppression of stage IV sleep in treatment of parasomnias	Oral	–	–	← 1–5mg →		1 (at bedtime)	
Relief of muscle spasm	Oral	–	DOSE BY WEIGHT <1 year 250 microgram/kg DOSE BY AGE >1 year 2.5mg	<5 years 2.5mg >5 years 5mg	10mg	2 2	For post-operative skeletal muscle pain and as initial doses for tension and irritability in cerebral spasticity.

CONTRA-INDICATIONS & WARNINGS

Parenteral and rectal use can depress respiration: caution with coexistent respiratory disease or myasthenia gravis. Potential for dependency in anxiety treatment - use for a few weeks only. Acute porphyria.

INTERACTIONS

Caution with other *CNS depressants*.

PREGNANCY

Benzodiazepines cross the placenta and there is risk of adverse effects in the fetus. If benzodiazepines are administered at high doses, during late pregnancy, or during labour, effects on the neonate such as hypothermia, hypotonia and moderate respiratory depression may occur.

Infants born to mothers who take benzodiazepines chronically during the latter stages of pregnancy may develop physical dependence and be at risk of developing withdrawal symptoms (irritability or difficulty with feeding) in the postnatal period. If a benzodiazepine is prescribed to a woman of childbearing potential, she should be advised to contact her physician regarding discontinuation of the drug if she intends to become, or suspects that she is, pregnant.

BREAST-FEEDING

Benzodiazepines are excreted in breast milk, and they can cause lethargy in infant. Contact local Medicines Information Centre for advice.

SIDE-EFFECTS

Drowsiness, ataxia, dysarthria, irritability, light-headedness and social disinhibition.

Withdrawal syndrome in long-term users: muscle and abdominal cramps, tremor, irritability, convulsions and perceptual distortions.

POISONING/TOXICITY

Benzodiazepines are remarkably safe when taken alone in overdosage. Serious toxicity is rare. Treatment is symptomatic and supportive. *Flumazenil* is used for the reversal of sedative effects of benzodiazepines in anaesthetic procedures. It should only be given to children if the features of benzodiazepine overdosage are such that the child may be at serious risk. It should only be used in an intensive care or emergency setting. Repeated doses of *flumazenil* may be needed as it has a short duration of action. *Flumazenil* may cause convulsions.

D

PHARMACOKINETIC PROPERTIES

Rapidly and completely absorbed from the gastrointestinal tract following oral administration; peak plasma concentrations occurring within 15-90 minutes in adults and 15-30 minutes in children. Diazepam has a half-life of 20-100 hours, and this is prolonged in neonates. It is extensively metabolised in the liver and excreted in the urine, mainly as metabolites.

EXCIPIENTS

Contact manufacturer's for further details.

LICENSED STATUS

Tablets and liquid licensed for use in children for night terrors and somnambulism, pre-medication, management of spasticity and control of muscle spasm in tetanus.

Injection licensed in children for status epilepticus, febrile convulsions and convulsions due to poisoning and pre-medication.

The rectal tubes are licensed for use in children >1 year of age for acute severe anxiety and agitation, epileptic and febrile convulsions, tetanus and sedation for procedures.

Diazoxide

Vasodilator, thiazide derivative; inhibits insulin release from the beta cells of the pancreas, stimulates glycogenolysis and enhances secretion of adrenaline.

USES

Resistant hypertension; intractable hypoglycaemia.

PRESENTATION

Injection: 15mg in 1mL, 20mL ampoule – Eudemine®.

Suspension: may be extemporaneously prepared (from powder – named patient).

Tablet: 50mg – Eudemine®.

DOSAGE

Seek expert advice before prescribing.

Indication	Route	Age				Frequency	Notes
		birth–1 month	1 month–2 years	2–12 years	12–18 years	(times daily)	
Intractable hypoglycaemia	Oral	←	1.7–5mg/kg		→	3	Initial dose to establish response. Thereafter, dose can be increased as
Resistant hypertension	Oral	←	1.7mg/kg		→	3	necessary. Usual maximum dose is 15mg/kg/**day**, although up to 20mg/kg/**day** has been used in hyperinsulinism of infancy.
Severe hypertension	IV bolus	–	← 1-3mg/kg (maximum of 150mg)		→	single dose	Repeat after 5–15 minutes if necessary. Monitor blood pressure closely. Maximum 4 doses in 24 hours.

ADMINISTRATION

IV: give as a rapid injection over 30 seconds or less. Never give by IM or SC routes as it is very irritant.

CONTRA-INDICATIONS & WARNINGS

Hypersensitivity to any component of the preparation or to other thiazides. In the treatment of hypoglycaemia use is contra-indicated in cases which are amenable to surgery or specific therapy. Monitor blood pressure regularly. Retention of sodium and water may necessitate therapy with a *diuretic*. In hypertensive encephalopathy a rapid reduction in blood pressure can result in blindness, watershed cerebral infarction or death. Diazoxide is not the drug of first choice for this condition. Caution in patients with severe renal impairment – maintain adequate urinary volumes with diuretic therapy. Causes local ischaemia and necrosis on extravasation.

Monitor white blood cell and platelet counts regularly when used over a prolonged period. In children, regularly assess growth, bone and psychological maturation.

INTERACTIONS
Oral hypoglycaemics can cause antagonism of hypoglycaemia effect. Enhanced hypotensive effect with *ACE inhibitors, anaesthetics, antihypertensives, diuretics, beta-blockers, anxiolytics, hypnotics, calcium-channel blockers* and *nitrates*. *NSAIDs* and *corticosteroids* antagonise the hypotensive effect. Diazoxide may reduce *phenytoin* levels – monitor closely. *Phenytoin* may reduce the effect of diazoxide.

PREGNANCY
Diazoxide crosses the placenta. Prolonged therapy in pregnancy can affect neonatal glucose homeostasis and has also been associated with neonatal alopecia and hypertrichosis. If given during labour it may affect uterine tone and delay labour unless oxytocin is prescribed also.

BREAST-FEEDING
Contact local Medicines Information Centre for advice.

SIDE-EFFECTS
Nausea (common in the first 2-3 weeks of therapy and may require relief with an antiemetic), extrapyramidal effects, sodium and water retention, tachycardia, hyperglycaemia. May cause hypertrichosis and blood disorders if used long-term.

POISONING/TOXICITY
Excessive dosage can result in hyperglycaemia which will respond to insulin, and/or hypotension which will necessitate maintenance of blood volume with IV fluids.

EXCIPIENTS
Contact manufacturer's for further details.

LICENSED STATUS
Tablets licensed for use in children and adults. Powder is unlicensed for use in the UK.

FURTHER INFORMATION
Powder is available via Medeva Pharma Ltd.

Dichloroacetate

USES
Anecdotal evidence of use in the treatment of lactic acidosis in patients with defects in pyruvate dehydrogenase complex. Has also been used in other disorders of pyruvate metabolism.

PRESENTATION
Solution: 50mg in 1mL – manufactured 'special'.

DOSAGE

Route	Age				Frequency (times daily)	Notes
	birth–1 month	1 month–2 years	2–12 years	12–18 years		
Oral	←		12.5mg/kg	→	4	Doses of up to 200mg/kg/day have been used without adverse effect.

CONTRA-INDICATIONS & WARNINGS
Chronic use has led to polyneuropathy.

INTERACTIONS
None known.

PREGNANCY/BREAST-FEEDING
No information available.

SIDE-EFFECTS
Polyneuropathy. Abnormalities in oxalate metabolism. Concomitant metabolic acidosis. Rise in glycerol in the CSF.

PHARMACODYNAMIC PROPERTIES
Activates pyruvate dehydrogenase which catalyses the oxidation of lactate and pyruvate which leads to decreased lactate levels.

LICENSED STATUS
Available as a 'special' and as such is unlicensed.

FURTHER INFORMATION
Plasma concentrations can be measured by the London Medical Toxicology Unit (National Poisons Information Service). The solution is prepared from powder which is available from Special Products Ltd.

Diclofenac

Non-steroidal anti-inflammatory drug (NSAID).

USES
Pain and inflammation including rheumatic disease (including juvenile idiopathic arthritis) and musculoskeletal disorders. Bone pain including metastatic cancer.

PRESENTATION
Capsule: (modified release) 75mg – Diclomax SR®, 100mg – Diclomax Retard®.
Capsule: 75mg (25mg as enteric coated; 50mg as modified release) – Motifene® 75mg.
Gel: 1% – Voltarol® Emulgel®.
Injection: 25mg in 1mL, 3mL ampoule – Voltarol® and non-proprietary.
Suppository: 12.5mg, 25mg, 50mg and 100mg – Voltarol®; 100mg – non-proprietary.
Tablet: (dispersible) 10mg – manufactured 'special', 50mg – Voltarol®.
Tablet: (enteric coated) 25mg and 50mg – Voltarol® and non-proprietary.
Tablet: (modified release) 75mg – Voltarol® 75mg SR, 100mg – Voltarol® Retard.

DOSAGE

Route	Age			Frequency (times daily)	Notes
	1 month–2 years	2–12 years	12–18 years		
Oral/ rectal	<6 months	← 300 microgram–1mg/kg →		3	Up to a maximum of 150mg/day.
	Not recommended				
	>6 months				
	300 microgram–1mg/kg			3	
IM/IV	<6 months	← 300 microgram–1mg/kg →		1- 2	Up to a maximum of 150mg/day and for a maximum of 2 days.
	Not recommended				
	>6 months				
	300 microgram–1mg/kg			1-2	
Topical	Not recommended	← small amount →		3-4	

D

ADMINISTRATION
Oral: the enteric coated tablets or capsules may be taken on an empty stomach. Modified release tablets or capsules should be taken with or after food to minimise gastrointestinal side-effects. The dispersible tablets are less completely absorbed when taken with food. However, these tablets should still be given with or after food to increase gastrointestinal tolerance.
IM: should be given IM by deep intragluteal injection into the upper outer quadrant. Alternate buttocks should be used for consecutive injections. IM therapy should not continue for more than 2 days.
IV: do not administer as an IV bolus injection. For IV infusion 75mg diclofenac should be diluted in 100–500mL of either NaCl 0.9% or glucose 5%. These solutions must first be buffered with sodium bicarbonate solution (0.5mL of 8.4% or 1mL of 4.2%). The dose should be infused over 30 minutes to 2 hours. IV therapy should not continue for more than 2 days.
Topical: do not treat a large area, and wash hands after use. Topical administration does not avoid systemic effects.

CONTRA-INDICATIONS & WARNINGS
Should not be given to patients with active peptic ulceration, and should be used with extreme caution in patients with a history of peptic ulceration. Also contra-indicated in patients who have previously shown hypersensitivity reactions (asthma, rhinitis, urticaria) to aspirin or other NSAIDs.
Use with caution in renal, cardiac or hepatic impairment. The topical preparations should not be applied to broken skin or mucosal surfaces. Keep away from the eyes. Diclofenac may trigger attacks of hepatic porphyria in susceptible patients.
The rectal route is contra-indicated in ulcerative or acute inflammatory conditions of the anus, rectum or sigmoid colon.
The IV route is contra-indicated with concurrent NSAID or anticoagulant use (including low dose heparin), a history of haemorrhagic diathesis, a history of confirmed or suspected cerebrovascular bleeding, operations which carry a high risk of haemorrhage, a history of asthma, moderate or severe renal impairment, hypovolaemia or dehydration.

INTERACTIONS
May decrease the elimination of *methotrexate*. May cause an increase in *digoxin* levels. Increased risk of nephrotoxicity when given with *ciclosporin (cyclosporin)* or *diuretics*. Increased risk of convulsions with *quinolones*.

PREGNANCY
NSAIDs should be avoided in the third trimester as they may cause constriction of the ductus arteriosus in utero leading to persistent pulmonary hypertension in the newborn. In addition, these drugs may inhibit labour if used close to delivery.

BREAST-FEEDING
Diclofenac enters breast milk in such small quantities that the amount ingested by the infant is likely to be insignificant, and no undesirable effects are to be expected.

SIDE-EFFECTS
Gastrointestinal discomfort, nausea, diarrhoea and occasionally bleeding and ulceration; headache, dizziness, vertigo; fluid retention; hypersensitivity reactions e.g. bronchospasm, rashes; local discomfort, burning or itching and occasionally bleeding may occur with NSAID suppositories.

POISONING/TOXICITY
Management of acute poisoning with NSAIDs essentially consists of supportive and symptomatic measures. There is no typical clinical picture resulting from diclofenac overdose, but hypotension, renal failure, gastrointestinal irritation, respiratory depression and convulsions can occur.

PHARMACOKINETIC PROPERTIES
Diclofenac is rapidly absorbed via any route. Peak plasma levels occur 10-20 minutes after IM administration, and 30-60 minutes after rectal administration. Oral administration gives peak levels after 1 hour for dispersible tablets, and between 1-4 hours for enteric coated preparations. Diclofenac has a plasma half-life of 2 hours.

EXCIPIENTS
Voltarol® dispersible tablets contain sodium saccharin. Voltarol® SR tablets and Diclomax® capsules contain sucrose. Voltarol® injection includes benzyl alcohol. Contact manufacturer's for further details.

LICENSED STATUS
All the 25mg enteric coated tablets and the 12.5mg and 25mg suppositories are licensed for use in juvenile idiopathic arthritis >1 year of age at a dose of 1–3mg/kg/day in divided doses. Volraman® 50mg EC tablets are the only 50mg tablets licensed for this age group for the same dose and indication. All other preparations containing ≥50mg diclofenac are not licensed for use in children. 10mg dispersible tablets are a 'special' and as such are unlicensed.

FURTHER INFORMATION
10mg dispersible tablets are available from Special Products Limited.

Dicycloverine (dicyclomine) hydrochloride

Tertiary amine, synthetic antimuscarinic with low anticholinergic effects and possible direct effect upon smooth muscle.

USES
Relief from gastrointestinal pain due to smooth muscle spasm.

PRESENTATION
Tablet: 10mg – Merbentyl®, 20mg – Merbentyl 20®.
Syrup: 10mg in 5mL – Merbentyl®.

DOSAGE

Route	Age			Frequency	Notes
	1 month–2 years	2–12 years	12–18 years	(times daily)	
Oral	>6 months 5–10mg	–		3–4	15 minutes before feeds/food.
	–	10mg	10 –20mg	3	

ADMINISTRATION
Oral: tablets may be divided or crushed.

CONTRA-INDICATIONS & WARNINGS
Not to be used in infants <6 months of age. Not to be used in paralytic ileus; may aggravate gastro-oesophageal reflux.

PREGNANCY
Avoid if possible, although studies have not shown teratogenicity.

BREAST-FEEDING
Not known if excreted in breast milk. Contact local Medicines Information Centre for advice.

SIDE-EFFECTS
Seldom occur but can include dry mouth, thirst and dizziness. Rarely, fatigue, sedation, blurred vision, constipation, rash, nausea, vomiting and headache.

POISONING
Symptoms include headache, dizziness, dry mouth, nausea, difficulty in swallowing, dilated pupils and hot dry skin. Treatment is symptomatic.

PHARMACOKINETIC PROPERTIES
Well absorbed after oral administration. Onset of effect 1-2 hours, effects can continue for up to 4 hours. Extensively metabolised and eliminated in the urine with only a small amount excreted as unchanged drug.

EXCIPIENTS
Syrup includes sugar.

LICENSED STATUS
Licensed for >6 months of age.

D

Didanosine (ddi, DDI)

Nucleoside reverse transcriptase inhibitor.

USES
Combination antiviral treatment of Human Immunodeficiency Virus (HIV) infected patients.

PRESENTATION
Powder for oral solution: 2g, 4g (to prepare a solution 10mg in 1mL) – named patient.
Tablet: 25mg, 100mg, 150mg and 200mg (chewable, dispersible and buffered) – Videx®.

DOSAGE

Route	Age				Frequency	Notes
	birth–1 month	1 month–2 years	2–12 years	12–18 years	(times daily)	
Oral	No information available	←	120mg/m²	→	2	
		←	90mg/m²	→	2	Dose if concurrent treatment with zidovudine.

Dose in renal impairment

Creatinine clearance (mL/minute/1.73m²)	Dose/dose frequency
30–59	60% of the normal total dose, daily in two divided doses.
10–29	40% of the normal total dose once daily.
<10	30% of the normal total dose once daily.

The total daily dose may be given once daily if there are practical problems with administration or compliance. Dose reduction may be appropriate when reintroduced following discontinuation due to pancreatitis or neuropathy and should be considered in patients with hepatic impairment.

ADMINISTRATION

Oral: as absorption is reduced in the presence of food, it is recommended that didanosine is taken at least 30 minutes (preferably 1 hour) before or 2 hours after meals.

Following reconstitution the oral solution must be diluted with antacid to prevent acid degradation in the stomach. Suitable antacids are Maalox®; Mylanta Maximum Strength® (unlicensed in the UK, but available through import) may be preferable in children due to palatability and less potential to induce diarrhoea. Tablets should be chewed, crushed or dispersed in water; do not mix with fruit juice or other acid-containing liquid.

CONTRA-INDICATIONS & WARNINGS

Hypersensitivity to the components. Use with caution if there is a previous history of pancreatic disease or elevation of pancreatic amylase or triglycerides. Suspend treatment if pancreatitis is suspected or pancreatic enzymes are raised significantly during treatment even if asymptomatic. The tablets contain phenylalanine (from aspartame) and caution is advised in patients with phenylketonuria; use in such patients only if clearly indicated. Retinal or optic nerve changes have been reported in children and regular eye examinations are recommended at least 6 monthly or if vision disturbance occurs. Suspend treatment if any of the following become clinically significant: peripheral neuropathy, hyperuricaemia, raised liver enzymes, rapidly elevating aminotransferase levels, progressive hepatomegaly, hepatitis or lactic acidosis of unknown origin.

INTERACTIONS

Buffers and antacids present in didanosine formulations may reduce absorption of some drugs such as *ciprofloxacin, itraconazole, ketoconazole* and *dapsone*. This occurs either by direct interaction with aluminium/magnesium in the antacids or due to the raising of gastric pH. Avoid taking such drugs within 2 hours of didanosine. Use with caution with other drugs that may be associated with pancreatic toxicity or peripheral neuropathy.

PREGNANCY

Consider use only if clearly indicated and the expected benefits to the mother outweigh potential risks to the fetus, as there are no data are available.

BREAST-FEEDING

No human studies but it is excreted in animal milk and the potential for toxicity means that breast-feeding should be avoided.

SIDE-EFFECTS

Pancreatitis and elevation of serum amylase and lipase have been reported. Pancreatitis, which may be fatal, is more frequent with high doses, in advanced HIV disease and if there is a previous history of pancreatitis. It usually appears at 1-6 months after the start of treatment and resolves within 3 weeks of discontinuation of didanosine. Peripheral neuropathy has been associated with didanosine and may require dose modification. Abnormal liver function tests have been reported. Rare reports of liver failure. Also rare reports of lactic acidosis and hepatomegaly with steatosis have been reported with other dideoxynucleoside antivirals. Asymptomatic hyperuricaemia has been reported which may require discontinuation if there is no response to measures aimed at reducing uric acid levels. Gastrointestinal symptoms such as nausea, vomiting, abdominal pain, diarrhoea, constipation and taste disturbance have been reported. Dry mouth may also occur. Sensitivity reactions such as rash, pruritus, allergic reactions and anaphylaxis have occurred. Haematological effects such as leucopenia, thrombocytopenia and anaemia may be more common in children. Retinal or optic nerve changes have been reported in children and regular eye examinations are recommended at least 6 monthly or if vision disturbance occurs. Rare reports of diabetes mellitus and hypokalaemia.

PHARMACOKINETIC PROPERTIES

Didanosine is rapidly degraded at an acidic pH. All oral formulations must contain buffering agents to increase gastric pH. Administration with meals significantly reduces absorption by as much as 50%. Oral bioavailability may be more variable in children than in adults. Penetrates into CSF attaining concentrations averaging 46% of those in the plasma. Plasma protein binding is less than 5%. Renal clearance represents about 60% of total body clearance. Glomerular filtration and active tubular secretion are responsible for renal elimination. Elimination half-life averages 48 minutes in children (compared to 1.4 hours in adults). Metabolism has not been fully evaluated but is presumed to follow similar pathways to the elimination of endogenous purines.

POISONING/TOXICITY
There is no specific antidote. Anticipated complications of overdose would be secondary to hyperuricaemia or, possibly, to hepatic dysfunction. Didanosine is not dialysable by peritoneal dialysis, although there is some clearance by haemodialysis (20-35% over 3-4 hours dialysis).

EXCIPIENTS
Tablets include aspartame. Contact manufacturer's for further details.

LICENSED STATUS
Tablets licensed for ≥3 months of age. Powder for oral solution is not licensed for use in the UK.

FURTHER INFORMATION
Powder for oral solution available from Bristol-Myers Squibb.

Diethylcarbamazine

Anthelmintic.

USES
Treatment of lymphatic filariasis (due to *Wuchereria bancrofti* [bancroftian filariasis], *Brugia malayi* or *B. timori*), loiasis, tropical pulmonary eosinophilia and toxocariasis (visceral larva migrans).

PRESENTATION
Tablet: 100mg – Notezine® (imported).

DOSAGE

Indication	Route	Age			Frequency (times daily)	Notes
		1 month– 2 years	2–12 years	12–18 years		
Lymphatic filariasis (due to *Wuchereria bancrofti* [bancroftian filariasis], *Brugi malayi*, or *B. timori*. Loiasis	Oral	Day 1 ← 300 microgram/kg → then increasing gradually over 3 days to 2mg/kg			3	While the manufacturer and *BNF* recommend treatment for 3 weeks, WHO recommends treatment for only 6-18 days depending on the type of filariasis.
Tropical pulmonary eosinophilia	Oral	← 2mg/kg →			3	Given for 21 days.
Toxocariasis (visceral larva–migrans)	Oral	Days 1–2 ← 160 microgram/kg → then increasing gradually over 3 days to 2mg/kg			3	Continue dose of 2mg/kg 3 times daily for 7-10 days.

ADMINISTRATION
Oral: administer after meals to lessen gastrointestinal disturbances.

CONTRA-INDICATIONS & WARNINGS
Hypersensitivity to diethylcarbamazine. Severe allergic reactions can occur especially in patients with onchocerciasis or *Loa loa* infection. In the event of severe hypersensitivity reaction, administration of a corticosteroid is recommended. Encephalitis may occur in patients with loiasis. Monitor for eye changes in patients with onchocerciasis. Impaired renal function: dose reduction may be required.

D

INTERACTIONS

Concurrent use of diethylcarbamazine with *corticosteroids* may reduce the antifiliarial activity of diethylcarbamazine. *Urinary alkalinizers* can reduce the loss of diethylcarbamazine in the urine, whereas *urinary acidifiers* can increase the loss.

PREGNANCY

In view of severe reactions that may follow diethylcarbamazine administration, it is advised to postpone treatment until after parturition.

BREAST-FEEDING

Contact local Medicines Information Centre for advice.

SIDE-EFFECTS

Headache, lassitude, weakness, general malaise are seen most commonly. Nausea, vomiting, skin rash, occasionally observed. Severe allergic phenomenon can occur in conjunction with the skin rash. In patients with onchocerciasis severe allergic reactions may occur. Facial oedema and pruritus, especially of the eyes, are often encountered.

POISONING/TOXICITY

Symptoms of overdose consist of nausea, vomiting, headache, dizziness and drowsiness.

Gastric lavage should be performed only if within 2 hours of ingestion. Adequate fluids should be given to ensure optimal diuresis, acidification of urine should enhance excretion and routine supportive measures given where necessary.

PHARMACOKINETIC PROPERTIES

Readily absorbed from gastrointestinal tract. Also absorbed through skin and conjunctiva. Metabolised in liver; excreted as unchanged drug and the N-oxide metabolite in the urine. Urinary excretion and hence plasma half-life is dependent on urinary pH.

EXCIPIENTS

Contact manufacturer for further details.

LICENSED STATUS

Not licensed for use in the UK.

FURTHER INFORMATION

Available from IDIS World Medicines.

Infants (usually <1 year), the elderly, pregnant women and the debilitated, especially those with cardiac or renal disease, are normally excluded when diethylcarbamazine is used in mass treatment schedules.

Diethylstilbestrol (stilboestrol)

A synthetic non-steroidal oestrogen.

USES

Priming the pituitary prior to growth hormone stimulation testing.

PRESENTATION

Tablet: 1mg and 5mg – non-proprietary.

DOSAGE/ ADMINISTRATION

Oral: 1mg twice a day, for 2 days before the test.

CONTRA-INDICATIONS & WARNINGS

Pregnancy, liver disease, hypertension, thrombo-embolism and porphyria.

INTERACTIONS

As for oestrogens in general.

PREGNANCY/ BREAST-FEEDING

Contra-indicated. Female offspring of mothers who received diethylstilbestrol during pregnancy have developed cervical and vaginal abnormalities including adenosis and adenocarcinoma.

SIDE-EFFECTS

Nausea, fluid retention, venous and arterial thrombosis, impotence, gynaecomastia.

EXCIPIENTS
Contact manufacturer for further details.

LICENSED STATUS
Not licensed for this indication.

Digoxin

Cardiac glycoside.

USES
Treatment of acute or chronic congestive cardiac failure, control of ventricular rate in atrial flutter or fibrillation, management of supraventricular tachycardia .

PRESENTATION
Tablet: 62.5 microgram – Lanoxin-PG® and non-proprietary; 125 microgram and 250 microgram – Lanoxin® and non-proprietary.
Elixir: 50 microgram in 1mL – Lanoxin-PG®.
Injection: 250 microgram in 1mL, 2mL ampoule – Lanoxin® and non-proprietary; 100 microgram in 1mL – manufactured 'special'.

DOSAGE
The doses stated are for patients who have not received cardiac glycosides in the preceding 2 weeks. If cardiac glycosides have been given in the 2 weeks preceding commencement, it should be anticipated that optimum loading doses will be less than those stated (levels should be checked before loading).
The dosage schedules are meant as guidelines and careful clinical observation and monitoring of serum digoxin levels should be used as a basis for adjustment of dosage.
In myocarditis, halve loading and maintenance doses, as the myocardium is more sensitive to cardiac glycosides.
Check the doses carefully because an overdose can cause death.
Maintenance dose should start 12 hours after loading ends.
* >10 years use doses at the lower end of the range in early adolescence and/or in underweight children.

LOADING DOSE
The loading dose (IV or oral) should be administered in divided doses over 12 hours. Give half the total loading dose immediately, a quarter of the total loading dose after 6 hours and the remainder after a further 6 hours, assessing the clinical response before giving each additional dose. Each IV dose should be given by slow IV injection over 10 minutes.

Intravenous loading dose

Age	Preterm newborn infant <1.5kg	Preterm newborn infant 1.5–2.5kg	Newborn infant – 2 years	2–5 years	5–10 years	*>10 years
Dose	10 microgram/kg over 10 minutes	15 microgram/kg over 10 minutes	← 17.5 microgram/kg over 10 minutes →		12.5 microgram/kg over 10 minutes (maximum 250 microgram)	250–500 microgram over 10 minutes
	then	then	then		then	then
	after 6 hours 5 microgram/kg over 10 minutes	after 6 hours 7.5 microgram/kg over 10 minutes	← after 6 hours 8.75 microgram/kg over 10 minutes →		after 6 hours 6.25 microgram/kg over 10 minutes (maximum 125 microgram)	after 6 hours 125–250 microgram over 10 minutes
	then after a further 6 hours 5 microgram/kg over 10 minutes	then after a further 6 hours 7.5 microgram/kg over 10 minutes	← then after a further 6 hours 8.75 microgram/kg over 10 minutes →		then after a further 6 hours 6.25 microgram/kg over 10 minutes	then after a further 6 hours 125–250 microgram over 10 minutes

Oral loading dose

Age	Preterm newborn infant <1.5kg	Preterm newborn infant 1.5-2.5kg	Newborn infant - 2 years	2-5 years	5-10 years	*>10 years
Dose	12.5 microgram/kg	15 microgram/kg	22.5 microgram/kg	17.5 microgram/kg	12.5 microgram/kg (maximum 375 microgram)	375-750 microgram
	then	then	then	then	then	then
	after 6 hours	after 6 hours	after 6 hours	after 6 hours	after 6 hours	after 6 hours
	6.25 microgram/kg	7.5 microgram/kg	11.25 microgram/kg	8.75 microgram/kg	6.25 microgram/kg	187.5-375 microgram
	then after	then after	then after	then after	then after	then after
	a further 6 hours	a further 6 hours	a further 6 hours	a further 6 hours	a further 6 hours	a further 6 hours
	6.25 microgram/kg	7.5 microgram/kg	11.25 microgram/kg	8.75 microgram/kg	6.25 microgram/kg (maximum 187.5 microgram)	187.5-375 microgram

Maintenance dose: IV or oral

Age	Preterm newborn infant <1.5kg	Preterm newborn infant 1.5-2.5kg	Newborn infant - 2 years	2-5 years	5-10 years	*>10 years	Frequency (times daily)	Notes
Dose	2.5 microgram/kg	3 microgram/kg	5 microgram/kg			3 microgram/kg (maximum 125 microgram)	–	2	The total daily dose may be given once a day.
	–	–	–	–		125-750 microgram	1	

Dose reduction in renal impairment

Grade	Serum creatinine micromol/L (approx)	Creatinine clearance mL/minute/1.73m^2	Dosage (loading and maintenance)
Mild	150-300	20-50	reduce dose by 50%
Moderate	300-700	10-20	reduce dose by 50%
Severe	>700	<10	reduce dose by 75%

ADMINISTRATION

Oral: there are no data regarding safety of crushing, dissolving or halving tablets as there is a liquid formulation available. Crushing the tablets may alter the bioavailability. The liquid formulation must not be diluted.

IV: the injection may be given undiluted if given slowly over 10 minutes. The injection may be diluted with a four-fold or greater volume of glucose 5% or NaCl 0.9%. Dilution should be carried out immediately before use and any unused solution discarded.

IM: the IM route is painful and associated with muscle necrosis and therefore cannot be recommended.

NB. The oral bioavailability of the liquid (80%) and tablets (70%) differs. Blood levels should be checked if the preparation is changed. When changing from the IV to the oral route the dose may require to be increased by 20% (liquid) or 30% (tablets) to maintain the same blood levels.

CONTRA-INDICATIONS & WARNINGS

Contra-indications: complete heart block, hypertrophic cardiomyopathy, children >2 years with accessory pathways e.g. Wolff-Parkinson-White syndrome and those with a hypersensitivity to digitalis glycosides. *Warnings/precautions:* a reduction in loading and maintenance doses is necessary in patients with renal impairment. Hypokalaemia, hypomagnesaemia and marked hypercalcaemia increase myocardial sensitivity to cardiac glycosides. Rapid IV injection can cause vasoconstriction leading to hypertension and/or reduced coronary flow. Slow IV rate is important in cases of hypertensive heart failure and acute myocardial infarction. The risk of provoking dangerous arrhythmias with direct DC conversion is greatly increased in the presence of digitalis toxicity. Caution should be exercised in treating patients with pre-existing bradycardia. May exacerbate sinus bradycardia in sick sinus syndrome. Care in patients with thyroid disease.

INTERACTIONS
Digoxin serum levels can be increased by *quinidine* and *amiodarone*. The dose of digoxin should be halved if using concurrently. Digoxin serum levels may also be increased by *flecainide, propafenone, spironolactone, tetracycline, erythromycin, verapamil* and *diltiazem*. Monitor for digoxin toxicity and if levels dictate, reduce dose accordingly. Digoxin levels are reduced by *rifampicin, phenytoin* and *St. John's Wort*. Increased risk of hypokalaemia if *corticosteroids* and digoxin are used concurrently. Digoxin toxicity can be increased if used with *amphotericin* or *diuretics which cause hypokalaemia*.

PREGNANCY
The use of digoxin in pregnancy is not contra-indicated, although the dosage and control may be less predictable. Contact local Medicines Information Centre for advice.

BREAST-FEEDING
Digoxin may be excreted in minute quantities in breast milk. Breast-feeding is not contra-indicated.

SIDE-EFFECTS
Cardiac: digoxin toxicity can cause various arrhythmias and conduction disturbances.
Gastrointestinal: anorexia, nausea, vomiting and diarrhoea.
Gynaecomastia: may occur with long-term administration.
Skin rashes: rarely urticaria or scarlatiniform reactions.
CNS: weakness, apathy, fatigue, malaise, headache, visual disturbances, depression and psychoses.
Other: rarely thrombocytopenia.

POISONING/TOXICITY
The effects of digoxin poisoning are potentially very severe/fatal. It is recommended that a National Poisons Information Centre is consulted for full details of management.
Signs/symptoms: see the side-effects section for details. In acute overdosage hyperkalaemia is common; in chronic overdosage the potassium level is likely to be normal or decreased.
Treatment: ingestion of 50 microgram/kg would be expected to raise the blood concentration above the upper therapeutic limit of 2 microgram/L. Any suspected ingestion above this range should be treated with gut decontamination (preferably with activated charcoal) and observation in Accident and Emergency (for at least 6 hours following ingestion). Monitor ECG and electrolytes, with particular attention to potassium concentration, and treat any abnormalities appropriately. Blood concentrations are not meaningful until about 6 hours after ingestion and should be interpreted with caution as the concentration may not correlate with the clinical effects. In severe cases, i.e. those patients not responding to supportive care, those with intractable arrythmias and/or hyperkalaemia >6mmol/L, digoxin specific antibodies (Digibind®) should be used. See digoxin-specific antibody fragments monograph for details. Woolf *et al* (1992) suggest the routine use of digoxin-specific antibody fragments in cases of ingestion of >300 microgram/kg.

PHARMACOKINETIC PROPERTIES
Oral bioavailability is dependent on oral dosage form and ranges from 66-90%. Digoxin is 20-30% bound to plasma proteins. Mostly excreted unchanged via the kidneys. The mean plasma half-life is much longer than in adults; child (range 15-72 hours), neonate (range 55-90 hours). Therapeutic plasma concentration range is 0.8-2 microgram/L (1-2.6 nanomol/L). Levels should be measured in a plasma sample taken at least 6 hours after an oral or IV dose. Approximate time to steady state is 5-10 days. In the newborn period concentrations may not stabilise for 10 days because of the neonatal half-life.

D

EXCIPIENTS
Contact manufacturer for further details.

LICENSED STATUS
Licensed for use in all ages.

FURTHER INFORMATION
100 micrograms in 1mL injection is available from BCM Specials.

Digoxin-specific antibody fragments (Fab)

Digoxin-specific antibody fragments bind to free (unbound) digoxin intravascularly and in extracellular fluid, thereby preventing and reversing the pharmacological and toxic affects of the glycoside.

USES
Treatment of digoxin or digitoxin toxicity.

PRESENTATION
Injection: 38mg – Digibind®.

DOSAGE
Each vial of digoxin-specific antibody fragments will bind to approximately 500 micrograms of digoxin.

Acute ingestion of a known quantity
Calculate the dose using the following formula:

$$\text{Dose (in number of vials)} = \frac{\text{total amount ingested (mg)} \times 0.8}{0.5}$$

Dose of digoxin (in mg)	Digoxin specific antibody fragment dose (number of vials)
6.25mg	10
12.5mg	20
18.75mg	30
25mg	40
37.5mg	60
50mg	80

Acute ingestion of an unknown quantity

Route	Weight		Frequency	Notes
	≤20 kg	>20 kg		
IV	Clinical judgement	10–20 vials	single dose	Recommend commencing with 10 vials followed by another 10 vials if required.

Toxicity during chronic therapy – steady state concentration known
Calculate the dose using the following formula:

$$\text{Dose (in number of vials)} = \frac{\text{serum digoxin concentration (nanogram/mL)} \times \text{body weight (kg)}}{100}$$

Toxicity during chronic therapy – steady state concentration unknown

Route	Weight		Frequency	Notes
	≤20 kg	>20 kg		
IV	1 vial	6 vials	single dose	Dose usually enough to reverse toxicity.

ADMINISTRATION
IV: each vial is reconstituted with 4mL Water for Injections and may be further diluted with NaCl 0.9% to a convenient volume and given by IV infusion over 30 minutes through a 0.22 micron membrane filter. Digoxin-specific antibody fragments can be given as a bolus injection if cardiac arrest seems imminent.

CONTRA-INDICATIONS & WARNINGS
Possibility of anaphylactic, hypersensitive or febrile reactions. Use with caution if known allergies to papain, chymopapain or other papaya extracts.

INTERACTIONS
Digoxin-specific antibody fragments interfere with standard cardiac glycoside assay procedures.

PREGNANCY
Animal reproduction studies have not been performed. It is not known whether digoxin-specific antibody fragments can cause fetal harm when given to pregnant women.

BREAST-FEEDING
It is not known whether digoxin-specific antibody fragments are distributed into milk.

SIDE-EFFECTS
Allergic reactions have been reported rarely and are more likely in patients known to be allergic to sheep protein who have received digoxin-specific antibody fragments previously. Hypokalaemia, hypertension and a worsening of low cardiac output and congestive heart failure have also been reported.

POISONING/ TOXICITY
Doses greater than those calculated to neutralise digoxin may subject patients to a large and prolonged antigenic stimulus and prolong the time before redigitalisation and accurate measurement of serum digoxin.

PHARMACOKINETIC PROPERTIES
Peak serum concentrations occur at the completion of IV infusion. The digoxin-specific antibody fragments appear to distribute rapidly throughout the extracellular space into both plasma and interstitial fluid. Patients usually respond within 1 hour of completion of administration, often sooner. Reversal of effects should be complete within 6 hours. The digoxin-specific antibody fragments are eliminated renally with an elimination half-life of 16-20 hours (with good renal function).

EXCIPIENTS
See manufacturer's SPC for further details.

LICENSED STATUS
Licensed for use in all ages.

Dihydrocodeine tartrate

Opioid analgesic less potent than morphine.

USES
Moderate to severe pain.

PRESENTATION
Oral solution: 10mg in 5mL – non-proprietary.
Injection: 50mg in 1mL – non-proprietary (controlled drug).
Tablet: 30mg – non-proprietary.

DOSAGE

Route	Age			Frequency	Notes
	1 month–2 years	2–12 years	12–18 years	(times daily)	
Oral/IM/ deep SC	≥1 year 500 microgram/kg	<4 years 500 microgram/kg >4 years 500 microgram – 1mg/kg	30mg (up to 50mg has been given IM/deep SC)	4–6 hourly	Repeated doses increase the risk of respiratory depression. Avoid IM injections if possible. Use SC/IM cannula placed while under GA or topical LA. Dihydrocodeine can cause severe constipation so prophylactic laxatives should always be prescribed.

Renal impairment/liver disease
Avoid or reduce dose in moderate to severe renal impairment, and in chronic liver disease (may precipitate coma).

ADMINISTRATION
Oral: solution may be diluted with unpreserved syrup BP or syrup BP preserved with parahydroxybenzoic acid. The resultant diluted liquid has a shelf life of 14 days at room temperature.
IV: not recommended due to increased risk of respiratory depression.

CONTRA-INDICATIONS & WARNINGS
Avoid in respiratory depression, cystic fibrosis, head injury or raised intracranial pressure. Reduce dose in hypothyroidism. High doses of dihydrocodeine are

pharmacologically very similar to small doses of morphine. If dihydrocodeine provides inadequate analgesia, major opioids such as morphine should be the next step.

INTERACTIONS
May enhance sedative effects of *anxiolytics* and *hypnotics*. Antagonises effect of *cisapride* and *metoclopramide*. Plasma levels increased by *cimetidine*. Absorption of *mexiletine* reduced.

PREGNANCY
Use of opioid analgesics in the third trimester depresses neonatal respiration. Contact local Medicines Information Centre for advice.

BREAST-FEEDING
Dihydrocodeine does not appear to be significantly excreted into breast milk.

SIDE-EFFECTS
Constipation (use of laxatives may be necessary), nausea and vomiting, headache, vertigo, urinary retention.

POISONING/TOXICITY
Effects include respiratory depression, coma and pinpoint pupils. The opioid antagonist *naloxone* may be required as an antidote.

PHARMACOKINETIC PROPERTIES
Analgesic effect felt after about 1 hour and lasts for approximately 3-4 hours.

EXCIPIENTS
Contact manufacturers for further details.

LICENSED STATUS
Licensed for use ≥4 years of age.

Diloxanide furoate

Dichloroacetamide derivative; a luminal amoebicide.

USES
Acute and chronic amoebiasis; drug of choice for asymptomatic amoebic intestinal carriage and as an adjunct to metronidazole or tinidazole in acute amoebiasis.

PRESENTATION
Tablet: 500mg (scored) – non-proprietary.

DOSAGE

Route	Age			Frequency (times daily)	Notes
	1 month–2 years	2–12 years	12–18 years		
Oral	← 6.6mg/kg →		500mg	3	For 10 days. Can be repeated if necessary.

ADMINISTRATION
Oral: the tablets can be crushed and suspended in standard suspending agent. Administer with food.

CONTRA-INDICATIONS & WARNINGS
Hypersensitivity to diloxanide furoate.

PREGNANCY/BREAST-FEEDING
Safety not established.

SIDE-EFFECTS
No serious side-effects have been reported. Flatulence, vomiting, urticaria and pruritus may occur.

POISONING/TOXICITY
Unlikely to constitute a hazard in overdose. No specific antidote. Symptomatic and supportive treatment as necessary.

PHARMACOKINETIC PROPERTIES
Diloxanide furoate is largely hydrolysed into diloxanide and furoic acid. After absorption diloxanide is very rapidly conjugated to form a glucuronide. In circulating blood it is present to about 99% as a glucuronide and 1% as free diloxanide. It is predominantly excreted in the urine. It is believed that the unabsorbed diloxanide is the active anti-amoebic substance, up to 10% remaining in the gut, which is subsequently excreted as diloxanide in the faeces.

EXCIPIENTS

EXCIPIENTS
Contact manufacturer for further details.

LICENSED STATUS
Licensed for use in children ≥25kg body weight and adults.

Diltiazem

Potent peripheral vasodilator, and has a mild depressor effect on AV conduction.

USES
Raynaud's phenomenon.

PRESENTATION
Capsule: (modified release over 12 hours) 90mg, 120mg and 180mg – Adizem–SR®; 60mg, 90mg and 120mg – Dilcardia SR®, Dilzem SR®.
Capsule: (modified release over 24 hours) 120mg, 180mg, 240mg and 300mg – Adizem–XL®, Slozem®, Zemtard ML; 240mg and 300mg – Angitil XL®; 120mg, 180mg and 240mg – Dilzem XL®; 200mg and 300mg – Tildiem LA®; 120mg, 180mg, 240mg, 300mg and 360mg – Viazem XL®.
Tablet: (modified release) 60mg – Tildiem® and non-proprietary.
Tablet: (modified release over 12 hours) 120mg – Adizem–SR®, Angitil SR®; 90mg and 120mg – Calcicard CR®, Tildiem Retard®.

DOSAGE

Route	Age			Frequency	Notes
	1 month–2 years	2–12 years	12–18 years	(times daily)	
Oral	← Not recommended →		30–60mg	2–3	Some sustained release preparations can be given once daily.

ADMINISTRATION
Oral: tablets and capsules should not be crushed or split. Patients should stay dedicated to one brand as differences in release characteristics exist between brands.

CONTRA-INDICATIONS & WARNINGS
Diltiazem is contra-indicated in patients with bradycardia, second or third degree heart block (unless fitted with a pacemaker), sick sinus syndrome, decompensated heart failure, and in patients with left ventricular dysfunction following myocardial infarction.

INTERACTIONS
Diltiazem may cause an increase in *carbamazepine, ciclosporin (cyclosporin)* and *theophylline* levels. *Cimetidine* and *ranitidine* may cause an increase in diltiazem levels. There is an increased risk of AV block, bradycardia and myocardial depression when diltiazem is given with *amiodarone*. Diltiazem levels are reduced by *rifampicin, phenobarbital (phenobarbitone)* and *phenytoin.* There is an increased risk of AV block and bradycardia when diltiazem is given with *beta-blockers. Digoxin* levels may be increased by diltiazem.

PREGNANCY
There is limited information available, but there may be an association between maternal exposure to diltiazem and cardiovascular defects in the child. Contact local Medicines Information Centre for advice.

BREAST-FEEDING
Diltiazem appears to be present in milk at concentrations similar to those found in the maternal serum. Breast-feeding should be avoided. Contact local Medicines Information Centre for advice.

SIDE-EFFECTS
Nausea, headache, skin rashes, oedema (particularly in the legs), flushing, hypotension, fatigue, bradycardia.

POISONING/TOXICITY
Acute intoxication may cause profound hypotension or collapse, sinus bradycardia with or without AV conduction defects, hyperglycaemia, metabolic acidosis, hypoxia and pulmonary oedema.
Gastric lavage and osmotic diuresis should be undertaken when appropriate, and activated charcoal should be administered. Bradycardia may be treated with *atropine, isoprenaline,* or occasionally temporary

D

cardiac pacing. Plasma volume expanders may be required for hypotension, along with IV *calcium gluconate* and *positive inotropes*.

PHARMACOKINETIC PROPERTIES
Diltiazem is a benzothiapine and is eliminated by hepatic metabolism.

EXCIPIENTS
Contact manufacturers for further details.

LICENSED STATUS
Diltiazem preparations are not licensed for use in children.

Dimeticone (dimethicone)

Antifoaming agent.

USES
Infantile colic, gripes and wind pain but evidence of benefit is uncertain. Symptomatic relief in infants in whom more serious pathology is not present.

PRESENTATION
Emulsion (colic drops): activated dimeticone, 21mg in 2.5mL – Dentinox®.
Liquid: activated dimeticone, 40mg in 1mL – Infacol®.
Oral drops: activated dimeticone, 20mg in 0.3mL – Woodward's Colic Drops®.

DOSAGE
Dentinox® – infant 2.5mL with or after each feed, maximum of 6 doses in 24 hours; may be added to bottle feeds.
Infacol® – infant 0.5–1mL before each feed.
Woodward's Colic Drops® – child <2 years 0.3-0.6mL 4 times daily before feeds.

ADMINISTRATION
Oral: give directly by spoon or Dentinox® may be added to bottle feeds. Improvement occurs over several days.

CONTRA-INDICATIONS, SIDE-EFFECTS
None known.

POISONING
Symptomatic treatment.

EXCIPIENTS
Dentinox® includes sucrose.
Infacol® includes saccharin and is sugar-free.
Woodward's Colic Drops® include saccharin.

LICENSED STATUS
Licensed for use in infants.

Dinoprostone (prostaglandin E2)

In newborn infants with a closing ductus arteriosus, prostaglandin E2 markedly relaxes and may re-open the ductus Thus in infants with congenital cardiopulmonary defects that restrict pulmonary or systemic blood flow, the drug improves cardiovascular status in 80% of patients by maintaining ductal patency until corrective or palliative surgery can be performed.

USES
To maintain patency of the ductus arteriosus in duct dependent congenital heart disease including: obstructive right heart lesions such as pulmonary atresia, severe Fallot's tetralogy and tricuspid atresia, obstructive left heart lesions such as interrupted aortic arch, juxtaductal and preductal coarctation of the aorta, hypoplastic left heart syndrome and critical aortic stenosis. Transposition of the great arteries in which mixing between the systemic and pulmonary circulation is essential for survival.

PRESENTATION
Injection: 1mg in 1mL, 0.75mL ampoule; 10mg in 1mL, 0.5mL ampoule – Prostin E2®.
NB. Only the 1mg in 1mL strength should be used.
Oral solution: may be extemporaneously prepared.

DOSAGE

Route	Dose	Notes
Oral	Initially 20–25 microgram/kg, hourly	This may be doubled if necessary. If treatment continues for more than 1 week the frequency and/or dosage may then be reduced.
IV infusion	Initially 5 nanogram/kg/minute	This may be increased to 10–20 nanogram/kg/minute in 5 nanogram/kg/minute increments until effective or serious side-effects occur. Monitor heart rate, respiratory rate, temperature and blood pressure in the arm and leg. Doses up to 100 nanogram/kg/minute have been used but are associated with an increased incidence of side-effects.

WHERE POSSIBLE DO NOT START OR STOP THIS THERAPY WITHOUT FIRST CONSULTING A CARDIOLOGIST
Facilities for intubation and ventilation must be immediately available before commencing therapy as prostaglandin E2 may cause apnoea.

ADMINISTRATION
IV: must be given by IV infusion and rate titrated against response.
Never allow a bolus of this solution to be injected. A separate line must always be used for other fluids and medications.
Dilute with glucose 5% or NaCl 0.9% only. Diluted solutions should be used within 24 hours.
Suggested method of infusion preparation: add 500 microgram dinoprostone to 500mL (or 50 micrograms in 50mL) of glucose 5% to obtain an infusion of a concentration of 1 microgram in 1mL. Then using this concentration, weight (kg) x 0.3 as mL/hour = 5 nanogram/kg/minute. Use the lowest dose for the shortest time to achieve the necessary clinical effect.
Oral: dose should be titrated downwards as soon as the clinical condition allows.

CONTRA-INDICATIONS & WARNINGS
Prostaglandin E2 may cause apnoea in neonates with congenital heart defects and should only be used when ventilatory assistance is immediately available.

SIDE-EFFECTS
Pyrexia, apnoea, bradycardia, seizures, hypotension, tachycardia, diarrhoea, cutaneous vasodilatation. Side-effects are more likely if the infant is of low birth weight, or dose >10 nanogram/kg/minute.

POISONING/TOXICITY
Overdosage may result in apnoea, bradycardia, pyrexia, hypotension, and flushing. If apnoea or bradycardia occur, the infusion should be temporarily discontinued, the infant intubated and ventilated and the infusion restarted with caution at a reduced dose. If pyrexia is observed reduce incubator temperature. If hypotension occurs reduce rate until symptoms subside and give dopamine 10 microgram/kg/minute if indicated.

PHARMACOKINETIC PROPERTIES
In adults following IV injection, rapid degradation occurs predominantly in the lungs and liver and less than 5% is still intact within 90 seconds. Due to the short half-life kinetic studies have been limited.

EXCIPIENTS
See manufacturers SPC for further details.

LICENSED STATUS
Not licensed for this indication (see further information section below).

FURTHER INFORMATION
Prosaglandin E1 (alprostadil) – Prostin VR® is the licensed preparation for this indication, but an identical dose of dinoprostone – Prostin E2® has been shown to be equally effective and is less expensive.

Sedative antihistamine.

USES
Night sedation and eczema.

PRESENTATION
Tablet: 25mg – Dreemon®, Nightcalm® and Nytol®; 50mg – Nytol®.
Syrup: 10mg in 5mL – Dreemon® and Medinex®.

DOSAGE

Route	Age		Frequency (times daily)	Notes
	2-12 years	**12-18 years**		
Oral	10–25mg	25–50mg	1 (at night)	

CONTRA-INDICATIONS & WARNINGS
Porphyria. Use with caution <1 year due to possible association with sudden infant death syndrome.

INTERACTIONS
Potentiates other *sedative medication*.

BREAST-FEEDING
Excreted into breast milk in levels not thought to be sufficiently high enough to affect an infant but due to the increased sensitivity of newborn or premature infants to antihistamines, manufacturers suggest avoiding use during breast-feeding.

SIDE-EFFECTS
Some antimuscarinic effects.

POISONING/TOXICITY
Signs and symptoms are deep sleep/coma. Treatment is supportive.

PHARMACOKINETIC PROPERTIES
Oral absorption >90%. Half-life in young adults is 9.2 ±2.5 hours and in children 5.4±1.8 hours. It is extensively metabolised, mainly in the liver and the main route of excretion is via the kidneys.

EXCIPIENTS
Contact manufacturers for further details.

LICENSED STATUS
Over the counter medicine, not licensed for use in children.

Diphtheria antitoxin

USES
Treatment of suspected or confirmed infections due to toxin-producing strains of *Corynebacterium diphtheriae*.

PRESENTATION
Injection: 10mL, 20mL vials of diphtheria antitoxin derived from the serum of hyperimmunised horses and containing not less than 1000 international units in 1mL.

DOSAGE & ADMINISTRATION
This depends on the type of diphtheria. There are variations in the suggested dose regimen and some authorities suggest that only half the recommended dose is given to children <10 years old.

Type of diphtheria	Route	Dosage (units)
Nasal	IM	10,000–20,000
Tonsillar	IM or IV	15,000–25,000
Pharyngeal or laryngeal	IM or IV	20,000 –40,000
Combined types or delayed diagnosis	IV	40,000–60,000
Severe diphtheria e.g. with extensive membrane and/or severe oedema ('bull-neck' diphtheria)	IV or part IV and part IM	40,000–100,000

CONTRA-INDICATIONS & WARNINGS

Because of the horse serum origin of the antitoxin there is a significant risk of a hypersensitivity reaction. Before treatment with antitoxin is started, a diluted test dose should be given intradermally. The antitoxin should not be given to someone known to be sensitive to equine serum.

INTERACTIONS

None known.

PREGNANCY/ BREAST-FEEDING

No data available, but must not be withheld if its use is indicated.

SIDE-EFFECTS

After IM use, local reactions such as pain, erythema and tenderness may occur at the site of injection. Fever, chills, facial flushing, headache and nausea may follow IV use.

Hypersensitivity reactions have been reported.

POISONING/TOXICITY

No data available.

PHARMACODYNAMIC PROPERTIES

The protective effect only lasts up to 15 days.

LICENSED STATUS

Not licensed for use in the UK but it is available on a named patient basis for England & Wales from the Health Protection Agency Communicable Disease Surveillance Centre; for Scotland from the Scottish Centre for Infection and Environmental Health and for Northern Ireland, from the Public Health Laboratory, Belfast City Hospital.

FURTHER INFORMATION

Should only be used after discussion with an appropriate expert. More detailed information is available in the *Immunoglobulin Handbook*, PHLS, 2002. http://www.phls.org.uk/advice/ImmunoglobulinHandbook.pdf
Store between 2-8°C and protect from light.

Diphtheria vaccine (adsorbed)

D

Single antigen diphtheria vaccine is now rarely indicated. Diphtheria toxoid would usually be given in combination with tetanus toxoid and possibly, depending on the age of the recipient, other antigens. When diphtheria toxoid alone is indicated, it will need to be obtained direct from the manufacturers.

USES

Active protection against diphtheria as part of the routine childhood immunisation schedule. It should be administered in combination with the other indicated vaccines. The primary course is usually given at 8, 12 and 16 weeks of age. This is followed by a booster three years later and another at 13–18 years of age. Subsequent boosters are only necessary if travelling to areas where diphtheria is common or if in contact with a case of diphtheria or a carrier of a toxigenic strain. Rarely would single antigen diphtheria vaccine be indicated (see relevant monographs for combination vaccines).

PRESENTATION

Injection: adsorbed diphtheria vaccine for children <10 years old (D) as a single dose suspension.
Each dose of vaccine for children (D) contains not less than 30 international units of the diphtheria formol toxoid adsorbed on an aluminium carrier.
Injection: adsorbed diphtheria vaccine for adults and adolescents (d) as a single dose suspension.
Each dose of vaccine for adults (d) contains not less than 2 international units (usually 4 international units) of the same toxoid adsorbed on an aluminium carrier.

DOSAGE

Children <10 years old should receive the standard strength vaccine (D) and children ≥10 years old, the low dose preparation (d) 0.5mL of the appropriate vaccine should be administered. If the standard dose preparation is unavailable, vaccine for adults and adolescents (d) can be used as a booster for children <10 years old in the rare circumstance that diphtheria vaccine alone is required.

ADMINISTRATION

Deep SC or IM.

CONTRA-INDICATIONS & WARNINGS
As for vaccines generally; however, if the individual has been in contact with a case of diphtheria or a carrier of a toxigenic strain, the vaccination should be given in spite of any intercurrent illness which may otherwise be a contra-indication.

INTERACTIONS
It can be given simultaneously with or at any interval before or after any other vaccine.

PREGNANCY/ BREAST-FEEDING
No information is available, but there are no grounds to believe it would be harmful. If indicated in the management of a contact of a case of diphtheria or a carrier of a toxigenic strain, the vaccine should be given.

SIDE-EFFECTS
Local reactions such as pain, redness and swelling at the injection site are relatively common. Systemic reactions, including headache, lethargy, malaise and pyrexia are much less common. Acute anaphylaxis and urticaria are rare. Although peripheral neuropathy has been reported following diphtheria vaccination on rare occasions, it has not been convincingly shown to be a result of the vaccination. Acute anaphylaxis and urticaria are rare. The incidence of reactions is greater with successive doses. Injection site granuloma due to the aluminium component is more likely to occur when the vaccine is not injected deep enough.

POISONING/TOXICITY
When teenagers were given standard dose vaccine, i.e. 30 international units of toxoid instead of 4 international units, they had an increased incidence of (and more severe) local and systemic reactions than would have been expected with the correct dose. However, no major adverse effects were noted.

PHARMACODYNAMIC PROPERTIES
Diphtheria vaccine produces humoral immunity due to the stimulation of antibodies to diphtheria toxin.

EXCIPIENTS
Aluminium phosphate or hydroxide and thiomersal.

LICENSED STATUS
Licensed for use as described.

FURTHER INFORMATION
Protect from light and store at 2–8°C, do not freeze.

Diphtheria, tetanus and pertussis (acellular) vaccine (adsorbed)

USES
Active immunisation against diphtheria, tetanus and whooping cough as part of the routine childhood immunisation schedule at (8, 12 and 16 weeks of age) only where whole cell pertussis vaccine is contra-indicated, or routinely as part of the pre-school booster. It should be administered at the same time as any other indicated vaccines, but must not be mixed with them. If pertussis vaccine, of whatever sort, is contra-indicated, DT vaccine should be given instead.

PRESENTATION
Injection: (suspension available as single doses) – Infanrix®.
Each dose of the vaccine contains not less than 30 international units of diphtheria toxoid; not less than 40 international units of tetanus toxoid; and not less than 25 microgram of pertussis toxoid, not less than 25 microgram of filamentous haemaglutinin (FHA) antibody and not less than 8 microgram of pertactin.

DOSAGE
0.5mL.

ADMINISTRATION
IM or deep SC.

CONTRA-INDICATIONS & WARNINGS
As for vaccines generally.

INTERACTIONS
It can be given simultaneously with or at any interval before or after any other vaccine.

PREGNANCY/ BREAST-FEEDING
No information is available.

SIDE-EFFECTS
Local reactions such as pain, redness and swelling at the injection site are relatively common. Systemic reactions, including headache, lethargy, malaise and pyrexia, episodes of pallor, cyanosis and limpness are much less common. Acute anaphylaxis and urticaria are rare. Although peripheral neuropathy has been reported following diphtheria vaccination on rare occasions, it has not been convincingly shown to be a result of the vaccination. Convulsions due to the DTP vaccine are very uncommon with the current schedule. Long-term neurological damage has not been conclusively linked with the vaccine. The incidence of reactions is greater with successive doses. Injection site granuloma due to the aluminium component is more likely to occur when the vaccine is not injected deep enough.

POISONING/TOXICITY
No major adverse effects were noted.

PHARMACODYNAMIC PROPERTIES
Diphtheria and tetanus vaccines produce humoral immunity due to the stimulation of antibodies to diphtheria and tetanus toxins. The relative contributions of cellular and humoral immunity to protection against pertussis is unclear.

EXCIPIENTS
Aluminium salts and 2-phenoxyethanol.

LICENSED STATUS
Licensed for use as described in children ≤6 years of age.

FURTHER INFORMATION
Previous advice was that the vaccine could be mixed with Hib vaccine. From February 2003, the Department of Health has advised that this is no longer the case as it may reduce the response to the Hib vaccine. It may be given at the same time.
Protect from light and store at 2–8°C, do not freeze. Materials of porcine and bovine origin are used in the manufacturing process. Trace amounts of the original material may be present in the final product, however, all such material is obtained from sources known to be free of BSE.

D

Diphtheria, tetanus and pertussis (whole cell) vaccine (adsorbed)

USES
Active protection against diphtheria, tetanus and whooping cough as part of the routine childhood immunisation schedule and would usually be given mixed with Hib vaccine. It should also be administered at the same time as the other indicated vaccines. The primary course is usually given at 8, 12 and 16 weeks of age.
If whole cell pertussis immunisation is contra-indicated, consideration should be given to using the acellular vaccine. If pertussis vaccine, of any sort, is contra-indicated, DT vaccine should be given instead.

PRESENTATION
Injection: (suspension available as single doses) Adsorbed Diphtheria, Tetanus and Pertussis Vaccine BP; DTP Vaccine BP®. Each dose of the vaccine contains not less than 30 international units of diphtheria toxoid; not less than 40 international units (DTP vaccine Behring) or not less than 60 international units (Adsorbed Diphtheria, Tetanus and Pertussis Vaccine BP from Aventis Pasteur MSD) of tetanus toxoid; and not less than 4 international units of inactivated *Bordatella pertussis* organisms.

DOSAGE
0.5mL.

ADMINISTRATION
Deep SC or IM. Some DTP and Hib preparations can be mixed in the same syringe immediately prior to administration. ACT-HIB® may be reconstituted with a single dose of Absorbed Diphtheria, Tetanus and Pertussis Vaccine BP. Hiberix® can be mixed with DTP Vaccine Behring or Trivax-AD (DTP) immediately prior to administration. Check manufacturers literature for further details.

CONTRA-INDICATIONS & WARNINGS
As for vaccines generally; but the Joint Committee on Vaccination and Immunisation (JCUI) also advises that when a severe local reaction occurs after the

administration of a dose of combined DTP and Hib vaccines, the vaccines should be given seperately. A severe systemic reaction resulting from the combined vaccines is likely to be due to the pertussis component. If the whole cell vaccine had been used, consideration should be given to using acellular pertussis vaccine instead.

INTERACTIONS
It can be given simultaneously with or at any interval before or after any other vaccine.

PREGNANCY/BREAST-FEEDING
No information is available.

SIDE-EFFECTS
Local reactions such as pain, redness and swelling at the injection site are relatively common. Systemic reactions, including headache, lethargy, malaise and pyrexia, episodes of pallor, cyanosis and limpness are much less common. Acute anaphylaxis and urticaria are rare. Although peripheral neuropathy has been reported following

diphtheria vaccination on rare occasions, it has not been convincingly shown to be a result of the vaccination. Convulsions due to the DTP vaccine are very uncommon (probably less than one in 50,000 doses) with the current schedule. A severe acute neurological illness occurs about one in 110,000 doses. Long-term neurological damage has not been conclusively linked with the vaccine. The incidence of reactions is greater with successive doses. Injection site granuloma due to the aluminium component is more likely to occur when the vaccine is not injected deep enough.

POISONING/TOXICITY
No major adverse effects were noted.

PHARMACODYNAMIC PROPERTIES
Diphtheria and tetanus vaccines produce humoral immunity due to the stimulation of antibodies to diphtheria and tetanus toxins. The relative contributions of cellular and humoral immunity to protection against pertussis is unclear.

EXCIPIENTS
DTP Vaccine Behring: aluminium phosphate, aluminium hydroxide, sodium thimerfonate, formaldehyde and sodium edetate.
Adsorbed Diphtheria, Tetanus and Pertussis Vaccine BP (Aventis Pasteur MSD): aluminium hydroxide and thiomersal.

LICENSED STATUS
Licensed for use as described.

FURTHER INFORMATION
Protect from light and store at 2-8°C, do not freeze.
Materials of porcine and bovine origin are used in the manufacturing process. Trace amounts of the original material may be present in the final product, however, all such material is obtained from sources known to be free of BSE.

Diphtheria and tetanus vaccine (adsorbed)

USES
Active protection against diphtheria and tetanus as part of the routine childhood immunisation schedule.
DTP/Hib vaccine would usually be given at 8, 12 and 16 weeks. If whole cell pertussis immunisation is contra-indicated, consideration should be given to using the acellular vaccine. If pertussis vaccine, of any sort, is contra-indicated, DT vaccine should be given instead, with Hib vaccine given in separate syringes. DTaP vaccine would usually be given at 3–5 years as a pre-school booster. If pertussis vaccine is contra-indicated, DT should be given alone.

When tetanus vaccine is given to children in the management of a wound, it should be combined with diphtheria and, if the primary course has not been completed, pertussis and Hib.

Td is given as part of the 'school leavers booster' at 13–18 years old. Subsequent boosters are only necessary if travelling to areas where diphtheria is common or where medical care may be delayed or of low standard, if in contact with a case of diphtheria or a carrier of a toxigenic strain, or after a tetanus-prone injury.

Single antigen tetanus and diphtheria vaccines are only indicated if there is history of a severe reaction to one of the components of the combined vaccine.
No further doses of tetanus toxoid are required for protection against tetanus in the presence of a tetanus prone injury, where there is a history of the administration of five doses of appropriately spaced tetanus containing vaccine. Human tetanus immunoglobulin may be necessary (see monograph).

PRESENTATION
Injection: (suspension as single and multiple doses) adsorbed diphtheria and tetanus vaccine BP (DT). This often known as the 'standard dose vaccine' as opposed to the 'low dose' preparation.
Each dose of the vaccine for children (DT) contains not less than 30 international units of the diphtheria formol toxoid and not less than 40 international units of tetanus formol toxoid, both adsorbed on an aluminium carrier.
Injection: (suspension as single doses) adsorbed diphtheria and tetanus vaccine for adults and adolescents (Td) – Diftavax®. This is often known as the 'low dose vaccine', as opposed to the 'standard' preparation.
Each dose of vaccine for adults and adolescents (Td) contains not less than 2 international units (usually 4 international units) of diphtheria formol toxoid and not less than 40 international units of tetanus formol toxoid, both adsorbed on an aluminium carrier.

DOSAGE
Children <10 years old should receive the standard strength vaccine and children ≥10 years old, the low dose preparation. 0.5mL of the appropriate vaccine should be administered. If the standard dose preparation is unavailable, vaccine for use in adults and adolescents can be used as a booster for children <10 years old in the rare circumstance that diphtheria vaccine alone is required.

ADMINISTRATION
Deep SC or IM.

CONTRA-INDICATIONS & WARNINGS
As for vaccines generally, however, if the individual has suffered a tetanus prone wound and has not had five doses of tetanus vaccine, or if diphtheria vaccination is indicated because of contact with a carrier, the vaccine should be given, in spite of any intercurrent illness.

INTERACTIONS
It can be given simultaneously with or at any interval before or after any other vaccine.

PREGNANCY/ BREAST-FEEDING
No information is available, but there are no grounds to believe it would be harmful. If indicated in the management of a contact of a case of diphtheria or a carrier of a toxigenic strain, or after a tetanus-prone wound in an incompletely immunised individual, the vaccine should be given.

SIDE-EFFECTS
Local reactions such as pain, redness and swelling at the injection site are relatively common. Systemic reactions, including headache, lethargy, malaise and pyrexia, are much less common. Febrile convulsions, hypotonic hyporesponsive episodes, acute anaphylaxis and urticaria are rare. The incidence of minor reactions is greater with successive doses. Injection site granuloma due to the aluminium component is more likely to occur when the vaccine is not injected deep enough.

POISONING/TOXICITY
When teenagers were given standard dose diphtheria vaccine, i.e. 30 international units of toxoid instead of 4 international units, they had an increased incidence of (and more severe) local and systemic reactions than would have been expected with the correct dose. However, no major adverse effects were noted.

PHARMACODYNAMIC PROPERTIES
Diphtheria and tetanus vaccines produce humoral immunity due to the stimulation of antibodies to diphtheria toxin.

EXCIPIENTS
Aluminium hydroxide and thiomersal (or sodium thimerfonate).

LICENSED STATUS
Licensed for use as described.

FURTHER INFORMATION
Protect from light and store at 2-8°C, do not freeze.
Materials of porcine and bovine origin are used in the manufacturing process. Trace amounts of the original material may be present in the final product, however, all such material is obtained from sources known to be free of BSE.

Diphtheria, tetanus, pertussis (acellular) and Hib vaccine (adsorbed)

In February 2003 the Department of Health recommended that DTaP and Hib vaccines should not be mixed, instead the separate vaccines should be used (see DTaP and Hib monographs).

USES

Active protection against diphtheria, tetanus, whooping cough and *Haemophilus influenzae* type b as part of the routine childhood immunisation schedule. It should be administered at the same time as any other indicated vaccines. The primary course is usually given at 8, 12 and 16 weeks of age.

If whole cell pertussis immunisation is contra-indicated, consideration should be given to using the acellular vaccine. If pertussis vaccine, of any sort, is contra-indicated, DT and Hib vaccines should be given instead. They can be given at the same time, but not mixed in the same syringe.

PRESENTATION

Injection: (single dose suspension of DTP used to reconstitute a freeze dried pellet of Hib vaccine) – ACT-HIB® DTP. Each dose of the vaccine contains not less than 30 international units of diphtheria toxoid; not less than 60 international units of tetanus toxoid; not less than 4 international units of inactivated *Bordatella pertussis* organisms; and not less than 10 micrograms of *Haemophilus influenzae* type b polysaccharide conjugated to tetanus protein.

DOSAGE

0.5mL.

ADMINISTRATION

IM or deep SC.

CONTRA-INDICATIONS & WARNINGS

As for vaccines generally; but the Joint Committee on Vaccination and Immunisation (JCUI) also advises that when a severe local reaction occurs after the administration of a dose of combined DTP and Hib vaccines, the vaccines should be given seperately. A severe systemic reaction resulting from the combined vaccines is likely to be due to the pertussis component. If the whole cell vaccine had been used, consideration should be given to using acellular pertussis vaccine instead.

INTERACTIONS

It can be given simultaneously with or at any interval before or after any other vaccine.

PREGNANCY

Limited experience of administering Hib Vaccine (polysaccharide and conjugate) to women in the third trimester has revealed no adverse effects on the mother, fetus or neonate. Until more research has taken place, its use in pregnancy cannot be recommended.

BREAST-FEEDING

No information is available.

SIDE-EFFECTS

Local reactions such as pain, redness and swelling at the injection site are relatively common. Systemic reactions, including headache, lethargy, malaise and pyrexia, episodes of pallor, cyanosis and limpness are much less common. Acute anaphylaxis and urticaria are rare. Although peripheral neuropathy has been reported following diphtheria vaccination on rare occasions, it has not been convincingly shown to be a result of the vaccination. Convulsions due to the DTP vaccine are very uncommon (probably less than one in 50,000 doses) with the current schedule. A severe acute neurological illness occurs about one in 110,000 doses. Long-term neurological damage has not been conclusively linked with the vaccine. The incidence of reactions is greater with successive doses. Injection site granuloma due to the aluminium component is more likely to occur when the vaccine is not injected deep enough.

POISONING/TOXICITY

No major adverse effects were noted.

PHARMACODYNAMIC PROPERTIES

Diphtheria, tetanus and Hib vaccines produce humoral immunity due to the stimulation of antibodies to diphtheria and tetanus toxins. Hib vaccine protects by stimulating the production of anti-PRP antibodies. The vaccine has been shown to reduce nasal carriage as well or prevent disease. The relative contributions of cellular and humoral immunity to protection against pertussis is unclear

EXCIPIENTS

Aluminium hydroxide, TRIS, sucrose and thiomersal.

LICENSED STATUS

Licensed for use as described in children <4 years of age.

FURTHER INFORMATION

Protect from light and store at 2–8°C, do not freeze.

Materials of bovine and sheep origin are used in the manufacturing process. Trace amounts of the original material may be present in the final product however, all such material is obtained from sources known to be free of BSE.

Diphtheria, tetanus, acellular pertussis and inactivated poliomyelitis vaccine (adsorbed)

This vaccine was made available for a short time when there were supply problems with other vaccines. However, it is now only available on a named patient basis from the manufacturer and would rarely be indicated.

USES
Active protection against diphtheria, tetanus, pertussis and poliomyelitis, as part of the routine childhood immunisation schedule when both the live attenuated oral polio vaccine and the whole cell pertussis vaccine are contra-indicated. The primary course is usually given at 8, 12 and 16 weeks of age, with a booster at 3-5 years of age.

PRESENTATION
Injection: (single dose suspension) – Tetravac®.
Each 0.5mL contains not less than 30 international units of diphtheria toxoid, not less than 40 international units of tetanus toxoid, 25 micrograms of purified pertussis toxoid, 25 micrograms of filamentous haemaglutinin, 40 units of inactivated type 1 (Mahoney) poliovirus D antigen, 8 units of inactivated type 2 (MEF-1) D antigen and 32 units of inactivated (Saukett) poliovirus D antigen. The polio viruses are reared on Vero cells and then inactivated with formaldehyde. Tetanus and diphtheria toxins are detoxified with formaldehyde. Pertussis toxin is detoxified with glutaraldehyde.

DOSAGE/ADMINISTRATION
IM or deep SC: 0.5mL. Three doses at monthly intervals. It should not be mixed with any other vaccine, including Hib vaccine.

CONTRA-INDICATIONS & WARNINGS
As for vaccines generally; the vaccine should be postponed if the child has an evolving neurological disorder.

INTERACTIONS
It can be given simultaneously with or at any interval before or after any other vaccine. It should not be mixed with Hib vaccine as this may reduce the protective response to Hib.

PREGNANCY/BREAST-FEEDING
Not indicated in this age group.

SIDE-EFFECTS
Local reactions such as pain, redness and swelling at the injection site are relatively common. Systemic reactions, including headache, lethargy, malaise and pyrexia, are less common. Acute anaphylaxis and urticaria are rare.

POISONING/TOXICITY
There is no experience of overdosage.

EXCIPIENTS
Aluminium hydroxide, formaldehyde, 2-phenoxyethanol and Medium 199 (complex of amino acids, mineral salts, vitamins and other substances).

LICENSED STATUS
Licensed for use as described.

FURTHER INFORMATION
Protect from light and store at 2–8°C, do not freeze.
Materials of porcine and bovine origin are used in the manufacturing process. Trace amounts of the original material may be present in the final product however, all such material is obtained from sources known to be free of BSE.

Dipyridamole

An antiplatelet drug which has an antithrombotic action based on its ability to modify platelet aggregation, adhesion and survival.

USES
Modification of platelet function. Prevention of clot formation in surgically created cardiac shunts. With specialist advice in Kawasaki disease for treatment of persistent coronary artery aneurysms.

PRESENTATION

Injection: 5mg in 1mL, 2mL ampoule – Persantin®.
Oral suspension: 50mg in 5mL – manufactured 'special'.
Tablet: 25mg and 100mg – Persantin® and non-proprietary.

DOSAGE

Indication	Route	Age			Frequency (times daily)	Notes
		1 month–2 years	2–12 years	12–18 years		
Antiplatelet	Oral	← 2.5mg/kg →			2	Give before food.
				100–200mg	3	Avoid use with *antacids*.
Kawasaki syndrome	Oral	← 1mg/kg →			3	
				-		

ADMINISTRATION

The injection can be given orally.

CONTRA-INDICATIONS & WARNINGS

There are no absolute contra-indications to the use of dipyridamole. It is a potent vasodilator.

INTERACTIONS

Adenosine: the effect of *adenosine* is enhanced and extended, as dipyridamole is a known inhibitor of *adenosine* uptake. Concurrent use is not recommended, but if considered essential reduce the *adenosine* dose to one quarter of the usual dose. *Anticoagulants:* mild bleeding can sometimes occur if *anticoagulants* and dipyridamole are used concurrently, without altering prothrombin time.

PREGNANCY

Inadequate evidence of safety in human pregnancy but has been used for many years without apparent ill consequence. Contact local Medicines Information Centre for advice.

BREAST-FEEDING

Contact local Medicines Information Centre for advice.

SIDE-EFFECTS

Nausea, diarrhoea, throbbing headache, hot flushes, hypotension, dizziness and myalgia.

POISONING/TOXICITY

Overdose may lead to headache, gastrointestinal symptoms and hypotension. Use general supportive measures.

PHARMACOKINETICS

Metabolised predominantly by the liver and mainly excreted as glucuronide in the bile.

EXCIPIENTS

Contact manufacturers for further details.

LICENSED STATUS

Licensed for antiplatelet action use in children, but not for Kawasaki disease. The oral suspension is a 'special' and as such is unlicensed.

FURTHER INFORMATION

Oral suspension available as a 'special' from Rosemont.

Disodium pamidronate

A bisphosphonate.

USES

Disodium pamidronate may have usefulness in the following conditions: steroid-induced osteoporosis, immobilisation osteoporosis e.g. high-spinal injury and cerebral palsy, idiopathic juvenile osteoporosis, hypercalcaemia in malignant disease, fibrous dysplasia of bone, juvenile idiopathic arthritis and osteogenesis imperfecta. Also used in bone pain due to metastasis or osteopenia.

PRESENTATION
IV infusion: 15mg, 30mg, 60mg and 90mg vials – non-proprietary; 15mg, 30mg and 90mg vials, with diluent – Aredia Dry Powder®.

DOSAGE
Experience of the use of bisphosphonates in children is very limited and expert advice should be sought. Their use is only justified when the potential benefits outweigh any risk.

ADMINISTRATION
IV infusion: disodium pamidronate must NEVER be administered by bolus injection. The reconstituted powder should be diluted in NaCl 0.9% to a concentration not exceeding 60mg in 250mL (240 microgram in 1mL). The resulting solution should be infused slowly, at a rate not exceeding 1mg per minute (60mg per hour). The infusion rate should be reduced in patients with impaired renal function: a maximum infusion rate of 20mg per hour is recommended. Incompatible with calcium-containing infusion solutions.

CONTRA-INDICATIONS & WARNINGS
Hypersensitivity to disodium pamidronate or other bisphosphonate drugs. Should not be given with other bisphosphonate drugs. Convulsions have occurred in some patients with tumour-induced hypercalcaemia due to the electrolyte changes associated with the condition and its treatment – the relative contribution of each is not established.

INTERACTIONS
Disodium pamidronate has been shown to have synergistic effects when given concurrently with *calcitonin*.

PREGNANCY
Avoid during pregnancy due to risk of adverse effects on bone formation in the fetus.

BREAST-FEEDING
As a consequence of animal experiments which indicate that disodium pamidronate is excreted in breast milk it is advised that mothers should not breast-feed while receiving this treatment.

SIDE-EFFECTS
Asymptomatic hypocalcaemia is relatively common (incidence >10%), as is a pyrexia of 1-2°C above normal body temperature which typically occurs within the first 48 hours of treatment. Symptomatic pyrexia is rare and the pyrexia normally resolves without treatment. The pyrexia may be accompanied by malaise, rigor, fatigue and flushes. Side-effects with an incidence of 1-10% include: local reactions at the infusion site (e.g. pain, redness, swelling, induration, phlebitis, thrombophlebitis), hypomagnesaemia, transient bone pain, arthralgia, myalgia, generalised pain, nausea and vomiting, headache, lymphocytopenia.
Side-effects with an incidence of 0.001-1% include: muscle cramps, anorexia, abdominal pain, diarrhoea, constipation, dyspepsia, agitation, confusion, dizziness, insomnia, somnolence, lethargy, anaemia, leucopenia, hypotension or hypertension, rash, pruritus, hyperkalaemia or hypokalaemia, hypernatraemia.
Isolated cases of the following have been reported (incidence <0.001%): gastritis, seizures, visual hallucination, thrombocytopenia, haematuria, acute renal failure, deterioration of pre-existing renal impairment, conjunctivitis, uveitis, scleritis, episcleritis, xanthopsia, reactivation of herpes simplex and herpes zoster, abnormal liver function tests.

POISONING/TOXICITY
Clinically significant hypocalcaemia should be treated with an infusion of an appropriate calcium salt.

PHARMACOKINETIC PROPERTIES
Plasma levels fall rapidly on completion of an infusion with an apparent plasma half-life of 0.8 hours and clearance of 180mL per minute. Pamidronate is taken up by the skeleton due to its high affinity for calcified tissue. Binding to plasma proteins is of the order of 54%. No significant hepatic or other metabolism appears to occur, and approximately 20-55% of the administered dose is recovered in the urine within 72 hours of administration as unchanged pamidronate.

EXCIPIENTS
Contact manufacturers for further details.

LICENSED STATUS
Not licensed for use in children.

USES
Sub-acute and chronic psoriasis including psoriasis of the scalp.

PRESENTATION
Cream: 0.1%, 0.25%, 0.5%, 1%, 2% – Dithrocream®; 1%, 3% in a lipid-stabilised basis – Micanol®; Dithranol in Lassar's paste can be extemporaneously prepared (usual strengths 0.1-1%).
Other preparations can also be extemporaneously prepared.

DOSAGE/ADMINISTRATION
Topical: apply on a daily basis, leaving on for 20–30 minutes depending on the preparation being used, then remove by washing off. Always commence treatment with 0.1% continuing for at least 1 week increasing if necessary to 0.25%, 0.5%, 1% and 2%. Build up gradually over 4 weeks to the highest tolerated strength that gives the best effect. Apply evenly and sparingly to lesions.

CONTRA-INDICATIONS & WARNINGS
Do not use on face or for acute or pustular psoriasis. Do not apply to folded skin areas, e.g. groin or beneath breasts. Keep away from eyes and mucous membranes.

PREGNANCY
No adverse effects reported.

SIDE-EFFECTS
Feeling of warmth is normal. Stop treatment if burning sensation experienced.

POISONING/TOXICITY
Accidental oral ingestion – remove by gastric lavage. Dithranol is a laxative.

PHARMACODYNAMIC PROPERTIES
Dithranol reduces DNA synthesis and thus results in an inhibition of mitochondrial function and cell division.

EXCIPIENTS
Contact manufacturers for further details.

LICENSED STATUS
Dithrocream® is licensed for use in children and adults. Micanol® is not licensed for use in infants and young children. Extemporaneously prepared products are unlicensed.

FURTHER INFORMATION
May stain clothing, bed linen and skin.

Dobutamine hydrochloride

A synthetic catecholamine with potent cardiac stimulating properties.

USES
To provide inotropic support in the treatment of low output cardiac failure associated with e.g. cardiac surgery, septicaemia. To improve myocardial contractility. Myocardial stress testing.

PRESENTATION
Injection: 12.5mg in 1mL, 20mL vial – Dobutrex®, 20mL ampoule – non-proprietary; 50mg in 1mL, 5mL ampoule – Posiject®.

DOSAGE

Route	Age				Frequency (times daily)	Notes
	birth–1 month	1 month–2 years	2–12 years	12–18 years		
IV infusion	←	2–10 microgram/kg/minute		→	continuous	Dose can be increased up to a maximum of 20 microgram/kg/minute in newborn infants (but side-effects more likely at this higher dose) and 40 microgram/kg/minute in older children and adults, if necessary.

ADMINISTRATION

IV: IV administration only. Solutions must be diluted before use. The dilution can vary but generally the maximum recommended concentration is 5mg in 1mL. Direct IV push is not recommended. Diluted solutions should be used within 24 hours. Must be administered by IV infusion only using an infusion pump to control the flow rate. Avoid extravasation as this may cause tissue sloughing and necrosis.

Closely monitor ECG, blood pressure, heart rate and cardiac output.

Solution may exhibit pink discolouration without loss of potency for up to 24 hours at room temperature.

Compatible with glucose 5% and NaCl 0.9%. Incompatible with alkaline solutions e.g. sodium bicarbonate.

Dopamine and dobutamine can be mixed together in glucose 5% or NaCl 0.9%.

CONTRA-INDICATIONS & WARNINGS

Idiopathic hypertrophic subaortic stenosis or other conditions associated with obstruction to ventricular filling or emptying. Known hypersensitivity to dobutamine, hypovolaemia, low cardiac filling pressure, cardiac arrhythmias. Particular care should be taken in patients with acute myocardial infarction.

Warnings: if an undue increase in heart rate or systolic blood pressure occurs or if an arrhythmia is precipitated the dose of dobutamine should be reduced or the drug temporarily discontinued. Dobutamine may precipitate or exacerbate ventricular ectopic activity. Because dobutamine increases atrioventricular conduction, patients with atrial flutter or fibrillation may develop a rapid ventricular response. Dobutamine will not improve haemodynamics in most patients with mechanical obstruction affecting ventricular filling or outflow. Inotropic response may be inadequate in patients with markedly reduced ventricular compliance. Hypovolaemia should be corrected before administration of dobutamine. Dobutamine should be used with caution in severe hypotension complicating cardiogenic shock. If blood pressure drops quickly, decreasing the dose or stopping the infusion typically results in a return to base-line values.

If arterial blood pressure remains low or decreases progressively despite adequate ventricular filling pressure and cardiac output, consideration may be given to the concomitant use of a peripheral vasoconstrictor agent e.g. *noradrenaline (norepinephrine)* or *dopamine*.

Some dobutamine preparations contain sodium metabisulphite. This may cause allergic-type reactions including anaphylaxis and life-threatening or less severe asthmatic episodes in certain susceptible individuals.

PREGNANCY

Safe use of dobutamine during pregnancy has not been established, and therefore it should not be used unless the possible benefits outweigh the risks. Contact local Medicines Information Centre for further advice.

BREAST-FEEDING

It is not known if dobutamine is excreted in human milk; however if a mother requires dobutamine, she is unlikely to be well enough to breast-feed.

SIDE-EFFECTS

Principal adverse effects are ectopic heartbeats, increased heart rate, angina, chest pain, palpitation and elevations in blood pressure, all of which are dose-related. Rarely dobutamine has caused ventricular tachycardia. Minor vasoconstriction has been observed in patients treated with beta-blocking drugs. Conversely, alpha-adrenergic blockade may make the beta-1 and beta-2 effects apparent, resulting in tachycardia and vasodilatation.

Less frequent adverse events include nausea, vomiting, tingling sensation, paresthesia, dyspnoea, headache, leg cramps, reactions indicative of hypersensitivity e.g. rash, fever, bronchospasm, phlebitis at the site of infusion. Decreases in serum potassium levels have been reported.

There is evidence that partial tolerance with infusions for longer than 72 hours may occur, therefore higher doses may be required to maintain the same effects.

POISONING/TOXICITY

The symptoms of toxicity may include anorexia, nausea, vomiting, tremor, anxiety, palpitations, headache, shortness of breath, fatigue and anginal non-specific chest pain. The positive inotropic and chronotropic effects may cause hypertension, tachyarrhythmias, myocardial ischaemia and ventricular fibrillation. Hypotension may result from vasodilation. The duration of action is short (half-life approximately 2 minutes). Temporarily discontinue dobutamine until the patient stabilises. The patient should be monitored and any resuscitative measures started immediately. Forced diuresis, peritoneal dialysis, haemodialysis or charcoal haemoperfusion have not been established as beneficial.

PHARMACOKINETIC PROPERTIES

Dobutamine is virtually inactive after oral administration because of extensive pre-systemic metabolism in the gastrointestinal mucosa and liver. The onset of action after IV administration is rapid (about 2 minutes).

Mean plasma half-life in adults is 2 minutes. Dobutamine is extensively and rapidly metabolised in the liver and excreted renally.

D

EXCIPIENTS
See manufacturers SPC for further details.

LICENSED STATUS
Not licensed for use in children.

Docusate sodium

Stimulant laxative and faecal softener.

USES
To prevent and treat chronic constipation and opioid-induced constipation; as an adjunct in abdominal radiological procedures.

PRESENTATION
Capsule: 100mg – Dioctyl®.
Oral solution: 12.5mg in 5mL – Docusol® paediatric oral solution; 50mg in 5mL – Docusol® adult oral solution.
Enema: docusate sodium 90mg, glycerol 3.78g in 5mL – Fletcher's Enemette®; docusate sodium 120mg in 10g – Norgalax Micro-enema®.

DOSAGE

Route	Age			Frequency (times daily)	Notes
	1 month–2 years	2–12 years	12–18 years		
Oral	>6 months 2.5mg/kg	2.5mg/kg	100mg	3	
Rectal (Fletcher's Enemette®)	–	≥3 years one enema	one enema	single dose	As required.
Rectal (Norgalax Micro-enema®)	–	–	one enema	single dose	

ADMINISTRATION
Rectal: remove protective cap, insert nozzle into the rectum, squeezing gently until the tube is empty.

CONTRA-INDICATIONS & WARNINGS
Dioctyl® capsules should not be taken in the presence of abdominal pain, nausea, vomiting or intestinal obstruction. Enemas should be used with caution in patients with intestinal obstruction.

INTERACTIONS
Should not be taken concurrently with mineral oil.
Anthraquinone derivatives (e.g. senna) should be taken in reduced doses if administered with docusate sodium as their absorption is increased.

PREGNANCY
There is inadequate evidence of safety in human pregnancy with Dioctyl® capsules but they have been in wide use for many years without apparent ill consequence. Use in pregnancy only if benefits outweigh potential risks. The enema may be used in pregnancy.

BREAST-FEEDING
Docusate sodium is excreted in breast milk following oral administration and should be used with caution in lactating mothers. The enema may be used with breast-feeding.

SIDE-EFFECTS
Anal or rectal burning and pain, diarrhoea, rash, congestion of the rectal mucosa may occur following rectal use.

POISONING/TOXICITY
In case of overdose – excessive loss of water and electrolytes should be treated by drinking plenty of fluid.

PHARMACOKINETIC PROPERTIES
Orally: exerts its effects by means of its physical surfactant properties; acts within 1-2 days; is absorbed from the gastrointestinal tract and excreted in bile.
Rectally: promotes peristalsis and evacuation of the lower bowel; acts within 20 minutes.

EXCIPIENTS
Docusol® oral solutions include sorbitol and are sugar-free. See manufacturers SPC for further details.

LICENSED STATUS
Dioctyl® not licensed for use in children.
Docusol® 12.5mg/5mL licensed for >6 months of age and 50mg/5mL not licensed for use in children.
Fletcher's enemette® licensed for use ≥3 years of age.
Norgalax Micro-enema® licensed for use ≥12 years of age.

Domperidone

Dopamine receptor antagonist principally active in gastrointestinal tract but with some central activity. Prokinetic effects in upper gut.

USES
Intractable vomiting of known cause. Gastro-oesophageal reflux resistant to dietary changes, thickeners and other simple measures.
Radiotherapy and chemotherapy induced nausea and vomiting.

PRESENTATION
Tablet: 10mg – Motilium® and non-proprietary.
Suspension: 5mg in 5mL – Motilium®.
Suppository: 30mg – Motilium®.

DOSAGE

Indication	Route	Age			Frequency (times daily)	Notes
		1 month–2 years	2–12 years	12–18 years		
Gastro-oesophageal reflux, gastric stasis	Oral	◄─200–400 microgram/kg─►		10–20mg	3-4	Not often used <2 years; little data but extrapyramidal effects can occur. Before food and at night.
Radiotherapy/chemotherapy induced nausea and vomiting	Oral	◄─200–400 microgram/kg─►		10–20mg	single dose	Give every 4-8 hours. Not often used <2 years; little data but extrapyramidal effects can occur.
	Rectal	–	15–30mg	30–60mg	single dose	Single dose approximately 1mg/kg. Can repeat doses as below: <25kg repeat twice. 25–35kg repeat 3 times. >35kg repeat 4 times.

D

ADMINISTRATION
Rectal: suppositories may be cut in half.

CONTRA-INDICATIONS/WARNINGS
Less effective in centrally-mediated nausea and vomiting than metoclopramide. Prolonged QT-intervals have been seen in neonates. It is recommended in neonates to check ECG prior to dosing and at regular intervals afterwards (2 weeks after starting).

INTERACTIONS
May enhance the absorption of concurrently administered drugs. Actions may be antagonised by *antimuscarinics* and *opioid analgesics*.

PREGNANCY
manufacturers advise avoidance.

BREAST-FEEDING
Amount probably too small to be harmful.

SIDE-EFFECTS
Acute dystonic reactions (less common than with metoclopramide). Occasional rashes.

PHARMACOKINETICS
Systemic bioavailability about 15% due to first pass metabolism. Terminal elimination half-life 7.5 hours.

EXCIPIENTS
Suspension includes saccharin, sorbitol and is sugar-free. See manufacturers SPC for further details.

LICENSED STATUS
Only licensed in children for the management of nausea and vomiting following radiotherapy or chemotherapy.

Dopamine hydrochloride

An endogenous catecholamine that is the immediate precursor of noradrenaline (norepinephrine). It stimulates adrenergic receptors of the sympathetic nervous system (beta 1, beta 2 and alpha). The effect is dose dependant.

USES
Treatment of low cardiac output states (e.g. following cardiopulmonary bypass surgery or chronic congestive cardiac failure) and shock due to other causes, septicaemia, very low birth weight infants.
The renal low dose use of dopamine is controversial.

PRESENTATION
Injection: 40mg in 1mL, 5mL and 10mL vial – Select-A-Jet® Dopamine; 5mL ampoule – non-proprietary.
Injection: 160mg in 1mL, 5mL ampoule – non-proprietary.
IV infusion: 400mg in 250mL glucose 5% (1.6mg in 1mL); dopamine 800mg in 250mL glucose 5% (3.2mg in 1mL) – non-proprietary.

DOSAGE

Route	Age				Frequency (times daily)	Notes
	birth–1 month	1 month–2 years	2–12 years	12–18 years		
IV infusion	← 1–5 microgram/kg/minute →				continuous	Low dose for renal effect. See monograph as some debate over its use.
IV infusion	Start at 3 microgram/ kg/minute increasing as clinically indicated to a maximum of 20 microgram/ kg/minute	← 5–20 microgram/kg/minute →			continuous	Direct inotropic effect but vasoconstriction may occur at higher doses.

ADMINISTRATION
IV: administer with an infusion pump. Closely monitor ECG, blood pressure and heart rate. It is preferable to dilute dopamine with NaCl 0.9% or glucose 5% before administration, although if fluid restricted the 40mg in 1mL injection can be administered undiluted via a syringe pump, via a central line.
Low doses may be infused peripherally, however, peripheral infusions of inotropic doses should be avoided as vasoconstriction and gangrene of the fingers or toes may occur. Use a dilute solution, not more than 1.6mg in 1mL, via a large vein. Monitor for signs of peripheral ischaemia.
Dopamine can NOT be mixed with sodium bicarbonate and other strongly alkaline solutions.
Dopamine and dobutamine can be mixed together in glucose 5% or NaCl 0.9%.
Do not use if discoloured.

CONTRA-INDICATIONS & WARNINGS

Contra-indicated in patients with phaeochromocytoma or hyperthyroidism, uncorrected arterial or ventricular tachyarrhythmias or ventricular fibrillation. Cyclopropane and halogenated hydrocarbon anaesthetics should be avoided, due to arrhythmogenic potential.

Warnings: hypovolaemia should be corrected where necessary prior to dopamine infusion. Low doses should be used in shock due to acute myocardial infarction. If a disproportionate rise in diastolic pressure (i.e. a marked decrease in pulse pressure) is observed, the infusion rate should be decreased and the patient observed carefully for further evidence of predominant vaso-constriction activity, unless such an effect is desired. Extravasation can cause dangerous ischaemia with necrosis and sloughing of the surrounding tissue. Ischaemia can be reversed by immediate infiltration of the affected area with 5-10mg phentolamine mesilate in 10-15mL NaCl 0.9% using a fine needle; use the smaller dose for infants and young children.

INTERACTIONS

Alpha and beta-blockers: the cardiac effects of dopamine are antagonised by beta-adrenergic blocking agents and the peripheral vasoconstriction caused by high doses of dopamine is antagonised by *alpha-adrenergic blocking agents.* Dopamine induced renal and mesenteric vasodilation is not antagonised by *alpha or beta-blocking agents. Phenytoin:* administration of IV *phenytoin* to patients receiving dopamine has resulted in hypotension and bradycardia.

PREGNANCY

The effect of dopamine on the human fetus is unknown and therefore it should be used only if expected benefits outweigh the risks. Contact local Medicines Information Centre for advice.

BREAST-FEEDING

It is not known if dopamine is excreted in breast milk but it is inactive when ingested by mouth.

SIDE-EFFECTS

More common reactions: ectopic beats, tachycardia, anginal pain, palpitation, hypotension, vasoconstriction, nausea, vomiting, headache and dyspnoea.
Less common reactions: aberrant conduction, bradycardia, widened QRS complex, hypertension and gangrene.

POISONING/TOXICITY

Excessive elevation of blood pressure and vasoconstriction can occur. This condition is rapidly reversed by dose reduction or discontinuation of therapy. If these measures fail, consider *phentolamine mesilate*. Ischaemia caused by local vasoconstriction (see precautions section for details of how to reverse).

PHARMACODYNAMIC PROPERTIES

Low doses of dopamine were thought to stimulate dopamine receptors and cause renal and mesenteric vasodilation with a resultant increase in glomerular filtration rate, renal blood flow, sodium excretion and urine output. This effect is now questionable. At intermediate infusion doses (2-10 microgram/kg/minute) dopamine stimulates beta 1 receptors in the myocardium producing an increase in cardiac output and heart rate. Total peripheral resistance is relatively unchanged because of peripheral vasoconstriction (alpha-adrenergic effect) and muscle vasodilation (beta-adrenergic effect). Blood pressure may rise and urinary output is further increased. In newborns, doses as high as 20 microgram/kg/minute have been used with improvements in mean arterial pressure and subsequent increases in urine output. The blunted inotropic response observed in neonates may be related to incomplete sympathetic innervation of the heart and reduced noradrenaline stores.

At higher doses (>20 microgram/kg/minute), dopamine has a predominately alpha-adrenergic effect resulting in vasoconstriction. There are further increases in cardiac output and total peripheral resistance; renal blood flow is maintained at levels higher than those obtained before therapy.

PHARMACOKINETIC PROPERTIES:

Following IV infusion, dopamine is rapidly distributed throughout the body. Steady state plasma levels are achieved within 5-10 minutes. Plasma protein binding is negligible.

Dopamine is extensively metabolised, largely in the liver, and unchanged drug and its metabolites are excreted in the urine. Less than 10% of the drug is recovered as the unchanged compound.

In one study in children aged between 3 months and 13 years the plasma half-life was found to be 26 minutes (+/-14 minutes).

D

EXCIPIENTS

Contact the manufacturer for further details.

LICENSED STATUS

Not licensed for use in children.

Dornase alfa (rhDNAse)

A genetically engineered human enzyme which, *in vitro*, hydrolyses DNA in sputum and greatly reduces the viscoelasticity of cystic fibrosis sputum.

USES
Mucolytic used in management of cystic fibrosis patients.

PRESENTATION
Nebuliser solution: 1000 units in 1mL (1mg in 1mL), 2.5mL vial – Pulmozyme®.

DOSAGE

Route	Age			Frequency (times daily)	Notes
	1 month–2 years	2–12 years	12–18 years		
Nebulised	–	≥5 years ⟶		1	Use under specialist supervision.
		2500 units (2.5mg)			

ADMINISTRATION
Nebulised: do not mix with other drugs or solutions in the nebuliser. Containment of the aerosol is not necessary. Manufacturer recommends that a compressor with an output of between 6-6.5L should be used. Wait for at least 1 hour after a dose is given before physiotherapy, as most benefit likely to be seen 1-3 hours after the dose.

CONTRA-INDICATIONS
Patients with known hypersensitivity.

INTERACTIONS
No known interactions.

PREGNANCY
Not recommended although evidence of teratogenicity, effects on development or impaired fertility have not been shown in animals.

BREAST-FEEDING
It is not known whether it is excreted into breast milk. Not recommended during breast-feeding but systemic absorption is very low.

SIDE-EFFECTS
Pharyngitis, hoarseness, laryngitis, rashes, urticaria.

POISONING/TOXICITY
No information available.

PHARMACOKINETIC PROPERTIES
Low systemic levels following inhalation.

EXCIPIENTS
See manufacturers SPC for further details.

LICENSED STATUS
Licensed for use ≥5 years of age.
Safety and efficacy has not been demonstrated in patients with FVC of less than 40% of predicted.

FURTHER INFORMATION
Store between 2-8°C (preferably in a refrigerator).

Dosulepin (dothiepin) hydrochloride

Tricyclic antidepressant.

USES
Depression. Bruxism (tooth-grinding).

PRESENTATION
Tablet: 75mg – Prothiaden® and non-proprietary.
Capsule: 25mg – Prothiaden® and non-proprietary.

DOSAGE

Route	Age	Frequency	Notes
	12–18 years	(times daily)	
Oral	50–75mg	1 (but see notes)	Initial dose. Given as a single dose at bedtime or in divided doses. Increase gradually as necessary to 150mg per day. Up to 225mg per day can be used in some circumstances (e.g. hospital use).

ADMINISTRATION
Oral: a suspension can be prepared but has strong local anaesthetic properties.

CONTRA-INDICATIONS & WARNINGS, INTERACTIONS, PREGNANCY, BREAST-FEEDING, SIDE-EFFECTS, POISONING/TOXICITY
See imipramine monograph.

PHARMACOKINETIC PROPERTIES
Readily absorbed from the gastrointestinal tract and extensively metabolised in the liver. Dosulepin is excreted in the urine, mainly in the form of metabolites; appreciable amounts are also excreted in the faeces. Half-life varies widely (11-40 hours) and is approximately 50 hours for dosulepin and its metabolites.

EXCIPIENTS
Prothiaden® tablets include sucrose and glucose. Contact manufacturers for further details.

LICENSED STATUS
Not licensed for use in children.

D

Doxapram

Stimulates all levels of the cerebrospinal axis. Increases minute volume and respiratory rate.

USES
Central respiratory stimulant.

PRESENTATION
Injection: 20mg in 1mL; 5mL ampoule – Dopram®.
IV infusion: 2mg in 1mL; in glucose 5%, 500mL bottle – Dopram®.

DOSAGE

Route	Age	Frequency	Notes
	birth–3 months	(times daily)	
IV loading dose	2.5mg/kg	loading dose	Give over at least 5-10 minutes.
IV infusion	300 microgram/kg/hour (maximum 1.5mg/kg/hour)	continuous	Watch for accumulation if high doses are infused for more than 36-48 hours.
Oral	6mg/kg	4	Give after an IV loading dose. Experience with oral administration is limited.

ADMINISTRATION
IV: dilute with glucose 5% or NaCl 0.9% to a concentration of 1mg in 1mL.
Oral: the injection is given orally, diluted in glucose 5% if necessary.

CONTRA-INDICATIONS & WARNINGS
High doses may cause convulsions.

INTERACTIONS
Sympathomimetics: risk of hypertension.
Theophylline: increased CNS stimulation.

PREGNANCY/BREAST-FEEDING
Contact local Medicines Information Centre for advice.

SIDE-EFFECTS
Side-effects are dose related. Oral doses may cause gastro-intestinal disturbances. High doses can cause convulsions. Tachycardia, hypertension, hyperpyrexia, laryngospasm.

POISONING/TOXICITY
See side-effects above. No specific antidote.

PHARMACOKINETIC PROPERTIES
Extensively metabolised and little excreted by the kidney.

LICENSED STATUS
Not licensed in children.

Doxorubicin hydrochloride

Cytotoxic anthracycline antibiotic.

USES
In combination therapy for treatment of: osteogenic sarcoma, non-Hodgkin lymphoma (NHL), Ewing tumour, Wilms tumour and some liver tumours.

PRESENTATION
Injection: powder for reconstitution, 10mg and 50mg vials – non-proprietary.
Injection: 2mg in 1mL; 10mg, 50mg and 100mg vials – non-proprietary.

DOSAGE
** Always consult the current treatment protocol for details of dosage and scheduling. **

ADMINISTRATION
IV: powder for reconstitution should be reconstituted with Water for Injections or NaCl 0.9% injection to a concentration of 2mg in 1mL.
Due to the vesicant properties of doxorubicin, it is strongly recommended that it is administered through a central venous line. For ease of administration and to reduce cardiotoxicity a schedule of doxorubicin by daily, 6 hour infusions is recommended.

CONTRA-INDICATIONS & WARNINGS
A baseline echocardiogram must be obtained prior to treatment. This should be repeated after alternate courses of doxorubicin up to total cumulative doses of 300mg/m², and before every course thereafter. If the left-ventricular fractional shortening (FS) is <29% *, doxorubicin therapy should be temporarily withdrawn. If subsequent testing shows an improvement in FS then a re-introduction of doxorubicin may be considered.
*A fall in FS by an absolute value of ≥10 percentile units but within an FS >29% may represent significant deterioration and the opinion of a cardiologist should be sought.
Dosage reduction should also be considered in cases of significant impairment of hepatic function.
Full blood count (to demonstrate haematological recovery) and renal function (U&Es) should be assessed prior to each course of therapy.

INTERACTIONS
Doxorubicin may interact with the following but the clinical significance of many of these interactions is unclear.
Dexrazoxane: to reduce cardiotoxicity.
Cardiac irradiation: to increase cardiac damage.
Actinomycin, mithramycin: cardiomyopathy.
Mercaptopurine: increased hepatotoxicity.
Mitomycin: increased late congestive cardiac failure.
Barbiturates: increased doxorubicin clearance.
Verapamil: increased doxorubicin plasma levels, reversal of doxorubicin resistance.
Propranolol: increased cardiotoxicity.
Ciclosporin (cyclosporin): increased doxorubicin plasma levels, modulation of doxorubicin resistance, increased myelotoxicity.
Carbamazepine, phenytoin and sodium valproate: altered anticonvulsant plasma levels.
Warfarin: increased warfarin effect.

Cimetidine, ranitidine: increased doxorubicin toxicity.
Interferon-alfa: altered doxorubicin disposition, doxorubicin dose reduction.

PREGNANCY
Although there is no conclusive evidence, there is experimental data which suggests that doxorubicin may harm the fetus and should, therefore, not be administered to pregnant women.

BREAST-FEEDING
Doxorubicin is excreted in milk. It should not be administered to breast-feeding mothers.

SIDE-EFFECTS
Common side-effects: nausea and vomiting, myelosuppression, alopecia, mucositis/enteritis, diarrhoea and severe tissue damage if extravasation occurs.

Occasional side-effects: increased bilirubin levels and acute/delayed cardiotoxicity.
Rare side-effects: hepatocellular necrosis, hyperpigmentation, renal damage and anaphylaxis.

POISONING/TOXICITY
Full supportive measures. Cardiotoxicity may be ameliorated by administration of a cardioprotective agent (dexrazoxane), or by prolonged infusion schedules. Weekly rather than 3 weekly treatment and administration of doxorubicin in liposomal formulation while increasingly advocated are not yet of proven use.

PHARMACOKINETIC PROPERTIES
Eliminated by hepatic metabolism and biliary excretion. Total plasma clearance in range of 500-1200mL/minute/m^2 with half-life of 30 hours. 75% protein bound in plasma.

EXCIPIENTS
Contact manufacturer for further details.

LICENSED STATUS
Licensed for use in children and adults.

Ear wax removal products

Almond oil or Olive oil

USES
Softening of earwax prior to syringing.

DOSAGE
2-3 drops into the ear.

ADMINISTRATION
Allow oil to warm to room temperature before administration. The patient should lie with the affected ear uppermost for 5-10 minutes after the drops are instilled.

LICENSED STATUS
Unlicensed.

FURTHER INFORMATION
Pharmaceutical grades are available. For reasons of hygiene do not use bottle for more than 28 days after first opening it.

Docusate sodium

USES
To aid removal of earwax.

PRESENTATION
Ear drops 0.5% – 15mL Molcer®; 10mL Waxsol®.

DOSAGE
Sufficient drops to fill the affected ear(s) on not more than 2 nights.

CONTRA-INDICATIONS & WARNINGS
Perforation or inflammation.

SIDE-EFFECTS
Rare transient stinging or irritation.

EXCIPIENTS
Molcer® includes propylene glycol.

LICENSED STATUS
Molcer® licensed for use in >6 years of age. Waxsol® licensed for use in children and adults.

FURTHER INFORMATION
For reasons of hygiene do not use bottle for more than 28 days after first opening it.

Cerumol®

USES
Collection of soft wax or hard wax plug occluding the external auditory meatus.

PRESENTATION
Ear drops: arachis (peanut) oil 57.3%, chlorbutol 5% and paradichlorobenzene 2%, 11mLs – Cerumol®.

DOSAGE

Route	Age				Frequency	Notes
	birth–1 month	1 month–2 years	2–12 years	12–18 years	(times daily)	
Locally into the ear	← 2 drops →		3–5 drops	5 drops	2	For 3 days.

ADMINISTRATION
Head is held inclined. Instil drops into ear and apply cotton wool plug moistened with Cerumol® before head returns to upright position. Wax may clear itself or allow easier and safer syringing.

CONTRA-INDICATIONS & WARNINGS
Otitis externa, eczema, perforation. Allergic reaction to arachis (peanut) oil not reported.

SIDE-EFFECTS
Tingling.

POISONING/TOXICITY
Oral ingestion of the contents of one bottle by a child may lead to sedation.

EXCIPIENTS
Include o-dichlorobenzene, turpentine oil and 3-methoxybutyl acetate.

LICENSED STATUS
Licensed for use in all ages.

FURTHER INFORMATION
For reasons of hygiene do not use bottle for more than 28 days after first opening it.

Econazole

Imidazole, topical antifungal.

USES
Fungal skin infections.

PRESENTATION
Cream: 1% – Ecostatin® and Pevaryl®.

DOSAGE/ADMINISTRATION
Apply 2-3 times daily continuing for 14 days after lesions have healed.

CONTRA-INDICATIONS & WARNINGS Avoid contact with eyes.	**SIDE-EFFECTS** Occasional skin irritation or sensitivity.
PREGNANCY No specific precautions, systemic absorption is likely to be negligible.	**POISONING/TOXICITY** Following accidental ingestion of large quantities, treatment, if necessary, is symptomatic.

EXCIPIENTS
See manufacturers SPC for further details.

LICENSED STATUS
Licensed for use in children and adults.

Edrophonium chloride

A very short-acting anticholinesterase.

USES
Diagnosis of myasthenia gravis.
Test to differentiate between under/over dosing of cholinergic drugs (e.g. neostigmine, pyridostigmine), i.e. to differentiate between cholinergic or myasthenic crisis. Antagonist to non-depolarising neuromuscular blockade.

PRESENTATION
Injection: 10mg in 1mL; 1mL ampoule – non-proprietary.

DOSAGE

Indication	Route	Age				Frequency	Notes
		birth– 1 month	1 month– 2 years	2–12 years	12–18 years		
Diagnosis of myasthenia gravis	IV	← 20 microgram/kg →			2mg	single dose	Initial dose, followed after 30 seconds (if no adverse reaction has occurred) by the remainder of dose as indicated.
		then			then	then	
		← 80 microgram/kg →			8mg	single dose	
Differentiation between under /overdosing of cholinergic drug	IV	–	20 microgram/kg		2mg	single dose	Give one hour after cholinergic. Underdosing – rapid, transient increase in muscle strength. Overdosing – transient decrease in muscle strength (increased weakness).
Antagonist to non-depolarising neuromuscular blockade	IV	–	← 500-700 microgram/kg → plus ← 7 microgram/kg → of atropine			single dose	Slow injection (over several minutes). If patient is bradycardic administer atropine first to ensure adequate rate before commencing edrophonium.

ADMINISTRATION
IV: test for myasthenia gravis – after the initial dose, the syringe is left in situ and then the remainder given as outlined in the table.

CONTRA-INDICATIONS & WARNINGS
Edrophonium should not be given to patients with mechanical intestinal or urinary obstruction. Use with extreme caution in patients with asthma. Care should be taken in patients with bradycardia, recent coronary occlusion, hypotension, peptic ulcer or epilepsy. Have atropine sulphate drawn up in a syringe before the test as edrophonium can cause profound bradycardia.
Test to differentiate between myasthenic or cholinergic crisis – the test should only be performed in

E

conjunction with someone skilled in intubation (since intubation and controlled ventilation may be required if the test provokes a cholinergic crisis).
Atropine should be given simultaneously when edrophonium is used as an antagonist to neuromuscular blockade. Edrophonium should not be given during *cyclopropane* or *halothane* anaesthesia.

INTERACTIONS
Atropine antagonises the muscarinic effects of edrophonium and this interaction is utilised to counteract the muscarinic symptoms of edrophonium (see poisoning/toxicity). Higher doses of edrophonium, as used to antagonise neuromuscular blockade, interact with depolarising muscle relaxants (e.g. *suxamethonium*) and prolonged apnoea may result.

PREGNANCY
Safety during pregnancy has not been established. However, experience in pregnant patients with myasthenia gravis has revealed no untoward effect of the drug on the course of the pregnancy.

BREAST-FEEDING
There is no information on the excretion of edrophonium in breast milk although only negligible amounts would be expected to be present.

SIDE-EFFECTS
These may include nausea and vomiting, increased salivation, diarrhoea, abdominal cramps and bradycardia.

POISONING/TOXICITY
Overdosage may give rise to bradycardia, arrhythmias, hypotension and bronchiolar spasm. Perspiration, gastro-intestinal hypermotility and visual disturbances may also occur. Artificial ventilation should be instituted if respiration is severely depressed. Atropine sulphate (20–40 microgram/kg in a child; 1–2mg in an adult) given slowly IV is an antidote to the muscarinic effects.

PHARMACOKINETIC PROPERTIES
Onset of effect occurs within 30-60 seconds following IV administration and lasts for around 2-15 minutes. Plasma half-life is 1.8 hours. Metabolised by plasma esterases and in the liver. The main route of excretion is in urine.

EXCIPIENTS
Contact manufacturer for further details.

LICENSED STATUS
Licensed for use in children and adults.

Emollients

USES
Emollients soothe, smooth and hydrate the skin and are indicated for all dry scaling disorders such as eczema.

PRESENTATION
There is a vast array of proprietary emollients, varying enormously in price. The generic emollients listed here will be suitable for most patients.

Preparations	Constituents
Aqueous Cream BP	Emulsifying ointment 30%, phenoxyethanol 1% in purified water.
Coconut oil	See separate monograph.
Emulsifying Ointment BP	Emulsifying wax 30%, white soft paraffin 50%, liquid paraffin 20%.
Hydrous ointment BP (oily cream)	Dried magnesium sulphate 0.5%, phenoxyethanol 1%, wool alcohols ointment. 50% in purified water
Liquid and White Soft Paraffin Ointment NPF	Liquid paraffin 50%, white soft paraffin 50%.
White Soft Paraffin BP (white petroleum jelly)	Semi-solid mixture of hydrocarbons obtained from petroleum.
Yellow Soft Paraffin BP (yellow petroleum jelly)	Semi-solid mixture of hydrocarbons obtained from petroleum.

DOSAGE
All ages – apply to the affected areas as required to prevent the skin from drying out. A child with a generalised dry skin disorder will need 250-500g per week.

ADMINISTRATION
Topical: emollients can be applied to the skin prior to and/or after a bath, to minimise drying of the skin. Emulsifying ointment and all emollient creams can also be used as a soap substitute or applied before bathing/showering. Other greasy emollients are less useful for this purpose having more of a barrier effect. The emollient should be applied at least 1-2 hours before or after treatment with a topical steroid.

CONTRA-INDICATIONS & WARNINGS
Hypersensitivity to an ingredient, particularly preservatives in creams. Care should be taken when bathing as emollients make the skin and bath surfaces slippery. Under no circumstances should emulsifying ointment be dissolved in the bath with boiling water, which could result in scalds.

SIDE-EFFECTS
Very rarely, sensitivity reactions of the skin and acne. Emollients, especially ointments, may cause rubber to perish, damaging self-suspending pyjama trousers or causing the rubber seal of a washing machine to warp and require replacement.

PHARMACODYNAMIC PROPERTIES
Emollients encourage hydration of the skin and have a mild anti-inflammatory effect. Creams are emulsions of oil and water; they are less greasy and easier to apply. Ointments are greasy preparations which are normally anhydrous and insoluble in water and are more occlusive than creams for dryer skin.

EXCIPIENTS
The following additives may be associated with sensitisation of eczematous skin: wool fat (lanolin), chlorocresol, fragrances, ethylenediamine, benzylalcohol, butylated hydroxyanisole, butylated hydroxytoluene, hydroxybenzoates, polysorbates, propyl glycol and sorbic acid. Details of whether they are contained in a preparation can be established by contacting the manufacturers for further details.

LICENSED STATUS
Licensed for use in all ages.

Enalapril

Angiotensin-converting enzyme (ACE) inhibitor.

USES
Hypertension (particularly secondary to hyperreninaemia); heart failure.

PRESENTATION
Solution: may be extemporaneously prepared.
Tablet: 2.5mg, 5mg, 10mg and 20mg – Innovace®.

DOSAGE

Route	Age				Frequency (times daily)	Notes
	birth–1 month	1 month–2 years	2–12 years	12–18 years		
Oral	40 microgram/kg	← 100 microgram/kg →		2.5mg	1	Initial dose. In neonates it may be necessary to give total dose in 2-3 divided doses due to variability in duration of action e.g. 5-10 microgram/kg/**dose** given 1-3 times daily.
	300–500 microgram/kg	← 300 –500 microgram/kg → (maximum 1mg/kg)		10–20mg (maximum 40mg)	1	Gradually increase dose according to response, up to Maintenance dose.

Renal failure
Use with caution in patients with renal impairment. If GFR is <20mL/minute give 50% of dose and then dose according to response.

ADMINISTRATION
Oral: tablets can be dispersed in water prior to administration.

CONTRA-INDICATIONS & WARNINGS, SIDE-EFFECTS, INTERACTIONS, PREGNANCY, BREAST-FEEDING, POISONING/TOXICITY
See captopril monograph. Avoid whenever possible in neonates, particularly preterm neonates, due to the risk of renal failure and hypotension. Severe hypotension may occur particularly following the first dose. Patient should be observed every 15 minutes for the first hour.

EXCIPIENTS
See manufacturers SPC for further details.

LICENSED STATUS
Not licensed for use in children.

FURTHER INFORMATION
Enalapril has been substituted for captopril on a basis of 1mg enalapril for every 7.5mg captopril.

Enoxaparin

A low molecular weight heparin (LMWH).

USES
Prophylaxis and treatment of thromboembolic disease.

PRESENTATION
Injection: 100mg (10,000 units) in 1mL; 20mg, 40mg, 60mg, 80mg and 100mg prefilled syringes – Clexane®.
Injection: 150mg (15,000 units) in 1mL; 120mg and 150mg prefilled syringes – Clexane®.

DOSAGE

Indication	Route	Age			Frequency (times daily)	Notes
		1 month–2 years	2–12 years	12–18 years		
Prophylaxis	SC	<2 months 750 microgram/kg	← 500 microgram/kg → (maximum dose 40mg)		2	
		>2 months 500 microgram/kg			2	
Treatment	SC	<2 months 1.5 mg/kg	← 1mg/kg →		2	
		>2 months 1mg/kg			2	

Experience of the use in children is limited.

Renal and hepatic impairment
In renal impairment no adjustment of the prophylaxis dose is required but patients with severe renal impairment should be closely monitored when receiving treatment doses. In the absence of clinical studies involving hepatic impairment caution should be exercised.

CONTRA-INDICATIONS & WARNINGS
Contra-indicated in patients with acute bacterial endocarditis; major bleeding disorders; thrombocytopenia in patients with a positive in-vitro aggregation test in the presence of enoxaparin; active gastric or duodenal ulceration; hypersensitivity to enoxaparin; stroke (unless due to systemic emboli); other patients with an increased risk of haemorrhage. Enoxaparin is to be used with extreme caution in patients with a history of heparin-induced thrombocytopenia with or without thrombosis. Enoxaparin injection, as with any other anticoagulant therapy, should be used with caution in conditions with

increased potential for bleeding, such as: impaired haemostasis, history of peptic ulcer, recent ischaemic stroke, uncontrolled severe arterial hypertension, diabetic retinopathy, recent neuro- or ophthalmologic surgery.

INTERACTIONS
It is recommended that agents which affect haemostasis should be discontinued prior to enoxaparin therapy unless their use is essential.

PREGNANCY
Should not be used in pregnant patients unless no safer alternative is available. There is no evidence that enoxaparin crosses the placental barrier during the second trimester of pregnancy. Contact local Medicines Information Centre for advice.

BREAST-FEEDING
It is not known whether unchanged enoxaparin is excreted in human breast milk. The oral absorption of enoxaparin is unlikely. Contact local Medicines Information Centre for advice.

SIDE-EFFECTS
Pain, haematoma and mild local irritation may follow subcutaneous injection, thrombocytopenia,hyperkalaemia may also occur. Although rare, cutaneous or systemic allergic reactions may occur as well as exceptional cases of skin necrosis.

POISONING/TOXICITY
Accidental overdose following parenteral administration may produce haemorrhagic complications. These may be largely neutralised by slow intravenous injection of protamine sulphate. However, even with high doses of protamine, the anti-Xa activity of enoxaparin is never completely neutralised (maximum about 60%).

EXCIPIENTS
See manufacturers SPC for further details.

LICENSED STATUS
Not licensed for use in children.

Ephedrine hydrochloride

Ephedrine is a sympathomimetic agent which constricts nasal blood vessels thereby decongesting the mucosa of the nose and neighbouring areas of the pharynx.

USES
Relief of nasal congestion.

PRESENTATION
Nasal drops: 0.5% and 1%, 10mL – non-proprietary.
Nasal drops: 0.25% may be extemporaneously prepared (see further information for details).

DOSAGE

Route	Age				Frequency (times daily)	Notes
	birth– 1 month	1 month– 2 years	2–12 years	12–18 years		
Intra-nasal	Not recommended	← 1–2 drops in each nostril →			3-4 times daily when required (15 minutes before feeds if appropriate)	Maximum of 7 days treatment. <u><3 months</u> use the 0.25% strength, if NaCl 0.9% nose drops are ineffective. <u>>3 months</u> use the 0.5% strength.

E

CONTRA-INDICATIONS & WARNINGS
Caution in children <3 months (no good evidence of effectiveness and irritation may narrow the nasal passages).

PREGNANCY
No fetal toxicity or fertility studies have been carried out in animals. In view of the potential vasoconstriction effect it is not advisable to use during pregnancy.

BREAST-FEEDING
Contact local Medicines Information Centre for advice.

SIDE-EFFECTS
Avoid excessive use since tolerance and rebound congestion can occur.

POISONING/TOXICITY
Ingestion of large quantities could cause systemic hypertension, excitement, restlessness, dilated pupils, tachycardia and hallucinations.

PHARMACOKINETIC PROPERTIES
Systemic absorption may occur following nasal application.

LICENSED STATUS
Licensed for use in ≥3 months of age.

FURTHER INFORMATION
0.25% drops can be prepared by dilution of the 0.5% drops with NaCl 0.9%. Discard after 1 week. For reasons of hygiene do not use 0.5% drops for more than 28 days after first opening.

Epirubicin hydrochloride

Cytotoxic anthracycline antibiotic.

USES
Combination chemotherapy (with vincristine, asparaginase and dexamethasone) for re-induction and consolidation of relapsed acute lymphoblastic leukaemia. Combination therapy for the treatment of newly diagnosed and relapsed rhabdomyosarcoma and other soft tissue tumours of childhood.

PRESENTATION
Injection: powder for reconstitution 10mg, 20mg and 50mg vials – Pharmarubicin® Rapid Dissolution.
Injection: 2mg in 1mL; 10mg and 50mg vials – Pharmarubicin® Solution for Injection.

DOSAGE
** Always consult the current treatment protocol for details of dosage and scheduling. **

ADMINISTRATION
IV: by continuous IV infusion over a minimum of 6 hours. Epirubicin is a vesicant drug and administration via a central venous line is recommended.

CONTRA-INDICATIONS & WARNINGS
In order to minimise cardiotoxicity, the general consensus is that administration should be by IV infusion over at least 6 hours. The cardiac toxicity ratio of epirubicin relative to doxorubicin is 1:1.8. On this basis, the cumulative dose of epirubicin in respect of cardiac toxicity ought to be approximately 80% greater than that for doxorubicin. A maximum cumulative dose of $0.9\text{-}1\text{g/m}^2$ is recommended in adults to avoid cardiotoxicity. Regular monitoring with echocardiography is mandatory both during and after therapy (see the contra-indications and warnings section of the doxorubicin monograph for monitoring details).

INTERACTIONS
No specific drug interactions are reported. However, in common with other anthracyclines, epirubicin has the potential to interact with other drugs (see doxorubicin monograph). The clinical significance of these has yet to be determined.

PREGNANCY/BREAST-FEEDING
There is no conclusive information as to whether epirubicin may adversely affect human fertility or cause teratogenicity. Experimental data, however, suggest that epirubicin may harm the fetus. It should not normally be administered to patients who are pregnant or to mothers who are breast-feeding.

SIDE-EFFECTS

Extravasation of epirubicin will result in severe tissue lesions and possibly necrosis. Aside from the expected myelosuppression (often prolonged in heavily pre-treated patients), alopecia and mucositis (often severe) have been documented along with significant gastrointestinal toxicity.

POISONING/TOXICITY

Extension of infusion time to 6 hours may also help reduce cardiotoxicity. There is not yet sufficient evidence to suggest that increasing infusion time above 6 hours is advantageous in further reducing toxicity.

PHARMACOKINETIC PROPERTIES

No specific data available for children. Following IV injection there is a rapid distribution phase followed by a slow terminal phase with a mean half-life of approximately 40 hours. Clearance is primarily by hepatic metabolism (hydroxylation and conjugation), followed by biliary excretion. Approximately 10% of the dose will be excreted in the urine in 48 hours. Epirubicin does not cross the blood-brain barrier.

EXCIPIENTS

See manufacturers SPC for further details.

LICENSED STATUS

Licensed for use in children and adults.

Epoetin (recombinant human erythropoietin)

Endogenous glycoprotein hormone that regulates red blood cell production.
Epoetin alfa and epoetin beta have identical amino acid sequences but different glycosylation patterns; the clinical efficacy is similar for both.

USES

Anaemia associated with chronic renal failure. Prevention of anaemias of prematurity in infants.

PRESENTATION

Epoetin alfa: Eprex® – solution containing 1000 international units in 0.5mL, 2000, 4000, 10,000 or 40,000 international units in 1mL in vials and 1000 or 2000 international units in 0.5mL pre filled syringes as well as pre filled syringes at a concentration of 10,000 international units per ml in sizes of 0.3mL, 0.4mL, 0.5mL, 0.6mL, 0.7mL, 0.8mL, 0.9mL and 1mL.
Epoetin beta: NeoRecormon® – multidose powder for reconstitution 50,000 and 100,000 international units vials (both with solvent). NeoRecormon® Reco-Pen (for SC use, double chamber cartridges containing epoetin beta and solvent) – 10,000, 20,000 and 60,000 international units cartridges, for use with Reco-Pen injection device. NeoRecormon® – prefilled syringes 500, 1000, 2000, 3000, 4000, 5000, 6000 and 10,000 international units.

DOSAGE

Indication	Route	Age	Frequency	Notes
		Infants of gestational age <34 weeks and a birth weight of 750g–1.5kg		
Prevention of anaemia of prematurity	SC	250 international units/kg (epoetin beta)	3 times per week	Treatment should be started as early as possible, preferably by day 3 of life and continued for 6 weeks. Premature infants who have had blood transfusions before epoetin are unlikely to benefit as much as untransfused infants.

E

Indication	Route	Ages		Frequency	Notes
		All Ages			
Renal anaemia in dialysis patients	SC	Treatment 20 international units/kg (epoetin beta) or 50 international units/kg (epoetin alfa) for 4 weeks		3 times weekly 2–3 times weekly	Increase by 20 international units/kg/dose (epoetin beta) or 25 international units/kg/dose (epoetin alfa) at monthly intervals until desired haemoglobin is achieved.
	IV injection (over 2 minutes)	40 international units/kg (epoetin beta) or 50 international units/kg (epoetin alfa)		3 times weekly	Both routes maximum weekly dose 720 international units/kg (epoetin beta) or 600 international units/kg (epoetin alfa).
	SC or IV	Maintenance Once the target haemoglobin is achieved (usually 9.5-12g/100mL) reduce the corrective dose by half, then adjust according to response at 1-2 week intervals.			

ADMINISTRATION
Vials (except multidose preparation) are for single use only. NeoRecormon® powder – use within 2 hours of reconstitution. NeoRecormon® multidose use within 1 month of reconstitution. Do not mix with other drugs.

CONTRA-INDICATIONS & WARNINGS
Contra-indicated in uncontrolled hypertension. All patients should receive adequate iron supplementation after evaluation of iron status. Other causes of anaemia e.g. B_{12} or folate deficiency should be excluded before starting treatment with epoetin. Use with caution in patients with a history of seizures, thrombocytosis, chronic liver failure and ischaemic vascular disease.

INTERACTIONS
No evidence exists that epoetin alters the metabolism of other drugs but since *ciclosporin (cyclosporin)* is bound by red blood cells there is potential for interaction. Blood levels of *ciclosporin* should therefore be monitored if the two are used concurrently.

PREGNANCY/BREAST-FEEDING
Only use if the benefits outweigh the risk, as experience in human pregnancy/lactation is inadequate.

SIDE-EFFECTS
Dose dependent aggravation of hypertension, influenza-like symptoms, rash, shunt thrombosis.

POISONING/TOXICITY
Epoetin has a very wide therapeutic index. Even at high serum levels no symptoms of poisoning have been observed.

PHARMACOKINETIC PROPERTIES
Half-life of approximately 6 hours in children (after multiple IV administration); after SC administration, 24 hours.

E

EXCIPIENTS
NeoRecormon® all preparations include phenylalanine and some include benzyl alcohol. See manufacturers SPC for further details.

LICENSED STATUS
In children both products are licensed for the treatment of anaemia associated with chronic renal failure in patients on haemodialysis (although Eprex® is not licensed for SC use). Epoetin beta is licensed for the treatment of anaemia of prematurity (although the licence varies between NeoRecormon® preparations e.g. multidose vial only licensed for children >3 years old).

Epoprostenol (prostacyclin)

Epoprostenol is a prostaglandin which is a potent inhibitor of platelets and a potent vasodilator.

USES
Pulmonary vasodilatation where tolazoline has failed and nitric oxide is not available. Pulmonary hypertension. Digital ischaemia. Platelet aggregation inhibitor.

PRESENTATION
Infusion: (as sodium salt) 500 microgram, with a 50mL vial of sterile diluent – Flolan®.

DOSAGE
Neonate (birth – 1 month)

Route	Age		Notes
	birth–1 month		
IV infusion	20 nanogram/kg/minute		Monitor for systemic hypotension.
	(up to 40 nanogram/kg/minute can be tried)		

Child

Route	Age			Frequency (times daily)	Notes
	1 month–2 years	2–12 years	12–18 years		
IV infusion	← 2 nanogram/kg/minute →			continuous	Monitor for systemic hypotension.
	increasing up to 40 nanogram/kg/minute				Doses of up to 120 nanogram/kg/minute
	if necessary				have occasionally been necessary.

ADMINISTRATION
IV: reconstitution and dilution should be carried out immediately prior to use.
The injection vial should be reconstituted using the diluent provided. Draw 10mL of the diluent into a syringe, inject into the epoprostenol vial and dissolve the contents completely. Draw all the epoprostenol solution back into the syringe and add the contents of the syringe to the remaining 40mL of diluent and mix well. This solution is referred to as the *concentrated solution* and contains 10 microgram/1mL epoprostenol.

For neonate (birth – 1 month): draw into a syringe 6mL of the *concentrated solution* for every kg the baby weighs. The filter provided should then be attached to the syringe and the *concentrated solution* is dispensed by filtration using firm but not excessive pressure. Dilute to 25mL with NaCl 0.9% and infuse at 0.5mL/hour to infuse 20 nanogram of epoprostenol per kg per minute.

For infants/children: the quantity of *concentrated solution* should then be drawn up into a syringe and the filter provided attached to the syringe so that the *concentrated solution* is dispensed by filtration using firm but not excessive pressure. The filtered, *concentrated solution* can then be further diluted with NaCl 0.9% (in general 10mL of the filtered, *concentrated solution* is added to 40mL of NaCl 0.9% to give 2 microgram/mL). The filtered, *concentrated solution* of 10 microgram/mL can be infused neat via a central line.

Do not dilute below 1.7 microgram/mL (i.e more than 1 in 6), or with any fluid other than NaCl 0.9%. Incompatible with glucose, do not infuse with any other drugs. Infusions may be used for up to 24 hours if loss of potency is allowed for (see further information) and doses titrated to response.

E

CONTRA-INDICATIONS & WARNINGS
Treat any hypovolaemia before using this drug. Monitor blood pressure.

INTERACTIONS
Possible potentiation of *heparin* and *oral anticoagulants*. Vasodilator effect may augment or be augmented by *other vasodilators*.

PREGNANCY
No information on exposed pregnancies available. Animal studies do not indicate direct or indirect harmful effects with respect to pregnancy, embryonal/fetal development, parturition or postnatal development. Contact local Medicines Information Centre for advice.

BREAST-FEEDING
No information available.

SIDE-EFFECTS
Hypotension, flushing and bradycardia.

POISONING/TOXICITY
The main feature of overdose is likely to be hypotension. Reduce the dose or discontinue the infusion and initiate appropriate supportive measures as necessary; for example, plasma volume expansion and/or adjustment to pump flow.

PHARMACOKINETIC PROPERTIES
Half-life is 3 minutes.

EXCIPIENTS
See manufacturers SPC for further details.

LICENSED STATUS
Not licensed for use in pulmonary hypertension and not licensed for use in children.

FURTHER INFORMATION
Epoprostenol loses potency after reconstitution, 10% every 12 hours.

Ergocalciferol (calciferol, vitamin D2)

USES
Rickets due to vitamin D deficiency.

PRESENTATION
Oral liquid: several strengths available – manufactured 'specials'.
Tablets: 250 micrograms (10,000 units) – non-proprietary.

DOSAGE

Route	Age			Frequency (times daily)	Notes
	1 month–2 years	2–12 years	12–18 years		
Oral	< 6 months 3000 units	6000 units	10,000 units	1	
	> 6 months 6000 units			1	

CONTRA-INDICATIONS & WARNINGS
Renal insufficiency. All patients receiving pharmacological doses of vitamin D should have their plasma calcium concentration checked regularly and when nausea and vomiting are present.

INTERACTIONS
Ergocalciferol is inactivated, probably through enzyme systems, by the continuous administration of *anticonvulsants*.

PREGNANCY
Ergocalciferol 250 micrograms may be given to women in the third trimester of pregnancy if justified on medical grounds. Contact local Medicines Information Centre for advice.

BREAST-FEEDING
Should not be given to lactating mothers. Contact local Medicines Information Centre for advice.

SIDE-EFFECTS
Excessive doses may give rise to anorexia, nausea, vomiting, diarrhoea, loss of weight, headache, polyuria, thirst, vertigo.

POISONING/TOXICITY
If hypervitaminosis occurs: discontinue treatment with ergocalciferol, reduce dietary calcium intake and correct dehydration and electrolyte disturbance. Hypercalcaemia may be corrected by the administration of hydrocortisone or calcitonin.

EXCIPIENTS
Contact manufacturers for further details.

LICENSED STATUS
Ergocalciferol 250 microgram tablets are licensed for use in children and adults for simple vitamin D deficiency, vitamin D deficiency caused by intestinal malabsorption or chronic liver disease, hypocalcaemia of hypoparathyroidism.

FURTHER INFORMATION
Several strengths of oral liquid are available from various hospital manufacturing units.

Macrolide antibiotic.

USES
Upper and lower respiratory tract infections (including whooping cough), skin and soft tissue infections, oral/dental infections, infections of external and middle ear, genitourinary infections, gastrointestinal and biliary infections, endocarditis (as an alternative to penicillin, in penicillin allergic patients) and topically in acne.

In cystic fibrosis patients – treatment of asymptomatic *Staphylococcus aureus* isolates or minor exacerbations and treatment of atypical infection e.g. mycoplasma; some centres use erythromycin as a long-term anti-staphylococcal drug.

PRESENTATION
Capsule: 250mg – Erymax® and non-proprietary.
IV infusion: (as lactobionate) 1g vial – non-proprietary.
Oral suspension: (as ethyl succinate) 125mg in 5mL, 250mg in 5mL and 500mg in 5mL – Erythroped® and non-proprietary.
Tablet: 250mg – non-proprietary; (as stearate) 250mg and 500mg – Erythrocin®; (as ethylsuccinate) 500mg – Erythroped A®.
Topical gel: 2% and 4%, in an alcoholic basis – Eryacne®.
Topical solution: 2% in an alcoholic basis – Stiemycin®.

DOSAGE
Newborn infant (birth to 1 month)

Route	Age	Frequency	Notes
	birth–1 month	(times daily)	
Oral/IV	12.5mg/kg	4	

Child

Indication	Route	Age			Frequency	Notes
		1 month–2 years	2–12 years	12–18 years	(times daily)	
Infection	Oral		2–8 years	500mg	4	Doses can be doubled in severe infections. Maximum single dose 1g.
		125mg	250mg			
			9–12 years		4	
			500mg			
	IV	←	12.5mg/kg	→	4	
	Topical		–	directly to affected area	2	Apply after washing to the affected area.
Cystic fibrosis patients	Oral	DOSE BY WEIGHT			2	Treatment of asymptomatic *S. aureus* isolates or minor exacerbations. Total daily dose can be given in four divided doses.
		←	25mg/kg	→		
		DOSE BY AGE				
			2–8 years		2	
		250mg	500mg	1g		
			8–12 years			
			1g		2	
Pneumococcal prophylaxis	Oral		2–8 years	500mg	2	Used in penicillin allergic patients.
		125mg	250mg			
			9–12 years			
			500mg		2	
Gastric stasis	Oral/IV	←	3mg/kg	→	4	

ADMINISTRATION
Oral: total daily dose may be given in 2 divided doses, but gastrointestinal side-effects can occur.
IV: to allow for displacement volume the vial contains extra drug and therefore addition of 20mL Water for Injections to 1g vial (total volume 20mL) gives 1g in 20mL (i.e. 50mg in 1mL). Dilute 10 times in NaCl 0.9% or neutralised glucose 5% (prepare by adding 5mL of sterile 8.4% w/v sodium bicarbonate to one litre glucose 5% infusion). Infuse over 60 minutes. Total daily dose may be continuously infused over 24 hours at a concentration of 1mg in 1mL (maximum 5mg in 1mL).

E

CONTRA-INDICATIONS & WARNINGS
Known hypersensitivity to erythromycin. Contra-indicated with *terfenadine, cisapride, astemizole, ergotamine* and *dihydroergotamine*. Concurrent topical acne therapy should be used with caution because a cumulative irritant effect may occur.

INTERACTIONS
Increased risk of cardiotoxicity with *terfenadine, cisapride* or *astemizole*. Increased serum concentrations of *carbamazepine, digoxin, warfarin, phenytoin, theophylline, ciclosporin (cyclosporin), disopyramide, midazolam* and *alfentanil*.

PREGNANCY
No evidence of hazard from erythromycin in human pregnancy.

BREAST-FEEDING
Excreted in breast milk in small amounts but this should not present a problem to breast-feeding mothers.

SIDE-EFFECTS
Nausea, abdominal pain, vomiting, diarrhoea. Reversible hearing loss with high doses. Allergic reactions – anaphylaxis is rare. Cardiac arrhythmias have been very rarely reported and isolated reports of chest pain, dizziness and palpitations. Venous irritation can occur with IV administration, but if the injection is diluted and given slowly as outlined above, pain and venous trauma are minimised.

POISONING/TOXICITY
Symptoms: hearing loss, severe nausea, vomiting and diarrhoea.
Treatment: general supportive measures.

EXCIPIENTS
Contact manufacturers for further details.

LICENSED STATUS
Licensed for use in all ages.

Etanercept

Recombinant human tumour necrosis factor (TNF) receptor: Fc fusion protein.

USES
Moderate to severe active polyarticular juvenile idiopathic arthritis (JIA) in children ≥4 years of age who have failed to respond to an adequate therapeutic trial of methotrexate (see British Paediatric Rheumatology Group Guidelines (BPRG) April, 2000).

PRESENTATION
Injection: 25mg powder and solvent in a prefilled syringe – Enbrel®.

DOSAGE
All patients should have their varicella antibody status measured before commencing treatment. Siblings should be considered for varicella immunisation prior to commencement of treatment of the patient. Patients in contact with varicella should be considered for treatment with varicella zoster immunoglobulin (VZIG) if their varicella titres are negative. Patients with a significant exposure to varicella should have their etanercept therapy temporarily discontinued.

Route	Age		Frequency (times daily)	Notes
	2–12 years	12–18 years		
SC injection	≥ 4 years 400 micrograms/kg	400 micrograms/kg	Twice weekly with an interval of 72-96 hours between doses	Up to a maximum of 25mg per dose.

No dosage adjustment is required in renal and hepatic impairment.

ADMINISTRATION
SC injection: reconstitute vial with 1mL Water for Injections (provided in prefilled syringe). Solutions prepared with Water for Injections should be administered as soon as possible and within 6 hours following reconstitution. Any unused solution should be discarded.

CONTRA-INDICATIONS & WARNINGS

Contra-indications: women who are pregnant or breast-feeding or who are sexually active but with inadequate contraception. Treatment with etanercept should not be initiated in patients with active infections including chronic or localised infections. Current or previous tuberculosis, previous or present sepsis of a prosthetic joint still in situ, malignancy or pre-malignancy states, immunodeficiency, hypersensitivity to the active substance or to any of the excipients.

Warnings: patients who develop a new infection while undergoing treatment with etanercept should be monitored closely. Administration of etanercept should be discontinued if a patient develops a serious infection. Caution should be exercised in patients with a history of recurring infections or with underlying conditions which may predispose patients to infections such as poorly controlled diabetes. Caution should be exercised in patients with pre-existing or recent onset of CNS demyelinating disease. Etanercept should be used with caution in patients with a history of allergies, asthma, or allergic-type phenomena associated with other drugs.

Vaccinations: live vaccines should not be given concurrently with etanercept. No data are available on the secondary transmission of infection by live vaccines in patients receiving etanercept. It is recommended that JIA patients, if possible, be brought up to date with all immunisations in agreement with current immunisation guidelines prior to initiating etanercept therapy.

INTERACTIONS

No interactions have been observed when etanercept was administered with *glucocorticoids, salicylates, NSAIDs, analgesics* or *methotrexate.*

PREGNANCY

The use of etanercept in pregnant women is not recommended.

BREAST-FEEDING

Immunoglobulins can be excreted in breast milk, therefore etanercept should not be given to breast-feeding mothers.

SIDE-EFFECTS

Common side-effects include erythema and/or itching, pain, or swelling at the injection site. These are not usually an indication to discontinue therapy. Other reported side-effects include upper respiratory infections ('colds'), rhinitis, pharyngitis, cough and sinusitis, nausea and vomiting, abdominal pain, headache, dizziness, asthenia and rash. Autoantibody production may occur but is not associated with the development of autoimmune disease. Very rarely, blood dyscrasias have been reported.

POISONING/TOXICITY

During clinical trials no dose-limiting toxicities were observed.

PHARMACOKINETIC PROPERTIES

In most adults receiving etanercept 25mg subcutaneously twice weekly, steady-state concentrations are expected to be achieved approximately 3 weeks after initiation of therapy. The metabolic fate of etanercept is yet to be determined.

EXCIPIENTS

See manufacturers SPC for further details.

LICENSED STATUS

Licensed for use ≥4 years of age for treatment of active polyarticular JIA. A condition of the licence is that all patients must be entered into the BPRG Biologics Registry.

FURTHER INFORMATION

All patients to be started on this drug in the UK and Ireland must be registered on the central register held by the BPRG. Clinicians prescribing etanercept must undertake to document the patient's disease activity every month, whilst measures of outcome, and episodes of toxicity and intercurrent illness should be recorded quarterly. It is anticipated that clinicians using this new therapy will be currently managing many patients with severe JIA.

Ethambutol

Antituberculous drug.

USES

Treatment of tuberculosis (if isoniazid resistance is suspected), in combination with other drugs.

PRESENTATION

Tablet: 100mg and 400mg – non-proprietary.
Oral liquid: may be extemporaneously prepared.

DOSAGE

Treatment should always be given in collaboration with a specialist experienced in tuberculosis therapy.

Route	Age			Frequency (times daily)	Notes
	1 month–2 years	2–12 years	12–18 years		
Oral	←	15mg/kg	→	1	*The dose given is that used in the standard 6 month regimen of tuberculosis treatment where once daily dosing is used. Maximum dose 1.5g/day.

Creatinine clearance (mL/minute/1.73m²)	Dosage
10–50	50% of normal dose.
10	25% of normal dose.

Dosage reduction in renal impairment
Ethambutol is only slightly dialysable (5–20%).

ADMINISTRATION

Oral: absorption is not significantly altered by administration with food.

CONTRA-INDICATIONS & WARNINGS

Patients known to be hypersensitive to the drug; patients with known optic neuritis unless clinical judgement determines that it may be used. Patients who cannot understand warnings about visual side-effects should, if possible, be given an alternative drug. In particular, ethambutol should be used with caution in children until they are at least 5 years old and capable of reporting symptomatic visual changes accurately. Patients should undergo a full ophthalmic examination before starting treatment. This should include visual acuity, colour vision, perimetry and ophthalmoscopy. Thereafter, routine ophthalmological examinations may be considered desirable when treating young children (for the reasons outlined above) and older children/adults should be informed of the importance of reporting any change in vision.

INTERACTIONS

Aluminium salts can decrease ethambutol levels.

PREGNANCY

Animal studies have shown some teratogenic potential. There have been several reports of the drug being administered during pregnancy without any untoward effect. Nevertheless, it is recommended that the possibility of such effects should be kept in mind when treating women of child-bearing age.

BREAST-FEEDING

Mothers can breast-feed normally while taking ethambutol.

SIDE-EFFECTS

Optic neuritis, red/green colour blindness, peripheral neuritis, rarely rash, pruritus, urticaria, thrombocytopenia. Gastrointestinal symptoms such as nausea, vomiting and diarrhoea have been reported in patients on multiple-drug antituberculous therapy but not in patients receiving ethambutol as sole therapy.

POISONING/TOXICITY

No specific antidote; treatment is symptomatic and supportive.

PHARMACOKINETIC PROPERTIES

Following oral administration, absorption is approximately 80%. The drug is well distributed throughout the body with high concentrations in kidneys, lungs, saliva and red blood cells. Half-life is approximately 2.5-3.6 hours but this can be up to 7 hours or longer with renal impairment. 20% metabolism in the liver to inactive metabolite. Approximately 50% excreted in the urine and 20% in the faeces as unchanged drug.

EXCIPIENTS

Contact manufacturers for further advice.

LICENSED STATUS

Licensed for use in children and adults.

FURTHER INFORMATION

*Dosage is that given in the 1998 recommendations for chemotherapy and management of tuberculosis in the United Kingdom, produced by a subcommittee of the Joint Tuberculosis Committee (JTC) of the British Thoracic Society.

Synthetic oestrogen.

USES
Priming the pituitary for testing with growth hormone. Induction and maintenance of sexual maturation in females. Prevention of unacceptable tall stature in females.

PRESENTATION
Tablet: 2 microgram – named patient; 10 microgram, 50 microgram and 1mg – non-proprietary.

DOSAGE

Indication	Route	Age		Frequency	Notes
		2–12 years	12–18 years	(times daily)	
Induction of puberty	Oral	–	2 micrograms	1	Increasing every 6 months to 5, 10, and then 20 micrograms. Add progestogen after 18-24 months (see guidelines).
Maintenance	Oral	–	20 micrograms	1	Combined with progestogen.
Prevention of tall stature	Oral	20-50 micrograms	–	1	Requires specialist advice.
Priming before growth hormone test in girls with bone age >10 years	Oral	Bone age >10 years 100 micrograms	100 micrograms	1	For 3 days prior to the test (diethylstilbestrol 1mg twice is an alternative for boys and girls).

CONTRA-INDICATIONS & WARNINGS
Contra-indicated in those with a history or family history of thromboembolism, moderate to severe hyperlipoproteinaemia, severe liver disease and porphyria.

INTERACTIONS
Enzyme-inducing drugs such as *rifampicin, phenobarbital (phenobarbitone), carbamazepine* and *phenytoin* can lower the level of ethinylestradiol by accelerating its metabolism. Through its effects on the coagulation system, ethinylestradiol may reduce the effects of anticoagulants such as *warfarin.* The doses of *insulin* or *hypoglycaemic* drugs may need to be adjusted due to a mild diabetogenic effect. The clearance of *theophylline* may be reduced due to the inhibition of its metabolism.

PREGNANCY & BREAST-FEEDING
Contra-indicated.

SIDE-EFFECTS
Nausea, vomiting, cholestatic jaundice, fluid retention, behaviour changes, headache, migraine, breast tenderness, thromboembolism, hypertension, thrombosis, rash, corneal discomfort in contact lens users, sodium and water retention, reduced glucose tolerance and changes in body weight, hypercalcaemia.

POISONING/TOXICITY
Acute overdose may cause nausea and vomiting and may result in withdrawal bleeding in females.

PHARMACOKINETIC PROPERTIES
It is rapidly absorbed from the gastro-intestinal tract but undergoes some first-pass metabolism in the gut wall. It is metabolised by the liver. Enzyme-inducing agents, antibiotics and cigarette smoking affect the rate of metabolism. The elimination half-life ranges from 5-16 hours.

E

EXCIPIENTS
Contact manufacturers for further details.

LICENSED STATUS
The 2 microgram tablet are unlicensed. The other tablets are licensed for gonadal dysgenesis but other indications are unlicensed.

FURTHER INFORMATION
The 2 microgram tablet can be obtained from Celltech.

Antiepileptic.

PRESENTATION
Capsule: 250mg – Zarontin® and Emeside®.
Syrup: 250mg in 5mL – Zarontin® and Emeside®.

USES
Second or third line treatment of absence seizures (after sodium valproate and lamotrigine) and third line treatment of myoclonic seizures.

DOSAGE/ADMINISTRATION

Route	Age				Frequency (times daily)	Notes
	birth–1 month	1 month–2 years	2–12 years	12–18 years		
Oral	–	← 5mg/kg →		250mg	2	Usual starting dose. Increase dose by 2.5mg/kg/dose, taking 2–3 weeks to reach maintenance dose.
	–	← 10–20mg/kg →		500–750mg (maximum 1g)	2	Usual target maintenance dose. Rarely, total daily dose may be divided into 3.

CONTRA-INDICATIONS & WARNINGS
Porphyria. Withdraw gradually. Caution in liver or renal disease, monitor plasma levels. Counsel on recognition of haematological adverse effects such as fever, sore throat, mouth ulcers, bruising, bleeding; perform blood count if clinically indicated.

INTERACTIONS
May increase plasma levels of *phenytoin*. Ethosuximide plasma levels may be decreased by *carbamazepine*, *phenobarbital (phenobarbitone)*, *primidone*, *phenytoin* and may be increased by *sodium valproate*, *vigabatrin* and *isoniazid*. Effects are antagonised by *antidepressants* and *antipsychotics*.

PREGNANCY
Congenital malformations possible. Contact local Medicines Information Centre for advice.

BREAST-FEEDING
Excreted into breast milk but unlikely to be harmful.

manufacturers recommend avoid breast-feeding. Contact local Medicines Information Centre for advice.

SIDE-EFFECTS
Dose dependent side-effects include gastrointestinal upset (diarrhoea, colic), nausea, anorexia, headache, lethargy. Chronic adverse effects include headache, behaviour changes, low white blood cell count.

POISONING/TOXICITY
Nausea, vomiting, respiratory and CNS depression may be seen. Contact UK National Poisons Information Service for advice.

PHARMACOKINETIC PROPERTIES
Peak plasma levels 1-7 hours after oral administration. Elimination half-life is approximately 30 hours in children; longer in adults. Monitor trough plasma levels at least one week after dosage change if clinically indicated, reference range 40-100mg/L (300-700 micromol/L).

EXCIPIENTS
Emeside® syrup and Zarontin® liquid include sucrose. See manufacturers SPC for further details.

LICENSED STATUS
Licensed for adults, children and infants.

Etoposide

Epipodophyllotoxin.

USES
Etoposide is employed extensively in the treatment of many solid tumours and leukaemias in children. It is used primarily in multi-drug regimens in which it is administered by IV infusion.

Examples: Stage 4 neuroblastoma, germ-cell tumours, rhabdomyosarcoma, soft-tissue sarcomas, relapsed Hodgkin disease, non-Hodgkin lymphoma and Ewing tumour. Neuroectodermal tumours (including medulloblastoma). Intracranial germ cell tumours.

PRESENTATION
Injection: 20mg in 1mL, 5mL, 10mL and 25mL vials – non-proprietary; 5mL vial – Vepesid®.
Capsule: 50mg and 100mg – Vepesid®.

DOSAGE
** Always consult the current treatment protocol for details of dosage and scheduling. **

ADMINISTRATION
IV: infusion in NaCl 0.9% injection at a concentration not exceeding 400 micrograms in 1mL over 1-4 hours. Physical stability of etoposide in aqueous solution is concentration dependent. Solutions should be carefully examined immediately prior to infusion and regularly whilst it is running for any visible signs of precipitation.

CONTRA-INDICATIONS & WARNINGS
Rapid administration associated with hypotensive reactions. Full blood count, renal function (U&Es) and hepatic function should be assessed before each course.

INTERACTIONS
Etoposide may displace *warfarin* from protein binding sites or alter metabolism leading to increased prothrombin time. Co-administration of *phenytoin* and *phenobarbital (phenobarbitone)* may increase etoposide clearance.

PREGNANCY/BREAST-FEEDING
There are no adequate controlled studies in pregnant women. Etoposide should not normally be administered to pregnant and breast-feeding women.

SIDE-EFFECTS
Alopecia, myelosuppression, nausea and vomiting are common. Rarely anaphylactic reactions, fever, headache, pruritus, pigmentation, mucositis/enteritis and increased risk of second malignancies.

POISONING/TOXICITY
Full supportive measures.

PHARMACOKINETIC PROPERTIES
Median (range) pharmacokinetic parameters:
Clearance: 26 (14-54) mL/minute/m^2.
Half-life: 132 (87-6/5) minutes.
AUC: 3.9 (1.8-7.3)mg/mL/minute/100mg/m^2.
Children tend to have shorter drug elimination half-life than adults because of better renal function and hence better renal clearance. Clearance can be increased in hypoalbuminaemic patients leading to reduced AUC. Clearance is independent of age and dose (90–250mg/m^2) but is more variable at doses 100mg/m^2 and therapeutic drug monitoring may be indicated.

EXCIPIENTS
Contact manufacturer for further details.

LICENSED STATUS
Not licensed for use in children.

Factor IX

A preparation of human coagulation factor IX.

USES
Congenital factor IX deficiency (haemophilia B).

PRESENTATION
Recombinant coagulation factor IX (nonacog alfa) – BeneFIX®.
Dried factor IX prepared from human plasma (high purity) – Mononine® and Replenine® – VF (Heat-Treated).

Recombinant factor IX should be used in preference to products derived from human plasma. If factor IX derived from human plasma is used then high purity products should always be used in preference to intermediate purity products.

DOSAGE/ADMINISTRATION

Should only be administered after specialist advice from a haemophilia centre.

Consult the United Kingdom Haemophilia Centre Directors' Organisation (UKHCDO) treatment guidelines. Dose should always be tailored to clinical effectiveness in each individual. The number of units needed and the duration of treatment depend on the condition being treated. See individual product information for full dosage/administration details.

CONTRA-INDICATIONS & WARNINGS

Disseminated intravascular coagulation (DIC). Administer with caution to patients with liver disease, neonates and to patients postoperatively and those at risk of thromboembolic phenomena.

PREGNANCY/BREAST-FEEDING

Based on the rare occurrence of haemophilia B in women, experience regarding the use of factor IX during pregnancy and breast-feeding is not available.

SIDE-EFFECTS

Allergic reactions, mild chills, fever, nausea, flushing, stinging at the infusion site. Potential risk of thromboembolic episodes.

POISONING/TOXICITY

In the event of overdose, the infusion should be stopped and the patient carefully monitored and supportive treatment given. The risk of DIC and thrombosis may be enhanced in patients susceptible to these complications.

PHARMACOKINETIC PROPERTIES

Median half-life 21 hours.

EXCIPIENTS

Contact manufacturers for further details.

LICENSED STATUS

Licensed for use in children and adults.

FURTHER INFORMATION

Recombinant factor IX and high purity factor IX products are not suitable for the reversal of anticoagulant overdose. The manufacturers warn that despite all the precautions taken by them it cannot be assumed that products prepared from human blood or plasma are totally free of infectious agents. Dried factor IX fraction may also contain clotting factors II, VII and X depending on the product.

Factor VIII

A constituent of normal plasma; forms part of the clotting process.

PRESENTATION

Recombinant human antihaemophilic factor VIII (octocog alfa) – Alphanate®, Helixate® NexGen, Kogenate®, Recombinate® and ReFacto®.

The recombinant products should be used in the treatment of haemophilia A in preference to dried factor VIII derived from human plasma. Government policy (February 1998) stated that all children <16 years of age and new patients with haemophilia A should receive recombinant factor VIII.

USES

Prevention and control of haemorrhage in haemophilia A. These products are not indicated for the treatment of von Willebrand disease as they have at most only trace amounts of von Willebrand Factor.

PRESENTATION

Dried factor VIII fraction prepared from human plasma – Fanhdi®, Hemofil M®, Liberate®, High Potency Factor VIII Concentrate, Monoclate-P® and Replenate®.

All patients receiving dried factor VIII derived from human plasma should receive high purity factor VIII. The manufacturers warn that despite all the precautions taken by them it cannot be assumed that products prepared from human blood or plasma are totally free from infective agents.

F

USES
Prevention and control of haemorrhage in haemophilia A.

DOSAGE
Should only be administered after specialist advice from a haemophilia centre. Consult the United Kingdom Haemophilia Centre Directors' Organisation (UKHCDO) treatment guidelines.
The dose and dosing schedule for factor VIII must be calculated and adjusted according to the needs of the individual patient, taking into account the patient's body weight, the degree of factor VIII deficiency, the site and extent of the bleeding, the titre of inhibitors, the factor VIII level desired and the clinical condition.

The required dosage may be estimated using the following formula as a guide:

Number of factor VIII units required = Body weight (kg) x desired increase in factor VIII x 0.5
(international units)   (% of normal)

ADMINISTRATION
Use aseptic technique during reconstitution and administration. Do not administer at a rate exceeding 10mL/minute by injection or infusion. See individual product information for full reconstitution administration details.

CONTRA-INDICATIONS & WARNINGS
Monitor plasma level of factor VIII during treatment. Intravascular haemolysis may occur after large or frequently repeated doses in patients with blood groups A, B or AB (less likely with high potency concentrates).

PREGNANCY/BREAST-FEEDING
Based on the very rare occurrence of haemophilia A in women, experience regarding the use of factor VIII during pregnancy is not available. It should only be used during pregnancy and the breast-feeding period if clearly necessary.

SIDE-EFFECTS
Allergic reactions including chills and fever. Rarely, transient erythema and rash at injection site, chest tightness, dizziness, mild hypotension and nausea. Development of factor VIII inhibitors has been observed, predominantly in previously untreated haemophiliacs. The presence of these antibodies requires specialist advice and clinical management.

POISONING/TOXICITY
Rarely, massive doses of factor VIII concentrates have resulted in acute haemolytic anaemia, increased bleeding tendency or hyperfibrinogenaemia.

PHARMACOKINETIC PROPERTIES
After injection, approximately two-thirds to three-quarters of factor VIII remains in the circulation. The achieved factor VIII activity in the plasma should be between 80-120% of the predicted values. Plasma factor VIII activity probably decreases by a two-phase exponential decay. Initial phase half-life is 3-6 hours. Subsequent phase half-life is 6.5-12 hours in adults. In children the factor VIII half-life is shorter than in adults, necessitating treatment at 8 hourly intervals rather than 12 hourly. Many people now use treatment by continuous infusion after surgery to maintain adequate levels but none of the products are licensed for this method.

EXCIPIENTS
Contact manufacturers for further details.

LICENSED STATUS
Licensed for use in children and adults.

F

Feed thickeners

Starch or cellulose based agents which thicken milk feeds. Speed of action, nutritional content and mode of use vary.

USES
Gastro-oesophageal reflux without complications.
Dumping syndrome (rapid post-prandial gastric emptying).

PRESENTATION
☐ Dry powder/flakes to be added to milk in bottle or to be given as a spoon feed (in water) to breast-fed babies.
☐ Standard infant formula containing a thickener, which works when the feed is in the stomach – Enfamil® AR (see Nutrition tables section page 755).

DOSAGE/ADMINISTRATION
As per manufacturers advice and then adjust to provide an appropriate increase in viscosity.
See Nutrition tables section (page 753-755) of the formulary for individual product dosage/administration details.

CONTRA-INDICATIONS & WARNINGS
Oesophagitis. Gastro-oesophageal reflux related to respiratory problems. Enfamil® AR not to be used for longer than a 6 month period and not to be used in conjunction with any other thickener or antacid product.

PREGNANCY/BREAST-FEEDING
No adverse effect.

LICENSED STATUS
These are not licensed drug products. They are ACBS listed for thickening feeds in the treatment of vomiting/dysphagia.

Fenofibrate

Fibric acid derivative; lipid-modulating agent.

USES
Hyperlipidaemia, including familial hypercholesterolaemia in patients in whom diet therapy and resins have been unsuccessful.

PRESENTATION
Capsule: 67mg, 200mg and 267mg – Lipantil® Micro.

DOSAGE/ ADMINISTRATION
Experience in children is limited; refer to lipidologist.

CONTRA-INDICATIONS & WARNINGS, INTERACTIONS, PREGNANCY, BREAST-FEEDING, SIDE-EFFECTS, POISONING/TOXICITY, PHARMACODYNAMIC PROPERTIES

See bezafibrate monograph.

EXCIPIENTS
See manufacturers SPC for further details.

LICENSED STATUS
Not licensed for use in children.

Fentanyl (controlled drug)

Synthetic opioid analgesic related to pethidine and with similar properties to morphine.

USES
Peri-operative analgesia; analgesia and respiratory depression in assisted ventilation; chronic intractable pain (transdermally). For palliative care, second line major opioid, usually in patients already stabilised on morphine.

PRESENTATION
Injection: (as citrate) 50 microgram in 1mL, 2mL and 10mL ampoule – Sublimaze® and non-proprietary.
Lozenge (with integral oromucosal applicator): (as citrate) 200 microgram, 400 microgram, 600 microgram, 800 microgram, 1.2mg and 1.6mg – Actiq®.
Patches: releasing over 72 hours – 25 microgram per hour, 50 microgram per hour, 75 microgram per hour and 100 microgram per hour – Durogesic®.

DOSAGE

Indication	Route	Age				Frequency	Notes
		birth–1 month	1 month–2 years	2–12 years	12–18 years		
Assisted ventilation or for anaesthesia	IV bolus	← 15 microgram/kg →			300 microgram – 3.5mg	single dose	Initial dose.
to be followed by assisted ventilation		then ← 1–3 microgram/kg →			then 100–200 microgram	single dose	Subsequent doses as necessary.
Spontaneous respiration, ventilator	IV bolus	← 3–5 microgram/kg →			50–200 microgram	single dose	Initial dose.
support should be available		then ← 1 microgram/kg →			then 50 microgram	single dose	Subsequent doses as necessary.
Assisted ventilation on ITU	IV infusion	← 1–3 microgram/kg/hour →			3–6 microgram/ kg/hour	continuous	Infusion rates should be titrated to individual patient response.
Analgesia	Epidural	–	500 nanogram – 1 microgram/kg/hour		–	continuous	Usually given in 0.1% bupivacaine at a concentration of 5 microgram fentanyl in 1mL, at a rate of 0.1–0.2mL/kg/hour.
Pre-medication analgesia	Transmucosal	–	–	← 15-20 → microgram/kg		single dose	For children >10kg. Maximum dose 400 micrograms.
Breakthrough pain	Transmucosal	–	–	← 15-20 → microgram/kg		single dose	For children >10kg. Maximum dose 400 micrograms.

Parenteral fentanyl should only be prescribed/administered by a trained anaesthetist or intensivist. It is not recommended for use outside the operating theatre or intensive care environment. Repeated doses or continuous infusion may result in accumulation, increasing risks of prolonged respiratory depression.

Renal impairment: use smaller doses in moderate renal impairment (increased cerebral sensitivity).
Liver disease: avoid or reduce dose in liver disease (may precipitate coma).

Analgesia and palliative care: transdermal delivery
For selected patients where oral analgesia is not tolerated and parenteral analgesia not appropriate or to provide background analgesia as a supplement to oral/ parenteral analgesia. Fentanyl can cause severe constipation so prophylactic laxatives should always be prescribed.

Oral morphine (mg/24 hours)	30–134mg	135–224mg	225–314mg	315–404mg	405–494mg
Fentanyl patches (microgram/hour)	25	50	75	100	125

Recommended conversion scheme for use in children
Dose titration and maintenance: wait 24 hours before evaluating analgesic effect when starting or changing dose as serum fentanyl concentrations gradually increase over this time. Phase out previous analgesia gradually over this induction period. Where dosage adjustment is required, use 25 microgram/hour increments, re-evaluated every 24–48 hours. Supplement with short-acting analgesia for breakthrough pain during the titration period. Fentanyl patches are replaced every 72 hours to maintain plasma concentrations of fentanyl. More than one patch may be worn at a time to achieve required dose. A new skin site should be used for each new patch and several days should elapse before the same site is used again.
Discontinuation: fentanyl levels decrease gradually after removal of patch without replacement. It may take 17 hours or more to reduce levels to 50%. Replacement analgesia must be introduced gradually, starting with low dose and increasing slowly.

F

Renal failure: the volume of distribution of fentanyl may be altered in patients on dialysis. Observe for signs of fentanyl toxicity. Reduce dose if necessary.
Liver failure: serum concentrations of fentanyl from patches may be higher in hepatic impairment. Observe for signs of fentanyl toxicity. Reduce dose if necessary.

ADMINISTRATION

IV: slow IV injection, diluted with NaCl 0.9% or glucose 5% as desired. If necessary fentanyl can be administered as IV infusion in NaCl 0.9% or glucose 5%. Fentanyl injection is compatible with most agents used in anaesthesia with the exception of thiopental (thiopentone) and methohexitone. IV infusions should be used within 24 hours of preparation.
Transdermal patches: a non-hairy area of skin should be chosen. If cleaning is required use only water. Do not use soaps, oils or lotions. The skin should be completely dry before application. After removal of the protective layer, the patch should be pressed in place with the palm of the hand for 30 seconds, ensuring complete contact, especially around the edges. In palliative care some children have needed to have the patch changed every 48 hours rather than every 72 hours.

CONTRA-INDICATIONS & WARNINGS
Contra-indications: acute respiratory depression, paralytic ileus and phaeochromocytoma.
Warnings: significant respiratory depression will occur following the administration of doses in excess of 200 micrograms. This may persist or recur in the early post-operative period. Significant increase in body temperature may increase delivery rate of fentanyl from patches, resulting in increased plasma levels and possibly shorter duration of action of patch. Avoid exposure of application site to heat packs, hot water bottles, electric blankets and other external heat source.
Cautions: use with caution in raised intracranial pressure or head injury, renal impairment, liver disease and myasthenia gravis; in infants <1 year because of an increased susceptibility to respiratory depression, obstructive airways disease.
In palliative care, fentanyl should always be accompanied by breakthrough doses of a major opioid such as morphine (dose is a fixed proportion of the total daily opioid dose, see monograph).

INTERACTIONS
Enhanced sedative effects with *anxiolytics* and *hypnotics*. Antagonises the gastrointestinal effect of *cisapride, metoclopramide* and *domperidone*. Increased plasma concentration with *cimetidine*.

PREGNANCY
Fentanyl crosses the placenta. If it is used during childbirth it may therefore reduce neonatal respiration. Contact local Medicines Information Centre for advice.

BREAST-FEEDING
Fentanyl is excreted into breast milk. manufacturers recommend that breast-feeding should not start within 24 hours of treatment.

SIDE-EFFECTS
Nausea, constipation, respiratory depression, hypotension. May cause chest wall or jaw muscle rigidity if given without muscle relaxants. When fentanyl is used with a neuroleptic, chills and/or shivering, restlessness, post-operative hallucinatory episodes and extra-pyramidal symptoms may occur. Local reactions such as rash, erythema and itching have been reported following the use of patches.

POISONING/TOXICITY
Symptoms of toxicity include respiratory depression, which can be reversed using *naloxone*, muscle rigidity (treated by administration of IV neuromuscular blocking agent), and hypotension.

PHARMACOKINETIC PROPERTIES
Fentanyl is short acting after a single dose but has a relatively long elimination half-life because of rapid redistribution followed by slower release from tissue deposits. It is metabolised by the liver. Metabolites and some unchanged drug are excreted mainly in the urine. Fentanyl is 80% bound to plasma proteins.

EXCIPIENTS
Patches – the drug reservoir contains ethyl alcohol and hydroxyethylcellulose; the adhesive is silicone medical adhesive. See manufacturers SPC for further details.

LICENSED STATUS
Injections licensed for use in children and adults. Lozenges and patches not licensed for use in children.

Local anaesthetic-type antiarrhythmic compound (Class Ic antiarrhythmic).

USES
Treatment of resistant re-entry supraventricular tachycardia (especially AV nodal reciprocating tachycardia or accessory pathway); treatment of ventricular ectopics or ventricular tachycardia, arrhythmias associated with Wolff-Parkinson-White syndrome, paroxysmal atrial fibrillation in patients with disabling symptoms, especially in cases resistant to other therapies.

PRESENTATION
Tablet: 50mg and 100mg (scored) – Tambocor®; 50mg and 100mg – non-proprietary.
Oral liquid: 25mg in 5mL – named patient.
Injection: 10mg in 1mL, 15mL ampoule – Tambocor®.

DOSAGE
Flecainide should only be used under the direct supervision of a paediatric cardiologist.

Route	Age			Frequency	Notes
	Birth-1 month	1 month-2 years	2-12 years	(times daily)	
Oral	←	4mg/kg	→	single dose	Loading dose.
	←	2mg/kg	→	2-3	Maintenance dose.
IV bolus	←	2mg/kg	→	single dose	Give over at least 10 minutes with ECG monitoring.
IV infusion	←	100–250 microgram/kg/hour	→	continuous infusion	Stop when arrhythmia is controlled.

Route	Age	Frequency	Notes
	12-18 years	(times daily)	
Oral	supraventricular arrhythmias 50mg	2	May be increased to a maximum of 300mg **daily** if required.
	ventricular arrhythmias 100mg	2	Maximum **daily** dose 400mg, reserved for patients where rapid control is required.
IV bolus	2mg/kg (maximum dose 150mg)	single dose	Give over at least 10 minutes, with ECG monitoring.
IV infusion	Initiate therapy as for IV bolus, then continue at the rates: First hour: 1.5mg/kg/hour Second and later hours: 100–250 microgram/kg/hour	continuous	It is not recommended that the infusion duration exceeds 24 hours but if this is considered necessary plasma level monitoring should be carried out. The maximum cumulative dose given in the first 24 hours should not exceed 600mg.

Renal impairment
Reduce dose and monitor plasma levels. In severe impairment (creatinine clearance <35mL/minute/1.73m^2) dose reductions of 25-50% may be required.
Hepatic impairment
Do not use in patients with significant hepatic impairment unless benefits clearly outweigh risks. Plasma level monitoring is strongly recommended.

F

ADMINISTRATION
Oral: do not crush or dissolve in water. Liquid formulations may have a local anaesthetic effect.
IV: ECG monitoring is recommended. Bolus doses must be given over at least 10 minutes. The dose may be diluted and given as a mini-infusion over 30 minutes. Dilute with glucose 5%. Do not use NaCl 0.9%. When necessary, continuous IV infusion may be employed for the minimum required time period. Plasma level monitoring is strongly recommended. Transition to oral therapy should be accomplished as soon as possible. Do not mix with any other drugs, phosphates, alkaline solutions or sodium-containing products (including NaCl 0.9%, which may cause precipitation).

CONTRA-INDICATIONS & WARNINGS

Contra-indications: cardiac failure; patients with long-standing atrial fibrillation and in patients with haemodynamically significant valvular disease; patients with sinus node dysfunction, atrial conduction defects, second degree or greater AV block, bundle branch block or distal block, unless pacing rescue is available.

Warnings: correct electrolyte disturbances before use. Do not use if significant hepatic impairment unless benefits outweigh risks. Monitor plasma levels. Flecainide can increase endocardial pacing thresholds. Use with caution in patients with pacemakers or pacing electrodes. Do not administer to patients with poor thresholds or non-programmable pacemakers unless pacing rescue is available. Flecainide has a minor negative inotropic effect which may assume importance in patients predisposed to cardiac failure. Use with caution in patients with acute onset of atrial fibrillation following cardiac surgery.

INTERACTIONS

Digoxin levels may increase slightly when given concurrently with flecainide; no specific action required but be alert for evidence of the interaction by monitoring levels. Additive negative inotropic effects may be observed with *beta-blockers and other cardiac depressants*. *Cimetidine* may cause an increase of 30% in plasma flecainide levels and prolong half-life by 10%. When given with *amiodarone*, the usual flecainide dosage should be reduced by 50%. Plasma level monitoring is recommended. When *propranolol* and flecainide are given concurrently, plasma levels of both drugs are increased, patients should be monitored for increased effects of both drugs and additive negative inotropic effects on the heart. *Phenytoin, phenobarbital (phenobarbitone)* and *carbamazepine* may reduce flecainide levels.

PREGNANCY

manufacturers have no evidence regarding drug safety in human pregnancy. Flecainide crosses the placenta to the fetus. Contact local Medicines Information Centre for further advice.

BREAST-FEEDING

Flecainide is excreted in human milk and appears in concentrations which reflect those in maternal blood. The risk to the nursing infant is minimal. The American Academy of Pediatrics considers flecainide to be compatible with breast-feeding.

SIDE-EFFECTS

Cardiac: pro-arrhythmic effects may occur most commonly in patients with structural heart disease and/or significant ventricular impairment. In patients with atrial flutter the use of flecainide has been associated with 1:1 AV conduction following initial atrial slowing with resultant ventricular acceleration.

Dermatological: isolated cases of photosensitivity, allergic skin reactions.

Gastrointestinal: occasionally nausea and vomiting.

Hepatic: a number of cases of reversible jaundice and elevated liver enzymes have been reported.

Neurological: transient dizziness and light-headedness.

Ophthalmological: transient visual disturbances.

Other: during long-term use peripheral neuropathy and ataxia have been reported. Rare cases of corneal deposits and pneumonitis reported.

POISONING/TOXICITY

Even therapeutic doses may induce or aggravate arrhythmias. In cases of overdose cardiac features predominate with delayed conduction through the myocardium and depression of myocardial contractility. Bradycardia and tachycardia have been reported. Other features include ECG abnormalities, hypoxia, metabolic acidosis, hypotension and convulsions. No specific antidote is known. Forced acid diuresis may be useful. Treatment may include therapy with an inotropic agent, IV calcium, circulatory assistance, intubation and ventilation or temporary pacing.

PHARMACOKINETIC PROPERTIES

Flecainide is rapidly and almost completely absorbed from the gastrointestinal tract following oral administration. Oral bioavailability is 90-100%. Flecainide is metabolised extensively most probably in the liver to two major metabolites. Both metabolites undergo extensive conjugation and are not considered to be pharmacologically active. Flecainide and its metabolites are excreted largely in urine with 25% of dose as unchanged drug. Plasma protein binding is approximately 40%. Median terminal half-life is 7.5 hours in paediatric patients following IV administration of flecainide and 7.9 hours following oral administration has been reported. The half-life in infants <1 year old is approximately 11-12 hours and 8 hours in children aged 1-12 years. Plasma flecainide concentrations of 200-800 microgram/L appear to be effective. Oral trough levels may be measured after 2-4 days.

EXCIPIENTS

Contact manufacturers for further details.

LICENSED STATUS

Licensed for ≥12 years of age.

FURTHER INFORMATION

The oral liquid is available from Penn Pharmaceuticals Ltd.

Antibacterial.

USES
Treatment of infections due to Gram-positive organisms, including beta-lactamase producing staphylococci.
In cystic fibrosis patients – continuous anti-staphylococcal therapy, treatment of asymptomatic *Staphylococcus aureus* isolates or minor exacerbations and IV treatment of more severe exacerbations caused by *Staphylococcus aureus*.

PRESENTATION
Capsule: 250mg and 500mg – Floxapen® and non-proprietary.
Injection: (sodium salt) 250mg, 500mg and 1g – Floxapen® and non-proprietary.
Oral solution: 125mg in 5mL – non-proprietary.
Syrup: 125mg in 5mL and 250mg in 5mL – Floxapen®.

DOSAGE
Newborn infant (birth to 1 month)

Route	Age	Dosage	Frequency (times daily)	Notes
IV/oral	<7 days	25–50mg/kg	2	Dose may be increased to 100mg/kg/dose IV in severe infection (meningitis, cerebral abscess, staphylococcal osteitis). Oral route only recommended for minor infection.
	7–21 days	25–50mg/kg	3	
	>21 days	25–50mg/kg	4	

Child

Route	Age			Frequency (times daily)	Notes
	1 month–2 years	2–12 years	12–18 years		
IV or IM bolus	←	12.5mg–25mg/kg	→	4	Maximum single dose 1g. Dose may be doubled in severe infection, maximum single dose 2g.
Oral	<1 year 62.5mg >1 year -125mg	<5 years 125mg >5 years 250mg	250mg	4 / 4	Doses may be doubled in severe infection.
Oral for cystic fibrosis patients	←	16–33mg/kg	→ / 1g	4	Continuous anti-staphylococcal therapy. To aid compliance usually given in two divided doses but ideally given four times daily.
	←	12.5–25mg/kg	→	4	Treatment of asymptomatic S. aureus isolates or minor exacerbations. Maximum single dose of 1g. Daily dose can be given in three divided doses if necessary.

In renal failure: if creatinine clearance is less than 10mL/minute/1.73m^2, increase the dosage interval to 8 hourly.

ADMINISTRATION
Oral: give at least 30 minutes before food. The powder can be shaken out of the capsule, for patients allergic to colours and preservatives. The syrup can be diluted with Syrup BP.
IM/IV: on reconstitution 250mg displaces 0.2mL. IM injection – add 1.3mL Water for Injections to 250mg vial to give 250mg in 1.5mL and 1.6mL to 500mg vial to give 500mg in 2mL. IV bolus – dilute reconstituted dose to 5-10mL with Water for Injections and give over 3-5 minutes. Do not mix with aminoglycosides; do not administer through the same line without adequate flushing in-between.

F

CONTRA-INDICATIONS & WARNINGS
Penicillin hypersensitivity.

INTERACTIONS
With *warfarin* prothrombin time may be increased.

PREGNANCY
No known teratogenic effects. Contact local Medicines Information Centre for advice.

BREAST-FEEDING
Trace quantities can be detected in breast milk. Contact local Medicines Information Centre for advice.

SIDE-EFFECTS
Gastrointestinal effects, particularly at high oral doses. Skin rash; treatment should be discontinued. Hepatitis and cholestatic jaundice; may occur up to several weeks after stopping treatment. Pseudomembranous colitis has been reported rarely in combination with other antibiotics.

POISONING/TOXICITY
Problems of overdosage are unlikely to occur; if encountered they may be treated symptomatically.

PHARMACOKINETIC PROPERTIES
Flucloxacillin is well absorbed from the gastrointestinal tract but absorption is reduced by the presence of food in the stomach. It is metabolised to a limited extent and excreted renally, mainly as unchanged drug.

EXCIPIENTS
Injection includes 2.26mmol of sodium in each 1g of powder.
Syrup includes sucrose. Contact manufacturers for further details.

LICENSED STATUS
Licensed for use in all ages.

Fluconazole

Triazole antifungal.

USES
Antifungal agent used in the treatment of susceptible localised and systemic fungal infections and in the prophylaxis of such infections in immunocompromised patients. Resistant strains of *Candida* and *Cryptococcus* are recognised.

PRESENTATION
Capsule: 50mg, 150mg and 200mg – Diflucan®.
Oral suspension: 50mg in 5mL and 200mg in 5mL – Diflucan®.
IV infusion: 2mg in 1mL in NaCl 0.9%; 25mL and 100mL bottle – Diflucan®.

DOSAGE
Newborn infant

Route	Age	Dose	Frequency	Notes
Oral/IV	<14 days	6–12mg/kg	every 72 hours	Systemic candidiasis and cryptococcal infection. Dose
	14–28 days	6–12mg/kg	every 48 hours	can be reduced to 3mg/kg with the same dosage
	>28 days	6–12mg/kg	every 24 hours	intervals to treat mucosal candidiasis. Well absorbed
				orally when gastrointestinal function is adequate.

Child

Route	Age			Frequency	Notes
	1 month–2 years	2–12 years	12–18 years	(times daily)	
Oral/IV	←	6mg/kg	→	single dose	Loading dose.
	←	then 3mg/kg	→	1	Mucosal candidiasis for 7-14 days.
	←	6–12mg/kg	→	1	Systemic candidiasis and cryptococcal infection; dose depends on severity. Maximum dose 400mg.
	←	3–12mg/kg	→	1	Prevention of fungal infection in immunocompromised patients; dose depends on extent and duration of neutropenia. Maximum dose 400mg.

Renal impairment – reduce dose in renal impairment
Give normal dose on day 1 to achieve levels then:

Creatinine clearance (mL/minute/1.73m²)	Dosage/dose frequency adjustment
11–50	Reduce dose by 50% or give normal dose every 48 hours.
<10	Reduce to one third of the normal dose or give normal dose every 72 hours.

ADMINISTRATION
IV: give as an IV infusion over 10-30 minutes.
Compatible with Ringer's solution, Hartmann's solution, sodium bicarbonate 4.2%, NaCl 0.9% or glucose solutions.

CONTRA-INDICATIONS & WARNINGS
Contra-indicated in known hypersensitivity to azole compounds. In some patients, particularly those with underlying serious diseases, such as HIV or malignancies, hepatic, renal, haematological and biochemical abnormalities may be exaggerated. Patients with AIDS are considered at higher risk of developing severe cutaneous reactions. Co-administration of *cisapride* or *terfenadine* contra-indicated.

INTERACTIONS
Fluconazole enhances effects or plasma levels of *warfarin, sulphonylureas, phenytoin, theophylline, zidovudine* and *rifabutin*. Potential increase in levels of *midazolam* and *ciclosporin (cyclosporin)* but less clear.
Plasma levels measured where appropriate. Plasma concentration of fluconazole reduced by *rifampicin*; 25% decrease in AUC and 20% shorter half-life. Consider dose increase.
Hydrochlorothiazide may increase plasma fluconazole concentration by up to 40%.
Due to potentially serious interactions with *terfenadine* and *cisapride* leading to significantly increased levels of these drugs and an increased risk of various cardiac adverse events, fluconazole combination with either of these drugs is contra-indicated.

PREGNANCY
Little experience and theoretical risk due to potential inhibition of oestrogen synthesis, particularly at high doses. Avoid use.

BREAST-FEEDING
Passes into breast milk achieving similar or higher levels to those in plasma. Dose transferred to average suckling infant estimated as 0.27-0.44mg/kg/day.
Although caution is advisable this is a small dose compared to therapeutic doses which are considered well tolerated in neonates. Changes in gut flora may occur.

SIDE-EFFECTS
Gastrointestinal: nausea, diarrhoea and flatulence. Headache, skin rashes, seizures, leucopenia rarely reported. Toxic epidermal necrolysis and Stevens-Johnson syndrome reported rarely. Occasional abnormalities in liver enzymes, usually mild and transient, reported in 5-7% of patients. Higher increases reported in 1% of patients. Eosinophilia, anaemia, thrombocytopenia rarely reported. Hypokalaemia has been reported (see warnings section).

POISONING/TOXICITY
Supportive measures and symptomatic treatment should be adequate. Removed by haemodialysis.

PHARMACOKINETIC PROPERTIES
Rapidly and almost completely absorbed from the gastrointestinal tract Oral bioavailability exceeds 90%. Peak plasma concentration attained in 1-2 hours after oral dose. Widely distributed into body tissues and fluids, including CSF, attaining concentrations similar to or higher than plasma concentration.
Eliminated principally by renal excretion with a half-life ranging from 15-25 hours in children. This is prolonged in renal impairment and in neonates, ranging from 24-88 hours, depending on gestation and post-natal age.

EXCIPIENTS
Oral suspension includes sucrose. See manufacturers SPC for further details.

LICENSED STATUS
Licensed for use in patients of all ages.

F

Flucytosine

Competitive inhibitor of uracil metabolism. Interferes with protein synthesis and may impair fungal DNA synthesis.

USES
Systemic yeast and fungal infections, monotherapy generally not recommended due to risk of resistance emerging.

Adjunct to amphotericin in systemic candidiasis or other severe infections; adjunct to amphotericin or fluconazole in cryptococcal meningitis. Aspergillus generally resistant but other fungal or yeast species may be sensitive particularly *Torulopsis glabrata* and *Hansenula*.

PRESENTATION
Tablet: 500mg – named patient.
Suspension: may be extemporaneously prepared.
IV infusion: 10mg in 1mL, 250ml infusion bottle – Ancotil®.

DOSAGE
Newborn infant (birth to 1 month)

Route	Age		Frequency	Notes
	Up to 7 days	Over 7 days	(times daily)	
Oral/IV	25mg/kg	–	4	Reduced dose frequency is likely to be necessary in very
	–	25-50mg/kg	4	low birth weight infants when plasma levels known.

Child

Route	Age			Frequency	Notes
	1 month-2 years	2-12 years	12-18 years	(times daily)	
Oral/IV	←	50mg/kg	→	4	
	←	25–35mg/kg	→	4	Dose if organism known to be extremely sensitive to reduce potential toxicity.

Dose reduction in renal impairment

Creatinine clearance (mL/minute/1.73m^2)	Dosage/dose frequency adjustment
20–40	Give usual dose twice daily.
10–20	Give usual dose once daily.
<10	Give single dose of 50mg/kg and adjust following serum concentration monitoring.

ADMINISTRATION
IV: administer as an IV infusion over 20-40 minutes through a 15 micron filter to remove potential particulate contamination. Compatible with glucose 5%, glucose 10% and NaCl 0.9%.

CONTRA-INDICATIONS & WARNINGS
Hypersensitivity to flucytosine or any excipients. Monitoring of blood count and liver enzymes advisable before and during therapy. Use with particular care in patients with pre-existing bone marrow depression.

INTERACTIONS
Cytarabine may reduce plasma flucytosine concentrations; plasma concentration monitoring advisable.

PREGNANCY
Teratogenic in rats but this effect may be species specific due to metabolism. Little human data – weigh potential benefit against hazards. A small proportion (<5%) may be metabolised to fluorouracil, a known teratogen in humans. Isolated reports of use in second or third trimester with no apparent harm. Contact local Medicines Information Centre for advice.

BREAST-FEEDING
No data available. Contact local Medicines Information Centre for advice.

SIDE-EFFECTS
Nausea, vomiting, diarrhoea and skin rash. Rarely, confusion, hallucinations, convulsions, sedation and headache. Generally, reversible elevations of liver enzymes have been reported although hepatitis and hepatic necrosis have occurred. Bone marrow depression with leucopenia, thrombocytopenia, agranulocytosis or aplastic anaemia has occurred, generally when plasma levels are high in renal impaired patients treated concurrently with *amphotericin*.
Other adverse effects: pyrexia, hypoglycaemia, hypokalaemia, muscle weakness, cardiac arrest and respiratory arrest. Side-effects more likely if serum level >100 microgram/mL.

F

POISONING/TOXICITY
Maintain adequate fluid intake. Removed by haemodialysis. Monitor for gastrointestinal haemorrhage, haematological and hepatic effects.

PHARMACOKINETIC PROPERTIES
Well absorbed from gastrointestinal tract with around 75-90% of a dose being absorbed. Widely distributed in body tissues and fluids, including CSF, reaching similar levels to plasma. Minimally bound to plasma proteins (2-4%). Minimal amounts metabolised in humans. About 90% of a dose is renally excreted as unchanged drug. Elimination half-life 2-6 hours increased in renal impairment, slightly prolonged to 4-8 hours in neonates. Steady state blood levels of 25-50 microgram/mL are normally effective. It is recommended that blood levels are monitored. Measure serum concentration after 48-72 hours. Peak and trough measurements are ideal but peak alone may be sufficient.
Therapeutic concentration: 60-80 microgram/mL measured 1 hour after start of IV infusion or 2 hours after an oral dose (peak). 30-40 microgram/mL measured immediately before a dose (trough). Do not exceed a peak of 80 microgram/mL. It is recommended that steady state serum concentrations should be >25 microgram/mL to avoid resistant strains emerging.

EXCIPIENTS
IV infusion contains 34.5mmol of Na^+ in 250mL. Contact manufacturers for further details.

LICENSED STATUS
IV infusion licensed for children and adults; unlicensed in neonates. Tablets are not licensed for use in the UK.

FURTHER INFORMATION
Tablets are available from Bell and Croyden.
If IV infusion stored below 18°C, precipitation may occur which should be redissolved by heating to 80°C for not more than 30 minutes. Prolonged storage above 25°C could lead to decomposition, resulting in the formation of 5-fluorouracil.

Fludarabine phosphate

Purine analogue. Inhibits DNA synthesis and repair by inhibition of ribonucleotide reductase and DNA polymerase.

USES
Poor prognosis/relapsed acute myeloid and relapsed acute lymphoblastic leukaemia. Conditioning prior to bone marrow transplantation.

PRESENTATION
Injection: powder for reconstitution, 50mg – Fludara®.
Tablet: 10mg (film-coated) – Fludara®.

DOSAGE
** Always consult the current treatment protocol for details of dosage and scheduling. **

ADMINISTRATION
IV: reconstitute the contents of a vial with 2mL Water for Injections to give 25mg in 1mL. Dilute the reconstituted solution to 100-125mL with NaCl 0.9% or glucose 5%. Infuse IV over 30 minutes. May also be given by IV bolus in 10mL NaCl 0.9%.
Oral: swallow whole with water. Do not chew or break.

F

CONTRA-INDICATIONS & WARNINGS
Contra-indications: should not be given to anyone with known hypersensitivity to the drug. Should not be given to patients with creatinine clearance of <30mL/minute. Fludarabine is also contra-indicated during pregnancy and lactation.
Precautions: when used at high doses fludarabine has been associated with severe neurologic effects, including blindness, coma and death. Patients should be closely observed for signs of neurologic side-effects. Use with caution in hepatic impairment. If creatinine clearance is between 30-70 mL/minute, the dose should be reduced by up to 50% and close haematological monitoring should be used to assess toxicity. Transfusion-associated graft-versus-host disease has been observed after transfusion of non-irradiated blood. Patients who require blood transfusion and who are undergoing, or who have received, treatment with

fludarabine should receive irradiated blood only. Tumour lysis syndrome may occur in patients with high tumour burden therefore adequate precautions should be taken to prevent this. *Warnings:* monitor patients for signs of autoimmune haemolytic anaemia.

INTERACTIONS
Do not use fludarabine with *pentostatin (deoxycoformycin)* as fatal pulmonary toxicity can result. Do not administer with *dipyridamole* or other *inhibitors of adenosine* uptake as therapeutic efficacy of fludarabine is reduced.

PREGNANCY
Fludarabine should not be administered to women who are, or who are likely to become pregnant.

BREAST-FEEDING
It is not known whether fludarabine is excreted in breast milk, therefore breast-feeding should be discontinued during therapy.

SIDE-EFFECTS
Body as a whole: infection, fever, fatigue, weakness, malaise, and chills have been commonly reported. *Haematological:* neutropenia, thrombocytopenia and anaemia have been reported in the majority of patients. Myelosuppression may be severe and cumulative. Autoimmune haemolytic anaemia, autoimmune thrombocytopenia, thrombocytopenic purpura, pemphigus, Evans syndrome have all been reported. Patients must be monitored closely for signs of haemolysis. *Neurological:* peripheral neuropathy has been commonly observed. Confusion is uncommon. Coma and agitation occur rarely. Visual disturbances are commonly reported. In rare cases, optic neuritis, optic neuropathy and blindness have occurred. *Gastrointestinal:* nausea and vomiting, diarrhoea, stomatitis, and anorexia are common events. Gastrointestinal bleeding, mainly related to thrombocytopenia has been reported. *Other:* tumour lysis syndrome has been reported. This complication may include hyperuricaemia, hyperphosphataemia, hypocalcaemia, metabolic acidosis, hyperkalaemia, haematuria, urate crystalluria, and renal failure. The onset of this syndrome may be heralded by flank pain and haematuria. Skin rashes are common.

POISONING/TOXICITY
High doses have been associated with irreversible CNS toxicity characterised by delayed blindness, coma and death and also with severe thrombocytopenia and neutropenia due to bone marrow suppression. There is no known antidote for fludarabine overdosage and treatment consists of drug discontinuation and supportive therapy.

PHARMACOKINETIC PROPERTIES
Peak levels are achieved immediately following IV infusion. Post maximum levels decay in three disposition phases with an initial half-life of approximately 5 minutes, an intermediate half-life of 1-2 hours and a terminal half-life of approximately 20 hours. Metabolised intracellularly with 40-60% eliminated by the kidneys within 24 hours. After oral dosing, bioavailability is 50-65% with peak plasma levels occurring 1-2 hours post-dose. Taking with food increases absorption.

EXCIPIENTS
See manufacturers SPC for further details.

LICENSED STATUS
Licensed for use in adults for chronic lymphocytic leukaemia only. Not licensed for use in children.

FURTHER INFORMATION
Non-vesicant. 25mg/m^2 IV is equivalent to 40mg/m^2 orally.

F

Fludrocortisone acetate

Mineralocorticoid.

USES
Mineralocorticoid replacement in salt wasting adrenocortical insufficiency, congenital adrenal hyperplasia and sweat test.

PRESENTATION
Tablet: (scored) 100 microgram – Florinef®.
Capsule: 1mg and 5mg – manufactured 'specials'.
Liquid: may be extemporaneously prepared.

DOSAGE

Indication	Route	Age				Frequency (times daily)	Notes
		birth–1 month	1 month–2 years	2–12 years	12–18 years		
Adrenal insufficiency	Oral	←	50-200 microgram		→	1	Replacement therapy. Adjust according to response.
Sweat test	Oral	←	3mg/m²		→	1	Two doses given on consecutive days prior to sweat test.

ADMINISTRATION

Oral: capsules may be opened and the contents sprinkled on jam or a small quantity of food; tablets may be crushed.

CONTRA-INDICATIONS & WARNINGS

No contra-indications for short-term use for sweat test. Use is contra-indicated in patients with systemic infection, unless specific anti-infective therapy is used. Also contra-indicated in patients vaccinated with live vaccines. Periodic checking of serum electrolyte levels is advised during prolonged therapy. Glucocorticoid side-effects may occur (see prednisolone monograph) but can be reduced by reducing the dosage. Suppression of the inflammatory response and immune function increases the susceptibility to infections and their severity. Caution is necessary when using corticosteroids in patients with any of the following conditions: X-ray indicative or history of tuberculosis, hypertension, congestive cardiac failure, hepatic or renal failure, diabetes mellitus, epilepsy. Growth and development of children on prolonged therapy should be monitored.

INTERACTIONS

Drugs which induce liver enzymes (such as *rifampicin, rifabutin, carbamazepine, phenobarbital (phenobarbitone), phenytoin, aminoglutethimide)* will increase the metabolism of corticosteroids and may decrease their effects. Corticosteroids antagonise the effects of *hypoglycaemic agents* (including *insulin), antihypertensives* and *diuretics.* The hypokalaemic effects of *acetazolamide, loop diuretics* and *thiazide diuretics* are enhanced.

PREGNANCY

Administration of corticosteroids to pregnant animals can cause abnormalities of fetal development including cleft palate/lip and effects on brain growth and development. However, in humans there is no convincing evidence that systemic corticosteroids cause an increased incidence of congenital abnormalities, such as cleft palate or lip. There is a theoretical risk of adrenal suppression in the neonate following pre-natal corticosteroid exposure. However, this usually resolves spontaneously after birth and is rarely clinically important.

BREAST-FEEDING

Corticosteroids are found in breast milk. Contact local Medicines Information Centre for advice.

SIDE-EFFECTS

Hypertension, potassium loss, sodium and water retention. Minimal with the two doses used for sweat test.

POISONING/TOXICITY

Monitor serum electrolyte levels. Contact National Poisons Information Centre for advice.

PHARMACOKINETIC PROPERTIES

Oral administration is followed by rapid and complete absorption.

EXCIPIENTS

Contact manufacturers for further details.

LICENSED STATUS

Florinef® tablets licensed for replacement therapy in all ages; but not licensed for sweat test. Capsules are a 'special' and as such are unlicensed.

FURTHER INFORMATION

Capsules available from Mandeville Medicines.

Flumazenil

Flumazenil is a specific competitive inhibitor of substances which act via the benzodiazepine receptors, specifically blocking their central effects.

USES
Reversal of acute benzodiazepine overdosage. Should not be used to diagnose benzopdiazepine overdosage.

PRESENTATION
Injection: 500 microgram in 5ml – Anexate®.

DOSAGE

Route	Age				Frequency (times daily)	Notes
	birth–1 month	1 month–2 years	2–12 years	12–18 years		
IV bolus over 15 seconds	10 microgram/kg	10 microgram/kg (maximum of 200 microgram dose)		200 microgram dose	single dose	Initial dose. If the desired effect is not achieved – repeat at 1 minute intervals to a maximum total dose of 40 microgram/kg (2mg dose).
IV infusion	← 2–10 microgram/kg/hour → (maximum of 400 microgram dose per hour)			100–400 microgram dose per hour	continuous	This should be individually adjusted to achieve the desired level of arousal.

There is limited experience of the use of flumazenil in children.

WARNING
1. The duration of action of flumazenil is much shorter than the half-life of the benzodiazepines commonly encountered in overdosage. Patients must therefore be kept under observation for a few hours in case toxicity recurs.
2. Flumazenil may precipitate:
   □ withdrawl syndrome in benzodiazepine-dependent patients
   □ convulsions in epileptics
   □ arrhythmias in patients who have taken cardiotoxic drugs.
3. Do NOT give flumazenil for combined tricyclic antidepressant and benzodiazepine overdosage as convulsions and cardiac arrest may be precipitated.

Hepatic/renal impairment
Flumazenil is extensively metabolised in the liver, therefore careful titration of the dose is necessary in hepatic failure. The initial dose remains the same but subsequent doses should be reduced in size or frequency. No dosage adjustments are necessary in renal impairment.

ADMINISTRATION
IV: initial dose is administered IV over 15 seconds. This may be repeated after 1 minute if desired level of consciousness is not obtained. Flumazenil may be diluted with glucose 5% or NaCl 0.9%.

F

CONTRA-INDICATIONS & WARNINGS
See warning above. Contra-indicated in patients who have been given a benzodiazepine for control of a life threatening condition. Use is not recommended in epileptic patients who have been receiving benzodiazepine treatment for a prolonged period. Use with caution in patients with head injury.

INTERACTIONS
The effects of non-benzodiazepines acting via the benzodiazepine receptor (e.g. zopiclone) are blocked by flumazenil.

PREGNANCY
Flumazenil should only be given in pregnancy when considered absolutely necessary. It is expected to cross the placenta although the total quantity would be small. Animal studies have shown no teratogenic potential.

BREAST-FEEDING
Emergency use of flumazenil during lactation is not contra-indicated.

SIDE-EFFECTS
Generally well tolerated. Nausea and vomiting are the most common adverse effects and dizziness is a common CNS effect. Rare reports of seizures, especially in epileptics. Benzodiazepine withdrawal symptoms may be experienced in patients who have received benzodiazepines for long periods. In mixed overdose, administration of flumazenil

may unmask adverse effects of other psychotropic drugs. Cardiac arrhythmias are reported rarely.

PHARMACOKINETIC PROPERTIES
Following IV administration flumazenil is extensively metabolised in the liver to the carboxylic acid form. Excretion is predominantly in the urine. The elimination half-life is 40-80 minutes. In patients with impaired hepatic function the clearance of flumazenil is decreased and there is a prolonged half-life.

LICENSED STATUS
Not licensed for use in children.

Flumetasone (flumethasone) and Clioquinol

USES
Anti-inflammatory where secondary infection suspected. Otorrhoea.

PRESENTATION
Ear drops: flumetasone pivalate 0.02% and clioquinol 1%, 7.5mL – Locorten-Vioform®.

DOSAGE

Route	Age		Frequency (times daily)	Notes
	2–12 years	12–18 years		
Locally into the ear	← 2–3 drops →		2	For 7–10 days.

CONTRA-INDICATIONS & WARNINGS
Hypersensitivity to any ingredient or iodine. Primary outer ear infections. Perforation of tympanic membrane. Children <2 years of age.

PREGNANCY
There is inadequate evidence of safety in human pregnancy.

BREAST-FEEDING
It is not known if the active substances or their metabolites pass into breast milk.

SIDE-EFFECTS
Local irritation or burning. Hair discolouration. Adrenal suppression in long-term therapy.

POISONING/TOXICITY
If accidental ingestion of large quantities occurs, symptomatic treatment should be administered as appropriate.

EXCIPIENTS
Polyethylene glycol.

LICENSED STATUS
Licensed for use in ≥2 years of age.

FURTHER INFORMATION
For reasons of hygiene do not use bottle for more than 28 days after first opening it.

Flunarizine

A calcium antagonist.

USES
Migraine prophylaxis.

PRESENTATION
Capsule: 5mg – named patient Sibelium® (imported).
Tablets: 10mg – named patient Sibelium® (imported).

F

DOSAGE
Child

Indication	Route	Age		Frequency (times daily)	Notes
		2–12 years	12–18 years		
Migraine prophylaxis	Oral	≥ 3 years 5mg	10mg	1	

Dose reduction is required in liver impairment.

CONTRA-INDICATIONS & WARNINGS
Use with caution in depressed patients and hepatic impairment.

INTERACTIONS
Avoid co-administration of other *calcium-channel blockers* and *amiodarone* – risk of sinus arrest and atrioventricular block. Prolonged bradycardia may occur with *adenosine*. Enhancement of neuro-muscular blockade with *non-depolarising agents*. Potentiation of central effects of *sedatives, hypnotics, antihistamines*.

PREGNANCY
Safety not established but caution advised in first 6 months of pregnancy.

BREAST-FEEDING
From animal studies concentration in breast milk is higher than plasma. No data on human breast milk but breast-feeding not recommended.

SIDE-EFFECTS
The most commonly occurring are drowsiness, headache, insomnia, asthenia, depression and increased appetite which may lead to increase in body weight. Serious extrapyramidal reactions have occurred mainly in elderly patients. Heartburn, nausea, dry mouth and gastralgia are less common.

POISONING/TOXICITY
Symptoms of overdosage may include sedation, agitation and tachycardia. No specific antidote recommended.

PHARMACOKINETIC PROPERTIES
Absorption is rapid and nearly complete (>95%). Peak plasma levels at 2-4 hours. Metabolised with a long half-life of 18 days. 99% bound but with a large volume of distribution, mean 43L/kg. These are all adult values.

EXCIPIENTS
Contact manufacturer for further details.

LICENSED STATUS
Not licensed for use in the UK.

FURTHER INFORMATION
Available from IDIS World Medicines.

Flunisolide

Synthetic corticosteroid.

USES
Prophylaxis and treatment of perennial and seasonal allergic rhinitis including hay fever.

PRESENTATION
Aqueous nasal spray: 25 microgram per metered spray – Syntaris®.

DOSAGE/ADMINISTRATION

Route	Age		Frequency (times daily)	Notes
	2–12 years	12–18 years		
Intra–nasal	≥ 5 years 1 spray (each nostril)	12–14 years 1 spray (each nostril)	up to 3	Once the desired clinical effect is obtained, the maintenance dose should be the smallest amount necessary to control symptoms. For some patients this may be as low as 1 spray to each nostril per day.
		>14 years 2 sprays (each nostril)	2-3	

Continuous treatment in children 5-10 years should be limited to 4 weeks.

CONTRA-INDICATIONS & WARNINGS
Untreated fungal, bacterial or viral infection of nose or eyes. Hypersensitivity to any ingredient.

PREGNANCY
Not recommended in the first trimester of pregnancy. It may be used in the second or third trimester if considered essential.

BREAST-FEEDING
Contact local Medicines Information Centre for advice.

SIDE-EFFECTS
After-taste and mild, transient nasal burning and stinging, nasal dryness, epistaxis, runny and stuffy nose.

Adrenal suppression, secondary infection and nasal mucosal atrophy in prolonged use.

POISONING/TOXICITY
Administration of large amounts over a short period may produce suppression of hypothalamic-pituitary-adrenal function. In such an event reduce to the recommended dosage immediately.

PHARMACOKINETIC PROPERTIES
After intra-nasal administration (of 100 micrograms approximately) extremely low plasma levels were detected within 10-30 minutes of dosing and these fell to undetectable levels within 4 hours.

EXCIPIENTS
Include benzalkonium chloride, butylated hydroxytoluene, disodium edetate, polysorbates and propylene glycol.

LICENSED STATUS
Licensed for use in ≥5 years of age.

FURTHER INFORMATION
For reasons of hygiene do not use bottle for more than 28 days after first opening it.
Syntaris® (prescription only medicine – except maximum pack size of 240 doses which can be sold 'over the counter' for use in patients >12 years old for seasonal allergic rhinitis).

Fluoride (sodium fluoride, stannous fluoride)

Fluoride ions are thought to exert their caries preventive effect by a variety of means: alteration in tooth morphology, reduction in enamel solubility and enzyme inhibition of acid production by plaque bacteria.

USES
Prophylaxis of dental caries.

PRESENTATION
Gel: stannous fluoride 0.4%, 100mL – FluoriGard® Gel-Kam.
Mouthwash: sodium fluoride 0.05% 250mL – En-De-Kay® Daily Fluoride Mouthrinse; 500mL – Fluorigard® Daily Dental Rinse; sodium fluoride 2% (for dilution prior to use) daily or weekly rinse 100ml – En-De-Kay® Fluorinse; sodium fluoride 0.2% weekly dental rinse 150mL – Duraphat®.
Oral drops: sodium fluoride 550 microgram (250 microgram F⁻) per 0.15mL ≡ 7 drops (36 microgram per drop), 60mL bottle – En-De-Kay® Fluodrops.
Tablet: sodium fluoride 1.1mg (500 microgram F⁻), sodium fluoride 2.2mg (1mg F⁻) – En-De-Kay® Fluotabs, Fluor-a-day®, FluoriGard®.

DOSAGE
Oral drops and tablets (where water fluoride concentration is less than 0.3ppm/300 micrograms/litre):
6 months - 3 years: 250 microgram F⁻ per day
3-6 years: 500 microgram F⁻ per day
≥6 years: 1mg F⁻ per day
Dose is expressed as fluoride ion (F⁻). At water fluoride concentrations between 0.3-0.7ppm, half the above dosages should be prescribed for children ≥3 years of age or for children <3 years of age no fluoride is required.

Gels (recommended for children >3 years)
The gel should be applied to a clean toothbrush and brushed on all tooth surfaces after normal cleaning with toothpaste. The gel should then be swished between the tooth surfaces for 1 minute before spitting out the excess. No food or drink should be consumed for at least 30 minutes after use, for maximum effect.

F

Mouthwash (in children >6 years)

10mL of the mouthwash should be rinsed around the mouth for 1 minute, daily for the 0.05% (225ppm) rinse and weekly for the 0.2% (900ppm) rinse, before spitting out.

En–De-Kay® Fluorinse (in children >8 years)

For daily use, dilute 5 drops to 10mL of water and for weekly use dilute 20 drops to 10mL before use.

ADMINISTRATION

The fluoride supplement (oral drops or tablets) should be administered daily during the period of tooth formation and at a dose dependent upon the fluoride level in the water supply. This will be decided after consultation with the child's dentist taking into account associated risk factors, such as diet, motivation and oral hygiene levels. Drops should be given from a spoon or mixed with food. Tablets should be allowed to dissolve slowly in the mouth and the child encouraged to move the tablet around the mouth. Mouthwashes and gel should be used on the recommendation of a dentist. En-De-Kay® Fluorinse for dilution is a Prescription Only Medicine.

CONTRA-INDICATIONS & WARNINGS

Supplements (oral drops and tablets) should not be administered in areas with a water supply containing more than 0.7ppm fluoride. Systemic fluoride supplements should be avoided in patients whose renal function is seriously compromised. Advice must be sought from a general dental practitioner on the appropriate concentration of fluoridated toothpaste to be used during the period of fluoride supplementation.

INTERACTIONS

Interacts with *calcium* to reduce the absorption of fluorides.

SIDE-EFFECTS

Occasional white flecking of the teeth, extending to brown/cream discoloration, if the recommended dosage is not adhered to. This is more likely if the concentration of fluoride in toothpaste used concurrently is too high. It is vital that consideration is given to the appropriate concentration of fluoride toothpaste to be used in conjunction with the supplement if mottling of the teeth is to be avoided. For children <6 years of age a toothpaste containing fluoride at a concentration no greater than 550ppm is advisable but due consideration should be given to other risk factors for caries such as diet and oral hygiene measures. Brown/black staining of arrested carious lesions may occur with stannous fluoride preparations. Likewise if brushing is inefficient, light staining of pellicle will be evident but can be removed by professional prophylaxis or conscientious use of conventional toothpaste prior to the application of gel.

POISONING/TOXICITY

Acute poisoning: this may occur at doses of around 5mg/kg body weight. Sodium fluoride has a corrosive effect by reaction with the hydrochloric acid naturally present in the stomach. Other effects are as a consequence of metabolic and/or electrolyte disturbances, such as hypocalcaemia. Systemic effects include nausea, vomiting, tetany, tremors, paraesthesia, respiratory arrest, convulsions, cardiac arrythmias, failure and shock. Death may supervene in 2-4 hours. In cases of suspected poisoning, an estimate of the quantity consumed should be made. Milk slows the absorption of fluoride. If the suspected intake exceeds 5mg/kg body weight, emergency admission to hospital is indicated with treatment to include emptying of gastric contents.

Chronic overdosage: may result in enamel fluorosis in teeth that have still to erupt. This can be contained by advising parents to supervise brushing and rinsing as well as dispensing a small pea-sized amount of paste onto the child's toothbrush.

PHARMACOKINETIC PROPERTIES

Fluoride is readily absorbed into the body, a process accelerated when the pH is reduced. In the presence of calcium, fluoride becomes bound and thus unavailable. Fluoride is excreted in the urine, lost through sweat and excreted in the faeces. The former is the principal route of excretion with, in a relatively unexposed individual, half a single dose excreted in the urine within 24 hours, the remainder being deposited within bone. In individuals who are actively laying down mineral, excretion is lower. Infants excrete 40% of an ingested dose.

EXCIPIENTS

Contact manufacturers for further details.

LICENSED STATUS

Gel licensed for use ≥3 years.

Mouthwash licensed for use ≥6 years except En-De-Kay® Fluorinse which is licensed for use ≥8 years.

Oral drops licensed for use in infants and children. 6 months – 3 years of age. Tablets 500 microgram F⁻ – licensed ≥2 years, 1mg F⁻ – licensed ≥4 years, but see dosage section for recommended dosages.

Selective serotonin re-uptake inhibitor (SSRI).

USES
Depression, obsessive-compulsive disorder (OCD), anxiety (including social phobia and selective mutism, trichotillomania and bulimia). Idiopathic musculoskeletal pain.

PRESENTATION
Capsule: 20mg – Prozac® and non-proprietary ; 60mg – Prozac®.
Liquid: 20mg in 5mL – Prozac®.

DOSAGE

Indication	Route	Age		Frequency	Notes
		2–12 years	12–18 years	(times daily)	
Depression	Oral	≥6 years 10mg	10mg	1	Initial dose. Gradually increase dose over 3 weeks to 20mg once daily.
Bulimia	Oral	-	60mg	1	
Obsessive compulsive disorder. Severe anxiety	Oral	6-8 years 10mg 8-12 years 20mg	20mg	1 1	Initial dose. Gradually increase by 10-20mg increments, about every 2 weeks. Maximum dose of 60mg/**day**.
Idiopathic musculoskeletal pain	Oral	≥8 years 10mg	20mg	1	

CONTRA-INDICATIONS & WARNINGS
Avoid in hepatic or renal insufficiency. Ensure 2 week interval after MAOIs. Caution in poorly controlled epilepsy (lowers seizure threshold).

INTERACTIONS
Increases plasma levels of *carbamazepine, phenytoin* and *haloperidol.* Enhances effect of *warfarin.* Increases CNS adverse effects of *lithium. Lithium* levels should be monitored. The plasma *flecainide* concentration is increased by fluoxetine.

PREGNANCY
Only use if potential benefit outweighs possible risk. No evidence of teratogenicity from animal studies, but full testing was limited by maternal toxicity. Contact local Medicines Information Centre for advice.

BREAST-FEEDING
Significant amounts in breast milk; avoid. Contact local Medicines Information Centre for advice.

SIDE-EFFECTS
Nausea and gastrointestinal symptoms generally. Headache, light-headedness, restlessness, anxiety and weight loss. Seizures, rash, urticaria, fever and even neuroleptic malignant syndrome. Social disinhibition and euphoria, even precipitation of mania. Diminished libido and anorgasmia.

POISONING/TOXICITY
Nausea, vomiting, agitation, seizures. Treat with oral activated charcoal and general supportive measures.

PHARMACOKINETIC PROPERTIES
Well absorbed from the gastrointestinal tract following oral administration. Long half-life (up to 6 days of fluoxetine and 16 days of active metabolite, norfluoxetine).

F

EXCIPIENTS
Liquid includes sucrose and a small amount of alcohol in the peppermint flavouring. Contact manufacturers for further details.

LICENSED STATUS
Not licensed for use in children.

FURTHER INFORMATION
Therapeutic effect in depression may be delayed for 4 weeks. Doses in anxiety and OCD are usually higher than those needed in depression.

A corticosteroid which decreases tissue inflammation and bronchial hyper-reactivity.

USES
Prophylaxis of asthma (especially if not fully controlled by bronchodilators); prophylaxis and treatment of allergic rhinitis; treatment of nasal polyps.

PRESENTATION
Aerosol inhalation: 25 microgram – Flixotide®; 50, 125 and 250 microgram – Flixotide Evohaler®.
Dry powder for inhalation: 50, 100, 250 and 500 microgram per blister – Flixotide® Accuhaler® and Flixotide® Diskhaler®.
Nebules: 250 microgram in 1mL, 2mL nebules and 1mg in 1mL, 2mL nebules – Flixotide® Nebules®.
Aqueous nasal spray: 50 microgram per metered spray – Flixonase®.

DOSAGE

Route	Age		Frequency	Notes
	2–12 years	**12–18 years**	**(times daily)**	
Inhaled	<u><4 years</u> 50–100microgram ≥4 years 50–200 micrograms	<u>12–16 years</u> 50–200 microgram ≥16 years 100 microgram - 1mg	2 2	<u>Asthma:</u> the starting dose should be appropriate to the severity of the disease. The dosage should be adjusted until control is achieved and then reduced to the minimal effective dose according to individual response.
Nebulised	1mg	<u>12–16 years</u> 1mg	2	<u>Asthma:</u> acute exacerbation of asthma.
	–	<u>≥16 years</u> 500 microgram–2mg	2	<u>Asthma:</u> prophylactic management of chronic severe asthma in patients requiring high dose inhaled or oral corticosteroid therapy.
Intra-nasal	≥4 years 50 micrograms (1spray) into each nostril	100 micrograms (2 sprays) into each nostril	1	<u>Allergic rhinitis:</u> twice daily dosing may be required.

ADMINISTRATION
Inhaler: fluticasone aerosol inhaler can be used via a large volume spacer (Volumatic®, Babyhaler®) and mask for infants and young children. Administration of doses above 500 micrograms twice daily from the Evohaler® should also be administered via a large volume spacer.
Nebulised: via a jet nebuliser. Preferably with a mouthpiece to avoid atrophic changes to facial skin which may occur with prolonged use of a facemask. If a facemask is used the exposed skin should be protected with a barrier cream or the face should be thoroughly washed after treatment.

CONTRA-INDICATIONS & WARNINGS
Hypersensitivity to any ingredient of the preparation. In children using licensed doses of fluticasone, adrenal function and adrenal reserve should remain normal. Systemic effects of inhaled corticosteroids may occur, particularly at high doses prescribed for prolonged periods. These may include adrenal suppression, growth retardation in children and adolescents, decrease in bone mineral density, cataract and glaucoma.

INTERACTIONS
Due to low plasma concentrations of fluticasone being achieved following inhaled doses, there is low potential for drug interactions. Use of fluticasone propionate in patients taking concurrent drugs which are potent inhibitors of the cytochrome P450 3A4 system, *e.g. ketoconazole* and protease inhibitors such as *ritonavir*, may be associated with increased systemic exposure of fluticasone propionate.

PREGNANCY
Very small risk of intra-uterine growth retardation and cleft palate. Use in pregnancy should only be considered if the expected benefit to the mother is greater than any possible risks to the fetus. Data on a limited number (200) of exposed pregnancies has indicated no adverse effects of Flixotide® Evohaler® on pregnancy or the health of the fetus/newborn child.

BREAST-FEEDING
Unlikely to be problematic.

SIDE-EFFECTS
Occasionally candidiasis of the mouth, hoarseness. Rare

reports of peripheral oedema and cutaneous hypersensitivity reactions. Very rare reports of nasal septum perforation with the nasal spray. Paradoxical bronchoconstriction should be treated immediately with a fast acting inhaled bronchodilator.

POISONING/TOXICITY
Acute: may lead to temporary suppression of adrenal function. Treatment with fluticasone should be continued at a reduced dose to control asthma. Adrenal function will recover in a few days.
Chronic: use in excess of licensed doses for prolonged periods may lead to adrenal suppression. Treatment should be continued at a dose sufficient to control asthma. Monitoring of adrenal reserve may be needed.

PHARMACOKINETIC PROPERTIES
Systemic absolute bioavailability of fluticasone propionate is estimated at 12-26% of an inhaled dose, dependent on presentation. Systemic absorption occurs mainly through the lungs and is initially rapid then prolonged. Any corticosteroid that reaches systemic circulation will be metabolised mainly in the liver, but also in the kidneys, and is excreted in the urine. The remainder of the dose may be swallowed. Absolute oral bioavailability is negligible (<1%) due to a combination of incomplete absorption from the gastrointestinal tract and extensive first-pass metabolism. The relative potency of fluticasone to beclometasone (beclomethasone) and budesonide is 2:1.

EXCIPIENTS
See manufacturers SPC for further details.

LICENSED STATUS
Flixotide® aerosol inhalation, aqueous nasal spray, Accuhaler® 50 and 100 micrograms, Diskhaler® 50 and 100 micrograms and Evohaler® 50 micrograms are licensed for use ≥4 years of age. Flixotide® Nebules® are licensed for use ≥16 years of age.
Flixotide® Accuhaler® 250 and 500 micrograms, Diskhaler® 250 and 500 micrograms and Evohaler® 125 and 250 micrograms are not licensed for use in children.

Fluticasone/salmeterol (Seretide®)

USES
Used in the regular treatment of asthma where use of a combination product (long-acting beta-2-agonist and inhaled corticosteroid) is appropriate i.e, patients not adequately controlled with inhaled corticosteroids and 'as needed' inhaled short-acting beta-2-agonists or patients already adequately controlled on both inhaled corticosteroids and long-acting beta-2-agonist.

PRESENTATION
Aerosol inhaler: (as xinafoate) 25 microgram of salmeterol and 50, 125 or 250 micrograms of fluticasone propionate – Seretide 50 Evohaler®, Seretide 125 Evohaler® and Seretide 250 Evohaler®.
Dry powder for inhalation: (as xinafoate) 50 microgram of salmeterol and 100, 250 or 500 micrograms of fluticasone propionate – Seretide 100 Accuhaler®, Seretide 250 Accuhaler® and Seretide 500 Accuhaler®.

DOSAGE

Route	Age		Frequency	Notes
	2–12 years	12–18 years	(times daily)	
Aerosol inhaler	–	2 inhalations	2	Preventor: for regular use.
Dry powder inhaler	≥ 4 years 1 blister of Seretide Accuhaler 100	1 blister (of all strengths)	2	

ADMINISTRATION
Inhalation: aerosol inhaler can be used with Volumatic® spacer.

F

CONTRA-INDICATIONS & WARNINGS
Hypersensitivity to any ingredient of the preparation. Seretide® should not be used to control acute asthma symptoms. Seretide® treatment should not be stopped abruptly.

INTERACTIONS, PREGNANCY, BREAST-FEEDING, SIDE-EFFECTS, POISONING/TOXICITY, PHARMACO-KINETIC PROPERTIES
See fluticasone and salmeterol individual monographs.

EXCIPIENTS
See manufacturers SPC for further details.

LICENSED STATUS
Seretide 100 Accuhaler® licensed for >4 years of age. Seretide 250 and 500 Accuhaler® licensed for ≥12 years of age. Seretide 50, 125 and 250 Evohaler® licensed for ≥12 years of age.

Fluvoxamine maleate

Selective serotonin re-uptake inhibitor (SSRI).

USES
Depression. Obsessive-compulsive disorder.

PRESENTATION
Tablet: 50mg and 100mg – Faverin® and non-proprietary.

DOSAGE

Route	Age	Frequency (times daily)	Notes
	12–18 years		
Oral	100mg	1	Increase if necessary to a maximum of 300mg per day. (Doses >100mg give in two divided doses).

CONTRA-INDICATIONS & WARNINGS
See fluoxetine monograph. Avoid concurrent *theophylline* or *aminophylline* (see interactions).

INTERACTIONS
See fluoxetine monograph. Increases plasma concentrations of *theophylline*. Where it is not possible to avoid concurrent use halve the *theophylline* dose and monitor plasma *theophylline* levels closely. Can increase plasma levels of *propranolol*.

PREGNANCY
Animal studies have not shown a direct teratogenic effect, but safety in human pregnancy not established. Contact local Medicines Information Centre for advice.

BREAST-FEEDING, SIDE-EFFECTS, POISONING/TOXICITY
See fluoxetine monograph.

PHARMACOKINETIC PROPERTIES
Rapidly and completely absorbed after oral administration. Half-life is approximately 15 hours during repeated dosing, when steady-state plasma levels are usually achieved in 10-14 days.

EXCIPIENTS
Contact manufacturers for further details.

LICENSED STATUS
Not licensed for use in children.

Folic acid

An essential factor for the synthesis of methionine and purines/pyrimidines.

USES
Folate deficiency, congenital haemolytic conditions. In juvenille idiopathic arthritis (JIA) to limit methotrexate associated nausea.

PRESENTATION
Tablet: 400 microgram and 5mg – non-proprietary.
Syrup: 400 microgram in 5mL – Folicare® and non-proprietary; 2.5mg in 5mL – Lexpec® and non-proprietary.

DOSAGE
Newborn infant (birth to 1 month)
Preterm babies fed heat-treated human milk may benefit from a 500 microgram supplement once a week unless a suitable breast milk fortifier is used. Supplementation has no impact on the risk of anaemia developing in other term or preterm breast or formula fed babies.

Indication	Route	Age				Frequency (times daily)	Notes
		birth–1 month	1 month–2 years	2–12 years	12–18 years		
Supplementation in folate deficiency in infants and children; co-factor in metabolic disorders e.g. homocystinuria	Oral	← 250 microgram/kg →			5–10mg	1	For 6 months if a correctable cause; for life if uncorrectable cause.
Treatment of megaloblastic anaemia due to folate deficiency	Oral	1mg	DOSE BY WEIGHT <1 year 500 microgram/kg DOSE BY AGE 1–2 years 5mg	← 5mg →		1 1 1	For up to 4 months. For maintenance therapy the treatment doses may be given at daily to weekly intervals.
Haemolytic anaemia	Oral	-	← 2.5–5mg →		10mg	1	Seek haematologist's advice.
In JIA to limit methotrexate associated side-effects	Oral	-	-	← 1mg →		1	Prescribe according to local policy. Dose may be omitted on the day child receives methotrexate. Doses of 5mg weekly or twice weekly are sometimes given.

CONTRA-INDICATIONS & WARNINGS
Before treating megaloblastic anaemia with folic acid, vitamin B_{12} deficiency must be excluded, as neuropathy may be precipitated.

INTERACTIONS
Folic acid may decrease serum *phenobarbital (phenobarbitone), phenytoin* and *primidone* concentrations.

PREGNANCY
Is safely used in pregnancy to reduce the occurrence/recurrence of neural tube defects. Women planning a pregnancy are advised to take folic acid as a supplement until week 12 of pregnancy, at a dose of 400 micrograms daily to prevent first occurrence and 5mg daily to prevent a recurrence.

BREAST-FEEDING
Enters breast milk which may be beneficial to the infant.

SIDE-EFFECTS
Generally well tolerated. Gastrointestinal disturbances and hypersensitivity reactions have been reported rarely.

POISONING/TOXICITY
Even extremely high doses are unlikely to cause harm.

PHARMACOKINETIC PROPERTIES
Well absorbed orally (even in malabsorptive states), therefore parenteral therapy is only necessary when the oral route cannot be used.

EXCIPIENTS
Contact the manufacturers for further details.

LICENSED STATUS
Licensed for use in all ages. Not licensed for use in JIA to limit methotrexate associated side-effects.

USES
Soak for large mosaic plantar warts.

PRESENTATION
Gel: 0.75% in a water-miscible gel basis – Veracur®.
Lotion: 3% – may be extemporaneously prepared.

DOSAGE/ADMINISTRATION
Lotion: apply topically at night as a soak.
Gel: apply twice daily directly to the wart and cover with plaster. Remove the outer dead layers with an emery board or pumice stone as the treatment progresses.

CONTRA-INDICATIONS & WARNINGS	SIDE-EFFECTS
Avoid broken skin. Do not apply to face, anogenital region or large area. Do not use in diabetes or if peripheral blood circulation impaired.	Skin irritation.

EXCIPIENTS
Contact manufacturers for further details.

LICENSED STATUS
The gel is licensed for use in children and adults. The lotion is extemporaneously prepared and as such is unlicensed.

Formoterol (eformoterol) fumarate

A direct acting beta-2 receptor stimulant which has a long duration of action.

USES
Treatment of reversible airways obstruction in patients requiring long-term regular bronchodilator therapy.

PRESENTATION
Dry powder for inhalation: 12 microgram per capsule – Foradil®.
Dry powder inhaler: 6 microgram per inhalation and 12 microgram per inhalation – Oxis® Turbohaler®.

DOSAGE

Route	Age		Frequency (times daily)	Notes
	2–12 years	12–18 years		
Inhaled Turbohaler	> 6 years 6-12 microgram	6-12 microgram	1-2	Preventor: for regular use. Increase up to 24 microgram twice a day in severe obstruction.
Dry powder inhalation	> 5 years 12 microgram	12 microgram	2	

ADMINISTRATION
Inhalation.

CONTRA-INDICATIONS & WARNINGS
Hypersensitivity to any ingredient of the preparation. Should not be used as an alternative to short acting beta agonists used 'on-demand'.

INTERACTIONS
Concomitant treatment with *xanthine derivatives, steroids* or *diuretics* may potentiate hypokalaemia.
Drugs such as *disopyramide* and *tricyclic antidepressants* may be associated with QT interval prolongation and increased risk of ventricular arrythmia. *Beta-blockers* may weaken or antagonise the effect of formoterol.

PREGNANCY
Use should only be considered if expected benefit to mother is greater than the risk to the fetus. Contact local Medicines Information Centre for advice.

BREAST-FEEDING
Unknown as to whether formoterol passes into breast milk (animal studies showed only small amounts of formoterol in maternal milk). Contact local Medicines Information Centre for advice.

SIDE-EFFECTS
Commonly headaches, palpitations, tremor. Less commonly agitation, restlessness, sleep disturbances, muscle cramps, tachycardia. Rarely rashes, itching bronchospasms, hypokalaemia and hyperkalaemia.

POISONING/TOXICITY
Use cardioselective beta-blockers, but with extreme caution in case bronchospasm is provoked. Monitor serum potassium.

PHARMACOKINETIC PROPERTIES
Inhaled formulation is rapidly absorbed. Peak plasma concentrations are seen after 15 minutes. Plasma protein binding is approximately 50%. Mostly eliminated via metabolism.

EXCIPIENTS
See manufacturers SPC for further details.

LICENSED STATUS
Foradil® is licensed for >5 years of age. Oxis® is licensed for >6 years of age.

Foscarnet sodium

Organic analogue of inorganic pyrophosphate. Inhibits replication of human herpes virus by inhibition of virus specific DNA polymerases and reverse transcriptases. Activity in vitro against Epstein Barr virus, HIV and varicella-zoster as well as herpes virus 6, herpes simplex virus types 1 and 2 and cytomegalovirus (CMV).

USES
Treatment of CMV retinitis in patients with AIDS. Induction therapy of aciclovir (acyclovir) unresponsive mucocutaneous herpes simplex virus (HSV) infections in immuno-compromised patients. May also be useful in treatment of aciclovir resistant varicella-zoster virus, though this is an unlicensed indication.

PRESENTATION
IV infusion: (as sodium hexahydrate) 24mg in 1mL, 250mL and 500mL – Foscavir®.

DOSAGE
All doses of foscarnet are expressed in terms of foscarnet sodium. Very limited data in children but the following doses have been used, usually in combination with ganciclovir.

Route	Age			Frequency	Notes
	1 month–2 years	2–12 years	12–18 years	(times daily)	
IV	←	60mg/kg	→	3	Induction therapy for CMV retinitis.
	←	40mg/kg	→	3	Induction therapy of mucocutaneous HSV infection.
	←	90mg/kg	→	1	Maintenance therapy.

Dose adjustment in renal impairment – dose must be adjusted in renal failure (see manufacturers SPC for details).

ADMINISTRATION
IV: IV infusion over 1-2 hours via central or peripheral line. If given via peripheral line foscarnet infusion should be diluted to at least 12mg in 1mL. Injection solution has pH 7.4. Compatible with NaCl 0.9% and glucose 5%. Incompatible with calcium or magnesium containing solutions as may chelate divalent metal ions. Foscarnet deposits in bone and tooth enamel in animals and may do so in children.

CONTRA-INDICATIONS & WARNINGS
Hypersensitivity to foscarnet. Monitor renal function regularly during treatment as renal impairment may occur. Ensure adequate hydration. Monitor serum calcium and magnesium as foscarnet may chelate divalent metal ions and lead to an acute decrease in ionised calcium/magnesium.

INTERACTIONS
Concurrent *nephrotoxic drugs* may cause additive renal toxicity. Drugs known to reduce serum calcium *(pentamidine, furosemide (frusemide)*, may potentiate hypocalcaemia).

F

PREGNANCY
Potential teratogen; avoid in pregnancy.

BREAST-FEEDING
Contra-indicated in breast-feeding.

SIDE-EFFECTS
Renal function impairment. Genital irritation or ulceration. Serum electrolyte changes including hypocalcaemia, hypomagnesaemia, hypophosphataemia, hypokalaemia, hyperphosphataemia, and reductions in serum iron and zinc. Hypocalcaemia may be acute, symptomatic and related to rate of infusion. Convulsions have occurred during foscarnet therapy and in some cases may be related to acute hypocalcaemia. Skin rashes may occur during treatment. Decrease in haemoglobin concentration has been observed. CNS effects such as paraesthesia, headache, dizziness, involuntary muscle contractions, tremor, ataxia and neuropathy may occur. Anorexia, anxiety, nervousness, confusion, psychosis and aggression have also been reported. Other less common adverse effects reported include gastrointestinal effects (nausea, vomiting, diarrhoea and constipation) pancreatitis, increases in serum amylase, alkaline phosphatase, hyponatraemia. Foscarnet is not generally myelosuppressive but monitoring of white cell count is advisable. Thrombocytopenia, increases in serum ALT, AST and gamma GT, ventricular arrhythmia and diabetes insipidus also reported rarely.

POISONING/TOXICITY
Pattern of adverse events reported in overdose is that expected from the adverse effect profile of the drug. Removed by haemodialysis.

PHARMACOKINETIC PROPERTIES
Adult data. Wide variation in pharmacokinetics in adults. Plasma concentrations achieved and CSF penetration are variable. Levels achieved in CSF are around 25% of plasma concentration after one dose and 66% at steady state. Deposited in bone and gradually released. Up to 20% of the cumulative dose may end up in bone and caution is advised in children where this may be even greater. Excreted unchanged in the urine. Terminal half-life up to 87 hours reported. Plasma protein binding 14-17%. *Child data –* little information available.

EXCIPIENTS
See manufacturers SPC for further details.

LICENSED STATUS
Not licensed for use in children.

Furazolidone

A nitrofuran derivative with antiprotozoal and antibacterial activity.

USES
Giardiasis; alternative to metronidazole or tinidazole; not the treatment of choice.

PRESENTATION
Tablet: 100mg (scored) – named patient (imported).
Oral suspension: 50mg in 15mL – named patient (imported).

DOSAGE

Route	Age			Frequency	Notes
	1 month–2 years	2–12 years	12–18 years	(times daily)	
Oral	← 1.5mg/kg →		100mg	4	For 7-10 days.

ADMINISTRATION
Oral: tablets may be crushed.

CONTRA-INDICATIONS & WARNINGS
Prior sensitivity to furazolidone. Furazolidone may cause mild, reversible intravascular haemolysis in G6PD deficient patients. Such patients should be closely observed and furazolidone treatment stopped if any evidence of haemolysis occurs. Furazolidone should not be given to infants <1 month of age (who have immature enzyme systems and glutathione instability) because of the possibility of producing haemolytic anaemia. Furazolidone is a monoamine oxidase inhibitor (MAOI) and the

cautions advised for MAOIs regarding the concomitant administration of other drugs, especially indirect acting sympathomimetic amines, and the consumption of food and drink containing tyramine should be observed; however there appear to be no reports of hypertensive crisis in patients receiving furazolidone. Darkening of the urine due to the presence of metabolites.

INTERACTIONS
Alcohol: a disulfiram like reaction has been reported in patients consuming *alcohol* whilst on furazolidone; *alcohol* should be avoided for the duration of treatment and for 4 days thereafter to prevent this reaction.

PREGNANCY
There have been no clinical reports of adverse effects of the drug on the fetus, nor have animal studies revealed evidence of teratogenicity but safety in pregnancy has not been established. Use should be restricted to those cases where the possible benefits outweigh the potential risks.

BREAST-FEEDING
The concentration in breast milk has not been determined and safe use in breast-feeding mothers has not been established.

SIDE-EFFECTS
Nausea and vomiting are the most common side-effects and abdominal pain, diarrhoea, headache and malaise occur occasionally. Hypersensitivity reactions including a fall in blood pressure, urticaria, fever, arthralgia, and a vesicular morbilliform rash have occurred in a small number of patients.

POISONING/TOXICITY
Symptoms: see side-effects above. Patients with G6PD deficiency are at risk of developing haemolysis. A disulfiram like reaction is also possible.
Treatment is symptomatic and supportive. There is no specific antidote.

PHARMACOKINETIC PROPERTIES
Following oral administration furazolidone is poorly absorbed. There may be rapid and extensive metabolism in the intestine. About 5-65% of an oral dose is excreted in the urine as unchanged drug and metabolites.

LICENSED STATUS
Not licensed for use in the UK.

FURTHER INFORMATION
Available from IDIS World Medicines.

Furosemide (frusemide)

Potent loop diuretic.

USES
To induce diuresis in cardiac or renal failure or fluid overload; hypertension.

PRESENTATION
Injection: 10mg in 1mL, 2mL ampoule – Lasix® and non-proprietary; 50mg in 5mL and 250mg in 25mL – non-proprietary.
Liquid: 1mg in 1mL – Lasix® Paediatric.
Oral solution: 20mg in 5mL, 40mg in 5mL and 50mg in 5mL –non-proprietary.
Tablet: 20mg, 40mg and 500mg – Lasix® (all scored) and non-proprietary.

F

DOSAGE

Route	Age				Frequency (times daily)	Notes
	birth–1 month	1 month–2 years	2–12 years	12–18 years		
Oral	500 microgram/kg – 1mg/kg	–		–	2	Larger doses sometimes necessary but do not exceed maximum single dose of 6mg/kg/dose. Repeat as necessary.
	–	← 1–2mg/kg →		20–40mg	2–3	
IV bolus	← 500 microgram/kg – 1mg/kg →			20–40mg	single dose	Single doses up to 4mg/kg have been used. Dose can be repeated every 8 hours.

DOSAGE continued

Route	Age				Frequency (times daily)	Notes
	birth–1 month	1 month–2 years	2–12 years	12–18 years		
IV infusion	–	100 microgram/kg/hour – 2mg/kg/hour		not exceeding 4mg/minute	continuous	IV infusion for paediatric post operative cardiac patients – an initial dose of 100 microgram/kg/hour is suggested, doubling the dose every 2 hours until urine output exceeds 1mL/kg/hour, up to a maximum dose of 2mg/kg/hour.

Renal Failure
Patients in renal failure may require higher than usual doses to induce diuresis.

Hepatic Insufficiency
Dosage adjustments may be necessary in patients with cirrhosis and in patients with combined hepatic and renal insufficiency. Higher doses than normal may be required.

ADMINISTRATION
IM: the IM route is rarely used.
IV: bolus doses must be administered slowly over at least 2 minutes. Some centres give bolus doses at slower rates (5-10 minutes) because of risk of ototoxicity, especially if the child is also on aminoglycosides. The manufacturer recommends that larger doses should be infused. Infusion rates should not exceed those outlined in the table.
Compatibility with infusion solutions: furosemide may be mixed with NaCl 0.9%. It is incompatible with glucose solutions.

CONTRA-INDICATIONS & WARNINGS
Established anuria, electrolyte deficiency especially hypokalaemia, precomatose states associated with liver cirrhosis, hypersensitivity to furosemide or sulphonamides.
Warnings: correct hypotension or hypovolaemia before commencing therapy. Latent diabetes may become manifest or the insulin requirements of diabetic patients may increase.

INTERACTIONS
NSAIDs may reduce the antihypertensive and diuretic effect. Loop diuretics may attenuate the effects of *antidiabetics.* Increased risk of hypokalaemia with other *loop diuretics, thiazides* and *corticosteroids.* Diuretic-induced hypokalaemia may increase the risk of arrhythmias with *cardiac glycosides.* A marked fall in blood pressure may be seen when *ACE inhibitors* are added to diuretic therapy. Increased risk of ototoxicity with *aminoglycosides* (avoid prescribing at the same time of day).

PREGNANCY
Should only be used in pregnancy if strictly indicated and for short-term treatment. Never use with *ACE inhibitors* in pregnancy (oligohydramnios and intrauterine fetal death association). Contact local Medicines Information Centre for advice.

BREAST-FEEDING
May inhibit lactation or may pass into breast milk. Use with caution in nursing mothers. Contact local Medicines Information Centre for advice.

SIDE-EFFECTS
Hypokalaemia, hypomagnesaemia, hyponatraemia, hyperuricaemia, hypocalcaemia, nephrocalcinosis has been reported in premature infants, transient increase in plasma urea and creatinine, increase in plasma triglyceride levels, gastrointestinal disturbances, skin rashes, headache, hypotension or muscle cramps due to electrolyte and water disturbance, ototoxicity (usually reversible), acute pancreatitis (isolated cases), bone marrow depression (rare).

PHARMACOKINETIC PROPERTIES
Oral bioavailability range 27-80%. Extensively plasma protein bound 96-98%. Mainly renal excretion of unchanged drug and some elimination by metabolism and faecal excretion which contribute almost equally to the total plasma clearance. Half-life in adults is 30-120 minutes. Half-life in healthy children is on average 28 minutes. Half-life is very variable in the neonatal period, and may be as much as 24 hours in the young preterm infant, but is closer to 8 hours in full term infants >1 week old.

POISONING/TOXICITY
In cases of overdose there is a danger of dehydration and electrolyte depletion due to excessive diuresis. Treatment should therefore be aimed at fluid replacement and correction of electrolyte imbalance.

EXCIPIENTS
Lasix® paediatric liquid includes sorbitol and saccharin sodium. See manufacturers SPC for further details.

LICENSED STATUS
Licensed for use in children and adults.

Antiepileptic.

USES
Drug of second or third choice for partial seizures with or without secondary generalised tonic-clonic seizures. Ineffective for myoclonic or typical absence seizures.

PRESENTATION
Capsule: 100mg, 300mg and 400mg – Neurontin®.
Tablet: 600mg and 800mg – Neurontin®.

DOSAGE

Route	Age				Frequency (times daily)	Notes
	birth–1 month	1 month–2 years	2–12 years	12–18 years		
Oral	–	–	10mg/kg	300mg	see notes	Starting dose. Give once daily on day one, twice daily day two and three times daily on day three, increasing to maintenance. Note: although manufacturers recommend daily increments in initial adult doses some children may not tolerate daily increments and up to weekly increases may be more appropriate.
	–	–	10–20mg/kg	300–800mg	3	Target maintenance dose. May be effective given twice daily. Doses up to 70mg/kg/day may be required.

Dose adjustment in renal impairment
If >12 years, see SPC for details of dose adjustment.
If <12 years, reduce dose interval as shown below.

Creatinine clearance (mL/minute/1.73m²)	Frequency of maintenance dose
30–60	twice a day.
15–30	once daily.
<15	once daily on alternate days.

Haemodialysis: 8–12mg/kg loading dose then 6–8mg/kg after each 4 hour dialysis period.

ADMINISTRATION
Oral: capsules can be opened but contents are very bitter and difficult to mask even with blackcurrant or cola drinks. Concomitant antacids reduce absorption. Absorption is unaffected by food.

CONTRA-INDICATIONS & WARNINGS
Avoid abrupt withdrawal. Reduce dose in renal impairment.

INTERACTIONS
Does not appear to interact with other antiepileptics or oral contraceptives. Oral absorption reduced by *magnesium/aluminium antacids*.

PREGNANCY/BREAST-FEEDING
Safety in pregnancy not established. Excreted in breast milk; effects on infant unknown. Contact local Medicines Information Centre for advice.

SIDE-EFFECTS
Dose dependent side-effects are uncommon and include somnolence, fatigue, dizziness and behavioural changes. As yet there is inadequate data on potential chronic adverse effects.

POISONING/TOXICITY
Life threatening toxicity not seen at doses up to 49g in adults. Drowsiness, dizziness, double vision and slurred speech may be observed. Contact UK National Poisons Information Service.

PHARMACOKINETIC PROPERTIES
Peak plasma levels occur about 2 hours after oral administration. Elimination half-life approximately

G

6 hours. No metabolism; elimination entirely renal. Capsules and tablets are bioequivalent. Correlation between plasma levels and clinical efficacy has not been established, so routine levels not recommended.

EXCIPIENTS
See manufacturer's SPC for further details.

LICENSED STATUS
Licensed for >6 years of age.

FURTHER INFORMATION
Gabapentin is not suitable for rectal administration.

Ganciclovir

Synthetic guanine analogue which inhibits replication of herpes viruses (sensitive viruses: cytomegalovirus(CMV), herpes simplex virus 1 and 2, Epstein Barr virus, varicella-zoster and herpes virus type 6).

USES
IV: treatment of life or sight threatening CMV infections in immunocompromised individuals. Also used in prevention of CMV disease in such patients.
Capsules: maintenance treatment of CMV retinitis in AIDS patients following 3 weeks of IV therapy.

PRESENTATION
Capsule: 250mg and 500mg – Cymevene®.
IV infusion: (as sodium salt) 500mg vial – Cymevene®.
Oral suspension: manufactured 'special'.

DOSAGE
Newborn infant (birth to 1 month)

Route	Age		Frequency (times daily)	Notes
	Up to 7 days	Over 7 days		
IV	← 5mg/kg →		2	Reduce frequency in renal impairment and very low birth weight infants.

Child

Route	Age			Frequency (times daily)	Notes
	1 month–2 years	2–12 years	12–18 years		
Oral	← 20–40mg/kg →		1g	3	Give with food to maximise absorption. Unlicensed in children <12 years.
IV	← 5mg/kg →			2	Induction regime for 14–21 days if treatment of CMV or 7–14 days if used in prevention of CMV in at risk patients.
	← 5mg/kg →			1	Maintenance. For 7 days a week.
	← or 6mg/kg →			1	For 5 days a week.

Dosage in renal impairment
IV induction

Creatinine clearance (mL/minute/1.73m^2)	Dose	Frequency (times daily)
50–80	2.5mg/kg	2
10–50	2.5mg/kg	1
10	1.25mg/kg	1

Haemodialysis patients should be given 1.25mg/kg every 24 hours. Doses should be given shortly after dialysis session as ganciclovir is removed by dialysis.

Maintenance
Manufacturer has no recommendation but the following have been used:

IV maintenance (all ages)

Creatinine clearance (mL/minute/1.73m²)	Dose	Frequency (times daily)
50–70	2.5mg/kg	2
25–49	2.5mg/kg	1
10–24	1.25mg/kg	1

Oral maintenance (12-18 years)

Creatinine clearance (mL/minute/1.73m²)	Dose	Frequency
50–69	1.5g	once daily
25–49	1g	once daily
10–24	500mg	once daily
<10	500mg	3 times weekly

ADMINISTRATION
IV infusion: reconstitute each vial with 10mL Water for Injections to give 50mg in 1mL. Displacement value is negligible. Infuse over 1 hour at a concentration of no more than 10mg in 1mL. Compatible with NaCl 0.9%, glucose 5%, compound sodium lactate. Caution is advised when handling ganciclovir as the reconstituted solution has a pH around 11 and is irritant. Ganciclovir is also potentially carcinogenic and teratogenic. Gloves and eye protection are recommended.
Intravitreal injection: a solution of 2mg in 0.1mL in NaCl 0.9% is used.

CONTRA-INDICATIONS & WARNINGS
Contra-indicated in those patients with a known hypersensitivity to ganciclovir or aciclovir. Contra-indicated in pregnancy and lactation. Ensure adequate hydration when using IV. Avoid if neutrophil count <500 cell per microlitre. Increased risk of thrombocytopenia if platelet count <25,000 per microlitre. Regular monitoring of white blood cell count is advised. Ganciclovir should be considered potentially mutagenic, carcinogenic and teratogenic.

INTERACTIONS
Drugs that inhibit replication of rapidly dividing cells: potential additive toxicity. Patients receiving *immunosuppressive agents* may require decreased doses or temporary withdrawal of these drugs to prevent excessive suppression of the bone marrow or immune system. *Dapsone, pentamidine, flucytosine, amphotericin, co-trimoxazole*; potential for additive toxicity. *Zidovudine;* severe neutropenia likely if used concurrently. Regular monitoring advised. *Probenecid* and other drugs that inhibit renal tubular secretion or reabsorption may reduce renal clearance of ganciclovir. *Imipenem-cilastatin;* seizures have been reported when used in combination with ganciclovir.

PREGNANCY
Teratogenic in animal studies. Avoid in pregnancy.

BREAST-FEEDING
Unclear if excreted in human breast milk but animal studies suggest adverse effects are likely. Nursing should not be resumed until 72 hours after the last dose of ganciclovir.

SIDE-EFFECTS
Leucopenia and thrombocytopenia occur in 10 to 40% of patients given IV ganciclovir. Anaemia, fever, rash and abnormal LFTs occur in up to 2% of patients. Chills, oedema, confusion ataxia, nervousness, paraesthesia, psychosis, tremor, hypotension, hypertension, cardiac arrhythmias, gastrointestinal effects including haemorrhage, eosinophilia, decreased blood glucose, alopecia, pruritus, urticaria, haematuria, increases in serum creatinine and urea also reported.

POISONING/TOXICITY
Dialysis and hydration may reduce plasma levels. Reported effects of overdose are bone marrow suppression, renal toxicity, hepatic toxicity and gastrointestinal symptoms.

PHARMACOKINETIC PROPERTIES
Poorly absorbed from gastrointestinal tract with absolute bioavailability of 5-9% maximised by taking dose with food. Plasma peak concentration from oral dose is 1 microgram per mL and minimum 0.2 microgram per mL. This compares with peak of 8 microgram per mL and minimum 0.05 microgram per mL for IV maintenance. In viral infected cells ganciclovir is phosphorylated slowly with 60-70% remaining intracellularly after removal from the extracellular fluid. Widely distributed to body tissues and fluids including intra-ocular fluid and lungs where concentrations sufficient to treat pneumonitis are likely to be achieved. Only 1-2% bound to plasma proteins. Eliminated by excretion of unchanged drug in the urine by glomerular filtration. Terminal half-life is 2.5-4 hours in normal renal function increasing to 30 hours in severe renal impairment.

G

EXCIPIENTS
Injection: sodium content 2mmol in each 500mg vial. See manufacturers SPC for further details.

LICENSED STATUS
Licensed for use in the treatment and prevention of CMV as described in the 'uses' section. Treatment of other potentially susceptible viral infections is unlicensed.
Injection is licensed for use in children, though manufacturer urges caution; unlicensed in neonates. The capsules are unlicensed for use <12 years. Oral suspension available as a 'special' and as such is unlicensed.

Gastrografin®

An iodine-containing x-ray contrast medium, with high osmolality.

USES
Treatment of uncomplicated meconium ileus and distal intestinal obstructive syndrome in patients with cystic fibrosis. Investigation of the gastrointestinal tract.

PRESENTATION
Aqueous solution: 10% sodium diatrizoate and 66% meglumine diatrizoate, 100mL bottles — Gastrografin®.

DOSAGE

Route	Age				Frequency	Notes
	birth–1 month	1 month–2 years	2–12 years	12–18 years	(times daily)	
Oral			15–25kg			Dilute well with water.
or	← 15–30mL →		50mL	100mL	single dose	Keep patient well hydrated.
rectal			>25kg			
			100mL		single dose	

ADMINISTRATION
Oral: For infants and young children it is recommended that Gastrografin® be diluted with 3 times its volume of water or fruit juice. For older children and adults dilute with twice its volume of water or fruit juice. Dose may be divided if not well tolerated.
Rectal: <5 years dilute with 5 times its volume of water.
      >5 years dilute with 4 times its volume of water.
Rectal administration should be carried out under radiological supervision to ensure required site is reached. Gastrografin® may cause the loss of a large amount of fluid into the intestines. Fluid intake should be encouraged for 3 hours after administration. Intravenous prehydration is essential in neonates and infants.

CONTRA-INDICATION & WARNINGS
Hypersensitivity to iodine-containing contrast media. Manifest hyperthyroidism. Caution in patients with thyroid disease, dehydrated patients and patients with electrolyte disturbances (correct first). Caution in patients with oesophageal fistulae as aspiration into the lungs can lead to pulmonary oedema.

PREGNANCY
Safety not established but has been used. Contact local Medicines Information Centre for advice.

BREAST-FEEDING
No data but Gastrografin® is only minimally absorbed from the gastrointestinal tract. Contact local Medicines Information Centre for advice.

SIDE-EFFECTS
Absorption is minimal and systemic effects are rare. Nausea and vomiting occur in exceptional cases. Urticarial skin reactions have been observed, while anaphylactoid reactions and shock are possible.
Owing to its hypertonicity, Gastrografin® may occasionally cause diarrhoea, but this ceases as soon as the intestine had been emptied. If prehydration is inadequate, hypovolaemia and hypotension may occur.

POISONING/TOXICITY
There are no specific antidotes to Gastrografin®. Treatment should be symptomatic.

G

EXCIPIENTS
See manufacturers SPC for further details.

LICENSED STATUS
Licensed for use in all ages for doses up to that stated on the SPC. Larger doses given here are routinely used in cystic fibrosis patients with good effect. Gastrografin® is licensed for use in meconium ileus but not licensed for distal intestinal obstructive syndrome.

FURTHER INFORMATION
Iodine content is 370mg/mL. At temperatures <7°C Gastrografin® can crystallise. This can be reversed by gentle warming without any adverse effect on the Gastrografin®.

Gaviscon®

Antacid/alginate mixture. Works principally as an antacid and thickens gastric contents. Alginate forms foamy 'raft' on gastric contents.

USES
Gastro-oesophageal reflux. Heartburn, dyspepsia and regurgitation.

PRESENTATION
Tablet: alginic acid 500mg, dried aluminium hydroxide 100mg, magnesium trisilicate 25mg, sodium bicarbonate 170mg; lemon or peppermint flavour – Gaviscon®.
Liquid: sodium alginate 250mg, sodium bicarbonate 133.5mg, calcium carbonate 80mg in 5mL; peppermint or aniseed flavour – Gaviscon®.
Suspension: sodium alginate 500mg, potassium bicarbonate 100mg in 5mL; aniseed or peppermint flavour – Gaviscon® Advance.
Oral powder (dual-sachets): sodium alginate 225mg, magnesium alginate 87.5mg per dose (half dual- sachet); also contains mannitol and colloidal silical – Gaviscon® Infant.

DOSAGE

Route	Age				Frequency	Notes
	birth–1 month	1 month–2 years	2–12 years	12–18 years		
Oral	≤4.5 kg 1 dose (half a dual-sachet) >4.5 kg 2 doses (1 dual-sachet)		1 tablet or 5–10mL liquid	1–2 tablets or 10–20mL liquid	single dose	Give infant sachets with/ after feeds to a maximum of 6 times per day. >2 years give liquid or oral tablets after meals and at bedtime.
Oral	–	–	–	5–10mL	single dose	≥12 years of age Gaviscon® Advance after meals and at bedtime.

ADMINISTRATION
Oral tablet: may be crushed, chewed or mixed with food/drink.
Oral powder: note that 1 dose is half a dual-sachet. Mix with part or all of milk feed. In the breast-fed infant add 5mL of boiled, cooled water to the powder in a glass, mix to a smooth paste, add 2 or more 5mL spoonfuls of water, mix and give from a spoon, during or after a feed. In the bottle-fed infant under 4.5kg (10lb) 1 dose to be mixed into not less than 115mL of each feed in the bottle and shaken well. Over 4.5kg (10lb), 2 doses to be mixed into not less than 225mL of each feed in the bottle and shaken well.

CONTRA-INDICATIONS & WARNINGS
Gavison® Infant should be used in all children <2 years since it contains less sodium than the other presentations. This is particularly important in preterm infants. Gaviscon® Infant should not be used in intestinal obstruction and diarrhoea. Do not use

G

Gaviscon® Infant with thickening agents or infant milk preparations containing a thickening agent as it could lead to over thickening of the stomach contents.

INTERACTIONS
None reported. Although large doses of antacids interfere with the absorption of some drugs, the amount of antacid in the recommended dose of Gaviscon® is unlikely to interact with other drugs.

PREGNANCY/BREAST-FEEDING
No known problems. Gaviscon® is indicated for heartburn in pregnancy.

POISONING
Overdose presents virtually no hazard. The only likely consequence is abdominal distension which is best treated conservatively.

EXCIPIENTS
Gaviscon® Tablets are gluten and sugar-free; sodium content 2mmol per tablet. Gaviscon® Infant is sugar-free; sodium content 0.92mmol per half dual-sachet. Gaviscon® Liquid is gluten and sugar-free; sodium content 3mmol per 5mL. Gaviscon® Advance is sugar-free; sodium content 2.3mmol per 5mL and potassium content is 1mmol per 5mL.

LICENSED STATUS
Gaviscon® Infant: licensed for infants and young children, but <1 year only under medical supervision.
Gaviscon® Liquid and Tablets: licensed for use in ≥2 years; age 2–6 years use only on medical advice.
Gaviscon® Advance licensed for use in >12 years.

G–CSF (granulocyte–colony stimulating factor)

Recombinent human G-CSF is a glycoprotein which regulates production and release of functional neutrophils from the bone marrow.

USES
Reduction in duration of neutropenia associated with cytotoxic chemotherapy, mobilisation of peripheral blood progenitor cells for harvesting and subsequent autologous infusion, neutropenia, cyclic neutropenia or idiopathic neutropenia. Glycogen storage disease (GSD), type 1b, 1c (GSD 1b, GSD 1c).

PRESENTATION
Filgrastim (unglycosylated rhG–CSF)
Injection: 30 million unit (300 microgram) in 1mL; 1mL vial and prefilled syringe; 48 million unit (480 microgram) 1.6mL vial and prefilled syringe – Neupogen®.
Lenograstim (glycosylated rhG–CSF)
Injection: 13.4 million unit (105 microgram) and 33.6 million unit (263 microgram); vial with 1mL Water for Injection and 1mL prefilled syringe – Granocyte®.

DOSAGE
Lenograstim

Indication	Route	Age			Frequency	Notes
		1 month–2 years	2–12 years	12–18 years	(times daily)	
Following bone-marrow transplantation	IV infusion over 30 minutes or SC infusion	–	←— 150 microgram/m² —→ equivalent to ←— 5 microgram/kg —→		1 1	Usually start the day after transplantation and continue until neutrophil count stable in the acceptable range (maximum 28 days), but check protocol.
Cytotoxic-induced neutropenia	SC injection	–	←—150 microgram/m² —→		1	Start the day after completion of chemotherapy and continue until neutrophil count stable in the acceptable range (maximum 28 days).

G

Lenograstim continued

Indication	Route	Age			Frequency (times daily)	Notes
		1 month–2 years	2–12 years	12–18 years		
Mobilisation of peripheral blood progenator cells after chemotherapy	SC injection	–	← 150 microgram/m² →		1	Start the day after completion of chemotherapy.
Mobilisation of blood progenator cells with no chemotherapy	SC injection	–	← 10 microgram/kg →		1	For 4–6 days.

Filgrastim

Indication	Route	Age				Frequency (times daily)	Notes
		birth–1 month	1 month–2 years	2–12 years	12–18 years		
Idiopathic or cyclic neutropenia	SC injection	–	← 5 microgram/kg →			1	The dose may be increased according to response but the long-term safety of doses >24 micrograms/kg/day has not been established.
Severe congenital neutropenia	SC injection	–	← 12 microgram/kg →			1	Adjusted according to response.
Mobilisation of peripheral blood progenitor cells after adjunctive chemotherapy	SC injection	–	← 5 microgram/kg →			1	First dose not less than 24 hours after chemotherapy; for up to 14 days.
Mobilisation of peripheral blood progenitor cells (alone)	SC injection or SC infusion over 24 hours	–	← 10 microgram/kg →			1	For 6 days.
Glycogen storage disease	SC injection	← 5 microgram/kg →				1	
Myeloblative therapy followed by bone marrow transplant	IV infusion over 30 minutes or SC/IV infusion over 24 hours	–	← 10 microgram/kg →			1	First dose usually not less than 24 hours after chemotherapy and within 24 hours of bone marrow infusion, but check protocol.
Cytoxic induced neutropenia	SC injection or IV infusion	–	← 5 microgram/kg →			1	

G

NB. 150 microgram/m^2 lenograstim in trials was therapeutically equivalent to 5 microgram/kg filgrastim.

Renal and hepatic impairment
Dose adjustment of filgrastim is not required in severe renal or hepatic impairment.

ADMINISTRATION
Filgrastim
Single dose use only. May be diluted in glucose 5%. Dilution to a final concentration of <2 microgram in 1mL is not recommended. If diluted to concentrations between 2-15 microgram in 1mL, Human Serum Albumin should be added to a final concentration of 2mg in 1mL. Diluted solution should be stored in a refrigerator (2-8°C). Use within 24 hours of reconstitution. Do not dilute with NaCl 0.9%.

Lenograstim
Single dose use only. Reconstitute with Water for Injections (do not shake vigorously). May dilute with NaCl 0.9%. The maximum diluted volume should not exceed 50mL for 1 vial of 13.4 million-unit or 100mL for 1 vial of 33.6 million units. The diluted solution should be stored in a refrigerator (2-8°C). Use within 24 hours of reconstitution.

CONTRA-INDICATIONS & WARNINGS
Seek expert advice before prescribing. Caution in tumours with myeloid characteristics. Monitoring of bone density may be required in patients with underlying osteoporotic bone disease who undergo long-term therapy.

INTERACTIONS
Rapidly dividing myeloid cells are sensitive to *cytotoxic chemotherapy*. Use is not recommended from 24 hours before *cytotoxic chemotherapy* administration until 24 hours after administration ends.

PREGNANCY
Contact local Medicines Information Centre for advice.

BREAST-FEEDING
It is not known whether G-CSF is excreted in human milk. Contact local Medicines Information Centre for advice.

SIDE-EFFECTS
Musculoskeletal pain, urinary abnormalities, transient hypotension, alopecia, disturbances in LFTs, thrombocytopenia, headache, diarrhoea, bone pain, injection site pain, adult respiratory distress syndrome (ARDS), allergic reactions (more common after IV infusion).

POISONING/TOXICITY
Effect of overdose not established. Discontinuation of therapy usually results in 50% decrease in circulating neutrophils within 24-48 hours, with a return to normal levels within 1-7 days. Doses up to 40 microgram/kg/day of lenograstim have not been associated with side-effects other than musculoskeletal pain.

PHARMACOKINETIC PROPERTIES
Clearance (after SC and IV administration) follows first order kinetics (serum elimination, half-life approximately 3 hours or shorter following repeated IV infusion).

EXCIPIENTS
See manufacturers SPC for further details.

LICENSED STATUS
Filgrastim licensed for use in children and adults.
Lenograstim licensed >2 years in bone marrow transplant (BMT).

Gelatin

A purified protein obtained by the partial hydrolysis of animal collagen, which in modified form in solution can be used as a plasma substitute.

USES
Plasma replacement in hypovolaemic shock, burns, cardiopulmonary bypass surgery.

PRESENTATION
IV infusion: succinylated gelatin 4% (modified fluid gelatin, average molecular weight 30,000) in NaCl 0.9%, 500mL and 1L – Gelofusine®; polygeline 3.5% (degraded and modified gelatin, average molecular weight 30,000) in NaCl 0.9%, 500mL – Haemaccel®.

G

DOSAGE
In hypovolaemic shock 10-20mL/kg bolus as rapidly as possible. Repeat as necessary.
In trauma these requirements may increase up to 40mL/kg. At this level, replacement with whole blood should be considered.

ADMINISTRATION
IV: preferably at blood temperature, at a rate determined by the condition of the patient.

CONTRA-INDICATIONS & WARNINGS Hypersensitivity reactions. Gelofusine® has less risk of producing anaphylaxis than Haemaccel®.	**PREGNANCY** Suitable for use if necessary.
	SIDE-EFFECTS Large volumes may lower serum albumin.
INTERACTIONS Due to calcium content caution in treatment of patients on *cardiac glycosides*. Haemaccel® may cause a slight temporary increase in erythrocyte sedimentation rate (ESR).	**PHARMACOKINETIC PROPERTIES** Half-life of Gelofusine® is 4 hours. Most eliminated in 24 hours by renal excretion.

EXCIPIENTS
Gelofusine® includes Na$^+$ 154mmol/L, Cl$^-$ 120mmol/L, Ca^{2+} trace.
Haemaccel® includes Na$^+$ 145mmol/L, K$^+$ 5.1mmol/L, Cl$^-$ 145mmol/L, Ca^{2+} 6.25mmol/L.

LICENSED STATUS
Licensed for use in all ages.

FURTHER INFORMATION
The products should not be mixed with citrated blood, but citrated blood can be given before or after gelatin infusion provided there is adequate flushing of the infusion site.

Gemfibrozil

Fibric acid derivative; lipid-modulating agent.

USES
Hyperlipidaemia, including familial hypercholesterolaemia in patients in whom diet therapy and resins have been unsuccessful.

PRESENTATION
Capsule: 300mg – Lopid® and non-proprietary.
Tablet: 600mg – Lopid® and non-proprietary.

DOSAGE/ ADMINISTRATION
Oral: experience in children is limited, refer to lipidologist.

CONTRA-INDICATIONS & WARNINGS, INTERACTIONS, PREGNANCY, BREAST-FEEDING, SIDE-EFFECTS, POISONING/TOXICITY, PHARMACODYNAMIC PROPERTIES	See bezafibrate monograph.

EXCIPIENTS
Contact manufacturers for further details.

LICENSED STATUS
Not licensed for use in children.

G

Aminoglycoside antibiotic.

USES
Generally, first-line aminoglycoside. Licensed for use in urinary tract infections (UTI), chest infections, bacteraemia, septicaemia, neonatal infections and other systemic infections.

In cystic fibrosis patients – nebulised treatment of *Pseudomonas aeruginosa* infections; treatment of early *Pseudomonas aeruginosa* infections not cleared by oral ciprofloxacin plus nebulised colistin and treatment of moderate to severe exacerbations, in combination with other antibiotics (e.g. third generation cephalosporins, anti-pseudomonal penicillins, beta-lactam antibiotics and polymyxins).

Note: tobramycin is recommended as it is more active against *Pseudomonas aeruginosa* than gentamicin.

Intrathecal injection: supplement to systemic therapy in bacterial meningitis, ventriculitis and CNS infections.

Ear drops: treatment of superficial ear infections caused by sensitive organisms.

PRESENTATION
Drops (for ear or eye): 0.3% – Garamycin® and Genticin®.

Injection: (as sulphate, all strengths stated as gentamicin base) 10mg in 1mL, 2mL – Cidomycin® Paediatric, 40mg in 1mL, 2mL – Cidomycin®, Genticin® and non-proprietary; 40mg in 1mL, 1mL and 6mL – non-proprietary.

Intrathecal injection: (as sulphate) 5mg in 1mL – Cidomycin®.

DOSAGE & ADMINISTRATION
Many dose regimens exist for aminoglycosides depending on target concentrations aimed for and patient groups treated. The dose regimens shown here are generally accepted initial doses and dose adjustments should be made in the light of serum concentration measurement.

Newborn infant (birth to 1 month)
Extended dosing regimen

Route	*Postconceptional age	Dose	Frequency (times daily)	Notes
IV	<32 weeks	4–5mg/kg	36 hourly	Plasma samples usually taken around the third dose aiming for a 1 hour post dose (peak) of 5–10mg/L and a pre dose (trough) level of <2mg/L If there is no change in the dosage regimen or renal function repeat levels every 3-4 days.
	>32 weeks	4–5mg/kg	24 hourly	

*Postconceptional age = gestational age plus postnatal age.

Neonates presenting with patent ductus arteriosus (PDA), prolonged hypoxia or treated with indometacin (indomethacin) may have impaired elimination of gentamicin due to reduced glomerular filtration rate (GFR) and increase in dosage interval may be necessary.

Newborn infant (birth to 1 month)
Intrathecal dose

Route	Age birth–1 month	Frequency (times daily)	Notes
Intrathecal	1–2mg	every 24 to 48 hours	Aim for CSF level of 5–10mg/L Only preservative free intrathecal preparation should be used.

Child
Divided daily dose regimen

Route	Age 1 month–2 years	2–12 years	12–18 years	Frequency (times daily)	Notes
IV/IM	← 2.5mg/kg →		1–2mg/kg	3	Plasma samples usually taken around the third or fourth dose aiming for a pre dose (trough) level of <2mg/L and a 1 hour post dose (peak) 5–10mg/L

G

Child
Divided daily dose regimen continued

Route	Age			Frequency (times daily)	Notes
	1 month–2 years	2–12 years	12–18 years		
Intrathecal or intra-ventricular	←	1mg	→	1	Assess MIC of infecting organism and adjust dose to ensure adequate levels are maintained. May be increased if necessary to 5mg. CSF level should not exceed 10mg/L Accompanied by systemic therapy.
Nebulised	40mg	<8 years 80mg >8 years 160mg	160mg	2 2	Use preservative-free (phenol-free) formulations. Administer after physiotherapy and bronchodilators.
IV for cystic fibrosis patients	←	3mg/kg	→	3	Starting dose. Monitor blood levels after the third dose. Aim for a trough of <2mg/L and 1 hour post dose (peak) of 8–12mg/L.

Child
Single daily dose regimen

Route	Age			Frequency (times daily)	Notes
	1 month–2 years	2–12 years	12–18 years		
IV	←	7mg/kg	→	1	Plasma samples are usually taken at 18-24 hours after the first dose aiming for a level <1mg/L If the levels are >1mg/L then the dosing interval is normally increased by 12 hours. 1 hour post dose (peak) levels can be taken with a target range of 16-20mg/L. If there is no change in the dosage regimen or in renal function repeat levels every 3–4 days.

ADMINISTRATION
IV: slow IV injection over 3-5 minutes injected neat or diluted in NaCl 0.9% or glucose 5%. IV infusion over 30-60 minutes for high dose 'child – single daily dose regimen' in an appropriate volume of fluid. Compatible with NaCl 0.9% and 0.45%, glucose 5% and 10% and glucose 4%/ NaCl 0.18%. In general, gentamicin injection should not be mixed with penicillins, cephalosporins, erythromycin, heparin or sodium bicarbonate. Adequate flushing or administration at separate sites is suggested.

Intrathecal: ONLY INTRATHECAL PREPARATION SHOULD BE USED.

Nebulised: optimum nebuliser volume is 3mL; make up volume with NaCl 0.9%. An active venturi nebuliser system with outlet is recommended so that exhaled antibiotic can be discharged via a window, otherwise an effective filter system should be used. May be mixed with colistin if time factor is crucial; add the gentamicin dose to the colistin vial immediately before use and then make up to 3mL with NaCl 0.9%.

Ear drops: 2-3 drops 3-4 times daily and at night; children and adults.

CONTRA-INDICATIONS & WARNINGS
Known hypersensitivity to gentamicin, myasthenia gravis. Patients should be well hydrated during therapy and renal function monitored. In patients with impaired renal function dosage and/or frequency of administration must be adjusted in response to serum drug concentrations and the extent of renal impairment. The 'child – single daily dose regimen', is not recommended in children with renal impairment. Ear drops should not be used if there is perforation of the ear drum.

G

Hearing tests are recommended for cystic fibrosis patients having repeated courses of aminoglycosides.

INTERACTIONS
Increased risk of ototoxicity and nephrotoxicity with *cephalosporins, vancomycin, ciclosporin (cyclosporin), cisplatin, diuretics such as furosemide (frusemide), amphotericin, indometacin (indomethacin)*. Enhances effects of *non-depolarising muscle relaxants. Calcium IV* may reverse this effect. May antagonise effects of *neostigmine* and *pyridostigmine*. Contra-indicated in myasthenia gravis. Aminoglycosides have a magnesium-like effect acting at the neuromuscular junction pre-junctionally to reduce transmitter release and post-junctionally to reduce receptor sensitivity.

PREGNANCY
Gentamicin crosses the placenta and it should only be used if the potential benefits outweigh the possible risks. There is a risk of fetal ototoxicity. If given, serum gentamicin level monitoring is essential.

BREAST-FEEDING
Gentamicin is excreted into breast milk but in the absence of any gastrointestinal inflammation the amount ingested by the infant is unlikely to result in significant blood levels.

SIDE-EFFECTS
Nephrotoxicity and ototoxicity can occur if optimum blood levels are exceeded; unlikely if nebulised. Bronchospasm can occur with nebulised gentamicin.

POISONING/TOXICITY
Haemodialysis will aid removal from the blood. Intravenous calcium salts may be used to counter neuromuscular blockade. Toxicity unlikely if nebulised. The oral ingestion of the contents of one bottle of ear drops is unlikely to cause any significant adverse effect.

PHARMACOKINETIC PROPERTIES
Gentamicin distributes similarly to amikacin. 50-93% is eliminated unchanged in the urine in 24 hours in patients with normal renal function. Topical application can result in some systemic absorption. There is little diffusion into the cerebrospinal fluid and even if the meninges are inflamed, effective concentrations may not be achieved. Plasma elimination half-life is 2-3 hours in children >1 year of age, 3-3.5 hours in 1 week to 6 months, 5.5 hours in full-term infants, 6 hours in premature infants >2kg, 8 hours in 1.5-2kg, 12 hours in <1.5kg.

EXCIPIENTS
Intrathecal injection is preservative free.
Ear drops: all preparations contain benzalkonium chloride.
Contact manufacturers for further details.

LICENSED STATUS
Licensed for use in all ages as divided dose regimen. Injection solution not licensed for nebulisation.

Glucagon

A polypeptide pancreatic hormone which acts on hepatic glycogen to release glucose into the bloodstream.

USES
Treatment of acute hypoglycaemia.
Hyperinsulinaemia (as an interim measure if IV access is a problem).
Pituitary function testing for growth hormone secretion.

PRESENTATION
Injection: powder for reconstitution 1mg vial with prefilled syringe containing Water for Injections – GlucaGen® HypoKit.

DOSAGE

Indication	Route	Age				Frequency (times daily)	Notes
		birth–1 month	1 month–2 years	2–12 years	12–18 years		
Severe hypo-glycaemia in the treatment of diabetes.	IM, SC or IV rapid bolus	20 microgram/kg	500 microgram	500 microgram – 1mg (< 25kg: 500 microgram) (> 25kg: 1mg)		single dose	Should be effective within 15 minutes. If not. give IV glucose 5-10%.

G

DOSAGE continued

Indication	Route	Age				Frequency (times daily)	Notes
		birth–1 month	1 month–2 years	2–12 years	12–18 years		
Hyper-insulinaemia	IV infusion	1-10 microgram/kg/hour		-	-	continuous	Adjust to other treatment. Also stimulates insulin release.
	IM/IV	← 1mg →		-	-	single dose	Also stimulates insulin release.
Growth hormone test	IM	-	← 100 microgram/kg (maximum dose 1mg) →			single dose	Must eat a meal before discharge as deaths reported from rebound hypoglycaemia.

ADMINISTRATION
IM, IV or SC: do not use if the solution contains fibrils or solid particles. Glucagon should not be added to infusion fluids containing calcium ions as this causes precipitation of the glucagon.

CONTRA-INDICATIONS & WARNINGS
Phaeochromocytoma. Ineffective in chronic hypoglycaemia, starvation and adrenal insufficiency.

PREGNANCY
Does not cross the placenta. Its use in pregnant women with diabetes has been reported and no harmful effects are known.

BREAST-FEEDING
As it is degraded in the gastrointestinal tract and cannot be absorbed in its intact form, it will not exert any metabolic effect in the child.

SIDE-EFFECTS
Nausea, vomiting, diarrhoea and hypokalaemia.

POISONING/TOXICITY
Has positive inotropic and chronotropic effects. The serum potassium may decrease.

PHARMACOKINETIC PROPERTIES
Should be effective within 10-15 minutes. Plasma half-life is 3-6 minutes.

EXCIPIENTS
Includes lactose. See manufacturers SPC for further details.

LICENSED STATUS
Licensed for use in all ages for severe hypoglycaemia, but not licensed for growth hormone tests or hyperinsulinaemia.

Glutamine

USES
In glutamine depletion as part of an intravenous PN regimen use as a supplement to amino acid solution or an amino acid containing infusion in hypercatabolic states as it improves gut integrity. After bowel surgery it also supports immune function.

PRESENTATION
Solution: N(2)-L-alanyl–L-glutamine 200mg/mL (providing L-alanine 82mg and L-glutamine 134.6mg), 50mL and 100mL – Dipeptiven®.
Sterile infusion: L-glutamine 2.5% (2.5g per 100mL Water for Injections), 160ml and 800mL – manufactured 'special'.

DOSAGE
Child: 250–500mg/kg/day of L-glutamine has been used.
Up to 2mL/kg Dipeptiven® can be used in adults; it has been used in children and 2mL/kg is approximately equivalent to 300mg/kg L-glutamine.

ADMINISTRATION
IV: infusion as part of a balanced PN regimen.

G

CONTRA-INDICATIONS & WARNINGS
Severe renal insufficiency with creatinine clearance
<25mL/minute/1.73m^2. Severe hepatic insufficiency,
severe metabolic acidosis, hypersensitivity.

INTERACTIONS
None noted to date.

PREGNANCY/BREAST-FEEDING
Not recommended. Contact local Medicines Information
Centre for further details.

SIDE-EFFECTS
None known with correct administration.

POISONING/TOXICITY
As with other infusions, chills, nausea and vomiting can
occur when infusion rates are exceeded – stop infusion
immediately in this case.

LICENSED STATUS
L-glutamine 2.5% is a 'special' and as such is unlicensed.
Dipeptiven® is not licensed for use in children.

FURTHER INFORMATION
L-glutamine 2.5% infusion is available from Oxford Nutrition; store in a freezer.
A moderately soluble L-glutamine powder for oral use is available from Oxford Nutrition in 2g, 5g and 10g sachets.

Glutaraldehyde

Virucidal agent with drying properties.

PRESENTATION
Solution: 10% – Glutarol®.

USES
Treatment of warts especially plantar warts.

DOSAGE/ADMINISTRATION
Topical: remove dead skin by gentle rubbing with pumice stone before applying twice daily. Allow each drop to dry
before next is applied.

CONTRA-INDICATIONS & WARNINGS
Not to be used on face, anal or perianal region. Protect
surrounding skin and avoid broken skin.

INTERACTIONS
None known.

PREGNANCY/BREAST-FEEDING
No special precautions.

SIDE-EFFECTS
Skin irritation.

POISONING/TOXICITY
Treat accidental oral ingestion immediately by gastric
lavage with 2-5% aqueous sodium bicarbonate solution.
Monitor fluid and electrolyte balance and provide
appropriate supportive measures. Symptoms are
headache, nausea, vomiting, diarrhoea and respiratory
depression.

EXCIPIENTS
See manufacturers SPC for further details.

LICENSED STATUS
Licensed for use in children and adults.

FURTHER INFORMATION
Flammable. Avoid inhaling vapour.

G

Rectal stimulant.

USES
Constipation.

PRESENTATION
Suppository: gelatin 140mg, glycerol 700mg, purified water to 1g; infants 1g, child 2g, adult 4g – non-proprietary.

DOSAGE

Route	Age			Frequency	Notes
	1 month–2 years	2–12 years	12–18 years		
Rectal	<1year 1g >1year 2g	2g	4g	single dose	Moisten with water before insertion.

Glyceryl trinitrate

Vasodilator; its principal action being relaxation of vascular smooth muscle. Therapeutic IV doses reduce systolic, diastolic and mean arterial blood pressure.

USES
Control of hypertension during and after cardiac surgery; to increase cardiac output and to decrease peripheral vascular resistance in cardiac failure especially post-operative cardiac surgery; myocardial ischaemia (coronary artery vasodilatation).

PRESENTATION
Injection: 1mg in 1mL, 5mL vial and 50mL vial – Nitronal®, 10mL ampoule and 50mL bottle – Nitrocine®; 5mg in 1mL – 5mL and 10mL ampoules – non-proprietary.

DOSAGE

Route	Age				Frequency (times daily)	Notes
	birth–1 month	1 month–2 years	2–12 years	12–18 years		
IV infusion	◄── 200 nanogram/kg/minute – 5 microgram/kg/minute ──►				continuous	This dose may be increased as necessary to a maximum of 10 microgram/kg/minute. Monitor blood pressure and heart rate. Tolerance may occur with prolonged infusion.

ADMINISTRATION
IV: ampoule and vial dosage forms are concentrated solutions of a potent drug. They are usually diluted prior to infusion but the 1mg in 1mL strength injection can be given undiluted.
Only glucose 5% or NaCl 0.9% may be used as diluents. The maximum recommended final concentration is 400 microgram in 1mL, though concentrations of 1mg in 1mL in 5% glucose have been used. Dilutions in glucose 5% or NaCl 0.9% are stable for 24 hours at room temperature. As nitrates are adsorbed onto PVC, administration should be via a syringe pump or a rigid burette set with non-PVC tubing e.g. polyethylene.

CONTRA-INDICATIONS & WARNINGS
Hypersensitivity to nitrates, hypotension, hypovolaemia, increased intracranial pressure, constrictive pericarditis, pericardial tamponade, severe anaemia, arterial hypoxaemia, obstructive hypertrophic cardiomyopathy. Use with caution in patients with hypothyroidism, severe hypothermia, predisposition to closed-angle glaucoma, severe impairment of hepatic and/or renal function.

G

INTERACTIONS
Orthostatic hypotension may occur with the combined use of *calcium-channel blockers, antihypertensive agents, phenothiazines* and *tricyclic antidepressants*.

PREGNANCY
Safety for use during pregnancy has not been established. Contact local Medicines Information Centre for advice.

BREAST-FEEDING
Safety for use in the nursing mother has not been established. Contact local Medicines Information Centre for advice.

SIDE-EFFECTS
Hypotension, tachycardia, nausea, vomiting, headache, dizziness, restlessness, muscle twitching, retrosternal discomfort, palpitations and paradoxical bradycardia.

POISONING/TOXICITY
Overdosage usually results in hypotension and tachycardia and can be reversed by elevating the legs or decreasing or terminating the infusion. In severe cases IV administration of phenylephrine is recommended. Hypoxia due to methaemaglobinaemia can lead to cyanosis, metabolic acidosis, coma, convulsions and cardiovascular collapse. Monitor arterial blood gases and methaemoglobin levels as indicated.

PHARMACOKINETIC PROPERTIES
Glyceryl trinitrate is widely distributed in the body and is rapidly metabolised to dinitrates and mononitrates with a short half-life, in adults estimated to be 1-4 minutes. This results in a low plasma concentration after IV infusion. Glyceryl trinitrate is also well absorbed from the gastrointestinal tract. At plasma concentrations of between 50-500 nanogram/mL, the binding of glyceryl trinitrate to plasma proteins is approximately 60% and 30% respectively. Glyceryl trinitrate is metabolised primarily in the liver and to a lesser extent in plasma. The products of metabolism are excreted in urine and bile.

EXCIPIENTS
Some glyceryl trinitrate IV preparations contain propylene glycol which can lead to lactic acidosis. It is recommended that the use of these preparations be restricted to not more than 3 successive days. Contact manufacturers for further details.

LICENSED STATUS
Not licensed for use in children.

Glycine

USES
Isovaleric acidaemia.

PRESENTATION
Powder: 100g.

DOSAGE

Route	Age				Frequency (times daily)	Notes
	birth–1 month	1 month–2 years	2–12 years	12–18 years		
Oral	←		50mg/kg		→ 3	Dose may be increased to 200mg/kg 3 times a day during acute episodes.

ADMINISTRATION
Glycine powder is freely soluble in water. It may be mixed with infant feeds or water before administration.

CONTRA-INDICATIONS & WARNINGS
Do not use glycine in anuric patients as therapy depends on excretion of isovaleric acid as isovalerylglycine. Use with caution in liver/renal impairment.

INTERACTIONS
Aspirin interferes with synthesis of isovalerylglycine and is therefore contra-indicated.

PREGNANCY/BREAST-FEEDING
No information available.

G

SIDE-EFFECTS
None known.

PHARMACODYNAMIC PROPERTIES
Forms isovalerylglycine, which has a higher urinary clearance, with excess isovaleric acid.

LICENSED STATUS
Not licensed for use in the UK.

FURTHER INFORMATION
Powder available from Scientific Hospital Supplies.

Glycopyrronium bromide

Antimuscarinic agent with peripheral effects similar to those of atropine.

USES
Premedication to decrease salivary, tracheobronchial and pharyngeal secretions and to reduce the acidity and volume of gastric contents in patients undergoing surgical procedures, and to decrease intra-operative bradycardia and hypotension induced by anaesthetic agents. Protection against peripheral muscarinic actions of anticholinesterase agents during reversal of residual non-depolarising neuromuscular block.

PRESENTATION
Tablet: 1mg and 2mg (both scored) – named patient.
Injection: 200 microgram in 1mL; 1mL and 3mL ampoule – Robinul®. 500 microgram in 1mL with neostigmine 2.5mg; 1mL ampoule – Robinul-Neostigmine®.

DOSAGE

Indication	Route	Age				Frequency (times daily)	Notes
		birth–1 month	1 month–2 years	2–12 years	12–18 years		
Premedication and intra-operative use	IM/IV	–	←	4-8 microgram/kg	→	single dose	Maximum dose 200 micrograms; larger doses may result in profound and prolonged antisialogogue effect.
Antagonism of neostigmine muscarinic effects	IV	–	←	10 microgram/kg	→	single dose	With 50 microgram/kg neostigmine using the combined preparation. Used for reversal of residual non-depolarising neuromuscular block.
Control of upper airway secretions	Oral	–	←	40–100 microgram/kg	→	3-4	Note: oral dose is 10 times the parenteral dose.

ADMINISTRATION
IM injection: use undiluted injection 30–60 minutes prior to anaesthetic.
IV injection: use undiluted injection at induction.
Oral: injection can be given orally. Tablets can be dispersed in water.

CONTRA-INDICATIONS & WARNINGS
Contra-indications: urinary tract obstruction, ileus, pyloric stenosis.
Cautions: not recommended in children <1 month, conditions characterised by tachycardia e.g. thyrotoxicosis, heart failure, unstable cardiovascular status, hypertension, obstructive disease of the gastrointestinal tract, severe ulcerative colitis, hepatic and renal disease, glaucoma, myasthenia gravis, asthma, pyrexial patients due to inhibition of sweating and in asthmatics. Infants with Down's syndrome may be hypersensitive to the antimuscarinic effects.

INTERACTIONS
Likely to counteract the gastrointestinal motility induced

G

by *cisapride, domperidone* and *metoclopramide*. Concurrent use with other *anticholinergics* may intensify the anti muscarinic effect.

PREGNANCY
Glycopyrrolate does not cross the placenta in significant amounts. It has been recommended as the anticholinergic agent of choice during anaesthesia for ECT in pregnant patients. There is a lack of information in human patients. Contact local Medicines Information Centre for advice.

BREAST-FEEDING
It may cause a decrease in lactation. Contact local Medicines Information Centre for advice.

SIDE-EFFECTS
CNS: drowsiness, headache, fever, restlessness, hallucinations, confusion, dizziness, insomnia, inhibition of sweating, tremor.
Cardiovascular: tachycardia, hypotension, cardiac arrhythmias.
Gastrointestinal: impaired gastrointestinal motility, constipation, dry mouth, oesophageal reflux.
Ophthalmic: blurred vision, pupilary dilation and raised intraocular pressure.

Skin: skin flushing, irritation at the injection site.
Genito-urinary: urinary retention.

POISONING/TOXICITY
Symptoms: tachycardia, rapid respiration, hyperpyrexia and CNS stimulation marked by restlessness, confusion, excitement, ataxia, incoordination, paranoid and psychotic reactions, hallucinations and delirium and occasionally seizures.
Treatment: an anticholinesterase such as neostigmine may be given by the parenteral route.

PHARMACOKINETIC PROPERTIES
Poorly and irregularly absorbed from gastrointestinal tract (approx 10-25%), though it has been used orally. Absorption following IM administration is rapid. Rapidly distributed. Excreted in bile and urine mostly as unchanged drug relatively slowly with quantifiable plasma levels remaining up to 8 hours after administration. Following IM or SC injection, peak effects occur within 30-45 minutes, following IV injection onset of action occurs within 1 minute. Vagal blocking effects persist for 2-3 hours and the antisialogogue effects persist for up to 7 hours.

LICENSED STATUS
Licensed for use in children and adults as pre medication and for reversal of neuromuscular block as the combined preparation with neostigmine. Tablets are not licensed for use in the UK.

FURTHER INFORMATION
Tablets available from IDIS World Medicines.

GM–CSF (molgramostim)

Recombinant human granulocyte macrophage-colony stimulating factor (rHu GM-CSF).

PRESENTATION
Injection: 1.67 million unit (150 microgram) vial, 3.33 million unit (300 microgram) vial and 4.44 million unit (400 microgram) vial – Leucomax®.

USES
Reduction of severity of neutropenia (and risk of infection) in cytotoxic chemotherapy; acceleration of myeloid recovery following bone marrow transplant (BMT); neutropenia in patients treated with ganciclovir in AIDS-related cytomegalovirus (CMV) retinitis; neutropenia in preterm neonates (very limited experience).

DOSAGE
Newborn infant (birth to 1 month)

Route	Age	Frequency	Notes
	birth–1 month	(times daily)	
IV infusion (over at least 2 hours)	5 microgram/kg	1	Very limited information on neonatal use. A small number of studies have been carried out in neutropenic preterm neonates. Consult expert opinion before prescribing.

Child

Indication	Route	Age			Frequency (times daily)	Notes
		1 month– 2 years	2–12 years	12–18 years		
Cytotoxic chemotherapy	SC injection	←	5–10 microgram/kg	→	1	Start treatment 24 hours after the last dose of chemotherapy and continue for 7-10 days.
BMT	IV infusion (over 4–6 hours)	←	10 microgram/kg	→	1	Start treatment the day after BMT and continue until the absolute neutrophil count is $\geq 1 \times 10^9$/L Maximum duration of treatment 30 days.
Adjunct in ganciclovir treatment	SC injection	←	5 microgram/kg	→	1	After the fifth dose adjust to maintain desirable absolute neutrophil and WBC count.

ADMINISTRATION
IV: reconstitute powder with Water for Injections. May be further diluted in NaCl 0.9% or glucose 5% (then stable for 24 hours in refrigerator). Final concentration must be >80,000 units (approximately 7 microgram) per mL.
Only compatible with certain infusion sets. See manufacturers SPC for details. In-line filter recommended for IV administration. Do NOT use with a Port-a-Cath (Pharmacia) system.

CONTRA-INDICATIONS & WARNINGS
Myeloid malignancy. Monitor FBC closely.

PREGNANCY/BREAST-FEEDING
Contact local Medicines Information Centre for advice.

SIDE-EFFECTS
Nausea, diarrhoea, vomiting, anorexia, dyspnoea, asthenia, fatigue, rash, fever, musculoskeletal pain, flushing, rigors, local reactions after SC injection. Serious reactions reported include anaphylaxis, cardiac failure, capillary leak syndrome, cerebrovascular disorders, confusion, convulsions, hypotension, cardiac rhythm abnormalities, intracranial hypertension, pericardial effusion, pulmonary oedema, pericarditis, pleural effusion, syncope.

POISONING/TOXICITY
Symptomatic treatment with frequent monitoring of vital signs and close observation of patient.

PHARMACOKINETIC PROPERTIES
Elimination half-life of 1-2 hours after IV administration and 2-3 hours after SC administration.

EXCIPIENTS
Include human albumin. See manufacturers SPC for further details.

LICENSED STATUS
Not licensed for use in children.

Gonadorelin (Gonadotrophin-releasing hormone; GnRH; LH–RH)

USES
Assessment of anterior pituitary function; assessment of delayed puberty; may be used in combination with protirelin (thyrotrophin releasing hormone; TRH) for a more complete evaluation of the hypothalamic-anterior pituitary-gonadal axis.

PRESENTATION
Injection: 100 microgram vial with diluent – HRF®.

DOSAGE

Route	Age				Frequency	Notes
	birth–1 month	1 month–2 years	2–12 years	12–18 years		
IV/SC	←	2.5 microgram/kg (maximum dose 100 microgram)	→	100 microgram	single dose	

G

ADMINISTRATION
IV/SC: reconstitute before use with the diluent provided. Can be given either by rapid IV injection or SC injection.

CONTRA-INDICATIONS & WARNINGS
Pregnancy. Do not use in children <1 year of age as diluent contains benzyl alcohol.

INTERACTIONS
Response to gonadorelin may be blunted by medicines causing a rise in prolactin e.g. *phenothiazines*, *metoclopramide* and *digoxin*.

PREGNANCY/BREAST-FEEDING
Manufacturer states it should not be administered in pregnancy or to nursing mothers.

SIDE-EFFECTS
Side-effects are rare but facial flushing, abdominal pain, headache and increased menstrual bleeding have occasionally been reported.

POISONING/TOXICITY
Overdose has never been reported – unlikely to be a problem.

EXCIPIENTS
HRF® diluent contains benzyl alcohol.

LICENSED STATUS
Licensed for >1 year of age. HRF® is a hospital-only product.

Goserelin

Gonadorelin analogue.

USES
Central precocious puberty.

PRESENTATION
Implant (depot): 3.6mg – Zoladex®.
Implant (sustained release depot): 10.8mg – Zoladex LA®.

DOSAGE
3.6mg every 4 weeks or 10.8mg every 12 weeks. Injections may need to be given more frequently (e.g. every 3 weeks or every 10 weeks) if patients show signs of failure of hormone suppression.

ADMINISTRATION
SC injection: given SC into the anterior abdominal wall. Injection sites should be rotated to prevent atrophy and nodule formation.

CONTRA-INDICATIONS
Known hypersensitivity of luteinising hormone-releasing hormone (LHRH) analogues.

PREGNANCY
Contra-indicated in pregnancy; exclude pregnancy before treatment and use non-hormonal contraception during treatment.

BREAST-FEEDING
Not recommended in breast-feeding.

SIDE-EFFECTS
Hypersensitivity reactions, hypotension or hypertension. Local reactions include mild bruising at the site of injection. Sweating and mood changes including depression have occurred.

POISONING/TOXICITY
Symptomatic management only

PHARMACODYNAMIC PROPERTIES
Goserelin is slowly absorbed over the first 8 days following injection, thereafter absorption is steady for the remainder of the course. Serum half-life is 4.2 hours.

G

EXCIPIENTS
See manufacturers SPC for further details.

LICENSED STATUS
Not licensed for use in children.

$5HT_3$ antagonist.

USES
Prevention and treatment of chemotherapy induced nausea and vomiting.

PRESENTATION
Tablet: 1mg, 2mg – Kytril®.
Liquid: 1mg in 5mL – Kytril®.
Injection: 1mg in 1mL; 1mL and 3mL ampoule – Kytril®.

DOSAGE

Route	Age			Frequency (times daily)	Notes
	1 month–2 years	2–12 years	12–18 years		
Oral	← 20 microgram/kg → (to a maximum of 1mg)		1mg	2	Give the first dose 1 hour prior to starting chemotherapy.
IV	← 40 microgram/kg → (to a maximum of 3mg)		3mg	single dose (immediately prior to chemotherapy)	One additional dose may be given within a 24 hour period.

ADMINISTRATION
IV: injection or by IV infusion over 5 minutes diluted in 10-30mL NaCl 0.9% or glucose 5%.

CONTRA-INDICATIONS & WARNINGS
Hypersensitivity to granisetron or similar substances. Potential need for dose reduction in hepatic impairment.

INTERACTIONS
No clinically apparent drug interactions recorded.

PREGNANCY
Animal studies have shown no teratogenic effect, but there is no experience in human pregnancy. Contact local Medicines Information Centre for advice.

BREAST-FEEDING
Contact local Medicines Information Centre for advice.

SIDE-EFFECTS
Headache and constipation.

POISONING/TOXICITY
Symptomatic supportive care as appropriate. No specific antidote to granisetron.

PHARMACOKINETIC PROPERTIES
Oral bioavailability reduced to about 60% as a result of first-pass metabolism. Clearance primarily by hepatic metabolism. Approximately 10% of the drug can be recovered unchanged in the urine within 48 hours of administration.

EXCIPIENTS
See manufacturers SPC for further details.

LICENSED STATUS
Injection and oral liquid are licensed for use in children and adults. Tablets are not licensed for use in children.

Griseofulvin

Antifungal agent for treatment of dermatophyte infections.

USES
Treatment of fungal infection especially of the nails.

PRESENTATION
Tablet: 125mg and 500mg – Grisovin®.
Suspension: 125mg in 5mL – (imported).

G

DOSAGE

Route	Age			Frequency (times daily)	Notes
	1 month–2 years	2–12 years	12–18 years		
Oral	← 10mg/kg →		500mg	1	Local resistance may require doses of up to 20mg/kg.

ADMINISTRATION
Oral: to be taken with or after food.

CONTRA-INDICATIONS & WARNINGS
Liver failure, lupus erythematosus, porphyria. Males should not father children within 6 months of treatment.

INTERACTIONS
Accelerates metabolism of *warfarin* and *oral contraceptives*. *Phenobarbital (phenobarbitone)* accelerates griseofulvin metabolism. Plasma *ciclosporin (cyclosporin)* levels may be reduced.

PREGNANCY
Avoid during treatment and for 1 month after.

BREAST-FEEDING
Safety not established. Contact local Medicines Information Centre for advice.

SIDE-EFFECTS
Headache, nausea, vomiting, rashes, photosensitivity, dizziness, fatigue, agranulocytosis and leucopenia.

POISONING/TOXICITY
Symptomatic treatment.

EXCIPIENTS
Contact manufacturers for further details.

LICENSED STATUS
Tablet licensed for use in children and adults. Suspension is not licensed for use in the UK.

FURTHER INFORMATION
Suspension is available from IDIS World Medicines.

Haemophilus influenzae type b vaccine (Hib)

USES
The main use is as part of the routine infant immunisation schedule when it is given at 8, 12 and 16 weeks of age mixed with diphtheria, tetanus and pertussis vaccines (DTP) and at the same time as polio and meningococcal C vaccines. Children of 13-48 months who have not been immunised need receive only one dose of vaccine to develop immunity.
Older patients who are actually or functionally asplenic are particularly susceptible to invasive haemophilus disease and should also be given one dose of the vaccine, if not previously immunised. Consideration should also be given to administering the vaccine to immunosuppressed individuals.

PRESENTATION
Injection: (freeze dried pellet made up to a single dose of 0.5mL) – ACT-HIB® and Hiberix®; (single dose suspension) – HibTITER®.
Each dose contains 10micrograms of purified capsular polysaccharide (polyribosylribitol phosphate – PRP) conjugated either to tetanus toxoid – ACT-HIB® and Hiberix® or a non-toxic variant of diphtheria toxoid (CRM_{197}) – HibTITER®.
Hib vaccine is also available in combination packs with DTP, to be reconstituted immediately prior to administration (ACT-HIB DTP®, see separate monograph).

DOSAGE/ADMINISTRATION
IM or deep SC: 0.5mL.
Some DTP and Hib preparations can be mixed in the same syringe immediately prior to administration. ACT-HIB® may be reconstituted with a single dose of Adsorbed Diphtheria, Tetanus and Pertussis Vaccine BP. Hiberix® can be mixed with DTP Vaccine Behring or Trivax-AD (DTP) immediately prior to administration (check manufacturers' literature for further details).

G

CONTRA-INDICATIONS & WARNINGS
As for vaccines generally; also the Joint Committee on Vaccination and Immunisation (JCVI) advises that when a severe local reaction occurs after the administration of a dose of combined DTP and Hib vaccines, the vaccines should be given separately. A severe systemic reaction resulting from the combined vaccines is likely to be due to the pertussis component. If the whole cell vaccine has been used, consideration should be given to using acellular pertussis vaccine instead.

INTERACTIONS
It can be given simultaneously with, or at any interval before or after any other vaccine. It should not be mixed with DTaP vaccine as this may reduce the protective response to Hib. The vaccines containing tetanus and CRM$_{197}$ conjugates can be used interchangeably.

PREGNANCY/BREAST-FEEDING
No information is available, but there are no grounds to believe it would be harmful.

SIDE-EFFECTS
Swelling and redness may appear at the site of injection within 3-4 hours and resolve within 24 hours. The incidence of these effects declines with subsequent doses.

POISONING/TOXICITY
No data available.

PHARMACODYNAMIC PROPERTIES
Protects by stimulating the production of anti-PRP antibodies. The vaccine has been shown to reduce nasal carriage as well as prevent disease.

EXCIPIENTS
ACT-HIB®: TRIS and sucrose.
Hiberix®: Lactose.

LICENSED STATUS
Licensed for use as described.

FURTHER INFORMATION
Only protects against Haemophilus influenzae type b, not other serotypes. Immunisation with a conjugate containing tetanus toxoid or CRM$_{197}$, does not reduce the need for diphtheria or tetanus vaccination. Store at 2-8°C and do not freeze.
From February 2003, the Department of Health has advised that the Hib and DTaP vaccines should not be mixed, but they can be given on the same occasion.
Materials of bovine origin may be used in the manufacturing process. Trace amounts of the original material may be present in the final product however, all such material is obtained from sources known to be free of BSE.

Haemorrhoidal preparations

Soothing haemorrhoidal preparations.

Containing mild astringents
May give symptomatic relief in haemorrhoids. May also contain lubricants, vasoconstrictors or mild antiseptics.

Containing local anaesthetics
Used to relieve pain associated with haemorrhoids and pruritus ani. Local anaesthetic ointments can be absorbed through the rectal mucosa, therefore excessive application should be avoided, particularly in infants and children. Use for short periods of a few days only since they may cause sensitisation of the anal skin.

Preparations on sale to the public include:
Anacal® (heparinoid, laureth '9')
Anodesyn® (allantoin, lidocaine (lignocaine))
Anusol® cream (bismuth oxide, Peru balsam, zinc oxide)
Anusol® ointment and suppositories (bismuth oxide, bismuth subgallate, Peru balsam, zinc oxide)
Germoloids® (lidocaine (lignocaine), zinc oxide)
Hemocane® (benzoic acid, bismuth oxide, cinnamic acid, lidocaine (lignocaine), zinc oxide)
Lanacane® cream (benzocaine, chlorothymol)
Nupercainal® (cinchocaine).

Compound haemorrhoidal preparations with corticosteroids

Betnovate® rectal ointment

Analgesic, anti-inflammatory and vasoconstrictor properties.

USES
Relief of symptoms of itching, irritation, discomfort or pain associated with local non-infective anal or peri-anal conditions such as external haemorrhoids.

PRESENTATION
Rectal ointment: betamethasone valerate 0.05%, lidocaine (lignocaine) hydrochloride 2.5% and phenylephrine hydrochloride 0.1%; with applicator.

DOSAGE

Route	Age			Frequency (times daily)	Notes
	1 month–2 years	2–12 years	12–18 years		
Topical	←	Small amount of ointment	→	2-3	Reduce to once daily when inflammation is subsiding. Limit course of treatment to 7 days.

ADMINISTRATION
Rectal: use applicator if internal administration required.

CONTRA-INDICATIONS & WARNINGS
Contra-indicated in primary cutaneous viral infections. Hypersensitivity to any component of preparation. Not indicated in treatment of primarily infected skin lesions caused by infection with fungi or bacteria or in dermatoses in children <1 year including dermatitis and nappy rash.

PREGNANCY
Inadequate evidence of safety.

SIDE-EFFECTS
If used for prolonged periods consider possibility of hypothalamic pituitary axis suppression. May cause local atrophic changes in skin. Reports of pigmentation changes and hypertrichosis with topical steroids.

POISONING/TOXICITY
Chronic overdosage – hypercortisolism may appear and treatment should be stopped.

LICENSED STATUS
No lower age limit.

Proctosedyl®

Cinchocaine (dibucaine) hydrochloride is a local anaesthetic which relieves pain and relaxes sphincteric spasm. Pruritus and inflammation are relieved by hydrocortisone, which also decreases serous discharge.

USES
Short-term relief (<7 days) of pain, irritation and pruritus associated with haemorrhoids and pruritus ani.

PRESENTATION
Ointment: cinchocaine (dibucaine) hydrochloride 0.5% and hydrocortisone 0.5%.
Suppository: cinchocaine (dibucaine) hydrochloride 5mg and hydrocortisone 5mg.

DOSAGE
Ointment: apply to affected area morning and evening and after each bowel evacuation (all ages).
Suppositories: insert 1 in the morning and evening and after each bowel evacuation (adults).

CONTRA-INDICATIONS & WARNINGS
Contra-indicated in known hypersensitivity to any of the ingredients. Not for use in presence of an infection.

PREGNANCY
Not to be used extensively i.e. not in large amounts or for long periods.

SIDE-EFFECTS
Skin rash can occur in persons sensitive to any of the ingredients. Can cause thinning and damage to skin. Consider possibility of systemic absorption.

LICENSED STATUS
Ointment licensed for all age groups. Suppositories not licensed for use in children.

Scheriproct®

Cinchocaine (dibucaine) hydrochloride is a local anaesthetic; prednisolone relieves pruritus and inflammation.

USES
Symptomatic relief of haemorrhoids and pruritus ani for 5-7 days only.

PRESENTATION
Ointment: cinchocaine (dibucaine) hydrochloride 0.5% and prednisolone hexanoate 0.19%.
Suppository: cinchocaine (dibucaine) hydrochloride 1mg and prednisolone hexanoate 1.3mg.

DOSAGE
Ointment: apply thin layer twice daily. For a rapid response apply 3-4 times daily on first day only.
Suppositories: insert 1 daily. In severe cases may need to repeat 2-3 times daily initially.

ADMINISTRATION
Suppository: insert suppositories after bowel evacuation.

CONTRA-INDICATIONS & WARNINGS
Contra-indicated in viral infections, primary bacterial or fungal infections in the treatment area. Also secondary infections of skin in absence of appropriate anti-infective therapy. Avoid long-term continuous use especially in infants.

PREGNANCY
Inadequate evidence of safety in human pregnancy. May be a very small risk to human fetus.

BREAST-FEEDING
Contact local Medicines Information Centre for advice.

SIDE-EFFECTS
Possible systemic absorption resulting in adrenal suppression. Skin atrophy with extensive therapy. Allergic skin reactions may occur.

LICENSED STATUS
No lower age limit.

Ultraproct®

Cinchocaine (dibucaine) hydrochloride is a local anaesthetic; fluocortolone relieves pruritus and inflammation.

USES
Symptomatic relief of haemorrhoids and of pruritus ani for 5-7 days.

PRESENTATION
Ointment: cinchocaine (dibucaine) hydrochloride 0.5%, fluocortolone hexanoate 0.095% and fluocortolone pivalate 0.092%.
Suppository: cinchocaine (dibucaine) hydrochloride 1mg, fluocortolone hexanoate 630 micrograms and fluocortolone pivalate 610 micrograms.

DOSAGE
Ointment: apply thin layer twice daily. To achieve rapid response apply 3-4 times daily on first day.
Suppository: insert 1 daily. In severe cases may need to repeat 2-3 times daily at the start of treatment.

ADMINISTRATION
Suppository: insert suppositories after bowel evacuation.

CONTRA-INDICATIONS & WARNINGS, PREGNANCY, BREAST-FEEDING, SIDE-EFFECTS   See Scheriproct®.

LICENSED STATUS
No lower age limit.

Xyloproct®

Lidocaine (lignocaine) hydrochloride is a local anaesthetic; hydrocortisone relieves pruritus and inflammation.

USES
Relief of symptoms such as anal and peri-anal pruritus, pain and inflammation associated with haemorrhoids, anal fissure and fistulas, proctitis; pruritus vulva.

PRESENTATION
Ointment: aluminium acetate 3.5%, hydrocortisone acetate 0.275%, lidocaine (lignocaine) 5% and zinc oxide 18%.

DOSAGE & ADMINISTRATION
Topical ointment: apply several times daily. Short-term use only.

CONTRA-INDICATIONS & WARNINGS
Known hypersensitivity to local anaesthetics of the amide type or any other ingredient. Use only for limited periods. Appropriate antibacterial, antiviral or antifungal therapy should be given if infection present at site. Discontinue if irritation or rectal bleeding develops.

INTERACTIONS
Lidocaine (lignocaine) should be used with caution in patients receiving *antiarrhythmic drugs* since the toxic effects are additive.

PREGNANCY
Contact local Medicines Information Centre for advice.

BREAST-FEEDING
Lidocaine (lignocaine) hydrochloride and hydrocortisone acetate are excreted into breast milk but in such small quantities that adverse effects on the infant are unlikely at therapeutic doses.

SIDE-EFFECTS
Local reactions: dermatitis. Systemic absorption may occur with large doses especially in infants and children and CNS effects e.g. convulsions can occur.

POISONING/TOXICITY
Excessive use of large amounts may result in systemic absorption. See side-effects.

LICENSED STATUS
No lower age limit.

Haloperidol

Butyrophenone neuroleptic/antipsychotic.

USES
Schizophrenia; mania, agitated, excited or violent behaviour; tic disorders including Tourette syndrome; intractable hiccup; nausea.

PRESENTATION
Capsule: 500 microgram – Serenace®.
Injection: 5mg in 1mL, 1mL ampoules – Haldol® and Serenace®; 10mg in 1mL, 2mL ampoules – Serenace®.
Oral liquid: 1mg in 1mL – Dozic®; 2mg in 1mL – Serenace® and Haldol®; 1mg in 5mL manufactured 'special'.
Tablet (scored): 500 microgram and 20mg – non-proprietary; 1.5mg, 5mg and 10mg – Serenace® and non-proprietary; 5mg and 10mg (both scored) – Haldol®.

DOSAGE

Indication	Route	Age		Frequency (times daily)	Notes
		2–12 years	12–18 years		
Schizophrenia Mania Tic disorders	Oral	12.5–25 microgram/kg	250 microgram –15 mg	2	2–12 years maximum 10mg per day. 12–18 years maximum 60mg per day.
Intractable hiccup	Oral	–	1.5 mg	3	Adjust according to response. Lower doses may be effective.
Nausea	Oral	–	500 microgram – 2mg	2–3	

CONTRA-INDICATIONS & WARNINGS
See chlorpromazine monograph. Avoid in basal ganglia disease.

INTERACTIONS, POISONING/TOXICITY
See chlorpromazine monograph.

PREGNANCY
Safety in human pregnancy is not established. Contact local Medicines Information Centre for advice.

BREAST-FEEDING
Excreted into breast milk; amounts probably too small to be harmful. Contact local Medicines Information Centre for advice.

SIDE-EFFECTS
See chlorpromazine monograph but less muscarinic and hypotensive and more extrapyramidal effects. Acute school phobia/separation anxiety.

PHARMACOKINETIC PROPERTIES
Rapidly and almost completely absorbed following oral administration. Haloperidol is subject to 35-40% pre-systemic metabolism in the liver. It is highly plasma protein bound (approx. 92%). The terminal elimination half-life averages at 20 hours, but there is considerable individual variation. It is extensively metabolised, primarily in the liver, but to a significant extent in the brain and other tissues and is excreted in the urine, as well as in the faeces via the bile.

EXCIPIENTS
Contact manufacturers for further details.

LICENSED STATUS
Licensed for use in children and adults, but the 1mg in 5mL oral liquid is a 'special' and as such is unlicensed.

FURTHER INFORMATION
1mg in 5mL oral liquid is available from Rosemont Pharmaceuticals Limited.

Heparin (standard or unfractionated)

Naturally occurring anticoagulant that potentiates inhibition of several activated clotting factors, including thrombin and factor X.

USES
Heparin: anticoagulant; prophylaxis or treatment of thromboembolic disease.
Heparin flushes: to maintain line patency. See further information section for details.

PRESENTATION
Heparin sodium
Injection: 1000 units in 1mL, 5mL amp - Pump-Hep®; 1mL and 5mL amps – Monoparin® and non-proprietary; 10mL and 20mL amps – Monoparin®, Pump-Hep® and non-proprietary; 5mL vial – Multiparin® and non-proprietary.
Injection: 5000 units in 1mL, 1mL and 5mL amp – Monoparin® and non-proprietary; 5mL vial – Multiparin® and non-proprietary.
Injection: 25,000 units in 1mL, 0.2mL – Monoparin®; 1mL – Monoparin® and non-proprietary, 5mL vial – Multiparin® and non-proprietary.

Subcutaneous only
Injection: heparin calcium 25,000 units in 1mL, 0.2mL amp – Monoparin Calcium®; 0.2mL and 0.5mL syringes – Calciparine®.
Injection: heparin sodium 25,000 units in 1mL, 0.2mL amp – Minihep®.

Heparin flushes
Solution: 10 units in 1mL, 5mL amp – Heplok®, Hepsal® and non-proprietary.
Solution: 100 units in 1mL, 2mL amp – Canusal®, Hep-Flush® and non-proprietary.

H

DOSAGE (HEPARIN)

Indication	Route	Age				Frequency	Notes
		birth–1 month	1 month–2 years	2–12 years	12–18 years	(times daily)	
Anticoagulant treatment	IV	<35 weeks postconceptional age: 50 units/kg >35 weeks postconceptional age: 75 units/kg	←	75 units/kg	→	single dose	Loading dose.
	IV infusion	25 units/kg/hour	<1 year as neonate >1 year as older child	← 20 units/kg/hour →		continuous	Initial maintenance dose. Adjust subsequent doses to achieve required APTT level.
	SC	-	←	250 units/kg	→	2	
Anticoagulant prophylaxis	SC	-	←	100 units/kg	→	2	Maximum single dose 5,000 units.

In severe renal or hepatic impairment
The risk of bleeding is increased and dose reduction should be considered.

ADMINISTRATION
IV infusion: dilute with glucose 5% or NaCl 0.9%.

CONTRA-INDICATIONS & WARNINGS
Haemophilia and other haemorrhagic disorders, thrombocytopenia, hyperkalaemia (monitor potassium levels regularly in at-risk patients), peptic ulcer, recent cerebral haemorrhage, severe hypertension, severe liver disease, after major trauma or recent surgery. Thrombocytopenia is a potentially serious adverse effect which may be associated with serious thrombotic events. Hence platelet counts are recommended for patients receiving heparin for greater than 5 days.

INTERACTIONS
Increased anticoagulant effect with *aspirin* and other drugs that interfere with platelet function. e.g. *dextran*, *dipyridamole*. Increased risk of haemorrhage with *ketorolac. Glyceryl trinitrate* infusion increases excretion (reduced anticoagulant effect).

PREGNANCY
Heparin is not contra-indicated in pregnancy. Heparin does not cross the placenta. The decision to use heparin in pregnancy should be taken after evaluation of the risk/benefit in any particular circumstances.

Reduced bone density has been reported with prolonged heparin treatment during pregnancy. Haemorrhage may be a problem during pregnancy or after delivery.

BREAST-FEEDING
Is not excreted into breast milk.

SIDE-EFFECTS
Haemorrhage, skin necrosis, thrombocytopenia, hyperkalaemia, hypersensitivity reactions.

POISONING/TOXICITY
Haemorrhage is the major clinical sign of overdose. Protamine is the antidote – see protamine monograph.

PHARMACOKINETIC PROPERTIES
Monitor Activated Partial Thromboplastin Time (APTT) and adjust dose to keep within therapeutic range. British Society for Haematology (BSH) guidelines suggest that common practice should be 1.5-2.5 times normal, but each hospital should establish its own therapeutic APTT range by monitoring this against known heparin levels.

EXCIPIENTS
Contact manufacturer for further details.

LICENSED STATUS
Heparin
Calciparine®, Monoparin®, Multiparin® licensed for use in children (for 'treatment') and adults. Minihep®, Monoparin Calcium®, Pump-Hep® not recommended for use in children; for adults only.

Heparin flushes
Heplok®, Hepsal® and Hep-Flush® are not licensed for use in children but Canusal® is.

FURTHER INFORMATION
Heparin flushes have a clear role to maintain patency of arterial catheters. For peripheral venous lines heparin flushes offer no advantage over NaCl 0.9%. Consult local guidelines for individual hospital protocols.

Hepatitis A vaccine

USES
For active protection against hepatitis A in high risk groups
Travellers: those going to areas where risk of infection is high (it has replaced the use of human normal immunoglobulin (HNIG) in travellers). Hepatitis A infection is not usually severe in young children and in the past the vaccine would rarely have been given to travellers <5 years old. However, even in this age group, the illness can be serious and may act as a source of infection for older individuals. For these reasons, many practitioners now recommend its use in younger children.
Patients with chronic liver disease: as the consequences of hepatitis A infection in such patients are potentially very serious, they should be considered for immunisation.
Haemophiliacs: factors VIII and IX concentrates have been implicated in the transmission of hepatitis A, so all haemophiliacs should be immunised.
Individuals in residential accommodation for those with severe learning disabilities: if the risk, based on local knowledge, is high, immunisation may be advised.
Outbreaks: in the past HNIG has been the preferred method of immunisation in outbreak control, however, with the shortage of suitable HNIG and concerns about blood products, it has largely been replaced by hepatitis A vaccine. The vaccine is most effective if given within 7 days of exposure. If the interval is greater, the use of HNIG should be considered (see separate monograph).

PRESENTATION
Injection: (single dose suspension) – Avaxim®; Havrix Monodose®; Havrix Junior Monodose®; Vaqta® Paediatric.

All preparations contain formaldehyde-inactivated virus grown in human diploid cells.
Avaxim® – GBM strain, contains 160 antigen units in 0.5mL.
Havrix Monodose® – HM 175 strain, contains at least 1440 ELISA units in 1mL.
Havrix Junior Monodose® – HM 175 strain, contains at least 720 ELISA units in 0.5mL.
Vaqta® Paediatric – 25 antigen units in 0.5mL.

The virus is initially grown on MRC-5 human diploid cells.

There is a combined preparation of inactivated hepatitis A and purified Vi polysaccharide typhoid vaccines and another of inactivated hepatitis A and hepatitis B vaccines – see separate monographs.

DOSAGE
Depends on the preparation and the age of the recipient.

Avaxim®: not licensed for use <16 years; ≥16 years a single dose of 0.5mL (160 antigen units).
Havrix Monodose®: ≥16 years a single dose of 1mL (1440 ELISA units).
Havrix Junior Monodose®: not licensed for use <1 year; 1-15 years a single dose of 0.5mL (720 ELISA units).
Vaqta® Paediatric: not licensed for use <2 years; 2-17 years a single dose of 0.5mL (25 antigen units).

For continuing protection, lasting at least 10 years, a booster dose should be given 6-12 months after the first dose.

ADMINISTRATION
IM: must not be given in the gluteal region (give SC in those with haemophilia).

CONTRA-INDICATIONS & WARNINGS
As for vaccines generally.

Although the resulting antibody levels may be lower, they provide adequate protection.

INTERACTIONS
HNIG may be given at the same time as the vaccine.

PREGNANCY
Although no information is available and there are no

H

grounds to believe it would be harmful, general principles suggest that it should only be used in pregnancy if the potential recipient is at either high risk of exposure or if the development of hepatitis A would be particularly hazardous.

BREAST-FEEDING
No information is available, but there are no grounds to believe it would be harmful.

SIDE-EFFECTS
Local effects such as mild tenderness, erythema and induration at the site of injection may occur. Less commonly fever, malaise, headache, nausea and lack of appetite have been reported. No serious reactions have been causally connected with the vaccine.

POISONING/TOXICITY
No data available.

PHARMACODYNAMIC PROPERTIES
Immunity is present within 2-4 weeks of the first dose.

EXCIPIENTS
Havrix Monodose®: aluminium hydroxide, 2-phenoxyethanol, polysorbate 20, amino acids for injection, disodium phosphate, monopotassium phosphate, NaCl 0.9%, potassium chloride, Water for Injections and a trace of neomycin B sulphate (the latter is not in the Junior preparation).
Avaxim®: aluminium hydroxide, 2-phenoxyethanol, formaldehyde and Medium 199 (a mixture of amino acids, mineral salts, vitamins and other components). The vaccine may also contain undetectable traces of neomycin.
Vaqta® Paediatric: aluminium hydroxide, sodium borate and sodium chloride.

LICENSED STATUS
Fully licensed for the uses indicated above. See individual product licence details in the dosage section.

FURTHER INFORMATION
Protect from light and store at 2–8°C, do not freeze.
Materials of bovine and sheep origin are used in the manufacturing process. Trace amounts of the original material may be present in the final product, however, all such material is obtained from sources known to be free of BSE.

Hepatitis A and Hepatitis B vaccine (combined)

USES
Indicated for non-immune patients who are at risk of both hepatitis A and hepatitis B infection (see monographs on hepatitis A and B).

PRESENTATION
Injection: (single dose suspension for injection) - Twinrix® Paediatric; Twinrix® Adult vaccine.
Each 0.5mL dose of Twinrix® Paediatric vaccine contains not less than 360 ELISA units of inactivated hepatitis A virus and 10 micrograms of recombinant HBsAg protein. Each 1mL dose of Twinrix® Adult vaccine contains not less than 720 ELISA units of inactivated hepatitis A virus and 20 micrograms of recombinant HBsAg protein.
The hepatitis A virus is initially grown on MRC-5 human diploid cells. Hepatitis B surface antigen is produced in yeast cells by a recombinant DNA technique.

DOSAGE
Primary vaccination schedule. This consists of 3 doses, the second being administered one month after the first dose and the third 6 months after the first dose (a dose is 0.5mL of the paediatric preparation for children 1-15 years and 1mL of the adult preparation for those ≥16 years). Once initiated, the primary course of vaccination should be completed with the same preparation.
Booster dose. There is increasing evidence that once a satisfactory serological response has been attained after hepatitis B vaccine, no boosters are necessary. Booster vaccination with the combined vaccine can be recommended from 5 years after initiation of the primary course. If the monovalent vaccines are used as boosters, they can be administered 5 years after initiation of the primary course for hepatitis B and 10 years after initiation of the primary course for hepatitis A.

ADMINISTRATION
IM or deep SC: preferably IM injection in the deltoid region in adolescents and children or in the anterolateral thigh in infants. It must not be given in the gluteal region as a suboptimal response may be obtained. It may be given SC in patients with thrombocytopenia or bleeding disorders. However, this route of administration has resulted in suboptimal immune response to the vaccine.

CONTRA-INDICATIONS & WARNINGS
As for vaccines generally.

INTERACTIONS
No data on concurrent administration of Twinrix® Paediatric or Twinrix® Adult with specific hepatitis A immunoglobulin or hepatitis B immunoglobulin have been generated. However, when the monovalent hepatitis A and hepatitis B vaccines were administered concurrently with specific immunoglobulins, no influence on seroconversion was observed although it may result in lower antibody titres.

PREGNANCY
Although no information is available, there are no grounds to believe it would be harmful. General principles suggest that it should be used during pregnancy only when there is a clear risk of both hepatitis A and hepatitis B.

BREAST-FEEDING
No information available, but there are no grounds to believe it would be harmful.

SIDE-EFFECTS
Pain, redness and swelling at the site of injection are the most common reactions. See monographs for the monovalent hepatitis A and hepatitis B vaccines for other reactions that have been reported.

POISONING/TOXICITY
No information available.

PHARMACODYNAMIC PROPERTIES
Protection against hepatitis A and hepatitis B develops within 2-4 weeks of the first dose; in clinical studies, specific humoral antibodies against hepatitis A were observed in approximately 89% of the subjects within one month of the first dose and in 100% one month after the third dose. Specific humoral antibodies against hepatitis B were observed in approximately 67% of the subjects after the first dose and in 100% after the third dose. It is expected that in most vaccinees the antibodies will persist for at least 4-5 years after the primary vaccination course. Even though the antibodies to hepatitis B decline with time, there is considerable evidence that protection does not diminish with time.

EXCIPIENTS
Aluminium hydroxide, aluminium phosphate, amino acids for injection, formaldehyde, neomycin sulphate, 2-phenoxyethanol, polysorbate 20, sodium chloride, residual tris and phosphate buffer and Water for Injections.

LICENSED STATUS
Fully licensed for the uses stated. Twinrix® Paediatric is indicated for use in children and adolescents from 1-15 years. Twinrix® Adult is indicated for use in adults and adolescents ≥16 years.

FURTHER INFORMATION
Store at 2-8°C, do not freeze.

Hepatitis A and Typhoid vaccine (combined)

USES
Indicated for non-immune patients who are at risk of both hepatitis A and typhoid infections (see monographs for separate vaccines).

PRESENTATION
Injection: (single dose suspension) – Hepatyrix®.
Each 1mL contains not less than 1440 ELISA units of formaldehyde-inactivated HM175 strain of hepatitis A virus grown in MRC-5 human diploid cells with 25 micrograms of Vi capsular polysaccharide prepared from *Salmonella typhi* Ty2 strain.
Injection: (single dose suspension of each antigen in a dual chamber syringe) – ViATIM®.
Each 1mL of mixed vaccine contains 160 antigen units of inactivated GBM strain of hepatitis A virus grown on MRC-5 human diploid cells with 25 micrograms of *Salmonella typhi* Ty2 strain.

DOSAGE
1mL for those aged ≥15 years (Hepatyrix®) or ≥16 years (ViATIM®).
For continuing protection, a booster dose of hepatitis A vaccine should be given after 6-12 months and a dose of typhoid polysaccharide vaccine after three years.

ADMINISTRATION
IM: must not be given in the gluteal region (give SC in those with haemophilia).
Ideally, it should be given at least 2 weeks prior to exposure to typhoid and 4 weeks prior to exposure to hepatitis A.

CONTRA-INDICATIONS & WARNINGS
As for vaccines generally.

INTERACTIONS
Experience is limited. Human normal immunoglobulin (HNIG) may be given at the same time as the vaccine. Although the resulting antibody levels may be lower, they will probably provide adequate protection.

PREGNANCY
Although no information is available and there are no grounds to believe it would be harmful, general principles suggest that it should only be used in pregnancy if the potential recipient is at either high risk of exposure or if the development of hepatitis A or typhoid would be particularly hazardous.

BREAST-FEEDING
No information is available, but there are no grounds to believe it would be harmful.

SIDE-EFFECTS
Local effects such as mild tenderness, erythema and induration at the site of injection may occur. Less commonly fever, malaise, headache, nausea and lack of appetite have been reported. No serious reactions, apart from anaphylaxis, have been causally connected with the vaccine.

POISONING/TOXICITY
No data available.

PHARMACODYNAMIC PROPERTIES
Immunity is present within 2-4 weeks of the first dose.

EXCIPIENTS
Hepatyrix®: aluminium hydroxide, 2-phenoxyethanol, polysorbate 20, amino acids for injection, sodium chloride, Water for Injections, trometamol and neomycin sulphate.
ViATIM®: sodium chloride, disodium phosphate dihydrate, sodium dihydgroen phosphate dihydrate, 2-phenoxyethanol, formaldehyde and Medium 199 Hanks (a complex mixture of amono acids, mineral salts, vitamins and other components, including glucose, diluted with water and with hydrochloric acid or sodium hydroxide as needed) and polysorbate 80.

LICENSED STATUS
Fully licensed for the uses indicated above.

FURTHER INFORMATION
Protect from light and store at 2–8°C, do not freeze.
Materials of bovine and sheep origin are used in the manufacturing process. Trace amounts of the original material may be present in the final product, however, all such material is obtained from sources known to be free of BSE.

Hepatitis B immunoglobulin (HBIG)

USES
For post–exposure prophylaxis in one of the following categories:
☐ Babies born to mothers who are hepatitis B surface antigen positive, with e antigen or no e markers.
☐ Babies born to mothers who have had acute hepatitis B during this pregnancy.

The baby should be given a single 200 international unit dose of specific hepatitis B immunoglobulin (HBIG). This should be done as soon as is reasonably possible after birth. The baby will also need a course of vaccine (see hepatitis B vaccine monograph).

The SPC has changed and now states that the dose for neonates is 40 international unit/kg, in line with the European core product sheet. As the immunoglobulin is only given to high risk neonates in UK and the original research used 200 international units, the advice from the Health Protection Agency is that the recommended dose for neonates is still 200 international units.

Other post–exposure prophylaxis: the circumstances requiring treatment are difficult to define exactly. Treatment depends on the immunisation status of the individual and whether the exposure is considered to be significant e.g. percutaneous needle-stick or other contaminated sharp object, a bite which causes bleeding or other visible skin puncture; mucocutaneous exposure to blood (contamination of non-intact skin, conjunctiva or mucous membrane); unprotected sexual intercourse by whatever route.

Hepatitis B virus (HBV) prophylaxis for reported exposure incidents

HBV prophylaxis for reported exposure incidents (source: *Communicable Disease Review* (1992) 2:R97-101)

Hepatitis B (HB) vaccination status of exposed person	Significant exposure*			Non-significant exposure	
	HBsAg positive source	**Source status unknown**	**HBsAg negative source**	**Continued risk**	**No further risk**
Received one dose of vaccine or none	Accelerated course of HB vaccine** HBIG x 1	Accelerated course of HB vaccine**	Initiate course of HB vaccine	Initiate course of HB vaccine	No HBV prophylaxis – reassure
Two or more doses of vaccine received (anti-HBs not known)	One dose of HB vaccine followed by a second dose 1 month later	One dose of HB vaccine	Finish course of HB vaccine	Finish course of HB vaccine	
Known responder to vaccine (anti-HBs ≥10 milli-international units/mL 2-4 months post vaccination)	Booster dose of HB vaccine	Consider booster dose of HB vaccine	Consider booster dose of HB vaccine	Consider booster dose of HB vaccine	
Known non-responder to vaccine (anti-HBs <10 milli-international units/mL 2-4 months post vaccination)	HBIG x 1 Consider booster dose of HB vaccine	HBIG x 1 Consider booster dose of HB vaccine	No HBIG Consider booster dose of HB vaccine	No HBIG Consider booster dose of HB vaccine	

*Significant exposure can be taken to be one of the following:
☐ Percutaneous - needle-stick or other contaminated sharp object, a bite which causes bleeding or other visible skin puncture.
☐ Mucocutaneous exposure to blood (contamination of non-intact skin, conjunctiva or mucous membrane).
☐ Unprotected sexual intercourse by whatever route.

**An accelerated course of vaccine consists of doses spaced at 0, 1 ,2 and 12 months. In some circumstances a 'super-accelerated' course has been recommended in adults. This comprises doses at 0, 7 and 21 days with a booster at 12 months.

PRESENTATION
Injection: not less than 100 international units in 1mL of this suspension prepared from the plasma of donors having high titres of antibody to hepatitis B surface antigen - 2mL, 5mL ampoules. Donors are tested for hepatitis B and C and HIV infections. All donors come from countries where there are no known cases of non variant Creutzfeldt-Jakob Disease.

DOSAGE
Age	Dose
0-4 years	200 international units
5-9 years	300 international units
≥10 years	500 international units

ADMINISTRATION
IM injection.

H

CONTRA-INDICATIONS & WARNINGS
Anaphylactic reaction to a previous dose.

INTERACTIONS
Can be given simultaneously with hepatitis B vaccine, but at a different site. It may reduce the immunogenicity of live vaccines other than those against yellow fever and typhoid. If the immunoglobulin is given first, an interval of at least three months should pass before giving a live vaccine other than those mentioned above. If the live vaccine is given first, at least 3 weeks should elapse before giving the immunoglobulin.

PREGNANCY
There is no reason to believe this product might be harmful. Limited experience has shown it to be safe. If it would normally be indicated, it should be given.

BREAST-FEEDING
There is no reason to believe that this product might be harmful to the breast-fed infant. If it would normally be indicated, it should be given.

SIDE-EFFECTS
Local reactions such as pain, redness and swelling at the injection site may occur.

POISONING/TOXICITY
No data available.

PHARMACOKINETIC STUDIES
Measurable antibody levels are present 20 minutes after injection. Peak levels are achieved after 2–3 days. Half-life is 21–22 days.

EXCIPIENTS
Sodium chloride, glycine, sodium acetate trihydrate and sodium hydroxide.

LICENSED STATUS
Licensed for use as described.

FURTHER INFORMATION
HBIG is in short supply. It should only be used for the indications described above and preferably after discussion with an appropriate expert.
Protect from light and store at 2-8°C, do not freeze.

Hepatitis B vaccine

USES
Active prevention of hepatitis B infection in those at high risk
☐ Babies born to mothers who are carriers of hepatitis B virus or who have had acute hepatitis B during pregnancy: when a baby is born in these circumstances, a course of vaccine should be given. Babies born to mothers with e antigen or no e markers, or to mothers who have had acute hepatitis B during pregnancy, should also be given a single 200 international unit dose of specific hepatitis B immunoglobulin (HBIG). This should be done as soon as is reasonably possible after birth.
☐ Close family contacts of a case or carrier of hepatitis B.
☐ Families adopting children from countries with a high prevalence of hepatitis B: children from some parts of Eastern Europe, South East Asia and South America are at relatively high risk of being hepatitis B positive. Unless a child to be adopted from one of these areas is known to be surface antigen negative, immunisation should be offered to all members of the adopting family.
☐ Haemophiliacs receiving, or likely to receive, blood or blood products.
☐ Patients with chronic renal failure; such individuals may proceed to haemodialysis at which stage their response to the vaccine may be poor. Immunisation is therefore indicated as soon as it is felt that haemodialysis may be required at some time in their illness.
☐ Individuals in residential accommodation for those with severe learning disabilities: surveys in the past have often shown a high incidence of carriage of hepatitis B in such institutions and so consideration should be given to immunising all new residents. Depending on local assessment, it may be appropriate to immunise children in day care settings and special schools for those with severe learning disabilities.
☐ Long stay travellers to areas of high endemicity.

H

☐ Individuals abusing intravenous drugs.
☐ Individuals engaged in prostitution or following sexual contact with known carriers or acute cases of hepatitis B.
☐ Post-exposure prophylaxis (apart from neonates of infected mothers): see section on HBIG for details of immunisation in these circumstances.

PRESENTATION
Injection: (single dose suspension) – HBVAXPRO®; Engerix B®.
Each contains hepatitis B surface antigen produced in yeast cells (*Saccharomyces cerevisiae*) by a recombinant DNA technique. HBVAXPRO® 5 microgram/0.5mL, 10 microgram/1mL or 40 microgram/1mL; Engerix B® 20 microgram/1mL.

DOSAGE
Babies born to infected mothers should receive an accelerated program of doses at 0, 1, 2 and 12 months. This may also be used in other circumstances where it is very important to attain immunity as soon as possible. Where it is not so important to gain a rapid response, the commonly used regime consists of doses at 0, 1 and 6 months. The size of each dose depends on the preparation and the age of the recipient.

Engerix B® (SmithKline Beecham)
0-15 years	10 microgram (0.5mL)
>15 years	20 microgram (1mL)

HBVAXPRO® (Aventis Pasteur MSD)
0-15 years	5 microgram (0.5mL of vaccine for children and adolescents)
≥16 years	10 microgram (1mL of vaccine for adults and adolescents)
≥16 years	on or prior to dialysis 40 microgram (1mL of vaccine for predialysis and dialysis patients)

In the UK, hepatitis B vaccine is usually only given to high risk groups at continuing risk of exposure. In such circumstances, antibody to surface antigen should be measured 2-4 months after immunisation. If the level of antibody is less than 100 milli-international units/L, up to 3 further doses of vaccine may be given until a satisfactory response is achieved. It is unclear as to whether routine boosters are necessary. There is strong evidence that once an initial antibody response of 100 international units/L has been attained symptomatic infection or carriage is unlikely to result from subsequent exposure in immunocompetent individuals. In those on dialysis and others known to be immunosuppressed, antibody levels to the surface antigen ought to be checked at intervals and a booster dose given if they fall below 10 international units/L.

ADMINISTRATION
IM or deep SC: the vaccine is not licensed for use by the intradermal route and may result in lower antibody responses. The vaccine should not be given in the gluteal region as the antibody response has been shown to be reduced in adults. There is evidence that this may not be the case in infants, but the gluteal region should still be avoided.

CONTRA-INDICATIONS & WARNINGS
As for vaccines generally; however, if the individual has been exposed to a high risk of hepatitis B, the vaccination should be given in spite of any intercurrent illness. With increasing age or the presence of any illness that may affect the immune system, there is a diminished response to the vaccine and it is particularly important that such individuals have their antibody levels assayed after the basic course of immunisation.

INTERACTIONS
HBIG may be given at the same time as, or within a few days of the vaccine, as long as a different site is used. There are no known interactions with other vaccines.

PREGNANCY
There is limited experience of the use of the vaccine, especially in the third trimester. No adverse effects have been noted on the mother, fetus, or infant. However, because experience is limited, vaccination should be postponed until after delivery, unless there is a high risk of exposure.

BREAST-FEEDING
If it would normally be indicated, the vaccine should be given.

SIDE-EFFECTS
Local reactions at the site of injection (pain and erythema) are usually mild. Fever, rash, malaise and an influenza-like syndrome of arthritis, arthralgia and myalgia can occur. Anaphylaxis has been reported rarely. Other serious side-effects have not been proven to be caused by the vaccine.

POISONING/TOXICITY
No data available.

EXCIPIENTS

Engerix B® : aluminium oxide, hydrated polysorbate 20, thiomersal, sodium chloride, disodium phosphate dihydrate, sodium dihydrogen phosphate.
HBVAXPRO® : sodium chloride and sodium borate.

LICENSED STATUS

Licensed for use as described above.

FURTHER INFORMATION

Universal immunisation is not policy in the UK. All pregnant women should be screened for hepatitis B surface antigen.
Full protective immunity is not attained until a course of 3 doses has been given.
Protect from light and store at 2–8°C, do not freeze.

Human Albumin Solution

A colloid – an aqueous solution of protein obtained from plasma.

Isotonic solutions

USES

Plasma replacement e.g. in hypovolaemic shock or burns.

PRESENTATION

IV infusion: 50mL, 100mL, 250mL and 400mL bottles – Human Albumin Solution 4.5%; 100mL, 250mL and 500mL bottles – Human Albumin Solution 5%; 100mL and 400mL bottles – ALBA® 4.5%; 250ml and 500ml bottles – Albutein® 5%; 50mL, 100mL, 250mL and 500mL bottles – Zenalb® 4.5.

DOSAGE

In hypovolaemic shock 10-20mL/kg bolus as rapidly as possible. Repeat as necessary.
In trauma these requirements may increase up to 40mL/kg. At this level, replacement with whole blood should be considered.

ADMINISTRATION

IV: preferably at room temperature, at a rate determined by the condition of the patient.

Concentrated solutions (20–25%)

USES

Diuretic-resistant oedema in nephrotic syndrome.

PRESENTATION

IV infusion: 50mL and 100mL bottles/vials – Human Albumin Solution 20%; 100mL vial – ALBA® 20%; 50mL and 100mL bottles – Albutein® 20%; 20mL, 50mL and 100mL vials – Albutein® 25%; 50mL and 100mL bottles – Zenalb® 20.

DOSAGE/ADMINISTRATION

500mg-1g/kg over 4 hours with close monitoring with pulse oximetry because of the risk of pulmonary oedema.

CONTRA-INDICATIONS & WARNINGS

Severe anaemia and cardiac failure. Administer with caution in patients with diminished cardiovascular function and in infants and young children. Extreme care in babies with congenital heart defects.

SIDE-EFFECTS

Nausea, vomiting, shivering, salivation and fever. Allergic reactions – urticaria through to anaphylactic shock.

POISONING/TOXICITY

Albumin overload may cause pulmonary oedema, raised blood pressure and raised central venous pressure. Stop infusion and treat symptomatically.

EXCIPIENTS

See individual bottles/vials (varies with each batch) for further details.

LICENSED STATUS
Licensed for use in all ages.

FURTHER INFORMATION
Authors (Cochrane Injuries Group Albumin Reviewers) of a review of human albumin administration in critically ill patients published in the *BMJ* July 1998 concluded that 'there is no evidence that albumin administration reduces mortality in critically ill patients with hypovolaemia, burns, or hypoalbuminaemia and a strong suggestion that it may increase mortality. These data suggest that the use of human albumin in critically ill patients should be urgently reviewed'.

Human cytomegalovirus (CMV) immunoglobulin

USES
Prophylaxis and treatment of CMV infection in patients following transplantation or with acute CMV disease.

PRESENTATION
Human CMV immunoglobulin: lyophilised preparation of immunoglobulin G, manufactured from human plasma collected from donors with an elevated titre of anti-CMV IgG, each vial contains 3g immunoglobulin G – named patient.

DOSAGE
Doses of CMV immunoglobulin G need to be individualised to suit the patient. Typical dosage regimens are shown below.
Prophylaxis: 200mg/kg pre-transplant; 100mg/kg on days 7, 21, 42 and 63.
Treatment: 200mg/kg on days 1 and 7, given with appropriate antiviral therapy.

ADMINISTRATION
IV: reconstitute a vial using the 60mL Water for Injections provided; follow the accompanying instructions carefully. This will produce a solution with a protein concentration of approximately 45g/L, and a sucrose concentration of approximately 90g/L. Rate of administration varies according to body weight and previous experience with the material.

Slow – 0.01mL/kg/minute ($\equiv$ 0.6mL/kg/hour).
Medium – 0.02mL/kg/minute ($\equiv$ 1.2mL/kg/hour).
Fast – 0.04mL/kg/minute ($\equiv$ 2.4mL/kg/hour).

The recommended infusion times and rates are as follows:
☐ First infusion - slow for 30 minutes, medium for 30 minutes, maximum to completion.
☐ Second infusion - slow for 15 minutes, medium for 30 minutes, maximum to completion.
☐ Third infusion - maximum from the start.

The recommended infusion rates should be followed closely since adverse reactions are related to the rate of infusion. Vital signs (pulse, blood pressure, temperature) should be monitored during each infusion of CMV immunoglobulin.

CONTRA-INDICATIONS & WARNINGS
Contra-indicated in those with a history of anaphylactic or severe systemic response to IM or IV immunoglobulin preparations, and in patients with selective IgA deficiency who possess antibody to IgA.
Appropriate medication for the management of acute allergic reactions should be available.

INTERACTIONS
Specific drug interactions and incompatibilities have not been studied.

PREGNANCY/BREAST-FEEDING
The safety of this product has not been established in controlled clinical trials and should only be given to pregnant or lactating women if clearly indicated.

SIDE-EFFECTS
Adverse reactions, if they occur, generally occur during the initial infusion and are uncommon in subsequent infusions. Adverse reactions may include chills, headache, muscle pain, malaise, joint pain, fever, nausea and flushing. If adverse effects occur, the infusion rate should be

H

reduced, or the infusion interrupted, until the symptoms subside. Appropriate medication should be given if necessary. The infusion may then be resumed at a rate which is tolerated by the patient when the physician in charge of the patient's treatment feels it is safe to do so.

POISONING/TOXICITY
Overdosage has not been reported but is unlikely to have any harmful effects.

EXCIPIENTS
Contact manufacturer for further details.

LICENSED STATUS
CMV immunoglobulin from Scottish National Blood Transfusion Service (SNBTS) is unlicensed.
Batches of normal immunoglobulin with a high CMV titre are available from Grifols for treatment and prophylaxis of CMV infections but this is not a licensed indication for use.

FURTHER INFORMATION
Despite all the precautions taken by the manufacturer in the preparation of the product, the risk of transmission of blood borne viruses by IV immunoglobulin preparations cannot be entirely excluded. The information given in the monograph is for the SNBTS product.

Human normal immunoglobulin (HNIG)

USES
For passive protection against a number of diseases where active immunisation is inappropriate, unavailable or has been omitted.

Measles Immunosuppressed individuals who come into contact with someone with measles should be given HNIG as soon as possible. It is of most value if given within 72 hours but may be effective if given up to 6 days after exposure. Consideration should also be given to its use in pregnant women born between 1970 and 1980 if in contact with a case of measles.
6-8 month old infants in contact with a case of measles.
Infants <6 months old in contact with a case of measles, if there is reason to think their mother may not be immune. Protection lasts about 3 weeks.

Hepatitis A In the past, HNIG has been used for short-term travellers to areas where hepatitis A is a significant risk, however shortage of supply, low levels of hepatitis A antibody in some preparations and concern to avoid the use of human products have meant that this is no longer an indication. Hepatitis A vaccine should be used instead for all those travelling to endemic areas. Hepatitis A vaccine has also largely replaced HNIG in the prevention of disease in contacts of cases of hepatitis A. Where more than 7 days have elapsed since exposure, hepatitis A vaccine is likely to be less effective and so HNIG should be used. It is effective at preventing disease if given up to 14 days after exposure, and may reduce disease severity even if given later.

Polio Although there is no evidence of its efficacy, HNIG should be given to immunocompromised people who are given oral polio vaccine (OPV) or who have contact with someone given OPV. It may reduce the risk of developing paralytic polio.

Rubella There is no evidence that the administration of HNIG to a susceptible pregnant woman exposed to rubella has any effect on the likelihood of the fetus being infected and/or developing the congenital rubella syndrome. If however termination of pregnancy is declined, some authorities would feel that HNIG is indicated. For further guidance see http://www.phls.co.uk/advice/rash.pdf.

Varicella–zoster When specific varicella-zoster immunoglobulin is not available, HNIG may be used for prevention of chickenpox in high risk contacts. Further advice should be sought if HNIG is indicated.

PRESENTATION
Injection: HNIG is prepared from the pooled plasma of many donors and contains approximately 16mg/mL of protein of which 90% is gammaglobulin, mainly IgG.
It is available from the Scottish National Blood Transfusion Service (SNBTS) and contains 250mg (1.7mL) with at least 100 international units/mL of hepatitis A antibody.

H

DOSAGE
This is dependent on the indication and the age of the recipient.

Indication	Age	Dose of HNIG from SNBTS by age
Measles	<1 year	250mg
	1-2 years	500mg
	≥3 years	750mg
Polio	<1 year	250mg
	1-2 years	500mg
	≥3 years	750mg
Hepatitis A (contact)	<10 years	250mg
	≥10 years	500mg
Rubella in pregnancy	–	750mg

ADMINISTRATION
IM injection.

CONTRA-INDICATIONS & WARNINGS
The only contra-indication is an anaphylactic reaction to a previous dose of HNIG.

INTERACTIONS
Measles, mumps and rubella vaccines should not be given within 3 weeks before or 3 months after HNIG as their efficacy may be reduced. The efficacy of *yellow fever, oral typhoid* and *booster polio vaccines* is unlikely to be affected. Administration of any *immunoglobulin preparation* may raise antibody levels to a number of microorganisms and this must be borne in mind when interpreting antibody assays within 2-3 months of such administration.

PREGNANCY
There is no systematic data on use in pregnancy but it has been used on numerous occasions and no adverse effects on the fetus have been recorded. If it is indicated, its use should not be withheld.

BREAST-FEEDING
There is no systematic data on use during breast-feeding but there are no theoretical grounds to believe it may adversely effect the breast-fed infant and no adverse effects have been recorded. If it is indicated, its use should not be withheld.

SIDE-EFFECTS
Occasionally, it may give rise to mild local reactions and sometimes the volume required can prove painful. Fever, chills and malaise arising 6-8 hours after immunisation and subsiding within 24 hours are unusual. Hypersensitivity reactions are very uncommon.

POISONING/TOXICITY
No data available.

EXCIPIENT
Glycine.

LICENSED STATUS
Licensed for use as detailed above.

FURTHER INFORMATION
HNIG is obtained from donors who are tested for hepatitis B, hepatitis C and HIV. The method of preparation should inactivate all viruses. Protect from light and store at 0-4°C or 2-8°C, depending on the source.

HNIG is in very short supply. The only proven indications are now the prevention of measles in the immunocompromised or prevention of secondary cases of hepatitis A when more than 7 days have elapsed from the time of contact with the index case. Other possible uses require consultation with an expert. Further information is available from *Immunisation of the Immunocompromised Child*, RCPCH 2002.
http://www.rcpch.ac.uk/publications/recent_publications/Immunocomp.pdf
and *Immunoglobulin Handbook*, PHLS, 2002.
http://www.phls.org.uk/advice/ImmunoglobulinHandbook.pdf

H

Vasodilator.

USES
Hypertension.

PRESENTATION
Injection: 20mg ampoule – Apresoline®.
Oral liquid: may be extemporaneously prepared.
Tablet: 10mg – (imported); 25mg – Apresoline® and non-proprietary; 50mg – non-proprietary.
Tablet: (dispersible) 10mg – manufactured 'special'.

DOSAGE

Route	Age				Frequency (times daily)	Notes
	birth–1 month	1 month–2 years	2–12 years	12–18 years		
Oral	← 250–500 microgram/kg →				2–3	Starting dose; increase gradually to a dose not exceeding 7.5mg/kg or 200mg daily.
				25mg	2	
Slow IV bolus over 20 minutes	← 100–500 microgram/kg →			5–10mg	single dose	Can be repeated up to a maximum of 4–6 times daily.
IV infusion	← 12.5–50 microgram/kg/hour →			3–9mg/hour	continuous	

Hepatic and renal impairment
In any degree of hepatic or renal impairment, start with a small dose or increase dosing interval and adjust according to clinical response.

ADMINISTRATION
Oral: injection can be given orally.
IV: the contents of the ampoule should be reconstituted by dissolving in 1mL of Water for Injections. This should be further diluted with NaCl 0.9% and given by slow IV injection over at least 5 minutes or infusion. Glucose solutions should not be used.

CONTRA-INDICATIONS & WARNINGS
High output heart failure, porphyria, idiopathic systemic lupus erythematosus (SLE) and related diseases. Severe tachycardia and heart failure with a high cardiac output, myocardial insufficiency due to mechanical obstruction, cor pulmonale, dissecting aortic aneurysm. Known hypersensitivity to hydralazine or dihydralazine.
Check acetylator status before increasing dose. Monitor for anti-nuclear factor and proteinuria every 6 months in long-term use.

INTERACTIONS
Enhanced hypotensive effect with *ACE inhibitors, anaesthetics, antihypertensives, diuretics, beta-blockers, anxiolytics* and *hypnotics, calcium-channel blockers, nitrates. Corticosteroids* and *NSAIDs* antagonise the hypotensive effect.

PREGNANCY
Use before the third trimester should be avoided, but it can be used in later pregnancy if there is no suitable alternative and there are risks to the mother and child from the disease itself e.g. pre-eclampsia and/or eclampsia.

BREAST-FEEDING
Passes into breast milk but reports available so far have not shown adverse effects on the infant.

SIDE-EFFECTS
Fluid retention, headache, tachycardia, palpitation are frequent side-effects. Occasional side-effects include, blood disorders e.g. anaemia, leucopenia, thrombocytopenia, neutropenia; prolonged treatment (>6 months) may provoke a lupus erythematosus-like syndrome.

POISONING/TOXICITY
Symptoms include hypotension, tachycardia, myocardial ischaemia, dysrrhythmias and coma. Supportive measures include IV fluids. If hypotension is present an attempt should be made to increase blood pressure without increasing the tachycardia and therefore adrenaline (epinephrine) should be avoided.

PHARMACOKINETIC PROPERTIES
Well absorbed after oral administration. Extensive hepatic metabolism. 80% excreted in urine, mostly as metabolites.

EXCIPIENTS
Contact manufacturers for further details.

LICENSED STATUS
Not licensed for use in children.

FURTHER INFORMATION
The 10mg dispersible tablets are available from Special Products Limited. The 10mg tablets are available via IDIS World Medicines.

Hydrochlorothiazide

Thiazide diuretic

USES
Oedema, hypertension, nephrogenic diabetes insipidus (in combination with amiloride or in infants and young children, indometacin (indomethacin)).

PRESENTATION
Tablet: 25mg and 50mg – Hydrosaluric®.
Oral suspension: may be extemporaneously prepared.

DOSAGE/ADMINISTRATION

Route	Age				Frequency (times daily)	Notes
	birth–1 month	1 month–2 years	2–12 years	12–18 years		
Oral	←	1.25mg/kg	→	12.5 25mg	2	Oedema/hypertension. Infants <6 months may need up to 4mg/kg/day. Maximum dose for: ≤2 years 37.5mg/day >2 years 100mg/day.
Oral	←	1mg/kg	→	12.5–25mg	3	Nephrogenic diabetes insipidus.

CONTRA-INDICATIONS & WARNINGS, INTERACTIONS, PREGNANCY, BREAST-FEEDING, SIDE-EFFECTS, POISONING/TOXICITY
See chlorothiazide monograph. Patients with renal failure usually refractory to hydrochlorothiazide. Doses should be given after dialysis in haemodialysis patients. Displaces bilirubin from albumin.

PHARMACOKINETIC PROPERTIES
Patients with hepatic, cardiac failure and renal disease may have decreased oral absorption.

EXCIPIENTS
See manufacturers SPC for further details.

LICENSED STATUS
Licensed for use in all ages.

Hydrocortisone

Corticosteroid.

USES
Anaphylaxis, emergency treatment of severe acute asthma, replacement therapy in adrenocortical disease, local injection to tendon sheaths and small joints. Intravenous hydrocortisone may be used for short-term therapy in juvenile idiopathic

H

arthritis (JIA), connective tissue diseases and vasculitis, when oral medication is not tolerated or not absorbed. Topical treatment of ulcerative colitis, proctosigmoiditis and granular proctitis. Refractory hypotension in the newborn.

PRESENTATION
Injection: (as sodium phosphate) 100mg in 1mL, 1mL and 5mL ampoule – Efcortesol®; (as sodium succinate) 100mg vial – Solu-Cortef®.
Injection (intra-articular/peri-articular/intra-tendon sheath): (as acetate) 25mg in 1mL, 1mL ampoule – Hydrocortistab®.
Oral liquid: 10mg in 5mL – manufactured 'special'; or a suspension can be extemporaneously prepared.
Pellet (lozenge): (as sodium succinate) 2.5mg – Corlan®.
Rectal foam: (as acetate) 10%, 20.8g aerosol (14 applications) – Colifoam®.
Tablet: (scored) 10mg and 20mg – Hydrocortone®.

DOSAGE
Joint/tendon sheath injections: 5-25mg hydrocortisone acetate is used, depending on the size of the joint and the size of the child.

Indication	Route	Age				Frequency	Notes
		birth–1 month	1 month–2 years	2–12 years	12–18 years	(times daily)	
Anaphylaxis. Emergency treatment of severe acute asthma	IV bolus/ IM/intra-osseous	2.5mg/kg then 2mg/kg	← 4mg/kg → (maximum 100mg) then ← 2-4mg/kg →		100–300mg then 100–300mg	single dose then 4	Maintenance dose may be repeated if necessary every 6 hours. May be given by intraosseous route if IV not possible.
Replacement therapy	Oral	← 4-5mg/m² →			–	3	Maintenance.
		← 5-6.6mg/m² →			–	3	Larger replacement dose in congenital adrenal hyperplasia
Topical treatment of ulcerative colitis, proctosigmoiditis, granular proctitis	Rectal	–	–	1 application ← 125mg →		1-2	Daily for 2-3 weeks then once on alternate days.
Refractory hypotension	IV	2.5mg/kg	–			4-6	Once stable wean gradually over 2-4 days. Monitor blood glucose and electrolytes.

ADMINISTRATION
Oral: take after food in order to minimise gastrointestinal side-effects. The tablets may be split or crushed and given with food. The Efcortesol® injection may be given orally, but it contains significant amounts of phosphate.
IV: bolus over 3-5 minutes. IV infusion dilute the prescribed dose in NaCl 0.9% or glucose 5%.
IM: it is likely to take longer to obtain a response when the drug is given by IM rather than IV injection.
Joint/tendon sheath injection: shake the ampoule well before use.
Rectal: fill canister as directed. Insert applicator tip into the rectum and push plunger fully into applicator to expel contents.

CONTRA-INDICATIONS & WARNINGS, INTERACTIONS, PREGNANCY/BREAST-FEEDING
See prednisolone monograph. Hydrocortisone should not be given via the intra-articular/peri-articular routes when the joint or surrounding tissues are infected.

SIDE-EFFECTS
See prednisolone monograph. IV administration of hydrocortisone sodium phosphate (Efcortesol®) may cause paraesthesia which is short-lasting and probably related to the rate of injection. Perineal irritation may occur following IV injection of hydrocortisone sodium phosphate (Efcortesol®).

POISONING/TOXICITY
There is no specific antidote. Treatment is symptomatic. Serum electrolytes should be monitored.

H

PHARMACOKINETIC PROPERTIES
Metabolised in the liver and, to a lesser extent, the tissues to biologically inactive metabolites. These are then excreted by the kidneys.

EXCIPIENTS
Contact manufacturers for further details.

LICENSED STATUS
Hydrocortone® tablets are licensed for the treatment of chronic adrenal insufficiency. Solu-Cortef® and Efcortesol® injections are licensed for IV use in children. Hydrocortistab® injection is licensed for use in children. Use in hypotension is not licensed. Colifoam® is licensed for use in children and adults. Oral liquid is a 'special' and as such is unlicensed.

FURTHER INFORMATION
If IV hydrocortisone therapy must be continued beyond 48-72 hours, hypernatraemia may occur. In this situation methylprednisolone may be a better choice in order to minimise sodium retention. Prophylactic antacid administration may be required with high dose, short-term IV therapy. Corlan® pellets are often used as a useful source of a smaller strength tablet for younger children but these are only licensed for local use in treating mouth ulcers and systemic absorption may be unreliable.

Withdrawal of corticosteroids: in patients who have received systemic corticosteroids for greater than 3 weeks, withdrawal should not be abrupt. However, abrupt withdrawal is appropriate in some patients treated for up to 3 weeks if it is considered that the disease is unlikely to relapse or that the dose has been such that abrupt withdrawal is unlikely to lead to clinically relevant hypothalamic-pituitary-adrenal axis suppression.

Hydrocortisone and Gentamicin

USES
Otitis externa (including prophylaxis). Chronic suppurative otitis externa. Post-operative local use in surgery to infected mastoid cavities.

PRESENTATION
Ear drops: hydrocortisone acetate 1% and gentamicin 0.3% (as sulphate), 10mL – Gentisone-HC®.

DOSAGE
Ear: 2-4 drops 3-4 times daily and at night. Alternatively, wicks medicated with the drops may be placed in the ear or mastoid cavity.

CONTRA-INDICATIONS & WARNINGS
Hypersensitivity to any ingredient. Known or suspected perforation of the drum is a contra-indication in otitis externa only.

PREGNANCY/BREAST-FEEDING
Contact local Medicines Information Centre for advice.

SIDE-EFFECTS
Theoretical risk of ototoxicity with topical application into middle ear but infection itself may cause hearing loss.

EXCIPIENTS
Include benzalkonium chloride and disodium edetate.

LICENSED STATUS
Licensed for use in children and adults.

FURTHER INFORMATION
For reasons of hygiene do not use bottle for more than 28 days after first opening it.

Hydrocortisone, Neomycin and Polymyxin

USES
Otitis externa due to or complicated by bacterial infection.

H

PRESENTATION
Ear drops: polymyxin B sulphate 10,000 units/mL, neomycin sulphate 3400 units/mL and hydrocortisone 1%, 5mL – Otosporin®.

DOSAGE/ADMINISTRATION
Ear: place 3 drops into the ear 3-4 times daily.

CONTRA-INDICATIONS & WARNINGS	SIDE-EFFECTS
Hypersensitivity to any ingredients. Known or suspected perforation.	Allergic hypersensitivity particularly to neomycin manifest as an eczematous exacerbation with reddening, scaling, swelling and itching. Stinging and burning.

EXCIPIENTS
Include cetostearyl alcohol, hydroxybenzoates (parabens) and polysorbate 20.

LICENSED STATUS
Licensed for use in children and adults.

FURTHER INFORMATION
For reasons of hygiene do not use bottle for more than 28 days after first opening it.

Hydroxocobalamin (vitamin B$_{12}$)

Readily converted into the active co-enzyme forms which are essential for cell growth and replication.

USES
Prophylaxis and treatment of vitamin B$_{12}$ deficiency. Inborn errors of metabolism responsive to hydroxycobalamin e.g. methylmalonic acidaemia, disorders of uptake or intracellular utilisation of cobalamins and homocystinuria due to remethylation defects.

PRESENTATION
Injection: 1mg in 1mL ampoule – non-proprietary; 5mg in 2mL – Hepavit®.
Powder: imported.

DOSAGE

Indication	Route	Age			Frequency	Notes
		1 month–2 years	2–12 years	12–18 years	(times daily)	
Confirmed vitamin B$_{12}$ deficiency	IM	← 250 microgram–1mg →			3 times weekly	For 2 weeks.
		then			then	
		← 250 microgram →			once weekly	Until blood count is normal.
		then			then every	
		← 1mg →			2-3 months	Maintenance dose.
Inborn errors of metabolism responsive to hydroxo-cobalamin (see indications)	IM	← initially 1mg →			once daily	Initial dose for 5 days, then assess. If responsive, the dose is reduced to a maintenance dose of up to 1mg IM once or twice a week.
	Oral	← up to 10mg →			once or twice weekly	May be given orally once the IM response established. However, some patients do not respond to oral use.

ADMINISTRATION
Oral: injection may be given orally, or an extemporaneous oral preparation can be made from the powder.

CONTRA-INDICATIONS & WARNINGS
Do not give until diagnosis fully established. Warnings: monitor plasma potassium during initial therapy; monitor FBC regularly during treatment. If no response to treatment further investigations are necessary.

PREGNANCY
Should not be used for the treatment of megaloblastic anaemia of pregnancy unless vitamin B$_{12}$ deficiency has been established.

BREAST-FEEDING
Excreted into breast milk but is unlikely to harm the infant.

SIDE-EFFECTS
Itching, exanthema, chills, fever, hot flushes, nausea, vomiting, dizziness, malaise.

POISONING/TOXICITY
Treatment of overdose unlikely to be needed.

LICENSED STATUS
1mg in 1mL injection licensed for use in children and adults with B$_{12}$ deficiency. Hydroxocobalamin powder and Hepavit® injection are not licensed for use in the UK. Inborn errors of metabolism is not a licensed use.

FURTHER INFORMATION
Hydroxocobalamin powder and Hepavit® injection are available via IDIS World Medicines.

Hydroxychloroquine

Reduces the function of lymphocytes and polymorphonuclear leucocytes, and reduces the production of interleukin-1.

USES
Juvenile idiopathic arthritis (JIA), porphyria, systemic and discoid lupus erythematosus and polymorphic light eruptions.

PRESENTATION
Tablet: 200mg – Plaquenil®.

DOSAGE

Route	Age			Frequency (times daily)	Notes
	1 month–2 years	2–12 years	12–18 years		
Oral	←	5–6.5mg/kg (maximum 400mg)	→	1	

Dosage should be adjusted according to plasma levels in severe renal or hepatic impairment.

ADMINISTRATION
Oral: tablets may be crushed, or a suspension can be made (formula available from Sanofi). Take with food or a glass of milk.

CONTRA-INDICATIONS & WARNINGS
Hydroxychloroquine is contra-indicated in pre-existing maculopathy of the eye. Regular ophthamological examination is not considered necessary when used at doses stated in rheumatological disorders. Caution in patients with hepatic or renal disease, severe gastrointestinal, neurological or blood disorders. Caution with G6PD, porphyria cutanea tarda and psoriasis.

INTERACTIONS
Plasma *digoxin* levels may be increased. *Digoxin* therapy should be closely monitored in patients receiving both drugs. Absorption of hydroxychloroquine may be reduced by *antacids*. A 4 hour interval should be observed between hydroxychloroquine and *antacid* dosing. Hydroxychloroquine may also be subject to the known interactions of chloroquine even though specific reports have not appeared.

PREGNANCY
Hydroxychloroquine crosses the placenta to the fetus. The drug has not been shown to be harmful to the fetus at doses used for malaria prophylaxis. However, the use of doses such as those used in the treatment of rheumatological conditions probably represents an increased risk. A chemically related compound, chloroquine phosphate, has been found to cause fetal cochlear damage when taken in high doses during

pregnancy. Contact local Medicines Information Centre for advice.

BREAST-FEEDING

Careful consideration should be given to using hydroxychloroquine when breast-feeding, during daily therapy with hydroxychloroquine, due to the risk of accumulation in the infant. It has been shown to be excreted in small amounts in human breast milk, and it is known that infants are extremely sensitive to the toxic effects of 4-aminoquinolines. Contact local Medicines Information Centre for advice.

SIDE-EFFECTS

Gastrointestinal disturbance, nausea, diarrhoea, anorexia, abdominal cramps. Visual disturbances, irreversible retinal damage, corneal opacities. Retinopathy is extremely rare at currently recommended dosages. Skin rashes, pigmentary changes, bleaching of hair and hair loss. Hydroxychloroquine may precipitate attacks of psoriasis.

POISONING/TOXICITY

Hydroxychloroquine is highly toxic in overdose and children are particularly susceptible to its toxic effects. Fatalities have occurred in infants at dosages of 1-2g (5-10 tablets). Symptoms of overdosage may include headache, visual disturbances, cardiovascular collapse, and convulsions, followed by sudden and early respiratory and cardiac arrest. Since these effects may appear soon after overdosage, early treatment is important. The stomach should be immediately evacuated, either by emesis or by gastric lavage. Activated charcoal in a dose at least 5 times that of the overdose may inhibit further absorption if introduced into the stomach by tube, following lavage and within 30 minutes of ingestion of the overdose. Consideration should be given to administration of parenteral diazepam in cases of overdosage as this has been shown to reverse chloroquine cardiotoxicity. Respiratory support may be needed. Patients should be closely observed for at least 6 hours.

PHARMACOKINETIC PROPERTIES

Hydroxychloroquine has an extremely long half-life (approximately 40 days in adults). This means it may take several months before steady-state concentrations are reached.

EXCIPIENTS

See manufacturers SPC for further details.

LICENSED STATUS

Hydroxychloroquine is licensed for use in children and adults.

Hydroxyethyl starches

USES

Plasma expansion.

PRESENTATION

IV infusion: hexastarch 6% in NaCl 0.9%, 500mL – eloHAES®.
IV infusion: pentastarch 6% in NaCl 0.9%, 500mL bag and pentastarch 10% in NaCl 0.9%, 500mL bag – HAES–steril® and Hemohes®.

DOSAGE/ADMINISTRATION

Use in children is probably best restricted to an intensive care setting. Consult a consultant intensivist for dosage details. Has been tried in controlled trial in paediatric cardiac surgery. Administration is by IV infusion.

CONTRA-INDICATIONS & WARNINGS

Severe haemorrhagic defects, severe congestive heart failure, renal failure with oliguria and anuria, allergy to starch or severe dehydration. No safety data available for children.

PREGNANCY

Do not use during early pregnancy. Contact local Medicines Information Centre for advice.

SIDE-EFFECTS

Possible anaphylaxis, allergic skin reactions, rise in heart rate and fall in systolic blood pressure, prolongation of bleeding time, increase of serum amylase levels during infusion.

LICENSED STATUS

Not licensed for use in children.

Sedative antihistamine with anxiolytic activity.

USES
Pruritis. Anxiety (short-term treatment).

PRESENTATION
Tablet: 10mg, 25mg – Atarax®.
Syrup: 10mg in 5mL – Ucerax®.

DOSAGE

Indication	Route	Age			Frequency (times daily)	Notes
		1 month– 2 years	2–12 years	12–18 years		
Pruritus	Oral	>6 months 5-15mg	2-6 years 5-15mg	25mg	Once at night	Initial dose Increase as necessary to the following maximum daily doses, given in 3-4
			7–12 years 15–25mg		Once at night	divided doses: 6 months – 6 years: 50mg/day 7–12 years: 50–100mg/day 12–18 years: 100mg/day.
Anxiety	Oral	–	–	50–100mg	4	

Renal impairment: the total daily dose should be reduced by half.

CONTRA-INDICATIONS & WARNINGS
Patients with previous hypersensitivity to hydroxyzine or components of the preparation. Early pregnancy. May impair ability to perform activities requiring mental alertness or physical co-ordination such as operating machinery or driving a vehicle. May enhance their response to alcohol, barbiturates and other CNS depressants.
Use with caution in patients with impaired renal function since it is uncertain whether the drug may accumulate or have other adverse effects in such patients.
Avoid in patients with acute porphyria. The sedative effect is inappropriate in hepatic failure.

INTERACTIONS
Alcohol, barbiturates and other *CNS depressants.*

PREGNANCY
Contra-indicated in early pregnancy; not recommended for use in later pregnancy, unless there is no safer alternative or when the disease itself carries risks for the mother or child (inadequate clinical data to establish safety in pregnancy).

BREAST-FEEDING
Not recommended for administration to nursing mothers.

SIDE-EFFECTS
Drowsiness, headache, dry mouth, confusion, dizziness, tremor, weakness, convulsions.

POISONING/TOXICITY
Hypersedation is the most common symptom of overdose. General supportive care is indicated. Hypotension may be controlled with IV fluids and noradrenaline (norepinephrine). *Adrenaline (epinephrine)* should not be used since hydroxyzine counteracts its pressor action. There is no specific antidote.

EXCIPIENTS
Atarax® tablets include lactose and sucrose. Ucerax® syrup includes sucrose and ethanol. See manufacturers SPC for further details.

LICENSED STATUS
Licensed for children ≥6 months of age for pruritus. Licensed for use in anxiety in adults only.

Anticholinergic.

USES
Relief of spasm of the gastrointestinal or genitourinary tracts. Palliative care.
Injection: also indicated in radiology for differential diagnosis of obstruction and to reduce spasm and pain in pyelography and other diagnostic procedures where spasm may be a problem.

PRESENTATION
Tablet: 10mg – Buscopan®.
Injection: 20mg in 1mL, 1mL ampoule – Buscopan®.

DOSAGE

Route	Age			Frequency	Notes
	1 month–2 years	2–12 years	12–18 years	(times daily)	
Oral	–	6–12 years 10mg		3	
			20mg	4	
Oral in palliative care	500 microgram/kg	2–4 years 5mg	10–20mg	3–4	Use in palliative care.
		5–12 years 10mg		3–4	
IV/IM	–	≤ 6 years 5mg	20mg	single dose	Repeat if necessary. <12 years usually up to 3 times per day. >12 years up to 4 times per day.
		6–12 years 5–10mg			
IV/IM in palliative care	500 microgram/kg	DOSE BY WEIGHT 2–4 years 500 microgram/kg	10–20mg	3–4	Use in palliative care.
		DOSE BY AGE 5–12 years 5–10mg		3–4	

ADMINISTRATION
Oral: swallow tablets whole with adequate water. Injection may be given orally. Once ampoule opened – may be stored for up to 24 hours in refrigerator.
IV: give as a bolus over at least 1 minute. Injection may be diluted with NaCl 0.9% or glucose 5%.
SC: in palliative care 24 hourly SC infusions have been used.

CONTRA-INDICATIONS & WARNINGS
Contra-indicated in patients with myasthenia gravis, megacolon and glaucoma or in patients with known sensitivity to hyoscine-N-butylbromide.
Caution in patients susceptible to intestinal or urinary outlet obstruction or in those inclined to tachycardia.

INTERACTIONS
Increased anticholinergic effect of *tricyclic antidepressants, antihistamines, quinidine, amantadine, phenothiazines, butyrophenones* and *disopyramide*. Concomitant treatment with *dopamine antagonists* such as *metoclopramide* may decrease effect of both drugs on gastrointestinal tract. Tachycardic effects of *beta-agonists* may be enhanced.

PREGNANCY
No evidence of adverse consequences but avoid, especially in first trimester, unless benefit to the mother thought to outweigh risk to the fetus.

BREAST-FEEDING
Contact local Medicines Information Centre for advice.

SIDE-EFFECTS
Anticholinergic side-effects, including dry mouth, visual accommodation disturbances, tachycardia, constipation, urinary retention. Allergic reactions e.g. skin reactions. Rare reports of dyspnoea in patients with a history of bronchial asthma or allergy.

POISONING/TOXICITY
Serious signs of poisoning following acute overdosage in man have not been reported but might expect anticholinergic effects. Gastric lavage with medicinal charcoal followed by magnesium sulphate (15%). Symptoms respond to parasympathomimetics. Additional supportive measures.

PHARMACOKINETIC PROPERTIES
Poorly absorbed from gastrointestinal tract and does not readily cross the blood-brain-barrier.

EXCIPIENTS
Tablets include sucrose. See manufacturers SPC for further details.

LICENSED STATUS
Tablets licensed in >6 years of age. Injection not licensed for use in children.

Hyoscine hydrobromide

Competitive antagonist to acetylcholine and other parasympathomimetic agents.

USES
For the control of drooling arising from muscular incoordination (e.g. in cerebral palsy). In palliative care as an antiemetic and for drying of excess secretions ('death rattle').

PRESENTATION
Patch: self-adhesive 2.5cm^2, 1.5mg; drug released at a rate of 1mg over 72 hours – Scopoderm TTS®, Transcop®.
Tablet: 150 micrograms – Kwells® Junior, Joy-rides®; 300 micrograms – Kwells®.
Injection: 400 microgram per 1mL, 1mL ampoule; 600 microgram per 1mL, 1mL ampoule – non-proprietary.

DOSAGES

Route	Age			Frequency (times daily)	Notes
	1 month–2 years	2–12 years	12–18 years		
Oral or sublingual	–	10 microgram/kg	300 microgram	4	Can use tablets or the injection orally.
Topical	1/4 patch	2–3 years 1/4 patch 3–9 years 1/2 patch 10–12 years 1 patch	1 patch	once every 72 hours	Apply to the dry, hairless skin behind the ear. Alternate sides each time a new patch is applied. Clean the skin well after patch is taken off to remove any residue. Wash hands after application. Tolerance may develop, so that patches need changing every 48 hours.
SC/IV bolus	← 10 microgram/kg →		400 microgram	4	
SC/IV infusion	← 40–60 microgram/kg/day →			continuous over 24 hours	This is compatible in a syringe with diamorphine.

ADMINISTRATION
Patch: apply to a clean, dry hairless area (e.g. behind ear). Patches may be cut if required, provided that they are cut along their full thickness with scissors and the membrane is not peeled away, the controlled release properties of the patch remain unaltered. Alternatively the portion of the patch that is not required, can be covered so that it is not in touch with the skin.
Tablet: can be sucked, chewed or swallowed.

CONTRA-INDICATIONS & WARNINGS
Hyoscine is contra-indicated in patients with glaucoma, hypersensitivity to hyoscine. Use with care in patients with pyloric stenosis, bladder outflow obstruction, intestinal obstruction, impaired renal or hepatic function. Drowsiness, confusion, dizziness, visual disturbances. Effects may persist for up to 24 hours after removal of the patch. Do not ride bicycles. Seizure frequency may be increased in epileptic patients.

INTERACTIONS
Use with care in patients on other *anti-cholinergic* or *CNS-acting drugs*.

SIDE-EFFECTS
Pupillary dilatation, glaucoma, irritation of eyelids, dry mouth, drowsiness. Rarely, memory and concentration impairment, restlessness, dizziness, skin rash, urine retention, disorientation, confusion and visual

H

hallucinations. After removal of patch, rarely headache, nausea, vomiting, disturbances of balance.

POISONING/TOXICITY
Symptoms: restlessness, excitation and confusion leading at higher doses to delirium, hallucinations and convulsions. At very high doses, coma and respiratory paralysis may occur.
Treatment: remove patch and administer physostigmine 500 microgram IV.

Diazepam may be used to counter excitation and convulsions; dissipate heat if hyperthermia ensues.

PHARMACOKINETIC PROPERTIES
Transdermal: equilibrium between absorption and excretion is reached within 6 hours. Plasma concentrations of hyoscine in the range 0.17-0.33 nanomol/litre are produced. After removal plasma concentrations are reduced by one-third over 24 hours as the drug continues to be released from the skin into the blood stream.

EXCIPIENTS
Kwells® include saccharin sodium. Contact manufacturers for further details.

LICENSED STATUS
Scopoderm TTS® patches are not licensed for the control of drooling but they are licensed for >10 years of age for motion sickness. Transcop® patches are not licensed for use in the UK. Tablets are licensed for ≥3 years of age for motion sickness.

FURTHER INFORMATION
Transcap® patches are available from IDIS World Medicines.

Hypostop®

USES
Hypoglycaemia.

PRESENTATION
Gel: glucose gel 40% (9.2g glucose per 23g oral ampoule, 32g glucose per 80g bottle) – Hypostop®.

DOSAGE/ADMINISTRATION
For all age groups massage half a tube into the buccal cavity. Repeat if there is no clinical response within 10 minutes.

CONTRA-INDICATIONS & WARNINGS
Do not use in unconscious patients. It may be used in semi-conscious patients in whom the swallowing reflex is preserved.

PHARMACOKINETIC PROPERTIES
Varies dependent on route of administration. Transmucosal route gives a more rapid rise in blood sugar than by swallowing. Absorption is enhanced by massage.

EXCIPIENTS
Contact manufacturer for further details.

LICENSED STATUS
'Borderline substance' hence no licence at present.

Ibuprofen

Non-steroidal anti-inflammatory drug (NSAID).

USES
Treatment of pyrexia and mild to moderate pain. Pain and inflammation in rheumatic disease including juvenile idiopathic arthritis (JIA) and other musculoskeletal disorders. Effective alternative to indometacin (indomethacin), for pharmacological closure of a patent ductus arteriosus (PDA) in a neonate (usually preterm). Anti-inflammatory use in patients with cystic fibrosis.

PRESENTATION
Capsule: (modified release) 300mg – Fenbid®.
Gel: 10% – Fenbid® Forte Gel, Ibugel®.

Granules: 600mg/sachet – Brufen®.
Injection: 5mg in 1mL, 2mL ampoules – named patient.
Oral suspension: 100mg in 5mL – non-proprietary.
Syrup: 100mg in 5mL – Brufen®.
Tablet: 200mg, 400mg and 600mg – Brufen® and non-proprietary; 800mg – Motrin®.
Tablet: (modified release) 800mg – Brufen Retard®.

DOSAGE

Indication	Route	Age			Frequency	Notes
		1 month–2 years	2–12 years	12–18 years	(times daily)	
Pyrexia, mild to moderate pain	Oral	DOSE BY WEIGHT ← 5mg/kg →		–	3–4	Maximum of 20mg/kg/day up to 2.4g/day.
		DOSE BY AGE		200-600mg		
		1–2 years 50mg	3–7 years 100mg		3–4	
			8–12 years 200mg		3–4	
JIA and other rheumatic diseases	Oral	← 10 mg/kg →			3–4	Can be given up to 6 times daily in systemic JIA only.
Rheumatic and muscular pain	Topical	Not recommended	← small amount →		2–3	
Anti-inflammatory in cystic fibrosis patients	Oral	← 20-30mg/kg →			2	Use only under expert supervision as dose titration is essential to ensure beneficial effect without the risk of side-effects. Adjust dose according to levels, aim for level of 50-100mg/L.

Closure of patent ductus arteriosus

Newborn infant (birth – 1 month)
Dose expressed as ibuprofen base and given at 24 hourly intervals.

First dose   10mg/kg
Second dose 5mg/kg
Third dose   5mg/kg

If the ductus arteriosus does not close 48 hours after the last injection or if it re-opens, a second course of three doses, as above, may be given.

ADMINISTRATION
Oral: take with or after food or milk. The tablets may be crushed or chewed except for the modified release preparations, which must be swallowed whole.
Topical: do not treat a large area, and wash hands after use. Topical administration does not avoid systemic effects.
IV: as a bolus or as a short infusion over 15 minutes. Can use NaCl 0.9% or glucose 5% to adjust the injection volume if necessary. Follow administration with a flush (1.5-2mLs) of either NaCl 0.9% or glucose 5%.

CONTRA-INDICATIONS AND WARNINGS
Should not be given to patients with active peptic ulceration, and should be used with extreme caution in patients with a history of peptic ulceration. Also contra-indicated in patients who have previously shown hypersensitivity reactions (asthma, rhinitis, urticaria) to aspirin or other NSAIDs. Use with caution in renal, cardiac or hepatic impairment. The topical preparations should not be applied to broken skin or mucosal surfaces. Keep away from the eyes.

When using ibuprofen for PDA closure in neonates, it is contra-indicated in life-threatening infection; active bleeding, especially intracranial or gastrointestinal haemorrhage; thrombocytopenia or coagulation defects and significant impairment of renal function. Careful monitoring of both renal function and gastrointestinal function is recommended during treatment. The risk of bilirubin encephalopathy in premature newborn infants may be increased.

INTERACTIONS
Increased risk of hyperkalaemia and renal damage with *ACE inhibitors,* nephrotoxicity with *ciclosporin (cyclosporin)* and *diuretics,* toxicity with *methotrexate, lithium* and *baclofen* due to reduced excretion, convulsions with *quinolones e.g. ciprofloxacin.* Effects of *warfarin* enhanced.

PREGNANCY
There is no evidence to support an association between the use of ibuprofen and congenital defects. Use during the last trimester should be avoided because of the risk of premature closure of the ductus arteriosus. Contact local Medicines Information Centre for advice.

BREAST-FEEDING
Ibuprofen enters breast milk in amounts too small to be harmful.

SIDE-EFFECTS
Gastrointestinal discomfort, nausea, diarrhoea and occasionally bleeding and ulceration. Headache, dizziness, vertigo, confusion, fluid retention, hypersensitivity reactions e.g. bronchospasm, rashes.

POISONING/TOXICITY
In children, ingestion of <100mg/kg body weight is unlikely to cause toxic effects while >400mg/kg may cause serious toxicity. For adults, ingested doses do not correlate well with symptoms developed. Nausea, vomiting, epigastric pain, tinnitus, headache, blurred vision and tachycardia are common symptoms. More serious symptoms include coma, convulsions, apnoea and bradycardia. Renal and liver function tests may become abnormal. Patients who have ingested less than 100mg/kg body weight or who are asymptomatic 4 or more hours after ingestion do not require treatment. Those who have taken larger amounts and those who are symptomatic should receive activated charcoal.

PHARMACOKINETIC PROPERTIES
Peak plasma concentrations occur approximately 2 hours after oral administration. Excretion is complete 24 hours after the last dose.

EXCIPIENTS
Contact manufacturers for further details.

LICENSED STATUS
Topical preparations, granules and 800mg SR tablets are not licensed for use in children.
Injection is formulated for use IV in PDA but is unlicensed. Liquid preparations and plain tablets vary in the minimum licensed age for use – check individual products for further information.

FURTHER INFORMATION
Injection available from Orphan Europe.

There is preliminary evidence to suggest that NSAIDs may prevent pulmonary deterioration in cystic fibrosis patients, with mild disease, by way of an anti-inflammatory action. Cochrane review concluded that routine use cannot be recommended. Should only be used under expert supervision.

Ifosfamide

Alkylating agent; oxazaphosphorine prodrug requiring hepatic activation to produce cytotoxic metabolites.

USES
Treatment of rhabdomyosarcoma, soft-tissue sarcomas, Ewing tumour and relapsed osteogenic sarcoma.

PRESENTATION
Injection: powder for reconstitution, 1g and 2g vials – Mitoxana®.

DOSAGE
Always consult the current treatment protocol for details of dosage and scheduling.

ADMINISTRATION
IV: reconstitute with Water for Injections (1g vial with 12.5mL, 2g vial with 25mL) to provide a solution containing 80mg in 1mL ifosfamide. Administer by IV infusion over 1-3 hours, with hydration and concurrent administration of the uroprotectant mesna. See protocol for details of IV hydration.

CONTRA-INDICATIONS & WARNINGS

Ifosfamide administration must not be undertaken without adequate hydration and mesna uroprotection. Low serum albumin associated with increased risk of encephalopathy. Presence of large pelvic tumour (ureteric obstruction) may increase toxicity. Prior cisplatin treatment may enhance renal toxicity. Prior pelvic irradiation may increase risk of urothelial damage during ifosfamide administration. Full blood count and assessment of renal function, both glomerular and tubular, should be obtained prior to each course of therapy.

INTERACTIONS

The concurrent use of ifosfamide with *anticoagulants*, especially *warfarin*, may result in increased anticoagulant effect. *Carbamazepine, phenytoin* and prolonged *steroid* treatment increase the clearance and metabolism of ifosfamide but the clinical significance of this is unknown. *Azole antifungals* and *nifedipine* may inhibit metabolism.

PREGNANCY

Ifosfamide should not be used during pregnancy, especially the first trimester, unless the expected benefit is thought to outweigh the substantial risk to the fetus.

BREAST-FEEDING

Ifosfamide is excreted in breast milk: mothers receiving the drug should not breast-feed.

SIDE-EFFECTS

Renal toxicity, especially tubular dysfunction, myelosuppression, emesis and alopecia, liver dysfunction and haemorrhagic cystitis if inadequate mesna prophylaxis; rarely, encephalopathy.

POISONING/TOXICITY

The most serious consequences are haemorrhagic cystitis and myelosuppression. If recognised early, IV hydration and diuresis, together with mesna, may minimise urothelial damage. Methylthioninium chloride (methylene blue) at an IV dose of 1mg/kg every 8 hours and diazepam have shown some activity in reversing ifosfamide encephalopathy.

PHARMACOKINETIC PROPERTIES

The pharmacokinetics of ifosfamide are complex and its pharmacological activity resides with its metabolites. Ifosfamide is highly metabolised with the major route of elimination for both unchanged drug and metabolites being the kidney. A high degree of inter and intra patient variation in metabolism and pharmacokinetics has been reported. Similarly, the clearance of ifosfamide depends upon its schedule of administration as it induces its own metabolism following continuous exposure. The following values in children should be interpreted with regard to schedule of administration and prior ifosfamide treatment:

Half-life: 1-7 hours.
Clearance: 3-8L/hour/m².
Volume of distribution   310-1100L/kg.
The CSF penetration of ifosfamide is almost complete.

LICENSED STATUS

Licensed for use in children and adults.

Iloprost

Prostacyclin analogue with vasodilator and anti platelet effects.

USES

Treatment of severe Raynaud's phenomenon where digital infarction is imminent.

PRESENTATION

Concentrate for infusion: 134 microgram in 1mL of iloprost trometamol (equivalent to 100 microgram iloprost per mL); 0.5mL and 1mL ampoules – named patient.

DOSAGE

Route	Age		Frequency (times daily)	Notes
	12–18 years			
IV infusion	← 0.5 nanogram/kg/minute →		Given over 6 hours on 3–5 consecutive days	Starting dose. Increase to maintenance dose over several hours.
	← 1–2 nanogram/kg/minute →			Maintenance dose.

ADMINISTRATION

IV: give as an IV infusion through a peripheral venous cannula for 6 hours daily for 3-5 consecutive days. Continuous infusion is not recommended. 1mL of the concentrated solution is diluted to 500mL with NaCl 0.9% or glucose 5% before infusing the appropriate dose. A solution 10 times as concentrated (i.e. 1mL diluted to 50mL) may be given via a syringe driver.

CONTRA-INDICATIONS & WARNINGS

Patients with conditions where the effects of the drug on platelets might increase the risk of haemorrhage e.g. active peptic ulcers, trauma and intracranial haemorrhage. Patients with any of the following: severe coronary heart disease or unstable angina; myocardial infarction within the last 6 months; acute or chronic congestive cardiac failure; cardiac arrhythmias; suspected pulmonary congestion.

INTERACTIONS

Iloprost may enhance the antihypertensive effects of *beta-adrenoceptor blocking drugs, calcium-channel blockers* and *ACE inhibitors*. There may be an increased risk of bleeding when used with *heparin* or *coumarin anticoagulants*. Platelet function may be further inhibited in patients receiving *aspirin, phosphodiesterase inhibitors* and *NSAIDs*.

PREGNANCY

Rodent studies have shown iloprost to cause abnormalities in the fetus. Do not use in pregnancy.

BREAST-FEEDING

There is no information available.

SIDE-EFFECTS

Facial flushing, headaches, nausea, vomiting, abdominal cramping, diarrhoea. Adverse effects are dose related, and the gastrointestinal effects can generally be avoided by titrating up to the dose which produces flushing and mild headache. Less common effects include malaise, sedation, fever, chills, confusion, altered blood pressure, tachycardia, arrhythmias, extrasystoles, restlessness, angina, reddening and pain at infusion site, reddening along the infusion vein.

POISONING/TOXICITY

Symptoms include facial flushing, headaches, vasovagal reaction with sudden blanching; sweating, nausea and vomiting; abdominal pain, diarrhoea, blood pressure changes, bradycardia and tachycardia.

PHARMACOKINETIC PROPERTIES

Iloprost is completely metabolised. Steady state levels are achieved 10-20 minutes after the start of the infusion, and the levels fall rapidly on stopping the infusion.

EXCIPIENTS

Contact manufacturers for further details.

LICENSED STATUS

Iloprost is not licensed in the UK.

FURTHER INFORMATION

Available from Schering Health Care Limited.

Imiglucerase

USES

Treatment of Type I & III Gaucher's disease.

PRESENTATION

Injection: powder for reconstitution, 200 unit and 400 unit vial – Cerezyme®.

DOSAGE

Indication	Route	Age				Frequency	Notes
		birth–1 month	1 month–2 years	2–12 years	12–18 years	(times daily)	
Type I disease	IV infusion	←	60 units/kg		→	every 2 weeks	Dosage should be individualised for each patient based on a comprehensive evaluation of the clinical manifestations of the disease. Initial doses as shown have produced improvement in haematological and visceral parameters within 6 months of initiating therapy.
Type III disease	IV infusion	←	120 units/kg		→	every 2 weeks	

ADMINISTRATION

IV: reconstitute each 200 unit and 400 unit vial with 5.1mL and 10.2ml of Water for Injections respectively, to give 40 units in 1mL. Dilute in NaCl 0.9% to a final volume of 100-200mL; infuse over 1-2 hours; in-line particulate filter recommended. Infusion rate should not exceed 1 unit per kg per minute. It is recommended that patients are monitored for the presence of antibodies to Cerezyme® prior to the first infusion (baseline) and at 3, 6, 9, 12 and 18 months after the start of therapy.

CONTRA-INDICATIONS & WARNINGS
Hypersensitivity to product.

INTERACTIONS
No information available.

PREGNANCY
Not recommended.

BREAST-FEEDING
Use with caution. Contact local Medicines Information Centre for advice.

SIDE-EFFECTS
Discomfort, burning, pruritus and swelling at injection site, slight fever, chills, abdominal discomfort, nausea and vomiting, fever, rigor and dizziness. Hypersensitivity has been noted in a limited number of patients.

PHARMACODYNAMIC PROPERTIES
Gaucher's disease is characterised by a functional deficiency in the enzyme ß-glucocerebrosidase, resulting in the accumulation of lipid glucocerebroside in tissue macrophages.
ß-glucocerebrosidase catalyses the hydrolysis of glucocerebroside to glucose and ceramide. Imiglucerase is a genetically engineered form of the enzyme.

LICENSED STATUS
Licensed for use in children with Gaucher's disease type I.

FURTHER INFORMATION
Available from Therapeutic Group Genzyme Therapeutics.

Imipenem with cilastatin

Carbapenem beta-lactam antibiotic with a broad spectrum of activity. Imipenem can cause renal toxicity, and because it is partially inactivated within the kidney it is always given in combination with cilastatin, a specific dehydropeptidase enzyme inhibitor which blocks imipenem's renal breakdown.

USES

Aerobic and anaerobic Gram-positive and Gram-negative infections. Generally inactive against methicillin-resistant *Staphylococcus aureus* (MRSA). Usually reserved for infections resistant to other antibiotics. Second-line treatment in cystic fibrosis patients – treatment of early *Pseudomonas aeruginosa* infections not cleared by ciprofloxacin plus colistin and of moderate to severe exacerbations, in combination with an aminoglycoside; treatment of more severe *Burkholderia cepacia* infections.

PRESENTATION

IV infusion: 500mg imipenem with 500mg cilastatin – Primaxin®.

DOSAGE
Newborn infants (birth – 1 month)

Route	Age Postnatal age (days)	Dose	Frequency (times daily)	Notes
IV	<7	20mg/kg	2	
	7-21	20mg/kg	3	
	>21	20mg/kg	4	

Child

Route	Age			Frequency (times daily)	Notes
	1 month–2 years	2–12 years	12–18 years		
IV	<3 months 20mg/kg >3 months 15mg/kg	15mg/kg	500mg	4 4	In children <12 years the maximum dose is 500mg. In children >12 years the dose may be doubled in severe infection to a maximum of 1g per dose.
IV for cystic fibrosis patients	22.5mg/kg	<40kg 22.5mg/kg >40kg 1g		4 3-4	Maximum single dose of 1g.

Dose adjustment in renal failure
manufacturers SPC states no experience in children with renal failure but recommends reduced dose frequency in adults as follows:

Creatinine clearance (mL/minute/1.73m²)	Dose	Frequency (times daily)
31-70	7mg/kg	4
21-30	7mg/kg	3
6-20	3.5-7mg/kg	2

In patients undergoing haemodialysis a dose should be given post-dialysis (as imipenem is removed) and then at 12 hourly intervals.

ADMINISTRATION
IV: administered by IV infusion over 20-30 minutes.
Reconstitute vials with NaCl 0.9% or glucose 5% to make a final concentration of 5mg/mL.

CONTRA-INDICATIONS & WARNINGS
Caution in beta-lactam allergy as partial cross-sensitivity has been demonstrated. Monitor LFTs carefully in patients with pre-existing liver disease.

INTERACTIONS
Use with caution with *nephrotoxic drugs*. May cause positive Coomb's test without haemolysis. *Probenecid* inhibits renal excretion of cilastatin. General seizures with *ganciclovir*. Little evidence of other interactions though no formal studies have been done.

PREGNANCY
Adverse effects have been shown in animal studies. Howeve, no studies have been performed in humans, contact local Medicines Information Centre for advice.

BREAST-FEEDING
Detected in human milk. Contact local Medicines Information Centre for advice.

SIDE-EFFECTS
Local irritation at injection site, skin rashes, gastrointestinal upset, pseudo-membranous colitis reported rarely, reversible neutropenia, thrombocytopenia, eosinophilia, and thrombocytosis reported, raised LFTs may occur. Adverse CNS effects such as seizures have been reported, particularly in patients with underlying CNS disorders, bacterial meningitis or poor renal function.

POISONING/TOXICITY
Treatment should be symptomatic. In normal individuals rapid renal elimination will occur; in those with renal impairment haemodialysis will remove imipenem.

PHARMACOKINETIC PROPERTIES
Both imipenem and cilastatin are removed by renal excretion. Half-life is approximately 1 hour in healthy older children, 1.5-2 hours in younger children and up to 3 hours in premature infants. Imipenem is widely distributed in many body tissues but levels are low in the CNS.

LICENSED STATUS
Licensed for >3 months of age.

Imipramine hydrochloride

Tricyclic antidepressant.

USES
Nocturnal enuresis; depression; neuropathic pain particularly where this prevents or interrupts sleep; hyperactivity.

PRESENTATION
Tablet: 10mg – non-proprietary; 25mg – Tofranil® and non-proprietary.

DOSAGE

Indication	Route	Age			Frequency	Notes
		1 month–2 years	2–12 years	12–18 years	(times daily)	
Nocturnal enuresis	Oral	–	>6 years 25mg	25–75mg	1 (30 minutes before bedtime)	Not likely to be used <6 years of age. Maximum period of treatment 3 months – review before further courses.
Hyper-activity	Oral	–	>6 years 25–75mg	50–75mg	1	Start at the lower doses and increase if necessary. Doses >1.5 mg/kg/day should be given in 2 divided doses to decrease risk of cardiotoxic effects.
Depression	Oral	–	–	25mg	1–3	Initial dose. Increase stepwise to 150–200mg daily. This should be maintained until definite improvement has occurred. Usual maintenance dose 50–150mg daily, determined individually.
Neuropathic pain	Oral	← 200–400 microgram/kg increasing gradually (50% increase every 2–3 days) to 1–3mg/kg →			1 (at night)	Start at the lower dose and increase as tolerated if necessary.

CONTRA-INDICATIONS & WARNINGS
Acute porphyria, hepatic impairment. Caution in presence of cardiac disease. Monitor doses above 150mg per day with ECG; changes from baseline to be discussed with a cardiologist.

INTERACTIONS
Allow 3 week interval after discontinuation of *MAOIs* before initiating imipramine. Plasma concentration reduced by *rifampicin* and *many anticonvulsants*. Plasma concentration increased by *phenothiazines, cimetidine, oral contraceptives, calcium-channel blockers, methylphenidate* and *SSRIs*. Will increase effect of any *antimuscarinics, sedatives, hypotensives* and *drugs which prolong QT interval*. Hypertension and cardiac dysrhythmias with *sympathomimetics* (but not local injection of adrenaline (epinephrine)).

PREGNANCY
Inadequate evidence of safety in human pregnancy. Neonates whose mothers had taken tricyclic antidepressants up until delivery developed dyspnoea, lethargy, colic, irritability, hypo- or hypertension, tremor or spasms during the first hours or days. If possible, withdraw gradually at least 7 weeks before calculated date of delivery.

BREAST-FEEDING
Small quantities excreted in breast milk, probably not enough to be harmful. However, manufacturers advise mothers to withdraw medication or cease breast-feeding.

SIDE-EFFECTS

Marked anticholinergic (antimuscarinic) effects, sedation, postural hypotension, cardiac dysrhythmias, tremor, sweating, increased appetite and weight gain, lowered seizure threshold, sexual dysfunction.

POISONING/TOXICITY

Tricyclics cause anticholinergic effects with features including hot dry skin, dilated pupils, tachycardia, arrhythmias, urinary retention, hypertonia, hyperreflexia, agitation, delirium, fits and coma.
Treatment includes support of the airway and breathing, activated charcoal*, alkalinisation to reduce the toxic effects on the heart by hyperventilation in intensive care to reduce $PaCO_2$ to 3.5kPa and sodium bicarbonate infusion 1mmol/kg. IV diazepam (200 microgram/kg) may be required for the control of convulsions (preferably in emulsion form).
*Give activated charcoal if >4mg/kg has been taken in a child, provided that the airway can be protected; give a second dose after 2 hours in patients with central features of toxicity.

PHARMACOKINETIC PROPERTIES

Rapidly and completely absorbed after oral administration. Half-life mean of 19 hours. Peak plasma concentrations within 1-2 hours. Peak antidepressant effect is usually seen after 2 weeks or more.

EXCIPIENTS

Contact manufacturers for further details.

LICENSED STATUS

Licensed for treatment of depression in adults, but not in children. Licensed for relief of nocturnal enuresis in >6 years of age. Not licensed for hyperactivity or neuralgic pain.

Immunoglobulin (intravenous)

USES

Replacement therapy for patients with congenital agammaglobulinaemia and hypogammaglobulinaemia. Treatment of idiopathic thrombocytopenic purpura (ITP) (not first-line unless there is severe bleeding), Kawasaki disease, juvenile dermatomyositis, intractable epilepsy where previous drug therapy has failed (myoclonic, atonic and tonic seizures) – use in highly selected cases. Prophylaxis of infection following bone marrow transplantation and in other primary and secondary humoral immunodeficiency disorders. Guillain-Barre syndrome.

PRESENTATION

Normal immunoglobulin for IV use: 0.5g, 2.5g, 5g and 10g – Flebogamma® (5%); 0.5g, 2.5g, 5g and 10g –Gammagard® S/D; 3g, 5g and 10g – Human Immunoglobulin (SNBTS); 2.5g, 5g and 10g – Octagam®; 2.5g, 5g and 10g – Vigam®Liquid; 2.5g and 5g – Vigam®S.
NB: products are not all equivalent.

DOSAGE

Indication	Route	Age				Frequency	Notes
		birth–1 month	1 month–2 years	2–12 years	12–18 years	(times daily)	
ITP	IV infusion	←	800mg/kg - 1g/kg		→	once daily	For 1-2 days. Courses should only be repeated in the presence of symptoms rather than according to platelet count.
Kawasaki Syndrome	IV infusion	–	← 2g/kg →		–	single dose	Give over 12 hours (if rate in the product SPC permits) as soon as possible after onset of disease. Consider second dose if still pyrexial 48 hours later.

Indication	Route	Age				Frequency (times daily)	Notes
		birth–1 month	1 month–2 years	2–12 years	12–18 years		
Replacement therapy in immuno-deficiency syndrome	IV infusion	–	←	400mg/kg	→	once every 3 weeks	Dose is initially determined by severity and frequency of infections as well as the serum IgG concentration.
Intractable epilepsy	IV infusion	←	400mg/kg		→	once every three weeks	For 3 doses. If >75% reduction in seizure frequency consider continuing treatment for 9–12 months and then re-evaluate.
Juvenile dermato-myositis	IV infusion	–	←	1g/kg	→	once daily	For 2 days, repeated as clinically indicated.
Guillain-Barré syndrome	IV infusion	–	←	400mg/kg	→	once daily	For 3–5 days depending on the severity of illness and rate to recover.

ADMINISTRATION

IV: initial infusion should start slowly and increase gradually if tolerated (see individual product information for complete infusion guidelines).

CONTRA-INDICATIONS & WARNINGS

Contra-indicated in patients with selective IgA deficiency who possess antibody to IgA. Avoid in immune deficient patients with acute bacterial infection. Despite all precautions taken by the manufacturers, the risk of transmission of blood-borne viruses cannot be entirely excluded.

INTERACTIONS

Active immunisation with *live vaccines* (especially *MMR*) should be postponed until 3 months after the last administration of immunoglobulin as the efficacy of the live virus may be impaired. If possible an interval of 3 weeks should be observed after administration of live virus vaccines prior to immunoglobulin administration (this does not apply to yellow fever vaccine since normal immunoglobulin does not contain antibody to this virus).

PREGNANCY/BREAST-FEEDING

Safety in pregnancy has not been established. Contact local Medicines Information Centre for advice

SIDE-EFFECTS

Commonly observed pyrexia, chills, nausea and vomiting, flushing of face, headache, fatigue, malaise, sweating, back pain. Other uncommon reactions include hypotension, dyspnoea and tightness of chest. Most adverse effects relate to the infusion rate; if they occur decrease infusion rate or halt infusion until symptoms subside.

POISONING/TOXICITY

Overdose is unlikely to have any harmful effects.

EXCIPIENTS

Contact manufacturers for further details.

LICENSED STATUS

Products differ on their licensed indications. Check individual product information carefully.

FURTHER INFORMATION

May contain traces of IgA and IgM. SNBTS is the Scottish National Blood Tranfusion Service.

Indometacin (indomethacin)

Non-steroidal anti-inflammatory drug (NSAID).

USES

Pain and moderate to severe inflammation in rheumatic disease and other acute musculoskeletal disorders;

pharmacological closure of a patent ductus arteriosus (PDA) in a neonate (usually preterm).
Nephrogenic diabetes insipidus (infants and young children) in conjunction with hydrochlorthiazide or chlorthiazide.

PRESENTATION
Capsule: 25mg and 50mg – Indocid®.
Capsule: (modified release) 25mg – Indomod®; 75mg – Indomax 75 SR®, Slo-Indo®, Indolar SR®, Indocid-R®, Indomod®; 100mg – Indolar SR®.
Injection: 1mg – Indocid PDA®.
Suspension: 25mg in 5mL - manufactured 'special', import.
Suppository: 100mg – Indocid®.
Tablet: (modified release) 25mg, 50mg and 75mg – Flexin Continus®.

DOSAGE

Indication	Route	Age				Frequency (times daily)	Notes
		birth– 1 month	1 month– 2 years	2–12 years	12–18 years		
Pain/ inflammation in rheumatic disease	Oral/ rectal	–	◄— 500 microgram–1mg/kg —►			2	(Maximum dose 50mg). If modified release, give in 2 divided doses or once only with the evening meal.
Nephrogenic diabetes insipidus	Oral	500 microgram–1mg/kg	–	–		2	Amiloride is used in older children.

Newborn infant (birth to 1 month): closure of patent ductus arteriosus.

Age at first dose	Intravenous dosage (microgram/kg)		
	1st dose	2nd dose	3rd dose
Less than 48 hours	200	100	100
2–7 days	200	200	200
Over 7 days	200	250	250

A course of therapy is defined as three IV doses given at 12-24 hour intervals. If anuria or marked oliguria (urinary output of 0.6mL/kg/hour) is evident at the time of the scheduled second or third dose, do not give until renal function has returned to normal. If the ductus arteriosus remains patent a second course of therapy may be given (doses unchanged).
Some neonatal units use a six dose protocol: 100 microgram/kg IV or orally daily for 6 days. In established symptomatic PDA the first dose is given as 200 microgram/kg IV followed by five further doses of 100 microgram/kg IV or orally at daily intervals (unlicensed doses).

ADMINISTRATION
Oral: tablets/capsules – take with or after food to minimise gastrointestinal side-effects.
IV: reconstitute vial with 1-2mL of NaCl 0.9% or Water for Injections. Preparations containing glucose must not be used. Further dilution with intravenous infusion is not recommended. Indometacin injection is not buffered and reconstitution at pH levels below 6 may cause precipitation of insoluble indometacin.

Amount of diluent used	Concentration achieved
1mL	100 microgram in 0.1mL
2mL	50 microgram in 0.1mL

The indometacin solution may be injected IV over 20 minutes. This recommendation is based on published reports which indicate that there is a transient reduction in cerebral blood flow velocity and cerebral blood flow when the injection is rapidly infused over 5 minutes. A syringe pump which delivers rates of 0.1-0.2mL per hour can be used. With small injection volumes, it is necessary to consider the priming volume of the tubing and flush through with a suitable volume of fluid, following the active injection, given at the same rate.

CONTRA-INDICATIONS & WARNINGS

Should not be given to patients with active peptic ulceration, and should be used with extreme caution in patients with a history of peptic ulceration. Also contra-indicated in patients who have previously shown hypersensitivity reactions (asthma, rhinitis, urticaria) to aspirin or other NSAIDs. Use with caution in renal, cardiac or hepatic impairment.

Indometacin suppositories should not be used in patients with a history of proctitis or recent rectal bleeding.

Indocid PDA® is contra-indicated in infants with established or suspected untreated infection, bleeding especially with active intracranial haemorrhage or gastro-intestinal bleeding, congenital heart disease in whom patency of the ductus arteriosus is necessary for satisfactory pulmonary or systemic blood flow, thrombocytopenia, coagulation defects, known or suspected necrotising enterocolitis, significant impairment of renal function. Discontinue if signs and symptoms consistent with liver disease develop in the neonate. May inhibit platelet aggregation. Premature babies should be observed for signs of bleeding.

INTERACTIONS

May decrease the elimination of *methotrexate*. May cause an increase in *digoxin* levels. Increased risk of nephrotoxicity when given with *ciclosporin (cyclosporin)*. *Diflunisal* may markedly increase indometacin levels. This combination should be avoided. *Probenecid* delays the excretion of indometacin, leading to increased indometacin levels. The antihypertensive and diuretic effects of *loop* and *thiazide diuretics* may be reduced by indometacin. The *diuretic* dose may need to be increased. The antihypertensive effects of *beta-blockers* may be reduced by indometacin. The *beta-blocker* dose may need to be increased. The co-administration of indometacin and *triamterene* can rapidly lead to acute renal failure. *Aminoglycoside* levels may be increased.

PREGNANCY

NSAIDs should be avoided in the third trimester as they may cause constriction of the ductus arteriosus *in utero* leading to persistent pulmonary hypertension in the newborn. In addition, these drugs may inhibit labour if used close to delivery.

Oliguric renal failure, haemorrhage, and intestinal perforation have been found in premature infants exposed immediately prior to delivery. The interaction between indometacin and beta-blockers (see interaction section) may be of particular importance in the management of pre-eclampsia, when this combination should be avoided.

BREAST-FEEDING

Indometacin is excreted in breast milk. There has been a single report of a breast-fed infant who developed seizures, possibly due to indometacin ingested in breast milk. Despite this, the American Academy of Pediatrics considers indometacin to be compatible with breast-feeding.

SIDE-EFFECTS

Gastrointestinal discomfort, nausea, diarrhoea, occasionally bleeding and ulceration. Headache, dizziness and vertigo. Fluid retention. Hypersensitivity reactions e.g. bronchospasm, rashes. Local discomfort, burning or itching and occasionally bleeding may occur with NSAID suppositories. Indometacin has also been reported to cause depression and behavioural changes. The following side-effects may occur with Indocid PDA®:

Haemorrhagic: gross or microscopic bleeding into the gastrointestinal tract; oozing from the skin after needle puncture; pulmonary haemorrhage; and disseminated intravascular coagulopathy.

Renal: renal dysfunction including one or more of the following: reduced urinary output; reduced urine sodium, chloride or potassium, urine osmolality, free water clearance, or glomerular filtration rate; uraemia; transient oliguria; and hypercreatininaemia.

Gastrointestinal: vomiting; abdominal distension; melaena; transient ileus; localised perforations of the small and/or large intestine.

Metabolic: hypersensitivity; hyponatraemia; elevated plasma potassium; elevated blood urea; hypoglycaemia.

Cardiovascular: pulmonary hypertension, intracranial bleeding.

Coagulation: decreased platelet aggregation.

General: weight gain (fluid retention); and exacerbation of infection.

POISONING/TOXICITY

There is no specific antidote. Activated charcoal may markedly reduce the absorption of the drug. Further treatment is symptomatic. Monitor for gastrointestinal bleeding for several days.

PHARMACOKINETIC PROPERTIES

Indometacin suppositories may give relief from pain and stiffness for 13-16 hours after administration. Therapeutic levels may be reached from 1-2 hours after oral administration. Absorption is more rapid when given rectally than orally. Oral absorption will be further delayed by the presence of food.

EXCIPIENTS

Contact manufacturers for further details.

LICENSED STATUS

None of the currently available oral or rectal preparations are licensed for use in children. Indocid PDA® is licensed for the closure of PDA in premature babies.

FURTHER INFORMATION
Although indometacin appears to be less well tolerated than some other NSAIDs, it may be particularly valuable in controlling symptoms in the spondyloarthropathies. Indometacin suspension 25mg in 5mL is available from IDIS World Medicines or as a 'special' from Eldon Laboratories.

Infliximab

Chimeric IgG1 monoclonal antibody.

USES
Treatment of severe, active Crohn's disease, in patients who have not responded despite a full and adequate course of therapy with a corticosteroid and an immunosuppressant; or who are intolerant to or have medical contra-indications for such therapies.
Treatment of fistulating Crohn's disease, in patients who have not responded despite a full and adequate course of therapy.

PRESENTATION
Injection: 100mg – Remicaide®.

DOSAGE
Child

Indication	Route	Age			Frequency (times daily)	Notes
		1 month–2 years	2–12 years	12–18 years		
Severe active Crohn's disease	IV infusion	←	5mg/kg	→	single dose	IV infusion give over 2 hours.
Fistulating Crohn's disease	IV infusion	←	5mg/kg	→	single dose	IV infusion give over 2 hours.

If the signs and symptoms of disease recur, infliximab can be re-administered within 14 weeks following the last infusion. Due to the potential risk of a delayed hypersensitivity reaction, re-administration of infliximab after a drug free interval of 15 weeks or more cannot be recommended.

ADMINISTRATION
Reconstitute each vial with 10mL Water for Injections. Gently swirl to dissolve; do not shake. Allow to stand for 5 minutes and check that the solution is colourless to light yellow and opalescent. As infliximab is a protein, the solution may develop a few fine translucent particles. Do not use if opaque particles, discolouration or other foreign particles are present. On reconstitution, vials contain 10mg in 1mL infliximab. Dilute total volume of reconstituted solution to 250mL with NaCl 0.9%. Administer over at least 2 hours (maximum rate 2mL/minute) using an infusion set with an in-line, sterile, non-pyrogenic, low protein-binding filter (pore size less than or equal to 1.2 microns – available from Schering-Plough). Commence infusion as soon as possible following reconstitution and dilution – the manufacturers recommend within 3 hours. If stored in the fridge, the infliximab infusion solution can be used within 24 hours.
Patients must be observed during and for at least 1-2 hours after the infusion. Acute infusion reactions are most likely to occur during the first and second infusion and may be related to the rate of infusion. If symptoms occur, consider reducing the rate of the infusion or interrupting until they subside and then restart at a slower rate.

CONTRA-INDICATIONS / WARNINGS
Infliximab is contra-indicated in any patient with tuberculosis or other severe infection, patients with moderate or severe heart failure or in patients with a history of hypersensitivity to infliximab, to other murine proteins or to any of the excipients.
Infliximab has been associated with acute infusion-related reactions including anaphylactic shock and delayed hypersensitivity reactions; anaphylaxis kit must be readily available. Monitor patients closely for

infections, including tuberculosis, before, during and after treatment with infliximab.

PREGNANCY
There is no experience of the use of infliximab in pregnant women. Due to its inhibition of TNF-alpha, infliximab administered during pregnancy could affect normal immune responses in the newborn. Administration of infliximab is not recommended during pregnancy and it is recommended that women of childbearing potential use adequate contraception to prevent pregnancy during and for 6 months after infliximab treatment.

BREAST-FEEDING
It is not known whether infliximab is excreted in human milk or absorbed systemically after ingestion. Because human immunoglobulins are excreted in milk, women must not breast-feed for at least 6 months after infliximab treatment.

SIDE-EFFECTS
Resistance mechanism: common – viral infections; uncommon – abscess, cellulitis, sepsis, impaired healing, bacterial and fungal infections.
Immune: uncommon – autoantibodies, lupus-like syndrome.
Blood: uncommon – anaemia, leucopenia, lymphadenopathy, lymphocytosis, neutropenia, thrombocytopenia.
Psychiatric: uncommon – depression, confusion, agitation, amnesia, apathy, nervousness, somnolence.
Central and peripheral nervous system: common –
headache, dizziness; uncommon – exacerbation of demyelinating disease suggestive of multiple sclerosis.
Vision and hearing: uncommon – conjunctivitis, endophthalmitis.
Cardiovascular: common – flushing; uncommon – hypertension, hypotension, bradycardia, palpitation, thrombophlebitis.
Respiratory system: common – upper and lower respiratory tract infection; uncommon – epistaxis, bronchospasm.
Gastrointestinal system: common – nausea, diarrhoea, abdominal pain, dyspepsia; uncommon– constipation, gastroesophageal reflux.
Liver and biliary system: common – abnormal hepatic function.
Skin: common – rash, pruritus, urticaria, increased sweating, dry skin; uncommon – fungal infections, eczema, rosacea, verucca, abnormal skin pigmentation, alopecia.
Musculo-skeletal system: uncommon – myalgia, arthralgia.
Urinary system: uncommon – urinary tract infection.
Body as a whole: common – fatigue, chest pain, infusion-related reactions, oedema, hot flushes, pain, chills/rigors, anaphylactic reaction.
Administration site: uncommon – injection site reactions.

POISONING / TOXICITY
No clinical experience of overdose.

PHARMACOKINETIC PROPERTIES
In most patients, infliximab can be detected in the serum for at least 8 weeks after the recommended single dose of 5mg/kg for Crohn's disease.

EXCIPIENTS
Include sucrose.

LICENSED STATUS
Licensed for >17 years of age.

Influenza vaccine (inactivated)

USES
Active protection of at risk groups against influenza infection. Annual immunisation is recommended for children with the following: chronic respiratory disease (including cystic fibrosis, bronchopulmonary dysplasia and severe asthma), chronic heart disease (including congenital cyanotic heart disease), chronic renal failure, diabetes mellitus, inborn errors of metabolism that would be destabilised by influenza infection, immunosuppression (including functional asplenia) and chronic neurodevelopmental problems, including Down's syndrome. The vaccine should also be given to children and young people in long-term residential care.

PRESENTATION
Injection: (single dose suspension) – Aggripal®, Begrivac®, Fluarix®, Fluvirin®, Inactivated Influenza Vaccine (Split Virion) BP, Inactivated Influenza Vaccine (Surface Antigen) Ph.Eur, Influvac®.

All vaccines contain haemagglutinin and neuraminidase antigens. The virus is grown in embryonated hens' eggs, chemically inactivated and then purified. 'Split Virion' (Inactivated Influenza Vaccine (Split Virion) BP, Fluarix® and Begrivac®) vaccines contain whole disrupted virus whereas the 'surface antigen' (Aggripal, Inactivated Influenza Vaccine (Surface Antigen) Ph. Eur, Influvac® and Fluvirin®) vaccines contain highly purified haemagglutinin and neuraminidase antigens derived from the disrupted virus. All contain material from two type A and one type B subtypes of virus. Subtypes are chosen each year on advice from the World Health Organisation.

DOSAGE

This depends on age and whether influenza vaccine has been given in previous years.

6-35 months	0.25mL
≥36 months	0.5mL

≤12 years, if receiving the vaccine for the first time, a second dose should be given after an interval of 4 weeks. The vaccine should be given yearly to all those at continuing risk. The different vaccines currently available can be used interchangeably.

ADMINISTRATION

IM or deep SC.

CONTRA-INDICATIONS AND WARNINGS

As for vaccines generally; also, the vaccine should not be given to those who have had an anaphylactic reaction to egg. Some vaccines contain trace amounts of neomycin, gentamicin, polymixin and gelatin and should not be given to children or young people who have had anaphylactic reactions to them.

INTERACTIONS

Some studies have suggested that the vaccine may enhance the effect of *warfarin, theophylline* and *phenytoin*. The data is inconclusive, but sufficient to justify caution when the vaccine is used with any of these medications. Clotting studies or drug levels should be considered. Following the vaccination, false positive results in serology tests using ELISA for HIV1, Hepatitis C and HTLV have been reported.

PREGNANCY

There is limited systematic data available on the use of the vaccine in pregnancy. What little there is suggests no adverse effect on the mother, fetus or neonate. In the USA it is recommended that the vaccine should be given to all pregnant women if the second or third trimester falls within the influenza season and to women in high-risk categories, at whatever stage of pregnancy. This is not policy in the UK.

BREAST-FEEDING

There is no data available on use of the vaccine during breast-feeding. As immunisation is almost always an elective procedure it should usually be postponed until after the baby is weaned.

SIDE-EFFECTS

Mild local reactions at the site of injection may occur. Fever, malaise and arthralgia may occur 6-12 hours after immunisation and last up to 48 hours. Urticaria, angio-oedema, bronchospasm and anaphylaxis have been reported rarely. Guillain-Barré syndrome very rarely has a causal association with the vaccination.

POISONING/TOXICITY

No data available.

PHARMACODYNAMIC PROPERTIES

The vaccine takes 10-14 days to produce protective antibody levels.

EXCIPIENTS

Aggripal®: formaldehyde, sodium chloride, potassium chloride, potassium dihydrogen phosphate, disodium phosphate dihydrate, magnesium chloride, calcium chloride and thiomersal.

Begrivac®: formaldehyde, diethylether, sodium chloride, potassium chloride, magnesium chloride hexahydrate, disodium phosphate dihydrate, potassium dihydrogen phosphate, sucrose, polysorbate 80 and polymixin B.

Fluarix®: thiomersal, sodium chloride, disodium phosphate dodecahydrated, potassium dihydrogen phosphate, potassium chloride, magnesium chloride hexahydrate, Polysorbate 80, octoxynol, α-tocopheryl hydrogen succinate, formaldehyde, sodium deoxycholate and gentamicin.

Fluvirin®: potassium dihydrogenphosphate, disodium hydrogenphosphate, sodium chloride, thiomersal, formaldehydebetapropiolactone, nonoxynol 9 neomycin and polymyxin.

Inactivated Influenza Vaccine (Split Virion) BP: thiomersal, sodium chloride, potassium chloride, disodium phosphate dihygrogen dihydrate, potassium dihydrogen phosphate, neomycin, formaldehyde and Octoxynol-9.

Influenza Inactivated Vaccine (Surface Antigen) Ph. Eur: betapropiolactone, nonoxynol 9, thiomersal, potassium dihydrogenphosphate, disodium hydrogenphosphate and sodium chloride.

Influvac®: potassium chloride, potassium dihydrogen phosphate, disodium phosphate dihydrate, sodium chloride, calcium chloride, magnesium chloride hexahydrate, thiomersal, sucrose, sodium deoxycholate, formaldehyde, cetyltrimethyl ammonium bromide, polysorbate 80 and gentamicin.

LICENSED STATUS
Licensed for use as described.

FURTHER INFORMATION
Each year the World Health Organisation makes recommendations as to the composition of the vaccine depending on the prevalent strains of wild virus. The vaccine should be given at such a time that protection is provided from the middle of November.

Protect from light and store at 2-8°C, do not freeze. Materials of bovine origin are used in the manufacturing process. Trace amounts of the original material may be present in the final product, however, all such material is obtained from sources known to be free of BSE.

Insulins

USES
Primary treatment for patients with type 1 diabetes and type 2 diabetes uncontrolled by other means.

PRESENTATION
Injection: vials, cartridges for use with reusable pens, prefilled pens. Not all insulins are available in all presentations.

DOSAGE

Route	Age				Frequency (times daily)	Notes
	birth–1 month	1 month–2 years	2–12 years	12–18 years		
IV infusion	←	0.1 units/kg/hour		→	Continuous	Adjust dose according to blood glucose level.
SC injection	←	0.5-0.7 units/kg/**day**	→	Up to 2 units/kg/**day**	-	See below for information on dividing the daily dose. NB an increased dose may be required during the pubertal growth spurt.

Dosage should be adjusted according to response. Dose may need to be increased as patients reach the pubertal growth spurt. Consult the diabetes section of the Endocrine guidelines for full details.

ADMINISTRATION
SC/IV: by SC injection or continuous IV infusion.

For IV infusion make up a solution of 1 unit per mL of human soluble insulin by adding 50 units (0.5mL) soluble insulin to 50mL NaCl 0.9% in a syringe, so that 0.1mL/kg/hour = 0.1 units/kg/hour.

CONTRA-INDICATIONS & WARNINGS
Loss of warning may occur with recurrent hypoglycaemia. Dosage may need to be reduced in severe renal impairment.

INTERACTIONS
Enhanced hypoglycaemic effect with *beta-blockers*, *loop* and *thiazide diuretics*, *nifedipine* and *corticosteroids*.

SIDE-EFFECTS
Hypoglycaemia, local reactions and fat hypertrophy at injection site (may be prevented by rotating injection site used).

EXCIPIENTS
Contact manufacturers for further details.

LICENSED STATUS
Licensed for use in all ages.

FURTHER INFORMATION
Insulin should be prescribed by trade name; all parents/patients should be counselled on which brand of insulin they should be using. Human insulins are produced in 4 different ways: from proinsulin synthesised by bacteria using recombinant DNA technology; by enzymatic modification of porcine insulin; from a precursor synthesised by yeast using recombinant DNA technology; human insulin analogue of rDNA origin. Insulin should be stored in the refrigerator, and once opened should be discarded after 3 months, but has a shelf-life of 1 month when stored at room temperature.

INSULIN

Rapid acting
Humalog® (insulin lispro, Lilly)
Available as vials, prefilled pens, 1.5mL and 3mL cartridges. Onset of action within 15 minutes. Duration of action approximately 2-5 hours.

NovoRapid® (insulin aspart, Novo Nordisk)
Available as vials, prefilled pens and 3mL cartridges.
Onset of action within 10-20 minutes. Duration of action 3-5 hours.

Short acting (soluble)
Human Velosulin® (Novo Nordisk)
Available as vials. Duration of action approximately 8 hours.

Human Actrapid® (Novo Nordisk)
Available as vials, prefilled pens, 1.5mL and 3mL cartridges. Duration of action approximately 8 hours.

Humulin S® (Lilly)
Available as vials, prefilled pens and 3mL cartridges. Duration of action approximately 12 hours.

Insuman® Rapid (Hoechst)
Available as vials, prefilled pens and 3mL cartridges. Duration of action 7-9 hours.

Medium acting (isophane)
Human Insulatard® ge (Novo Nordisk)
Available as vials, prefilled pens, 1.5mL and 3mL cartridges. Duration of action approximately 24 hours.

Humulin I® (Lilly)
Available as vials, prefilled pens, 3mL cartridges. Duration of action approximately 22 hours.

Insuman® Basal (Hoescht)
Available as vials, prefilled pens and 3mL cartridges. Duration of action 11-20 hours.

Medium acting (insulin zinc suspension)
Human Monotard® (Novo Nordisk)
Available as vials only. Duration of action approximately 24 hours.

Humulin Lente® (Lilly)
Available as vials only. Duration of action approximately 23 hours.

Long acting (crystalline zinc suspension)
Human Ultratard® (Novo Nordisk)
Available as vials only. Duration of action approximately 24-28 hours.

Humulin Zn® (Lilly)
Available as vials only. Duration of action approximately 25 hours.

Lantus® (insulin glargine, Aventis)
Available as vials, prefilled pens and 3mL cartridges. Duration of action approximately 15-30 hours.

Biphasic (soluble and isophane)
Speed of onset of the combination products is proportional to the amount of soluble insulin.

Human Mixtard® (Novo Nordisk)
Available as 10/90, 20/80, 30/70, 40/60 and 50/50 mixtures, in prefilled pens, 1.5 and 3ml cartridges. Only the 30/70 and 50/50 mixtures are available in vials. Total duration of action approximately 24 hours.

Humulin M® (Lilly)
Available as M2 (20/80) in prefilled pens and 3mL cartridges; M3 (30/70) in vials, prefilled pens and 3mL cartridges; M5 (50/50) in vials. Total duration of action approximately 22 hours.

Insuman® Comb (Hoechst)
Available as 15/85, 25/75 and 50/50 mixtures, in prefilled pens, 3mL cartridges and vials. Total duration of action is approximately 12-18 hours.

Biphasic (rapid acting and protamine suspension)
Speed of onset is proportional to the amount of rapid acting insulin.

Humalog® Mix (Lilly)
Available as Mix25 (25/75) mixture, in prefilled pens and 3mL cartridges. Also Mix50 (50/50) mixture, in prefilled pens. Onset of action within 15 minutes. Duration of action up to 15 hours.

NovoMix® 30 (Lilly)
Available as 30/70 mixture, in prefilled pens and 3mL cartridges.

All the above insulins are classed as human; beef and pork insulin products are also available.

Interferon alfa

USES
Treatment of chronic active hepatitis B and C infection.
Seroconversion from e-antigen positivity to e-antibody positivity.
To induce the early regression of life-threatening corticosteroid resistant haemangiomata of infancy.

PRESENTATION

Preparation	Interferon	Form	Concentration
Intron A®	Interferon alfa–2b	Injection solution	25 million units in 2.5mL
		Powder for reconstitution	10 million units
		Multidose injection pen (1.2mL)	15, 25 and 50 million units in 1mL
Roferon-A®	Interferon alfa–2a	Pre-filled syringe	3, 4.5, 6 and 9 million units in 0.5mL
		Injection solution	18 million units in 1mL
		Pen cartridge	18 million units in 0.6mL
Viraferon®	Interferon alfa–2b	Injection solution	18 million units in 3mL
		Multidose injection pen (1.2mL)	15 and 25 million units in 1mL

DOSAGE

Route	Age				Frequency (times daily)	Notes
	birth–1 month	1 month–2 years	2–12 years	12–18 years		
SC injection	← 3 million units/m^2 →		← 3–10 million units/m^2 →		Usually 3 times per week, but it is given daily in haemangiomata of infancy	Experience in children is limited. Specialist advice should always be sought. Usual duration of treatment is 4–6 months.

DOSAGE continued

Route	Age				Frequency (times daily)	Notes
	birth–1 month	1 month–2 years	2–12 years	12–18 years		
SC injection in chronic hepatitis B	–		←— 5–10 million units/m² —→ (Intron A® and Viraferon®)		3 times per week (every other day)	For chronic hepatitis B.
	–		←— 2.5–5 million units/m² —→ (Roferon-A®)		3 times per week (every other day)	For chronic hepatitis B. Up to 10 million units/m² of Roferon-A® has been used in children.

CONTRA-INDICATIONS & WARNINGS

Roferon-A® should not be used in the neonatal period, due to possibility of fatal reactions to the benzylalcohol excipient.

Hypersensitivity to interferon alfa or any component of the individual formulation. Severe pre-existing cardiac disease, severe renal, hepatic or myeloid dysfunction. Epilepsy, and/or compromised CNS function. Patients with pre-existing psychiatric condition or history of severe psychiatric disorder. Chronic hepatitis with advanced cirrhosis or decompensated hepatic disease. Chronic hepatitis in patients currently or recently treated with immunosuppressive agents (excluding corticosteroids). Autoimmune hepatitis, or history of autoimmune disease. Immunosuppressed transplant recipients and patients for whom allogenic bone marrow transplantation is planned or possible in the immediate future. Thyroid disease unless well controlled.

Caution should be exercised in: patients with debilitating conditions, including pulmonary disease, diabetes mellitus prone to ketoacidosis, coagulation disorders, mild to moderate renal, hepatic or myeloid disease. Patients with chronic hepatitis B, with evidence of deteriorating synthetic function. Clinical decompensation may follow a flare of aminotransferases and the risks of treatment should be weighed against the possible benefits. Patients with a history of congestive heart failure and/or previous or current arrhythmic disorders should be closely monitored. A baseline ECG is advised, with monitoring as appropriate throughout treatment. Cardiac arrhythmias, usually supraventricular, respond to conventional therapy but may necessitate discontinuation of interferon alfa. Adequate hydration must be maintained to prevent fluid depletion and hypotension.

INTERACTIONS

Narcotic drugs, hypnotics and *sedatives* should be used with caution due to the risk of interferon affecting CNS function. May interfere with oxidative metabolism; concurrent use of drugs metabolised by this route, such as *theophylline*, should be undertaken with caution. Monitor serum *theophylline* levels. May reduce the activity of the cytochrome P-450 enzyme system. Drugs metabolised by this enzyme system, including *cimetidine, phenytoin, diazepam, propranolol, warfarin, cyclophosphamide* and *doxorubicin* should be used with caution due to a risk of enhanced effects and/or toxicity.

Concurrent administration with *vinblastine* or *busulphan* may produce severe myelosuppression. Concurrent administration with *aciclovir* may enhance the risk of progressive renal failure, although the combination is reported as beneficial in hepatitis B infection.

PREGNANCY

Interferon alfa crosses the placenta in humans and enters the fetal circulation. It has demonstrated abortifacient properties in rhesus monkeys at dose levels of 90–180 times that recommended. It should only be used in pregnant women where the benefits outweigh any risk to the fetus.

BREAST-FEEDING

Given the potential for adverse reactions in the infant a decision should be made as to whether breast-feeding or interferon should be stopped.

SIDE-EFFECTS

The most commonly reported adverse effects are flu-like symptoms such as fever, fatigue, headache and myalgia. These acute side-effects tend to diminish with continued therapy or dose reduction and can be reduced by administration of paracetamol. Other common adverse effects include rigors, anorexia and nausea. Less common effects include vomiting, diarrhoea, arthralgia, asthenia, somnolence, dizziness, dry mouth, alopecia, back pain, malaise, increased sweating, altered taste, insomnia, impaired concentration and hypotension. Abnormalities of liver function, hypo- and hyperthyroidism and ocular adverse effects have occurred rarely. Baseline assessment of liver and thyroid function and visual acuity is recommended. Pulmonary infiltrates, pneumonitis and pneumonia have been observed rarely and may lead to fatality. Any patient developing fever, cough, dyspnoea or other respiratory symptoms should be investigated. If chest X-ray shows evidence of pulmonary infiltrates or impairment of function the patient should be closely monitored and discontinuation considered. A wide variety of other adverse effects have been reported rarely; see manufacturers SPC for further details.

POISONING/TOXICITY
Overdosage has not been reported. There is no specific antidote. Symptomatic and supportive treatment should be given as appropriate. Repeated high-dose therapy has been associated with profound lethargy, prostration and coma.

PHARMACODYNAMIC PROPERTIES
The antiviral properties of interferon alfa are due to induction of two enzymes, 2-5A oligoadenylate synthetase and a protein kinase, both of which affect the translation of viral and cellular messenger RNA. They also have immunomodulatory effects, suppressing antibody formation through an effect on ß-lymphocytes and inhibiting the development of delayed hypersensitivity. Macrophage activity is also enhanced.

PHARMACOKINETIC PROPERTIES
Pharmacokinetic parameters are linear over a wide dose range. The following data refers to Roferon-A$^®$: fraction absorbed after SC/IM injection: >80%, elimination half-life of 3.7-8.5 hours (mean 5.1 hours), volume of distribution is 0.223-0.748L/kg (mean 0.4L/kg) at steady state. Interferon alfa is excreted in the urine, reabsorbed by the proximal tubules and undergoes lysosomal degradation in these cells.

EXCIPIENTS
Intron A$^®$ and Viraferon$^®$ include human albumin. Roferon-A$^®$ includes benzyl alcohol.

LICENSED STATUS
Not licensed for use in children. Viraferon$^®$ is only licensed for hepatitis.

Interferon gamma-1b (immune interferon)

USES
Adjunct therapy to reduce the frequency of serious infections in patients with chronic granulomatous disease (CGD).

PRESENTATION
Injection: recombinant human interferon gamma-1b 200 micrograms in 1mL, 0.5mL vial – Immukin$^®$.

DOSAGE

Route	BSA <0.5m^2	BSA >0.5m^2	Frequency	Notes
SC	1.5 micrograms/kg	50 micrograms/m^2	3 times a week	For example given on Monday, Wednesday and Friday.

Not recommended for children <6 months.

ADMINISTRATION
SC: preferably administered in the evening. Optimum sites for injection are the right and left deltoid and the anterior thigh.

CONTRA-INDICATIONS & WARNINGS
Contra-indicated in patients who have hypersensitivity to interferon gamma or known hypersensitivity to closely related interferons.
Cautioned in seizure disorders and/or compromised CNS function; pre-existing cardiac disease (including ischaemia, congestive heart failure and arrhythmias); severe hepatic or renal impairment. Monitor before and during treatment: haematological tests (including FBC, differential white cell count and platelet count), blood chemistry tests (including renal and liver function tests) and urinalyis.

INTERACTIONS
Simultaneous administration of interferon gamma-1b with other heterologous serum protein preparations or immunological preparations (e.g. vaccines) should be avoided because of the risk for unexpected amplified immune response.

PREGNANCY
Safety in pregnancy has not been established. The manufacturers of Immukin$^®$ only recommend using it, in pregnancy, if the potential benefit justifies the potential risk to the fetus. Contact local Medicines Information Centre for advice.

BREAST-FEEDING
Not known whether interferon gamma-1b is excreted into human milk. Contact local Medicines Information Centre for advice.

SIDE-EFFECTS
Fever, headache, chills, myalgia or fatigue; nausea and vomiting, arthralgia, rashes and injection-site reactions.

POISONING/TOXICITY
CNS adverse reactions including decreased mental status, gait disturbance and dizziness have been seen but usually reversed within a few days of dose reduction or discontinuation of therapy. Reversible neutropenia, elevations of hepatic enzymes and of triglycerides; thrombocytopenia has also been observed.

PHARMACOKINETIC PROPERTIES
Slowly cleared after SC administration. With the subcutaneous dose of 50 microgram/m² the mean elimination half-life was 4.9 hours and the mean residence time was 2.5 hours. Time to reach maximum plasma concentration ranged from 4-14 hours.

EXCIPIENTS
See manufacturers SPC for further details.

LICENSED STATUS
Not licensed for children <6 months.

FURTHER INFORMATION
Vials must be stored in a fridge between 2-8°C.

Iodine

USES
Thyrotoxicosis (pre-operative). Neonatal thyrotoxicosis.

PRESENTATION
Oral solution: iodine 5%, potassium iodide 10% in purified water (total iodine 130mg in 1mL) – Aqueous Iodine Oral Solution (Lugol's solution).

DOSAGE

Route	Age				Frequency (times daily)	Notes
	birth–1 month	1 month–2 years	2–12 years	12–18 years		
Oral	1 drop	–	–	–	3	Neonatal thyrotoxicosis.
	← 0.1–0.3mL →				3	Thyrotoxicosis (pre-operative).

ADMINISTRATION
Oral: dilute well with milk or water.

CONTRA-INDICATIONS & WARNINGS
Breast-feeding. Not for long-term treatment.

PREGNANCY
Neonatal goitre and hypothyroidism could occur. Contact local Medicines Information Centre for advice.

BREAST-FEEDING
Contra-indicated as danger of neonatal goitre and hypothyroidism; appears to be concentrated in milk.

SIDE-EFFECTS
Hypersensitivity reactions including coryza-like symptoms, headache, lachrymation, conjunctivitis, pain in salivary glands, laryngitis, bronchitis, rashes.

POISONING/TOXICITY
The symptoms of acute poisoning from ingestion of free iodine (Lugol's solution) are mainly due to its corrosive effects on the gastrointestinal tract (mean lethal dose = 40-80mL); a disagreeable metallic taste, vomiting, abdominal pain, and diarrhoea occur also. Renal failure and anuria may occur 1 to 3 days later; death may be due to circulatory failure, oedema of the epiglottis resulting in asphyxia, aspiration pneumonia, or pulmonary oedema. Oesophageal stricture may occur if the patient survives the acute stage. Treatment includes copious amounts of milk or starch mucilage, activated charcoal and sodium thiosulphate solution 1% or 5% to reduce iodine to iodide.

LICENSED STATUS
Licensed for use in all ages.

Ipratropium bromide

Anticholinergic bronchodilator, which affects airway function via the parasympathetic nervous system blocking anticholinergic receptors on smooth muscle in the lungs.

USES
Treatment of chronic reversible airways obstruction. May be used with a beta-2 agonist in the treatment of severe, acute asthma.

PRESENTATION
Aerosol inhalation: 20 and 40 microgram – Atrovent®.
Breath-actuated aerosal inhalation: 20 microgram – Atrovent Autohaler®.
Dry powder for inhalation: 40 microgram – Atrovent® Aerocaps®, for use with Atrovent Aerohaler®.
Nebuliser solution: 250 microgram in 1mL, 500 microgram in 2mL – Atrovent®, Ipratropium Steri-Neb®, Respontin® and non-proprietary.

DOSAGE

Route	Age				Frequency (times daily)	Notes
	birth–1 month	1 month–2 years	2–12 years	12–18 years		
Inhaled	←	20 microgram up to 120 microgram		→	4	RELIEVER for symptom relief only.
Dry powder inhalation	–	–	–	40 microgram (1 capsule)	3-4	RELIEVER for symptom relief only.
Nebulised	25 microgram/kg	<1 year 62.5 microgram	<5 years 125-250 microgram	500 microgram	single dose	Can be repeated every 20-30 minutes in the first 2 hours in acute severe asthma.
		>1 year 125-250 microgram	>5 years 250-500 microgram		single dose	Reduce dose frequency as clinical improvement occurs.

ADMINISTRATION
Nebuliser: dilute to suitable volume with NaCl 0.9%. The nebuliser solution can be mixed with salbutamol, budesonide and terbutaline nebuliser solutions.
Inhaler: aerosol inhaler can be used via Nebuhaler® spacer with mask for infants and young children, or Volumatic® spacer.

CONTRA-INDICATIONS & WARNINGS
Care if known hypersensitivity to atropine. Avoid accidental spraying into the eyes. On rare occasions bronchospasm may be made worse.

PREGNANCY
There is no definite evidence of ill consequences of the use of ipratropium bromide during pregnancy.

BREAST-FEEDING
Contact local Medicines Information Centre for advice.

SIDE-EFFECTS
Rarely dry mouth, urinary retention, constipation and worsening of bronchospasm.

POISONING/TOXICITY
Inhaled doses of 5mg produce an increase in heart rate and palpitations.

PHARMACOKINETIC PROPERTIES
Following inhalation, uptake into plasma is minimal. A peak blood concentration is obtained 1-3 hours after inhalation. Excretion is mainly via the kidneys.

EXCIPIENTS
See manufacturers SPC for further details.

LICENSED STATUS
All presentations are licensed for use in all ages; however, the doses given here exceed those recommended by the manufacturers.

Iron

Iron is an essential constituent of the body necessary for haemoglobin formation.

USES
Iron-deficiency anaemias, prophylaxis of iron deficiency in low birth weight infants and breast-fed infants.

PRESENTATION

The elemental iron content represents the amount of available iron and is given below for each product. All mg doses are expressed as elemental iron.

Oral Preparations

Ferrous Sulphate
Tablet: 200mg (65mg iron) – non-proprietary.
Tablet (modified release): 150mg (47mg iron) – Feospan®; 325mg (105mg iron) – Ferrograd® and 160mg (50mg iron) – Slow-Fe®.
Oral solution: Paediatric BP – may be extemporaneously prepared.

Sodium Ironedetate (sodium feredetate)
Elixir: 27.5mg iron in 5mL – Sytron®.

Ferrous Glycine Sulphate
Syrup: 25mg iron in 5mL – Plesmet®.

Ferrous Gluconate
Tablet: 300mg (35mg iron) – non-proprietary.

Ferrous Fumarate
Capsule: 305mg (100mg iron) – Galfer®.
Tablet: 322mg (100mg iron) – Fersaday®.
Tablet: 210mg (68mg iron) – Fersamal®.
Syrup: 45mg iron in 5mL – Fersamal® and Galfer®.

Injectable Preparations
Injection: iron sucrose 20mg iron in 1mL, 5mL ampoule – Venofer®.

DOSAGE
Newborn infant (birth to 1 month)
All mg doses are expressed as elemental iron.

Indication	Route	Age		Frequency	Notes
		birth–1 month		(times daily)	
Prophylaxis of iron deficiency in low birth weight (<2.5 kg), breast-fed infants	Oral	5 mg of elemental iron or 1mL Sytron® elixir		1 / 1	Usually started at 28 days postnatal age and continued until mixed feeding is established. There is no good evidence that formula fed babies require further supplementation after discharge (unless they are on Osterprem®). Current practice varies throughout the UK; refer to local policy as doses may differ from those stated.

Child
All mg doses are expressed as elemental iron.

Indication	Route	Age			Frequency	Notes
		1 month– 2 years	2–12 years	12–18 years	(times daily)	
Treatment of iron deficiency anaemia	Oral	>3 months ← 2.5mg/kg → of elemental iron		–	2	Calculate dose in terms of elemental iron, specifying prescribing in terms of elemental iron or convert the dose to the iron salt preparation required and specify prescribing in terms of the specific salt with for example the dose given in mLs.
		–		60mg of elemental iron	3	

See under administration for injectable preparations.

ADMINISTRATION
Oral: tablets too hard to halve accurately, so use liquid preparation when necessary. Take with food to reduce gastrointestinal irritation. All preparations can be given once or twice daily if tolerated.
IV: Venofer® must be administered IV by drip infusion, by slow injection or directly into the venous limb of a dialyser. It is not suitable for IM use. The manufacturers SPC must be consulted for calculation of the total dose required and details of test doses. It has been used in doses of 3-7mg iron/kg/day.

CONTRA-INDICATIONS & WARNINGS
Haemochromatosis, haemosiderosis, anaemia not caused by iron deficiency. Parenteral iron is contra-indicated in untreated pyelonephritis and acute liver disease.

INTERACTIONS
Absorption of oral iron decreased by *antacids, milk, tetracycline, trientene, zinc.*
Absorption of *ciprofloxacin, levofloxacin, norfloxacin, ofloxacin, tetracycline, levodopa, entacapone, penicillamine* is decreased by oral iron. Parenteral iron preparations should not be administered concomitantly with oral iron preparations, since this decreases the unsaturated iron binding capacity of the blood – see manufacturers SPC for further information.

PREGNANCY
Iron is widely used – safe to use in pregnancy.

BREAST-FEEDING
Safe to use. Iron salts are excreted into breast milk, which may be beneficial. Venofer® unlikely to be excreted into milk, therefore should not be a risk to the child.

SIDE-EFFECTS
Gastrointestinal irritation: nausea, epigastric pain, diarrhoea, constipation. With parenteral iron, also taste disturbances, dizziness, flushing, pain or discolouration at injection site. May discolour stools.

POISONING/TOXICITY
Nausea and vomiting, diarrhoea, haematemesis, rectal bleed, lethargy, cardiovascular collapse, hyperglycaemia and metabolic acidosis. Antidote is desferrioxamine – see desferrioxamine monograph for dosage.

PHARMACOKINETIC PROPERTIES
Iron is irregularly and incompletely absorbed from the gastrointestinal tract. Absorption is aided by acid secretion of the stomach and a state of iron deficiency or fasting.
Haemoglobin measurement will give an indication of response to iron therapy. A positive response to treatment is demonstrated by a rise of at least 1g/100mL over a week.

EXCIPIENTS
Sytron® contains sorbitol solution. Contact manufacturers for further details.

LICENSED STATUS
Feospan® licensed for >1 year of age. Ferrograd® licensed for >12 years of age. Fersamal® and Sytron® liquid licensed for use in all ages. Galfer® and Plesmet® syrup licensed for use in children and adults. Slow-Fe® licensed for >6 years of age. Venofer® not licensed for use in children.

FURTHER INFORMATION
Modified release iron preparations have no therapeutic advantage over standard preparations and should not be used. They are likely to carry the iron past the first part of the duodenum into an area of the gut where conditions for iron absorption are poor.

Iron chloride injection

USES
As an iron supplement for infants and children on long-term PN. Iron supplementation is not usually necessary before age 3 months.

PRESENTATION
Injection: 100 micrograms of iron ($\equiv$1.79 micromol) per mL, 10mL ampoule – manufactured 'special'.

DOSAGE/ADMINISTRATION
1mL/kg as part of a balanced PN regimen.

CONTRA-INDICATIONS & WARNINGS
Risk of long-term accumulation of iron especially if the patient has multiple blood transfusions. Low transferrin levels in malnourished patients can lead to toxicity.

SIDE-EFFECTS
None likely at the dosage suggested above.

POISONING/TOXICITY
As for other iron preparations – see oral iron monograph.

PHARMACOKINETIC PROPERTIES
Iron is bound to transferrin and transported to the bone marrow where it is incorporated into haemaglobin. Little iron is excreted and most is re-used by the body.

LICENSED STATUS
Unlicensed product; manufactured by QMC Nottingham for Pharmacia; the product has a manufacturers licence as opposed to a product licence.

FURTHER INFORMATION
Not all units with long-term PN patients add iron. The addition of iron chloride may cause stability problems with lipid containing regimes. The maximum amount of iron chloride added to a bag must be calculated using the volume of the aqueous phase only. Exceeding the recommended maximum can lead to precipitation of iron phosphate and possibly other salts, plus causing damage to the lipid emulsion.

Isoniazid

Antituberculous drug.

USES
Treatment of tuberculosis, in combination with other drugs. Prophylaxis of tuberculosis.

PRESENTATION
Elixir: 50mg in 5mL – manufactured 'special'.
Injection: 25mg in 1mL, 2mL ampoule – non-proprietary.
Tablet: 50mg and 100mg – non-proprietary.

DOSAGE
Treatment should always be given in collaboration with a specialist experienced in tuberculosis therapy.

Route	Age				Frequency (times daily)	Notes
	birth–1 month	1 month–2 years	2–12 years	12–18 years		
Oral/IM/IV	5mg/kg	←	10mg/kg (maximum 300mg)	→	1	See guidelines for further information. Doses may be doubled in tuberculosis meningitis.

ADMINISTRATION
IV: it is recommended that IV administration is by slow bolus of the undiluted injection, although the injection may be diluted with water if required and given immediately.

CONTRA-INDICATIONS & WARNINGS
Should not be given to patients with a history of isoniazid sensitivity. Baseline LFTs and then monitor hepatic function in all patients, use with caution in hepatic impairment. Use with caution in renal impairment; dosage adjustments are generally not necessary until creatinine clearance falls to 10mL/minute/1.73m^2; such patients, and patients with slow acetylator status may require a dose reduction to maintain trough plasma levels of 1mg/L.

INTERACTIONS
The metabolism of *phenytoin, carbamazepine* and *diazepam* may be reduced by isoniazid. The absorption of isoniazid may be reduced by concurrent administration of *antacids*. Corticosteroid effects of *prednisolone* may be enhanced.

PREGNANCY

There is conflicting evidence that isoniazid, taken in pregnancy, may be teratogenic, but there is nothing to suggest that treatment should be withheld in pregnancy on this account. There is, however, a potential risk of neuropathy and, to counteract this, pregnant women are generally advised to take 10mg pyridoxine daily while on treatment.

BREAST-FEEDING

Mothers can breast-feed normally while taking isoniazid. Substantial quantities of isoniazid (and its main metabolite) appear in the milk of nursing mothers but toxic symptoms have not been seen in the breast-fed baby. Nevertheless it would be prudent to monitor the baby for possible toxicity. Theoretical risk of convulsions and neuropathy.

SIDE-EFFECTS

Isoniazid is generally well tolerated; the only common side-effect is peripheral neuropathy which is more likely to occur if there are pre-existing risk factors such as malnutrition, chronic renal failure, diabetes and HIV infection. In children supplemental pyridoxine is not necessary, except for breast-fed infants and malnourished children. When given, the daily pyridoxine prophylaxis dosage in neonates is 5mg, children 5-10mg, adults 10mg.

The following have been reported less frequently; nausea, vomiting, optic neuritis, convulsions, psychotic episodes, hypersensitivity reactions, allergic skin reactions, hyperglycaemia, hepatitis. Although hepatitis occurs only rarely, patients and their carers should be told how to recognise signs of liver disorder and to seek medical attention if symptoms such as persistent nausea, vomiting, malaise or jaundice develop.

PHARMACOKINETIC PROPERTIES

Absorption following oral and IM administration is rapid and complete. Metabolism is by the liver with decay rate determined genetically by acetylation phenotype. The half-life is approximately 30-100 minutes in fast acetylators and 2-5 hours in slow acetylators. The half-life may be prolonged in patients with impaired hepatic function and severe renal impairment. Excreted in the urine (75-95%), faeces and saliva.

POISONING/TOXICITY

In severe poisoning the main risk is of epileptiform convulsions. In addition, any of the side-effects listed above may occur together with metabolic acidosis and hyperglycaemia. Treatment should be directed to the control of the convulsions and large doses of pyridoxine may limit the occurrence of other effects. Metabolic acidosis may require sodium bicarbonate infusion. The drug is removed by dialysis.

EXCIPIENTS

Contact manufacturers for further details.

LICENSED STATUS

Licensed for use in all ages but the oral liquid is an unlicensed 'special'.

Isoprenaline

Synthetic catecholamine that is a very potent beta-adrenoceptor agonist with almost no action on alpha-adrenoceptors. Continuous IV infusion can increase cardiac output through its inotropic and chronotropic action and increase in cardiac venous return.

USES

Severe bradycardia including complete heart block; cardiogenic shock; evaluation of congenital cardiac defects e.g. sub-aortic stenosis.

PRESENTATION

Injection: (as hydrochloride) 20 microgram in 1mL, 10mL syringe – Min-I-Jet® Isoprenaline; (as sulphate) 2.25mg in 2mL ampoule and other strengths available – manufactured 'special'.
NB isoprenaline sulphate 2.25mg ≡ isoprenaline hydrochloride 2mg.

DOSAGE

ECG monitoring is recommended.

Route	Age				Frequency (times daily)	Notes
	birth–1 month	1 month–2 years	2–12 years	12–18 years		
IV infusion	20-300 nanogram/ kg/minute	20 nanogram /kg/minute– 1 microgram/kg/minute		1–4 microgram/ minute	continuous	Prescribed in terms of hydro-chloride salt, see Presentation for equivalence of sulphate salt. Use the lowest possible effective dose.

ADMINISTRATION
IV: compatible with glucose 5% or NaCl 0.9%. May decompose rapidly at pH >6. Separate administration of alkaline solutions e.g. sodium bicarbonate is advised. The maximum recommended rate of IV administration of isoprenaline is 1 microgram/kg/minute.

CONTRA-INDICATIONS & WARNINGS
Contra-indicated in patients prone to episodes of ventricular fibrillation or tachycardia secondary to their slow rate and those with hypersensitivity to isoprenaline. Use with caution in patients with hyperthyroidism or diabetes. Isoprenaline may precipitate ventricular extrasystoles and arrhythmias especially in patients who may be hypersensitive to the drug. In such cases the infusion rate should be reduced or possibly discontinued.

INTERACTIONS
May induce arrhythmias when administered with *halothane, cyclopropane* and *trichloroethylene*. Care is required when given simultaneously with *adrenaline (epinephrine)* or *other sympathomimetics* that are capable of stimulating beta-adrenoceptors because their effects will be additive and this may be dangerous in patients with cardiovascular disease. The risk of cardiac arrhythmias may be increased if patients are taking *digitalis glycosides*.

PREGNANCY/BREAST-FEEDING
Safety during pregnancy or lactation has not been established. Contact local Medicines Information Centre for advice.

SIDE-EFFECTS
Palpitations, tremor, precordial pain, sweats, facial flushing and headaches.

POISONING/TOXICITY
Symptoms of overdosage are as listed in the side-effects section. Fatality may also occur in cases of serious overdoses. A beta-adrenergic blocking drug may diminish toxic effects and should be accompanied by monitoring of heart rhythm.

PHARMACOKINETIC PROPERTIES
Plasma protein binding 62-74%. Metabolised in the liver, lungs and other tissues. Plasma half-life phase 1:2.5-5 minutes and phase 2:3-7 hours. It has been reported that children between 6-16 years of age appeared to metabolise IV isoprenaline much more quickly than adults.

EXCIPIENTS
Contact manufacturers for further details.

LICENSED STATUS
Licensed for use in children and adults, but the 'specials' are unlicensed.

FURTHER INFORMATION
Injection 'specials' are available from various NHS manufacturing units and Martindale Pharmaceuticals Ltd.

Isotretinoin

Isomer of tretinoin (the acid form of vitamin A); reduces sebum secretions.

USES
Oral: treatment of severe chronic acne under the supervision of a consultant dermatologist.
Topical: mild to moderate acne.

PRESENTATION
Capsule: 5mg, 20mg – Roaccutane® and non-proprietary.
Gel: 0.05% – Isotrex®.

DOSAGE

Route	Age		Frequency	Notes
	12–18 years		(times daily)	
Oral	500 microgram/kg		1	Initial dose for 4 weeks, if good response continue for further 8–12 weeks. If little response give up to 1mg/kg for 8–12 weeks. If intolerant, reduce dose to 100–200 microgram/kg daily. Dose may be given in 2 divided doses.
Topical	Apply thinly		1–2	Apply over the whole affected area.

ADMINISTRATION
Capsule: take with food.
Gel: apply thinly 1-2 times daily.

CONTRA-INDICATIONS & WARNINGS
Hypersensitivity to isotretinoin or excipients.
Contra-indicated in hepatic and renal impairment and hyperlipidaemia. Pregnancy must be excluded before therapy and contraceptive measures taken in women of child-bearing potential. Topical preparations: avoid contact with eyes, nostrils, mouth and mucous membranes. Do not use simultaneously with peeling agents. Do not use ultraviolet lamps (minimise exposure to sunlight). Use with care in diabetes and depression.

INTERACTIONS
Reduced anticoagulant effect with *warfarin*. Plasma concentration of *carbamazepine* may be reduced. Increased plasma concentration of *methotrexate* and increased risk of hepatotoxicity. *Tetracyclines* – increased risk of benign intracranial hypertension. *Topical:* concomitant topical medications and toiletry preparations should be used with care.

PREGNANCY/BREAST-FEEDING
Contra-indicated in pregnancy – major fetal abnormalities reported. Limited data available for use in breast-feeding so should be avoided.

SIDE-EFFECTS
Skin: dryness of skin, epidermal fragility, hyperpigmentation.
Eye: dryness of conjunctiva, rarely keratitis, visual disturbances.
Blood: thrombocytopenia, neutropenia and anaemia.
Other: hyperlipidaemia, depression.
Topical use: irritation, erythema and peeling. See manufacturers SPC for extensive list and further details.

POISONING/TOXICITY
Symptoms of hypervitaminosis A – severe headache, nausea and vomiting, drowsiness, irritability and pruritus. Reversible – no need for treatment.

PHARMACOKINETIC PROPERTIES
Peak serum levels after 1-4 hours. Duration of activity is 3-5 days.

EXCIPIENTS
See manufacturers SPC for further details.

LICENSED STATUS
Not for pre-pubertal children (affects epiphyseal closure). Capsules: prescription must be initiated by consultant dermatologist. Only available to hospitals and specified retail pharmacies.

FURTHER INFORMATION
Liver function and blood lipids (fasting values) should be measured at the start of oral treatment, after 1 month and thereafter 3 monthly intervals.

Ispaghula husk

Bulk-forming laxative.

USES
Effective remedy for constipation. Also indicated for the treatment of diarrhoea, irritable bowel syndrome and the management of patients with a colostomy. Indicated in habitual constipation, including cases due to spastic colon, dietary insufficiencies in patients with haemorrhoids or diabetes. Can be used to normalise bowel movement in patients with mucous or ulcerative colitis.

PRESENTATION
Granules: 3.5g sachet – Fybogel® plain, lemon or orange flavour; 200g – Isogel®.
Powder: 6g sachet – Konsyl® Sugar Free; 3.4g sachet – Konsyl® Orange; 3.4g sachet – Regulan® lemon/lime or orange flavour.

DOSAGE

Product	Route	Age			Frequency (times daily)	Notes
		1 month– 2 years	2–12 years	12–18 years		
Fybogel®	Oral	1/2 –1 level 5mL spoonful		1 sachet	2	Morning and evening, preferably after meals.
Isogel®	Oral	1 x 5mL spoonful		2 x 5mL spoonful	1-2	Preferably at mealtimes.
Konsyl®	Oral	1/2 sachet (or less)		1 sachet	1-3	Before or after meals.
Regulan®	Oral	1/2 - 1 level 5mL spoonful		1 sachet	1-3	

ADMINISTRATION
Oral: stir required quantity briskly into half a glass of water. Swallow at once. Do not take immediately before going to bed.

CONTRA-INDICATIONS & WARNINGS
Do not give to patients with intestinal obstruction. Fybogel® and Regulan® contain aspartame and should not be given to patients with PKU.

PREGNANCY
No known adverse effects. Ispaghula is not absorbed from the gastrointestinal tract.

BREAST-FEEDING
No adverse effects in lactation.

SIDE-EFFECTS
Flatulence and bloating may be experienced during the first few days of treatment.

POISONING/TOXICITY
Abdominal discomfort and flatulence can occur. Maintain adequate fluid intake, particularly if the granules have been taken without water.

EXCIPIENTS
Fybogel® contains aspartame and is gluten-free. Konsyl® is gluten-free and sugar-free. Regulan® contains aspartame; is gluten-free and sugar-free.

LICENSED STATUS
Licensed for ≥6 years of age. If <6 years on medical advice only.

FURTHER INFORMATION
Each 6g sachet of Konsyl® Sugar Free contains almost twice as much ispaghula husk as the 3.4g sachet of Konsyl® Orange.

Itraconazole

Broad-spectrum antifungal agent.

USES
Treatment of fungal infections. Oral liquid in treatment of allergic bronchopulmonary aspergillosis (ABPA) in cystic fibrosis – use is not well established, but thought to have some effect as a steroid-sparing agent after frequent relapses.

PRESENTATION
Capsule: 100mg – Sporanox®.
Oral liquid: 50mg in 5mL – Sporanox®.

DOSAGE

Route	Age			Frequency	Notes
	1 month–2 years	2–12 years	12–18 years	(times daily)	
Oral	← 3–5mg/kg →		100mg	1	Tinea corporis and tinea cruris – treat for 15 days. Tinea pedis and tinea manuum – treat for 30 days. Oropharyngeal candidiasis – treat for 15 days.
	← 1.5–2.5mg/kg →			2	For ABPA – use the oral liquid.

ADMINISTRATION

Oral: capsules – take immediately after a meal; liquid – take without food and refrain from eating for 1 hour after administration. If acid-reducing drugs are being taken they should be taken at least 2 hours after itraconazole. If patient is on a proton pump inhibitor or H_2-antagonist take the itraconazole dose with a cola drink.

CONTRA-INDICATIONS & WARNINGS

Avoid in liver disease. For treatment longer than 1 month, liver function tests required. Caution with renal disease – decreased bioavailability. Absorption reduced in AIDS and neutropenia. Discontinue if peripheral neuropathy occurs.

INTERACTIONS

Increased plasma levels of *terfenadine, astemizole* and *cisapride* – risk of serious arrhythmias, avoid concurrent use. Increased plasma levels of *midazolam* – prolonged sedation, concurrent oral use contra-indicated. Increased levels of *digoxin, warfarin* and *ciclosporin (cyclosporin)* have been reported – monitor levels. *Phenytoin, rifampicin* and *carbamazepine* greatly reduce the oral bioavailability of itraconazole.

PREGNANCY

Contra-indicated – toxicity in animal studies.

BREAST-FEEDING

Small amounts excreted in breast milk. Contact local Medicines Information Centre for advice.

SIDE-EFFECTS

Nausea, abdominal pain, dyspepsia, constipation (diarrhoea with oral liquids). Headache, dizziness, raised hepatic enzymes, menstrual disorders. Allergic reactions including pruritus, rash, urticaria and angio-oedema.

POISONING/TOXICITY

Treat symptomatically with supportive measures.

PHARMACOKINETIC PROPERTIES

Peak plasma concentration of 1 microgram/mL is measured 1.5-3 hours after administration. Half-life is 20 hours. Monitoring of levels is recommended in severe infection/immunocompromised. Blood levels greater after administration of oral liquid compared to capsules.

EXCIPIENTS

Capsules include sugar. Oral liquid includes saccharin sodium and sorbitol. See manufacturers SPC for further details.

LICENSED STATUS

Not licensed for use in children. Not licensed for use in ABPA.

Ivermectin

Anthelmintic.

USES

Onchocerciasis; drug of choice as it reduces the microfilarial load without producing unacceptable reactions. It has also been used in lymphatic filariasis (ideal dose schedule not yet established) and in chronic *Strongyloides stercoralis*.

PRESENTATION

Tablet: 3mg – named patient.

DOSAGE

Safety in children <5 years of age or weighing <15kg has not been established.

Indication	Route	Age		Frequency	Notes
		2–12 years	12–18 years		
Chronic *Strongyloides stercoralis*	Oral	≥5 years ← 200 microgram/kg →		single dose	Take for 2 days in chronic cases. Repeat every 6–12 months if necessary.
Onchocerciasis	Oral	≥5 years ← 150 microgram/kg →		single dose	Repeat every 6–12 months.

Doses of 200 microgram/kg for *Strongyloides stercoralis* approximate to:

Body weight	Dose
15-24kg	3mg
25-35kg	6mg
36-50kg	9mg
51-65kg	12mg
66-79kg	15mg
>80kg	200 micrograms/kg

Doses of 150 microgram/kg for onchocerciasis approximate to:

Body weight	Dose
15-25kg	3mg
26-44kg	6mg
45-64kg	9mg
65-84kg	12mg
>85kg	150 micrograms/kg

ADMINISTRATION

Oral: no food should be taken for 2 hours before or after the dose.

CONTRA-INDICATIONS & WARNINGS

Contra-indications: history of hypersensitivity to ivermectin; children <5 years of age; severe concurrent illness (delay treatment); pregnancy.
Cautions: individuals with CNS disorders e.g. epilepsy, meningitis or trypanosomiasis; nursing mothers. Monitor for ophthalmic and other hypersensitivity reactions when onchocerciasis is being treated.

PREGNANCY

Safety not established. Pregnant women excluded from mass treatment schedules with ivermectin.

BREAST-FEEDING

Ivermectin is excreted into breast milk in small amounts. Contact local Medicines Information Centre for advice.

SIDE-EFFECTS

Fever, pruritus, arthralgia, myalgia, postural hypotension, oedema, lymphadenopathy, gastrointestinal symptoms, sore throat, cough and headache. It is thought these reactions result from hypersensitivity reaction to the dying microfilaria. Less severe than those occurring with diethylcarbamazine.

POISONING/TOXICITY

Emesis, mydriasis and sedation were reported in a human subject receiving overdose of about 8mg/kg body weight. No human deaths reported to be associated with ivermectin. Treat symptomatically with supportive measures.

PHARMACOKINETIC PROPERTIES

Readily absorbed after oral administration. Extensively metabolised and excreted chiefly in the faeces. Less than 1% of the drug is excreted in the urine. Less than 2% is excreted in breast milk. Plasma half-life is about 12 hours.

EXCIPIENTS

Contact manufacturer for further details.

LICENSED STATUS

Not licensed for use in the UK.

FURTHER INFORMATION

Available free of charge from MSD, telephone: 01992 452 052.

USES
Active protection against Japanese encephalitis in those ≥1 year old. The vaccine may be appropriate for those travelling, usually for more than 1 month, to rural areas of some parts of the Indian subcontinent, South East Asia and the Far East. The risk to travellers seems to be greatest in areas where rice growing and pig farming co-exist and when travel takes place towards the end of the monsoon season (i.e. about June to September). Most holiday-makers to these regions will not require the vaccine.

PRESENTATION
JE-VAX®: injection (single dose pellets for reconstitution with Water for Injections). Multidose vials are also available.
Japanese Encephalitis (JE) Vaccine: single dose injection.

Both preparations contain formalin-inactivated whole cell vaccine derived from mouse brains infected with the Nakayama–NIH strain of virus. The potency is no less than that of the JEV Reference vaccine (J-NIH).

DOSAGE
There are 2 possible schedules; a two dose schedule and a three dose schedule. The two dose schedule should be reserved for those resident in an endemic area.

Primary course	Timing of doses	Reinforcing doses
3 doses of 1mL (0.5mL if <3 years old)	0, 7 and 14–30* days	Booster after 2–4 years.
2 doses of 1mL (0.5mL if <3 years old)	0 and 7 days	Booster after 6 months.

*30 days is preferable, but the third dose may be given earlier if time is short.

The three dose schedule is indicated for those not native to areas where the disease is endemic. The necessity for subsequent boosters is not known, but one dose may be given after 2 years.

ADMINISTRATION
Deep SC.

CONTRA-INDICATIONS & WARNINGS
As for vaccines generally; also not advised in children <1 year old, as there is insufficient data on its use at this age.

INTERACTIONS
Although no significant interactions have been recorded, in view of its potential for side-effects, it probably ought not to be given with other vaccines.

PREGNANCY
Japanese encephalitis virus infection during pregnancy may cause fetal infection and intrauterine death. No data is available on the use of the vaccine and therefore travel to an endemic area should be postponed until after delivery. If this is not possible, the advisability of administering the vaccine should be discussed with an expert in the field.

BREAST-FEEDING
No data available but there is no reason to believe it might be harmful. If the risk to the breast-feeding mother is significant, the vaccine should not be withheld.

SIDE-EFFECTS
Hypersensitivity reactions such as urticaria, angioneurotic oedema, hypotension and dyspnoea may occur within minutes or up to 2 weeks after receiving the vaccine. It is recommended that recipients should be kept under observation for 30 minutes and departure to anywhere without good medical facilities should not take place until at least 10 days have elapsed.

POISONING/TOXICITY
No data available.

PHARMACODYNAMIC PROPERTIES
Evidence suggests that the vaccine protects against disease but not against infection.

EXCIPIENTS
Thiomersal, formaldehyde, polysorbate 80, mouse serum protein and gelatin.

LICENSED STATUS
Not licensed in UK, but it is recommended in the Department of Health's book *Immunisation against Infectious Disease 1996* which reflects the advice of the Joint Committee on Vaccinations and Immunisation.
Available on a named patient basis from Pasteur Mérieux.

FURTHER INFORMATION
The vaccine should be given at least 4 weeks before potential exposure as immunity may take this long to develop. Recent evidence suggests that some anaphylactic reactions to the vaccine may be due to gelatin. It is suggested that international travel is delayed for 10 days to ensure that adequate medical help is available in case of a delayed adverse reaction. Protect from light and store at 2-8°C. Once reconstituted, it should be used within 8 hours.

Potent analgesic and a dissociative anaesthetic.

USES
Induction and maintenance of anaesthesia. Analgesia/sedation for painful procedures e.g. bone marrow aspiration, lumbar puncture, painful dressing changes. Non-ketotic hyperglycinaemia (anecdotal evidence of use). Neuropathic pain in palliative care.

PRESENTATION
Injection: (as hydrochloride) 10mg in 1mL, 20mL vial; 50mg in 1mL, 10mL vial; 100mg in 1mL, 10mL vial – Ketalar®; preservative-free 10mg in 1ml, 5ml ampoule – (imported).
Oral solution: manufactured 'special'.

DOSAGE

Route	Age				Frequency (times daily)	Notes
	birth–1 month	1 month–2 years	2–12 years	12–18 years		
Intermittent IV injection	←	1–2mg/kg	→	1–4.5mg/kg	single dose	Induction dose. Maximum initial dose 4.5mg/kg. Maintenance doses titrated according to response (usually half the full induction dose) or give by infusion.
IV infusion	←	500 microgram – 2mg/kg	→		single dose	Induction dose.
	8.33 microgram/kg/minute (500 microgram/kg/hour)	←	10–45 microgram/kg/minute (600 microgram–2.7mg/kg/hour)	→	continuous	Maintenance. Rate adjusted according to response. Note: in palliative care, sub-anaesthetic doses of 100-300 micrograms/kg/hour (maximum 1.5mg/kg/hour) have been used for neuropathic pain.
IM injection	4mg/kg	←	4–10mg/kg	→	single dose	Induction dose. 10mg/kg will usually produce surgical anaesthesia. 4mg/kg is normally sufficient for di-agnostic procedures or proce-dures not involving intense pain. Additional doses for maintenance titrated accord-ing to response.
Oral	-	←	6–10mg/kg	→	single dose	Pre-medication prior to in-vasive or painful procedures.
Rectal		←	7–10mg/kg	→	single dose	Pre-medication prior to minor surgery.
IV/oral	←	250 microgram/kg –7.5mg/kg	→		4	Non-ketotic hyperglycinaemia.
Caudal (epidural)	-	←	500 microgram/kg	→	single dose	Peri-operative analgesia. Must be 'preservative free'.

Should only be prescribed/administered by a trained anaesthetist or intensivist.

ADMINISTRATION
Oral: injection can be given orally. It should be mixed with a flavoured soft drink to mask the bitter flavour.
IV: give injection over at least 1 minute.
IV infusion: a solution containing 1mg in 1mL ketamine in glucose 5% or NaCl 0.9% is suitable for infusion.

Rectal: the preservative-free injection can be used neat or diluted and given rectally.

Ketamine injection is chemically incompatible with barbiturates and diazepam. These therefore should not be mixed in the same syringe or infusion fluid.

CONTRA-INDICATIONS & WARNINGS
Contra-indications: systemic hypertension, severe coronary or myocardial disease, cerebrovascular accident or cerebral trauma.
Warnings: ketamine may produce laryngospasm, particularly in infants. It should therefore be given only by a trained anaesthetist or intensivist able to deal safely with acute upper airway obstruction. Fasting, as before general anaesthesia, is necessary before it is used.
Cautions: children with pulmonary hypertension, patients prone to hallucinations or psychiatric disorders.

INTERACTIONS
Prolonged recovery times have occurred with concurrent use of barbiturates and/or opioids.

PREGNANCY
Do not use in eclampsia or pre-eclampsia. Ketamine rapidly crosses the placenta but if given in induction doses during caesarian section does not sedate the baby. There are no reports of teratogenicity attributable to ketamine.

BREAST-FEEDING
Although it is likely to be excreted in breast milk, this is unlikely to be of clinical relevance. Contact local Medicines Information Centre for advice.

SIDE-EFFECTS
Ketamine may produce laryngospasm in infants. Temporary elevation of blood pressure and pulse rate is frequently seen. Depression of respiration and apnoea may occur following too rapid IV administration. It can produce nightmares and hallucinations during recovery, especially in older children (>15 years). Pre-medication with diazepam, lorazepam or midazolam may help to prevent this. Causes local pain at injection site, which can be alleviated by premixing lidocaine (lignocaine) 200 microgram/kg with the ketamine injection.

POISONING/TOXICITY
Respiratory depression can follow overdose of ketamine. Supportive ventilation should be employed.

PHARMACODYNAMIC PROPERTIES
The mechanism of action of ketamine is unclear. In non-ketotic hyperglycinaemia the NMDA channel is stimulated by glycine to cause seizures and irritability. It is thought that ketamine antagonises this channel.

PHARMACOKINETIC PROPERTIES
After IV injection onset of action is rapid (within 1 minute). This anaesthetic effect will last for 5-10 minutes. IM injection acts within 3-4 minutes and the effect lasts 12-25 minutes. Ketamine is rapidly dispersed into perfused tissues including, brain and placenta. Termination of anaesthesia is partly by redistribution and partly by metabolism. Elimination half-life approximately 2-3 hours. Excretion is via the kidney mostly as conjugated metabolites.

EXCIPIENTS
Ketalar® injections include benzethonium chloride.

LICENSED STATUS
All strengths of Ketalar® injection are licensed for use in children and adults. Injection is not licensed for oral or rectal administration, for the treatment of non-ketotic hyperglycinaemia and for neuropathic pain in palliative care. Preservative-free injection is not licensed for use in the UK.

FURTHER INFORMATION
Preservative-free injection available from IDIS World Medicines.

Ketoconazole

Broad-spectrum antifungal agent.

USES
Seborrhoeic dermatitis and dandruff, pityriasis versicolor.

PRESENTATION
Shampoo: 2% – Nizoral®.

DOSAGE
Pityriasis versicolor: use daily for a maximum of 5 days.
Seborrhoeic dermatitis and dandruff: use twice weekly for 2-4 weeks.

ADMINISTRATION
Use as shampoo, leaving in contact for 3-5 minutes before rinsing thoroughly.

CONTRA-INDICATIONS & WARNINGS
Hypersensitivity to any of ingredients. When stopping long-term topical corticosteroids, use the topical corticosteroid with the shampoo and then gradually withdraw the steroid therapy over 2-3 weeks. Keep out of eyes.

PREGNANCY/BREAST-FEEDING
No specific precautions.

SIDE-EFFECTS
Local burning sensation, itching, irritation and oily/dry hair. Discolouration of chemically damaged hair observed.

POISONING/TOXICITY
If accidental ingestion occurs, only supportive measures should be carried out. To avoid aspiration, emesis and gastric lavage should not be instigated.

LICENSED STATUS
Licensed for use in children and adults.

Labetalol

Non-cardioselective alpha-blocker with additional beta-blocking properties.

USES
Hypertension and hypertensive crises.

PRESENTATION
Injection: 5mg in 1mL, 20mL ampoule – Trandate®.
Oral solution: may be extemporaneously prepared.
Tablet: 50mg – Trandate®, 100mg, 200mg and 400mg – Trandate® and non-proprietary.

DOSAGE

Route	Age				Frequency (times daily)	Notes
	birth–1 month	1 month–2 years	2–12 years	12–18 years		
IV bolus	–	←— 250–500 microgram/kg —→		50mg	single dose	Loading dose.
IV infusion	500 microgram/kg/hour up to a maximum of 4mg/kg/hour	←— 1–3mg/kg/hour —→		120 mg/hour	continuous	Start at low dose and titrate according to response, until the blood pressure has been reduced to an acceptable level.
Oral	–	←— 1–2mg/kg —→		50–200mg (maximum 300mg)	3-4	

Renal impairment
No dose adjustment necessary.

ADMINISTRATION
Oral: injection can be given orally with juice.
IV infusion: in glucose 5%, NaCl 0.9% or glucose 4%/NaCl 0.18% at a concentration of 1mg in 1mL. Can be infused undiluted in fluid restricted patients.
IV bolus: give over at least 1 minute.

CONTRA-INDICATIONS & WARNINGS
See propranolol monograph. Liver damage: severe hepatocellular damage reported after both short-term and long-term treatment. Appropriate laboratory testing needed at first symptom of liver dysfunction and if laboratory evidence of damage (or if jaundice) labetalol should be stopped and not restarted. Avoid in liver disease. May cause hypoglycaemia in dialysis patients.

INTERACTIONS, PREGNANCY, BREAST-FEEDING, SIDE-EFFECTS, POISONING/TOXICITY
See propranolol monograph.

PHARMACOKINETIC PROPERTIES
Half-life 3-9 hours, 50% protein bound.

EXCIPIENTS
See manufacturers SPC for further details.

LICENSED STATUS
Not licensed for use in children.

FURTHER INFORMATION
There is limited information on the use of labetalol in paediatric patients. It should be used with caution and with careful dosage adjustment and BP monitoring.

Lactulose

A semi-synthetic disaccharide which is not absorbed from the gastrointestinal tract. Osmotic laxative.

USES
Constipation; hepatic encephalopathy (portal systemic encephalopathy); hepatic coma.

PRESENTATION
Solution: lactulose 3.1-3.7g in 5mL (depending on the brand) – non-proprietary.

DOSAGE

Indication	Route	Age			Frequency	Notes
		1 month–2 years	2–12 years	12–18 years	(times daily)	
Constipation	Oral	<1 year 2.5mL	≤5 years 5mL	15mL	2	Initial dose. Then adjust to suit patient.
		1–2 years 5mL	5–10 years 10mL		2	
			10–12 years 15mL		2	
Hepatic encephalo-pathy	Oral	–	–	30–50mL	3	Initial dose. Then adjust the dose to produce 2-3 soft stools a day.

ADMINISTRATION
Oral: solution may be taken with water or other drinks. Relatively ineffective in opioid-induced constipation as primarily an osmotic rather than a stimulant laxative.

CONTRA-INDICATIONS & WARNINGS
Galactosaemia; where there is evidence of gastrointestinal obstruction.

PREGNANCY
Suitable for use within recommended dosage regimen.

BREAST-FEEDING
No data available, but it is almost completely unabsorbed from the gastrointestinal tract.

SIDE-EFFECTS
Flatulence may occur; this usually disappears within a few days. Diarrhoea may occur especially when using higher doses; adjust dose to obtain 2-3 formed stools per day. Can cause colicky abdominal pain.

POISONING/TOXICITY
No specific antidote; symptomatic treatment.

PHARMACODYNAMIC PROPERTIES
Broken down in the large bowel by bacteria, to simple organic compounds which results in increased faecal bulk and stimulation of peristalsis. In patients with hepatic encephalopathy large doses of lactulose are used; a significant reduction in the pH of the colonic contents results, which reduces markedly the formation and absorption of ammonium ions and other nitrogenous toxins into the portal circulation.

EXCIPIENTS
Contact manufacturers for further details.

LICENSED STATUS
Licensed for constipation in all age groups. Not licensed for hepatic encephalopathy in children.

FURTHER INFORMATION
Soft stool formed and normal bowel action encouraged without irritation or direct interference with the gut mucosa. May take up to 48 hours before effects are obtained. 15mL per day ≡ 58kJ (14kcal), therefore unlikely to affect diabetics.

Lamotrigine

Antiepileptic.

USES
First or second line treatment of tonic-clonic, absence, atonic and myoclonic seizures; third line treatment of partial seizures and infantile spasms [NB: myoclonic seizures may worsen in children with severe myoclonic epilepsy].

PRESENTATION
Tablet: 25mg, 50mg, 100mg and 200mg – Lamictal®.
Tablet: (dispersible) 2mg, 5mg, 25mg and 100mg – Lamictal®.

DOSAGE

Indication	Route	Age		Frequency	Notes
		2–12 years	12–18 years	(times daily)	
When given with sodium valproate (with/without any other antiepileptics)	Oral	150 microgram/kg*	-	1	Weeks 1 and 2.* If the calculated dose is 2.5-5mg (i.e. patients weighing between 17-33kg), then 5mg may be taken on alternative days for weeks 1 and 2.
		-	25mg	alternate days	
		300 microgram/kg	25mg	1	Weeks 3 and 4. Total dose may be given as two divided doses.
		500 microgram/kg - 2.5mg/kg (maximum 100mg)	50-100mg	2	Usual target maintenance dose. To achieve maintenance increase every 1-2 weeks by: - 150 microgram/kg/dose (2-12 years) - 12.5-25mg/dose (12-18 years) Total daily dose may be given as a single dose.
When given with enzyme inducing antiepileptics other than sodium valproate	Oral	300 microgram/kg	-	2	Weeks 1 and 2.
		-	25mg	2	
		600 microgram/kg	50mg	2	Weeks 3 and 4.
		2.5-7.5mg/kg (maximum 200mg)	100-200mg	2	Usual target maintenance dose. To achieve maintenance increase every 1-2 weeks by: - 600 microgram/kg/dose (2-12 years) - 50mg/dose (12-18 years)
Monotherapy	Oral	-	25mg	1	Weeks 1 and 2.
		-	50mg	1	Weeks 3 and 4. Total dose may be given as two divided doses.
		-	100-200mg	1	Usual target maintenance dose. To achieve maintenance increase the daily dose by 50-100mg every 1-2 weeks. Total dose may be given as two divided doses.

L

The manufacturers dosage recommendations as above minimise the incidence of rash. There are several different regimens used to introduce lamotrigine gradually and some differ from the manufacturers current recommendation.

ADMINISTRATION
Oral: dispersible tablets are to be chewed or dissolved in water. Tablets can be crushed and mixed with syrup or jam just before administration.

CONTRA-INDICATIONS & WARNINGS
Caution in renal failure, glucuronide metabolite accumulates. Do not withdraw abruptly. Reduce initial doses in liver disease and titrate to response. Counsel on recognition of haematological and skin adverse effects.

INTERACTIONS
Sodium valproate and lamotrigine may be synergistic in absence (typical and atypical), tonic-clonic and myoclonic seizures. *Ethosuximide* and lamotrigine may be synergistic in absence (typical and atypical) seizures. Lamotrigine may increase the risk of *carbamazepine*-induced adverse effects whilst *sodium valproate* increases the risk of adverse effects of lamotrigine. Inducers of liver enzymes, including *carbamazepine, phenytoin, phenobarbital (phenobarbitone), primidone* may enhance metabolism of lamotrigine and increase dose requirement.

PREGNANCY
Increased risk of neural tube defects and other malformations especially if more than one antiepileptic used. Specialist counselling, management and screening required. Administer folate supplements before and during pregnancy.

BREAST-FEEDING
Excreted in breast milk. Contact local Medicines Information Centre for advice.

SIDE-EFFECTS
Dose dependent side-effects include 'measles-like' skin rash (particularly if used in conjunction with sodium valproate) usually within first 8 weeks of commencing therapy; rarely Stevens-Johnson syndrome, nausea/vomiting, headache, fever, ataxia. Insufficient data available on chronic adverse effects.

POISONING/TOXICITY
Sedation, ataxia, diplopia, nausea and vomiting may occur. Treatment is supportive. Contact UK National Poisons Information Service.

PHARMACOKINETIC PROPERTIES
Peak plasma levels approximately 2.5 hours after oral administration; timing delayed but extent not affected by food. Elimination half-life 24-35 hours in adults; shorter in children and greatly influenced by interacting drugs. Extensively metabolised in the liver. Blood target range 4-18 micromol/litre.

EXCIPIENTS
Dispersible tablets include saccharin sodium. See manufacturers SPC for further details.

LICENSED STATUS
Licensed for ≥2 years of age. Licensed for monotherapy in children ≥12 years of age.

FURTHER INFORMATION
On theoretical grounds lamotrigine can be absorbed by the rectal route. The dispersible tablets may be used.

L

Lassar's paste (Zinc and Salicylic Acid Paste BP)

USES
Removal of scale in psoriasis.

PRESENTATION
Paste: zinc oxide 24%, salicylic acid 2%, starch 24% and white soft paraffin 50%.

DOSAGE/ADMINISTRATION
Topical: apply twice daily.

CONTRA-INDICATIONS & WARNINGS
Sensitivity. Avoid applying to large areas; salicylate toxicity may result. Avoid broken or inflamed skin.

SIDE-EFFECTS
Excessive drying, irritation.

FURTHER INFORMATION
Lassar's paste is commonly used as a vehicle for dithranol due to it's stability.

Gonadorelin analogue.

USES
Central precocious puberty.

PRESENTATION
Injection (depot): 3.75g – Prostap®SR.
Injection (sustained release depot): 11.25mg – Prostap®3.

DOSAGE
3.75mg every 4 weeks or 11.25mg every 12 weeks. Injections may need to be given more frequently (e.g. every 3 weeks or every 10 weeks) if patients show signs of failure of hormone suppression.

ADMINISTRATION
Prostap®SR: the vial of powder should be reconstituted with the sterile vehicle provided. Given IM or SC, injection sites should be rotated to prevent atrophy and nodule formation.
Prostap®3: the vial of powder should be reconstituted with the sterile vehicle provided. Given SC, injection sites should be rotated to prevent atrophy and nodule formation.

CONTRA-INDICATIONS
Known hypersensitivity of luteinising hormone-releasing hormone (LHRH) analogues.

PREGNANCY
Contra-indicated in pregnancy; exclude pregnancy before treatment and use non-hormonal contraception during treatment.

BREAST-FEEDING
Should not be used in breast-feeding.

SIDE-EFFECTS
Hypersensitivity reactions, local reactions include mild bruising at the site of injection. Peripheral oedema, fatigue, arthralgia, dizziness, paraesthesia and palpitations, thrombocytopenia and leucopenia have been reported.

POISONING/TOXICITY
Symptomatic management only.

PHARMACODYNAMIC PROPERTIES
Prostap®SR: an initial high plasma level is achieved within 3 hours of injection, which drops over 24-48 hours to maintenance levels, and a slow decline thereafter. Effective levels persist for 30-40 days.
Prostap®3: an initial high plasma level is achieved within 3 hours of injection, followed by a decrease to maintenance levels in 7-14 days. Effective levels are maintained for up to 117 days.

EXCIPIENTS
See manufacturers SPC for further details.

LICENSED STATUS
Not licensed for use in children.

Levamisole

Anthelmintic.

USES
Ascariasis lumbricoides (roundworm) and *ancylostomiasis* (hookworm) infections. Nephrotic syndrome.

PRESENTATION
Tablet: 50mg – Ergamisol® (imported).

DOSAGE
There is little information on use as an anthelmintic in children <2 years of age.

Indication	Route	Age			Frequency	Notes
		1 month–2 years	2–12 years	12–18 years		
Ascaris lumbricoides (large round-worm)	Oral	← 2.5–3mg/kg →		150mg	single dose	
Ancylostomiasis (hookworm)	Oral	← 2.5mg/kg →		150mg	single dose	Repeat after 7 days if severe infection. In adults 300mg dose over 1–2 days may be given.
Nephrotic syndrome	Oral	← 2.5mg/kg →			alternate days	Seek expert nephrologist advice before prescribing.

CONTRA-INDICATIONS & WARNINGS

Contra-indicated in patients demonstrating previous hypersensitivity to levamisole. Also patients with pre-existing blood disorders. Caution in rheumatoid arthritis, Sjogren syndrome, epilepsy and liver disease where dose adjustment may be necessary.

INTERACTIONS

Warfarin and *phenytoin* – some evidence that levamisole can increase effects of these drugs but clinical importance uncertain. There have been reports that levamisole can produce a disulfiram-like reaction with *alcoho*l.

PREGNANCY

No well controlled teratogenic studies evaluating effect of levamisole in pregnant women. Animal studies have shown levamisole is embryotoxic in doses up to 180mg/kg. Therefore only consider use in pregnancy if potential benefit outweighs potential risk to fetus.

BREAST-FEEDING

Contact local Medicines Information Centre for advice.

SIDE-EFFECTS

When given in single doses for the treatment of worm infestations it is generally well tolerated and side-effects are limited to nausea, vomiting, diarrhoea, abdominal pain, dizziness and headache (affects approximately 1% of patients). When given for longer periods for other indications (immunostimulant effect) may get more serious side-effects including hypersensitivity reactions, haematological reactions (consult an expert nephrologist for advice on monitoring blood counts during treatment).

POISONING/TOXICITY

At high doses levamisole exhibits positive inotropic and chronotropic properties on heart muscle as well as convulsant properties. General supportive measures are recommended.

PHARMACOKINETIC PROPERTIES

Rapidly absorbed from gastrointestinal tract. Maximum plasma concentrations within 1.5-4 hours. Extensively metabolised in the liver. Excreted mainly in the urine as metabolites. Only 3-5% excreted unchanged in urine.

EXCIPIENTS

Contact manufacturer for further details.

LICENSED STATUS

Not licensed for use in the UK.

FURTHER INFORMATION

Available from IDIS World Medicines.

Levobupivacaine hydrochloride

Local anaesthetic of the amide type (S-isomer of bupivacaine).

USES

Local anaesthesia by infiltration; regional anaesthesia by epidural or intrathecal routes or peripheral nerve block; acute pain management.

PRESENTATION
Injection: 2.5mg in 1mL, 10mL ampoule; 5mg in 1mL, 10mL ampoule and 7.5mg in 1mL, 10mL ampoule – Chirocaine®.

DOSAGE

Indication	Route	Age				Frequency	Notes
		birth–1 month	1 month–2 years	2–12 years	12–18 years	(times daily)	
Ilioinguinal/ iliohypogastric nerve block	Local infiltration	←	1.25–2.5mg/kg	→	–	single dose	

The above is the only licensed indication for levobupivacaine in children, but its local anaesthetic properties are equivalent to racemic bupivacaine. It is therefore expected that other indications and doses will be as for bupivacaine.

Intrathecal or epidural administration should be carried out by, or under the supervision of, a consultant anaesthetist. A test dose of lidocaine (lignocaine) with adrenaline (epinephrine) should be given before commencing epidural block with levobupivacaine to detect inadvertent intravascular administration.

Liver disease: as levobupivacaine is metabolised in the liver the manufacturers advise caution in patients with liver disease.

ADMINISTRATION
Levobupivacaine may be diluted with NaCl 0.9%.
Clonidine 8.4 microgram/mL, morphine 50 microgram/mL and fentanyl 4 microgram/mL have been shown to be compatible with levobupivacaine in NaCl 0.9%.

CONTRA-INDICATIONS & WARNINGS
Contra-indications: hypersensitivity to local anaesthetics of the amide type, intravenous regional anaesthesia (Biers block), severe hypotension, hypovolaemia, paracervical block in obstetrics, 7.5mg/mL solution in obstetrics.
Caution: liver disease, epilepsy, impaired cardiovascular function, respiratory impairment.
Warnings: accidental IV injection of levobupivacaine may cause immediate toxic reactions (see poisoning/toxicity), IV access should always be established before treatment with levobupivacaine.

INTERACTIONS
Possible increased myocardial depression with *antiarrhythmics.*

PREGNANCY
Manufacturer advises avoid in first trimester if possible. Reproductive toxicity has been shown in animal studies. Use of large doses for epidural block in labour may cause neonatal respiratory depression, hypotonia and bradycardia.

BREAST-FEEDING
Likely to be excreted in breast milk, but risk to infant minimal at therapeutic doses.

SIDE-EFFECTS
Accidental intrathecal injection can lead to very high spinal anaesthesia possibly with apnoea, severe hypotension and loss of consciousness. Systemic adverse effects are likely to occur following accidental IV administration or following excessive dosage. See poisoning/toxicity below.

POISONING/TOXICITY
In the event of overdose peak plasma concentration may not be reached until 2 hours after administration depending upon the injection site. Signs of toxicity may therefore be delayed and the effects prolonged.
CNS: symptoms – numbness of the tongue, light headedness, dizziness, blurred vision and muscle twitch followed by drowsiness, convulsions, unconsciousness and possible respiratory arrest; treatment – convulsions should be treated immediately with IV thiopental (thiopentone) or diazepam titrated as necessary.
Cardiovascular: symptoms – hypotension, bradycardia, cardiac arrhythmia, and ventricular fibrilation; treatment – hypotension may be prevented or attenuated by pretreatment with a fluid load and/or use of vasopressors. If hypotension occurs it should be treated with intravenous crystalloids or colloids and/or incremental doses of a vasopressor such as ephedrine. Atropine should be used to counter severe bradycardia. Ventricular fibrillation should be treated by cardioversion.

PHARMACOKINETICS
The pharmacokinetics of levobupivacaine are similar to those of bupivacaine. It has a slow onset of action, taking up to 30 minutes for full effect and a long duration of action. It is extensively metabolised in the liver with conjugated metabolites being excreted mainly in the urine.

EXCIPIENTS
See manufacturers SPC for further details.

LICENSED STATUS
Levobupivacaine is licensed in children <12 years for analgesia (ilioinguinal/iliohypogastric block).

FURTHER INFORMATION
Shelf-life after dilution: chemical stability has been demonstrated for 7 days at 20-22°C. Stability with clonidine, morphine or fentanyl has been demonstrated for 40 hours at 20-22°C.

Levonorgestrel

A progestogen.

USES
Induction of sexual maturity, in combination with an oestrogen.

PRESENTATION
Tablet: 30 microgram – Microval® and Norgeston®.

DOSAGE/ADMINISTRATION
Oral: 30 micrograms once daily for the last 7 days of a 28 day cycle.

CONTRA-INDICATIONS & WARNINGS
Pregnancy, liver disease, hypertension, thromboembolism, porphyria.

INTERACTIONS
Tricyclic antidepressants, anticoagulants and *corticosteroids.*

PREGNANCY
Contra-indicated.

BREAST-FEEDING
A small fraction of the progestogen has been identified in the milk of mothers receiving the drug. Contact local Medicines Information Centre for advice.

SIDE-EFFECTS
Headache, slight weight gain, nausea, skin disorders and breast tenderness.

EXCIPIENTS
See manufacturers SPC for further details.

LICENSED STATUS
Not licensed for this indication.

Levothyroxine (thyroxine) sodium

Thyroid hormone.

USES
Hypothyroidism; including congenital hypothyroidism and juvenile myxoedema.

PRESENTATION
Capsule: 12.5 microgram – manufactured 'special'.
Suspension: may be extemporaneously prepared.
Tablet: 25 microgram, 50 microgram and 100 microgram – non-proprietary.

DOSAGE

Route	Age				Frequency	Notes
	birth–1 month	1 month–2 years	2–12 years	12–18 years	(times daily)	
Oral	10–15 microgram/kg	5–10 microgram/kg	5 microgram/kg	50–100 microgram	1	Initial dose.

L

Infants may be treated with crushed tablets, allowing dosage increments of 12.5 micrograms. Treatment aims in congenital hypothyroidism are to correct free thyroxine to >20pmol/L within 2 weeks, and thyroid stimulating hormone (TSH) to <10 milliunits/L within 4 weeks. Thyroid function should be monitored at 2 weekly intervals until target levels, followed by diminishing frequency guided by progress and compliance.

In older children, dosage changes are made in increments of 25 micrograms and are guided by tests at 4-8 weeks until normal adult ranges are reached, after which biochemical monitoring may be reduced to 6-12 monthly.

ADMINISTRATION
Oral: tablets may be halved and crushed.

CONTRA-INDICATIONS & WARNINGS
Thyrotoxicosis. A number of drugs may affect thyroid function tests and this should be borne in mind prior to initiation of therapy. Caution in conditions predisposing to adrenal insufficiency (initiate corticosteroid therapy before giving levothyroxine in these cases).

INTERACTIONS
Decreased levels with *rifampicin, carbamazepine, phenobarbital (phenobarbitone), phenytoin* and *colestyramine (cholestyramine)*. Enhances *warfarin* and reduces *propranolol* effectiveness. May increase requirement for *hypoglycaemic drugs and insulin*.

PREGNANCY
Monitor maternal serum thyrotrophin levels - dose adjustment may be necessary. Contact local Medicines Information Centre for advice.

BREAST-FEEDING
Excreted into breast milk in low concentrations. It is contentious whether this may interfere with neonatal screening programs.

SIDE-EFFECTS
The following are indicative of excessive dose and usually disappear on dose reduction or withdrawal of treatment for a few days: excitability, sweating, cramps, headache, tachycardia, cardiac arrhythmias, palpitations and diarrhoea.

POISONING/TOXICITY
Symptoms: exaggeration of side-effects; the following may also occur: agitation, confusion, hyperactivity, tachypnoea, pyrexia and convulsions. The appearance of clinical hyperthyroidism may be delayed for up to 5 days.
Treatment: symptomatic.

PHARMACOKINETIC PROPERTIES
Incompletely and variably absorbed from the gastrointestinal tract. Half-life is approximately 7 days in a normal person but this may be shortened in hyperthyroid states and prolonged in hypothyroid states due to altered rate of metabolism. Largely bound to plasma proteins; extensively metabolised in the thyroid, liver, kidney and anterior pituitary and excreted in the urine and faeces, partly as free drug and partly as conjugates and deiodinated metabolites.

EXCIPIENTS
Contact manufacturers for further details.

LICENSED STATUS
Tablets licensed for use in all ages. Capsules and suspension are unlicensed.

FURTHER INFORMATION
Capsules are available from Martindale Pharmaceuticals.

Lidocaine (lignocaine) hydrochloride

Antiarrhythmic, local anaesthetic.

USES
Antiarrhythmic (as an alternative to amiodarone during CPR). Local anaesthetic.
Prevention of pain during dental operative procedures. May be used in conjunction with general anaesthesia when good post-operative pain relief is required.

PRESENTATION
Dental injection: a large variety of lidocaine injections, plain or with adrenaline (epinephrine) or noradrenaline (norepinephrine), is also available in dental cartridges under the names of Lignostab A®, Lignospan®, Rexocaine®, Xylocaine® or Xylotox®.

Gel: 1% in 15mL tube – non-proprietary; 2% in 15mL tube - non-proprietary.
Gel: 2% with chlorhexidine gluconate 0.25%, 6mL and 11mL disposable syringes – Instillagel®.
Infusion: 0.1% (1mg/mL) or 0.2% (2mg/mL) in glucose 5%, 500mL container – non-proprietary.
Injection: 0.5% (5mg in 1mL), 10mL ampoule – non-proprietary.
Injection: 1% (10mg in 1mL), 2mL, 5mL, 10mL and 20mL ampoule – non-proprietary; 10mL disposable syringe – Min-I-Jet® Lignocaine.
Injection: 2% (20mg in 1mL), 2mL, 5mL, 10mL and 20mL ampoule – non-proprietary; 5mL disposable syringe – Min-I-Jet® Lignocaine.
Injection: 0.5% with adrenaline (epinephrine) 1 in 200,000, 20mL vial – non-proprietary.
Injection: 1% with adrenaline (epinephrine) 1 in 200,000, 20mL vial – non-proprietary.
Injection: 2% with adrenaline (epinephrine) 1 in 200,000, 20mL vial – non-proprietary.
Ointment: 5% in 15g tube – Xylocaine®.
Pump spray: 10% – Xylocaine®.
Topical solution: 4% in 30mL bottle – Xylocaine®.

DOSAGE

Indication	Route	Age				Frequency	Notes
		birth–1 month	1 month–2 years	2–12 years	12–18 years		
Anti-arrhythmic	IV bolus	← 500 microgram – 1mg/kg →			50–100mg then infusion (as shown below)	single dose	Loading dose: in the 12–18 year age group give 50mg in lighter patients or those whose circulation is severely impaired.
		then					
	IV infusion	← 10–50 microgram/kg/**minute** → (600 microgram – 3mg/kg/hour)			4mg/minute for 30 minutes then 2mg/minute for 2 hours then 1 mg/minute reducing concentration further if infusion is continued beyond 24 hours	continuous	Maintenance dosing: ECG monitoring with infusion.
VF or pulseless tachycardia	IV/IO	← 1mg/kg → (maximum dose100mg)			50–100mg	single dose	Repeat every 5 minutes if needed to a total maximum of 3mg/kg. In the 12–18 year age group give 50mg in lighter patients or those whose circulation is severely impaired.
Local anaesthetic	Local infiltration	← up to 3mg/kg →			up to 200mg	single dose	Not more often than every 4 hours. Use fine needles (27–29) gauge.
	Intra-urethral	← 3–4mg/kg →				single dose	Prior to urinary catheterisation. Warm the solution to body temperature and inject it very slowly to reduce local stinging.
Dental	Topical	–	Apply sparingly to dried oral mucosa at the proposed site of injection.			single dose	2% gel.
	Infiltration	–	← 1mL →			single dose	2% solution with adrenaline (epinephrine) 1:80,000.
	Nerve block	–	← 1.5–2mL →			single dose	

ADMINISTRATION

IV: compatible with glucose 5% or NaCl 0.9%.

L

CONTRA-INDICATIONS & WARNINGS
AV block, sino atrial disorders, severe myocardial depression and porphyria. Use with caution in patients with bradycardia, epilepsy, hypokalaemia, renal or liver impairment, congestive cardiac failure, severe respiratory depression. Local anaesthetics should not be given into inflamed or infected tissues. The excessive use of topical anaesthetics in the mouth may interfere with swallowing and increase the dangers of aspiration of foods. Patients and parents must be strongly warned against any behaviour likely to traumatise anaesthetised tissue. Great care must be taken to avoid intravascular injection. Careful surveillance for toxic effects is necessary for the first 30 minutes following oral injection.

INTERACTIONS
Increased myocardial depression with *antiarrhythmics* or *beta-blockers;* hypokalaemia antagonises lidocaine (lignocaine) effect. *Propranolol* and *cimetidine* may reduce the renal and hepatic clearance of lidocaine (lignocaine). Effect of *suxamethonium* prolonged by lidocaine (lignocaine).

PREGNANCY
Not applicable in a life support situation. With large doses neonatal respiratory depression, hypotonia and bradycardia after epidural block are possible.

BREAST-FEEDING
Lidocaine (lignocaine) enters the mothers' milk, but in such small quantities that there is generally no risk of affecting the child at therapeutic levels.

SIDE-EFFECTS
Dizziness, paraesthesia, drowsiness, fitting, blurred or double vision, sensation of heat, cold, numbness. Hypersensitivity reactions (extremely rare). Anaphylactic shock. Respiratory depression, cardiovascular collapse.

POISONING/TOXICITY
Overdose may lead to CNS excitation, muscle twitching, convulsions, heart block, severe hypotension and cardiac arrest. Treatment involves close monitoring of cardiovascular and respiratory functions and electrolytes. Toxic effects associated with local anaesthetics are usually a result of excessively high plasma concentrations, whether associated with acute or cumulative overdose or with accidental intravascular injection.

PHARMACOKINETIC PROPERTIES
Metabolised mainly by the liver. The metabolites have a weaker antiarrhythmic action and are excreted renally. As an IV injection it has a short duration of action of 15–20 minutes. Local anaesthetics do not rely upon uptake by the circulation to transport them to their site of action, but uptake into the general circulation is important in terminating their action. Following most regional anaesthetic procedures, maximum arterial plasma concentrations of anaesthetic develop within about 10-25 minutes.

EXCIPIENTS
Contact manufacturers for further details.

LICENSED STATUS
Use as an antiarrhythmic is unlicensed. Local anaesthetic and dental use licensed in children and adults.

L

Lidocaine (lignocaine) and prilocaine cream – EMLA®

Lidocaine and prilocaine are local anaesthetics of the amide type.

USES
Surface anaesthesia prior to venepuncture or procedures such as split skin grafting.

PRESENTATION
Cream: lidocaine 2.5% and prilocaine 2.5% – Emla®.

DOSAGE

Indication	Route	Age				Frequency	Notes
		birth–1 month	1 month–2 years	2–12 years	12–18 years		
Minor procedures e.g. venepuncture, IV cannulation	Topical	Not recommended	Approx. 2g for a minimum of 1 hour and a maximum of 5 hours (under an occlusive dressing)			single dose	Smaller amounts may be adequate for small children and infants. Not adequate for heel prick sampling.

DOSAGE continued

Indication	Route	Age				Frequency	Notes
		birth–1 month	1 month–2 years	2–12 years	12–18 years		
Procedures to larger areas e.g. split skin grafting	Topical	Not recommended	Approx. 1.5 –3g per 10cm² for a minimum of 2 hours and a maximum of 5 hours (under an occlusive dressing)			single dose	Smaller amounts may be adequate for small children and infants.

ADMINISTRATION
Topical: analgesic efficiency may decline if the application time is greater than 5 hours. Procedures on intact skin should begin soon after the removal of the occlusive dressing. The duration of analgesia after an application of time 1-2 hours is at least 2 hours after removal of the dressing.

CONTRA-INDICATIONS & WARNINGS
Contra-indication: known hypersensitivity to local anaesthetics of the amide type.
Cautions: not to be applied to wounds, mucous membranes, areas of atopic dermatitis and genital mucosa in children. Avoid use near eyes or middle ear. Although systemic absorption is low, caution should be exercised in patients with anaemia, congenital or acquired methaemoglobinaemia or on concurrent therapy known to produce such conditions.

INTERACTIONS
Methaemoglobinaemia may be accentuated in patients already taking drugs known to induce this condition e.g. *sulphonamides.*

PREGNANCY
Topical application during pregnancy is unlikely to be a risk.

BREAST-FEEDING
Both lidocaine and prilocaine are excreted in breast milk in quantities too small to be harmful.

SIDE-EFFECTS
Transient paleness, redness and oedema have been reported.

POISONING/TOXICITY
Systemic toxicity is unlikely to be seen after application to intact skin but may occur if accidentally ingested or following absorption from mucous membranes, broken skin or higher vascular areas. Symptoms include light-headedness followed by sedation, circumoral paraesthesia and twitching, convulsions and cardiovascular system depression.

EXCIPIENTS
See manufacturers SPC for further details.

LICENSED STATUS
Licensed for >1 year of age.

L

Liothyronine sodium (L-Tri–iodothyronine sodium)

Thyroid hormone.

USES
Hypothyroidism when use of levothyroxine (thyroxine) is inappropriate, e.g. IV formulation required or urgent correction of hypothyroid coma.

PRESENTATION
Injection: 20 microgram ampoule – Triiodothyronine®.
Tablet: (scored) 20 microgram – Tertroxin®.

DOSAGE
20 micrograms liothyronine = 100 micrograms levothyroxine.
See levothyroxine monograph for further details.

CONTRA-INDICATIONS & WARNINGS
Caution in conditions predisposing to adrenal insufficiency. Liothyronine is contra-indicated in patients with cardiovascular disorders. Give with extreme caution in myxoedema coma as too large a dose may precipitate heart failure.

INTERACTIONS
Decreased levels with *rifampicin, carbamazepine, phenobarbital (phenobarbitone), phenytoin* and *colestyramine (cholestyramine)*. Enhances *warfarin* and reduces *propranolol* effectiveness. May increase requirement for hypoglycaemic drugs and insulin.

PREGNANCY, BREAST-FEEDING, SIDE-EFFECTS, POISONING/TOXICITY
As for levothyroxine.

PHARMACODYNAMIC PROPERTIES
Liothyronine is more rapidly metabolised and has a more rapid effect than levothyroxine. Its effects develop after a few hours and disappear within 24-48 hours. Liothyronine is less readily bound to plasma proteins than levothyroxine, the half-life in blood is about 1-2 days in euthyroidism.

EXCIPIENTS
See manufacturers SPC for further details.

LICENSED STATUS
Not licensed for use in children.

Liquid paraffin

Faecal softener.

USES
Constipation.

PRESENTATION
Oral emulsion: liquid paraffin 5mL, vanillin 5mg, chloroform 0.025mL, benzoic acid solution 0.2mL, methylcellulose – 20 200mg, saccharin sodium 500 microgram, water to 10mL – Liquid Paraffin Oral Emulsion BP.

DOSAGE

Route	Age		Frequency	Notes
	2–12 years	12–18 years	(times daily)	
Oral	>3 years 0.5–1mL/kg	10–30mL	single dose	At night, as required but not immediately before going to bed.

CONTRA-INDICATIONS & WARNINGS
Avoid prolonged use. Do not use when abdominal pain, nausea or vomiting are present. CSM contra-indicates use in children <3 years.

SIDE-EFFECTS
Anal seepage of paraffin, anal irritation after prolonged use, granulomatous reactions caused by absorption of small quantities of liquid paraffin (especially from the emulsion), lipoid pneumonia following aspiration, and interference with the absorption of fat soluble vitamins.

LICENSED STATUS
Licensed for >3 years of age.

Lithium

USES
Prophylaxis of recurrent unipolar or bipolar affective disorder; treatment of acute mania; reduction of aggressive or self-injurious behaviour; prophylaxis of Kleine-Levin syndrome.

PRESENTATION
Oral solution: (all as citrate) 509mg in 5mL and 1.018g in 5mL – Li-Liquid®; 520mg in 5mL – Priadel®.
Tablet: (as carbonate, scored) 250mg – Camcolit 250®.
Tablet (modified release): (all as carbonate, all scored) 200mg – Priadel®; 400mg – Camcolit 400® and Priadel®; 450mg – Liskonum®.

DOSAGE

Route	Age	Frequency	Notes
	12–18 years	(times daily)	
Oral	200 – 800mg	2	Usual dose range for lithium carbonate (citrate is a higher dose, citrate 509mg=200mg carbonate). Dose should be sufficient to maintain a plasma level of 0.4–1mmol/L 12 hours after last dose (monitor 3 monthly once stable).

CONTRA-INDICATIONS & WARNINGS
Renal insufficiency, thyroid disease, adrenocortical deficiency. Do not prescribe unless monitoring available. Check blood pressure, electrolytes, renal and thyroid function before commencing treatment and 6 monthly thereafter.

INTERACTIONS
Diuretics (sodium depletion); concurrent high dose *haloperidol* can cause encephalopathy; potentiation of *neuroleptics; NSAIDs* can increase lithium level. Neurotoxic syndrome with *carbamazepine*.

PREGNANCY
There is epidemiological evidence that lithium may be harmful to the fetus in human pregnancy. Should the use of lithium be unavoidable, close monitoring of serum concentrations should be made throughout pregnancy and during parturition.

BREAST-FEEDING
Excreted in breast milk, monitor infant for possible intoxications. Low incidence of adverse effects but increased by continuous ingestion; good control of maternal plasma concentrations minimises risk.

SIDE-EFFECTS
Fine tremor, nephrogenic diabetes insipidus, mild gastrointestinal effects. Thyroid dysfunction with long-term treatment.

POISONING/TOXICITY
There is no antidote to lithium poisoning. In the event, lithium treatment should be stopped and levels measured every 6 hours. May be precipitated by dehydration/sodium depletion in pyrexial illness or gastrointestinal upset. At blood level >1mmol/L vomiting, diarrhoea, ataxia, nystagmus, dysarthria, drowsiness, muscle twitching, seizures, coma. Treat initially by maintenance of fluid and electrolyte balance. If plasma level >4 mmol/L, haemodialysis is probably required.

PHARMACOKINETIC PROPERTIES
Well absorbed after oral administration. Half-life is 8-45 hours. Eliminated unchanged by the kidneys.

L

EXCIPIENTS
Li-Liquid® includes sorbitol and glucose. See manufacturers SPC for further details.

LICENSED STATUS
Not licensed for use <12 years of age.

Lofepramine

Tricyclic antidepressant.

USES
Depression.

PRESENTATION
Tablet: 70mg – Gamanil® and non-proprietary.
Oral liquid: 70mg in 5mL – non-proprietary.

DOSAGE

Route	Age		Frequency	Notes
	12–18 years		(times daily)	
Oral	35–105mg		2	

CONTRA-INDICATIONS & WARNINGS
As imipramine but safer in overdose.

INTERACTIONS, PREGNANCY, BREAST-FEEDING, SIDE-EFFECTS, POISONING/TOXICITY
See imipramine monograph.

PHARMACOKINETIC PROPERTIES
Rapidly absorbed following oral administration with peak plasma concentrations being reached within 1 hour and a half-life of 5 hours. It is almost completely metabolised before excretion, which is mainly in the urine and faeces.

EXCIPIENTS
Oral liquid includes ethanol, sorbitol and liquid maltitol; sugar-free. Contact manufacturers for further details.

LICENSED STATUS
Not licensed for use in children.

FURTHER INFORMATION
Reputedly less dangerous in overdose than other tricyclic antidepressants.

Loperamide

Antimotility drug.

USES
Acute diarrhoea, chronic diarrhoea; short bowel syndrome.

PRESENTATION
Capsule: 2mg – Imodium® and non-proprietary.
Syrup: 1mg in 5mL – Imodium®.
Tablet: 2mg – Norimode®.

DOSAGE/ADMINISTRATION

Indication	Age			Frequency	Notes
	1 month–2 years	2–12 years	12–18 years	(times daily)	
Chronic diarrhoea e.g. short bowel syndrome	<1 year 200 microgram/kg			30 minutes before feeds	Doses of up to 2mg/kg/day have occasionally been required <1year.
	1–2 years 100–200 microgram/kg	As for 1–2 years	2–4mg	3–4	
Acute diarrhoea	Not recommended for acute diarrhoea In children.		4mg then	initial dose	Usual total daily dose of 6–8 mg. Maximum daily dose 16mg.
			2mg	after each loose stool	Up to 5 days only.

CONTRA-INDICATIONS & WARNINGS
Should not be used when inhibition of peristalsis is to be avoided (e.g. in ileus or constipation), if abdominal distension develops, in patients with acute ulcerative colitis, in pseudomembranous colitis associated with broad-spectrum antibiotics. Do not use alone in acute dysentry. Use with caution when hepatic function (necessary for the drugs metabolism) is defective as this might result in a relative overdose.

PREGNANCY
Studies in animals have not demonstrated any teratogenic effects but safety in humans not established. Not advisable to use in pregnancy.

BREAST-FEEDING

Very low amount of loperamide secreted in human milk, but still caution if loperamide is administered to a nursing mother.

SIDE-EFFECTS

Paralytic ileus, abdominal cramps and bloating. Other side-effects observed are skin reactions (including urticaria), nausea, vomiting, constipation, tiredness, drowsiness, dizziness and dry mouth.

POISONING/TOXICITY

Overdosage: constipation, ileus and neurological symptoms (miosis, muscular hypertonia, somnolence and bradypnoea). If intoxication is suspected, naloxone may be given as an antidote. Effects may last for up to 48 hours. Children and patients with hepatic dysfunction may be more sensitive to CNS effects. Gastric lavage or induced emesis and/or enema or laxatives may be recommended.

PHARMACOKINETIC PROPERTIES

Well absorbed from gut but almost completely extracted and metabolised by liver where it is conjugated and excreted via bile. Due to its high affinity for gut wall and its high first pass metabolism, very little loperamide reaches systemic circulation. Half-life is 9-14 hours. 97% plasma protein bound. Following oral administration, action occurs within 30-60 minutes.

EXCIPIENTS

Syrup includes sodium saccharin, a negligible amount of alcohol and is sugar-free.

LICENSED STATUS

Not licensed for use in children <4 years of age for acute diarrhoea (but note that it is not recommended for acute diarrhoea in children even though it is licensed!). Not licensed for the treatment of chronic diarrhoea in children.

Loratadine

Non-sedative antihistamine.

USES

Symptomatic relief of allergic reactions, where central sedative or anticholinergic side-effects are undesirable.

PRESENTATION

Syrup: 5mg in 5mL – Clarityn®.
Tablet: 10mg – non-proprietary.

DOSAGE

Route	Age		Frequency (times daily)	Notes
	2–12 years	12–18 years		
Oral	2–5 years	10mg	1	Safety and efficacy in children under 2 years not established.
	5mg			
	6–12 years		1	
	10mg			

L

CONTRA-INDICATIONS & WARNINGS

Hypersensitivity or idiosyncrasy to components of loratadine preparations.

INTERACTIONS

Cimetidine, erythromycin, ketoconazole, quinidine, fluconazole, fluoxetine all inhibit cytochrome P450 enzymes and therefore could elevate plasma loratadine levels, which could theoretically result in adverse effects. Clinically this is not believed to be significant.

PREGNANCY

Contra-indicated in pregnancy since it is possible that at high doses it may have effects on embryo.

BREAST-FEEDING

Contra-indicated in lactation by manufacturers. Low levels of loratadine pass into breast milk. Allow breast-feeding under close supervision.

SIDE-EFFECTS

Fatigue, nausea, headache, tachycardia, syncope,

alopecia, anaphylaxis, abnormal hepatic function, supraventricular tachycardias, all reported but incidence of each is rare.

POISONING/TOXICITY
Following overdosage treatment is symptomatic and supportive. Loratadine is not dialysed out in haemodialysis.

EXCIPIENTS
Clarityn® syrup includes sucrose. Contact manufacturers for further details.

LICENSED STATUS
Licensed for use ≥2 years.

Lorazepam

Short-acting benzodiazepine with anxiolytic, sedative, hypnotic, anticonvulsant and muscle relaxant properties.

USES
Premedication. Status epilepticus. In palliative care, for the relief of dyspnoea, particularly associated with panic.

PRESENTATION
Injection: 4mg in 1mL – Ativan®.
Tablet: 1mg and 2.5mg – non-proprietary.
Suspension: various strengths available – manufactured 'specials'.

DOSAGE

Indication	Route	Age				Frequency	Notes
		birth– 1 month	1 month– 2 years	2–12 years	12–18 years		
Pre-medication	Oral	–	50-100 microgram/kg (maximum 4mg)		1–4mg	single dose	Give at least one hour before surgery. Round dose to the nearest 500 micrograms .
Pre-medication	IV/IM	–	← 50-100 microgram/kg → (maximum 4mg)			single dose	IV give 30–45 minutes before surgery. IM give 60-90 minutes before surgery. IV is the preferred parenteral route.
Status epilepticus	IV Rectal Sublingual	← 100 microgram/kg → (maximum dose 4mg)			4mg	single dose	Generally given as a single dose; may be repeated once if initial dose is ineffective. Limited experience in neonates.

Renal Impairment
In severe renal impairment use 50% of dose (increased cerebral sensitivity). Risk of coma in liver disease.

ADMINISTRATION
IV or IM: injection should usually be diluted with an equal volume of NaCl 0.9% or Water for Injections before IM or IV administration. IV injections should be given slowly at a rate not exceeding 50 microgram/kg over 3-5 minutes into a large vein. In neonates dilute to 100 microgram/mL for IV use and 1mg/mL for IM use.
Oral: in palliative care, oral preparation has been used sublingually.
Rectal/buccal/sublingual: IV injection can be given rectally, buccally or sublingually.

CONTRA-INDICATIONS & WARNINGS
Contra-indications: pre-existing CNS depression, coma, acute pulmonary insufficiency or sleep apnoea. Encephalopathy may be precipitated in patients with severe hepatic insufficiency. Ensure that lorazepam injection is not administered intra-arterially as arteriospasm and gangrene may occur.
Cautions: chronic pulmonary insufficiency, patients with muscle weakness, impaired liver or kidney function. Use with caution in neonates, especially preterm where

neurotoxicity and myoclonus have been reported. *Warnings:* Apnoea, bradycardia, hypertension, hypotension and cardiac arrest have occurred following rapid IV injection, respiratory support must be available and extreme care taken when administering to very ill patients, those with limited pulmonary reserve and patients in status epilepticus. Injection includes propylene glycol and benzyl alcohol excipients which are potentially toxic to the baby.

INTERACTIONS
Enhanced sedation or respiratory and cardiovascular depression may occur if benzodiazepines are given with other drugs that have CNS depressant properties e.g. *anaesthetics, opioids, antihistamines, baclofen, barbiturates, antipsychotics, anxiolytics, antidepressants.* Aminophylline may antagonise the sedative effects of benzodiazepines. There have been discordant reports of *benzodiazepines* antagonising or increasing the effects of neuromuscular blocking agents, therefore caution is required.

PREGNANCY
Use in the first trimester has been associated with various congenital malformations in the infant but no clear causal relationship has been established. Chronic use may cause physical dependence and withdrawal symptoms in the neonate. Use in the third trimester and during labour seems to be associated in some infants with neonatal withdrawal symptoms and CNS depression. Respiratory depression, hypothermia, lethargy, hypotonia, apnoea, impaired metabolic response to cold stress and poor feeding have all been observed when mothers are given high dose medication shortly before delivery. The manufacturers do not recommend use in pregnancy, especially the first and last trimesters as fetal damage may be caused.

BREAST-FEEDING
Lorazepam is excreted into breast milk in low concentrations. It may be a safe premedication in breast-feeding mothers, but chronic use may lead to sedation, feeding difficulties and weight loss in the infant. The manufacturers do not recommend use in breast-feeding mothers.

SIDE-EFFECTS
CNS: drowsiness, sedation and ataxia are the most frequent adverse effects. High dosage or parenteral administration can cause respiratory depression and hypotension. Paradoxical reactions have been seen such as restlessness, agitation, irritability, aggressiveness and psychoses and may be more likely in children. Occasionally, confusion, hangover, headache, dizziness, blurred vision, depression, hallucinations.
Haematological: blood dyscrasias and increased liver enzymes have been reported.
Other: pain, venous thrombosis and phlebitis at the injection site; physical dependence with prolonged use.

POISONING/TOXICITY
Symptoms: impairment of consciousness is fairly rapid, deep coma or other manifestations of severe depression of brainstem vital functions are rare; more common is a sleep-like state from which the patient can be temporarily roused by appropriate stimuli. There is usually little or no respiratory depression, and cardiac rate and rhythm remain normal in the absence of anoxia or severe hypotension. Since tolerance to benzodiazepines develops rapidly, consciousness is often regained while concentrations of drug in the blood are higher than those which induced coma. Anxiety and insomnia can occur during recovery from acute overdosage.
Treatment: flumazenil may be indicated in emergencies, and may also be useful in the diagnosis of benzodiazepine overdose. May precipitate convulsions in some patients with epilepsy. Several cases of rhythmic myoclonic jerking have occurred in preterm neonates receiving lorazepam for sedation. There have been reports of toxicity presumed to be due to polyethylene glycol or propylene glycol following prolonged parenteral administration.

PHARMACOKINETIC PROPERTIES
Readily absorbed from the gastrointestinal tract following oral administration, with a bioavailability of about 90%, onset of action is 20-30 minutes, duration is approximately 8 hours, peak plasma concentrations occurring about 2 hours after an oral dose. The absorption profile following IM injection is similar to that following administration by mouth. If given IV it acts within 2-5 minutes and lasts 4-6 hours. The elimination half-life has been reported to range from 10-20 hours; this is increased to 30-50 hours in the neonatal period. It is about 85% bound to plasma protein. It is metabolised in the liver to the inactive glucuronide, and excreted in urine.

EXCIPIENTS
Injection contains polyethylene glycol 400, propylene glycol and benzyl alcohol, which may be hazardous to infants. Contact manufacturers for further details.

LICENSED STATUS
Tablets licensed for ≥5 years of age for premedication. Injection licensed for ≥12 years of age for premedication. Injection licensed in children for treatment of status epilepticus. Rectal administration of the injection is off label.

FURTHER INFORMATION
Suspension available from BCM Specials.

USES
Hypomagnesaemia.

PRESENTATION
Tablet: approximately 1g of magnesium glycerophosphate equivalent to 4mmol (approximately 97mg) magnesium and 4mmol phosphate – manufactured 'special'.
Tablet: (dispersible) 4mmol – manufactured 'special'.
Oral liquid: may be extemporaneously prepared.

DOSAGE

Route	Age			Frequency	Notes
	1 month–2 years	2–12 years	12–18 years	(times daily)	
Oral	← 0.2mmol/kg →		4–8mmol	3	Usual starting dose; adjust according to plasma level of magnesium.

ADMINISTRATION
Oral: the tablets can be swallowed whole, crushed, chewed or dispersed in water immediately prior to administration. The dispersible tablets can be dispersed in water immediately prior to administration.

CONTRA-INDICATIONS & WARNINGS
Do not use in patients with hyperphosphataemia. Caution in patients with renal failure as accumulation of magnesium may occur. In patients taking large doses of magnesium or in renal failure, deep tendon reflexes should be examined regularly and magnesium levels monitored.

INTERACTIONS
Magnesium salts in antacids have been shown to lower the serum levels of *tetracyclines* and *quinolones*. It is possible that magnesium glycerophosphate may do the same. If concurrent administration is necessary separate their administration by 4 hours.

PREGNANCY/BREAST-FEEDING
No information.

SIDE-EFFECTS
Diarrhoea, usually dose dependent, is less common than with other magnesium salts. Possibility of hypermagnesaemia with large doses (see poisoning/toxicity).

POISONING/TOXICITY
Hypermagnesaemia; symptoms vary depending on serum magnesium level and include nausea and flushing at levels >2mmol/L; loss of deep tendon reflexes, depression of muscle tone and drowsiness at levels >3mmol/L and voluntary muscle paralysis and respiratory arrest at levels >5mmol/L. Cardiac effects range from bradycardia and hypotension, to all forms of heart block and eventually asystole at very toxic concentrations.

EXCIPIENTS
Contact manufacturer's for further details.

LICENSED STATUS
Available as 'specials' and as such are unlicensed.

FURTHER INFORMATION
The tablet is available via IDIS World Medicines. The dispersible tablet is available from Special Products Limited.

Magnesium salts

Osmotic laxative.

USES
Constipation, rapid bowel evacuation.

PRESENTATION/DOSAGE

Andrews Original Salts
Effervescent powder containing citric acid 19.5%, magnesium sulphate 17.4% and sodium bicarbonate 22.6%.

Constipation dose
<3 years   not recommended
>3 years   5mL in a glass of water before breakfast or at bedtime.
Adults   10mL in a glass of water before breakfast or at bedtime.

Phillips Milk of Magnesia Liquid
Mint or raspberry flavoured suspension containing magnesium hydroxide 415mg per 5mL.

Constipation dose
<3 years   not recommended
>3 years   5-10mL at bedtime (repeat nightly reducing dose until constipation relieved).
Adults   30-45mL at bedtime (repeat nightly reducing dose until constipation relieved).

CONTRA-INDICATIONS & WARNINGS
Contra-indicated in acute gastrointestinal conditions. Caution in renal impairment as risk of magnesium accumulation. Use of magnesium salts should be avoided in patients with hepatic coma if at risk of renal failure.

INTERACTIONS
Antacids may reduce the absorption of *gabapentin, phenytoin, itraconazole, ketoconazole, some antibacterials, phenothiazines* and *bisphosphonates.*

SIDE-EFFECTS
Colic.

LICENSED STATUS
Licensed for ≥3 years of age.

Magnesium sulphate

High serum magnesium levels are sedative, causing muscle relaxation and significant vasodilatation.

USES
Symptomatic hypocalcaemia in the newborn (a serum calcium <1.7mmol/L). The intramuscular route was used in all the research work concerned with treating neonatal hypocalcaemia. Most cases of symptomatic hypocalcaemia are associated with hypomagnesaemia, thus the use of magnesium sulphate for this indication.
Persistent pulmonary hypertension in ventilated neonates (to promote pulmonary vasodilatation).
Magnesium supplement in deficiency (also consult magnesium glycerophoshate monograph for oral magnesium doses in hypomagnesaemia).

PRESENTATION
Injection: 10% (100mg in 1mL, 0.4mmol Mg^{2+} in 1mL) 5mL and 10mL ampoules – manufactured 'special'.
Injection: 20% (200mg in 1mL, 0.8mmol Mg^{2+} in 1mL) 20mL syringe – from Aurum Pharmaceuticals.
Injection: 50% (500mg in 1mL, 2mmol Mg^{2+} in 1mL) 2mL, 5mL and 10mL ampoules; 10mL prefilled syringe – non-proprietary.

DOSAGE
Newborn infant (birth to 1 month)

Indication	Route	Dose	Frequency (times daily)	Notes
Neonatal hypocalcaemia	IM	← 100mg/kg →	2	Two doses will control most cases of late neonatal hypocalcaemia. One further dose may be necessary in a minority of cases.

DOSAGE
Newborn infant continued

Indication	Route	Dose	Frequency (times daily)	Notes
Hypo-magnesaemia	IV/IM	← 100mg/kg →	single dose	Repeat after 6–12 hours if necessary.
Persistent pulmonary hypertension	IV infusion	← 200mg/kg → (2mL/kg of 10% solution)	single loading dose	If a response occurs once the plasma level exceeds 3.5mmol/L consider a continuous infusion.
	IV infusion	← 20–75mg/kg/hour → (0.2–0.75mL/kg/hour of 10% solution)	continuous	Try to maintain a plasma magnesium level between 3.5-5.5mmol/L Can be given for 2-5 days.

Child

Route	Age			Frequency (times daily)	Notes
	1 month–2 years	2–12 years	12–18 years		
IV slow injection over at least 10 minutes	← 0.2mmol/kg → (50mg/kg or 0.5ml/kg of 10% solution)		4mmol	single dose	Supplement in deficiency. Can be repeated every 12 hours if necessary.

ADMINISTRATION
IM: to give a 100mg/kg dose use 0.2mL/kg of a 50% solution by deep IM.
IV: dilute to 10% (100mg in 1mL) or less with glucose 5% or NaCl 0.9%. If fluid restricted, maximum concentration is 20% (200mg in 1mL). For persistent pulmonary hypertension give the loading dose by infusion over 20-30 minutes using a 10% (100mg in 1mL) solution.

CONTRA-INDICATIONS & WARNINGS
High magnesium levels cause sedation and muscle relaxation.

INTERACTIONS
Effect of *non-depolarising muscle relaxants* enhanced by parenteral magnesium.

PREGNANCY
Mothers treated with magnesium (for pre-eclampsia or to inhibit preterm labour) may have levels high enough to cause hypotonia, respiratory depression and reduced gastrointestinal motility in their newborn babies.

BREAST-FEEDING
Magnesium sulphate enters breast milk and may cause diarrhoea in breast-fed infants. Contact local Medicines Information Centre for advice.

POISONING/TOXICITY
High magnesium levels cause sedation and muscle relaxation. Hypermagnesaemia can cause muscular weakness, respiratory depression and cardiac arrhythmias.

LICENSED STATUS
10% ampoules are manufactured 'specials' and as such are unlicensed. 20% injection is licensed for use in children and adults. 50% injection – licence data does not specify ages.

FURTHER INFORMATION
The 10% ampoules are available from some NHS manufacturing units.

Malathion

Organophosphate parasiticidal agent.

USES
Scabies, head lice.

PRESENTATION
Liquid: 0.5% in aqueous basis – Derbac-M®, Quellada-M®.
Lotion: 0.5% in an alcoholic basis – Prioderm®, Suleo-M®.

DOSAGE/ADMINISTRATION
Topical: medical supervision is required for children <6 months of age.
Scabies – apply to whole body excluding head and neck, allow to dry, wash off after 24 hours. Children <2 years should have a thin film applied to scalp, face and ears, avoiding eyes and mouth. If hands or any other part are washed the treatment must be reapplied.
Head lice – rub liquid gently into dry hair until all hair is thoroughly moistened. Comb and allow to dry naturally, away from heat or sunshine. A contact time of 12 hours or overnight is recommended. Repeat after 7 days only if live lice are found again.

CONTRA-INDICATIONS & WARNINGS Avoid contact with eyes. Do not use on broken or secondarily infected skin. Do not use more than once a week for 3 weeks at a time. Alcoholic lotion not recommended for headlice in severe eczema, asthma or in small children. **PREGNANCY/BREAST-FEEDING** Use with caution.	**SIDE-EFFECTS** Skin irritation. **POISONING/TOXICITY** Treat by gastric lavage, assisted respiration, and in the case of massive ingestion, administration of atropine with pralidoxime.

EXCIPIENTS
See manufacturers SPC for further details.

LICENSED STATUS
Licensed for use in children and adults, but medical supervision required <6 months of age.

FURTHER INFORMATION
Treat all affected members of family/household on the same day.

Mannitol

Mannitol is a relatively inert hexahydric alcohol, used as an osmotic diuretic.

USES
Treatment of oedematous states, including ascites and treatment of raised intracranial pressure.

PRESENTATION
IV infusion: 10% and 20% – non-proprietary.

DOSAGE
A test dose may be given (to assess adequate renal function): 200mg/kg (maximum 12.5g) over 3-5 minutes (to produce a urine flow of at least 1mL/kg/hour for 1-3 hours); then doses as in table below.

M

Route	Age				Frequency	Notes
	birth–1 month	1 month–2 years	2–12 years	12–18 years		
IV infusion over 30 minutes	500 mg/kg - 1g/kg (2.5 -5mL/kg of 20% solution)	◄— 500mg/kg - 1.5g/kg (2.5mL - 7.5 mL/kg of a 20% solution) —►			single dose	Cerebral and ocular oedema. May be repeated once or twice after an interval of 4–8 hours if necessary (if serum osmolality <310mOsm/L).
IV infusion over 2-6 hours	-	◄— 1–2g/kg —►			single dose	Peripheral oedema and ascites.

ADMINISTRATION

Do not mix with any other drugs. The 20% solution is supersaturated; warming will dissolve any crystals that form, or give through a filter to trap any small crystals.

CONTRA-INDICATIONS & WARNINGS

Known hypersensitivity to mannitol; pulmonary oedema or congestive heart failure; inadequate urine flow; dehydration and/or acidosis; intracranial bleeding.

INTERACTIONS

Aminoglycosides: mannitol potentiates ototoxic effects. *Lithium:* renal excretion of lithium may be increased. *Neuromuscular-blocking drugs:* effect of tubocurarine and other competitive or depolarising neuromuscular blockers may be enhanced. *Oral anticoagulants:* mannitol may reduce the effect of anticoagulant drugs by concentrating circulating clotting factors secondary to dehydration. *Digoxin:* increased risk of digoxin toxicity if mannitol administration produces hypokalaemia. *Cisplatin:* mannitol reduces the renal toxicity of cisplatin. *Potassium chloride, sodium chloride,* other electrolytes, or drugs should not be added to mannitol solutions due to risk of precipitation.

PREGNANCY

Safety in pregnant women is not established. Contact local Medicines Information Centre for advice.

BREAST-FEEDING

Contact local Medicines Information Centre for advice.

SIDE-EFFECTS

Administration of hypertonic mannitol solutions in therapeutic amounts may produce severe fluid and electrolyte imbalance. Pulmonary oedema, water intoxication, convulsions and hypertension or hypotension may result. Irreversible crenation of red blood cells may occur if mannitol is administered too quickly. Long-term use of mannitol results in hypernatraemia and dehydration. Hyperkalaemia and acidosis may occur and depend on the dose, rate of administration and insulin response. Hypokalaemia may occur due to increased urine flow and hyperaldosteronism associated with extracellular fluid expansion. Hypersensitivity reactions, including urticaria. Extravasation may cause oedema, inflammation, skin necrosis and thrombophlebitis. Thirst, headache, dizziness, chills, fever, tachycardia, chest pain, nausea and vomiting, urinary retention and blurred vision have all been reported.

POISONING/TOXICITY

Overdosage with mannitol produces CNS toxicity including lethargy, confusion, stupor, coma and death. These signs are accompanied by fluid overloading, severe hyponatraemia and a large osmolarity gap. Treatment is haemodialysis with removal of mannitol and sodium replacement. Peritoneal dialysis may also be used. In less severe cases symptomatic treatment directed at correction of fluid and electrolyte disturbance.

PHARMACOKINETIC PROPERTIES

Oral absorption is negligible. Plasma half-life is 2.17 hours (range 2-36 hours). Volume of distribution is 0.16-0.27L/kg. After IV administration, 80% of mannitol is excreted in the urine unchanged. Very little metabolism of mannitol occurs, with unchanged mannitol also being excreted in bile, particularly in renal failure.

LICENSED STATUS

Mannitol is not licensed for use in children <12 years of age.

FURTHER INFORMATION

Mannitol should not be used as a vehicle for IV drug administration.

Measles vaccine

There is no indication for the use of a single antigen measles vaccine, and there is no available vaccine licensed for use in the UK. The MCA permits the importation of single measles antigen to complete a course of measles, mumps and rubella vaccination that has already been started with one of the other single vaccines, or where there is a medical contra-indication to the combined vaccine. There is no scientific basis to either of these indications. MMR can be used to complete a course when any of the single antigens has been given. There is no contra-indication to the MMR that does not also contra-indicate the single measles vaccine.

Licensed measles vaccine is only available in the UK in combination with mumps and rubella vaccines (MMR vaccine).

Anthelmintic.

USES
Enterobius vermicularis (threadworm/pinworm), *Trichuris trichiuria* (whipworm), *Ascaris lumbricoides* (large roundworm), *Ancylostoma duodenale* (common hookworm) and *Necator americanus* (American hookworm).

PRESENTATION
Tablet: 100mg (chewable) – Vermox® (scored) and non-proprietary.
Suspension: 100mg in 5mL – Vermox®.

DOSAGE

Indication	Route	Age			Frequency	Notes
		1 month–2 years	2–12 years	12–18 years	(times daily)	
Threadworm	Oral	≥6 months 100mg	← 100mg →		single dose	It is strongly recommended that all family members be treated simultaneously. If re-infection is suspected, a second dose is recommended after 2-3 weeks.
Whipworm, large roundworm, common hookworm	Oral	≥1 year 100mg	← 100mg →		2	Take for 3 consecutive days.

Liver disease/renal impairment: doses may need adjusting in liver impairment. No reduction of dose is necessary in impaired renal function.

CONTRA-INDICATIONS & WARNINGS
Contra-indications: pregnancy, breast-feeding of children <2 years of age and in patients with known hypersensitivity to the product or its components.

INTERACTIONS
Increased plasma mebendazole concentration with *cimetidine*. Plasma concentrations may be lowered with concurrent administration of *phenytoin* or *carbamazepine*.

PREGNANCY
Mebendazole has been shown to have embryotoxic and teratogenic activity in rats at single oral doses. No such findings reported in the rabbit, dog, sheep or horse. No reports of human teratogenicity due to mebendazole have been located, but since there is a risk mebendazole could produce fetal damage it is contra-indicated in women who are thought to be or may be pregnant.

BREAST-FEEDING
There are no data available on the passage of mebendazole into human milk, however, since only about 2–10% of an oral dose is absorbed, it is doubtful that the drug is excreted into milk in significant quantities. Contact local Medicines Information Centre for advice.

SIDE-EFFECTS
Rarely, transient abdominal pain and diarrhoea – only reported in cases of massive infestation and expulsion of worms. Hypersensitivity reactions e.g. exanthema, rash, urticaria and angiooedema. Rare reports of convulsions in children <1 year.

POISONING/TOXICITY
Symptoms: abdominal cramps, nausea, vomiting and diarrhoea, rare reports of reversible liver function disturbances, hepatitis and neutropenia in patients on large doses for prolonged periods for hydatid disease.
Treatment: treat symptomatically with supportive measures and gastric lavage with activated charcoal if necessary.

PHARMACOKINETIC PROPERTIES
Poorly absorbed from gastrointestinal tract. Undergoes extensive first pass metabolism. Metabolised in liver; eliminated in bile as unchanged drug and metabolites and excreted in the faeces. Only 2% of drug dose excreted unchanged or as metabolites in the urine. Highly protein bound.

EXCIPIENTS
Vermox® tablets include saccharin. Vermox® suspension includes sucrose. See manufacturers SPC for further details.

LICENSED STATUS
Licensed for use >2 years of age.

Direct relaxant of intestinal smooth muscle.

USES

Relief from gastrointestinal pain due to smooth muscle spasm. Symptomatic treatment of irritable bowel syndrome and related conditions (colicky abdominal pain and cramps, persistent non-specific diarrhoea plus alternating constipation, flatulence).

PRESENTATION

Tablet: 135mg – Colofac® and non-proprietary.
Capsules: 200mg modified release – Colofac MR®.
Liquid: (as embonate) 50mg in 5mL – Colofac®.
Compound granules: ispaghula husk 3.5g and mebeverine 135mg – Fybogel® Mebeverine (contains 7mmol potassium per sachet).

DOSAGE

Presentation	Route	Age		Frequency	Notes
		2–12 years	12–18 years	(times daily)	
Tablets/liquid	Oral	>3 years: 25mg	1 tablet	3	20 minutes before meals.
		4–8 years: 50mg	or	3	
		9–10 years: 100mg	15mL liquid	3	
		> 10 years			
		1 tablet or 15mL liquid		3	
Modified release capsule	Oral	–	200mg	2	20 minutes before meals.
Compound granules	Oral	–	1 sachet	2–3	Usually morning and evening, 30 minutes before meals. An additional sachet may be taken before the midday meal if necessary.

ADMINISTRATION

Oral: compound granules must be taken dispersed in a glass of water. Not advised immediately before going to bed. Capsules should be swallowed whole without chewing, preferably 20 minutes before meals.

CONTRA-INDICATIONS & WARNINGS

Use with caution in children. Experience limited in younger children. Not to be used in paralytic ileus.

PREGNANCY

Caution advised. Animal studies have failed to show any teratogenic effects.

BREAST-FEEDING

Amount in breast milk too small to be harmful.

POISONING

CNS excitability may occur. No specific antidote, treatment is symptomatic.

EXCIPIENTS

Colofac®: tablets include lactose and sucrose; liquid is sugar-free. Compound granules include sodium saccharin. Contact manufacturers for further details.

LICENSED STATUS

Tablets and liquid licensed for ≥10 years of age. Compound granules and capsules licensed for ≥12 years of age.

USES
In the treatment of chronic eczema where occlusion is indicated.

PRESENTATION

Bandage	Proprietary name
Zinc paste BP	Steripaste® (15%), Zincaband® (15%), Viscopaste PB7® (10%).
Zinc paste and Calamine	Calaband®.
Zinc paste, Calamine and Clioquinol BP	Quinaband®.
Zinc paste and Ichthammol BP	Ichthaband® (15/2%), Ichthopaste® (6/2%).

DOSAGE
To be applied once daily or as frequently as required in the clinical circumstances.

ADMINISTRATION
The medicated bandage should be covered by an additional bandage or dressing to prevent soiling of clothes.

CONTRA-INDICATIONS & WARNINGS
Care should be taken if it is decided to apply topical steroid preparations under the bandage as their absorption may be increased.

SIDE-EFFECTS
Hypersensitivity to an ingredient of the paste.

EXCIPIENTS
Contact manufacturers for further details.

LICENSED STATUS
Licensed for use in all ages.

Mefloquine

Antimalarial drug that essentially destroys the asexual blood form of the malarial pathogens that affect humans.

USES
Treatment and prophylaxis of malaria.
Treatment: *P. falciparum* malaria resistant to other antimalarial agents; chloroquine-resistant vivax malaria.
Prophylaxis: travel to malarious areas in which multiple resistant *P. falciparum* strains occur.

PRESENTATION
Tablet: 274.09mg mefloquine hydrochloride, equivalent to 250mg mefloquine base – Lariam®.

DOSAGE
Curative treatment

Patient category	Weight/dose		Notes
Non-immune adult patients	Up to 60kg 3 tablets (750mg) 2 tablets (500mg) –	Over 60kg 3 tablets (750mg) 2 tablets (500mg) 1 tablet (250mg)	Loading dose. After 6–8 hours. After a further 6–8 hours.
Children, irrespective of immunity status	< 45kg 25mg/kg (≡ 1 tablet per 10kg ≡ quarter tablet per 2.5kg)		Single dose. May be given in 2–3 divided doses if necessary to reduce side-effects.

M

Malaria prophylaxis

Route	Age	Weight	Dose mg	Dose tablets	Notes
Oral	12 weeks - 11 months	6-9.9kg	62.5mg	1/4 tablet	Stated dose to be given once weekly, always on the same day for a minimum of 6 weeks.
	1-3 years	10-15.9kg	62.5mg	1/4 tablet	
	4-7 years	16-24.9kg	125mg	1/2 tablet	First dose 1 week before arrival in malarious area (may be started 2-3 weeks prior to travel to ensure mefloquine is tolerated).
	8-12 years	25-44.9kg	187.5kg	3/4 tablet	
	>13 years	>45kg	250mg	1 tablet	Further doses at weekly intervals during and for 4 weeks after visiting the malarious area.

ADMINISTRATION
Oral: take with food and a suitable liquid or water. Tablets may be crushed.

CONTRA-INDICATIONS & WARNINGS
Contra-indications: prophylactic use in patients with renal insufficiency or severe impairment of liver function; a history of psychiatric disturbances or convulsions. Known hypersensitivities to mefloquine or related products e.g. quinine. Because of lack of experience, prophylactic use in young children (body weight of <5kg) is not recommended. In patients with epilepsy, mefloquine should be used only for curative treatment and only if compelling reasons exist. Avoid pregnancy during and for 3 months after taking mefloquine.
Cautions: mefloquine should be taken with caution in patients suffering from cardiac conduction disorders.

INTERACTIONS
Mefloquine must not be administered concurrently with *quinine* or related compounds, e.g. *chloroquine*, since this could increase the risk of convulsions and ECG changes. In severe cases, however, patients may be treated initially for one or more days with quinine given IV, and subsequently with mefloquine after a period of 12 hours. Because of the danger of a potentially fatal prolongation of the QTc interval, *halofantrine* must not be given simultaneously with or subsequent to mefloquine. Concomitant use of mefloquine with *anticonvulsants* may reduce seizure control by lowering the plasma levels of the *anticonvulsant*. For *oral live typhoid vaccines,* attenuation of the immunisation induced by such vaccines cannot be excluded. Therefore vaccination should be completed at least 3 days before the first intake of mefloquine, keeping in mind that mefloquine prophylaxis should be started 1 week before arrival in a malarious area. Increased risk of cardiotoxicity with *digoxin, beta-blockers, calcium-channel antagonists, amiodarone* and *pimozide.*

PREGNANCY
Use only if there are compelling medical reasons.

BREAST-FEEDING
Mefloquine is excreted into breast milk in small amounts, the activity of which is unknown. Mothers should not breast-feed while taking mefloquine.

SIDE-EFFECTS
At the doses given for acute malaria, adverse reactions to mefloquine may not be distinguishable from symptoms of the disease itself. Because of the long half-life of mefloquine, adverse reactions may occur or persist up to several weeks after the last dose. Obtain medical advice before the next weekly dose if any concerning or neuropsychiatric symptoms develop. Discontinuation should be considered, particularly if neuropsychiatric reactions occur. Common side-effects include nausea, vomiting, dizziness or vertigo, loss of balance, headache, somnolence, sleep disorders (insomnia, abnormal dreams), loose stools or diarrhoea and abdominal pain.

POISONING/TOXICITY
In cases of overdosage, the symptoms mentioned under side-effects may be more pronounced. Monitor cardiac function (if possible by ECG) and neuropsychiatric status for at least 24 hours.

PHARMACOKINETIC PROPERTIES
The maximum plasma concentration is reached within 2-12 hours after a single oral dose. The average half life is 21 days. Excretion is primarily via the bile and faeces.

EXCIPIENTS
See manufacturers SPC for further details.

LICENSED STATUS
Licensed for use in patients ≥3 months or ≥5kg.

Trivalent arsenical derivative.

USES
Trypanosomiasis; late disease with CNS involvement.

PRESENTATION
Injection: 3.6% solution w/v in propylene glycol – named patient (imported).

DOSAGE
Children: usual initial doses have been 0.36mg/kg/day, increasing gradually to a maximum 3.6mg/kg/day at intervals of 1-5 days for a total of 9-10 doses (18–25mg/kg total over 1 month).
Adults: 2–3.6mg/kg/day for 3 days; after 1 week, 3.6mg/kg/day for 3 days, then repeated again after 10-21 days (1.3g total over 1 month).
The dose should be determined based on clinical status as opposed to body weight alone. Lower doses are suggested in frail or severely ill patients. Up to 180mg/day has been used in adults.

ADMINISTRATION
It should be given by slow IV injection; the patient should be supine and fasting and remain so for at least 5 hours after the injection. Melarsoprol injection is very irritant and additional care should be taken during administration to avoid extravasation.

Renal and hepatic impairment
In renal or hepatic impairment the potential exists for increased toxicity; these patients should be closely monitored during therapy. Although there are no supportive data in the literature, empirical dose reductions should be considered.

CONTRA-INDICATIONS & WARNINGS
The drug should be used with caution in patients with hypertension, arrhythmias, myocardial ischaemia, heart failure, pre-existing nervous system disorders (e.g. epilepsy, neuropathy), leprosy, G6PD deficiency.

PREGNANCY
Treatment of pregnant women with trypanosomiasis should be deferred until after delivery.

BREAST-FEEDING
Contact local Medicines Information Centre for advice.

SIDE-EFFECTS
Adverse effects are common and may be severe. The greatest risk is from reactive encephalopathy which has been reported in about 10% of patients treated with melarsoprol. Symptoms include fever, headache, tremor, slurring of speech, convulsions and coma; death has occurred in up to 5% of patients treated with melarsoprol. Other toxic effects include fever, peripheral neuropathy, hypertension, arrhythmias, myocardial damage, abdominal pain, vomiting, nephrotoxicity, hepatotoxicity, skin reactions and hypersensitivity.

POISONING/TOXICITY
Symptoms: parenteral overdose – see side-effects. Acute oral ingestion of arsenic compounds generally produces symptoms within 30 minutes but may be delayed for several hours if ingested with food. Dehydration, intense thirst, vomiting, diarrhoea, fluid-electrolyte disturbances and hypovolaemia are common.
Treatment: following oral or parenteral exposure: no specific antidote; gastric lavage and activated charcoal may be indicated. Monitor liver, renal and cardiac function and fluid/electrolyte status. Maintain high urine output. Consult a source of information on arsenic poisoning for full details.

PHARMACOKINETIC PROPERTIES
After IV administration of 3.6mg/kg melarsoprol, serum levels range from 5-6 microgram/mL at 30 minutes and decline to <2 microgram/mL at 24 hours; cerebrospinal fluid levels have been 50–fold lower than serum concentrations. It is excreted in urine and possibly bile, and an elimination half-life of 35 hours has been reported.

EXCIPIENTS
Contact manufacturer for further details.

LICENSED STATUS
Not licensed for use in the UK.

FURTHER INFORMATION
Available from IDIS World Medicines.

Endogenous hormone produced by pineal gland.

USES
Treatment of sleep disorders in children with visual impairment or blindness, learning difficulties, cerebral palsy, autism.

PRESENTATION
Capsule: 1mg, 2mg, 2.5mg, 3mg, 5mg and 10mg – named patient.
Capsule (sustained release): 3mg – named patient.
Lozenge (sub-lingual tablet): 3mg – named patient.

DOSAGE

Route	Age			Frequency	Notes
	1 month–2 years	2–12 years	12–18 years		
Oral	←	2–3mg	→	30–60 minutes before bedtime	Doses from 500 microgram to 10mg at bedtime have been used. Usual starting dose is 2–3mg in all ages of children. Dose may be increased to 4–6mg if insufficient benefit after 1–2 weeks. In rare circumstances 9–10mg can be tried. Doses higher than this are not considered to be of greater efficacy and may cause increased side-effects. If no benefit is seen after 2 weeks on the higher dose then melatonin should be stopped.

Dose in hepatic insufficiency.
Clearance is reduced significantly and half-life prolonged in cirrhotic patients. Relevance in terms of dose adjustments in patients with liver disease is unclear.

ADMINISTRATION
Powder from capsule may be dispersed in water, milk or orange juice.

CONTRA-INDICATIONS & WARNINGS
Cautions: liver disease, history of cerebrovascular disease, history of neurological disorders, depression.

INTERACTIONS
Bioavailability may be increased by *fluvoxamine.* Blood pressure control may be affected in patients maintained with *nifedipine.* Rarely patients on *multiple drug therapy* have shown less response, possibly due to unidentified interactions.

PREGNANCY
Not recommended due to lack of information of effects on the fetus. Contact local Medicines Information Centre for advice.

BREAST-FEEDING
Not recommended due to lack of information of effects on the infant. Contact local Medicines Information Centre for advice.

SIDE-EFFECTS
Cardiovascular: tachycardia been reported rarely.
CNS: increased seizure activity in some children with epilepsy. Occasional withdrawal syndromes including dyskinesias have been reported. High doses can reduce body temperature and induce daytime fatigue, headache, dizziness and increase irritability in some subjects following repeated treatments with pharmacological doses. There have been anecdotal reports of restlessness, confusion, tachycardia, pruritis and nausea possibly due to impurities in some formulations.

POISONING/TOXICITY
There are theoretical possibilities of unwanted modification to reproductive function e.g. hypogonadism, delayed puberty, precocious puberty. Signs of excessive sedation/fatigue may warrant dose reduction.

PHARMACOKINETIC PROPERTIES
Peak plasma concentrations occur within 20-120 minutes following immediate release oral tablet ingestion, and in 2-4 hours following sustained release tablets. Onset of action is usually within 30-120 minutes. Melatonin undergoes significant first pass metabolism (up to 60% of an oral dose). Bioavailability may be higher when ingested with food. Inactivation occurs in the liver, where it is converted to inactive 6-hydroxymelatonin and N-acetyl serotonin by the P-450-dependent microsomal enzyme system. Most of these metabolites are excreted in the urine and faeces as sulphate conjugates. The elimination half-life is 30-50 minutes.

EXCIPIENTS
Contact manufacturer for further advice.

LICENSED STATUS
Available on a named patient basis and as such are unlicensed.

FURTHER INFORMATION
Available from IDIS World Medicines or Penn Pharmaceuticals.
Immediate release formulations may be more effective in inducing sleep, sustained-release formulations may be better for maintenance of sleep. Melatonin treatment is likely to be more successful when combined with strict environmental sleep structuring. It may be possible to withdraw the drug after 2-3 months when a regular sleep pattern has been established.

Meloxicam

Non-steroidal anti-inflammatory drug (NSAID) that shows preference for inhibition of cyclooxygenase-2 (COX-2).

USES
Treatment of pain and inflammation in rheumatic diseases including juvenile idiopathic arthritis (JIA) and other musculoskeletal disorders in adolescents intolerant to other NSAIDs.

PRESENTATION
Tablet: (scored) 7.5mg and 15mg – Mobic®.
Suppository: 7.5mg and 15mg – Mobic®.

DOSAGE

Route	Age		Frequency (times daily)	Notes
	2–12 years	12–18 years		
Oral/rectal	–	<50kg		Patients with increased risks for adverse effects should start treatment with 7.5mg/day. In terminal renal failure a daily dose of 7.5mg must not be exceeded.
		7.5mg	1	
		>50kg		
		15mg	1	

ADMINISTRATION
Oral: tablets may be crushed and will disperse in water.

CONTRA-INDICATIONS & WARNINGS
Although there may be less gastrointestinal intolerance than other NSAIDs, meloxicam should not be given to patients with active peptic ulceration, and should be used with extreme caution in patients with a history of peptic ulceration. Also contra-indicated in patients who have previously shown hypersensitivity reactions (asthma, rhinitis, urticaria) to aspirin or other NSAIDs. Hypersensitivity to the active substance or to any of the excipients. Use with caution in renal, cardiac or hepatic impairment.

INTERACTIONS
Increased risk of: ulcers and gastrointestinal bleeding with other *NSAIDs* including high doses of *salicylates,* bleeding with *oral anticoagulants, heparin* and *ticlopidine,* toxicity with *methotrexate* and *lithium* due to reduced excretion, nephrotoxicity with *ciclosporin (cyclosporin)* and *diuretics*. Efficacy of *intrauterine contraceptive devices* is decreased.

PREGNANCY
The use of meloxicam in pregnant women is not recommended. NSAIDs should be avoided in the third trimester as they may cause constriction of the ductus arteriosus in utero leading to persistent pulmonary hypertension in the newborn. In addition, these drugs may inhibit labour if used close to delivery. Contact local Medicines Information Centre for advice.

BREAST-FEEDING
NSAIDs are excreted into breast milk, therefore meloxicam should not be used whilst breast-feeding. Contact local Medicines Information Centre for advice.

SIDE-EFFECTS
Gastrointestinal discomfort, nausea, diarrhoea, abdominal pain and more rarely gastrointestinal bleeding. Disturbances of blood count have been described in patients taking meloxicam. Headache, dizziness, vertigo, drowsiness, fluid retention, hypersensitivity reactions e.g. rashes and including anaphylactoid reactions.

POISONING/TOXICITY
Although there is no known antidote evidence was found in one clinical trial of acceleration of the elimination of meloxicam by colestyramine (cholestyramine).

PHARMACOKINETIC PROPERTIES
The bioavailability of meloxicam following oral administration is 89%. Steady state is reached in 5 days. The mean elimination half-life is approximately 20 hours. Meloxicam is extensively metabolised.

EXCIPIENTS
See manufacturers SPC for further details.

LICENSED STATUS
Licensed ≥15 years of age.

Melphalan

Bifunctional alkylating agent.

USES
Use only as part of an intensive high-dose consolidation therapy (alone or in combination with other drugs, mIBG or TBI).

PRESENTATION
Injection: powder for reconstitution (as hydrochloride), 50mg vial and 10mL solvent-diluent – Alkeran®.

DOSAGE
** Always consult the current treatment protocol for details of dosage and scheduling. **

ADMINISTRATION
IV: (fast) injection into established large-bore IV access. IV boluses of reconstituted, but not further diluted, melphalan must be administered within 30 minutes of preparation. Or if the melphalan is further diluted, the shelf-life can be extended to 2 hours, so it can be infused over 1.5 hours (maximum) if diluted to a concentration of 400 microgram in 1mL in NaCl 0.9%. Hydration must be established ($3L/m^2$/day) with good urine output prior to administration of melphalan and continued for at least 12 hours afterwards.

CONTRA-INDICATIONS AND WARNINGS
Ensure adequate renal function (GFR >30mL/minute/1.73m²). Adequate hydration and urine output at time of administration. Adequate 'rescue' available (marrow or stem cells). *Cyclophosphamide* 'prime' of 300mg/m², 5-9 days prior to single agent melphalan therapy may help minimise gastrointestinal tract toxicity.

INTERACTIONS
Co-administration of *nalidixic acid* has been reported to result in severe gastrointestinal tract toxicity in children.

PREGNANCY
Avoid use whenever possible during pregnancy, especially during the first trimester.

BREAST-FEEDING
Mothers receiving melphalan should not breast-feed.

SIDE-EFFECTS
Nausea and vomiting (severe and immediate). Profound myelosuppression, mucositis/enteritis, alopecia and sterility (in boys). Occasional haemorrhagic diarrhoea, amenorrhoea, encephalopathy and hypersensitivity. Rarely veno-occlusive disease, pulmonary fibrosis/pneumonitis, secondary leukaemia and dermatitis.

POISONING/TOXICITY
Full supportive measures.

PHARMACOKINETIC PROPERTIES
Melphalan is cleared primarily by chemical degradation. Urinary excretion of intact melphalan <20%. There is a weak relationship between glomerular filtration rate and melphalan clearance in adults but this cannot be used to adjust dose.
Median (and range) pharmacokinetic parameters:
Clearance: 331 (306-443) mL/minute/m².
Half-life: 62 (38-180) minutes.

M

EXCIPIENTS
See manufacturers SPC for further details.

LICENSED STATUS
Licensed for use in children and adults.

USES
Active protection against systemic disease due to groups A and C meningococci. The vaccine is only indicated in the following high-risk groups.

Travel: those travelling in sub-Saharan Africa and some parts of the Indian subcontinent, especially if staying longer than a month.

Saudi Arabia used to require it for people coming to the annual Haj pilgrimage, irrespective of their country of origin, but this has now been replaced by a requirement for the quadrivalent vaccine (meningococcal A, C, W_{135} and Y).

Contacts and outbreak control: immediate family and close contacts of cases of group A or C meningococcal disease should be offered vaccination. In some outbreaks, vaccination may also be appropriate for more distant contacts. This should only be undertaken after consultation with the local CCDC.

Functional asplenia: these patients are at increased risk of meningococcal disease. However, because the protection from the vaccine is probably short lived, it is unclear whether 'routine' immunisation should be offered. It should certainly be given if a patient also falls into one of the other high-risk groups noted above.

In adults and older children, protection lasts from 3-5 years. There is evidence of tolerance and the value and timing of booster doses is unclear.

PRESENTATION
Injection: (single dose freeze-dried pellet to be reconstituted to 0.5mL) – AC Vax®; Mengivac (A+C)®.
Both contain not less than 50 micrograms of polysaccharide from each of groups A and C *Neisseria meningitidis* in each 0.5mL dose.

DOSAGE/ADMINISTRATION
IM & deep SC: 0.5mL of reconstituted vaccine.

CONTRA-INDICATIONS & WARNINGS
As for vaccines generally. In children <18-24 months, protection against meningococcal C disease is very poor. At any age, where protection against meningococcal C disease is required, the conjugate meningococcal C vaccine should be used.

INTERACTIONS
If a plain polysaccharide meningococcal vaccine is given and then followed by the conjugate vaccine, an interval of 6 months should be left between the two, unless the recipient is <5 years old, in which case the interval may be shortened to 2 weeks. If the conjugate vaccine is given first, an interval of only 2 weeks is necessary.
Apart from this, the vaccine can be given simultaneously with, or at any interval before or after any other vaccine.

PREGNANCY
No adverse effects were reported after the vaccine was given to pregnant women during an epidemic in Brazil. However, it should not normally be given to a pregnant woman.

BREAST-FEEDING
No information is available, but there are no grounds to believe it would be harmful.

SIDE-EFFECTS
Erythema, slight induration and tenderness at the site of injection may occur. Fever is much less common.

POISONING/TOXICITY
No information available.

PHARMACODYNAMIC PROPERTIES
Protection is present within 2-3 weeks of injection.

EXCIPIENTS
Lactose.

LICENSED STATUS
Licensed for use as described.

FURTHER INFORMATION
There is little response to the group A polysaccharide in infants <3 months and to the group C polysaccharide in those <18 months.

Also available are a plain polysaccharide vaccine against meningococcal A, C, W_{135} and Y strains and conjugate meningococcal C vaccines (see separate monographs). The conjugate vaccine is part of the routine vaccination programme. If travelling to an area where meningococcus A is endemic, the A and C polysaccharide vaccine should be given, even if the conjugate vaccine has been received previously. For travel to Saudi Arabia the A, C, W_{135} and Y vaccine may be required.

Store at 2-8°C and protect from light. Use within 1 hour of reconstitution.

Materials of bovine origin are used in the manufacturing process. Trace amounts of the original material may be present in the final product, however, all such material is obtained from sources known to be free of BSE.

USES

This vaccine is primarily for use in those going to Saudi Arabia for the annual Haj pilgrimage, irrespective of their country of origin. W_{135} is also seen in some African countries and so the vaccine would be indicated for travel to these areas as well. It is also indicated for those in contact with a case of meningococcal disease due to serotype W_{135}.

In adults and older children, protection lasts from 3-5 years. There is evidence of tolerance and the value and timing of booster doses is unclear.

PRESENTATION

Injection: (single dose freeze-dried pellet for reconstitution to 0.5mL) – ACWYVax®. Multidose vials of 10 or 50 doses are available.

Each 0.5mL contains not less than 50 micrograms of polysaccharide from each of groups A, C, W_{135} and Y *Neisseria meningitidis*.

DOSAGE/ADMINISTRATION

Deep SC or IM: 0.5mL of reconstituted vaccine.

CONTRA-INDICATIONS & WARNINGS

As for vaccines generally; also, the vaccine should not be used in children <2 months. The vaccine does not stimulate a protective response to serogroup C in children <2 years old. The responses of children <5 years old to serogroups A, W_{135} and Y are adequate but short-lived. Children in this age group may need re-vaccination after 2-3 years if at continued risk.

INTERACTIONS

A gap of 6 months should be left between the administration of this vaccine and the subsequent administration of the meningococcal C conjugate vaccine, except in children <5 years old. In this age group, children may receive the conjugate vaccine at least 2 weeks after the plain polysaccharide vaccine. If the conjugate vaccine is given first, a minimum interval of 2 weeks should be left before administering the plain polysaccharide preparation. Otherwise the vaccine can be given simultaneously with, or at any interval before or after, any other vaccine.

PREGNANCY

Limited experience of administering the vaccine to women in pregnancy has revealed no adverse effects on the mother, fetus or neonate. However, until more research has taken place, its use in pregnancy cannot be recommended.

BREAST-FEEDING

No information is available, but there are no grounds to believe it would be harmful.

SIDE-EFFECTS

Erythema, slight induration and tenderness at the site of injection may occur. Fever is much less common.

POISONING/TOXICITY

No information available.

PHARMACODYNAMIC PROPERTIES

Protection is present within 2-3 weeks of injection.

EXCIPIENTS

Lactose.

LICENSED STATUS

Licensed for use as described.

FURTHER INFORMATION

Store at 2-8°C and protect from light. Use within 1 hour of reconstitution.

Also available are a plain polysaccharide vaccine against meningococcal A and C strains and a conjugate meningococcal C vaccine (see separate monographs). The conjugate vaccine is part of the routine vaccination programme.

Meningococcal C conjugate vaccine

USES

To provide active immunity against systemic disease due to group C meningococci. It is given as part of the routine childhood immunisation schedule at 8, 12 and 16 weeks. The vaccine was introduced in November 1999 in the UK and over the following 12 months it was offered to all children and young people <18 years old. From January 2002, it has also been offered to all those <25 years old. It should be offered to all students, irrespective of age, in their first year of higher education if they have not previously been immunised with it.

PRESENTATION

Injection: there are three vaccines available.

Meningitec® – a suspension containing 10 micrograms of meningococcal group C oligosaccharide conjugated to approximately 15 micrograms of *Corynebacterium diphtheriae* CRM$_{157}$ protein in each dose.

Menjugate® – a freeze dried powder containing 10 micrograms of meningococcal group C oligosaccharide conjugated to approximately 15 micrograms of *Corynebacterium diphtheriae* CRM$_{157}$ protein in each dose.

NeisVac-C® – a suspension containing 10 micrograms of meningococcal group C polysaccharide conjugated to 10-20 micrograms of tetanus toxoid protein in each dose.

DOSAGE/ADMINISTRATION

IM or deep SC: 0.5ml. The number of doses depends on the age of the recipient. When the course is commenced with the primary immunisations at 8, 12 or 16 weeks, three doses should be given each separated by 4 weeks; if started at older than 16 weeks, but <1 year old, two doses at an interval of 4 weeks is appropriate; for children >12 months only one dose is necessary.

CONTRA-INDICATIONS & WARNINGS

As for vaccines generally. Meningitec® and Menjugate® should not be given to someone with known hypersensitivity to diphtheria toxoid. NeisVac-C® should not be given to someone with known hypersensitivity to tetanus toxoid.

INTERACTIONS

The vaccine can be given at the same time as OPV, HBV, DTP-Hib, DT, Td and MMR vaccines. It should be given at a different site. If a plain polysaccharide meningococcal vaccine is given before the conjugate vaccine, an interval of 6 months should be left before giving the conjugate vaccine unless the recipient is <5 years old, in which case the interval may be shortened to 2 weeks. If the conjugate vaccine is given first, an interval of only 2 weeks is necessary.

PREGNANCY

In mice it has shown no evidence of teratogenicity. There is no experience in humans and its use should be avoided in pregnancy. There is, however, no reason to believe that it would have a deleterious effect on the fetus or mother.

BREAST-FEEDING

There is no experience of its use during breast-feeding and its use should be avoided. There is, however, no reason to believe that it would have a deleterious effect on the suckling infant.

SIDE-EFFECTS

These are similar to those seen with Hib vaccine. See table below.

POISONING/TOXICITY

There is no experience of overdosage.

PHARMACODYNAMIC PROPERTIES

The vaccine produces humoral immunity due to the production of protective levels of antibodies in >98% of recipients of a course appropriate for their age.

Side-effects of vaccine

Age group	Local redness >3 cm	Systemic reactions*	
		Fever	Headaches/irritability
<12 months	2–4%	2–4%	Irritability – 50%
12–17 months	2–3%	5%	Irritability – 19%
4–11 years	29%	1.1%	Headaches – 10%
12–18 years	26%	2.5%	Headaches – 14%

*On the whole, these rates are no higher than the background rates seen with other routinely administered vaccines. It would appear that the vaccine causes little additional effect. Headaches in older children may be related to the vaccine.

EXCIPIENTS

Meningitec®: sodium chloride, aluminium phosphate.
NeisVac-C®: sodium chloride, aluminium hydroxide.
Menjugate®: mannitol, sodium phosphate monobasic monohydrate, sodium phosphate dibasic heptahydrate, aluminium hydroxide and sodium chloride. The multidose vial also contains 2-phenoxyethanol.

LICENSED STATUS

All are licensed for use as described.

FURTHER INFORMATION

Combined meningococcal A and C polysaccharide vaccines are available as is a vaccine against meningococcal A, C, W_{135} and Y strains (see separate monographs). Because of their limitations they should be reserved primarily for use in travellers. If travelling to an area where meningococcus A is endemic, the A and C polysaccharide vaccine should be given, even if the conjugate vaccine has been received previously. For travel to Saudi Arabia the A, C, W_{135} and Y vaccine may be required.

There is evidence that the vaccine reduces nasal carriage of meningococcus C in adolescents.

Storage – keep at 2-8°C. Do not freeze.

Material of bovine origin is used in the manufacturing process. There should be none of the original material present in the final product, however, all such material is obtained from sources known to be free of BSE.

Mepacrine hydrochloride

USES

Pigment that can be taken by mouth for photosensitive disorders. No longer used to treat malaria. Chiefly effective against wavelengths which cause sunburn.

PRESENTATION

Tablets: 100mg – manufactured 'special'.

DOSAGE

Route	Age	Frequency	Notes
	12–18 years	(times daily)	
Oral	100mg	1-2	

CONTRA-INDICATIONS & WARNINGS

Avoid in psoriatic patients. Caution with history of psychosis.

INTERACTIONS

Mild disulfiram like effect with alcohol.

SIDE-EFFECTS

Dizziness, headache, nausea and vomiting. Reversible yellow discolouration of skin and urine, ocular toxicity and chronic dermatoses during long-term administration. Transient acute toxic psychosis and convulsions at high dose. Rarely hepatotoxicity and aplastic anaemia.

EXCIPIENTS

Contact manufacturer for further details.

LICENSED STATUS

Available as a 'special' and as such is unlicensed.

FURTHER INFORMATION

Available from BCM Specials as a 'special'.

Mercaptamine (cysteamine)

Reduces cystine accumulation in some cells of nephropathic cystinosis patients and, when started early, delays the development of renal failure.

USES

Management of nephropathic cystinosis and eye symptoms from cystine crystals in cystinosis.

PRESENTATION

Capsule: 50mg and 150mg mercaptamine base (as mercaptamine bitartrate) – Cystagon®.
Eye drops: (as hydrochloride) 0.11%, 10mL – manufactured 'special'.

DOSAGE

Route	Age				Frequency (times daily)	Notes
	birth–1 month	1 month–2 years	2–12 years	12–18 years		
Oral	← 2–3mg/kg →			100mg	4	Initial dose; gradually increased over 4–6 weeks to avoid intolerance.
	← 12.5mg/kg →			500mg	4	Maintenance dose.
Topical	← 1 drop in each eye →				4–6	

Doses are based on mercaptamine free base.
Starting doses should be one quarter to one sixth of the expected maintenance dose.

ADMINISTRATION
Oral: for children unable to swallow capsules, the capsule should be opened and the contents sprinkled onto food or mixed in a strongly flavoured drink. Avoid mixing with acidic drinks as powder does not mix well and may precipitate out. Mercaptamine has a very unpleasant taste and smell.

CONTRA-INDICATIONS, WARNINGS & MONITORING
Hypersensitivity to any mercaptamine salt or to penicillamine. Monitor leucocyte cystine levels. A trough blood level should be taken and checked frequently when initiating therapy (e.g. monthly) and then every 3-4 months when on a stable dose.

INTERACTIONS
None known.

PREGNANCY
No safety data available on use during pregnancy. Mercaptamine is not recommended during pregnancy. The effect of untreated cystinosis on pregnancy is also unknown.

BREAST-FEEDING
Mercaptamine must not be used during breast-feeding.

SIDE-EFFECTS
Mercaptamine causes an unpleasant smell on the breath and body odour. It can also cause nausea, vomiting, diarrhoea, lethargy, fever and rash. It may also cause anaemia, leucopenia, raised liver enzymes and rarely gastrointestinal ulceration and bleeding. Temporary suspension of mercaptamine therapy and gradual re-introduction may be effective in improving tolerance.

POISONING/TOXICITY
Symptoms would include nausea and vomiting. Seizures and lethargy have been reported at high doses. Treatment is symptomatic and supportive.

PHARMACOKINETIC PROPERTIES
Mercaptamine reacts with cystine to form cysteine and a cysteine-mercaptamine mixed disulphide. The disulphide complex structurally resembles lysine and uses its lysosome transport system for removal.
The mean time to peak plasma levels is 1.5 hours and the half-life is approximately 5 hours.

EXCIPIENTS
Contact manufacturers for further details.

LICENSED STATUS
Mercaptamine bitartrate capsules are licensed for use in children of all ages but initiation of therapy should be under the supervision of a physician experienced in the treatment of cystinosis. Supply is dependent on completion of the company's surveillance forms. The eye drops are unlicensed.

FURTHER INFORMATION
Mercaptamine does not contain phosphate, therefore if changing from phosphocysteamine, phosphate supplements may need to be initiated or increased.
Eye drops are available from Guy's and St Thomas' Hospital as a 'special'.

Mercaptopurine

An antimetabolite which interferes with the synthesis of nucleic acids in proliferating cells.

USES
Acute lymphoblastic leukaemia/lymphoma; T-non-Hodgkin Lymphoma (T–NHL).
Inflammatory bowel disease e.g. corticosteroid dependent/intractable Crohn's disease (experience limited).

PRESENTATION
Tablet: 50mg (scored) – Puri-Nethol®.
Capsule: 10mg - manufactured 'special'.
Suspension: 100mg in 5mL – manufactured 'special'.

DOSAGE
Leukaemia/lymphoma/T–NHL
** Always consult the current treatment protocol for details of dosage and scheduling. **
The dosage should be carefully adjusted according to blood counts.

Inflammatory bowel disease

Route	Age			Frequency	Notes
	1 month–2 years	2–12 years	12–18 years	(times daily)	
Oral	–	← 1–1.5mg/kg →		1	Experience limited; seek expert advice. Initial maximum dose of 50mg once daily. May be increased, as necessary, to a maximum of 75mg once daily.

ADMINISTRATION
Oral: tablets are administered as a single daily dose.

CONTRA-INDICATIONS & WARNINGS
Contra-indications: there are no absolute contra-indications to its use. Patients who exhibit hypersensitivity to any of the components should not take mercaptopurine tablets.
Warnings: treatment with mercaptopurine causes bone marrow suppression and full blood counts must be taken daily during remission induction and careful monitoring of haematological parameters should be conducted during maintenance therapy.
The leucocyte and platelet counts continue to fall after treatment is stopped, so at the first sign of an abnormally large fall in the counts, treatment should be interrupted immediately.
Mercaptopurine is hepatotoxic and liver function tests should be monitored weekly during treatment. More frequent monitoring may be advisable in those with pre-existing liver disease or receiving other potentially hepatotoxic therapy. The patient should be instructed to discontinue mercaptopurine immediately if jaundice becomes apparent.
Cautions: there are individuals with an inherited deficiency of the enzyme thiopurine methyltransferase (TPMT) who may be unusually sensitive to the myelosuppresive effect of mercaptopurine and prone to developing rapid bone marrow depression following the initiation of treatment. This problem could be exacerbated by coadministration with drugs that inhibit TPMT, such as olsalazine, mesalazine or sulphasalazine.
During remission induction when rapid cell lysis is occurring, uric acid levels in blood and urine should be monitored as hyperuricaemia and/or hyperuricosuria may develop, with the risk of uric acid nephropathy.

INTERACTIONS
Allopurinol inhibits mercaptopurine conversion to inactive metabolite. If allopurinol is given concurrently, the dose of mercaptopurine must be reduced to a quarter of the original dose. Inhibition of the anticoagulant effect of *warfarin* has been reported.

PREGNANCY
The use of mercaptopurine should be avoided whenever possible during pregnancy, particularly during the first trimester. Normal offspring have been born after mercaptopurine therapy during human pregnancy, but abortion, prematurity and malformation have been reported. In any individual case the potential hazard to the fetus must be balanced against the expected benefit to the mother.
As with all cytotoxic chemotherapy, adequate contraceptive precautions should be advised if either partner is receiving mercaptopurine tablets.

BREAST-FEEDING
Mothers receiving mercaptopurine should not breast-feed.

SIDE-EFFECTS
Haematological: the main side-effect is bone marrow suppression leading to leucopenia and thrombocytopenia.
Hepatobiliary: mercaptopurine is hepatotoxic in animals and man causing hepatic necrosis and biliary stasis. The incidence of hepatotoxicity varies considerably and can occur with any dose but more frequently when the recommended dose of 2.5mg/kg bodyweight daily or 75mg/m^2 body surface area per day is exceeded.
Gastrointestinal: anorexia, nausea and vomiting have occasionally been noted. Oral ulceration has been reported during mercaptopurine therapy and rarely intestinal

ulceration has occurred. Pancreatitis has been reported in association with the unlicensed use of mercaptopurine in the treatment of inflammatory bowel disease.

Other: rare complications are drug fever and skin rash.

POISONING/TOXICITY

Symptoms: gastrointestinal effects, including nausea, vomiting and diarrhoea and anorexia may be early symptoms of overdosage. The principal toxic effect is on the bone marrow, resulting in myelosuppression. Haematological toxicity is likely to be more profound with chronic overdosage than with a single ingestion. Liver dysfunction and gastroenteritis may also occur.

Treatment: as there is no known antidote the blood picture should be closely monitored and general supportive measures, together with appropriate blood transfusion, instituted if necessary. Active measures (such as the use of activated charcoal or gastric lavage) may not be effective in the event of mercaptopurine overdose unless the procedure can be undertaken within 60 minutes of ingestion. Mercaptopurine is 30% protein bound but the drug is dialysable.

PHARMACOKINETIC PROPERTIES

Mercaptopurine exhibits first-pass metabolism and the bioavailability shows considerable inter-individual variability (ranging from 5-37%). The elimination half-life of 6-mercaptopurine is 90 +/- 30 minutes, but the active metabolites have a longer half-life (approximately 5 hours) than the parent drug. The apparent body clearance is 4832 +/- 2562 mL/minute/m². There is low entry of mercaptopurine into the cerebrospinal fluid.

The main method of elimination for mercaptopurine is by metabolic alteration. The kidneys eliminate approximately 7% of mercaptopurine unaltered within 12 hours of the drug being administered. Xanthine oxidase is the main catabolic enzyme of mercaptopurine and it converts the drug into the inactive metabolite, 6-thiouric acid. This is excreted in the urine. Individual variation in thiopurine methyltransferase (TPMT) which produces an inactive metabolite, will influence the level of active metabolites and thus efficacy and toxicity.

LICENSED STATUS

Puri-Nethol® tablets are licensed for use in children and adults. The oral suspension and capsules are 'specials' and as such are unlicensed. Inflammatory bowel disease is not a licensed indication.

EXCIPIENTS

Contact manufacturers for further details.

FURTHER INFORMATION

Cross resistance usually exists between mercaptopurine and thioguanine.

Nova Laboratories (manufacturing unit Leicester Royal Infirmary Tel: 0116 2230100) can manufacture capsules or a 100mg in 5mL oral suspension. Other suspension strengths are available on request.

Meropenem

Carbapenem beta-lactam antibiotic with a broad spectrum of activity.

USES

Aerobic and anaerobic Gram-positive and Gram-negative infections. Generally inactive against methicillin-resistant *Staphylococcus aureus* (MRSA). Usually reserved for infections resistant to other antibiotics.

In cystic fibrosis patients – second-line treatment of early *Pseudomonas aeruginosa* infections not cleared by ciprofloxacin plus colistin and of moderate to severe exacerbations in combination with an aminoglycoside; treatment of more severe *Burkholderia cepacia* infections, discuss with local microbiology department.

PRESENTATION

Injection: (as trihydrate salt) 500mg and 1g vial – Meronem®.

DOSAGE
Newborn infant (birth to 1 month)

Route	Age Postnatal age (days)	Dose (mg/kg/dose)	Frequency (times daily)	Notes
IV	<7	20mg/kg	2	Double dose in meningitis or severe infection.
	>7	20mg/kg	3	

Child

Route	Age			Frequency (times daily)	Notes
	1 month–2 years	2–12 years	12–18 years		
IV	←	10mg/kg	→	3	UTI, gynaecological, skin and skin structure infections. Maximum single dose 500mg.
	←	20mg/kg	→	3	Pneumonia, peritonitis, neutropenia, septicaemia. Maximum single dose 1g.
	←	40mg/kg	→	3	Cystic fibrosis patients. Meningitis and life threatening infections. Maximum single dose 2g.

Dose adjustment in renal failure

Creatinine clearance (mL/minute/1.73m²)	Dose	Dosage interval
25–50	100%	12 hours
10–25	50%	12 hours
<10	50%	24 hours

ADMINISTRATION

IV: administered by slow IV injection over 5 minutes or by IV infusion over 20-30 minutes.

Each 250mg displaces 0.22mL of water on reconstitution. For slow IV injection a concentration of 50mg in 1mL should be used. May be further diluted with glucose 5% or 10%, or NaCl 0.9% to provide a solution between 1-50mg in 1mL for IV infusion.

CONTRA-INDICATIONS & WARNINGS

Caution in beta-lactam allergy as partial cross-sensitivity between penicillins and cephalosporins has been demonstrated. Monitor LFTs carefully in patients with pre-existing liver disease.

INTERACTIONS

Use with caution with nephrotoxic drugs. May cause positive Coomb's test without haemolysis. *Probenecid* inhibits renal excretion of meropenem. Little evidence of other interactions though no formal studies have been done.

PREGNANCY

No adverse effects shown in animal studies. No studies have been performed in humans. Contact local Medicines Information Centre for advice.

BREAST-FEEDING

Present in very low concentrations in animal breast milk. No data available in humans. Meropenem is inactivated by gastric acid.

SIDE-EFFECTS

Local irritation at injection site, skin rashes, gastrointestinal upset, pseudo-membranous colitis reported rarely, reversible neutropenia, thrombocytopenia, eosinophilia, and thrombocythaemia reported, raised LFTs may occur, adverse CNS effects such as seizures have been reported particularly in patients with underlying CNS disorders, bacterial meningitis or poor renal function.

POISONING/TOXICITY

Treatment should be symptomatic. In normal individuals rapid renal elimination will occur; in those with renal impairment haemodialysis will remove meropenem and its metabolite.

PHARMACOKINETIC PROPERTIES

Half-life is approximately 1 hour in healthy older children, 1.5-2 hours in younger children and up to 3 hours in premature infants. 70% of dose excreted in urine over 12 hours. Metabolised to inactive metabolite. 2% plasma protein bound. Penetrates well into most body fluids and tissues including CSF in bacterial meningitis.

EXCIPIENTS

Each 1g of powder includes 3.9mmol of sodium. See manufacturers SPC for details.

LICENSED STATUS

Licensed for >3 months of age.

Mesalazine is the active component of sulfasalazine (sulphasalazine), an aminosalicylate.

USES
Treatment of mild to moderate acute exacerbations of ulcerative colitis (suppositories and enema particularly appropriate in distal disease). Maintenance of ulcerative colitis remission (tablets and suppositories). For the maintenance of remission in Crohn's ileo-colitis.

PRESENTATION
Tablet: 250mg (enteric coated) – Salofalk®; 400mg (enteric coated) – Asacol®; 500mg (slow release) – Pentasa®.
Suppository: 250mg – Asacol®; 500mg – Asacol® and Salofalk®; 1g – Pentasa®.
Enema: 1g per metered application – Asacol®; 1g in 100mL – Pentasa®; 2g in 59mL – Salofalk®.
Granules: 1g per sachet (modified release) – Pentasa®.

DOSAGE
There is very little published data on the use of mesalazine in children. The table gives oral doses which have been used in some centres. Rectal doses are given for ≥12 years only.

Preparation	Indication	Route	Age		Frequency (times daily)	Notes
			2–12 years	12–18 years		
Asacol® and Salofalk®	Acute treatment	Oral	>5 years 15–20mg/kg	2 tablets	3	In the 12-18 year age group a dose for an acute episode may be 2 tablets and a maintenance dose 1-2 tablets of either brand. However, do not interchange preparations/brands.
	Maintenance	Oral	>5 years 10mg/kg	1-2 tablets	2-3	
Pentasa® slow-release and granules	Acute treatment	Oral	>5 years 15–20mg/kg	2 tablets	3	≥15 years can have up to 4g **daily** in 2-3 divided doses.
Pentasa® slow-release	Maintenance	Oral	>5 years 10mg/kg		2-3	
				500mg	3	
Pentasa® granules	Maintenance	Oral	>5 years 10mg/kg		2-3	
				500mg-1g	2	
Asacol® enema	Acute attack recto-sigmoid region	Rectal	–	1g enema (1 metered application)	daily	For 4-6 weeks.
	Acute attack descending colon	Rectal	–	2g enema (2 metered applications)	daily	For 4-6 weeks.
Pentasa® and Salofalk® enema		Rectal	–	1 enema	bedtime	
Asacol® suppository		Rectal	–	1-2 x 250mg suppository	3	Maximum 3 x 500mg **daily**. Last suppository should be inserted at bedtime.
Pentasa® suppository		Rectal	–	1 x 1g suppository	daily	For 2-4 weeks.
Salofalk® suppository	Acute attack	Rectal	–	1-2 x 500mg suppository	2-3	

ADMINISTRATION
Oral: swallow tablets whole. Pentasa® tablets can be dispersed in water before swallowing but do not completely dissolve. Not advised to mix with fruit juice as this may affect the slow release formulation. Pentasa® tablets can be halved and quartered, but do not chew.

Mesalazine is highly unstable in solution and also in light. It has a direct action on the colon. If crushed or chewed and the matrix is broken, the drug will be absorbed from the upper gastrointestinal tract and will not reach the site at which it is needed. Therefore it is not possible to make a suspension with mesalazine. Pentasa® granules should be placed on the tongue and washed down with water or orange juice without chewing. A Pentasa® granules 1g sachet weighs (with excipients etc.) 2g, so part doses can be weighed out immediately before use and the remaining granules discarded.

Enema: Asacol® – shake can, push applicator on the spout of the can and hold can upside down with the dome pointing downwards. Insert applicator into the rectum and to administer a dose fully depress the dome once and release. The foam will not come out of the can until the dome is released. To administer a second dose, press and release the dome again. Wait 15 seconds before withdrawing the applicator. Salofalk® – action is enhanced if patient lies on the left side while introducing the enema.

CONTRA-INDICATIONS & WARNINGS
Contra-indicated in patients with a history of sensitivity to salicylates or renal sensitivity to sulfasalazine (sulphasalazine). Severe renal impairment (GFR <20mL/minute). Serious blood dyscrasias have been reported very rarely with mesalazine; haematological investigations should be performed if the patient develops unexplained bruising, purpura, anaemia, fever or sore throat. Contra-indicated in severe hepatic impairment.

Although data in children is limited, because release of mesalazine in the small bowel results in greater absorption of the drug and nephrotoxicity may be a concern, renal function should be regularly assessed, especially in children receiving large oral doses. In addition to routine blood counts and liver function tests, blood urea nitrogen and serum creatinine determinations and a urinalysis should be performed at least monthly for 3 months, then every 3-6 months.

INTERACTIONS
Should not be given with *lactulose* or similar preparations which lower stool pH and may prevent release of mesalazine.

PREGNANCY
Only negligible quantities cross the placenta.

BREAST-FEEDING
The amount excreted in breast milk is small but there has been a report of watery diarrhoea in an infant whose mother had used suppositories 500mg twice daily. Avoid unless essential.

SIDE-EFFECTS
Predominantly gastrointestinal; nausea, diarrhoea and abdominal pain. Headache. Rare reports of blood dyscrasias, pancreatitis, hepatitis, allergic lung reactions, lupus erythematous-like reactions and rash, interstitial nephritis and nephrotic syndrome (with oral therapy). Renal failure.

POISONING/TOXICITY
Tablet ingestion – gastric lavage and IV transfusion of electrolytes to promote diuresis. No specific antidote.

PHARMACOKINETIC PROPERTIES
Oral preparations are formulated to release the drug in the terminal ileum and colon, where it is thought to exert a mainly local action. The specific release characteristics differ somewhat between formulations. The absorbed portion is almost completely acetylated in the gut wall and in the liver. The elimination half-life is approximately 1 hour; the acetylated metabolite has a half-life of 10 hours.

EXCIPIENTS
Asacol® tablets include lactose. See manufacturers SPC for further details.

LICENSED STATUS
Asacol® is not licensed for use in children. Asacol® preparations are licensed for the treatment of mild to moderate acute exacerbations of ulcerative colitis in adults. Asacol® tablets and suppositories are licensed for maintenance of remission of ulcerative colitis in adults. Asacol® tablets are licensed for maintenance of remission of Crohn's ileo-colitis in adults.
Pentasa® slow release tablets are licensed for the treatment of mild to moderate acute exacerbations of ulcerative colitis ≥15 years of age. Pentasa® granules are licensed for the treatment of mild to moderate acute exacerbations of ulcerative colitis ≥12 years of age.
Pentasa® retention enema is licensed for the treatment of ulcerative colitis affecting the colon and rectum ≥15 years of age.
Pentasa® suppositories are licensed for the treatment of ulcerative proctitis ≥15 years of age.
Salofalk® not licensed for use in children and contra-indicated in babies and infants. Salofalk® is licensed for the treatment of mild to moderate acute exacerbations of ulcerative colitis and maintenance of remission of ulcerative colitis in adults.

Mesna (sodium mercaptoethane sulphonate)

Non-cytotoxic. Mesna reacts specifically with urotoxic urinary metabolites of cyclophosphamide and ifosfamide.

USES
Specific uroprotectant administered with the oxazaphosphorines cyclophosphamide and ifosfamide, to ameliorate urothelial toxicity. In cystic fibrosis patients, it is used occasionally when other mucolytic agents fail.

PRESENTATION
Injection: 100mg in 1mL, 4mL and 10mL ampoules – Uromitexan®.
Nebule: 200mg in 1mL, 3mL ampoule – Mistabron®.

DOSAGE

Uroprotectant
Injection: Mesna doses vary but in practice doses greater than 100% (mg:mg) of the total daily oxazaphosphorine dose are used. **Always consult the current treatment protocols for details of dosage and scheduling.**

Mucolytic
Nebule: 3-6mL of a 20% solution twice daily. Maximum of 24mLs per day.

ADMINISTRATION
IV: IV bolus, or continuous IV infusion in conjunction with IV hydration.
Nebule: Use neat or diluted with an equal volume of NaCl 0.9%.

CONTRA-INDICATIONS AND WARNINGS
Known hypersensitivity to mesna or other thiol compounds.

INTERACTIONS
Possible false positive test for urinary ketones. Possible interference with dipstick test for erythrocytes in urine. Urinary microscopy recommended.

PREGNANCY
No evidence of embryotoxic or teratogenic effects. Should a patient be undergoing oxazaphosphorine therapy during pregnancy then mesna should be given. Contact local Medicines Information Centre for advice.

BREAST-FEEDING
Lactation is a contra-indication to cytostatic treatment and consequently mesna is not likely to be used under these circumstances.

SIDE-EFFECTS
Nausea after rapid IV administration. Skin rashes. Pseudoallergic reactions.

POISONING/TOXICITY
No evidence of major toxic effects after high doses. No specific antidote to mesna.

PHARMACOKINETIC PROPERTIES
After IV injection, mesna is oxidised in the plasma to its sole unreactive metabolite, dimesna. Both mesna (half-life 22 minutes) and dimesna (half-life 70 minutes) are excreted rapidly from the vascular compartment by glomerular filtration. A significant proportion of the dimesna excreted is absorbed by the renal tubular cells and re-oxidised to mesna, which is then re-excreted into the urine. This sequence of events results in a 'time-to-peak' free-mesna concentration in the urine after IV injection of approximately 60 minutes.

EXCIPIENTS
See manufacturers SPC for further details.

LICENSED STATUS
Injection licensed for use in children and adults. Nebule is unlicensed for use in the UK.

Metformin hydrochloride

A biguanide.

USES
Type 2 diabetes, when diet has failed, as an adjunct to insulin in insulin resistance.

PRESENTATION
Tablet: 500mg and 850mg – Glucophage® and non-proprietary.
Suspension: may be extemporaneously prepared.

DOSAGE

Route	Age		Frequency (times daily)	Notes
	2–12 years	12–18 years		
Oral	–	500mg	2-3	Initial dose May be increased to 1g twice a day if required.

CONTRA-INDICATIONS & WARNINGS
Hypersensitivity, ketoacidosis, impairment of renal function, chronic liver disease, cardiac failure and a history or states associated with lactic acidosis and conditions associated with hypoxaemia.

CAUTIONS
Regular monitoring of renal function is advised. Intravascular contrast studies with iodinated materials can lead to acute alteration of renal function and have been associated with lactic acidosis in patients receiving metformin. Therefore metformin should be discontinued prior to the procedure and withheld for 48 hours afterwards and reinstituted only after renal function has been found to be normal. Patients receiving continuous metformin therapy should have their vitamin B12 levels monitored annually.

INTERACTIONS
Cimetidine reduces the renal clearance of metformin and *anticoagulant therapy* may require adjustment.

LICENSED STATUS
Not licensed for use in children.

PREGNANCY
Not advised in pregnancy.

BREAST-FEEDING
Present in milk in animal studies. Contact local Medicines Information Centre for advice.

POISONING/TOXICITY
Hypoglycaemia may occur when metformin is taken in conjunction with alcohol. Lactic acidosis may develop and supportive therapy should be given.

SIDE-EFFECTS
Gastro-intestinal effects, including anorexia, lactic acidosis.

PHARMACOKINETIC PROPERTIES
Metformin is excreted unchanged in the urine, with a half-life of 1.7-5.4 hours in adults with normal renal function.

Methionine

Methionine is an essential amino acid. It enhances the synthesis of glutathione and is used to prevent hepatic damage in the treatment of paracetamol poisoning.

USES
Treatment of paracetamol overdosage presenting within 8 hours of ingestion.

PRESENTATION
Tablet: 250mg – non-proprietary.
Capsules: manufactured 'special'.

DOSAGE

Route	Age		Frequency	Notes
	<6 years	≥6 years	(times daily)	
Oral	1g	2.5g	4 hourly	Total of 4 doses. <6 years total daily dose 4g. ≥6 years total daily dose 10g.

Methionine:
☐ Should be started within 8 hours of a paracetamol overdose
☐ Cannot be administered after activated charcoal
☐ Is unsuitable for unconscious patients.

ADMINISTRATION
Tablet: too hard and brittle to be crushed.
Capsule: may be opened and contents sprinkled onto food.
Liquid: cannot be prepared as methionine hydrolyses rapidly.

CONTRA-INDICATIONS & WARNINGS
Should not be used in patients with acidosis. May aggravate metabolic acidosis and may precipitate acute reactions in schizophrenic patients. May aggravate hepatic damage in patients with established liver insufficiency. Should be used with caution in patients with severe liver disease.

INTERACTIONS
The effects of *levodopa* can be reduced by methionine.

PREGNANCY
In pregnancy, the mother is always treated.

SIDE-EFFECTS
Nausea, vomiting, drowsiness and irritability may occur. Large doses can cause neurological changes and precipitate encephalopathy in patients with hepatic cirrhosis, particularly in the presence of portal hypertension. May provoke an acute exacerbation of symptoms in schizophrenic patients.

POISONING/TOXICITY
Systematic toxicity studies have not been carried out with methionine. Methionine depletes hepatic adenosine triphosphate (ATP) and in large doses it causes metabolic acidosis through conversion to inorganic sulphate.

PHARMACOKINETIC PROPERTIES
Methionine is converted to homocysteine via 5-adenosylmethionine and about 80% is sequentially metabolised to cystathionine, cysteine, taurine and inorganic sulphate. Cysteine serves as a precursor for the synthesis of glutathione.

EXCIPIENTS
Contact manufacturer for further details.

LICENSED STATUS
Tablets are licensed for use in children and adults. Capsules are available as 'specials' and as such are unlicensed.

FURTHER INFORMATION
Capsules are manufactured as 'specials' in some hospital pharmacies.

Methotrexate

Antimetabolite, immunosuppressant.

USES
Treatment of solid tumours, non-Hodgkin's lymphoma (NHL), intracranial germ-cell tumours and some CNS tumours; infant brain tumours. In combination therapy in treatment of leukaemia.
Juvenile idiopathic arthritis (JIA), other connective tissue disorders (including juvenile dermatomyositis), vasculitis and uveitis.

PRESENTATION
Tablet: 2.5mg, 10mg – non-proprietary.
Oral solution: 10mg in 5mL – manufactured 'special'.
Injection: (as sodium salt) equivalent to 5mg in 2mL, 50mg in 2mL, 200mg in 8mL, 500mg in 20mL, 1g in 10mL, 1g in 40mL, 5g in 50mL and 5g in 200mL of methotrexate per vial. All solutions are preservative-free.

DOSAGE

Malignancy
** Always consult the current treatment protocol for details of dosage and scheduling. **

By intravenous infusion: dosage determined by protocol and staging, with folinic acid rescue.

By intrathecal injection: may include combination therapy with cytarabine and hydrocortisone. The maximum intrathecal dose is 15mg.

Indication	Route	Age			Frequency	Notes
		1 month–2 years	2–12 years	12–18 years	(times daily)	
Juvenile idiopathic arthritis	Oral/SC/IM/IV	←	10–15mg/m²	→	once weekly	Starting dose
	Oral/SC/IM/IV	←	up to 25mg/m²	→	once weekly	Maintenance dose Increase dose only if necessary and tolerated.

ADMINISTRATION

Methotrexate can be given by the oral, IM, IV (bolus and infusion), intrathecal, intra-arterial and intraventricular routes. With parenteral administration bioavailability may be greater than when administration is by the oral route.

Oral: the tablets are given as a single dose once a week. More frequently prescribed doses should always be queried with the prescriber.

Intrathecal: only the low volume preparations should be used (without preservative).

IV: standard dose IV bolus. High dose by IV infusion over 3 hours or 24 hours depending on protocol.

To prevent renal damage and systemic toxicity, IV hydration and alkalinisation is given before methotrexate is commenced and continued until plasma methotrexate levels are 0.1-0.2 micromol/L (depending on protocol). See protocol for details of IV hydration.

At the methotrexate dosages used in these protocols folinic acid must be written up at the same time as the methotrexate is prescribed. IV folinic acid is commenced 24 hours or 36 hours after the start of the methotrexate and continued until plasma methotrexate levels are 0.1-0.2 micromol/L (depending on protocol). See protocol for details of folinic acid rescue. Folinic acid may be given orally if the child is not vomiting.

CONTRA-INDICATIONS & WARNINGS

Consider dose reduction, or avoid use in renal impairment when GFR 60mL/minute/1.73m^2. Ensure that renal function is not deteriorating, even though a value obtained before starting the infusion is normal i.e. the trend in renal function should always be improving or stable prior to methotrexate. Pre-treatment full blood counts, U&Es and liver function tests should be taken. When treating JIA, full blood counts should be taken fortnightly for the first 4 weeks of therapy and at this frequency after any dose increase. If stable after this period, full blood counts may be taken monthly thereafter. Follow the recommendations in the treatment protocol when treating malignancy. An immediate blood count should be carried out if neutropenia or thrombocytopenia is suspected due to symptoms such as a sore throat, glossitis, buccal ulceration, or easy bruising or bleeding. Abrupt discontinuation may lead to a flare in JIA.

INTERACTIONS

Drugs which compromise renal function e.g. *aminoglycosides* and *cisplatin* can decrease clearance of methotrexate and lead to systemic toxicity. Avoid concurrent use of *salicylates* and *sulphonamides*. *NSAIDs* may alter methotrexate pharmacokinetics, resulting in the potential for increased toxicity in patients receiving the combination. The low weekly methotrexate dose taken by rheumatology patients does not necessitate discontinuation of *NSAIDs*. Large doses of *penicillin* may interfere with the active renal tubular secretion of methotrexate. Prophylactic *co-trimoxazole* must be stopped 1 week before methotrexate therapy.

PREGNANCY

Methotrexate is contra-indicated in pregnancy. It has been shown to be teratogenic and to cause fetal death and/or congenital abnormalities in humans.

BREAST-FEEDING

Contra-indicated.

SIDE-EFFECTS

Skin rashes, mild nausea and vomiting, myelosuppression, mucositis, enteritis, pneumonitis. Rarely, acute renal failure, hepatotoxicity and neurotoxicity. Osteopenia has been reported.

POISONING/TOXICITY

Although high doses of methotrexate are generally well tolerated, unpredictable life threatening toxicity can occur. For patients who have markedly delayed clearance of methotrexate secondary to renal dysfunction, therapeutic options are few and of limited efficacy. Carboxypeptidase-G2 (CPDG-2) inactivates methotrexate by hydrolysing the C-terminal glutamate residue. CPDG-2 may be used to rescue patients with renal dysfunction and delayed methotrexate excretion. CPDG-2 must be administered under expert supervision in a paediatric oncology unit. UK contact to obtain CPDG-2: Dr Roger Melton. Enact Pharma. Tel: 01980 613754, fax: 01980 613713.

PHARMACOKINETIC PROPERTIES

Intravenous dosing: after IV bolus, plasma half-lives

Phase	Value
A. Tissue distribution	2-8 minutes
B. Excretion and metabolism	0.9-2 hours
C. Methotrexate release from cells	5.5-11 hours

Between 40-50% of methotrexate is bound to plasma protein, primarily albumin. At methotrexate concentrations >5 x 10^{-5}M binding is saturated, resulting in increased concentrations of the free drug. Dose-dependent methotrexate pharmacokinetics have been demonstrated over a dose range of 0.5-33.6g/m^2/24 hours. There is a significant correlation between dose and steady-state concentration (Css) but increase in dose is accompanied by a disproportionate increase in Css. Higher doses result in a shorter half-life, lower volume of distribution at steady-state and slower systemic clearance.

Third space distribution into pleural or ascitic fluid after methotrexate may provide a source of prolonged release which can extend the terminal phase of drug excretion.

Age dependence: children aged 1-4 years show significantly lower plasma steady-state levels, faster systemic clearance and higher volume of distribution.

EXCIPIENTS
Contact individual manufacturers for details.

LICENSED STATUS
Licensed for use in children and adults for treatment of malignancy. JIA, other connective tissue diseases and vasculitis are not licensed indications. The oral suspension is a 'special' and as such is unlicensed.

FURTHER INFORMATION
Suspension available from Nova Laboratories.

Methoxsalen

Systemic antipsoriatic.

USES
Psoralen agent used to enhance ultra violet light therapy of psoriasis (PUVA).

PRESENTATION
Tablet: 10mg – named patient, Puvasoralen-8®.

DOSAGE

Route	Age	Frequency	Notes
	12–18 years	(times daily)	
Oral	600 microgram/kg (maximum dose 70mg)	1	Dose is given with every treatment, 2-3 hours before UVA. Treatment usually 1-3 times a week. Treatment should not be given more than once every other day. Give with food or milk.

CONTRA-INDICATIONS & WARNINGS
Only for use in specialised centres. The potential benefits must be weighed against the risks of premature skin ageing and carcinogenicity. Avoid if hypersensitive to psoralens. Avoid sunbathing. Protect eyes with wraparound UVA blocking glasses for first 1-2 days. Over-exposure may result in severe burning/blistering. Contra-indicated in patients with actinic damage, skin cancer, hepatic insufficiency and diseases associated with photosensitivity such as porphyria, acute lupus erythematosus, hydroa and polymorphic light eruptions, or other risk factors for skin cancer e.g. immunosuppressed.
Liver function tests should be performed monthly for the first few months and less frequently thereafter.

Avoid using with any agent with photosensitising properties. Contra-indicated for patients on anticoagulant therapy.

INTERACTIONS
Concurrent use of *fosphenytoin* and *phenytoin* may make treatment ineffective.

PREGNANCY/BREAST-FEEDING
Contra-indicated: contraception during treatment recommended for men and women as necessary.

SIDE-EFFECTS
Nausea, nervousness, insomnia, pruritis, erythema, skin pain and headache.

LICENSED STATUS
Unlicensed. Not recommended for children <12 years.

FURTHER INFORMATION
Available on a named patient basis only from: Crawford Pharmaceuticals, Furtho House, 20 Towcester Road, Old Stratford, Milton Keynes, Buckinghamshire, MK19 6AQ. A fact sheet is available on request.

Bulk-forming laxative and faecal softener.

USES
Control of colostomy, ileostomy and diarrhoea. Management of diverticular disease. Management of simple constipation. Aid to appetite control and as an aid to the management of obesity.

PRESENTATION
Tablet: 500mg (scored) – Celevac®.
Oral mixture: 9% methyl cellulose, may be extemporaneously prepared.

DOSAGE

Route	Age			Frequency (times daily)	Notes
	1 month–2 years	2–12 years	12–18 years		
Oral	–	50mg/kg	1.5–3g (3–6 tablets)	2	Do NOT take immediately before going to bed.

ADMINISTRATION
Oral: for constipation, take with a good quantity of liquid. In diarrhoea, ileostomy and colostomy control, minimise liquid intake for 30 minutes before and after the dose.

CONTRA-INDICATIONS & WARNINGS
Do not use in conditions where it is believed there is a pathological cause for diarrhoea which would render the condition unsuitable for symptomatic medical treatment e.g. infective bowel disease or bowel obstruction.

PREGNANCY
No evidence of ill consequence during human pregnancy but use with caution.

BREAST-FEEDING
No adverse effects.

POISONING/TOXICITY
Not absorbed. Overdose features would be abdominal distension which may be followed by intestinal obstruction. Gastric lavage may be appropriate. Fluids given. Intestinal obstruction – rectal washout may be necessary.

EXCIPIENTS
Tablets include lactose.

LICENSED STATUS
SPC gives no indication as to specific licensing status in children.

Methyldopa

Centrally acting antihypertensive.

USES
Refractory hypertension.

PRESENTATION
Suspension: 250mg in 5mL – may be extemporaneously prepared.
Tablet: 125mg, 250mg, 500mg – Aldomet® and non-proprietary.

DOSAGE

Route	Age				Frequency (times daily)	Notes
	birth–1 month	1 month–2 years	2–12 years	12–18 years		
Oral	←	2.5 mg/kg	→		3	Initial dose. Increase at
				250mg	2–3	intervals of 2 or more days to a maximum of 15mg/kg 3 times daily in neonates; 65mg/kg/day or 3g/day (whichever is less) in older children and adults.

Renal impairment
GFR 10-20mL/minute increase dosing interval to 12 hourly, GFR <10mL/minute increase to 24 hourly, titrate according to response. Administer after haemodialysis.

CONTRA-INDICATIONS & WARNINGS
Active liver disease, phaeochromocytoma, porphyria.

INTERACTIONS
When used with other *antihypertensives* potentiation of the antihypertensive action may occur. *NSAIDs* antagonise the antihypertensive effect.

PREGNANCY
Methyldopa has been used under close medical supervision for the treatment of hypertension during pregnancy, with no clinical evidence of fetal abnormality.

BREAST-FEEDING
Appears in breast milk, probably in amounts too small to be harmful. The baby should be watched for any possible adverse effects.

SIDE-EFFECTS
Dry mouth, sedation (usually transient during initial period of therapy or when dose is increased), drowsiness, diarrhoea, fluid retention, haemolytic anaemia, rashes.

POISONING/TOXICITY
Acute overdosage may produce acute hypotension with other responses attributable to brain and gastrointestinal malfunction (excessive sedation, weakness, bradycardia, dizziness, light-headedness, constipation, distension, flatus, diarrhoea, nausea, and vomiting). There is no specific antidote. Methyldopa is dialysable. Treatment is symptomatic. Infusions may be helpful to promote urinary excretion. Special attention should be directed towards cardiac rate and output, blood volume, electrolyte balance, paralytic ileus, urinary function and cerebral activity. Administration of sympathomimetic agents may be indicated.

PHARMACOKINETIC PROPERTIES
Oral absorption is variable and incomplete. The way in which the half-life varies with age is not well defined, but it is probably about 2 hours. Most of the drug is eliminated by the kidney.

EXCIPIENTS
See manufacturers SPC for further details.

LICENSED STATUS
Tablets licensed for use in children and adults.

Methylphenidate hydrochloride (controlled drug)

CNS stimulant.

USES
Hyperkinetic/attention-deficit hyperactivity disorder (ADHD). Narcolepsy.

PRESENTATION
Tablet: 5mg, 10mg and 20mg (all scored) – Equasym®; 10mg (scored)– Ritalin®.
Tablets (modified release): 18mg and 36mg – Concerta® XL.

DOSAGE

Route	Age		Frequency	Notes
	2–12 years	12–18 years	(times daily)	
Oral	≥6 years 5mg	5mg	1 or 2	Initial dose Increase if necessary by weekly increments of 5–10mg daily. Maximum of 60mg **per day** given in 2–4 divided doses.
Oral (Concerta XL®)	≥6 years 18mg	18mg	1 (morning)	Initial dose Increase if necessary by weekly increments of 18mg daily, according to response. Maximum of 54mg **daily**.

When switching from Equasym® or Ritalin® each total dose of 15mg daily is considered equivalent to 18mg daily of Concerta® XL.

ADMINISTRATION
Oral: Equasym® and Ritalin® tablets can be halved, but unreliable dose if quartered. If anorexia is a problem give dose after breakfast and lunch. If rebound hyperactivity occurs in the latter part of the day the dose can be given in more divided doses. Methylphenidate can cause insomnia so the last dose should not usually be given any later than 4pm.

CONTRA-INDICATIONS & WARNINGS
Psychosis. Concurrent or recent (last 14 days) MAOI. Substance misuse. Eating disorder. Proceed with care when concomitant poorly controlled seizure disorder, severe tic disorder, anxiety, cardiovascular disease, pervasive development disorder. *Caution*: monitor growth in children, as growth retardation has been reported.

INTERACTIONS
Increases plasma concentration of *phenytoin* and delays intestinal absorption of *phenytoin, phenobarbital (phenobarbitone), ethosuximide.* Inhibits metabolism of *tricyclic antidepressants* and *warfarin*.

PREGNANCY
There is no evidence of risk to the fetus but experience during pregnancy is limited.

BREAST-FEEDING
It is not known whether methylphenidate and/or its metabolites passes into breast milk. Mothers taking methylphenidate should avoid breast-feeding.

SIDE-EFFECTS
Insomnia, anxiety, dysphoria, decreased appetite, growth retardation, headache, abdominal pain (usually transitory), tics. Increased blood pressure, tachycardia, palpitations, auditory hallucinations, paranoid psychosis and occasional rebound hyperactivity after each dose (dependence not a problem in treatment of childhood hyperactivity).

POISONING/TOXICITY
Acute overdose may result in agitation, tremor, hyperreflexia, twitching, hyperpyrexia, tachycardia, seizures, hallucinations, delirium, sweating, flushing, headache, cardiac arryhthmias, hypertension. There is no specific antidote.
In the presence of severe intoxication, a carefully titrated dose of a short-acting barbiturate can cautiously be given. Intensive care should be provided to maintain adequate circulation and respiratory exchange; external cooling procedures may be required for hyperpyrexia.

PHARMACOKINETIC PROPERTIES
Mean plasma half-life is 2 hours. Main effect lasts only about 3 hours. Ingestion with food accelerates absorption, but has no influence on the amount absorbed.

EXCIPIENTS
See manufacturers SPC for further details.

LICENSED STATUS
Licensed for use in children ≥6 years.

FURTHER INFORMATION
Treatment must be under the supervision of a specialist in childhood behavioural disorders and should be part of a comprehensive treatment programme for ADHD.

Glucocorticoid.

USES
Severe systemic juvenile idiopathic arthritis (JIA), severe life-threatening connective tissue diseases and vasculitis; graft rejection.

PRESENTATION
IM depot injection: (as acetate) 40mg in 1mL, 1mL, 2mL and 3mL vial – Depo-Medrone®.
IV injection: (as sodium succinate) 40mg and 125mg – Solu-Medrone®; 500mg, 1g and 2g – Solu-Medrone® and non-proprietary.

DOSAGE

Indication	Route	Age			Frequency	Notes
		1 month–2 years	2–12 years	12–18 years		
Severe JIA, connective tissue diseases	IV	←	30mg/kg	→	once daily	Give daily for 3 days. Maximum 1g/**day**.
Graft rejection	IV	←	10–20mg/kg	→	once daily	
Demyelinating disorders	IV	←	500mg →	1g	once daily	

Dosage may have to be reduced in patients with hepatic impairment. The lowest effective dose should be used.
Prophylactic antacid administration may be required with high dose, short-term IV therapy.
If a patient is receiving oral steroids then these are usually stopped on the days that methylprednisolone is given.

ADMINISTRATION
IM: dosage must be individualised and depends on the condition being treated and its severity.
IV: give over at least 30 minutes. It may be diluted with NaCl 0.9% or glucose 5%.

CONTRA-INDICATIONS & WARNINGS, INTERACTIONS, PREGNANCY, BREAST-FEEDING
See prednisolone monograph.

SIDE-EFFECTS
See prednisolone monograph. During IV infusion, transient increases or decreases in blood pressure, metallic taste, flushing, headache and mood change may occur.

POISONING/TOXICITY
There is no specific antidote. Treatment is symptomatic. Serum electrolytes should be monitored.

PHARMACOKINETIC PROPERTIES
Methylprednisolone is eliminated by hepatic metabolism.

EXCIPIENTS
Contact manufacturers for further details.

LICENSED STATUS
Depo-Medrone® licensed for intra-articular, IM, intrabursal, intralesional and periarticular injections, and injections into the tendon sheath in children and adults. Solu-Medrone® licensed in children up to maximum dose of 1g per day, IV or IM.

Metoclopramide hydrochloride

Dopamine antagonist with prokinetic effect upon the gut and antiemetic properties. Also active in the CNS.

USES
Prophylaxis and treatment of vomiting associated with chemotherapy/radiotherapy.
Intractable vomiting of known cause. Gastro-oesophageal reflux.
Premedication for jejunal biopsy and small bowel intubation, to assist passage through pylorus.
In palliative care, as prokinetic for chronic or opioid-induced constipation.

PRESENTATION
Tablet: 5mg (scored) – Maxolon®, 10mg (scored) – Maxolon® and 10mg - non-proprietary.
Oral solution: 5mg in 5mL – non-proprietary.
Syrup: 5mg in 5mL – Maxolon®.
Paediatric liquid: 1mg in 1mL – Maxolon®.
Injection: 5mg in 1mL, 2mL ampoule – Maxolon® and non-proprietary.

DOSAGE

Route	Age				Frequency (times daily)	Notes
	birth–1 month	1 month–2 years	2–12 years	12–18 years		
Oral, IM, slow IV bolus	←	100 microgram/kg	→		2–3	Higher doses may be needed with chemotherapy but <12 years of age the **total daily dose** should not exceed 500 microgram/kg (maximum 10mg) per **day**. Can be given more frequently with chemo-therapy.
				<60kg		
				5mg	3	
				>60kg		
				10mg	3	

Dosage in renal impairment – see contra-indications and warnings

ADMINISTRATION
IV: as a slow bolus injection over at least 5 minutes or for doses over 10mg at a suggested concentration of 200 micrograms per mL over 15-30 minutes. Dilute in NaCl 0.9% or glucose 5% if required. For diagnostic procedures, IV dose is given 10-20 minutes before procedure.

CONTRA-INDICATIONS & WARNINGS
In mild to moderate renal impairment use 75% of dose, and in severe impairment 25-50% of dose. Reduce dose in severe liver disease.

INTERACTIONS
Antimuscarinics and *opioid analgesics* antagonise the effect of metoclopramide on gastrointestinal activity. *Paracetamol* and *aspirin* give an enhanced effect. *Antipsychotics* increase risk of extrapyramidal effects.

PREGNANCY
Not known to be harmful, but not advisable unless compelling need.

BREAST-FEEDING
Amount in milk small, but avoid unless essential. Metoclopramide stimulates prolactin secretion from the anterior pituitary and has been used in a dose of 8-15mg three times daily to enhance lactation.

SIDE-EFFECTS
Extrapyramidal side-effects, dystonic reactions including oculogyric crises; more common in children and young adults. Treat with an anticholinergic e.g. *benzatropine (benztropine)*, *procyclidine*. Drowsiness, diarrhoea, restlessness.

POISONING
Acute dystonic reactions (see above).

PHARMACOKINETICS
Rapidly absorbed from the gastrointestinal tract. Variable bioavailability, average 75%. Terminal elimination half-life of 4-6 hours. Excreted in the urine. 20-30% unchanged, the rest as metabolites.

EXCIPIENTS
Maxolon® syrup and paediatric liquid include saccharin sodium and are sugar-free.

LICENSED STATUS
Licensed for use in children and adults (tablets only licensed for ≥15 years); however, use <20 years should be restricted to the uses outlined in the monograph.

Thiazide diuretic.

USES
Oedema resistant to loop diuretics. Addition of metolazone can induce a profound diuresis.

PRESENTATION
Tablet: 5mg – Metenix 5®.
Suspension: may be extemporaneously prepared.

DOSAGE

Route	Age			Frequency (times daily)	Notes
	1 month–2 years	2–12 years	12–18 years		
Oral	← 100–200 microgram/kg →		5–10mg	1	Usually given once daily but may be given twice daily in children.

ADMINISTRATION
Tablets may be crushed and mixed with water immediately before use.

CONTRA-INDICATIONS & WARNINGS, INTERACTIONS, PREGNANCY, BREAST-FEEDING, SIDE-EFFECTS, POISONING/TOXICITY
See chlorothiazide monograph. Profound diuresis occurs when given with furosemide (frusemide). Thiazides are usually ineffective in patients with moderate/severe renal failure, however, metalozone may still be effective at GFR rates as low as 20mL/minute. Can cause profound hypokalaemia so potassium should be monitored regularly.

PHARMACOKINETIC PROPERTIES
Diuresis and saluresis begin within 1 hour of administration reaching a maximum in 2 hours, continuing for 12- 24 hours depending on dose.

EXCIPIENTS
See manufacturers SPC for further details.

LICENSED STATUS
Not licensed for use in children.

Metoprolol

Beta-blocker.

USES
Hypertension.

PREPARATIONS
Solution: may be extemporaneously prepared.
Tablet: 50mg and 100mg – Betaloc®, Lopressor® and non-proprietary.

DOSAGE

Indication	Route	Age			Frequency (times daily)	Notes
		1 month–2 years	2–12 years	12–18 years		
Hypertension	Oral	← 1mg/kg →		-	2	Usual starting dose <12 years. Increase to a maximum of 8mg/kg/**day**. Daily dose may be given in 4 divided doses.
		-		100mg	1	Usual starting dose ≥12 years. Increase by 100mg/day at weekly intervals. If not controlled with a single dose use twice daily regimen. Maximum dose 400mg/**day**.

Renal impairment
No dose adjustment should be required but start with a small dose if GFR is <20mL/minute.

Liver impairment
Dose reduction required.

CONTRA-INDICATIONS & WARNINGS
Metoprolol is relatively cardioselective but can still have an effect on airways resistance. Therefore it should be avoided in patients with a history of asthma. Caution in heart failure.

INTERACTIONS, SIDE-EFFECTS, POISONING/TOXICITY
See propranolol monograph.

PREGNANCY
Avoid use in pregnancy, however, has been used under close supervision for the treatment of hypertension after 20 weeks gestation.

BREAST-FEEDING
There are no significant beta-blocking effects with normal therapeutic doses.

PHARMACOKINETIC PROPERTIES
Oral administration takes 1 hour to achieve a response. Mainly eliminated by hepatic metabolism. Half-life of 3-4 hours.

EXCIPIENTS
See manufacturers SPC for further details.

LICENSED STATUS
Not licensed for use in children.

Metronidazole

Antimicrobial with high activity against anaerobic bacteria and protozoa.

USES
Prophylaxis and treatment of infection caused by anaerobic bacteria and protozoa, including *Trichomonas vaginalis, Entamoeba histolytica, Balantidium coli* and *Giardia lamblia* which are sensitive to metronidazole. Adjunct in the eradication of *Helicobacter pylori* in patients with duodenal ulcers. Disorders of propionate metabolism (propionic and methylmalonic acidaemia).

PRESENTATION
IV infusion: 5mg in 1mL, 20mL ampoule and 100mL container – non-proprietary; 100mL bag – Flagyl® and Metrolyl®.
Suspension: (as benzoate) 200mg in 5mL – Flagyl S® and non-proprietary.
Suppository: 125mg, 250mg – manufactured 'specials'; 500mg and 1g – Flagyl® and Metrolyl®.
Tablet: 200mg and 400mg – Flagyl® and non-proprietary; 500mg – non-proprietary.

DOSAGE
Newborn infant (birth to 1 month)

Route	Age	Frequency	Notes
	birth–1 month	(times daily)	
IV	15mg/kg	single dose	Loading dose followed 24 hours later by twice daily dosing as below.
	7.5mg/kg	2	Oral therapy may be used when absorption considered normal.

Child

Route	Age			Frequency (times daily)	Notes
	1 month-2 years	2-12 years	12-18 years		
Oral	← 7.5mg/kg → (maximum 400mg)		400mg	3	Anaerobic infections. Oral route has excellent bioavailability; reserve IV route for serious infections or when oral route is not available. Disorders of propionate metabolism.
IV	← 7.5mg/kg → (maximum 500mg)		500mg	3	
Rectal	**DOSE BY WEIGHT** ← 7.5mg/kg → OR **DOSE BY AGE** <1 year 1-5 years 5-12 years 125mg 250mg 500mg		1g	3 3	Anaerobic infections. Substitute oral therapy as soon as possible. 3 times daily for 3 days; twice daily thereafter.
Oral	← 40mg/kg → (maximum 2g)			1	Giardiasis for 3 days.
Oral	← 5mg/kg →		300mg or 400mg or 2g	3 2 single dose	Trichomoniasis for 7 days. For 7 days.
Oral	← 10mg/kg →		400-800mg	3	Amoebiasis – for 5–10 days. Balantidiasis – for 5 days.
Oral for *H. pylori*	>1 year 100mg	2-6 years 100mg 6-12 years 200mg	400mg	3 3	Treatment for 14 days with amoxicillin and omeprazole.
	>1 year 100mg	2-6 years 100mg 6-12 years 200mg	400mg	2 2	Treatment for 14 days with clarithromycin and omeprazole.

Dose adjustment in renal and hepatic impairment.
Increase dose interval to 12 hourly in severe renal impairment (creatinine clearance $<20\text{mL/minute}/1.73\text{m}^2$).
Reduce dose in severe liver disease. Avoid in hepatic encephalopathy.

ADMINISTRATION
Oral: tablets should be swallowed whole with or after food. Suspension should be administered 1 hour before food to maximise the bioavailability of benzoate salt.
IV: infuse over 20-30 minutes. Maximum rate 25mg per minute. Compatible with glucose 5%, NaCl 0.9%, glucose 4%/NaCl 0.18% or potassium infusions (20-40mmol/L).

CONTRA-INDICATIONS & WARNINGS
Use with caution and reduce dose in severe hepatic impairment. In patients with pre-existing blood dyscrasia leucocyte counts are advised.

INTERACTIONS
Potentiates anticoagulant effect of *warfarin*. No effect on *heparin*. Increased levels of *lithium* may lead to lithium toxicity. Increased levels of *phenytoin* may occur and levels should be monitored. *Cimetidine* reduces hepatic metabolism of metronidazole leading to increased serum levels and potentially increased incidence of side-effects. *Phenobarbital (phenobarbitone)* may significantly decrease serum levels. Possible potentiation of *vecuronium* action has been reported. Disulfiram reaction may occur with *alcohol* and the alcohol content of concurrently administered medication should be considered.

PREGNANCY

Metronidazole readily crosses the placenta. Mutagenicity of metronidazole has been demonstrated in some bacterial systems. Tests for embryotoxicity and teratogenicity in animal models have shown negative results. No adverse human fetal effects have been reported. A meta-analysis conducted could find no evidence for any relationship between metronidazole and birth defects. However, it would still be wise to avoid metronidazole, particularly large doses, in the first trimester.

BREAST-FEEDING

Distributes into milk in concentrations equal to plasma concentrations. May give the milk a bitter taste and discourage suckling. Worries about mutagenicity in bacterial test systems and tumours induced in animal models are probably unfounded and no direct evidence has been found in humans. However, metronidazole, as with all drugs, should not be used unnecessarily in lactating mothers and the infant should be monitored for adverse effects. Breast-feeding probably requires interruption only following large maternal doses over 1g orally.

SIDE-EFFECTS

Nausea, vomiting, unpleasant taste and gastrointestinal disturbances are most common, and darkening of urine may occur. CNS effects such as drowsiness, dizziness, headache and ataxia occur rarely. Skin rashes, urticaria, myalgia and arthralgia have been reported. During intensive or prolonged therapy, seizures or peripheral neuropathy have occurred. Mild leucopenia and thrombocytopenia have also been reported rarely.

POISONING/TOXICITY

Treatment should be symptomatic and supportive, aimed at reversing dehydration and correcting electrolyte imbalance, particularly hyperkalaemia.

PHARMACOKINETIC PROPERTIES

Metronidazole has excellent oral bioavailability (approximately 80%) and is not significantly influenced by food. There is a linear relationship between dose and plasma concentration. Rectal administration results in levels around 50 to 60% of that achieved orally. It is widely distributed into most body tissues and fluids including CNS. Tissue levels approach serum levels. 40% to 80% of a dose is metabolised in the liver.

The normal plasma half-life of 6-8 hours is prolonged in patients with impaired hepatic function and neonates.

EXCIPIENTS

Contact manufacturers for further details.

LICENSED STATUS

Licensed for use in children and adults. Not licensed for use in neonates. The manufactured 'specials' are unlicensed.

FURTHER INFORMATION

Manufactured 'specials' available from some hospital manufacturing units.

Metyrapone

A competitive inhibitor of 11ß-hydroxylation in the adrenal cortex.

USES

Limited role in the assessment of suspected adrenocorticotrophic hormone (ACTH) dependent Cushing syndrome (seek specialist advice). Specialist management of Cushing syndrome e.g. in preparation for surgery.

PRESENTATION

Capsule: 250mg – Metopirone®.

DOSAGE

Route	Age			Frequency	Notes
	1 month–2 years	2–12 years	12–18 years		
Oral	←— 15mg/kg —→ (minimum 250mg)		750mg	4 hourly	Test for Cushing syndrome. For 6 doses on day 3 of the test. First 2 days serve as a control period. Follow hospital protocol for taking samples etc.

CONTRA-INDICATIONS & WARNINGS
Primary adrenocortical insufficiency, hypersensitivity to metyrapone or any of the excipients in the product.

INTERACTIONS
Anticonvulsants, antidepressants, and *neuroleptics, hormones* that affect the hypothalamo-pituitary axis and *anti-thyroid agents* may influence the results of the test.

PREGNANCY/BREAST-FEEDING
Should not be administered during pregnancy since the drug can impair the biosynthesis of fetal-placental steroids. It is not known whether metyrapone passes into the breast milk, therefore nursing mothers should refrain from breast-feeding their infants during treatment with metyrapone.

SIDE-EFFECTS
Occasional nausea, vomiting, dizziness, headache, hypotension, sedation; rarely, abdominal pain, allergic skin reactions, hypoadrenalism, hirsutism.

POISONING/TOXICITY
Symptoms: gastrointestinal symptoms and acute adreno-cortical insufficiency. Signs and symptoms may be aggravated or modified in patients receiving insulin or antidiabetic drugs.
Treatment: no specific antidote; treatment is symptomatic and supportive; also give a large dose of hydrocortisone and IV sodium chloride and glucose. Measure blood pressure and monitor fluid and electrolyte balance for a few days.

PHARMACOKINETIC PROPERTIES
Rapidly absorbed and eliminated from the plasma; peak plasma levels usually occur 1 hour after ingestion; half-life of elimination from the plasma is 20-26 minutes.

EXCIPIENTS
See manufacturers SPC for details.

LICENSED STATUS
Licensed for use in children and adults.

Miconazole

Broad-spectrum antifungal.

USES
Fungal skin infections. Prevention and treatment of oral candidiasis.

PRESENTATION
Cream: 2% – Daktarin® and non-proprietary.
Oral gel: 24mg in 1mL; 15g and 80g tube – Daktarin®.

DOSAGE

Indication	Route	Age				Frequency (times daily)	Notes
		birth–1 month	1 month–2 years	2–12 years	12–18 years		
Fungal skin infections	Topical	← apply to affected area →				2	Continue for 10 days after the lesions have healed.
Oral candidiasis	Topical and then swallowed	1–2mL	2.5mL	2–6 years 5mL		2	Use in the mouth after food or feeds and retain as long as possible before swallowing. For localised infection, apply directly to affected area.
				6–12 years 5mL	5–10mL	4	

PREGNANCY
Use with caution if strictly necessary, although only small amounts are absorbed following topical administration.

BREAST-FEEDING
It is not known if miconazole is excreted into breast milk. Contact local Medicines Information Centre for advice.

SIDE-EFFECTS
Occasional skin irritation or sensitivity.

POISONING/TOXICITY
Not highly toxic; vomiting and diarrhoea may occur; treatment is symptomatic and supportive.

LICENSED STATUS
Licensed for use in all age groups.

Midazolam

Short-acting benzodiazepine with hypnotic, anxiolytic, amnesic, muscle relaxant and anticonvulsant activity.

USES
Premedication, sedation prior to short procedures and in intensive care situations, anticonvulsant, induction of general anaesthesia. In palliative care, for relief of anxiety (including for sedation during acute terminal haemorrhage), dyspnoea, intractable seizures and terminal agitation.

PRESENTATION
Injection: (as hydrochloride) 10mg in 2mL and 10mg in 5mL – Hypnovel®; 1mg in 1mL, 50mL – non-proprietary; 5mg in 1mL, 2mL, 5mL, 10mL and 18mL – non-proprietary.
Syrup (buccal liquid): 10mg in 1mL – Epistat (manufactured 'special').
Syrup: 2.5mg in 1mL – Amsed (manufactured 'special').

DOSAGE
Newborn infant (birth to 1 month)

Indication	Route	Age	Frequency	Notes
		birth–1 month		
Sedation	IV infusion	1 microgram/kg/minute for the first 24 hours then decrease to 500 nanograms/kg/minute in babies <33 weeks post-conceptional age to avoid accumulation.	continuous	Can be used for up to 4 days with apparent safety in the ventilated newborn baby.

Child

Indication	Route	Age			Frequency	Notes
		1 month–2 years	2–12 years	12–18 years		
Premedication	IM	← 70–100 microgram/kg →			single dose	Administer 30–60 minutes prior to surgery. Monitor from time of administration.
	Oral	← 500 microgram/kg → (maximum dose 15mg)			single dose	
Sedation for procedures	IV bolus	–		2mg	single dose	If after 2 minutes sedation is not adequate, incremental doses of 500 microgram – 1mg can be given. Doses >5mg are rarely needed.
	IV bolus or IM	50–100 microgram/kg		–	single dose	Doses up to 300 microgram/kg may be needed.
	Oral	← 500 microgram/kg → (maximum dose 15mg)			single dose	
	Rectal	← 500–750 microgram/kg →			single dose	
	Intranasal	← 200–300 microgram/kg →			single dose	Half the dose should be given into each nostril.

Child continued

Indication	Route	Age			Frequency	Notes
		1 month–2 years	2–12 years	12–18 years		
Sedation in intensive care	IV bolus (over 3-5 minutes)	← 30–300 microgram/kg →			single dose	This may not be needed if the patient is already receiving morphine, or is sedated post-op. Reduce the dose in hypovolaemia, vasoconstriction and hypothermia. Low doses may be adequate if the patient is also receiving an opiate. Adjust according to response.
	IV infusion	then 500 nanogram - 3.3 microgram/kg/minute			continuous	
Induction of anaesthesia	Slow IV bolus	–	>7 years 150 microgram/kg	200–300 microgram/kg	single dose	In adults the dose should be titrated against individual response. Young fit unpremedicated patients may require at least 300 microgram/kg. Those premedicated with an opiate usually only require a dose of 200 microgram/kg.
Status epilepticus	IV bolus	← 150-200 micrograms/kg →			single dose	Initial bolus. Follow with infusion as below.
	IV infusion	1 microgram/kg/minute increasing by 1 microgram/kg/minute every 15 minutes until the seizure stops Maximum of 5 microgram/kg/minute			continuous	Start with the initial bolus above before commencing the infusion. Not yet an established drug in this area. Most experience in PICUs.
	Buccal/intranasal	DOSE BY WEIGHT <6 months 300 microgram/kg	1-4 years 5mg 5-9 years 7.5mg	10mg	single dose single dose	Buccal administration is the preferred route over intranasal administration.
		DOSE BY AGE ≥6 months 2.5mg	>10 years 10mg		single dose	
Intractable seizures in palliative care	IV infusion/SC infusion	← 5mg/24 hours →			continuous	<u>Initial dose</u> can be titrated up to 40mg/24 hours.
Anxiety in palliative care	IV infusion/SC infusion	← 2.5mg/24 hours →			continuous	

Dose adjustment in renal and liver disease: dose should be reduced in severe renal impairment and liver failure.

ADMINISTRATION
Buccal/intranasal/oral: syrup (buccal liquid) may be given intranasally. Injection can be given bucally, intranasally or orally. Nasal route of administration is unpleasant, but has a rapid onset of action (5–15 minutes). Bitter taste when injection given orally may be disguised by administration in e.g. apple or blackcurrant juice, or chocolate sauce.
IV/IM: injection may be diluted in NaCl 0.9% or glucose 5%.
Rectal: injection can be given rectally.

Patient should be supine and remain so throughout any procedures. It is recommended that patients should remain under medical supervision for at least an hour after receiving midazolam.

CONTRA-INDICATIONS & WARNINGS

Caution: following IV bolus, profound hypotension and apnoea have been seen in neonates and children already receiving opiates. Paediatric patients with chronic respiratory insufficiency, hepatic or renal dysfunction, severe fluid/electrolyte imbalance, congestive heart failure or cardiovascular instability require special caution when receiving parenteral midazolam – lower doses and continuous monitoring are recommended. *Warnings:* Administration by IV bolus is not recommended in neonates. Avoid intra-arterial injection and extravasation. Loss of efficacy has been reported in some patients receiving long-term sedation in ICU, physical dependence may develop resulting in withdrawal symptoms if treatment is abruptly terminated. Safety after 14 days of use is not established.

INTERACTIONS

Erythromycin and other *macrolide antibiotics, quinupristin/dalfopristin* and *cimetidine* inhibit the metabolism of midazolam resulting in reduced clearance, prolonged half-life, and increased volume of distribution producing raised and prolonged plasma midazolam concentrations resulting in profound sedation. *Itraconazole, ketoconazole* and possibly *fluconazole* markedly raise the plasma concentration of midazolam thereby increasing the sedative and amnesic effects, as do antivirals including *efavirenz, nelfinavir, saquinavir, indinavir,* and *ritonavir.*
Diltiazem and *verapamil* markedly increase the plasma levels and the effects of midazolam. *Grapefruit juice* can increase the bioavailability of oral midazolam by as much as 50%. *Theophylline, carbamazepine* and *phenytoin* may antagonise the sedative effects of benzodiazepines. Larger doses of midazolam are likely to be needed to produce sedation in *theophylline* treated patients. Respiratory depression may occur if *theophylline* is discontinued without reducing the midazolam dose. Enhancement of central depressive effect may occur when midazolam is used concomitantly with *opiates, anticonvulsants, sedative antihistamines, antipsychotics, antidepressants* and other *anxiolytic/sedative agents.*

PREGNANCY

Midazolam crosses the placenta. Small risk cannot be excluded but there is no indication that the risk of congenital anomalies in the children of women treated with midazolam during pregnancy is likely to be great. Use during labour has been reported to cause irregularities in fetal heart rate, hypotonia, hypothermia, poor sucking and respiratory depression and use immediately prior to caesarian section has caused severe respiratory depression in the neonate requiring active resuscitation. Not recommended by manufacturer unless considered essential and not recommended at all in the last trimester.

BREAST-FEEDING

Midazolam should be used with caution in lactating mothers, as the drug is known to be excreted in breast milk. A WHO working group on Drugs and Human Lactation concluded that the use of this drug for a short period while breast-feeding is probably safe. It does seem to be controversial, however, the American Academy of Pediatrics state that the effects of midazolam on the nursing infant are unknown but may be of concern. The manufacturers do not recommend the use of midazolam in breast-feeding mothers.

SIDE-EFFECTS

CNS: drowsiness, prolonged sedation and ataxia are the most frequent adverse effects. Paradoxical reactions such as agitation, involuntary movements, hyperactivity, hostility, aggressiveness and excitement have been seen in children. Convulsions or abnormal movements have been seen in neonates and encephalopathic withdrawal symptoms have been encountered after 1-2 days use in neonates. There have been reports of life-threatening and fatal adverse respiratory and cardiovascular events occurring after IV administration. Facilities for resuscitation should always be available and respiratory and cardiac function continuously monitored. Treatment beyond 1-2 weeks, especially at large doses has been associated with an acute benzodiazepine withdrawal syndrome. Infusions should be gradually reduced over several days. When treatment has been given for several days and gradually withdrawn, patients may be awake but sedated for a further 12-24 hours reducing their ability to cough and expectorate. Diazepam is the treatment of choice for withdrawal symptoms. Dependence may develop after regular use even in therapeutic doses for short periods.
GI: nausea, vomiting, constipation, dry mouth and hiccup.
Local: intranasal use can cause irritation of the mucous membranes, which may be severe in some patients. Pain, tenderness and thrombophlebitis have occurred following IV administration.

POISONING/TOXICITY

Symptoms: overdosage can cause CNS depression and coma or paradoxical excitation. Long-term use such as in the intensive care situation has been suggested to be associated with drug accumulation and development of a severe encephalopathic illness in infants, with drowsiness, dystonic posturing, and choreoathetosis developing 1-2 days after treatment is stopped and persisting for a week or more.
Treatment: the effects of midazolam can be reversed by flumazenil. This may precipitate convulsions in patients with epilepsy.

PHARMACOKINETIC PROPERTIES

Absorption of midazolam from oral, buccal, intranasal and IM sites is rapid.

Approximate time to onset of effect:

	Time to onset	Duration of effect
Buccal	5 minutes	
IM	5-15 minutes	1-6 hours
Intranasally	5-10 minutes	45-60 minutes
Oral/rectal	10-30 minutes	20-90 minutes
IV	2-3 minutes	30-60 minutes

Extensive first pass metabolism results in a low systemic bioavailability (<50%) after oral administration. Midazolam is extensively bound to plasma proteins, about 96%. Bioavailability is higher but variable after IM injection. Although supplied as the water-soluble acid salt, at physiological pH midazolam becomes highly lipophilic and rapidly crosses the blood brain barrier. It has a large volume of distribution and an elimination half-life of 2-5 hours. Elimination is prolonged in neonates (3-12 hours - mean 6 hours) and in patients with liver disorders. Elimination half-life is shorter in children 3-10 years of age (1-1.5 hours). Metabolism is in the liver, the major metabolite being less active than midazolam with a half-life of approximately 1 hour. Metabolites are excreted in the urine mainly as glucuronide conjugates. Metabolism also occurs in the intestinal mucosa to a significant extent following oral administration.

EXCIPIENTS

Contact manufacturers for further details.

LICENSED STATUS

Hypnovel® 10mg/2mL is licensed in children for sedation in intensive care units, for premedication before induction of anaesthesia in children and conscious sedation before and during diagnostic or therapeutic procedures with or without local anaesthesia. Amsed and Epistat are 'specials' and as such are unlicensed. Other routes and indications are not licensed.

FURTHER INFORMATION

Oral midazolam has been prepared by mixing injectable midazolam in apple juice, raspberry and cherry syrups and carbonated cola beverages though little stability data is available for these formulations. Amsed and Epistat syrups are available from Special Products Limited.

Milrinone lactate

A phosphodiesterase III inhibitor with positive inotropic and vasodilator properties. Administration of milrinone results in an increase in cardiac output, stroke volume, decreased intra-cardiac filling pressure, and decreased systemic resistance with no significant change in heart rate or myocardial oxygen consumption.

USES

Treatment of congestive heart failure. Treatment of low cardiac output states following cardiac surgery. Treatment of patients refractory to escalating doses of catecholamines. Prophylaxis in patients at high risk of developing low cardiac output syndrome following cardiac surgery.

PRESENTATION

Injection: 1mg in 1mL, 10mL ampoule – Primacor®.

DOSAGE

Route	Age				Frequency (times daily)	Notes
	birth–1 month	1 month–2 years	2–12 years	12–18 years		
IV injection	← 50-75 microgram/kg →			50 microgram/kg	1	Loading dose. Given over 60 minutes.
IV infusion	← 250-750 nanogram/kg/minute →				continuous	Maintenance infusion. Dose titrated according to haemodynamic and clinical response. Maximum dose 1 microgram/kg/minute.

Renal impairment
Data obtained from patients with severe renal impairment but without heart failure have demonstrated that the presence of renal impairment significantly increases the terminal half-life of milrinone. Doses should be reduced by 25-50%. The infusion should be adjusted to haemodynamic and clinical response.

ADMINISTRATION
IV: IV administration only. Due to long half-life, a loading dose administered over 10 minutes is usually followed by a continuous infusion. Dilute to a concentration of 200 micrograms in 1mL (though concentrations of 400 micrograms in 1mL have been used) and give as a continuous infusion using a syringe pump or other apparatus to control flow rate. NaCl 0.45%, NaCl 0.9% or glucose 5% may be used as diluents.
In congestive cardiac failure, patients have been maintained on infusion for up to 5 days, although usual period is 48-72 hours.
Furosemide (frusemide) or bumetanide should not be administered in IV lines containing milrinone injection since precipitation occurs on admixture. Sodium bicarbonate IV infusion should not be used for dilution.

CONTRA-INDICATIONS & WARNINGS
Hypersensitivity to milrinone or other ingredients of the preparation. Not recommended for use immediately following acute myocardial infarction. Careful monitoring should be maintained during milrinone injection therapy, including blood pressure, heart rate, clinical state, electrocardiogram, fluid balance, electrolytes, and renal function. In patients with severe obstructive aortic or pulmonary valvular disease or hypertrophic subaortic stenosis, milrinone should not be used in place of surgical relief of the obstruction. In these conditions it is possible that a drug with inotropic/vasodilator properties might aggravate outflow obstruction.
Supraventricular and ventricular arrhythmias have been observed in the high-risk population. In some patients an increase in ventricular ectopy including non-sustained ventricular tachycardia has been observed which did not affect patient safety or outcome.
There is a possibility of an increased ventricular response rate in patients with uncontrolled atrial flutter/fibrillation, since milrinone produces a slight enhancement in AV node conduction. Patients should be closely monitored for arrhythmias during infusion and the infusion stopped if arrhythmias develop.
Use with caution in patients who are hypotensive prior to treatment. If prior vigorous diuretic therapy is suspected of having caused significant decreases in cardiac filling pressure, milrinone should be cautiously administered while monitoring blood pressure, heart rate and clinical symptomatology.

PREGNANCY
Although animal studies have not revealed evidence of drug induced fetal damage or other deleterious effects on reproductive function, the safety of milrinone in human pregnancy has not been established. Contact local Medicines Information Centre for advice.

BREAST-FEEDING
Not known whether milrinone is excreted in human milk. Contact local Medicines Information Centre for advice.

SIDE-EFFECTS
Ventricular ectopic activity, supraventricular and ventricular arrhythmias have been reported. An increase in ventricular response rate in patients with atrial fibrillation may occur. The incidence of arrhythmias has not been related to dose or plasma levels of milrinone. These arrhythmias are rarely life threatening. If present, they are often associated with underlying factors such as pre-existing arrhythmias, metabolic abnormalities (e.g. hypokalaemia), abnormal digoxin levels and catheter insertion. Very rarely cases of torsades de pointes have been reported. Other reported side-effects include hypotension, angina/chest pain, headaches, hypokalaemia, tremor, bronchospasm and anaphylactic shock.
Thrombocytopenia has been reported and is more common at higher doses. Skin reactions such as rash, and abnormality in liver function tests have been observed.

POISONING/TOXICITY
Overdose may produce hypotension and cardiac arrhythmia. If this occurs, administration should be reduced or temporarily discontinued until the patient's condition stabilises. No specific antidote is known, but general measures for circulatory support should be taken.

INTERACTIONS
Beta-blockers: combination with *beta-blockers* may potentiate hypotension or cardiac arrhythmias.
Calcium-channels antagonists: theoretically, *calcium antagonists* could impair the response to milrinone, but a clinically important interaction has not been established. Increased inotropic activity with *other inotropes* and increased vasodilatory effects with *other vasodilators*.

PHARMACOKINETIC PROPERTIES
Pharmacokinetic studies have suggested that steady state plasma concentrations of milrinone are lower in children than in adults given similar doses, and that milrinone clearance is faster in children.
There is a linear relationship between creatinine and milrinone clearance. The half-life is increased in patients with impaired renal function. In patients with heart failure, clearance is reduced. Milrinone is about 70% protein bound. Elimination occurs mainly via the urine: about 83% of a dose is excreted as unchanged drug.
The plasma half-life of milrinone varies depending on

age, renal function and in congestive heart failure. The half-life reported in healthy adults is 0.83 hours, in adults with congestive heart failure the half-life increases to 1.5-2.6 hours. In adults with renal impairment, half-life increases to 3.24 hours. The median half-life reported in children with septic shock is 1.5 hours.

EXCIPIENTS
See manufacturers SPC for further details.

LICENSED STATUS
Not licensed for use in children.

Minocycline

A tetracycline antibiotic.

USES
Treatment of acne.

PRESENTATION
Capsule: 50mg and 100mg – non-proprietary.
Capsule (modified release): 100mg – Minocin MR®.
Tablet: 50mg and 100mg – non-proprietary.

DOSAGE

Route	Age	Frequency	Notes
	12–18 years	(times daily)	
Oral	50mg	2	Minimum 6 week course.
Oral modified release preparation	100mg	1	

Dosage in renal impairment
May be used at normal dosage in mild to moderate renal impairment. In severe renal insufficiency reduce dose and monitor renal function.

CONTRA-INDICATIONS & WARNINGS
Contra-indicated in children <12 years. Avoid in complete renal failure. Use with caution in patients with hepatic dysfunction.

INTERACTIONS
With *oral contraceptives* possibility of contraceptive failure. Do not use with *penicillins*. Reduced doses of concomitant *anticoagulants* may be necessary. Absorption impaired by *antacids, iron, calcium, magnesium, aluminium* and *zinc salts.*

PREGNANCY
Contra-indicated due to effect on tooth development.

BREAST-FEEDING
Contra-indicated.

SIDE-EFFECTS
Gastrointestinal: nausea, vomiting, diarrhoea.
Skin: severe exfoliative rashes; photosensitivity – hyperpigmentation. Hypersensitivity reactions including urticaria, anaphylaxis, SLE.
Blood: haemolytic anaemia, thrombocytopenia, neutropenia and eosinophilia.
CNS: dizziness and vertigo.

POISONING/TOXICITY
Overdosage: no specific antidote; treatment is symptomatic and supportive.

EXCIPIENTS
Contact manufacturer for further details.

LICENSED STATUS
Not licensed for use in children <12 years of age.

FURTHER INFORMATION
Warn patients about dizziness – avoid driving or cycling if affected.

Vasodilator.

USES
Severe hypertension, in addition to a diuretic and a beta-blocker.

PRESENTATION
Suspension: may be extemporaneously prepared.
Tablet: 2.5mg, 5mg and 10mg – Loniten®.

DOSAGE

Route	Age			Frequency	Notes
	1 month–2 years	2–12 years	12–18 years	(times daily)	
Oral	← 200 microgram/kg →		5mg	1 (but see notes)	Initial dose. Incremental increases every 3 days of 100–200 microgram/kg/day in those <12 years to a maximum of 1mg/kg/day and >12 years incremental increases every 3 days of 5–10 mg/day to a maximum of 100mg/day (seldom necessary to exceed 50mg/day). The total daily dose can be given in 2 divided doses.

Renal impairment
Use lower doses and titrate according to response.

CONTRA-INDICATIONS & WARNINGS
Phaeochromocytoma. Use with caution in porphyria.

INTERACTIONS
The effect of minoxidil may be additive to concurrent antihypertensive agents.

PREGNANCY
Safety in human pregnancy is not established, and it should only be used if considered essential. Neonatal hirsutism has been reported. Contact local Medicines Information Centre for advice.

BREAST-FEEDING
Minoxidil is excreted into breast milk, but it is not known to be harmful. The American Society of Pediatrics considers minoxidil to be compatible with breast-feeding.

SIDE-EFFECTS
Sodium and water retention, weight gain, tachycardia, hypertrichosis, rashes. Hypertrichosis generally reversible after 1-3 months of stopping.

POISONING/TOXICITY
Exaggerated hypotension in association with residual sympathetic nervous system blockade (guanethidine–like effects or alpha-adrenergic blockade) can occur. The recommended treatment is IV administration of NaCl 0.9%. Sympathomimetic drugs should be avoided. *Phenylephrine, angiotensin II* and *vasopressin*, which reverse the effect of minoxidil should only be used if inadequate perfusion of a vital organ is evident.

PHARMACOKINETIC PROPERTIES
About 90% of an oral dose is absorbed from the gastrointestinal tract. Maximum hypotensive effect usually occurs after 2-3 hours. Action may persist for up to 75 hours. Plasma half-life is about 4.2 hours.
Minoxidil is not bound to plasma proteins. It is extensively metabolised in the liver primarily via glucuronidation and is excreted in the urine mainly in the form of metabolites.

EXCIPIENTS
See manufacturers SPC for further details.

LICENSED STATUS
Licensed for use in children and adults.

Analogue of naturally occurring prostaglandin E1. It protects the gastroduodenal mucosa by inhibiting basal, stimulated and nocturnal acid secretion, reducing the volume of gastric secretions, the proteolytic activity of the gastric fluid, and increasing bicarbonate and mucus secretion.

USES
Prevention or treatment of non-steroidal anti-inflammatory drug (NSAID) induced gastroduodenal damage e.g. in children with juvenile idiopathic arthritis (JIA). To improve fat absorption in children with cystic fibrosis on pancreatic enzyme therapy.

PRESENTATION
Tablet: 200 microgram (scored) – Cytotec®.

DOSAGE

Indication	Route	Age				Frequency (times daily)	Notes
		birth–1 month	1 month–2 years	2–12 years	12–18 years		
Prophylaxis of NSAID induced gastroduodenal damage	Oral	-	-	-	200 microgram	4	Should be taken at the same time as the NSAID with or after food.
Treatment of NSAID induced gastroduodenal damage	Oral	-	-	5 micro-gram/kg	-	2	With breakfast (or main meals) and at bedtime.
		-	-	-	200 microgram	2-4	
To improve fat absorption in CF patients	Oral	-	-	← 100 microgram →		4	

ADMINISTRATION
Give tablets with meals. manufacturers advise not to crush or dissolve in water. Misoprostol is very unstable in solution. Tablets have been crushed and dissolved in 20mL of sterile water immediately before administration via a nasogastric tube. Rinse the tube with 20mL of sterile water.

CONTRA-INDICATIONS & WARNINGS
Known allergy to prostaglandins. Do not give to patients who are pregnant or who may become pregnant because it can cause uterine contractions. Use with caution in cardiovascular disease.
No dosage adjustment is needed in liver or renal impairment.

INTERACTIONS
Increased risk of CNS toxicity with *phenylbutazone*.

PREGNANCY
Do not use in pregnancy or in women planning a pregnancy. Misoprostol increases uterine tone and contraction during pregnancy.

BREAST-FEEDING
It is not known if the active metabolite of misoprostol is excreted in breast milk. Manufacturers advise not to use during breast-feeding.

SIDE-EFFECTS
Diarrhoea, occasionally severe and prolonged, which may necessitate withdrawal of the drug. It is less likely if the dose is restricted to 200 micrograms, is taken with food and concurrent use of *antacids* containing magnesium is avoided.
Abdominal pain with or without dyspepsia and diarrhoea. Dyspepsia, flatulence, nausea and vomiting. Increased uterine contractility and abnormal vaginal bleeding, includes menorrhagia and intermenstrual bleeding. Skin rashes, headache and dizziness. Hypotension rare at recommended doses.

POISONING
Intensification of the pharmacological effects may occur. Symptomatic and supportive therapy should be given.

PHARMACOKINETICS
Rapidly absorbed and metabolised to its active form, misoprostol acid. Administration with food reduces the rate but not the extent of absorption. Metabolised by oxidation in a number of body organs and excreted mainly in the urine. Plasma elimination half-life 20-40 minutes.

EXCIPIENTS
See manufacturers SPC for further details.

LICENSED STATUS
Not licensed for use in children.

Mitoxantrone (mitozantrone) hydrochloride

Antineoplastic – an intercalating agent and inhibitor of DNA topoisomerase II.

USES
A variety of solid tumours, non-Hodgkin lymphoma and adult acute non-lymphocytic leukaemia. Has been used in acute myeloid leukaemia in paediatrics.

PRESENTATION
Injection: 2mg in 1mL; 10mL, 12.5mL and 15mL vials — Novantrone®, Onkotrone®.

DOSAGE
** Always consult the current treatment protocol for details of dosage and scheduling. **
Careful supervision is recommended when treating patients with severe hepatic insufficiency.

ADMINISTRATION
IV: dilute the required volume of mitoxantrone injection to at least 50mL in any of the following IV infusions – NaCl 0.9%, glucose 5%, or NaCl 0.18% and glucose 4%. Administer the resulting solution over not less than 3 minutes via the tubing of a freely running IV infusion of the above fluids. In paediatrics usually given over 6 hours, via a central line.
Dilutions for infusion should be used or discarded within 24 hours. Mitoxantrone dilutions will maintain potency for 24 hours at room temperature in PVC or glass containers.

CONTRA-INDICATIONS & WARNINGS
Contra-indications: NOT for intrathecal use. Mitoxantrone should not be given to anyone with known hypersensitivity to the drug.
Warnings: mitoxantrone should be used with caution in patients with myelosuppression or poor general condition. Cases of functional cardiac changes, including congestive heart failure and decreases in left ventricular ejection fraction have been reported. The majority of these cardiac events have occurred in patients who have had prior treatment with *anthracyclines*, prior mediastinal/thoracic radiotherapy, or with pre-existing heart disease. It is recommended that patients in these categories are treated with mitoxantrone at full cytotoxic dosage and schedule. However, added caution is required in these patients and careful regular cardiac examinations are recommended from the initiation of treatment. As experience of prolonged treatment with mitoxantrone is presently limited, it is suggested that cardiac examinations also be performed in patients without identifiable risk factors during therapy exceeding a cumulative dose of 160mg/m^2.

INTERACTIONS
Nil of note.

PREGNANCY
As with other antineoplastic agents, patients and their partners should be advised to avoid conception for at least 6 months after cessation of therapy. Mitoxantrone should not normally be administered to patients who are pregnant.

BREAST-FEEDING
Novantrone® is excreted in human milk and significant concentrations have been reported for 28 days after the last administration. Because of the potential for serious adverse reactions in infants, breast-feeding should be discontinued before starting treatment.

SIDE-EFFECTS
Haematopoietic: myelosuppression.
Gastrointestinal: stomatitis, nausea and vomiting, diarrhoea or constipation.
Renal: raised creatinine and urea.
Hepatic: raised liver enzyme levels.
Cardiovascular: evidence of cardiotoxicity includes decreased left ventricular ejection fraction, ECG changes and acute arrhythmia. Congestive heart failure has been reported and has generally responded well to treatment with digitalis and/or diuretics.
Genitourinary: blue/green colouration of urine.
Skin and appendages: blue/green colouration of skin

and nails. Alopecia may occur, but is most frequently of minimal severity and reversible on cessation of therapy. Tissue necrosis following extravasation has been reported rarely.

Other side-effects: occasionally reported allergic reactions, amenorrhoea, anorexia, dyspnoea, fatigue and weakness, fever, gastrointestinal bleeding, mucositis/conjunctivitis and non-specific neurological side-effects such as somnolence, confusion, anxiety and mild paraesthesia.

Topoisomerase II inhibitors, including mitoxantrone, in combination with other antineoplastic agents, have been associated with the development of acute leukaemia.

POISONING/TOXICITY
Symptoms: haemopoietic, gastrointestinal, hepatic or renal toxicity may be seen depending on dosage given.
Treatment: there is no known antidote and treatment consists of symptomatic and supportive therapy.

PHARMACOKINETIC PROPERTIES
Following administration, mitoxantrone rapidly distributes to most tissues, but does not cross the blood-brain barrier to any appreciable extent. Distribution into testes is also relatively low. Elimination of the drug is slow with a mean half-life of 12 days. Mitoxantrone is excreted via the renal and hepatobiliary systems. Metabolites are inactive.

EXCIPIENTS
See manufacturers SPC for further details.

LICENSED STATUS
Licensed for adults only for treatment of advanced breast cancer, non-Hodgkin lymphoma and adult acute non-lymphocytic leukaemia. It has also been used in the palliation of non-resectable primary hepatocellular carcinoma.

FURTHER INFORMATION
Store at controlled room temperature (15°-25°C). Do not freeze.
Mitoxantrone is non-vesicant.
Dexrazoxane may be given with mitoxantrone to potentially reduce cardiotoxicity.

MMR (measles, mumps and rubella) vaccine

USES
To provide active protection against measles, mumps and rubella infections. It is given as part of the routine childhood immunisation programme at 12–15 months. A second dose should be given after at least 3 months have elapsed, usually at the same time as the preschool booster of DTaP and OPV, at between 3-5 years old. This second dose of MMR is not a 'booster', but is intended to provide immunity to those not protected after the first dose. If given within 72 hours of exposure to a case of measles, it may prevent infection in a susceptible contact.

PRESENTATION
Injection: (single dose freeze dried pellet for reconstitution to 0.5mL).
The measles and mumps viruses are grown in chick embryo tissue. The rubella virus is grown on a human diploid cell line, MRC5, which originates from cells taken from a fetus aborted for medical reasons in 1966. The rubella virus itself originates from a different fetus aborted because the mother was infected with rubella during pregnancy.
Two vaccines are currently available:
MMR 11® (Pasteur Mérieux MSD) which contains measles virus (Enders' attenuated Edmonston strain) at least 1000 $TCID_{50}$, mumps virus (Jeryl Lynn strain) at least 20,000 $TCID_{50}$, rubella virus (Wistar RA27/3 strain) at least 1000 $TCID_{50}$.
Priorix® (SmithKline Beecham) which contains measles virus (attenuated Schwarz strain) at least 1000 $CCID_{50}$, mumps virus (RIT 4385 derived from the Jeryl Lynn strain) at least 5000 $CCID_{50}$, rubella virus (Wistar RA27/3 strain) at least 1000 $CCID_{50}$.

DOSAGE/ADMINISTRATION
IM or deep SC: 0.5mL of reconstituted vaccine.

CONTRA-INDICATIONS & WARNINGS

As for vaccines generally. Also MMR should not be given to anyone who is severely immunosuppressed. It should be given to HIV positive children. Children who have had an anaphylactic reaction to egg can be safely immunised. However, if a parent is concerned about this, it could be administered under medical supervision. Other lesser reactions to egg are not important. Individuals who develop ideopathic thrombocytopenic purpura (ITP) within 6 weeks of receiving a first dose of MMR, should have serology against measles, mumps and rubella checked by PHLS prior to when the second dose is due. If they are not immune to all three viruses, they should be given a second dose of MMR.

INTERACTIONS

As it is a live vaccine it may be given at the same time as other *live vaccines* or after a minimum interval of 3 weeks. It should not be given within a period of 3 weeks before and 3 months after human immunoglobulin and blood or plasma transfusions. The vaccine should not be given to children <1 year old, as maternal antibodies may interfere with the response. The vaccine may temporarily convert someone who would have had a positive response to a tuberculin test to a non-responder. A tuberculin test should ideally be postponed until 4 weeks have elapsed since immunisation. If this would significantly hamper the management of a patient, the test can be done, but a negative result should be interpreted with caution.

PREGNANCY

While there is evidence of fetuses becoming infected with rubella virus after inadvertent rubella vaccination during pregnancy, no cases of congenital rubella syndrome have been reported. As immunisation is likely to be an elective procedure, immunisation with a rubella containing vaccine should not be carried out during pregnancy and pregnancy should be avoided for a month after the vaccine has been administered.

BREAST-FEEDING

No information is available, but there are no grounds to believe it would be harmful and rubella vaccine has been used extensively in breast-feeding women.

SIDE-EFFECTS

Local reactions, such as tenderness and redness may occur. About 5–10 days after immunisation, the recipient may experience a mild attack of measles with rash, fever, malaise, cough, coryza and headaches. Febrile convulsions due to the vaccine occur at a rate of 1 per 3000 doses and it is said that the rate of encephalitis due to the vaccine is 1 per million doses. This may be no higher than the background rate.

Research suggesting a causal link between measles vaccine and Crohn's disease has not been replicated and there are no scientific data to connect the vaccine with autism. A paper in *the Lancet* in early 1998 described a series of children with bowel and behavioural symptoms. In two thirds of cases the parents or child's physician associated the onset of symptoms with the child being given MMR. The flaws in this paper have been pointed out and all the evidence available suggests there is no link between MMR, inflammatory bowel disease and autism. A meeting of relevant experts on 23rd March 1998 confirmed the government's recommendation that the combined vaccine should continue to be given. Research conducted since 1998 to look for an association between autism and/or bowel disease and MMR vaccine has found no link.

Occasionally a mild form of mumps may develop about 3 weeks after immunisation. Meningoencephalitis has not been shown to follow the Jeryl Lynn strain. Mild transient symptoms of rubella may occur 1-3 weeks after immunisation. These include fever, sore throat, lymphadenopathy, arthralgia and arthritis. Joint symptoms are much less common in children than adults. Thrombocytopenic purpura, usually self-limiting, has been shown to be caused by MMR at a frequency of approximately 1 in every 32,000 doses. Individuals who develop ITP within 6 weeks of receiving a first dose of MMR, should have serology against measles, mumps and rubella checked by PHLS prior to when the second dose is due. If they are not immune to all three viruses, they should be given a second dose of MMR.

POISONING/TOXICITY

No data available.

EXCIPIENTS

MMR 11®: neomycin sulphate, sorbitol, sodium phosphate (monobasic and dibasic), sodium carbonate, Medium 199 (a mixture of amino acids, mineral salts, vitamins and other components, including glucose), Minimum Essential Medium – Eagle (a mixture of amino acids, mineral salts, vitamins and other components), phenol red, photasium phosphate (monobasic and dibasic), monosodium l-glutamate, human albumin and porcine gelatin.
Priorix®: neomycin, sorbitol, human albumin, lactose, mannitol and various amino acids.
In both cases the human albumin is derived from donors in countries free of BSE.

LICENSED STATUS
Licensed for use as described above.

FURTHER INFORMATION
An MMR vaccine (Triviraten Berna®) free of chicken-related antigens is available from Switzerland. This vaccine is not licensed for use in the UK. As the strain of mumps virus in this vaccine ('Rubini') has been shown to be very poorly protective and there is no indication for its use, this vaccine cannot be recommended.

Materials of bovine and sheep origin are used in the manufacturing process. Trace amounts of the original material may be present in the final product, however, all such material is obtained from sources known to be free of BSE.

If given within 3 days of exposure to measles it may prevent the disease developing as the induced antibody appears more quickly than the infection.

Protect from light and store at 2–8°C, do not freeze. Should be used within 1 hour of reconstitution.

Montelukast

Leukotriene receptor antagonist.

USES
Add-on therapy in patients with mild to moderate persistent asthma, inadequately controlled on inhaled corticosteroids and in whom 'when required' short-acting beta-agonists do not control asthma adequately.

Prophylaxis of asthma in which the predominant component is exercise-induced bronchoconstriction.

PRESENTATION
Tablet: 4mg and 5mg (both chewable) – Singulair Paediatric®.
Tablet: 10mg – Singulair®.

DOSAGE

Route	Age		Frequency (times daily)	Notes
	2–12 years	12–18 years		
Oral	2–5 years	12–14 years		Taken at bedtime.
	4mg	5mg	1	
	6–12 years	>14 years		
	5mg	10mg	1	

ADMINISTRATION
Oral: the 4mg or 5mg chewable tablet should be taken 1 hour before or 2 hours after food. The 10mg tablet can be taken with or without food.

CONTRA-INDICATIONS & WARNINGS
Avoid administration if there has been any previous sensitivity to montelukast. Do not use to treat acute asthma attacks. Do not substitute for inhaled or oral corticosteroids. Possible (although not established) link to Churg-Strauss syndrome. Monitor for eosinophilia, vasculitic rash, worsening of pulmonary symptoms, cardiac complications and neuropathy.

INTERACTIONS
Montelukast is metabolised by CYP 3A4 and if it is co-administered with CYP 3A4 inducers such as *phenytoin, phenobarbital (phenobarbitone)* and *rifampicin*, plasma levels of montelukast may be decreased.

PREGNANCY/BREAST-FEEDING
There have not been any controlled studies using montelukast in pregnant or nursing women. It should not be used in such patients unless considered clearly essential. Montelukast has been shown to cross the placental barrier and is excreted in breast milk of animals.

SIDE-EFFECTS
These appear to be mild but may include abdominal pain, headache, skin rashes, fever and gastrointestinal disturbance.

POISONING/TOXICITY
There is no information regarding the treatment of overdosage.

PHARMACOKINETIC PROPERTIES
Rapidly absorbed orally, with peak plasma levels occurring approximately 3 hours after administration. It is 99% protein bound and is extensively metabolised in the liver. Montelukast and its metabolites are mainly excreted via the bile. No dosage adjustment is necessary in patients with renal impairment.

EXCIPIENTS
Chewable tablets contain aspartame. See manufacturers SPC for further details.

LICENSED STATUS
Licensed for use in patients aged ≥2 years.

Morphine sulphate (controlled drug)

Opioid analgesic with agonist activity mainly at μ-opioid receptors.

USES
Relief of acute/post-operative pain, peri-operative pain and sedation and analgesia in intensive care, relief of severe pain in chronic pain, palliative care: relief of dyspnoea.

PRESENTATION
Injection: 10mg in 1mL, 15mg in 1mL, 20mg in 1mL and 30mg in 1mL; 1mL and 2mL ampoules – non-proprietary. 10mg in 1mL, 1mL prefilled syringe – non-proprietary. 1mg in 1mL, 50mL vial and 2mg in 1mL, 50mL vial – non-proprietary. Other strengths of injection, including preservative-free, are available as manufactured 'specials'.
Oral solution: 10mg in 5mL – Oramorph® and Sevredol®.
Concentrated oral solution: 100mg in 5mL – Oramorph® and Sevredol®.
Suppository: 5mg – manufactured 'special'; 10mg, 15mg, 20mg and 30mg – non-proprietary.
Suspension (modified release): 20mg, 30mg, 60mg, 100mg and 200mg per sachet – MST Continus®.
Tablet: 10mg, 20mg and 50mg – Sevredol®.
Tablet/capsule (modified release): 5mg, 10mg, 15mg, 20mg, 30mg, 50mg, 60mg, 90mg, 100mg, 120mg, 150mg and 200mg – Morcap® SR, MST Continus®, MXL® and Zomorph®.

DOSAGE
Newborn infant (birth to 1 month)

Route	Age	Frequency	Notes
	birth–1 month	(times daily)	
Slow IV bolus	40–100 microgram/kg	6 hourly	Give over at least 5-10 minutes.
IV infusion (preterm)	25–50 microgram/kg	single dose	Loading dose.
	then		
	5 microgram/kg/hour	continuous	
IV infusion (term)	50–100microgram/kg	single dose	Loading dose.
	then		
	10–20 microgram/kg/hour	continuous	Doses up to a maximum of 40 microgram/kg/hour have been used.

Note: Newborn infants show an increased susceptibility to respiratory depression and therefore appropriate monitoring should be undertaken. Respiratory support should be available for non-ventilated patients.

Child

Prophylactic laxatives should always be prescribed when commencing major opioids.

Premedication and analgesia for acute/post-operative pain

Route	Age			Frequency (times daily)	Notes
	1 month–2 years	2–12 years	12–18 years		
IM/SC injection	100–200 microgram/kg	200 microgram/kg	5–20mg	≤6 months up to 4 times in 24 hours	Respiratory monitoring is mandatory. Give IV over at least 5–10 minutes. <1 year use the lower stated dose and consider oxygen saturation monitoring.
IV bolus	◄— 100–200 microgram/kg —►		2.5–10mg	>6 months up to 6 times in 24 hours	
IV infusion	◄— 10–30 microgram/kg/hour —► ≤6 months initial rate is 10 microgram/kg/hour >6 months initial rate is 20 microgram/kg/hour			continuous	Use IV bolus as loading dose first.
SC infusion	1–3 months 10 microgram/kg/hour >3 months 20 microgram/kg/hour	◄— 20 microgram/kg/hour —►		continuous	Use 24 gauge cannula over deltoid or abdominal wall. Change rate and change sites every 48–72 hours.

Note: For patient controlled analgesia follow local hospital protocols.

Analgesia and sedation in ventilated and other ITU patients

Use IV bolus and infusion doses as shown in the table above as loading and maintenance doses.

Dose adjustment in renal impairment

In renal failure use 75% of dose if creatinine clearance is 10-50mL/minute/1.73m^2 and 50% if it is <10mL/minute/1.73m^2.

Chronic pain/palliative care

Route	Age			Frequency (times daily)	Notes
	1 month–2 years	2–12 years	12–18 years		
Oral or rectal	<1 year 80 microgram/kg >1 year 200–400 microgram/kg	200–500 microgram/kg	10–15mg	up to 6 times in 24 hours	Starting doses which should be reviewed regularly and adjusted according to the patient's response (see note following table). Doses for relief of dyspnoea in palliative care approximately 50% of those used for analgesia.
SC/IM	150–200 microgram/kg	200 microgram/kg	5–20 mg	up to 6 times in 24 hours	Use with caution if poor peripheral perfusion. Avoid IM injections if possible. Use SC/IM cannula placed under GA or topical LA.

Increase dose in increments of 50% initially until optimum dosages are achieved. Transfer to modified release preparation can then be made. Dose of modified release morphine equals total 24 hour requirement divided by two and given 12 hourly or total requirement given once daily depending on product selected. One sixth of daily requirement can be prescribed as oral liquid or non-modified release preparation for control of breakthrough pain. Diamorphine is preferred parenterally because of its higher solubility.

10mg oral morphine salts approximately equivalent to 3mg diamorphine hydrochloride (IM/IV).

ADMINISTRATION

Oral: tablets may be halved. Modified release preparations should not be chewed or crushed.

Injection: stable for at least 24 hours when diluted in glucose 5%, 10% or NaCl 0.9%.

It is recommended that preservative-free morphine injections are used if possible for continuous infusion to decrease the incidence of phlebitis.

CONTRA-INDICATIONS AND WARNINGS

Contra-indications: paralytic ileus, acute respiratory depression and liver failure (may precipitate coma). *Cautions:* raised intracranial pressure or head injury, biliary colic, hypothyroidism or moderate renal impairment (see notes under dosage). There is less information about admixing than for *diamorphine*. The latter is preferred for infusions where multiple medications are to be used.

INTERACTIONS

Enhanced sedative effect with *anxiolytics* and *hypnotics*, antagonism of gastrointestinal effect of *cisapride, metoclopramide* and *domperidone*. Possibly increased plasma levels with *cimetidine*.

PREGNANCY

Use in the third trimester depresses neonatal respiration. Withdrawal effects are seen in neonates of dependant mothers.

BREAST-FEEDING

Therapeutic doses unlikely to affect infant.

SIDE-EFFECTS

Nausea and vomiting, constipation and drowsiness. Larger doses produce respiratory depression and hypotension. Histamine release with IV therapy may provoke hypotension and tachycardia. Neonates and children <1 year show an increased susceptibility to respiratory depression. Pruritis can be managed using topical agents, antihistamines or by changing to an alternative major opioid such as fentanyl.

POISONING/TOXICITY

Signs of morphine toxicity and overdose include pinpoint pupils, respiratory depression and hypotension. Circulatory failure and coma may occur in more severe cases. Assisted ventilation may be required. *Naloxone* may be used to treat morphine overdose. Modified release preparations remaining in the intestine will continue to release morphine for a number of hours.

PHARMACOKINETIC PROPERTIES

Morphine salts are well absorbed from the gastrointestinal tract but undergo extensive first pass metabolism. They are conjugated with glucuronic acid in the liver and gut. Up to 10% of a dose may be excreted through the bile into the faeces; the remainder is excreted in the kidneys. The pharmacokinetics of morphine in children are similar to adults, with an elimination half-life of about 2 hours following IV administration. Neonates exhibit an increased elimination half-life probably because of immature renal function and reduced metabolic capacity. The half-life in the preterm baby is 6-12 hours and very variable but related to gestational age at birth.

EXCIPIENTS

Oramorph® oral solution 10mg in 5mL includes sugar and alcohol. Contact manufacturers for further details.

LICENSED STATUS

The 5mg suppositories are a 'special' and as such are unlicensed. Morcap® and Zomorph® are not licensed for use in children. Sevredol® tablets are licensed in children >3 years of age. Sevredol® and Oramorph® oral morphine solution and MXL® are licensed for >1 year of age. MST Continus® is licensed for children with severe cancer pain.

M   Mouthwash solution – tablets

USES

To make a mouthwash suitable for dental purposes.

PRESENTATION

Tablets: containing antimicrobial, colouring and flavouring agents in a suitable soluble effervescent base – Tellodont®.

DOSAGE

1 tablet dissolved in a tumblerful of warm water.

ADMINISTRATION

Use as required during dental treatment.

EXCIPIENTS
Contact manufacturer for further details.

LICENSED STATUS
Not a licensed drug product.

Multivitamins

USES
Prevention of vitamin deficiency.

PRESENTATION
Capsule/tablet: see table, Multivitamins BPC -non-proprietary.
Oral drops: see table – Abidec®, Dalivit® and Children's Vitamin Drops (Department of Health).
Liquid/tablet: see table – Ketovite®.

DOSAGE
All preparations in this table given by the oral route. In neonates requirements vary depending on the quantity of feed per day and the type of feed. Infants discharged on a nutrient enriched feed e.g. Nutriprem 2 do not require supplements. Contact a dietitian for further advice.

All preparations in this table given by the oral route

Preparation	Age				Frequency (times daily)	Notes
	birth–1 month	1 month–2 years	2–12 years	12–18 years		
Abidec drops	0.3mL	<1year 0.3mL	← 0.6 mL →		1	Supplement for prevention of deficiency states.
0.6 mL contains:		>1 year				
Vitamin A 1333 units		0.6mL			1	
Vitamin D 400 units						
Vitamin C 40mg	0.6mL	0.6mL	–		1	Premature babies. Dependent on
B vitamins						feed - see under dosage above.
Dalivit drops	–	<1 year 0.3mL	← 0.6 mL →		1	Supplement for prevention of deficiency states.
0.6 mL contains:						
Vitamin A 5000 units		>1 year				
Vitamin D 400 units		0.6 mL			1	
Vitamin C 50mg	–	<1year 0.6mL	← 1mL →		1	Cystic fibrosis supplement.
B vitamins		>1 year 1mL			1	
Children's Vitamin drops (DOH)	0.2mL	–	–		1	Deficiency of prematurity in babies <2.5kg. Continue until on full milk feeds at home.
0.2mL contains:						
Vitamin A 1000 units	0.4mL	–	–		1	Bronchopulmonary dysplasia require extra vitamin A.
Vitamin D 400 units						
Vitamin C 30mg						
Multivitamins BPC	–	← 1 capsule or tablet →		2 capsules or tablets	1	Supplement for prevention of deficiency states.
each capsule or						
tablet contains:	–	2 capsules or tablets	2–3 capsules or tablets		1	Cystic fibrosis supplement.
Vitamin A 2500 units						
Vitamin D 300 units						
Vitamin C 15mg						
B vitamins						

Ketovite® preparations given by the oral route.

Preparation	Age			Frequency (times daily)	Notes
	1 month–2 years	2–12 years	12–18 years		
Ketovite liquid *5mL contains:* Vitamin A 2500 units Vitamin D 400 units Choline chloride 150mg Vitamin B$_{12}$ 12.5 microgram	←	5mL liquid	→	1	Tablets and liquid must both be given for complete supplementation.
Ketovite tablets *Each tablet contains:* Thiamine 1mg Riboflavine 1mg Pyridoxine 330 microgram Vitamin C 16.6mg Vitamin E 5mg Nicotinamide 3.3mg Calcium pantothenate 1.16mg Biotin 170 microgram Folic acid 250 microgram Inositol 50mg Acetomenaphthone 500 microgram	←	1 tablet	→	3	

ADMINISTRATION

Oral: Ketovite® tablets may be crushed if necessary. Ketovite® liquid can be mixed with milk, cereal or fruit juice.
Cystic fibrosis patients who are pancreatic insufficient should administer vitamin supplements with food and pancreatic enzymes.

CONTRA-INDICATIONS & WARNINGS
Hypersensitivity.

INTERACTIONS
No interactions known.

PREGNANCY
Large doses of vitamin A during first trimester may be teratogenic.

BREAST-FEEDING
Vitamin D may cause hypercalcaemia in infants.

SIDE-EFFECTS
No side-effects known.

POISONING/TOXICITY
Most vitamins are virtually non-toxic in a single acute overdose. However, ingestion of more than 3.6mg/kg (12,000 international units/kg) vitamin A would be expected to cause symptoms such as vomiting, dizziness, drowsiness, irritability within 8-12 hours of ingestion.

EXCIPIENTS
Abidec® drops include 45mg sucrose in 0.6mL. Dalivit® drops include 120mg sucrose in 0.6mL. Ketovite® liquid includes saccharin; sugar-free. See manufacturers SPC for further details.

LICENSED STATUS
All presentations are licensed but cystic fibrosis doses given here are unlicensed. The area of vitamin supplementation in cystic fibrosis patients is one of active research and current recommendations are under review.

FURTHER INFORMATION
Cystic fibrosis patients should have serum concentrations of vitamin A and D monitored at least annually and supplements adjusted accordingly.

There is no indication for a single antigen mumps vaccine, and there is no available vaccine licensed for use in the UK. The MCA permits the importation of single mumps antigen to complete a course of measles, mumps and rubella vaccination that has already been started with one of the other single vaccines or where there is a medical contra-indication to the combined vaccine. There is no scientific basis to either of these indications. MMR can be used to complete a course when any of the single antigens has been given. There is no contra-indication to the MMR that does not also contra-indicate the single mumps vaccine.

Licensed mumps vaccine is only available in the UK in combination with mumps and rubella vaccines (MMR vaccine).

Mupirocin

Topical antibacterial active against organisms commonly responsible for skin infections.

USES
Cream: secondarily infected traumatic lesions.
Nasal ointment: elimination of nasal carriage of staphylococci, including methicillin-resistant *Staphylococcus aureus* (*MRSA*).
Ointment: bacterial skin infections e.g. impetigo.
Elimination of perineal candida infection.

PRESENTATION
Cream: 2% – Bactroban®.
Nasal ointment: 2% – Bactroban Nasal®.
Ointment: 2% – Bactroban®.

DOSAGE & ADMINISTRATION
Topical: cream – apply to affected area 3 times daily for up to 10 days; nasal ointment – apply to the inner surface of each nostril 2-3 times a day for 5-7 days; ointment – apply to affected area 2-3 times daily for up to 10 days.

CONTRA-INDICATIONS & WARNINGS
Hypersensitivity to mupirocin or constituents. Avoid application to the eyes. Ointment (not nasal ointment) contains polyethylene glycol (PEG) which may be absorbed from open wounds and damaged skin. PEG is excreted renally and caution is needed in moderate or severe renal impairment, in neonates and burns patients. Prolonged use may result in overgrowth of non-susceptible organisms.

PREGNANCY
No teratogenic effects reported. Contact local Medicines Information Centre for advice.

BREAST-FEEDING
Manufacturer recommends breast-feeeding be discontinued during mupirocin therapy. However, it is unlikely that clinically significant concentrations would appear in breast milk following topical application to normal skin. Contact local Medicines Information Centre for advice.

SIDE-EFFECTS
Rarely minor local irritation reactions, hypersensitivity.

POISONING/TOXICITY
Toxicity low; symptomatic treatment.

PHARMACOKINETIC PROPERTIES
Small amounts absorbed topically – rapidly metabolised to monic acid.

EXCIPIENTS
See manufacturers SPC for further details.

LICENSED STATUS
Licensed for use in children and adults.

FURTHER INFORMATION
Bacterial resistance has emerged, particularly during long-term treatment.

Monoclonal antibody.

USES
Acute graft rejection in renal, hepatic and cardiac transplant.

PRESENTATION
Injection: 1mg in 1mL, 5mL ampoule – Orthoclone OKT3®.

DOSAGE

Route	Age			Frequency	Notes
	1 month–2 years	2–12 years	12–18 years	(times daily)	
IV	← 50 micrograms/kg →			stat	First dose
	DOSE BY WEIGHT PER KG ← 100 micrograms/kg →			1	Maintenance dose. Maximum dose of 5mg/day.
	DOSE BY WEIGHT RANGE/AGE ≤30kg / >30kg 2.5mg / 5mg			1	Treat for 4–14 days. Check with local protocol as may use different doses.

Adjust dose to maintain CD3+ count at 25cells/mm^3 or drug serum concentration at >800 nanogram/mL.

Renal impairment
No dose adjustment necessary.

ADMINISTRATION
IV: bolus over less than 1 minute. The injection should be drawn into syringe via a 0.2 micron filter.

CONTRA-INDICATIONS & WARNINGS
Contra-indicated in hypersensitivity to any product of murine origin, uncompensated heart failure, fluid overload and seizures. Resuscitation facilities should be available when giving Muromab-CD3.

SIDE-EFFECTS
Most patients develop an acute clinical syndrome ranging from flu-like symptoms to less frequently life-threatening shock-like reactions. This syndrome usually occurs 30-60 minutes after administration and may persist for several hours. More commonly seen are rigors, fever, nausea/vomiting, muscle aches, abdominal pain and tremor. During the first 3 days of treatment some patients may have a decrease in urine output and a transient decrease in GFR with resulting increase in plasma creatinine. Severe pulmonary oedema has occurred in patients with fluid overload and in those who appeared to be normovolaemic. Less frequently reported side-effects include minor dermatological reactions and a spectrum of often serious cardiorespiratory and neuropsychiatric events. Anaphylaxis and other serious hypersensitivity reactions have been reported.

Muromab is usually added to immunosuppressive regimens thereby augmenting the degree of immunosuppression and altering the spectrum and severity of infectious complications.

PREGNANCY
Use in pregnancy is contra-indicated.

BREAST-FEEDING
There is no information about Muromab-CD3 use in breast-feeding therefore avoid.

EXCIPIENTS
Contact manufacturers (Janseen-Cilag) for further details.

LICENSED STATUS
Not licensed for use in children.

Multivitamins for infusion.

USES
Multivitamin supplement in children receiving PN.

PRESENTATION
Solution: powder for reconstitution – MVI Paediatric.
Each vial contains:

Alpha tocopheryl acetate	7mg
Ascorbic Acid	80mg
Biotin	20 microgram
Cyanocobalamin	1 microgram
Dexpanthenol	5mg
Ergocalciferol	10 microgram
Folic acid	140 microgram
Niacinamide	17mg
Phytomenadione	200 microgram
Pyridoxine	1mg
Retinol	700 microgram
Riboflavin	1.4mg
Thiamine	1.2mg

DOSAGE
The dose in the table below provides daily multivitamin maintenance for children up to 11 years of age.

Dosage when reconstituted with 5mL of the diluent.

Body weight	Volume of MVI daily
<1kg	1.5mL
1–3kg	3.25mL
>3kg	5mL

ADMINISTRATION
IV: dissolve in 5mL Water for Injections, NaCl 0.9% or glucose 5%. Dilute into a PN solution of amino acids, NOT into fat emulsions, to a minimum volume of 5mL in 100mL fluid. Infuse over 2-24 hours and complete the infusion within 24 hours.

CONTRA-INDICATIONS & WARNINGS
Hypersensitivity to any vitamin especially thiamine and vitamin K. Blood samples for megaloblastic anaemia may not show deficiencies of folate and cyanocobalamin while receiving this preparation due to MVI contents. Preparations containing polysorbate 80 have been associated with renal and hepatic toxicity in low birth weight infants.

INTERACTIONS
The folic acid component may be inactivated by *calcium salts*. Physically incompatible in solution with *acetazolamide, chlorothiazide, aminophylline, ampicillin, tetracycline* or other alkaline IV infusions. Drugs affected by folate levels should be monitored e.g. *phenytoin*. Pyridoxine may reduce the effects of *levodopa*. Vitamin K may reduce the effects of *coumarin anticoagulants*.

SIDE-EFFECTS
Isolated reports of rash, erythema pruritus, dizziness, anxiety, headache, diplopia, urticaria, periorbital and digital oedema.

EXCIPIENTS
Contact manufacturer for further details.

LICENSED STATUS
Not licensed for use in the UK.

FURTHER INFORMATION
Available via IDIS World Medicines.

Mycophenolate mofetil is metabolised to mycophenolic acid, a cytotoxic immunosuppressant.

USES
Immunosuppression in cardiac, renal and liver transplant recipients, in conjunction with ciclosporin or tacrolimus and corticosteroids for prophylaxis of acute rejection.

PRESENTATION
Tablet: 500mg – CellCept®.
Capsule: 250mg – CellCept®.
Oral suspension: 1g in 5ml – CellCept®.
Infusion solution: 500mg vial (as hydrochloride) – CellCept®.

DOSAGE

Transplant	Route	Age			Frequency (times daily)	Notes
		1 month–2 years	2–12 years	12–18 years		
Renal	Oral	←	600mg/m²	→	2	The initial dose should be given within 72 hours following transplantation. Maximum total daily dose of 2g.
Liver	Oral	←	10mg/kg increasing to	→	2	
		←	20mg/kg (maximum 1g)	→	2	

ADMINISTRATION
Oral: give before food. Due to teratogenic effects demonstrated in animals it is recommended that the capsule should not be opened or the tablet/capsule crushed. Inhalation or direct contact between the powder contained within the capsule and skin or mucous membranes should be avoided. Contamination should be promptly removed by washing with soap and water. Eyes should be rinsed with plain water.
IV: reconstitute each 500mg vial with 14mL glucose 5% and further dilute the contents of the vial to a concentration of 7.14mg/mL with a compatible infusion solution. Infuse over 2 hours.

CONTRA-INDICATIONS AND WARNINGS
Hypersensitivity to mycophenolate mofetil or any of the excipients. In common with other immunosuppressive treatments, patients treated with mycophenolate are at increased risk of developing lymphomas, and other malignancies, particularly of the skin. Patients should avoid exposure to strong sunlight. Severe neutropenia (<0.5 x 10⁹/L) occurs in approximately 0.5% of adult patients treated with 2g daily. Close monitoring of patients is advised with dose reduction or drug withdrawal as appropriate.
Administer with caution in patients with active gastrointestinal disease. Gastrointestinal haemorrhage is reported in approximately 1.5% of adult patients treated with 2g daily. Gastrointestinal perforation has been reported. Concurrent treatment with *azathioprine* should be avoided due to a lack of study data on the combination.

INTERACTIONS
Food reduces the peak plasma level but does not reduce total absorption. *Colestyramine (cholestyramine)* significantly impairs the absorption of mycophenolate. Absorption is impaired if given at the same time as *antacids* containing *magnesium* or *aluminium hydroxides*. A sufficient interval should be allowed between giving each drug. Concurrent administration with *aciclovir* and *ganciclovir* can result in higher plasma concentrations of all three drugs.

PREGNANCY
Mycophenolate mofetil is teratogenic when administered to pregnant rats and rabbits at dose levels 50% less than anticipated when human patients are treated with 2g daily. There is no current data on effects on the human fetus. Mycophenolate should only be used in pregnancy when the benefits outweigh the risk to the fetus. A negative pregnancy test should be obtained before commencing mycophenolate in women of childbearing age, and patients should be advised to seek medical advice if they become pregnant. Effective contraception is advised for women on treatment and for 6 weeks after discontinuation.

BREAST-FEEDING
Excreted into breast milk in rats. No data in humans. The continuation of mycophenolate therapy in nursing

mothers should only follow an evaluation of the relative risks to mother and baby.

SIDE-EFFECTS
The following adverse effects were seen at a frequency of ≥10% in patients treated in Phase III studies.

Whole body: sepsis (particularly CMV viraemia), infection, fever, chest, back, abdominal and generalised pain, headache, asthenia.

Haematological system: anaemia, hypochromic anaemia, leucopenia, leucocytosis, thrombocytopenia.

Urogenital system: urinary tract infection and other disorders, renal tubular necrosis, haematuria.

Cardiovascular: hypertension.

Metabolic system: hypo- and hyperkalaemia, hyperglycaemia, hypophosphataemia, hyper-cholesterolaemia, peripheral oedema, oedema.

Gastrointestinal system: diarrhoea, nausea, vomiting, constipation, dyspepsia, oral moniliasis.

Respiratory system: pneumonia, infection, dyspnoea, bronchitis, pharyngitis, increased cough.

Skin: Herpes simplex, acne.

Nervous system: dizziness, insomnia, tremor.
The overall adverse effect profile is difficult to establish due to the patient's underlying condition and the multiplicity of concurrent drug therapy.

POISONING/TOXICITY
There is no current data on overdosage. *Colestyramine (cholestyramine)* may be of value in reducing secondary re-absorption. Haemodialysis is unlikely to be of benefit.

PHARMACOKINETIC PROPERTIES
Mycophenolic acid is well absorbed orally with a mean bioavailability of 94%. Approximately 97% bound to plasma albumin. Metabolised principally to the glucuronide, which is not pharmacologically active. Enterohepatic re-circulation is significant and produces a secondary peak in plasma mycophenolic acid levels 6-12 hours after administration. Urinary excretion of active drug is negligible. 87% of the administered dose is excreted in urine as the glucuronide.

EXCIPIENTS
See manufacturers SPC for further details.

LICENSED STATUS
Licensed for ≥2 years of age for renal transplant recipients. Licensed in adults for cardiac and hepatic transplantation.

Nabilone

Synthetic cannaboid with anti-emetic properties.

USES
Control of nausea and vomiting caused by cytotoxic chemotherapy, unresponsive to conventional anti-emetic treatment.

PRESENTATION
Capsules: 250 microgram – manufactured 'special'; 1mg – Cambridge.

DOSAGE

Indication	Route	Age		Frequency	Notes
		2–12 years	12–18 years	(times daily)	
Emetogenic chemotherapy	IV/oral	<u><18kg</u> 500 micrograms	-	2	Start the night before chemotherapy.
		<u>18-36kg</u> 1mg	-	2	Give throughout chemotherapy and for up to 48 hours after the last dose of each cycle.
		<u>>36kg</u> 1mg	-	3	
			1-2mg	2	

ADMINISTRATION
The first dose should be taken the night before initiation of cytotoxic treatment and the second dose 1-3 hours before the first dose of cytotoxic drug.

CONTRA-INDICATIONS & WARNINGS
Not recommended in severe hepatic impairment. Caution in patients with hypertension and heart disease. Patients receiving nabilone should be observed in an in-patient setting. Adverse effects on the mental state can persist for 48-72 hours after stopping.

INTERACTIONS
Administer with caution to patients on other *psychoactive drugs* or *CNS depressants*.

PREGNANCY/BREAST-FEEDING
Laboratory studies have shown no evidence of teratogenicity, but there are no adequate and well-controlled studies of the use of nabilone in pregnant women. The use of nabilone in breast-feeding is not recommended. Contact local Medicines Information Centre for advice.

SIDE-EFFECTS
Drowsiness, vertigo/dizziness, euphoria, dry mouth, ataxia, visual disturbance, concentration difficulties, sleep disturbance, dysphoria, hypotension, headache and nausea. Also reported confusion, disorientation, hallucinations, psychosis, depression, decreased co-ordination, tremors, tachycardia, decreased appetite and abdominal pain.

POISONING & TOXICITY
Signs and symptoms are an extension of the psychotomimetic and physiological effects of nabilone. Overdosage may be considered to have occurred, even at prescribed dosages, if disturbing psychiatric symptoms are present. Vital signs should be monitored, since hypertension, hypotension and tachycardia have occurred. See nabilone SPC for further details.

PHARMACOKINETIC PROPERTIES
Absorbed from the gastrointestinal tract. Primarily excreted by biliary route. Plasma elimination half-life of approximately 2 hours.

EXCIPIENTS
Contact manufacturers for further details.

LICENSED STATUS
Not licensed for use in children <18 years of age.

FURTHER INFORMATION
250 microgram capsule made by Cambridge Laboratories as a 'special'.

Naloxone

Naloxone is a pure opioid antagonist.

USES
Reversal of opioid induced central and respiratory depression.

PRESENTATION
Injection: 400 microgram in 1mL, 1mL ampoule – Narcan® and non-proprietary; 20 microgram in 1mL, 2mL ampoule – Narcan Neonatal® and non-proprietary.
Pre-filled syringe: 400 microgram in 1mL, 1mL and 2mL disposable syringe – Min-I-Jet® Naloxone.

DOSAGE
Newborn infant (birth to 1 month)
☐ Do not administer to newborns whose mothers are suspected of narcotic abuse, as a withdrawal syndrome may be precipitated.
☐ Always establish and maintain adequate ventilation before administration of naloxone.

N

Route	Age		Frequency	Notes
	birth-1 month		(times daily)	
IV bolus, IM or SC	10 microgram/kg		single dose	May be repeated using doses up to 100 microgram/kg as required, at 2-3 minute intervals.
IV infusion	5-20 microgram/kg/hour		continuous	

☐ Naloxone is specifically indicated for the reversal of respiratory depression in a newborn infant whose mother has received narcotics within 4 hours of delivery. It is generally preferred to give an IM injection for a prolonged effect.

Route	Age		Frequency	Notes
	birth-1 month		(times daily)	
IM	100 microgram/kg		single dose	Use 400 microgram/mL naloxone preparation. Gradual onset of action (3-4 minutes) but the effect is prolonged.

Child

Route	Age			Frequency	Notes
	1 month-2 years	2-12 years	12-18 years	(times daily)	
IV bolus	← 10 microgram/kg →		10 microgram/kg (maximum dose 800 microgram)	single dose	Initial dose followed by a higher dose if no response. Due to short half-life of naloxone, repeat doses as necessary to maintain opioid reversal. Observe for recurrence of CNS and respiratory depression.
	then		then		
	← 100 microgram/kg → (maximum dose 2mg)		2mg	single dose	
IV infusion	← 5-20 microgram/kg/hour →		Infuse a solution of 4 microgram/mL at a rate adjusted according to response.	continuous	

If no response is observed after the second dose has been administered, the diagnosis of opioid-induced toxicity should be questioned. Another CNS depressant or brain damage may be present.

ADMINISTRATION
IV: infusion concentration 2mg in 500mL glucose 5% or NaCl 0.9% i.e. 4 microgram in 1mL. Any solution not used within 12 hours should be discarded and a fresh solution prepared.

CONTRA-INDICATIONS & WARNINGS
Hypersensitivity to naloxone. Use with caution in patients dependent on opioids. See under dosage for neonates whose mothers may be dependent. Use with caution in patients with cardiac problems or those receiving cardiotoxic drugs.

PREGNANCY
Safety in pregnancy has not been established. Naloxone crosses the placenta.

BREAST-FEEDING
No data available, but no theoretical contra-indication.

SIDE-EFFECTS
Nausea and vomiting. Reports of hypotension, hypertension, cardiac arrhythmias and pulmonary oedema.

POISONING/TOXICITY
No reports of respiratory depression or psychotomimetic effects.

PHARMACOKINETIC PROPERTIES
Naloxone is highly lipid soluble and is rapidly distributed throughout the body. High concentrations occur in the brain, kidney, lung, heart and skeletal

N

muscle. High CNS levels after IV bolus injection are short-lived as rapid redistribution takes place and this accounts for the relatively short duration of action seen clinically. Naloxone undergoes extensive biotransformation in the liver. The metabolites are excreted largely in the urine. The effects of renal and hepatic failure on the metabolism and distribution of naloxone have not been studied.

LICENSED STATUS
Licensed for use in all ages.

Naproxen

Non-steroidal anti-inflammatory drug (NSAID).

USES
Relief of symptoms (arthralgia, joint stiffness and fever) in inflammatory arthritis and treatment of acute musculoskeletal syndromes.

PRESENTATION
Suppository: 500mg – import.
Suspension: 125mg in 5mL – import.
Tablet: 250mg and 500mg – Naprosyn® and non-proprietary.
Tablet: (enteric coated) 250mg and 500mg – Naprosyn EC®, Nycopren® and non-proprietary; 375mg – Naprosyn EC® and non-proprietary.
Tablet: (as naproxen sodium equivalent to 250mg naproxen) 275mg – Synflex®.

DOSAGE

Route	Age			Frequency (times daily)	Notes
	1 month–2 years	2–12 years	12–18 years		
Oral/rectal	←	5–10mg/kg	→	2	Maximum 1g/day.
Oral	←	10–15mg/kg	→	2	In severe disease. Doses greater than 10mg/kg twice daily should be used for a few weeks only.

Renal impairment
Use with caution in patients with renal impairment, monitoring serum creatinine and/or creatinine clearance. Avoid use in those with a creatinine clearance <20 mL/minute/1.73m^2.

ADMINISTRATION
Oral: the enteric coated and modified release tablets may be taken on an empty stomach but must be swallowed whole. The plain tablets may be crushed or chewed. These tablets and the suspension should be taken with or after food to minimise gastrointestinal complaints.

CONTRA-INDICATIONS AND WARNINGS
Naproxen should not be given to patients with active peptic ulceration, and should be used with extreme caution in patients with a history of peptic ulceration. Also contra-indicated in patients who have previously shown hypersensitivity reactions (asthma, rhinitis, urticaria) to aspirin or other NSAIDs. Use with caution in renal, cardiac or hepatic impairment

INTERACTIONS
May decrease the elimination of *methotrexate*. Increased risk of nephrotoxicity when given with *ciclosporin (cyclosporin)*. *Probenecid* delays the excretion of naproxen, leading to increased naproxen levels.

PREGNANCY
NSAIDs should be avoided in the third trimester as they may cause constriction of the ductus arteriosus in utero leading to persistent pulmonary hypertension in the newborn. In addition, these drugs may inhibit labour if used close to delivery. Contact local Medicines Information Centre for advice.

N

BREAST-FEEDING
Excreted into breast milk in small quantities, but the amount ingested by the infant is likely to be insignificant.

SIDE-EFFECTS
Gastrointestinal discomfort, nausea, diarrhoea and occasionally bleeding and ulceration. Headache, dizziness, vertigo. Fluid retention. Hypersensitivity reactions e.g. bronchospasm, rashes. Local discomfort, burning or itching and occasionally bleeding may occur with NSAID suppositories. Pseudoporphyria, other skin rashes and confusion have been reported.

POISONING/TOXICITY
There is no specific antidote. Activated charcoal may markedly reduce the absorption of the drug. Further treatment is symptomatic.

PHARMACOKINETIC PROPERTIES
Peak plasma concentrations occur 2-4 hours after oral administration, but this may be delayed with the enteric coated preparations. Half-life of 12-15 hours. May be more rapidly absorbed as the sodium salt.

EXCIPIENTS
Contact manufacturers for further details.

LICENSED STATUS
Nycopren® 250mg and 500mg EC tablets are licensed for use in juvenile idiopathic arthritis (JIA) for patients >50kg in weight. Naprosyn® tablets are licensed for the treatment of JIA >5 years of age, at a dosage of 5mg/kg twice a day. Naprosyn® SR and Synflex® are licensed ≥16 years of age. Suspension and suppositories are not licensed in the UK.

FURTHER INFORMATION
Suppository and suspension available from IDIS World Medicines.

Nedocromil sodium

An anti-allergic agent that acts mainly by inhibiting release of inflammatory mediators.

USES
Prophylaxis in bronchial asthma not fully controlled by bronchodilators alone.

PRESENTATION
Aerosol inhalation: 2mg per metered inhalation   Tilade®.

DOSAGE

Route	Age		Frequency (times daily)	Notes
	2–12 years	12–18 years		
Inhalation	←——— >6 years 4mg ———→		4	Initial treatment.
	←——— >6 years 4mg ———→		2	Maintenance treatment.

ADMINISTRATION
Inhalation: can be used with Syncroner® spacer device.

CONTRA-INDICATIONS & WARNINGS
Hypersensitivity to any constituent of the formulation.

INTERACTIONS
None known.

PREGNANCY
Appears not to be a problem in pregnancy based on animal studies.

BREAST-FEEDING
Unlikely to be problematic.

N

SIDE-EFFECTS
Headache, upper gastrointestinal symptoms (nausea, vomiting, dyspepsia, abdominal pain), cough, bronchospasm.

POISONING/TOXICITY
No evidence to suggest toxic effects of nedocromil sodium at high dosage. Treatment should be supportive, and directed towards control of the relevant symptoms.

PHARMACOKINETIC PROPERTIES
Poorly absorbed from the gastrointestinal tract. Rapidly absorbed from the lungs following inhalation, and is then excreted unchanged into the urine and bile. Half-life of 1.5-3 hours.

EXCIPIENTS
Include saccharin sodium. See manufacturers SPC for further details.

LICENSED STATUS
Licensed for use in patients aged >6 years.

Neostigmine

A cholinesterase antagonist which potentiates the effect of naturally occurring acetylcholine.

USES
Myasthenia gravis and reversal of non-depolarising muscle relaxants.

PRESENTATION
Tablet: (as bromide) 15mg (scored) – non-proprietary.
Oral liquid: may be extemporaneously prepared.
Injection: 2.5mg in 1mL, 1mL ampoule – non-proprietary.

DOSAGE
Newborn Infant (birth to 1 month)

Indication	Route	Age	Frequency	Notes
		birth–1 month	(times daily)	
Myasthenia gravis	Oral	1–2mg	single dose	Initial dose. Give at least 30 minutes before feed is due.
		1–5mg	6	Subsequent doses. Dose will require regular adjustment according to symptoms.
	IM	100 microgram	single dose	Initial dose.
	IM or SC	50–250 microgram	6	Subsequent doses. Dose requires adjustment according to symptoms. 2-3mg IM or SC is equivalent to 30mg orally.
Reversal of non-depolarising neuromuscular blockade	IV bolus over 1 minute	80 microgram/kg (plus 20 microgram/kg atropine)	single dose	Dose when used with drugs other than atracurium.
		50 microgram/kg (plus 20 microgram/kg atropine)	single dose	Dose when used with atracurium.

N

Child

Indication	Route	Age			Frequency	Notes
		1 month–2 years	2–12 years	12–18 years		
Myasthenia gravis	Oral	7.5mg	2–5 years 7.5mg 6–12 years 15mg	15–30mg	single dose single dose	Initial dose: then the same dose is repeated at suitable intervals through-out the day. Adjust according to response. Usual daily dose: 1 month–12 years: 15–90mg 12–18 years: 75–300mg.
	IM or SC	← 200-500 microgram →		1–2.5mg	as required	Given at suitable intervals throughout the day. 2-3 mg IM or SC is equivalent to 30mg orally.
Reversal of non-depolarising neuromuscular blockade.	IV bolus over 1 minute	← 80 microgram/kg → ← (maximum 2.5mg) → (maximum 5mg) (see notes section re: atropine dose)			single dose	Dose when used with drugs other than atracurium. Plus 20 microgram/kg atropine (minimum dose atropine 100 micrograms and maximum dose atropine 600 micrograms).
		← 50 microgram/kg → ← (maximum 2.5mg) → (maximum 5mg) (see notes section re: atropine dose)			single dose	Dose when used with atracurium. Plus 20 microgram/kg atropine (minimum dose atropine 100 micrograms and maximum dose atropine 600 micrograms).

Consider dose reduction in mild renal impairment. Reduce to 50% in moderate and to 25% in severe renal impairment.

ADMINISTRATION
When used in a conscious child with myasthenia gravis, neostigmine may cause severe gastrointestinal pain. Simultaneous administration of atropine (20 microgram/kg) may prevent the muscarinic side-effects.

CONTRA-INDICATIONS & WARNINGS
Neostigmine should not be given to patients with mechanical gastrointestinal or urinary obstruction. Do not use in conjunction with depolarising muscle relaxants (*suxamethonium*) due to prolonged apnoea. Extreme caution when administered to patients with bronchial asthma, bradycardia, recent coronary occlusion, hypotension, peptic ulceration or epilepsy. Post-thymectomy patients may have a reduced dose requirement.

INTERACTIONS
Effects of neostigmine are antagonised by *aminoglycosides, chlorpromazine, clindamycin, colistin, imipenem/cilastatin, lithium, procainamide* and *quinidine*. Drugs that may worsen myasthenia and thus diminish the effect of neostigmine are *acetazolamide, ampicillin, aspirin, chloroquine, dipyridamole, erythromycin, hydroxychloroquine, ketoprofen* and *penicillamine*. *Beta-blockers* can worsen bradycardia. Effect of *suxamethonium* is enhanced but that of *atracurium, tubocurarine, pancuronium* and *vercuronium* are antagonised. The use of *steroids* or *immunosuppressants* can increase the response to neostigmine.

PREGNANCY
Safety in pregnancy has not been established. Although the possible hazards to the mother and child must therefore be weighed against the potential benefits in every case, experience in pregnant patients with myasthenia gravis has revealed no untoward effect of the drug on the course of the pregnancy. As severity of myasthenia gravis often fluctuates considerably, particular care is required to avoid cholinergic crisis, due to overdosage of the drug, but otherwise management is no different from that in non-pregnant patients.

BREAST-FEEDING
Safety during lactation has not been established but only negligible amounts of drug are excreted in breast milk. Contact local Medicines Information Centre for advice.

SIDE-EFFECTS
May include nausea and vomiting, increased salivation, diarrhoea and abdominal cramps and bradycardia.

POISONING/TOXICITY
Signs of overdosage due to muscarinic effects may include abdominal cramps, increased peristalsis, diarrhoea, nausea and vomiting, increased bronchial

N

secretions, salivation, sweating, involuntary defaecation and urination, bradycardia, hypotension and miosis. Nicotinic effects consist of involuntary twitching, muscular cramps, and general weakness. Artificial respiration should be instituted if respiration is severely depressed. *Atropine sulphate* (20-40 microgram/kg in a child, 1-2mg in an adult) given IV is an antidote to the muscarinic effects.

Peak plasma concentrations occur at 1-2 hours after an oral dose if patient fasted, and delayed by 90 minutes if taken with food. Duration of action 2-4 hours. Metabolism is by plasma esterases and elimination is by renal and non-renal mechanisms. After oral administration 20% is eliminated by the kidneys and after an intramuscular dose this increases to 80%, 50% as unchanged. Plasma half life is 1-2 hours in adults but is known to be shorter in children.

PHARMACOKINETIC PROPERTIES
Poorly absorbed orally, estimated bioavailability 1-2%.

EXCIPIENTS
Contact manufacturer for further details.

LICENSED STATUS
Licensed for use in all age groups.

FURTHER INFORMATION
Extemporaneous formulation e.g. Nova Laboratories using Suspension Diluent A (xanthan gum 1%) as a suspending agent. Shelf life 14 days stored at room temperature.
Approximate equivalent doses: 500 microgram IV ≡ 1-1.5mg IM or SC ≡ 15mg orally.

Netilmicin

Aminoglycoside antibiotic.

USES
Serious Gram-negative infections resistant to gentamicin; less active against *Pseudomonas*.

PRESENTATION
Injection: (as sulphate) 15mg in 1.5mL, 50mg in 1mL, 100mg in 1mL, 150mg in 1.5mL and 200mg in 2mL expressed as netilmicin base – Netillin®.

DOSAGE
Many dose regimens exist; those outlined below are generally accepted initial doses and dose adjustments should be made in the light of serum concentration measurement.

Divided daily dose regimen
Newborn infant (birth to 1 month)

Route	Age		Frequency	Notes
	birth–1 month			
IV	3mg/kg		12 hourly	Increase to 8 hourly for term neonates >1 week old. Monitor after the third dose aiming for a 1 hour post dose (peak) of 8-12mg/L and a trough level of <3mg/L

Prolongation of the dosage interval is recommended in newborn infants presenting with patient ductus arteriosus (PDA), prolonged hypoxia or concurrent treatment with indometacin (indomethacin).

N

Extended daily dose regimen
Newborn infant (birth to 1 month)

Route	*Postconceptional age	Dose	Dose Frequency	Notes
IV	<32 weeks	6mg/kg	36 hourly	Plasma samples usually taken around the third dose aiming for a pre -dose trough level of <3mg/L. If there is no change in the dosage regimen or renal function repeat levels every 3-4 days.
	>32 weeks	6mg/kg	24 hourly	

*Postconceptional age = gestational plus postnatal age.

Divided daily dose regimen
Child

Route	Age			Frequency (times daily)	Notes
	1 month-2 years	2-12 years	12-18 years		
IV or IM	← 2.5mg/kg →		2mg/kg	3	Monitor after the third dose aiming for a 1 hour post dose (peak) of 8-12mg/L and a pre -dose trough level of <3mg/L
Intra-peritoneal	concentrations of 7.5-10mg/L in peritoneal dialysis fluid without elevation of serum levels				

Dose adjustment in renal impairment.

In patients with impaired renal function dosage and/or frequency of administration must be adjusted in response to serum drug concentrations and the extent of renal impairment. There are various methods to determine dosage and a wide variation in dosage recommendations. See manufacturers SPC recommendations.

Single daily dose regimen
Child

Route	Age			Frequency (times daily)	Notes
	1 month-2 years	2-12 years	12-18 years		
IV	← 7.5mg/kg →			1	Plasma levels usually taken at 18-24 hours after the first dose. Aiming for a trough level of <1mg/L If levels are >1mg/L then the dosing interval is normally increased by 12 hours. 1 hour post dose (peak) levels may be measured aiming for a target of >20mg/L If there is no change in the dosage regimen or renal function repeat levels every 3-4 days.

At least pre-dose levels must be monitored in children with impaired renal function.

ADMINISTRATION

IV: slow IV injection over 3-5 minutes injected neat or diluted in NaCl 0.9% or glucose 5%. IV infusion over 30-60 minutes for high dose 'child – single daily regimen' in an appropriate volume of fluid. Physically compatible with NaCl 0.9%, glucose 5% and 10%. Should not be mixed with penicillins, cephalosporins, erythromycin, heparin, sodium bicarbonate. Adequate flushing or administration at separate sites is suggested.

CONTRA-INDICATIONS & WARNINGS
Hypersensitivity to other aminoglycosides. Contra-indicated in myasthenia gravis. Aminoglycosides have a magnesium-like effect acting at the neuromuscular junction pre-junctionally to reduce transmitter release and post-junctionally to reduce receptor sensitivity.

INTERACTIONS
Increased risk of ototoxicity and nephrotoxicity with *cephalosporins, vancomycin, ciclosporin (cyclosporin), cisplatin, diuretics* such as *furosemide (frusemide), amphotericin*. Enhances effects of *non-depolarising muscle relaxants. Calcium IV* may

N

reverse this effect. Antagonises effects of *neostigmine and pyridostigmine*.

PREGNANCY
See amikacin monograph.

BREAST-FEEDING
Netilmicin is excreted into breast milk in low concentration and since oral absorption is poor the potential for toxicity is low in the nursing infant.

SIDE-EFFECTS
As with all aminoglycosides nephrotoxicity and ototoxicity can occur if optimum blood levels are exceeded. May be a more potent neuromuscular blocking agent.

POISONING/TOXICITY
Removed by haemodialysis and peritoneal dialysis.

PHARMACOKINETIC PROPERTIES
Netilmicin distributes into tissues, sputum, pericardial, synovial and peritoneal fluids. Only small amounts are excreted in the bile. CSF penetration is poor. In normal renal function 74% of a dose is excreted in 24 hours.
Bolus IV injections over 3-5 minutes may produce peak serum concentrations up to twice as high as those following a 30 minute infusion. Therefore, for once daily treatment, the infusion is recommended.

LICENSED STATUS
Licensed for use in all ages.

Nicardipine

Calcium-channel blocker.

USES
Hypertensive crisis.

PRESENTATION
Injection: 2.5mg in 1mL, 10mL ampoule – named patient (Cardene®).

DOSAGE

Route	Age				Frequency	Notes
	birth–1 month	1 month–2 years	2–12 years	12–18 years		
IV infusion	← 500 nanogram/kg/minute →				continuous	Initial dose. Titrate according to response.
	← 1–4 microgram/kg/minute →				continuous	Usual maintenance dose.

ADMINISTRATION
IV: infuse IV in glucose 5% or NaCl 0.9% at a concentration of 100 micrograms in 1mL. To minimise the risk of peripheral venous irritation the site of infusion should be changed every 12 hours.

CONTRA-INDICATIONS & WARNINGS
Contra-indicated in aortic stenosis, calcium-channel blocker hypersensitivity. Caution in liver impairment, extensively metabolised by liver. May cause decrease in GFR, use with caution in moderate renal impairment.
Blood pressure will fall to about 50% of its ultimate decrease in 45 minutes and does not reach steady state for approximately 50 hours.

PREGNANCY
Use only if the benefits outweigh the risks. Contact local Medicines Information Centre for advice.

BREAST-FEEDING
Contact local Medicines Information Centre for advice.

INTERACTIONS, SIDE EFFECTS, POISONING/TOXICITY
See nifedipine monograph.

EXCIPIENTS
Contact manufacturers for further details.

LICENSED STATUS
Not licensed for use in the UK.

FURTHER INFORMATION
There is limited information on the use of nicardipine in paediatric patients. It should be used with caution and with careful dosage adjustment and blood pressure monitoring. Injection only currently available by importing USA products.

Anthelmintic.

USES
Anthelmintic (not first line) for treatment of tapeworm infections: *Taenia saginata* (beef tapeworm), *Taenia solium* (pork tapeworm), *Diphyllobothrium latum* (fish tapeworm) and *Hymenolepis nana* (dwarf tapeworm).
No effect in cysticercosis and echinococcosis due to cestode larvae lodging in extra-intestinal tissue.

PRESENTATION
Tablet: 500mg (imported).

DOSAGE

Indication	Route	Age			Frequency	Notes
		1 month–2 years	2–12 years	12–18 years		
Pork, beef, fish tapeworms	Oral	500mg	2–6 years 1g	2g	single dose	In the case of beef and fish tapeworms, the dose may be divided, half being taken after breakfast, and the re-mainder one hour later.
			7–12 years 2g		single dose	
Dwarf tapeworm	Oral	500mg	2–6 years 1g	2g	single dose (day 1)	
			7–12 years 2g			Treat for a total of 7 days.
		then	then	then		
		250mg	2–6 years 500mg	1g	single dose (days 2–7)	
			7–12 years 1g			

ADMINISTRATION
Oral: tablets should be chewed thoroughly before washing down with water or fruit juice. In the case of small children, crush tablets before administration. Doses should be taken after a light breakfast. Acidic fruit juice such as orange juice can be very beneficial in the elimination of tapeworms.

CONTRA-INDICATIONS & WARNINGS
Contra-indications: hypersensitivity to niclosamide.
Warnings: in infection with *Taenia solium* there is always a danger of cysticercosis. A drastic purge is therefore recommended to eject the lower segment of the tapeworm containing mature eggs. For other warnings refer to the manufacturers SPC.

INTERACTIONS
Alcohol may possibly increase the side-effects of niclosamide.

PREGNANCY
Avoid in first trimester of pregnancy. Experimental studies in rats showed no embryotoxic or teratogenic effects.

BREAST-FEEDING
As niclosamide is only minimally absorbed from the gastrointestinal tract, excretion of the drug in breast milk would not appear to be a significant problem for breast-feeding infants. However, no specific data is available.

SIDE-EFFECTS
Mild transient gastrointestinal effects e.g. nausea, retching and abdominal pain, light-headedness, pruritis.

POISONING/TOXICITY
Niclosamide is not absorbed and no cases of overdose have occurred. In the event of overdose a fast acting laxative and enema may be given. Vomiting should not be induced.

PHARMACOKINETIC PROPERTIES
Not significantly absorbed from the gastrointestinal tract; eliminated in the faeces.

N

EXCIPIENTS
Contact manufacturer for further details.

LICENSED STATUS
Not licensed for use in the UK.

FURTHER INFORMATION
Available from IDIS World Medicines.

Nifedipine

Calcium-channel blocker.

USES
Hypertension; management of angina pectoris due to coronary artery disease in Kawasaki disease or progeria; Raynaud's phenomenon.

PRESENTATION
Capsule: 5mg and 10mg – Adalat®, non-proprietary.
Capsule: (modified release) 10mg and 20mg – Coracten SR®; 30mg – Coracten XL®.
Oral liquid: 2% (20mg in 1mL, 1mg per 0.05mL drop) – named patient.
Tablet: (modified release) 10mg – Nifedipress® MR; 10mg and 20mg – Adalat® Retard, Adipine® MR, Cardilate MR®, Tensipine MR®' Hypolar® Retard 20; 20mg – Coroday MR®, Nifedipress® Retard, Slofedipine®; 30mg and 60mg – Slofedipine®; 40mg – Fortipine LA 40®; 20mg, 30mg and 60mg – Adalat® LA.

DOSAGE

Indication	Route	Age			Frequency	Notes
		1 month–2 years	2–12 years	12–18 years	(times daily)	
Hypertensive crisis/angina	Oral	← 250–500 microgram/kg →			single dose	Bite the capsules releasing the contents into the mouth and then swallow.
Hypertension/angina	Oral	← 200–300 microgram/kg →		5–20mg	3 (but see notes)	Dose frequency depends on preparation used eg. some modified release preparations are given once daily and others are given twice daily. Maximum dose of 3mg/kg/**day** or 100mg/**day**.
Raynaud's phenomenon	Oral	< 2 years Not recommended	← 2.5–10mg →		2–4 (but see notes)	Start at a low dose at night and build up gradually to avoid postural hypotension.

Hepatic/renal impairment
Nifedipine is metabolised in the liver. In patients with hepatic impairment use the lower stated dose and monitor carefully. Patients with renal impairment should not require adjustment of dosage. Give dose after dialysis.

ADMINISTRATION
Oral: if liquid preparation required for young children, liquid can be aspirated from capsules using a syringe. However, different brands of nifedipine 10mg capsules contain different amounts of liquid: IVAX capsules contain 10mg nifedipine in 0.45mL; Bayer and APS capsules contain 10mg nifedipine in 0.34mL; Alpharma capsules contain 10mg nifedipine in 0.36mL; Hillcross capsules contain 10mg in 0.28mL.
Aspirated liquid dose should be covered in foil and administered immediately as nifedipine is very light sensitive. Rather than remove liquid from capsules, some paediatric units crush the nifedipine retard tablets and administer immediately; this may alter the modified release action. Some units have found that the retard tablets may require three times daily dosing, even if swallowed whole.

N

CONTRA-INDICATIONS & WARNINGS
Pregnancy. Use with caution in patients whose cardiac reserve is poor. Lowering blood pressure too rapidly may cause cerebral or coronary ischaemia.

INTERACTIONS
Beta-blockers may increase cardiovascular adverse effects. *Cimetidine* may increase nifedipine serum concentration. Nifedipine may increase *digoxin* serum concentration; monitor *digoxin* levels and if necessary reduce *digoxin* dose. Reduced levels of nifedipine with *rifampicin;* do not use together as effective levels of nifedipine may not be reached. Nifedipine helps ameliorate the nephrotoxicity of *ciclosporin (cyclosporin),* but exacerbates gum hyperplasia. Bioavailability is increased if taken with *grapefruit juice.*

PREGNANCY
May inhibit labour. Contact local Medicines Information Centre for advice.

BREAST-FEEDING
Excreted in breast milk in levels too small to be harmful, but manufacturers advise avoidance.

POISONING/TOXICITY
Severe hypotension due to vasodilatation, tachycardia or bradycardia, hyperglycaemia, metabolic acidosis, heart block and cardiogenic shock with pulmonary oedema. Treat by elevation of extremities, plasma expanders. If ineffective consider *calcium gluconate* and addition of *beta-sympathomimetic* and *vasoconstrictor.* Bradycardia may be treated with *atropine* or temporary cardiac pacemaker.

SIDE-EFFECTS
Headache, flushing, tachycardia, palpitations, dizziness, rash, gum hyperplasia. May increase intracranial pressure.

PHARMACOKINETIC PROPERTIES
Onset of action: oral – within 20 minutes; sublingual – within 1-5 minutes. Absorption is slowed by administration with food.

LICENSED STATUS
Not licensed for use in children.

EXPCIPIENTS
Contact manufacturers for further details.

FURTHER INFORMATION
Nifedipine should be prescribed by generic name, strength, form AND trade name as all products are not bioequivalent. Oral liquid available via IDIS World Medicines.

Nitrazepam

Benzodiazepine, antiepileptic.

USES
Second-line treatment of infantile spasms; also used in treating myoclonic seizures and periodic epileptic spasms occurring outside infancy.

PRESENTATION
Tablet: 5mg – non-proprietary.
Liquid: 2.5mg in 5mL – Somnite®; 5mg in 5mL – manufactured 'special'.

DOSAGE/ADMINISTRATION

Route	Age				Frequency (times daily)	Notes
	birth–1 month	1 month–2 years	2–12 years	12–18 years		
Oral	← 125 microgram/kg →			–	2	Usual starting dose.
	← 250 microgram/kg → (maximum 500 microgram/kg)			–	2	Usual target maintenance dose. Total daily dose may be divided into 3.

Dose adjustment
Target maintenance dose should be reached over 2-3 weeks. Consider need to reduce dose in severe renal impairment or liver disease.

N

CONTRA-INDICATIONS & WARNINGS
Porphyria; respiratory disease; muscle weakness. Contra-indicated in respiratory depression, acute pulmonary insufficiency, severe hepatic impairment, myasthenia gravis, sleep apnoea syndrome.

INTERACTIONS
Enzyme inhibitors (e.g. cimetidine) may enhance the effects and *enzyme inducers (e.g. rifampicin)* may reduce the effects of nitrazepam.

PREGNANCY
Manufacturer states safety in pregnancy not established. Heart irregularities in the fetus and hypotonia, poor suckling, hypothermia reported in neonates when taken in the third trimester.

BREAST-FEEDING
Nitrazepam is excreted into breast milk. Breast-feeding is appropriate if maternal dose is normal.

SIDE-EFFECTS
Dose dependent side-effects include sedation, irritability. Chronic adverse effects include tachyphylaxis, behaviour changes, cognitive dysfunction.

POISONING/TOXICITY
Drowsiness, dizziness, ataxia, slurred speech, coma may be seen. Flumazenil is a benzodiazepine antagonist but will also reduce anticonvulsant effect in patients with epilepsy.

PHARMACOKINETIC PROPERTIES
Peak plasma levels occur 2-3 hours after oral administration of Somnite® and elimination half-life is approximately 24 hours in adults.

EXCIPIENTS
Somnite® includes sucrose. Contact manufacturers for further details.

LICENSED STATUS
Not licensed for the above uses. The 5mg in 5mL liquid is a 'special' and as such is unlicensed.

FURTHER INFORMATION
The 5mg in 5mL liquid is available from Rosemont.

Nitric oxide

Stimulates production of cyclic GMP. Rapidly inactivated by haemoglobin producing methaemoglobin.

USES
Used by inhalation to produce selective pulmonary vasodilatation of ventilated lung.

PRESENTATION
Gas cylinder: available in cylinders at a concentration of 400 parts per million (ppm).

DOSAGE
The maximum recommended dose is 20ppm.

>33 weeks gestation: start at 20ppm. If this produces a rise in post ductal pO_2 of at least 3kPa (while ventilator parameters remain unchanged), reduce the dose after an hour to the lowest dose capable of producing a sustained response.

≤33 weeks gestation: start with a dose of 5ppm and consider increasing in stages to a maximum of 40ppm. If this produces no response return to 5ppm and give this for 12 hours. If still no response – stop.

Tailing off: always try to use the lowest effective dose, failure to do so may result in increasing dependency. Try to reduce the dose further every 12 hours. Drop the concentration by 10% every 3 minutes but reverse any reduction that causes the arterial saturation to drop by more than 2%.

ADMINISTRATION
Special equipment for delivering and scavenging is required in addition to specialised circuit and environmental monitoring equipment.

N

CONTRA-INDICATIONS & WARNINGS
Oxidises readily to NO_2 which is toxic. Contact time between NO and O_2 should be minimal. NO_2 levels should be monitored.

SIDE-EFFECTS
Methaemoglobinaemia, NO_2 toxicity (pulmonary oedema).

PHARMACOKINETIC PROPERTIES
Biological half-life is 3-6 seconds.

EXCIPIENTS
Nitrogen (ensure adequate ventilation).

LICENSED STATUS
Licensed ≥34 weeks gestation – maximum licensed dose 20ppm.

FURTHER INFORMATION
Infants receiving nitric oxide are extremely sensitive to its sudden loss so a spare cylinder must be available, and any hand ventilation system must also contain the same concentration of nitric oxide.

Nitrofurantoin

A broad-spectrum antibacterial agent, active against the majority of urinary pathogens.

USES
Treatment and prophylaxis of urinary tract infection (not indicated for pyelonephritis).

PRESENTATION
Capsule: 50mg and 100mg – Macrodantin®.
Capsule (modified release): 100mg – Macrobid®.
Suspension: 25mg in 5mL – Furadantin®.
Tablet: 50mg and 100mg – Furadantin® (scored) and non-proprietary.

DOSAGE

Route	Age				Frequency (times daily)	Notes
	birth–1 month	1 month–2 years	2–12 years	12–18 years		
Oral	contra-indicated	<3 months contra-indicated	750 microgram/kg	50–100mg	4	Treatment.
		>3 months 750 microgram/kg			4	
	–	–	–	100mg	2	Treatment (modified release capsule).
	contra-indicated	<3 months contra-indicated	1mg/kg	50–100mg	1 (at night)	Prophylaxis.
		>3 months 1mg/kg			1 (at night)	

Dosage in renal impairment
Do not use if creatine clearance is less than $60mL/minute/1.73m^2$.

ADMINISTRATION
Oral: take with food or milk to minimise gastrointestinal reactions. The modified release capsules should be swallowed whole.

N

CONTRA-INDICATIONS & WARNINGS
Nitrofurantoin should not be given to infants <3 months of age or to pregnant patients at term (during labour and delivery) because of the theoretical possibility of haemolytic anaemia in the fetus or the newborn infant due to immature erythrocyte enzyme systems. It is also contra-indicated in patients with a creatinine clearance less than 60mL/minute/1.73m^2 and in anyone with hyper-sensitivity to nitrofurantoin or other nitrofurans. Contra-indicated in patients with G6PD deficiency.

INTERACTIONS
Concurrent administration with *magnesium trisilicate* reduces absorption. *Uricosuric drugs* such as *probenecid* and *sulphinpyrazone* may inhibit renal tubular secretion of nitrofurantoin; the resulting increase in serum levels may increase toxicity and decreased urinary levels could lessen the efficacy of nitrofurantoin as a urinary tract antibacterial. There may be decreased antibacterial activity in the presence of *carbonic anhydrase inhibitors* and *urine alkalinising agents*.

PREGNANCY
Animal studies have shown no teratogenic effects and suitability of nitrofurantoin in human pregnancy has been well documented. It should not be given during labour and delivery for the reasons outlined in the contra-indications section.

BREAST-FEEDING
Although only small amounts appear in breast milk these may be sufficient to produce haemolysis in G6PD deficient infants so contra-indicated in breast-feeding mothers.

SIDE-EFFECTS
Gastrointestinal: nausea, anorexia and less commonly vomiting, abdominal pain and diarrhoea.
Respiratory: acute and chronic pulmonary reactions (may be associated with lupus erythematosus-like syndrome).
Hepatic: rarely cholestatic jaundice and hepatitis.
Neurological: peripheral neuropathy reported infrequently.
Haematological: agranulocytosis, leucopenia, granulocytopenia, haemolytic anaemia, thrombocytopenia, G6PD deficiency, megaloblastic anaemia and eosinophilia have occurred.
Hypersensitivity: allergic skin reactions including pruritus; exfoliative dermatitis and erythema have been reported rarely.
Other: benign intracranial hypertension, transient alopecia. Superinfections by fungi or resistant organisms such as *Pseudomonas* may occur; limited to the genito-urinary tract.

POISONING/TOXICITY
Signs and symptoms of overdosage include gastric irritation, nausea and vomiting. There is no specific antidote and treatment is symptomatic. Monitoring of full blood count, liver function tests and pulmonary function are recommended. A high fluid intake should be maintained to promote urinary excretion of the drug. Nitrofurantoin is removed by haemodialysis.

PHARMACOKINETIC PROPERTIES
95% orally absorbed. Half-life is 0.3-1 hour. 60-77% protein bound. Rapidly and extensively excreted in the urine.

EXCIPIENTS
Contact manufacturers for further details.

LICENSED STATUS
Capsules, suspension and tablets are licensed for ≥3 months of age. The modified release capsules are licensed for use ≥12 years of age.

FURTHER INFORMATION
Suspension available from IDIS World Medicines.

Nitrous oxide

Analgesic in sub-anaesthetic concentrations administered by inhalation.

USES
To produce sedation and analgesia without loss of consciousness e.g. for dressing changes, wound debridement, suturing, removal of pins, wires or drains; for relative analgesia in dentistry.

PRESENTATION
Compressed medical gas: mixture of nitrous oxide and oxygen, 50% of each gas – Entonox® and Equanox®. Contained in cylinders with a blue body, and blue and white shoulder.

N

DOSAGE & ADMINISTRATION

Inhalation: nitrous oxide is administered with oxygen to avoid the hypoxia which would otherwise occur.

Doses may be self-regulated in most cases by the use of a face-mask connected through a demand valve to the cylinder. The valve is operated by the act of inhalation by the patient and closes when the patient ceases to inhale. This will generally only be possible with children aged about 5 years and over. It should be administered only by personnel trained in its use. Dose adjustments are not necessary in renal or hepatic disease.

CONTRA-INDICATIONS & WARNINGS

Contra-indications: patients with an air-containing closed space since nitrous oxide will diffuse into such a space with a resulting increase in pressure. This effect may be dangerous in the presence of a pneumothorax or air embolus which may enlarge to compromise respiration. It should not be used for analgesia in patients with head injuries with impairment of consciousness, maxillofacial injuries or those heavily sedated.

Cautions: patients with acute intestinal obstruction, hypotension, coronary artery disease and pulmonary hypertension. Administration more frequently than every 4 days should be accompanied by routine blood cell counts for evidence of megaloblastic change in red cells and hypersegmentation of neutrophils.

Warnings: thorough ventilation or scavenging of waste gases is necessary to reduce operating theatre or treatment room levels of ambient nitrous oxide to a level below 100ppm.

INTERACTIONS

Respiratory and cardiac depression may occur if given concurrently with other *CNS depressants,* e.g. *opiates.*

PREGNANCY

Single acute maternal exposure to nitrous oxide during pregnancy at the doses used to produce anaesthesia is unlikely to pose a substantial teratogenic risk, although data are insufficient to state there is no risk.

SIDE-EFFECTS

CNS: signs and symptoms of hypoxia include headache, dizziness and excitation proceeding to possible CNS depression. Raised intracranial pressure and peripheral neuropathy with prolonged use have been reported. Malignant hyperthermia has been reported rarely.

Cardiovascular: hypotension and cardiac arrhythmias may be seen.

Respiratory: respiratory irritation.

Gastrointestinal: nausea and /or vomiting.

POISONING/TOXICITY

There should be no risk of overdose with Entonox® used as patient-controlled analgesia since light anaesthesia will supervene if the patient continues to inhale and the mask will fall away. The main complications following the use of nitrous oxide are those caused by varying degrees of hypoxia due to rapid excretion of nitrous oxide (diffusion hypoxia). Exposure to patients for prolonged periods, either by continuous or intermittent administration may result in megaloblastic anaemia and neuropathies. Leucopenia, thrombocytopenia and severe megaloblastic anaemia may also occur following chronic intermittent inhalation.

PHARMACOKINETIC PROPERTIES

Rapidly absorbed on inhalation. Onset of action is within 3-5 minutes. Duration of action is for 3–5 minutes after discontinuation of inhalation. Most is rapidly eliminated through the lungs although small amounts diffuse through the skin.

LICENSED STATUS

Licensed for these indications for all age groups of children and adults.

FURTHER INFORMATION

Cylinders should be protected from the cold to prevent separation of the gases. If exposed to temperatures less than -6°C they should be stored horizontally for 24 hours at a temperature not less than 10°C before use to ensure thorough mixing. If this is not practical, before use cylinders must be maintained at a temperature above 10°C for at least 2 hours and then completely inverted 3 times, or alternatively placed in warm water at body temperature for 5 minutes and then completely inverted 3 times.

Noradrenaline (norepinephrine)

Infusing produces alpha-adrenergic receptor mediated vaso-constriction with an increase in total peripheral resistance and elevation of both diastolic and systolic blood pressure. This is accompanied by a vagal-mediated reflex fall in heart rate. Cardiac output is unchanged or reduced. Peripheral vascular resistance increases in most vascular beds and the blood flow through the kidney, liver and skeletal muscle is decreased.

N

USES
As a positive myocardial inotrope in states of low cardiac output e.g. following cardiac surgery.
As an emergency measure for blood pressure restoration in acute hypotension.

PRESENTATION
Injection: 2mg in 1mL (as acid tartrate ≡ 1mg in 1mL noradrenaline (norepinephrine) base in 2mL, 4mL and 20mL ampoules, also referred to as 1:1000 noradrenaline (norepinephrine) – non-proprietary.

DOSAGE
2mg of noradrenaline (norepinephrine) acid tartrate contains 1mg of noradrenaline (norepinephrine) base. The drug is always best prescribed in terms of the amount of base to be given to prevent ambiguity, as in the table below.

Route	Age				Frequency	Notes
	birth–1 month	1 month–2 years	2–12 years	12–18 years		
IV infusion	← 20 nanogram – 100 nanogram/kg/minute →				continuous	Dose should be titrated according to response to a maximum of 1 microgram/ kg/minute. Monitor ECG and haemodynamic status.

ADMINISTRATION
IV: must be diluted and given as an IV infusion via a central venous catheter, using a syringe pump or other apparatus to control the flow rate. Infuse in glucose 5% or NaCl 0.18%/glucose 4%. For continuous infusion dilute to 4-16 microgram in 1mL. Solutions containing the equivalent of 40 micrograms of the base in 1mL have also been used. Stable in solutions of pH 3.6–6. Above pH 6, significant loss of potency may occur. Discard solutions if precipitation or brown discolouration occurs.

CONTRA-INDICATIONS & WARNINGS
Should be used only in conjunction with appropriate blood volume replacement.

The use of pressor amines during *cyclopropane* or *halothane* anaesthesia may cause serious cardiac arrhythmias. Because of the possibility of increasing the risk of ventricular fibrillation, norepinephrine should be used with caution in patients receiving these or any other *cardiac sensitising agent* or who exhibit profound hypoxia or hypercarbia.

When infusing, the blood pressure and blood flow should be checked regularly to avoid hypertension. Extravasation of the solution may cause local tissue necrosis. The infusion site should be checked frequently. If extravasation occurs, the area should be infiltrated with 5-10mg of *phentolamine mesilate* in 10–15mL NaCl 0.9% using a fine needle, without delay (the lower dose should be used in infants and small children).

INTERACTIONS
Halogenated anaesthetic agents: serious cardiac arrhythmias may be precipitated during concomitant use with noradrenaline (norepinephrine). *Digoxin and other drugs which sensitise the myocardium:* concomitant administration with noradrenaline (norepinephrine) may increase the risk of arrhythmias. Risk of hypertension with *beta-blockers, tricyclic antidepressants, doxapram* and *MAOIs.*

PREGNANCY
May impair placental perfusion and induce fetal bradycardia. It may also exert a contractile effect on the pregnant uterus and lead to fetal asphyxia in late pregnancy. These possible risks to the fetus should be weighed against the potential benefit to the mother.

BREAST-FEEDING
Since noradrenaline (norepinephrine) does not achieve pharmacologically active levels after oral administration, breast-feeding should not present any hazard to the infant.

SIDE-EFFECTS
Hypertension may occur, which may be associated with bradycardia as well as headache and peripheral ischaemia including gangrene of the extremities. Prolonged administration may lead to plasma volume depletion. Extravasation of noradrenaline (norepinephrine) during infusion leads to sloughing and necrosis around the infusion site.

POISONING/TOXICITY
Overdose may result in severe hypertension, reflex bradycardia, marked increase in peripheral resistance and decreased cardiac output. These may be accompanied by violent headache, photophobia, retrosternal pain, pallor, intense sweating and vomiting. In the event of overdose, treatment should be withdrawn and appropriate corrective treatment initiated.

N

PHARMACOKINETIC PROPERTIES
Rapidly and extensively metabolised in the gut and liver and consequently ineffective after oral administration. It cannot be given by IM or SC injection because it is such a powerful vasoconstrictor. Metabolism is extensive and rapid; stable concentrations are reached within 10-15 minutes of starting an infusion. Plasma half-life is 2-2.5 minutes. Clearance is not influenced by renal function. Plasma protein binding is approximately 50%.

EXCIPIENTS
Some noradrenaline (norepinephrine) preparations may contain sodium metabisulphite. Contact manufacturers for further details.

LICENSED STATUS
Not licensed for use in children.

Norethisterone

A progestogen.

USES
Induction of sexual maturity, in combination with an oestrogen.
Postponement of menstruation.

PRESENTATION
Tablet: 5mg – Primolut N®, Utovlan® and non-proprietary.

DOSAGE/ADMINISTRATION
Induction of sexual maturity
Oral: 5mg once daily for the last 7 days of a 28 day cycle.

Postponement of menstruation.
Oral: 5mg three times a day, starting 3 days before the expected onset of menstruation.

CONTRA-INDICATIONS & WARNINGS
Pregnancy, liver disease, hypertension, thromboembolism, porphyria. When used for postponement of menstruation, if menstrual bleeding fails to occur following the end of treatment, pregnancy must be excluded before a further course is given.

PREGNANCY
Contra-indicated.

BREAST-FEEDING
Higher doses may suppress lactation and alter milk composition. Contact local Medicines Information Centre for advice.

SIDE-EFFECTS
Nausea and rarely jaundice.

POISONING
Overdosage may be manifested by nausea, vomiting, breast enlargement and later, vaginal bleeding. Treatment should be symptomatic. Gastric lavage may be employed if the overdose is large and the patient is seen within 4 hours.

PHARMACOKINETIC PROPERTIES
Oral bioavailability is approximately 60% due to high first pass metabolism. Elimination half-life is 5-12 hours.

EXCIPIENTS
See manufacturers SPC for further details.

LICENSED STATUS
Licensed for the postponement of menstruation. Not licensed for induction of sexual maturation.

N

Tricyclic antidepressant.

USES
Nocturnal enuresis. Depression. Hyperactivity.

PRESENTATION
Tablet: 10mg and 25mg (scored) – Allegron®.

DOSAGE

Indication	Route	Age		Frequency (times daily)	Notes
		2–12 years	12–18 years		
Nocturnal enuresis	Oral	≥ 6 years 20–25kg 10mg	25–35mg	1 (at night)	Not likely to be used <6 years of age. Maximum period of treatment 3 months – review before further courses.
		25–35kg 10–20mg		1 (at night)	
		35–54kg 25–35mg		1 (at night)	
Depression	Oral	–	30–100mg	1 (see notes)	Can be given as a single dose at night or in divided doses. Use low dose initially increased as necessary to 100mg.

CONTRA-INDICATIONS & WARNINGS, PREGNANCY, BREAST-FEEDING, SIDE-EFFECTS
See imipramine monograph.

INTERACTIONS
See imipramine monograph. Great caution with patients receiving *levothyroxine (thyroxine)* (risk of cardiac tachyarrhythmias).

POISONING/TOXICITY
See imipramine monograph with risk of agitation, confusion and restlessness and sub-coma state.

PHARMACOKINETIC PROPERTIES
Rapidly and completely absorbed from the gastrointestinal tract. Pre-systemic metabolism is approximately 40-50%. Plasma steady state levels are reached in 1-2 weeks.

EXCIPIENTS
See manufacturers SPC for further details.

LICENSED STATUS
Not licensed for depression in children. Licensed for nocturnal enuresis ≥6 years.

NTBC (2-[2-nitro-4-trifluoro-methylbenzoyl]-1,3-cyclohexanedione) (nitisinone)

Inhibitor of enzyme, 4-hydroxyphenylpyruvate dioxygenase, which is required in an early step in the catabolism of tyrosine; thus preventing formation of toxic metabolites, which lead to acute porphyria-like crisis, liver and kidney damage.

USES
Treatment of Tyrosinaemia type I.

PRESENTATION
Capsule: 2mg, 5mg and 10mg – named patient.

DOSAGE

Route	Age			Frequency (times daily)	Notes
	1 month–2 years	2–12 years	12–18 years		
Oral	← 500–750 microgram/kg →			1	Initial dose. Larger doses up to 2mg/kg/day may be required. The daily dose may be given as 2 divided doses.

N

CONTRA-INDICATIONS AND WARNINGS
Treatment with NTBC should be combined with a diet low in both tyrosine and phenylalanine in order to avoid increases in tyrosine levels which may result in crystal deposition in the cornea and skin lesions, as is seen in Tyrosinaemia type II. Plasma tyrosine levels should be kept below 600 micromol/L, if possible.

INTERACTIONS
No information available.

PREGNANCY
In vitro experiments indicate that NTBC may have weak mutagenic and/or genotoxic properties. Safety in pregnant women is not established.

BREAST-FEEDING
No information available.

SIDE-EFFECTS
Transient leucopenia and thrombocytopenia.

PHARMACODYNAMIC PROPERTIES
The primary defect in Tyrosinaemia type I is a deficiency of the enzyme fumarylacetoacetase, which catalyses the final step in the catabolism of tyrosine. The deficiency results in the accumulation of toxic metabolites, including succinylacetone, which are responsible for the renal and hepatic damage associated with the disorder. NTBC inhibits the enzyme 4-hydroxyphenylpyruvate dioxygenase (HPPD) which is active at an early stage in the catabolism of tyrosine. By preventing the formation of toxic metabolites, the acute porphyria-like crises characteristic of the disease are prevented. If started shortly after birth NTBC appears to prevent or delay the development of progressive liver disease, and possibly hepatoma. Patients with severe established disease are unlikely to benefit. Therapeutic plasma concentration of NTBC is 25-50 micromol/L.

PHARMACOKINETIC PROPERTIES
Limited information available from animal studies. Apparently well absorbed orally. Limited biotransformation, but present in plasma mainly as unchanged drug. Excreted in both urine and faeces.

LICENSED STATUS
Not licensed for use in the UK.

FURTHER INFORMATION
Available from Orphan Europe.

Nystatin

Antifungal.

USES
Prevention and treatment of candida infections of the oral cavity, oesophagus and intestinal tract. Prophylaxis against oral candidiasis in infants born to mothers with vaginal candidiasis and, if indicated, in other patient groups.

PRESENTATION
Cream: 100,000 units/g – Nystan®.
Ointment: 100,000 units/g – Nystan®.
Oral suspension: 100,000 units in 1mL – Nystan® and non-proprietary.
Pastille: 100,000 units – Nystan®.
Tablet: 500,000 units – Nystan®.

DOSAGE
Newborn Infant (birth to 1 month)

Route	Age	Frequency	Notes
	birth–1 month	(times daily)	
Oral	1mL	3	Prophylaxis administered after feeds.
	1mL	4	Treatment administered after feeds.

N

Child

Route	Age			Frequency (times daily)	Notes
	1 month–2 years	2–12 years	12–18 years		
Oral	1mL	← 1mL or 1 pastille →		4	Intestinal or oral candidiasis.
	1mL	← 1mL or 1 pastille →		4–6	Oral candidiasis in the immunocompromised.
	5mL	← 5mL or 1 tablet →		4–6	Oesophageal/intestinal candidiasis in the immunocompromised.

Continue for 48 hours after clinical cure to prevent relapse.

Topical candidiasis
Apply cream or ointment 2-4 times a day. Continue for 7 days after lesions have healed.

ADMINISTRATION
Oral: in infants and children drop suspension into the mouth. In older children retain for one minute before swallowing. Pastilles are dissolved in the mouth. Administer after meal or feed.

CONTRA-INDICATIONS & WARNINGS
Hypersensitivity to nystatin has been reported. Some nystatin oral suspension preparations contain sugar and are unsuitable for children with disaccharide intolerance. Use sugar-free brands.

INTERACTIONS
None known.

PREGNANCY/BREAST-FEEDING
Although caution is advised as no information exists, nystatin is not absorbed orally and risks are negligible.

SIDE-EFFECTS
Infrequent and generally mild and transient: nausea, vomiting, gastrointestinal distress, diarrhoea; very rarely rashes and Stevens-Johnson syndrome.

POISONING/TOXICITY
Since oral absorption is negligible no systemic toxicity is likely.

PHARMACOKINETIC PROPERTIES
Absorption from the gastrointestinal tract is negligible. Excreted in faeces.

EXCIPIENTS
Sugar is included in some brands of oral suspension; Nystan® oral suspension contains ethanol. Pastilles include dextrose monohydrate, gelatin, liquid glucose and sugar. Contact manufacturers for further details.

LICENSED STATUS
Licensed in all ages.

Octreotide

A long-acting analogue of somatostatin. It inhibits the secretion of peptides of the gastro-pancreatic endocrine system and of growth hormone.

USES
Treatment of bleeding oesophageal and gastric varices; hyperinsulinacmia (if glucagon, diazoxide and chlorothiazide fail).

PRESENTATION
Injection: 50 microgram in 1mL, 100 microgram in 1mL and 500 microgram in 1mL, 1mL ampoules; 1mg in 5mL multidose vial – Sandostatin®.

N

DOSAGE

Indication	Route	Age			Frequency	Notes
		1 month–2 years	2–12 years	12–18 years		
Varices	IV infusion	← 1 microgram/kg/hour →			continuous	Initial dose: significantly higher doses may be given to obtain control of bleeding (increases up to 3 microgram/kg/hour have been used). Wean the infusion over 24 hours before stopping to avoid rebound bleeding.
Hyper-insulinaemia	SC	← 1 microgram/kg →			4 hourly	Initial dose: increased to a maximum of 40 microgram/kg/day dependent on response.

Dosage in renal impairment
No dose adjustment required, although clearance is significantly reduced.

ADMINISTRATION
Allow the injection solution to reach room temperature before commencing administration.
IV infusion: give as a continuous IV infusion in NaCl 0.9% diluted to a ratio of not less than 1:1 and not more than 1:9. Prepared infusion should be used within 8 hours of preparation. Incompatible with glucose solutions.
Can also be given by the SC route. Administer between meals or at bedtime. Do not give around meal times.

CONTRA-INDICATIONS & WARNINGS
Contra-indications: hypersensitivity to octreotide or any excipient.
Warnings: may reduce the requirement for insulin or oral hypoglycaemic agents in patients with diabetes mellitus; inhibits gall bladder motility, bile acid secretion and bile flow. A worsening of liver disease in patients whose disease stems from biliary obstruction might be anticipated. There is a clear association between octreotide therapy and the formation of gallstones (incidence may be up to 20%) but this is unlikely to be problematic during short-term therapy. Monitor thyroid function on long-term therapy.

INTERACTIONS
Octreotide is reported to reduce the absorption of *ciclosporin (cyclosporin)*, and to delay that of *cimetidine*.

PREGNANCY
Studies in animals demonstrate transient growth retardation of the fetus, but no fetotoxic or teratogenic effects. Octreotide should not be given during pregnancy other than in the most compelling circumstances.

BREAST-FEEDING
Not recommended.

SIDE-EFFECTS
Do not appear to be dose related. Local reactions include pain, a sensation of stinging, tingling or burning at the injection site, redness and swelling (rarely lasting more than 15 minutes). Gastrointestinal effects include anorexia, nausea, abdominal pain, bloating, flatulence, loose stools, diarrhoea and steatorrhoea. In rare cases gastrointestinal symptoms may resemble those of obstruction, with progressive abdominal distension, severe epigastric pain, abdominal tenderness and guarding. Octreotide may impair post-prandial glucose tolerance. Persistent hyperglycaemia has been reported associated with chronic administration.
Hepatic dysfunction has been reported rarely. The picture is one of acute hepatitis, without cholestasis, with normalisation of transaminases on drug withdrawal, or slow development of hyper-bilirubinaemia, associated with elevations of alkaline phosphatase, gamma-glutamyl transferase, and, to a lesser extent, transaminases.

POISONING/TOXICITY
No life-threatening reactions have been reported after acute overdosage. In one case report, an IV bolus of 1mg resulted in the adult patient experiencing a brief drop in heart rate, facial flushing, abdominal cramps, diarrhoea, an empty feeling in the stomach and nausea. Signs and symptoms resolved within 24 hours. Management should be symptomatic.

PHARMACOKINETIC PROPERTIES
Octreotide is poorly absorbed orally. It is rapidly absorbed after SC and IV injection, with peak plasma

O

levels occurring after 30-60 minutes and 4 minutes respectively. Plasma protein binding 65%. Volume of distribution 0.27L/kg. There is evidence of extensive hepatic metabolism. Elimination half-life 72-98 minutes (IV). Total body clearance 11.4L/hour. Reduced to 4.5L/hour in renal failure. 11% is excreted as unchanged drug in urine, with 2% unchanged in faeces.

EXCIPIENTS
Multidose vials contain phenol. See manufacturers SPC for further details.

LICENSED STATUS
Not licensed for use in children.

Olanzapine

Atypical antipsychotic.

USES
Treatment of schizophrenia and mania.

PRESENTATION
Tablets: 2.5mg, 5mg, 7.5mg, 10mg and 15mg – Zyprexa®.
Orodispersible tablet: 5mg, 10mg and 15mg – Zyprexa® Velotab®.

DOSAGE

Route	Age		Frequency	Notes
	12–18 years			
Oral	5-20mg		1	Initial dose. Titrate from initial dose up to the usual dose of 10mg once daily.

ADMINISTRATION
Velotab® can be placed on tongue and allowed to dissolve, or dispersed in water, orange juice, apple juice, milk or coffee.

CONTRA-INDICATIONS & WARNINGS
May exacerbate, possibly precipitate, diabetes mellitus, low white blood cell count or liver dysfunction. Caution in galactosaemia and phenylketonuria due to excipients.

INTERACTIONS
Carbamazepine induces metabolism and lowers blood levels. CYP1A2 inhibitors (e.g. *fluvoxamine, ciprofloxacin, ketoconazole*) raise blood levels of olanzapine.

PREGNANCY
Contra-indicated on general grounds as no specific information.

BREAST-FEEDING
Manufacturer advises against.

SIDE-EFFECTS
Drowsiness and weight gain are relatively common. Postural hypotension and peripheral oedema less so. Blood dyscrasias, seizures, hyperglycaemia, extra-pyramidal syndromes, neuroleptic malignant syndrome rare.

POISONING/TOXICITY
Agitation, tachycardia and extrapyramidal symptoms leading to sedation. No specific antidote. Activated charcoal reduces bioavailability. ECG monitoring advisable. Avoid sympathomimetics.

PHARMACOKINETIC PROPERTIES
Rapidly absorbed. Peak plasma concentrations reached within 5-8 hours. Hepatic metabolism to inactive glucuronide through cytochrome P450 channels. Elimination half-life approximately 33 hours.

EXCIPIENTS
Velotab® includes aspartame. See manufacturers SPC for further details.

LICENSED STATUS
Not licensed for use in children.

Olsalazine sodium

Aminosalicylate.

USES
Treatment of acute mild ulcerative colitis and the maintenance of remission.

PRESENTATION
Capsule: 250mg – Dipentum®.
Tablet: 500mg – Dipentum®.

DOSAGE

Route	Age			Frequency (times daily)	Notes
	1 month–2 years	2–12 years	12–18 years		
Oral (acute ulcerative colitis)	–	← 500mg →		2	Initial dose. The dose may be titrated upwards over 1 week to a maximum of 3g per **day** in divided doses. A single dose should not exceed 1g.
Oral (maintenance)	–	← 250-500mg →		2	

ADMINISTRATION
Oral: take at end of a meal to reduce risk of loose stools and diarrhoea. Capsules can be opened and the contents sprinkled onto food.

CONTRA-INDICATIONS & WARNINGS
Hypersensitivity to salicylates. Serious blood dyscrasias have been reported very rarely.

PREGNANCY
Only use if potential benefit outweighs risk to fetus, experience in human pregnancy is limited.

BREAST-FEEDING
Contact local Medicines Information Centre for advice.

SIDE-EFFECTS
Gastrointestinal side-effects most common e.g. diarrhoea (can be controlled by taking with meal, reducing dose or dose titration). Arthralgia, rash, blood dyscrasias have been reported.

POISONING/TOXICITY
No specific antidote. Treatment should be supportive.

PHARMACOKINETIC PROPERTIES
Systemic absorption is minimal. 99% of an oral dose will reach the colon. Converted to 5-aminosalicylic acid (5-ASA) in the colon, which acts topically on colonic mucosa

LICENSED STATUS
Not licensed for use in children.

FURTHER INFORMATION
Can be used concomitantly with corticosteroids. Since olsalazine acts locally at the target site and the action is not systemic there is no logical reason to reduce the adult dose in children.

Omeprazole

Suppresses gastric acid secretion by inhibiting the parietal cell H^+/K^+ ATP pump.

USES
Treatment of oesophageal reflux disease.
Prophylaxis against bleeding from oesophageal and gastric varices.
Acid related problems resistant to ranitidine.
Helicobacter pylori eradication in patients with duodenal ulcers.
Persistant fat malabsorption despite optimal use of enzyme replacement in cystic fibrosis.

O

PRESENTATION
Capsule: 10mg, 20mg and 40mg – Losec® and non-proprietary.
Tablet: 10mg, 20mg and 40mg – non-proprietary.
Tablet: 10mg, 20mg and 40mg (all dispersible) – Losec® MUPS®.
Injection: 40mg vial (with 10mL solvent) – Losec®.
Intravenous infusion: 40mg – Losec®.

DOSAGE

Route	Age			Frequency	Notes
	1 month–2 years	2–12 years	12–18 years	(times daily)	
Oral	initially				Dose should preferably be rounded to
	← 700 microgram/kg →		20–40mg	1	the nearest oral dose form. Initial dose
	increasing as necessary to			1	is given once daily; higher doses may
	3mg/kg/day				be given in 2 divided doses.
Oral for *H. pylori*	>1 year				Treatment for 14 days with amoxicillin
	← 1-2mg/kg →		40mg	1	and clarithromycin, or amoxicillin and
	rounded to nearest 10mg to				metronidazole, or clarithromycin and
	a maximum of 40mg				metronidazole (see individual drug monographs for doses).
IV infusion/ IV injection	initially				*There is limited data on IV
	← 500 microgram/kg →		40mg	1	administration in children. Initial dose is
	increasing as necessary to				given once daily; higher doses may be
	2mg/kg/day				given in 2 divided doses if necessary.

* The IV dose given above is based on the relative bioavailability by the oral and IV routes. There is very limited published information on IV doses in children.

ADMINISTRATION
Oral: if capsules cannot be swallowed whole then they can be opened and the intact enteric coated granules mixed in an acidic drink e.g. orange or apple juice and then swallowed without chewing. Alternatively the MUPS® tablets can be dispersed in water, fruit juice or yogurt. For narrow bore nasogastric or PEG tubes the MUPS® tablets should be dispersed in a large volume of water or a suspension can be made using the granules as follows: add the enteric-coated granules to 10mL of sodium bicarbonate 8.4% and leave to stand for about 10 minutes until a turbid suspension is formed. Administer the suspension immediately and flush the tube with water. The patient may be pre-treated with a solution of sodium bicarbonate 8.4%, to buffer the pH of the stomach. This is not necessary for administration via a jejunostomy tube as the jejunostomy pH is already alkaline.
Injection: slow IV bolus over at least 2.5-5 minutes at a rate not exceeding 2mL per minute. The IV solution should be used within 4 hours of reconstitution.
Infusion: the vial of omeprazole powder should be dissolved in 100mL of NaCl 0.9% or glucose 5% for infusion. No other solutions should be used. The infusion should then be given at a suitable rate. The infusion should be complete within 12 hours of reconstitution if NaCl 0.9% is used and within 3 hours if glucose is used.

NB. Preparations for infusion and injection are distinct and separate.

CONTRA-INDICATIONS AND WARNINGS
Treatment with omeprazole may mask the symptoms of other gastric disease. Caution should be exercised in patients with hepatic impairment since both bioavailability and half-life may increase. Patients transferred from capsules to tablets should be monitored for any reports of 'flare up' of disease symptoms.

INTERACTIONS
Omeprazole may delay the excretion of *diazepam*, *phenytoin* and *warfarin*. Close monitoring of *phenytoin* and *warfarin* levels is advised, with dose adjustment as necessary. Plasma concentrations of both omeprazole and *clarithromycin* are increased during concurrent treatment for *H. pylori* eradication. The bioavailability of *digoxin* is increased by omeprazole due to raised gastric pH. Absorption of *ketoconazole* and *itraconazole* may be reduced.

PREGNANCY
Safety in pregnant women is not established. Animal studies have revealed no teratogenic effect, but reproduction studies have revealed reduced litter weight. Contact local Medicines Information Centre for advice.

BREAST-FEEDING
Contact local Medicines Information Centre for advice.

SIDE-EFFECTS
Side-effects are generally mild.
CNS: headache.
Dermatological: rash, urticaria and pruritus.
Gastrointestinal: diarrhoea, nausea and vomiting, flatulence, abdominal pain.
An increased frequency of gastric glandular cysts has been noted on prolonged treatment. These are considered to be a physiological response to prolonged inhibition of gastric acid secretion. The cysts are benign and apparently reversible. Isolated cases have been reported of irreversible visual impairment in critically ill patients who have received IV omeprazole, particularly at high doses. No causal relationship has been established.

POISONING/TOXICITY
Doses of ten times the normal dose do not result in any apparent change to the elimination mechanisms, and supportive treatment only is indicated, as required.

PHARMACOKINETIC PROPERTIES
Adults: oral absorption 50-65% (capsules and tablets are bioequivalent); pre-systemic metabolism (faecal excretion): 20%; plasma half-life 1 hour (range 0.5-1.5 hours); volume of distribution 0.3-0.4L/kg; plasma protein binding (albumin) 95%; almost completely metabolised to 6 inactive metabolites, which are excreted in the urine.

EXCIPIENTS
See manufacturers SPC for further details.

LICENSED STATUS
Capsules and tablets licensed in children ≥ 2 years of age for the treatment of severe ulcerating reflux oesophagitis. The injection and the infusion are not licensed for use in children.

Ondansetron

$5HT_3$ receptor antagonist.

USES
Chemotherapy and radiotherapy induced nausea and vomiting.
Post-operative nausea and vomiting (PONV).
Pruritus.

PRESENTATION
Injection: 2mg in 1mL, 2mL and 4mL ampoules – Zofran®.
Oral lyophilisates: 4mg and 8mg – Zofran Melt®.
Syrup: 4mg in 5mL – Zofran®.
Tablet: 4mg and 8mg – Zofran®.

DOSAGE

Indication	Route	Age			Frequency (times daily)	Notes
		1 month–2 years	2–12 years	12–18 years		
Emetogenic chemotherapy	IV	← 5mg/m² → (maximum 8mg)		8mg	single dose (immediately prior to chemotherapy)	Can be repeated every 8–12 hours during chemotherapy and for at least 24 hours after chemotherapy. or
	Oral	then ← 4mg →		8mg	2-3	Give orally after initial IV dose. Continue oral treatment for up to 5 days after a course of chemotherapy.

O

DOSAGE continued

Indication	Route	Age			Frequency (times daily)	Notes
		1 month– 2 years	2–12 years	12–18 years		
PONV	IV slow injection	–	100 microgram/kg (maximum 4mg)	4mg	single dose	For prevention >12 years give at induction of anaesthesia; for 2–12 years give prior to, or after, induction of anaesthesia. The same dose can be used for the treatment of established PONV.
Pruritus	Oral	← 2-4mg →		4–8mg	2	
Palliative care	IV or SC infusion	← 5mg/m² →			continuous over 24 hours	Used for antiemesis and pruritis in palliative care.

ADMINISTRATION
Oral: the melt tablets melt in the mouth; no water required, but they must be swallowed (not bucally absorbed).
IV: injection over 2-5 minutes; infusion over 15 minutes diluted in glucose 5% or NaCl 0.9%.

NB. In palliative care ondansetron has been administered as a 24 hourly SC or IV infusion.

CONTRA-INDICATIONS AND WARNINGS
Hypersensitivity to any component of the preparation.

INTERACTIONS
No specific interactions reported.

PREGNANCY
Ondansetron is not teratogenic in animals, but there is no experience in human pregnancy therefore use only if expected benefit to patient outweighs potential risk to fetus.

BREAST-FEEDING
Not recommended; ondansetron passes into breast milk.

SIDE-EFFECTS
Headache, constipation.

POISONING/TOXICITY
Symptomatic and supportive measures as required.

PHARMACOKINETIC PROPERTIES
Disposition after oral and IV dosing is similar. Clearance and volume of distribution are age-dependent. Clearance 300mL/minute at 12 years, falling to 100mL/minute at 3 years. Volume of distribution 75L at 12 years falling to 17L at 3 years. Clearance is primarily by hepatic metabolism and in patients with marked hepatic impairment clearance is significantly reduced. In patients with severe renal impairment the pharmacokinetics of ondansetron are essentially unchanged.

EXCIPIENTS
Oral solution includes sorbitol. Melt tablets include aspartame. See manufacturers SPC for further details.

LICENSED STATUS
Licensed for use in children and adults. Not licensed for pruritis.

FURTHER INFORMATION
Ondansetron dosage and scheduling is often dictated by local policy and treatment guidelines. It is often administered as a component of a multi-drug anti-emetic regime dictated by the emetic potential of the chemotherapy. The late-emesis characteristic of some highly emetogenic chemotherapy regimes may require continued treatment with IV or oral ondansetron. There is published evidence that ondansetron may not be the best anti-emetic for delayed nausea and vomiting; domperidone alone or in combination may be superior.

Oral rehydration salts

When reconstituted with water these form isotonic solutions of glucose and sodium which stimulate intestinal water absorption.

USES
Correction of fluid and electrolyte loss in diarrhoea.

O

PRESENTATION

Dioralyte® oral powder blackcurrant or citrus flavoured or natural
Each sachet contains:
Sodium chloride 470mg
Potassium chloride 300mg
Glucose 3.56g
Disodium hydrogen citrate 530mg

Dioralyte® effervescent tablets blackcurrant or citrus flavoured
Each tablet contains:
Sodium chloride 117mg
Potassium chloride 186mg
Anhydrous glucose 1.62g
Citric acid anhydrous 384mg
Sodium bicarbonate 336mg

Dioralyte® relief oral powder apricot, blackcurrant or raspberry flavoured. Rice based product with lower osmolarity than glucose based products
Each sachet contains:
Cooked rice powder 6g
Sodium chloride 350mg
Potassium chloride 300mg
Sodium citrate 580mg

Diocalm Junior® orange
Each sachet contains:
Sodium chloride 350mg
Potassium chloride 300mg
Sodium citrate 590mg
Anhydrous glucose 4g

Electrolade® banana, blackcurrant, melon or orange flavoured or plain
Each sachet contains:
Sodium chloride 236mg
Potassium chloride 300mg
Sodium bicarbonate 500mg
Anhydrous glucose 4g

Rehidrat® oral powder blackcurrant, lemon and lime or orange flavour
Each sachet contains:
Sodium chloride 440mg
Potassium chloride 380mg
Sodium bicarbonate 420mg
Citric acid 440mg
Glucose 4.09g

Lemon and lime or orange flavour also contain:
Fructose 70mg
Sucrose 8.07g

Blackcurrant flavour also contains:
Fructose 10mg
Glucose 4.13g
Sucrose 8.17g

DOSAGE/ADMINISTRATION
According to fluid loss
Infant: 1-1.5 times the usual 24 hour feed volume or 150mL/kg/**day** given in divided doses.
Child: 200mL solution after each loose motion.
Adult: 200-400mL solution after each loose motion.

O

Powder in sachets: reconstitute the sachets with the quantity of water recommended i.e. 250mL for Rehidrat®, 200mL for other preparations. Use sterile or freshly boiled and cooled water for infants.
Effervescent tablets: dissolve 2 tablets in 200mL of water. Only use for ≥1 year of age.

CONTRA-INDICATIONS & WARNINGS
Inappropriate in intestinal obstruction requiring surgical intervention, renal failure with oliguria or anuria, intractable vomiting and severe dehydration or severe infantile diarrhoea where parenteral therapy is required. Care should be taken when used in patients with severe renal or hepatic impairment who have underlying electrolyte disturbances.

PREGNANCY/BREAST-FEEDING
Not contra-indicated.

POISONING/TOXICITY
In significant overdose monitor serum electrolytes and correct as necessary.

LICENSED STATUS
Licensed for all ages; except Dioralyte® effervescent tablets which are licensed for use ≥1 year of age.

FURTHER INFORMATION
In initial stage of diarrhoea, all foods including cow's milk and artificial milk formulas should be stopped. Breast milk should not be stopped – give oral rehydration fluid then put to breast until satisfied. Return to normal diet gradually once rehydrated. If patient also vomiting take small amounts of oral rehydration solution.
Once prepared, solutions can be refrigerated for up to 24 hours. Do not prepare a weaker or stronger solution than that recommended.

Oxandrolone

A synthetic androgenic anabolic steroid.

USES
Androgen replacement in constitutional delayed growth and puberty in boys.
Turner syndrome in girls (sometimes used particularly in late presentation in combination with growth hormone – not standard management).

PRESENTATION
Tablet: 2.5mg – named patient.

DOSAGE/ADMINISTRATION
Oral: 1.25-2.5mg once daily, generally for about 3-6 months, but has been used occasionally for up to 1 year; evidence suggests using doses as low as 625 micrograms for Turner syndrome, in combination with growth hormone – seek expert advice before prescribing.

CONTRA-INDICATIONS & WARNINGS
Contra-indicated in severe hepatic impairment. Caution in patients with a history of diabetes, malignancy, cardiac, hepatic or renal impairment. Monitor skeletal maturation in young patients.

INTERACTIONS
Warfarin: effect may be enhanced.

PREGNANCY/BREAST-FEEDING
Not applicable.

POISONING/TOXICITY
No information.

SIDE-EFFECTS
Sodium retention with oedema, virilisation, premature epiphyseal closure; jaundice can occur if given for long periods.

PHARMACOKINETIC PROPERTIES
Rapidly absorbed from the gastrointestinal tract following oral administration. It is excreted mainly in the urine as metabolites and unchanged oxandrolone; small amount excreted in faeces.

LICENSED STATUS
Not licensed for use in the UK

FURTHER INFORMATION
Available via IDIS World Medicines.

Antiepileptic.

USES
Monotherapy and adjunctive therapy for partial seizures with or without secondary generalised tonic-clonic seizures.

PRESENTATION
Tablet: (scored) 150mg, 300mg and 600mg – Trileptal®.

DOSAGE
See table

Route	Age		Frequency	Notes
	2–12 years	12–18 years	(times daily)	
Oral	≥6 years 4–5mg/kg	–	2	Initial dose in adjunctive and monotherapy: increase dose by a maximum of 5mg/kg/dose twice daily, at weekly intervals. Adjunctive therapy: maximum dose of 15mg/kg twice daily. Monotherapy: Maximum dose of 23mg/kg twice daily.
	–	4–5mg/kg (maximum initial dose 300mg)	2	Initial dose. Increase by 300mg/dose twice daily at weekly intervals. Usual dose range 300mg -1.2g twice daily. NB in adjunctive therapy, patients may require dose reduction of concomitant antiepileptics when using high doses of oxcarbazepine.

ADMINISTRATION
Doses of other anticonvulsants may require reduction with higher doses of oxcarbazepine. No dose adjustment required in mild to moderate liver disease. No information for severe renal impairment. Decrease starting dose by 50% in mild impairment (< 30ml/minute/1.73m^2) and adjust cautiously according to response.

CONTRA-INDICATIONS AND WARNINGS
Hypersensitivity to *carbamazepine* (although not an absolute contra-indication to using oxcarbazepine as there is a 30-50% cross-reactivity). Caution in liver and renal disease, hyponatraemia, heart failure and cardiac conduction disorders. Counsel patients on recognition of blood, hepatic and skin disorders. Avoid use within 2 weeks of *MAOIs* including the antibacterial *linezolid*. Avoid abrupt withdrawal.

PREGNANCY
Increased risk of neural tube defects and other malformations. Refer for specialist counselling and screening. Administer folate supplements before and during pregnancy. Administer vitamin K during last weeks of pregnancy and to newborn to prevent bleeding disorders in the newborn.

BREAST-FEEDING
Excreted in breast milk; manufacturer advises to avoid breast-feeding. Contact local Medicines Information Centre for advice.

SIDE-EFFECTS
Gastrointestinal, CNS, skin, visual, hyponatraemia.

Severe blood, liver and skin disorders or hypersensitivity reactions may occur. Some patients cross react with *carbamazepine*.

INTERACTIONS
May increase plasma levels of *phenobarbital* (*phenobarbitone*) and *phenytoin*. May decrease levels of *carbamazepine* and increase metabolite levels. May reduce effect of *oral contraceptives*. Levels of oxcarbazepine active metabolite may be decreased by *carbamazepine, phenobarbital, phenytoin* and *sodium valproate*.

PHARMACOKINETICS
After oral administration oxcarbazepine is completely absorbed and extensively metabolised to its pharmacologically active metabolite (the monohydroxy derivative, (MHD)). The apparent volume of distribution of MHD is 49 litres. Approximately 40% of MHD is bound to plasma proteins. Oxcarbazepine is cleared from the body mostly in the form of metabolites predominantly via the kidneys. The plasma half-life of oxcarbazepine varies between 1.3-2.3 hours and the plasma half-life of MHD averages 9.3 ± 1.8 hours. Steady-state plasma concentrations of MHD are reached within 2-3 days in twice daily dosing.

O

POISONING

No specific antidote. Symptomatic and supportive treatment should be administered as appropriate. Removal of the drug by gastric lavage and/or inactivation by administering activated charcoal should be considered.

EXCIPIENTS

See manufacturers SPC for further details.

LICENSED STATUS

Licensed for ≥6 years of age.

Oxybutynin

Antimuscarinic agent.

USES

Urgency; urinary frequency and incontinence; nocturnal enuresis; neurogenic bladder instability.

PRESENTATION

Elixir: 2.5mg in 5mL – Ditropan®.
Oral solution: 5mg in 5mL – manufactured 'special'.
Intravesical instillation: 5mg in 30mL – named patient.
Tablet: 2.5mg – Ditropan® and non-proprietary; 3mg – Cystrin® and non-proprietary; 5mg – Cystrin®, Ditropan® and non-proprietary.

DOSAGE

Route	Age			Frequency	Notes
	2–12 years		12–18 years	(times daily)	
Oral	<5 years	>5 years			12–18 years
	1.25–2.5mg	2.5–5mg	5mg	2–3	Maximum dose of 5mg four times daily.
Intravesical instillation	5mg		5mg	2–3	

ADMINISTRATION

Intravesical: administer into the bladder if side-effects from oral administration cannot be tolerated.

CONTRA-INDICATIONS & WARNINGS

Significant bladder outflow obstruction, intestinal atony, severe ulcerative colitis, toxic megacolon and glaucoma.

INTERACTIONS

Potentiation of anticholinergic effect is possible if administered with other *anticholinergic agents.*

PREGNANCY

There is no experience of the use of oxybutynin in human pregnancy. Use only if considered essential. Contact local Medicines Information Centre for advice.

BREAST-FEEDING

Passes into breast milk, but effect on the infant not known. Contact local Medicines Information Centre for advice.

SIDE-EFFECTS

Dry mouth, constipation, blurred vision, nausea, abdominal discomfort, facial flushing, headache, dizziness, diarrhoea.

POISONING/TOXICITY

Symptoms: progress from intensification of usual side-effects of CNS disturbances (from restlessness and excitement to psychiatric behaviour), circulatory changes (flushing, fall in blood pressure, circulatory failure etc.), respiratory failure, paralysis and coma. Contact National Poisons Information Centre for advice.

EXCIPIENTS
Elixir includes sorbitol and sucrose. Oral solution includes sorbitol and saccharin sodium. Contact manufacturers for further details.

LICENSED STATUS
Ditropan® and Cystrin® are licensed >5 years of age for nocturnal enuresis and neurogenic bladder disorders. The intravesical preparation and the oral solution are unlicensed products.

FURTHER INFORMATION
The intravesical preparation should be stored in the refrigerator. Oral solution available from Rosemont Pharmaceuticals.

Oxygen

USES
To correct hypoxia, to reduce pulmonary vascular tone and treatment of carbon monoxide poisoning.

PRESENTATION
Piped hospital supply, cylinders of varying capacity, oxygen concentrators, liquid oxygen.

DOSAGE
Dependent on condition. In some conditions (e.g. bronchopulmonary dysplasia), very low flow rates (e.g. 0.1L/minute) may maintain oxygen saturation.

ADMINISTRATION
Inhalation: nasal prongs, face mask, tracheostomy adapter. With or without humidification.

CONTRA-INDICATIONS & WARNINGS
In infants the amount of oxygen (as a percentage) each baby is breathing should be recorded regularly and adjusted as necessary. Caution in hypercapnia – titrate dose carefully to avoid hypoventilation secondary to abolition of hypoxic respiratory drive.

PREGNANCY/BREAST-FEEDING
No problems associated with use in pregnancy or breast-feeding.

SIDE-EFFECTS
Retinopathy of prematurity in newborn infants.

POISONING/TOXICITY
Prolonged high concentrations can be toxic to the pulmonary epithelium and hyperbaric oxygen can cause convulsions.

FURTHER INFORMATION
Special low flow meters and regulators are available. Portable cylinders and portable liquid oxygen reservoirs are available if mobility is required. Cylinders, concentrators and liquid oxygen are available for home use.

Oxytetracycline

A tetracycline antibiotic.

USES
Treatment of acne, alternative to macrolides in infections due to mycoplasma and chlamydia, also brucellosis and Lyme-disease.

PRESENTATION
Tablet: 250mg – non-proprietary.

O

DOSAGE

Indication	Route	Age		Frequency	Notes
		12–18 years		(times daily)	
Acne	Oral	250–500mg		12 hourly	
Infection	Oral	250–500mg		6 hourly	See guidance section.

ADMINISTRATION

Oral: swallow with plenty of liquid. Avoid taking milk, iron or indigestion remedies at the same time of day as oxytetracycline. Best taken an hour before food, or on an empty stomach.

CONTRA-INDICATIONS & WARNINGS
Avoid in liver or renal impairment. Contra-indicated in children <12 years as it adversely affects tooth development (discolouration and enamel hypoplasia).

INTERACTIONS
Absorption may be impaired by *aluminium, calcium, magnesium, zinc* or *iron salts*. Long-term therapy depresses plasma prothrombin activity so *anticoagulant* dose may need to be reduced. Concurrent use of *oral contraception* – possibility of reduced contraceptive effect.

PREGNANCY/BREAST-FEEDING
Contra-indicated.

SIDE-EFFECTS
Gastrointestinal: nausea, vomiting, diarrhoea. *Skin:* maculopapular and erythematous rashes. *Photosensitivity:* discontinue if erythema occurs. *Hypersensitivity reactions:* urticaria, anaphylaxis. *Blood:* haemolytic anaemia, thrombocytopenia, neutropenia and eosinophilia.

POISONING/TOXICITY
Overdosage: supportive treatment.

PHARMACOKINETIC PROPERTIES
Oxytetracycline is readily absorbed orally. 40-70% is excreted unchanged in urine. Half-life is 6-10 hours. Concentrates in hepatic system, excreted in bile and faeces.

EXCIPIENTS
Contact manufacturer for further details.

LICENSED STATUS
Not licensed for use in children <12 years of age.

Palivizumab (humanised respiratory syncytial virus (RSV) monoclonal antibody)

USES
For passive protection against lower respiratory tract infection caused by RSV in children born at <36 weeks gestation and <6 months of age at the beginning of the RSV season, or in children <2 years of age and who had bronchopulmonary dysplasia within the last 6 months.

PRESENTATION
Injection: (powder for reconstitution) 50mg and 100mg – Synagis®.

DOSAGE
15mg/kg once monthly, starting just prior to the beginning of the RSV season, for a total of 5 doses.

ADMINISTRATION
IM: injection preferably in the anterolateral aspect of the thigh. Slowly add 0.6mL of Water for Injections for the 50mg vial or 1mL for the 100mg vial along the inside of the wall of the vial to minimise foaming. Tilt vial slightly and rotate gently for 30 seconds. DO NOT SHAKE the vial. Allow reconstituted solution to stand at room temperature for 20 minutes until the solution clarifies. Administer within 3 hours of reconstitution and discard any remaining after use.

CONTRA-INDICATIONS/WARNINGS
The only contra-indication is an anaphylactic reaction to a previous dose of this preparation, its constituents or any other humanised monoclonal antibody. Care should be taken in patients with thrombocytopenia or any coagulation disorders due to the IM route of administration.

INTERACTIONS
As the antibody is specific to RSV, there is no interaction with active vaccines.

SIDE-EFFECTS
Occasionally it may give rise to mild local reactions, fever and irritability.

POISONING/TOXICITY
No medical consequences were seen in three patients who received greater than recommended doses.

PHARMACOKINETIC PROPERTIES
Mean half-life of 20 days in paediatric studies.

EXCIPIENTS
See manufacturers SPC for further details.

LICENSED STATUS
Licensed for use as detailed above.

FURTHER INFORMATION
While undoubtedly safe and effective (reduces admissions by about 50%), it is unclear whether this preparation is cost-effective. More work on this aspect is needed.

Pancreatin

USES
Treatment of pancreatic insufficiency.

PRESENTATION
Capsule: enteric-coated microspheres in capsules.

Preparation	Protease units	Amylase units	Lipase units
Creon 10000®	600	8000	10,000
Creon 25000®	1000	18,000	25,000
Pancrease®	330	2900	5000
Pancrease HL®	1250	22,500	25,000
Pancrex V®	430	9000	8000
Pancrex V '125'®	160	3300	2950
Nutrizym GR®	650	10,000	10,000
Nutrizym 10®	500	9000	10,000
Nutrizym 22®	1100	19,800	22,000

Granules: enteric-coated microspheres.

Preparation	Protease units	Amylase units	Lipase units
Creon® Micro	200 per 100mg	3600 per 100mg	5000 per 100mg

Creon® Micro: 20g – named patient.

Tablet: enteric-coated, sugar-coated.

Preparation	Protease units	Amylase units	Lipase units
Pancrex V®	110	1,700	1,900
Pancrex V forte®	330	5,000	5,600

Powder

Preparation	Protease units	Amylase units	Lipase units
Pancrex V®	1400/g	30,000/g	25,000/g

P

DOSAGE
Dose varies widely and should be tailored to each individual patient according to symptoms, stool type and abdominal findings; should not exceed 10,000 lipase units per kg body weight per day.

ADMINISTRATION
Capsules may be swallowed whole immediately prior to eating or opened and contents sprinkled on soft food, which should be swallowed immediately without chewing.
Powder can be given mixed in with each feed in newborn infants although this is not routinely done in practice – it is preferred to mix the enteric-coated granules with a small amount of bottle or breast milk and administer from a spoon.

CONTRA-INDICATIONS & WARNINGS
Contra-indicated in early acute stages of pancreatitis and in patients with history of hypersensitivity to porcine proteins.

INTERACTIONS
No interactions known.

PREGNANCY
Inadequate evidence of safety during pregnancy. Contact local Medicines Information Centre for advice.

BREAST-FEEDING
Contact local Medicines Information Centre for advice.

SIDE-EFFECTS
Nausea and vomiting, abdominal discomfort, hyperuricaemia and hyperuricosuria, hypersensitivity, oral and rectal irritation (consider using a barrier cream).

POISONING/TOXICITY
Perianal irritation. Colonic stricture has been reported with high doses.

EXCIPIENTS
See manufacturer's SPC for further details.

LICENSED STATUS
All preparations licensed for use in all age groups, except Creon® Micro which is unlicensed for use in the UK.

FURTHER INFORMATION
Creon® Micro is available from Solvay Healthcare.
The CSM has advised of data associating the high strength pancreatin preparations Nutrizym 22® and Pancrease HL® with the development of fibrosing colonopathy in children with cystic fibrosis aged between 2-13 years. No association was found with Creon 25000®.
The following was recommended: Pancrease HL® and Nutrizym 22® should not be used in children ≤15 years of age with cystic fibrosis. The total dose of pancreatic enzyme supplements used in patients with cystic fibrosis should not usually exceed 10,000 units of lipase per kg body weight per day. If a patient on any pancreatin preparation develops new abdominal symptoms (or change in existing symptoms) the patient should be reviewed to exclude the possibility of colonic damage. It is important to ensure adequate hydration at all times in patients receiving higher strength pancreatin preparations.

A competitive non-depolarising muscle relaxant with a medium duration of action.

USES
Neuromuscular blockade for ventilation and surgical procedures.

PRESENTATION
Injection: 2mg in 1mL, 2mL ampoule – non-proprietary.

DOSAGE
Newborn infant (birth to 1 month)

Route	Age		Frequency	Notes
	birth–1 month		(times daily)	
IV loading	100 microgram/kg		single dose	
IV maintenance	50 microgram/kg		4–6	As need arises.

Child

Route	Age			Frequency	Notes
	1 month–2 years	2–12 years	12–18 years	(times daily)	
IV	← 60–100 microgram/kg →			single dose	Initial dose. Subsequent doses 10-20 microgram/kg – adjusting dose and interval as required.

ADMINISTRATION
IV: bolus administration. Can be diluted in NaCl 0.9% or glucose 5% if needed.

CONTRA-INDICATIONS & WARNINGS
Use with caution in severe renal impairment as duration of action is prolonged. Since pancuronium causes relaxation of the respiratory muscles, respiration must be assisted in all patients.

PREGNANCY
There is insufficient data available to assess potential harm to the fetus; very little crosses the placenta. Studies have shown its safety for use in caesarian section.

BREAST-FEEDING
There is no available evidence that breast-feeding after a mother has been given pancuronium, has any adverse effects on the baby.

INTERACTIONS
Effects enhanced by *procainamide, quinidine, aminoglycosides, polymyxin, propranolol, nifedipine, verapamil, lithium, magnesium salts, clindamycin* and *baclofen*. Antagonised by *cholinergics*.

SIDE-EFFECTS
Mild sustained increase in heart rate and blood pressure. Joint contractures responsive to gentle physiotherapy have been reported in a few chronically paralysed babies.

POISONING/TOXICITY
Reversed by atropine (20 microgram/kg) followed by IV neostigmine (80 microgram/kg).

PHARMACOKINETIC PROPERTIES
Major elimination by the kidney, reduced clearance in renal failure.

EXCIPIENTS
Contact manufacturer for further details.

LICENSED STATUS
Licensed for use in all ages.

P

Analgesic and antipyretic.

USES
Mild to moderate pain, pyrexia.

PRESENTATION
Oral solution: 120mg in 5mL – non-proprietary.
Oral suspension: 120mg in 5mL and 250mg in 5mL – non-proprietary.
Suppository: 60mg, 120mg, 125mg, 240mg, 250mg and 500mg -non-proprietary. 30mg and 1g – manufactured 'special'.
Tablet: 500mg – non-proprietary.
Tablet (dispersible): 120mg and 500mg – non-proprietary.

DOSAGE/ADMINISTRATION
Analgesic/antipyretic/post-operative pain relief – newborn infant (birth to 1 month)

Route	Age			Frequency	Notes
	preterm 28–32 weeks	preterm 32–36 weeks	birth–1 month	(times daily)	
Oral loading dose	←	20mg/kg	→	single dose	
Oral maintenance dose	15mg/kg	–		12 hourly	Maximum **daily** dose 30mg/kg.
	–	← 20mg/kg	→	8 hourly	Maximum **daily** dose 60mg/kg.
Rectal loading dose	20mg/kg	← 30mg/kg	→	single dose	
Rectal maintenance dose	15mg/kg	–		12 hourly	Maximum **daily** dose 30mg/kg.
	–	← 20mg/kg	→	8 hourly	Maximum **daily** dose 60mg/kg.

Child – analgesic/antipyretic

Route	Age			Frequency	Notes
	1 month–2 years	2–12 years	12–18 years	(times daily)	
Oral loading dose	← 20mg/kg	→	–	single dose	
Oral maintenance dose	**DOSE BY WEIGHT** ← 1–3 months → 20mg/kg ← > 3 months → 15mg/kg		– –	8 hourly 4–6 hourly	Maximum total dose in 24 hours: <3 months: 60mg/kg >3 months–12 years: 90mg/kg >12 years: 4g.
	DOSE BY AGE 1–3 months ← 30–60mg → 3 months – 1 year ← 60–120mg → 1–5 years ← 120–250mg → 6–12 years ← 250–500mg →		500mg - 1g	8 hourly 4–6 hourly 4–6 hourly 4–6 hourly	
Rectal loading dose	1–3 months ← 30mg/kg → > 3 months ← 40mg/kg →		–	single dose single dose	

DOSAGE/ADMINISTRATION continued

Route	Age			Frequency	Notes
	1 month–2 years	2–12 years	12–18 years	(times daily)	
Rectal maintenance dose	DOSE BY WEIGHT ← 20mg/kg →		-	see by age below	Maximum total dose in 24 hours: <3 months: 60mg/kg
	DOSE BY AGE				>3 months-12 years: 90mg/kg
	1-3 months				>12 years: 4g.
	← 30-60mg →			8 hourly	
	3 months - 1 year				
	← 60-125mg →			4-6 hourly	
	1-5 years				
	← 125-250mg →			4-6 hourly	
	6-12 years				
	← 250-500mg →	500mg - 1g		4-6 hourly	

Note: the maximum dose should be reviewed after 48 hours for < 3 months old and after 72 hours for > 3 months old.

Post–operative pain relief (over 3 months)
The total daily dose may be increased to 90mg/kg/**day** (maximum 4g) orally or rectally, for 48 hours. Give loading dose of 20mg/kg then 15mg/kg orally or 30mg/kg then 20mg/kg rectally up to 4 hourly. Give regular doses for first 24–48 hours.

Renal failure
Dose interval not <6 hours in moderate impairment (creatinine clearance 10–50mL/min/1.73m^2) and not <8 hours in severe impairment (creatinine clearance <10mL/minute/1.73m^2). Significantly removed by haemodialysis; give dose after haemodialysis. Not significantly removed by CAPD.

Liver failure
Dose-related toxicity: avoid large doses.

CONTRA-INDICATIONS & WARNINGS
Cautions: renal failure and liver failure – see dosage section. Use with care in patients taking other drugs that affect the liver.

INTERACTIONS
Prolonged, regular use may prolong prothrombin time with *warfarin; metoclopramide* and *domperidone* enhance and *colestyramine (cholestyramine)* reduces absorption of paracetamol. Increased risk of neutropenia with *zidovudine* (possibly due to reduced metabolism).

PREGNANCY
There is no evidence that paracetamol in therapeutic dosage is associated with any specific problems during pregnancy despite placental transfer. It is recommended as the mild analgesic of choice.

BREAST-FEEDING
Amount excreted into breast milk is too small to be harmful.

SIDE-EFFECTS
Side-effects are rare but rashes and blood disorders have been reported.

POISONING/TOXICITY
Most children who accidentally ingest paracetamol do not require active treatment. They seldom seem to ingest sufficient to be at risk of liver damage and they may also metabolise the drug differently from adults. Significant paracetamol poisoning in childhood is usually intentional. Paracetamol in acute overdosage is hepatotoxic and nephrotoxic but toxicity takes 3–4 days to reach a peak. The only early features of poisoning are nausea and vomiting and these usually settle within 24 hours. The time interval since ingestion is critical in assessing whether treatment is required, but is often difficult to establish. Patients/carers often give inaccurate histories. If there is doubt about the timing or the need for treatment, treat. The treatment lines on the accompanying graph are estimates of risk based on the best available clinical evidence. They are critically dependent upon the accuracy of the history with respect to time of overdose ingestion. Beyond 15 hours the risk estimates are even less reliable and clinical judgement becomes more important in management.

Management within 4 hours of ingestion
If more than 150mg/kg has been taken: consider activated charcoal. There is little evidence that gastric lavage will be of benefit in a child in whom paracetamol is known to have been the only substance ingested. Wait until 4 hours from ingestion have elapsed then take a

P

venous blood sample for measurement of the plasma paracetamol concentration; if there is absolute certainty that a single dose of paracetamol <150mg/kg body weight has been ingested or <75mg/kg in children at enhanced risk of developing severe liver damage, this can reasonably be considered unnecessary and the child may be discharged. Plasma concentration measured less than 4 hours post-ingestion cannot be interpreted. If the serum level is on or above the paracetamol graph treatment line (see graph page 473) then acetylcysteine should be given (see monograph page 4 for dosing schedule). The high risk treatment line should be used if the child has existing liver disease, is malnourished, is on enzyme-inducing drugs (e.g. *carbamazepine*, *phenobarbital (phenobarbitone)*, *phenytoin*, *rifampicin*) or is HIV positive, as these patients are at higher risk of liver damage. A child need not be admitted if the plasma paracetamol concentration is below the relevant line on the graph and the history is consistent with <150mg/kg body weight of paracetamol having been ingested.

Management 4–8 hours post ingestion

It is too late for gastric emptying or activated charcoal to be of value. Measure the plasma paracetamol concentration as soon as possible. If the result will be known within 8 hours of ingestion wait for result to determine need for acetylcysteine. If the plasma paracetamol concentration will not be known within 8 hours of ingestion give acetylcysteine immediately if >150mg/kg has been taken; do not wait for results. When the result is received refer to the paracetamol graph to determine if acetylcysteine should be continued, stopped or started. When acetylcysteine is started within 8 hours of the overdosage it is reasonable to expect patients to be declared fit for discharge from medical care on completion of its administration. However, INR, plasma creatinine and ALT should be checked for normality on completion of treatment and before discharge. Advice should be given to return to hospital if vomiting or abdominal pain develop or recur.

Management 8–15 hours post ingestion

Give acetylcysteine immediately if the patient has taken >150mg/kg body weight. DO NOT WAIT for the result of the plasma paracetamol concentration. The efficacy of acetylcysteine declines rapidly during this period and must therefore be given urgently. Measure the plasma paracetamol concentration. When the result is received refer to the graph to determine if acetylcysteine should be continued, stopped or started. Those being treated with acetylcysteine should also have their INR, plasma creatinine and ALT measured at the end of the infusion. If any of these are abnormal or the patient is symptomatic, further monitoring is required and advice should be sought from a National Poisons Information Centre.

Management 15–24 hours post ingestion

Give acetylcysteine to all patients unless convinced that <150mg/kg has been taken. Measure the plasma paracetamol concentration. Measure the INR, plasma creatinine and ALT concentrations at the end of the acetylcysteine infusion. The patient may be discharged medically if there are no symptoms and the INR, plasma creatinine and ALT are normal. They should be advised to return to hospital if vomiting or abdominal pain develop. If the INR, plasma creatinine or ALT are abnormal, liver and renal function should be monitored for 72–96 hours post ingestion and damage managed conventionally.

Management >24 hours post ingestion

Measure the INR, plasma creatinine and ALT. Discuss case with a specialist liver unit especially if any of the above are abnormal, encephalopathy or hypotension is present or there is pre-existing liver disease.

Staggered overdosage

In patients who have taken several overdoses of paracetamol over a short period of time (staggered overdose), the plasma paracetamol concentration will be meaningless in relation to the treatment graph. Such patients should be considered to be at serious risk and treated with acetylcysteine. They can be discharged after acetylcysteine treatment or 24 hours from the last paracetamol dose provided they are asymptomatic and the INR, plasma creatinine and ALT are normal.

Oral methionine (refer to methionine monograph) can be given for suspected poisonings where delay prior to IV acetylcysteine therapy is anticipated e.g. in remote areas. Once the patient reaches hospital the need to continue treatment must be assessed. It may also be given if a patient has ingested >150mg/kg paracetamol and presents within 4 hours of ingestion. It can however cause vomiting in which case it will not be known if the entire dose has been absorbed; anti-emetic drugs can help prevent this. The patient will still need to have plasma paracetamol levels taken 4 hours after ingestion and acetylcysteine given if indicated.

PHARMACOKINETIC PROPERTIES

Paracetamol is readily absorbed from the gastrointestinal tract with peak plasma concentration occurring about 10-60 minutes after oral administration with adequate levels maintained for 2-4 hours. It crosses the blood-brain barrier and placenta. Absorption from the rectum is slow, irregular and prolonged in older children but similar to oral in neonates and infants. It is metabolised predominantly in the liver and the metabolites excreted in the urine. Clearance is slower in premature neonates and initially in term neonates but quickly approaches that of older children and adults.

Paracetamol is metabolised in the liver by three main pathways, sulphation, glucoronidation and oxidation. The products of sulphation and glucoronidation are non-toxic but that of oxidation is highly reactive. It is rendered non-toxic by preferential conjugation with glutathione. The relative capacities of these systems and the ability to synthesise glutathione varies with age. In neonates sulphation is the most important pathway for paracetamol metabolism. The ratio of glucoronidation to sulphation increases with age. Neonates have a greater ability to synthesize glutathione than adults. This may explain the lower incidence of liver failure due to paracetamol overdose in young children than in adults.

P

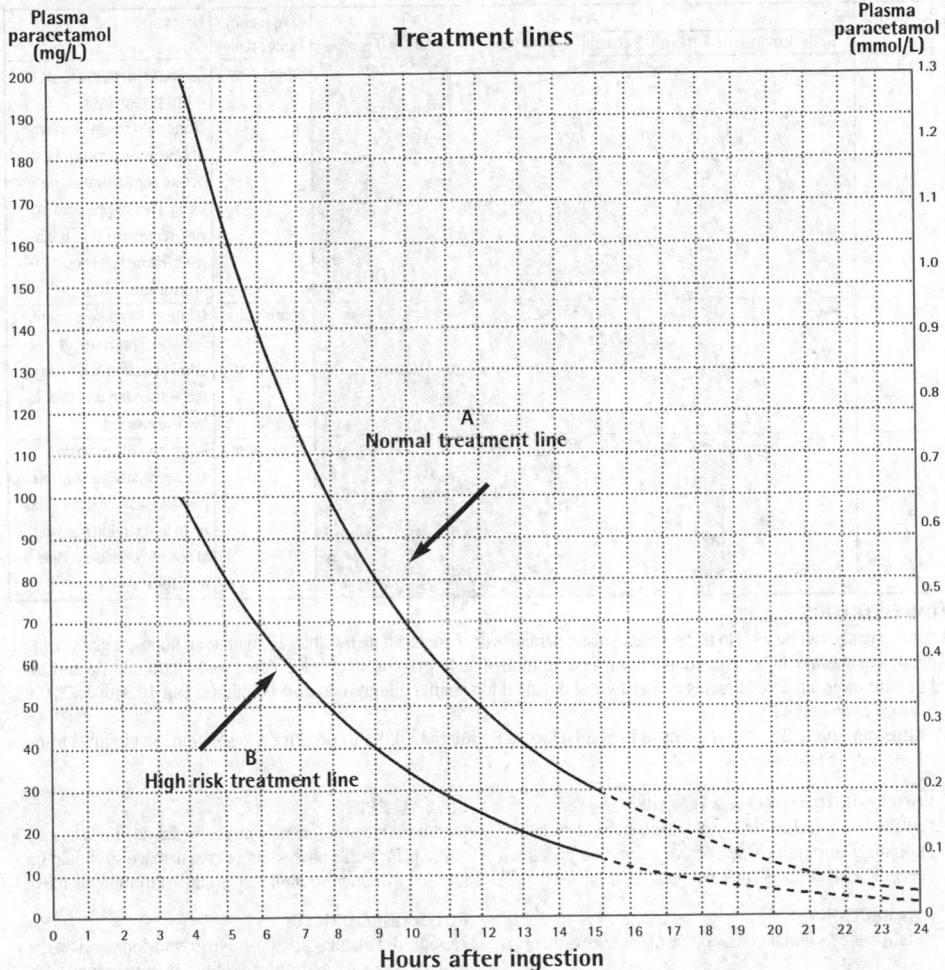

Treatment lines

Plasma paracetamol (mg/L)

Plasma paracetamol (mmol/L)

A — Normal treatment line

B — High risk treatment line

Hours after ingestion

EXCIPIENTS
Contact manufacturers for further details.

LICENSED STATUS
The 30mg and 1g suppositories are 'specials' and as such are not licensed. All other preparations are licensed >2 months for post immunisation pyrexia and >3 months as an antipyretic and analgesic.

Antiepileptic.

USES
Treatment of convulsive status epilepticus (see status epilepticus algorithm).

PRESENTATION
Enema: equal parts paraldehyde and olive oil – may be extemporaneously prepared or manufactured 'special'.
Injection: 5mL ampoules – non-proprietary.

DOSAGE

Route	Age				Frequency (times daily)	Notes
	birth–1 month	1 month–2 years	2–12 years	12–18 years		
Rectal	← 0.4mL/kg →			5–10mL	single dose	Doses stated in mL/kg or as mL of paraldehyde. Dilute with an equal volume of olive or sunflower oil before administration, or if using a ready-prepared 'special', remember that it is already diluted and dose accordingly.
IV infusion	← 1–4 mL/kg/hour of 5% solution →				continuous	Dilute to 5% before administration. This route of administration is no longer recommended and should be discouraged.
IM	0.2mL/kg	← 0 .1–0.15mL/kg →		5–10mL	single dose	IM use should be avoided whenever possible. May cause pain and sterile abscess. Maximum 5mL (1mL in neonates) at one site. Consider adding hyaluronidase 150 units.

ADMINISTRATION
A plastic syringe can be used to measure/administer paraldehyde if contact time less than 10 minutes, if not use a glass syringe.
Rectal: enema may be extemporaneously prepared immediately prior to use, using equal parts paraldehyde and olive oil or sunflower oil; avoid arachis oil because of potential for peanut allergy. Can also be diluted 1 in 10 with NaCL 0.9% and given as an enema.
IV infusion: dilute 2.5mL paraldehyde in 50mL glucose 5% or NaCl 0.9% to produce 5% solution. Stable for 24 hours (but see note in table above).

CONTRA-INDICATIONS & WARNINGS
Caution in respiratory or hepatic disease. Avoid rectal use in colitis. Old paraldehyde (brown coloration and smell of acetic acid) is dangerous and must never be used.

INTERACTIONS
Sedative effects enhanced by other *CNS depressants*.

PREGNANCY
No information on congenital abnormality. Crosses the placenta and may cause neonatal depression. Contact local Medicines Information Centre for advice.

BREAST-FEEDING
Excreted in breast milk. Contact local Medicines Information Centre for advice.

SIDE-EFFECTS
Rectal administration may cause irritation. IM use may cause pain, sterile abscess and nerve damage so should be avoided. IV administration may produce thrombophlebitis.

POISONING/TOXICITY
Laboured breathing, acidosis, liver and kidney damage may be seen. Use supportive therapy and contact UK National Poisons Information Service.

PHARMACOKINETIC PROPERTIES
Metabolised extensively in the liver, excreted unchanged through the lung. Variable, prolonged half-life in neonates of up to 27 hours, 7 hours in children.

EXCIPIENTS
Contact manufacturers for further details.

LICENSED STATUS
Injection licensed for status epilepticus in children and adults but by IM and rectal routes only. Enema is a 'special' or prepared extemporaneously and as such is unlicensed.

FURTHER INFORMATION
Avoid prolonged contact of undiluted paraldehyde with rubber and plastics.

Paromomycin sulphate

P

Aminoglycoside antibiotic which is used as a luminal or contact amoebicide.

USES
Amoebiasis; asymptomatic intestinal carriage.
Cutaneous leishmaniasis: topically as an ointment.

PRESENTATION
Tablet: 250mg paromomycin base – named patient (imported).
Oral syrup: 125mg paromomycin base in 5mL – named patient (imported).
Ointment: paromomycin 15% plus methylbenzethonium chloride 12% – named patient (imported).

DOSAGE

Indication	Route	Age			Frequency (times daily)	Notes
		1 month– 2 years	2–12 years	12–18 years		
Intestinal amoebiasis	Oral	–	← 8.3–11.6mg/kg →		3	For 5–10 days.
Cutaneous leishmaniasis	Topical	–	← Apply as necessary →		2	For 10 days or longer.

ADMINISTRATION
Oral: give with or after meals.

CONTRA-INDICATIONS & WARNINGS
Patients with a known hypersensitivity to the drug. Patients with intestinal obstruction. Use with caution in renal impairment and in those with ulcerative intestinal lesions. During treatment monitor renal function and hearing in order to quickly detect signs of ototoxicity or nephrotoxicity. Not to be used in the treatment of extra-intestinal amoebiasis as paromomycin is only active against intestinal protozoa.

INTERACTIONS
Do not give with other *ototoxic* or *nephrotoxic* drugs in order to avoid any additive effects.

PREGNANCY
Because paromomycin is poorly absorbed from the gastrointestinal tract it may be useful in the treatment of intestinal infections during pregnancy; nevertheless only use when considered essential.

BREAST-FEEDING
Excretion in human milk is not expected as paromomycin is not absorbed systemically after oral dosing. Poor lipid solubility also limits its passage into milk.

SIDE EFFECTS
Nausea, vomiting, diarrhoea, abdominal cramps. Rash, headache and dizziness occasionally. Rarely nephrotoxicity and ototoxicity due to inadvertent absorption.

POISONING/TOXICITY
Symptoms: nausea, vomiting and diarrhoea; nephrotoxicity and ototoxicity can occur.
Treatment: symptomatic and supportive.

PHARMACOKINETIC PROPERTIES
Poorly absorbed from the gastrointestinal tract; most of an oral dose is excreted unchanged in the faeces. Impaired gastrointestinal motility or lesions in the intestines facilitate absorption of the drug which is then slowly excreted in the urine.

EXCIPIENTS
Gabboral® syrup includes saccharin sodium and sorbitol.

LICENSED STATUS
Not licensed for use in the UK.

FURTHER INFORMATION
Available from IDIS World Medicines.

Paroxetine

Selective serotonin re-uptake inhibitor (SSRI).

USES
Obsessive-compulsive disorder (OCD). Panic and anxiety disorder, including social phobia. Idiopathic musculoskeletal pain.

PRESENTATION
Tablet: 20mg and 30mg – Seroxat®.
Liquid: 10mg in 5mL – Seroxat®.

DOSAGE

Indication	Route	Age		Frequency (times daily)	Notes
		2–12 years	12–18 years		
Obsessive compulsive disorder	Oral	–	20mg (maximum 60mg)	1	Initial doses. Increase gradually if necessary, in weekly increments of 10mg, to the maximum dose. Give as a single morning dose.
Panic disorder	Oral	–	10mg (maximum 40mg)	1	
Idiopathic musculoskeletal pain	Oral	≥ 8 years 10mg	20mg	1	

CONTRA-INDICATIONS & WARNINGS, INTERACTIONS, PREGNANCY, BREAST-FEEDING, POISONING/TOXICITY
See fluoxetine monograph.
The MHRA advise that paroxetine should not be used in children and adolescents under the age of 18 years with major depressive disorder.

SIDE-EFFECTS
See fluoxetine monograph. May be relatively higher rate of extrapyramidal side-effects and agitated confusion on withdrawal. Can exacerbate symptoms of panic disorder initially.

PHARMACOKINETIC PROPERTIES
Well absorbed following oral administration and undergoes first-pass metabolism. The elimination half-life is variable but is generally about 24 hours. Steady state systemic levels are attained by 7-14 days after starting treatment. Extensively metabolised by the liver with only 1-2% excreted unchanged in the urine.

EXCIPIENTS
Liquid includes sorbitol and saccharin sodium. See manufacturers SPC for further details.

LICENSED STATUS
Not licensed for use in children.

P

USES
As part of a complete IV nutrition regimen providing a source of trace elements for children <40kg.

PRESENTATION
Solution: trace elements (traces of Zn^{2+}, Mn^{2+}, Cu^{2+}, Se^{4+}, F⁻ and I⁻), 10mL vial – Peditrace® (see manufacturers SPC for further details).

DOSAGE
1mL/kg up to a maximum dose of 15mL.

ADMINISTRATION
IV: maximum concentration 6mL in 100mL of compatible fluid (glucose IV infusions) administered over at least 8 hours. Usually administered as part of an IV feed (e.g. Vaminolact®, Vamin® 14 Electrolyte-Free) over 24 hours. In this case the maximum concentration is 1mL in 100mL of solution.

CONTRA-INDICATIONS & WARNINGS
Injection should not be given undiluted. Record baseline whole blood and serum manganese level within or below the normal range and normal liver function before administering Peditrace® for >1 month. Monitor manganese levels and liver function monthly for patients on long-term PN. Caution in impaired renal and hepatic function (monitor manganese levels).

SIDE-EFFECTS
Impaired renal or hepatic excretion may lead to chronic overdose of one or more trace elements.

PHARMACOKINETIC PROPERTIES
Excretion both biliary and renal.

LICENSED STATUS
Licensed for use in children and infants.

Pegaspargase

Oncospar® pegaspargase is a pegylated form of E. coli asparaginase.

Asparaginase inhibits protein synthesis in tumour cells dependent on exogenous asparagine, a non-essential amino acid in humans.

USES
Acute lymphoblastic leukaemia.

PRESENTATION
Injection: 3750 international unit, 5mL vial – Oncospar®.

DOSAGE
** Always consult the current treatment protocol for details of dosage and scheduling. **

ADMINISTRATION
IM: maximum volume at a single site is 2mL.
IV: give over 1-2 hours in 100mL NaCl 0.9% or glucose 5% via the side arm of a fast running drip.

CONTRA-INDICATIONS & WARNINGS
Contra-indications: previous serious allergic reaction to pegaspargase. Patients with pancreatitis or previous history of pancreatitis. Patients who have had significant haemorrhagic events associated with prior L-asparaginase.

INTERACTIONS
Depletion of serum proteins by pegaspargase may increase the toxicity of other drugs that are protein bound. Pegaspargase may interfere with drugs such as *methotrexate* which require cell replication for their lethal effects. Caution should be taken when administering any concurrent anticoagulant therapy such as w*arfarin, heparin, dipyridamole, aspirin* or *NSAIDs* due to imbalances in coagulation factors noted with pegaspargase.

P

PREGNANCY
It is not known whether pegaspargase causes fetal harm or affects reproductive capacity, therefore it should not be administered to pregnant women.

BREAST-FEEDING
There are no reports of pegaspargase being given to women who are breast-feeding and safety is not established. A decision must be made whether to continue breast-feeding or discontinue the drug given the importance of the drug to the mother.

SIDE-EFFECTS
Hypersensitivity reactions: may be acute or delayed and include acute anaphylaxis, bronchospasm, dyspnoea, urticaria, arthralgia, erythema, induration, oedema, pain, tenderness, hives, chills, fever and rash.
Gastrointestinal: pancreatitis, sometimes fulminant and fatal. Increased serum amylase and lipase have also occurred. Anorexia, constipation, diarrhoea, indigestion, flatulence, mucositis, colitis, nausea and vomiting have been observed.
Hepatic: elevations of enzymes and bilirubin, jaundice, ascites and hypoalbuminaemia associated with peripheral oedema. These are usually reversible. Fatty changes in the liver and liver failure have also been observed.
Haematological: hypofibrinogenemia, prolonged prothrombin time (PT) and activated partial thromboplastin time (APTT). Thromboses, leucopenia, agranulocytosis, pancytopenia and thrombocytopenia, disseminated intravascular coagulation, haemolytic anaemia and anaemia have been observed.
Metabolic: hyperglycaemia, hypoglycaemia, uric acid nephropathy, hyperuricaemia, hypoproteinaemia and peripheral oedema have been observed. Hypoalbuminaemia, proteinuria, weight loss and metabolic acidosis have occurred. Blood ammonia may increase due to conversion of L-asparagine to aspartic acid.
Neurological: status epilepticus, temporal lobe seizures, somnolence, coma, malaise, dizziness, headache, paraesthesias, mood changes, night sweats and Parkinson-like syndrome have occurred. These are usually reversible.
Renal: increased blood urea nitrogen (BUN), creatinine, urine frequency, haematuria (due to thrombocytopenia), haemorrhagic cystitis, renal dysfunction and renal failure.
Respiratory: cough, epistaxis, bronchospasm and upper respiratory tract infection (URTI).
Skin: itch, alopecia, blisters, purpura, hand whiteness, nail changes, erythema and rash are reported. Injection site reactions include pain, swelling and redness.

POISONING/TOXICITY
Facilities should be available to manage anaphylaxis and patients should be observed for 1 hour after administration. Reactions during infusion may be managed by administration of an antihistamine and slowing the infusion down. No specific measures are recommended in overdose.

PHARMACOKINETIC PROPERTIES
Apparent volume of distribution is equal to plasma volume. Plasma half-life is 5.8 days. After administration, L-asparaginase is measurable in plasma for at least 15 days.

EXCIPIENTS
See manufacturers SPC for further details.

LICENSED STATUS
Not licensed for use in the UK. It is licensed in Germany for treatment of children and adults.

FURTHER INFORMATION
Oncospar® can be purchased from Medac (UK) via UDG Ltd (tel: 0177 3510 123).

Penicillamine

Inhibits T-cell function and impairs antigen presentation.
Therapy may result in marked decrease in IgM and rheumatoid factor. Reduces copper concentrations by chelating copper which is then excreted in the urine.

USES
Systemic sclerosis; Wilson's disease.

PRESENTATION
Tablet: 125mg and 250mg – Distamine®, Pendramine® and non-proprietary.

DOSAGE

Indication	Route	Age			Frequency	Notes
		1 month–2 years	2–12 years	12–18 years	(times daily)	
Systemic sclerosis	Oral	← 1.25–2.5mg/kg → increased gradually to 7.5–10mg/kg		62.5–125mg increased gradually to 250–375mg	2 2	Initial dose: dose is increased at 4 weekly intervals over a period of 3–6 months.
Wilson's disease	Oral	← 2.5mg/kg →		750mg–1g	2	Start with 2.5mg/kg twice daily to avoid precipitating neurological decompensation. Increase every 1-2 weeks to 20mg/kg/day.

Full blood count (FBC), platelet count and urinalysis should be performed prior to treatment with penicillamine. Urinalysis and FBC should be carried out monthly during treatment. Caution should be exercised in patients with renal insufficiency, and modification of the dosage may be necessary. Renal function should be assessed monthly. An immediate blood count should be carried out if neutropenia or thrombocytopenia are suspected due to symptoms such as a sore throat, glossitis, buccal ulceration, easy bruising or bleeding. If any abnormal results are found, treatment should be withheld and discussed with the clinician responsible for the child's care. Severe dyspepsia or taste disturbances may necessitate dosage reduction.

ADMINISTRATION
Oral: tablets should be taken half to one hour before food.

CONTRA-INDICATIONS & WARNINGS
Patients who have previously experienced agranulocytosis or severe thrombocytopenia due to penicillamine, patients with systemic lupus erythematosus.

INTERACTIONS
Sucralfate, antacids and *iron preparations* may substantially reduce the absorption of penicillamine. Separate their administration by at least 2 hours. *Digoxin* levels may be reduced by penicillamine. Monitor *digoxin* levels during concomitant therapy. Concomitant use of penicillamine and *gold salts* may release *gold* from tissues leading to bone marrow suppression and rashes, even many months after *gold therapy* has been discontinued.

PREGNANCY
Penicillamine crosses the placenta to the fetus. Most reports do not support an association between the drug and significant teratogenic effects. Although there is a lack of consensus, most references recommend avoiding penicillamine during pregnancy if possible, or at least reducing the daily dose to 500mg or less. Contact local Medicines Information Centre for advice.

BREAST-FEEDING
There are no reports of the use of penicillamine while breast-feeding and it is not known how much the drug is excreted in the milk. In view of the lack of data, penicillamine should not be used to treat mothers who wish to breast-feed. Contact local Medicines Information Centre for advice.

SIDE-EFFECTS
Nausea, vomiting, epigastric discomfort, diarrhoea, allergic reactions (urticaria, erythema, hyperpyrexia), loss or impairment of taste (usually resolves spontaneously), thrombocytopenia, neutropenia, aplastic anaemia, proteinuria, stomatitis.

POISONING/TOXICITY
There is no specific antidote. Treatment of penicillamine overdosage is symptomatic. Withdrawal of the drug is necessary if serious side-effects (as listed above) occur.

PHARMACOKINETIC PROPERTIES
Penicillamine is rapidly absorbed from the gastrointestinal tract, with peak concentrations in blood seen 1-3 hours after administration.

EXCIPIENTS
See manufacturers SPC for further details.

LICENSED STATUS
Licensed for use in children and adults.

FURTHER INFORMATION
Consider co-administration of pyridoxine to prevent deficiency secondary to penicillamine.

Aromatic diamidine and an antiprotozoal agent.

USES
Pneumocystis carinii pneumonia (PCP); antimony resistant visceral and cutaneous leishmaniasis; trypanosomiasis (Gambian disease).

PRESENTATION
Injection: powder for reconstitution, 300mg vial – Pentacarinat®.
Nebuliser solution: 300mg in 10mL – Pentacarinat®.

DOSAGE

Indication	Route	All ages	Frequency	Notes
Treatment of PCP	IV infusion/IM	4mg/kg	once daily	Continue for 14–21 days.
	Inhalation	600mg	once daily	
Prophylaxis of PCP	Inhalation	300mg	once monthly	Ongoing.
Leishmaniasis – visceral	IM (deep)	4mg/kg	alternate days	To a maximum of 10 injections. May repeat if necessary.
Leishmaniasis – cutaneous	IM (deep)	4mg/kg	once or twice weekly	Ongoing until condition resolves.
Trypanosomiasis (Gambian disease)	IV infusion/ IM (deep)	4mg/kg	once daily or on alternate days	To a total of 7-10 injections.

Renal insufficiency
Life threatening cases of PCP dose once daily for 7–10 days, then alternate days to complete a course of at least 14 doses.

ADMINISTRATION
Reconstitute in a vertical laminar flow cabinet or fume cupboard.
IM injection: 1 vial should be dissolved in 3mL of Water for Injections and the necessary dose administered by deep IM injection.
IV infusion: 1 vial should be reconstituted with 3–5mL Water for Injections and the necessary dose may later be further diluted in 50–250mL of glucose 5% or NaCl 0.9% and given over at least 60 minutes with the patient supine.
Inhalation: reconstitute 300mg vial with 4-6mL Water for Injections and administer using a suitable nebuliser in a vacated, well ventilated room. Do not mix with other drugs.

Displacement value: 300mg pentamidine isetionate displaces approximately 0.15mL of water.

CONTRA-INDICATIONS & WARNINGS
Adverse effects are relatively common and are life threatening. Protect personnel during handling and administration.
Caution and careful monitoring of the following is needed:
Hypotension: baseline blood pressure; dose administration supine; monitor blood pressure during infusion.
Hypoglycaemia: fasting blood glucose daily during therapy, weekly after therapy.
Cardiac arrhythmias: ECG twice weekly.
Acute pancreatitis: amylase weekly.
Renal insufficiency: urea, creatinine and electrolytes daily; urine analysis daily.
Hepatic dysfunction: bilirubin, enzymes daily during therapy, weekly after therapy.
Leucopenia: FBC twice weekly.
Hypocalcaemia: calcium weekly.

INTERACTIONS
Avoid concomitant use with other nephrotoxic drugs – *aminoglycosides, amphotericin B, foscarnet.* Caution with other drugs that can cause hypoglycaemia, e.g. *foscarnet.* Increased risk of ventricular arrhythmias if given with *amiodarone.* Increased risk of pancreatitis with *didanosine, stavudine, lumivudine.*

PREGNANCY/BREAST-FEEDING
No information available. Contact local Medicines Information Centre for advice.

SIDE-EFFECTS
See under warnings above; also bronchospasm with inhalation route which may be prevented by prior use of bronchodilators.

POISONING
Symptomatic treatment of effects as cited under warnings.

PHARMACOKINETICS
Rapidly distributed to body tissues after IV administration followed by a prolonged elimination phase. Half-life after IV administration is about 6 hours and about 9 hours after IM administration.

EXCIPIENTS
See manufacturers SPC for further details.

LICENSED STATUS
Pentacarinat® injection is licensed for use in children and adults; Pentacarinat® nebuliser solution is licensed for use in adults only.

FURTHER INFORMATION
All bystanders, including medical personnel, are advised to minimise exposure to atmospheric pentamidine from nebulisers. 1.74mg pentamidine isetionate ≡ 1mg pentamidine base.

Peppermint

Direct relaxant of intestinal smooth muscle.

USES
Relief from gastrointestinal pain due to smooth muscle spasm.
Infantile colic (peppermint water).

PRESENTATION
Capsule: 0.2mL peppermint oil – Colpermin®, Mintec®.
Peppermint water: may be extemporaneously prepared. See further information.

DOSAGE

Preparation	Route	Age			Frequency (times daily)	Notes
		1 month–2 years	2–12 years	12–18 years		
Peppermint water (see further information)	Oral	3-6 months 2.5mL <u>6 months –2 years</u> 5mL	10-40mL	–	4	20 minutes before feeds/ food. Dilute well with water. Do not give to infants < 3 months of age.
Peppermint oil capsules	Oral	–	–	<u>12-15 years</u> 1 capsule <u>>15 years</u> 1-2 capsules	3 \n\n 3	Swallow whole with water 30-60 minutes before meals.

ADMINISTRATION
Capsules should not be broken or chewed because peppermint oil may irritate the mouth or oesophagus.

CONTRA-INDICATIONS & WARNINGS
May aggravate gastro-oesophageal reflux. Not to be used in paralytic ileus. Colpermin® capsules contain refined peanut (arachis) oil. A double blind placebo controlled trial of administration of refined peanut oil to patients known to be sensitive to peanuts did not result in allergic reactions.

INTERACTIONS
Antacids should not be taken at the same time of day as peppermint oil capsules.

SIDE-EFFECTS
Peppermint oil capsules: occasional heartburn, perianal irritation; allergic reactions to menthol, which are rare

but include erythematous skin rash, headache, bradycardia, muscle tremor and ataxia.

PREGNANCY
No data to establish safety in pregnancy.

BREAST-FEEDING
Significant levels of menthol in breast milk unlikely.

POISONING/TOXICITY
Peppermint oil capsules: in the event of overdosage patients should be observed and symptomatic and supportive treatment carried out if necessary. Symptoms can include a burning sensation in the mouth and throat, hypersalivation, vomiting, diarrhoea, CNS stimulation, excitement and convulsions. If a substantial quantity of peppermint oil capsules have been recently ingested, gastric lavage may be undertaken (within 1 hour of ingestion) if the airway can be protected.

EXCIPIENTS
Colpermin® capsules contain peanut (arachis) oil. Contact manufacturers for further details.

LICENSED STATUS
Colpermin® capsules are licensed ≥15 years of age.
Mintec® capsules are licensed for adults.

FURTHER INFORMATION
Peppermint Water BP 1973 is the preparation for which dosages are given in this monograph. This constitutes a 1 in 40 dilution of Concentrated Peppermint Water BP 1973. Deaths have occurred with the wrong dilution.
To prepare Peppermint Water BP 1973, 2.5mL of Concentrated Peppermint Water should be diluted to 100mL with freshly boiled and cooled water.
The Concentrated Peppermint Water (which is 40 times as strong as Peppermint Water BP 1973) should be **NEVER** be given undiluted.

Permethrin

Parasiticidal agent.

USES
Treatment of scabies and head lice.

PRESENTATION
Dermal cream: 5% – Lyclear® Dermal Cream.
Cream rinse: 1% – Lyclear® Creme Rinse.

DOSAGE/ADMINISTRATION
Scabies (dermal cream)
Single topical application of up to:
1 tube for children >12 years.
Half a tube for children aged 6-12 years.
A quarter of a tube for children aged 1-5 years.
An eighth of a tube for children aged 2 months – 1 year.

Medical supervision required for children <2 years of age. If necessary a second application may be given not less than 7 days after the initial application.

Apply to whole body excluding head. Wash off after 8-12 hours. Children <2 years old should also have the cream applied to the face, neck, scalp and ears. If hands or any part are washed, the treatment must be reapplied.

Head lice (cream rinse)
Apply to clean damp hair, leave on for 10 minutes, rinse and dry. Not affected by chlorine in swimming pools.

CONTRA-INDICATIONS & WARNINGS
Avoid contact with eyes. Do not use on broken or secondarily infected skin.

INTERACTIONS
None known.

PREGNANCY
Use only if clearly needed.

BREAST-FEEDING
Not known if excreted. The low concentrations that theoretically will be in breast milk are unlikely to present any risk.

SIDE-EFFECTS
Pruritus, erythema, and stinging.

POISONING/TOXICITY
Gastric lavage should be considered if within 2 hours of ingestion.

PHARMACOKINETIC PROPERTIES
0.5% of applied permethrin is absorbed in first 48 hours.

EXCIPIENTS
See manufacturers SPC for further details.

LICENSED STATUS
Licensed for use in children, but medical supervision required <2 years of age for scabies treatment with the dermal cream and <6 months of age for head lice treatment with the cream rinse.

Pertussis vaccine

Single antigen pertussis vaccine, whether whole cell or acellular, is no longer available in the UK. Both are available in combination with diphtheria and tetanus toxoids (DTwP and DTaP). They are also available combined with diphtheria, tetanus and Hib (DTwP-Hib) and the acellular vaccine with diphtheria, tetanus and inactivated polio (DTaP-IPV). If one or more doses of pertussis vaccine were omitted from the primary course and it is desired to complete a course of three doses of pertussis vaccination diphtheria/ tetanus/ pertussis vaccine should be used. The Department of Health has provided the following recommended schedule.

Age group	Scenario		Advice
	DT immunisation history (DTaP, DTwP or DT)	P immunisation history (DTaP, DTwP or aP)	DTaP = diphtheria, tetanus, acellular pertussis vaccine. DTwP = diphtheria, tetanus, whole cell pertussis vaccine.
Infants and children to 3 1/2 years	3 of 3 doses of DT primary course	No immunisation against pertussis	☐ DTwP# at around first birthday or at least 6 months after the third dose of DT.
	3 of 3 doses of DT primary course	1 dose of a pertussis- containing vaccine	
	3 of 3 doses of DT primary course	2 doses of a pertussis- containing vaccine	☐ DTaP as a preschool booster, at least 1 year after the third dose of DT.
	2 of 3 doses of DT primary course	No immunisation against pertussis	☐ DTwP# at least one month after previous dose of DT. ☐ And DTwP# at around first birthday or at least 6 months after the previous dose of DTP. ☐ DTaP as a pre-school booster, at least 1 year after the third dose of DT.
	2 of 3 doses of DT primary course	1 dose of a pertussis containing vaccine	☐ DTwP# at least one month after previous dose of DT/P. ☐ And DTwP# at around first birth-day or at least 6 months after the previous dose of DTP. ☐ DTaP as a preschool booster, at least 1 year after the 3rd dose of DT.

P

Age group	Scenario		Advice
	DT Immunisation history DTaP, DTwP or DT)	P immunisation history (DTaP, DTwP or aP)	DTaP = diphtheria, tetanus, acellular pertussis vaccine. DTwP = diphtheria, tetanus, whole cell pertussis vaccine.
Infants and children to 3 1/2 years	1 of 3 doses of DT primary course	No immunisation against pertussis	☐ 2 doses of DTwP# one month apart and at least one month after last dose of DT. ☐ And DTwP# at around first birthday or at least 6 months after the previous dose of DTP. ☐ DTaP as a preschool booster, at least 1 year after the 3rd dose of DT.
Children 3 1/2-7 years	Child has had no primary doses of DT or P		☐ Give 3 doses of DTaP one month apart and a 4th dose of DTaP as a preschool booster at least 1 year after the 3rd dose of DTP.
	Child has not completed DT or P primary courses and presents for pre-school booster		☐ Give DTaP as a pre-school booster and one further dose of DTaP, one year later, to complete 4 doses of P where possible and 5 doses of DT.
	Child has completed DT primary course (3 doses) and presents for pre-school booster with no or incomplete pertussis immunisation		☐ Give DTaP as a pre-school booster and one further dose of DTaP, one year later, to complete 4 doses of P where possible and 5 doses of DT.
Children >7 years*	Child presents with no or incomplete pertussis immunisation		☐ There is currently no pertusssis containing vaccine licensed for immunisation of this group. Immunisation with DT or Td should be completed according to the age of the child.

☐ The current DTaP preparation (Infanrix®) is licensed for use in children up to and including 6 years of age.

☐ DTaP# should be used as appropriate when a severe reaction to DTwP has occurred (Department of Health. *Immunisation against infectious disease*. London: HMSO, 1996).

After two doses of pertussis vaccine a child is likely to be protected against serious disease.
Note: This is general guidance. In special circumstances further advice should be sought.

Pethidine hydrochloride (controlled drug)

Synthetic opioid analgesic.

USES
Moderate to severe acute pain.

PRESENTATION
Tablet: 50mg – non-proprietary.
Injection: 50mg in 1mL; 1mL and 2mL ampoules; 10mg in 1mL, 5mL and 10mL ampoules – non-proprietary.

DOSAGE

Route	Age				Frequency	Notes
	birth–1 month	1 month–2 years	2–12 years	12–18 years	(times daily)	
Oral	500 microgram –1mg/kg	← 500 microgram–2mg/kg →		50–100mg	single dose	≤ 2 months: can be repeated every 10-12 hours.
SC/IM	500 microgram –1mg/kg	500 microgram–2mg/kg		25–100mg	single dose	≥2 months: can be repeated every 4-6 hours.
IV bolus	← 500 microgram–1mg/kg →			25– 50mg	single dose	Neonates and infants <1 year show an increased susceptibility to respiratory depression.
IV infusion	–	← 1mg/kg then →			loading dose	Ventilated patients may require higher doses. Adjust according to response.
		← 100–400 microgram/kg/hour →			continuous infusion	

Renal impairment
Avoid in severe impairment. Accumulation of the metabolite norpethidine may induce seizures. Accumulation of this metabolite may also occur in sickle cell crisis and prolonged infusions.

Liver disease
Avoid as may precipitate coma.

ADMINISTRATION
IV: for IV infusion dilute with NaCl 0.9% or glucose 5% to required volume. Solutions are physically stable for at least 24 hours. For IV bolus dilute to 10mg in 1mL with Water for Injections and give over 2-5 minutes.
Solutions of pethidine hydrochloride are acidic and are incompatible with a large number of drugs. It is best to avoid mixing with other IV drugs unless compatibility has been confirmed.
Oral: injection can be given orally.

CONTRA-INDICATIONS & WARNINGS
Contra-indications: severe renal impairment (see notes under dosage), paralytic ileus, acute respiratory depression.
Cautions: hepatic impairment, increased intracranial pressure, head injury.
Warnings: histamine release may provoke hypotension and tachycardia.

INTERACTIONS
Enhanced sedative effects with *anxiolytics* and *hypnotics*; antagonism of gastrointestinal effects of *cisapride, metoclopramide* and *domperidone*; increased plasma concentration with *cimetidine* and *ritonavir* (risk of toxicity); CNS excitation or depression with *MAIO's*; hyperpyrexia and CNS toxicity with *selegiline*.

PREGNANCY
Use in the third trimester depresses neonatal respiration. Peak incidence occurs 2-3 hours after maternal IM injection. Feeding may be slow and some babies show impaired behavioural responses and EEG abnormalities for 2-3 days after birth. There is no evidence of teratogenicity.

BREAST-FEEDING
Pethidine is excreted into the breast milk but no adverse effects have been reported.

SIDE-EFFECTS
Respiratory depression, nausea and constipation (less constipating than *morphine*). Convulsions may be precipitated by repeated administration or overdose. IV administration may result in an increased heart rate.

POISONING/TOXICITY
Symptoms of toxicity include respiratory depression, pinpoint pupil, hypotension and convulsions (mainly attributed to norpethidine). Respiratory depression can be reversed by use of the opioid antagonist *naloxone*. Convulsions may need treatment with short acting muscle relaxant, intubation and controlled respiration.

PHARMACOKINETIC PROPERTIES
Only 50% of an oral dose reaches systemic circulation because of first pass metabolism. Pethidine is metabolised in the liver and the metabolites excreted in the urine. Only small amounts are excreted unchanged. Peak plasma concentrations 1-2 hours after oral administration. Plasma half-life of pethidine 3-6 hours, norpethidine approximately 20 hours. In babies <3 months, clearance of pethidine is much slower, average duration 11 hours (range 3-60 hours).

EXCIPIENTS
Contact manufacturers for further details.

LICENSED STATUS
Licensed for use in all ages.

Phenobarbital (phenobarbitone)

Antiepileptic.

USES
Epilepsy (most seizure types as third line antiepileptic drug). Convulsive status epilepticus (see status epilepticus algorithm). Neonatal hyperbilirubinaemia. Pruritis. Cerebral irritation (e.g. following acute cerebral event), intractable seizures in terminal period.

PRESENTATION
Tablet: 15mg, 30mg and 60mg – non-proprietary.
Oral liquid: various strengths available – may be extemporaneously prepared or manufactured 'special'.
Elixir: 15mg in 5mL; contains alcohol and is not recommended.
Injection: (as sodium salt) 200mg in 1mL – Gardenal Sodium® and non-proprietary; other strengths e.g. 60mg in 1mL – manufactured 'specials'.

DOSAGE

Indication	Route	Age				Frequency	Notes
		birth–1 month	1 month–2 years	2–12 years	12–18 years	(times daily)	
Antiepileptic	Oral	Give an IV loading dose	← 1-1.5mg/kg →		60-180mg	2	Starting dose.
		2.5-5mg/kg	← 2.5-4mg/kg →			2*	Usual target maintenance dose.
					60-180mg	1	
Status epilepticus	IV slow bolus	← 20mg/kg then →			20mg/kg then	single dose then	Loading dose then
		← 2.5-5mg/kg →			300mg dose	2*	maintenance.
Pruritus	Oral	← 3-5mg/kg →				1	Usually at night.
Neonatal hyperbili-rubinaemia	Oral	5-8mg/kg	–			1	For 2-7 days. Not widely used as phototherapy usually suffices.

* The plasma half-life is long in the neonatal period (2–4 days) and therefore once daily dosing may be adequate but it decreases with age and is halved after 1–2 weeks of medication because the drug acts to induce liver enzymes.

Dose adjustment
See basic principles in epilepsy introduction. Increase oral dose in increments of 2mg/kg/day as required. Dose may occasionally be given once daily in children; in adults often given as one dose at night. Higher doses have been used in ventilated patients.

ADMINISTRATION
Oral: tablets may be crushed.
IV: all injection formulations can be diluted 1 in 10 with Water for Injections. In fluid restriction injection strengths lower than 200mg in 1mL, should be adequately diluted e.g. 30mg in 1mL ampoules often diluted with an equal quantity of Water for Injections (giving a solution of 15mg in 1mL) and used in neonates. Give no faster than 1mg/kg/minute. Avoid umbilical artery cannula injection in neonates. Avoid extravasation of the alkaline injection.
Rectal: phenobarbital sodium injection solution has been administered as a rectal retention enema. Total daily dose should be similar to oral dose.

CONTRA-INDICATIONS & WARNINGS
Porphyria. Respiratory depression.
Reduce dose and monitor levels in renal and liver disease. Warn of drowsiness particularly at start of treatment and not to cease therapy without advice. Drowsiness is enhanced by alcohol.

INTERACTIONS
Enzyme inducer. Reduces plasma concentration of *carbamazepine, clonazepam, lamotrigine, sodium valproate* and sometimes *ethosuximide*. May reduce or increase *phenytoin* levels. Increases metabolism and reduces effect of many other drugs including *anticoagulants, calcium-channel blockers* such as *nifedipine, corticosteroids, ciclosporin (cyclosporin)* and *oral contraceptives*. Anticonvulsant effect antagonised by *antidepressants* and *antipsychotics*.

PREGNANCY
Possible increased risk of neural tube defects especially if more than one antiepileptic used. Specialist counselling, management and screening required. Administer folate supplements before and during pregnancy. Blood levels may be altered. Administer vitamin K during last weeks of pregnancy and to newborn to prevent bleeding disorders in the newborn. Neonatal enzymes may be induced. Withdrawal effects may be seen in the neonate as plasma levels decrease.

BREAST-FEEDING
Excreted in breast milk and drowsiness may occur.

SIDE-EFFECTS
Dose dependent adverse effects include sedation, ataxia, cardio-respiratory depression. Chronic adverse effects include cognitive dysfunction, behaviour changes.

POISONING/TOXICITY
Drowsiness, coma, respiratory depression, hypotension and hypothermia. Contact UK National Poisons Information Service. Measure levels.

PHARMACOKINETIC PROPERTIES
Usual target concentration is trough level at 7-14 days 10-25mg/L. Higher levels may be used especially in status epilepticus when the patient is ventilated.
Phenobarbital sodium as solution intended for injection containing propylene glycol is slowly but well absorbed from the rectum.

EXCIPIENTS
200mg in 1mL injection contains 90% propylene glycol. Elixir contains 38% alcohol and should not be used. Contact manufacturers for further details.

LICENSED STATUS
Controlled drug. Only 200mg in 1mL injection and tablets are licensed for use in children and adults. Preparations available as 'specials' or extemporaneously prepared are unlicensed. Neonatal hyperbilirubinaemia and pruritis are not licensed indications.

FURTHER INFORMATION
For therapeutic purposes phenobarbital and phenobarbital sodium may be considered equivalent in effect.

Phenoxybenzamine hydrochloride

Long-acting, non-competitive, alpha-adrenoceptor blocker.

USES
Treatment of severe shock in the presence of adequate circulating blood volume, including post-operative cardiac surgery. Management of hypertension due to phaeochromocytoma.

PRESENTATION
Capsule: 10mg – Dibenyline®.
Injection: 50mg in 1mL, 2mL ampoule – non-proprietary.
Oral liquid: may be extemporaneously prepared.

P

DOSAGE

Route	Age			Frequency (times daily)	Notes
	1 month–2 years	2–12 years	12–18 years		
Oral	←	500 microgram–1mg/kg	→	2	
IV infusion over at least 2 hours	←	500 microgram–1mg/kg	→	1	Give over at least 2 hours (one third of the dose in the 1st hour and two–thirds in the 2nd hour) or by continuous infusion over 24 hours if required. When used post-cardiac surgery an initial dose of 1mg/kg can be followed if necessary by 500 microgram/kg (over 2 hours) every 12 hours with dose titrated according to response.

ADMINISTRATION

Oral: capsules may be opened and the contents administered orally.

IV: the IV route only must be used. Dilute before use, using NaCl 0.9%, and infuse over 2 hours as outlined in the dosage table above. Solutions must be prepared immediately before use. Any that remains 4 hours after dilution should be discarded because of reduced potency.

The patient should be recumbent. Blood pressure must be determined every few minutes during administration. Facilities for rapid infusion of IV fluid must be available. The phenoxybenzamine infusion should be slowed or stopped if there is a precipitous fall in blood pressure. This usually indicates an inadequate circulating blood volume, but occasionally may occur in the presence of an adequate blood volume in hypertensives or in patients with carbon dioxide retention, and in these cases is relatively unresponsive to the administration of IV fluids. Nevertheless, if severe hypotension does occur, treatment can be attempted (see SPC for details).

Care should be taken to avoid extravasation, as the diluted solution is irritant to muscle tissue.

Avoid contact with skin/hands as contact sensitisation can occur.

CONTRA-INDICATIONS & WARNINGS

Do not use in the presence of hypovolaemia in patients with severe shock.

Do not use in patients who have had a cerebrovascular accident or in the recovery period (usually 3-4 weeks) after acute myocardial infarction.

Use with great caution in patients in whom a fall in blood pressure and/or tachycardia may be undesirable such as those with severe heart disease, congestive heart failure, cerebrovascular disease or renal damage. Phenoxybenzamine is carcinogenic in the rat and has shown mutagenic activity in the bacterial Ames test and the mouse lymphoma assay. It should therefore be used only after careful consideration of the risks in children for whom alternative treatment is inappropriate. The adrenergic blocking effect may aggravate symptoms of respiratory infections.

INTERACTIONS

Adrenaline (epinephrine): hypotension can be exacerbated due to unopposed beta-2 stimulation which will also tend to exacerbate the reflex tachycardia. *Anaesthetic agents:* profound hypotension may be precipitated. Volume replacement is helpful in correcting it. *Alpha sympathomimetics* may be ineffective if used concurrently with phenoxybenzamine. Care should be taken if phenoxybenzamine is used concurrently with *myocardial depressants e.g. beta-blockers* and *anti-arrhythmics.*

PREGNANCY/BREAST-FEEDING

There is little evidence regarding the safety of phenoxybenzamine in pregnancy/breast-feeding, therefore it should not be used unless considered to be essential. However there are reports of successful use of phenoxybenzamine, during pregnancy and labour in the management of phaeochromocytoma. Contact local Medicines Information Centre for advice.

SIDE-EFFECTS

Phenoxybenzamine, given IV, has a sedative effect and patients may become more drowsy and less responsive during the infusion. Convulsions have been reported after rapid infusion. Some fall in blood pressure is a normal response but an idiosyncratic profound hypotensive effect can occur, usually within 5 minutes of starting the infusion.

Other side-effects include orthostatic hypotension with dizziness and compensatory tachycardia, miosis, dry mouth, nasal congestion and gastrointestinal upset.

POISONING/TOXICITY
Oral: the main effect of overdosage is profound hypotension which may last several hours, tachycardia and collapse. Treatment of oral overdosage consists of the induction of vomiting and/or gastric lavage together with appropriate symptomatic and supportive measures.
IV: there may be a precipitous fall in blood pressure, even at the recommended dosage. Facilities for the rapid infusion of IV fluid should therefore be available and in the event of such a severe hypotensive episode, the infusion should be slowed or stopped.
Treat hypotension with plasma expanders and the 'head down' position. *Noradrenaline (norepinephrine)* is of little value when alpha-adrenergic receptors are blocked. *Adrenaline (epinephrine)* should not be used since stimulation of beta-adrenergic receptors will further decrease blood pressure.

PHARMACOKINETIC PROPERTIES
Phenoxybenzamine is incompletely absorbed orally. Only 20–30% appears in the active form after an oral dose. It is effective when given parenterally but is irritant and should therefore only be given intravenously in a diluted form. The mean plasma half-life in adults is 24 hours but the effect is not related to plasma concentration and lasts much longer. Plasma protein binding is negligible. Phenoxybenzamine is metabolised in the liver and excreted in faeces and urine.

EXCIPIENTS
Injection includes absolute ethyl alcohol and propylene glycol. Contact manufacturers for further details.

LICENSED STATUS
Not licensed in children.

Phenoxymethylpenicillin (Penicillin V)

An acid-stable penicillin for oral administration.

USES
Tonsillitis, otitis media, erysipelas, rheumatic fever and pneumococcal infection prophylaxis. It should not be used for serious infections because absorption can be unpredictable and plasma concentrations variable.

PRESENTATION
Tablet: 250mg – non-proprietary.
Oral solution: 125mg in 5mL and 250mg in 5mL – non-proprietary.

DOSAGE

Route	Age			Frequency	Notes
	1 month–2 years	2–12 years	12–18 years	(times daily)	
Oral	<1 year 62.5mg 1–2 years 125mg	2–5 years 125mg 6–12 years 250mg	500mg (750mg in severe infection)	4 4	Treatment doses.
	<1 year 62.5mg 1–2 years 125mg	2–5 years 125mg 6–12 years 250mg	500mg	2 2	Pneumococcal infection prophylaxis.
	← 250mg →			2	Rheumatic fever prophylaxis.

ADMINISTRATION
Oral: take an hour before food or on an empty stomach or 2 hours after food.

CONTRA-INDICATIONS & WARNINGS
Penicillin hypersensitivity.

INTERACTIONS
Guar gum – reduced absorption of phenoxymethylpenicillin; *probenecid* – reduced excretion of penicillins; *oral contraceptives* – possibility of reduced contraceptive effect.

PREGNANCY
Penicillins are not known to be harmful.

BREAST-FEEDING
Only trace amounts excreted in breast milk.

SIDE-EFFECTS
Hypersensitivity reactions including urticaria, fever, joint pains, rashes, angioedema, anaphylaxis, serum sickness-like reactions, haemolytic anaemia, and interstitial nephritis, neutropenia, thrombocytopenia, coagulation disorders and central nervous system toxicity reported (especially with high doses or in severe renal impairment); paraesthesia with prolonged use; diarrhoea and antibiotic-associated colitis have also been reported.

PHARMACOKINETIC PROPERTIES
Absorption is usually rapid, although variable, about 60% of an oral dose being absorbed. The effect of food on absorption generally appears to be slight. Plasma half-life is about 30–60 minutes and may be increased to about 4 hours in severe renal failure. Approximately 80% protein bound. Metabolised in the liver and unchanged drug and metabolites are excreted rapidly in the urine.

EXCIPIENTS
Contact manufacturers for further details.

LICENSED STATUS
Licensed for use in all age groups.

Phenytoin

Antiepileptic.

USES
Epilepsy (third or fourth line oral antiepileptic drug). The drug may exacerbate typical absence and myoclonic seizures. Used IV in status epilepticus (see status epilepticus algorithm) and for treating acute symptomatic seizures associated with head trauma or neurosurgery.
Neuropathic pain and also in paroxysmal kinesigenic choreoathetosis or symptomatic myotonia; slightly lower doses can often be used in these non-epileptic disorders.
Cardiac arrhythmias where first-line therapy is not effective, especially if digoxin-induced or in post-operative patients following repair of Tetralogy of Fallot.

PRESENTATION
Tablet: phenytoin sodium 50mg and 100mg – non-proprietary.
Tablet: (chewable, scored) phenytoin base 50mg – Epanutin Infatabs®.
Capsule: phenytoin sodium 25mg – Epanutin®; 50mg and 100mg – Epanutin® and non-proprietary; 300mg – Epanutin®.
Suspension: phenytoin base 30mg in 5mL – Epanutin®; 90mg in 5mL – manufactured 'special'.
Injection: phenytoin sodium 50mg in 1mL, 5mL ampoule – Epanutin Ready Mixed Parenteral® and non-proprietary.

DOSAGE

Indication	Route	Age				Frequency	Notes
		birth–1 month	1 month–2 years	2–12 years	12–18 years	(times daily)	
Antiepileptic	Oral	Use IV loading dose	←——1.5–2.5mg/kg——→		75–150mg	2	Starting dose.
		2–4mg/kg	←—— 2.5–5mg/kg ——→		150–200mg	2	Usual target maintenance dose.
		7.5mg/kg	←—— 7.5mg/kg ——→		300mg	2	Usual maximum dose.
	IV	20mg/kg	←—— 18mg/kg ——→			single dose	Loading dose (over 30–45 minutes)
		←—— 2.5–5mg/kg ——→			–	2	Usual maintenance dose
		–			100mg	3–4	(over 30 minutes).
Anti–arrhythmic	IV	–	←—— 18mg/kg ——→			single dose	

Dose adjustment
See basic principles in epilepsy introduction. Increase oral dose by no more than 1mg/kg/day. Measure phenytoin blood level after 1 week and as required. Loading IV dose only to be given if patient not on phenytoin or if blood level less than 2.5mg/L. If blood level is 10-20mg/L 2 hours after loading dose completed, start maintenance dose 12 hours after loading dose complete. If blood level is <10mg/L 2 hours after loading dose is completed, give a further loading dose of 5mg/kg over 20 minutes at once and commence maintenance dose after 8 hours.
Reduce dose in liver disease. In renal disease dose adjustment may be required.

Note: different preparations contain the different forms, phenytoin base or phenytoin sodium. 100mg phenytoin sodium is equivalent to 90mg phenytoin base on a molecular weight basis, but this is not necessarily biologically equivalent. Exercise care when changing the dosage form and monitor plasma levels.

ADMINISTRATION
Oral: tablets are coated but Infatabs® are scored and may be chewed. Bioavailability may be reduced by enteral feeds and/or nasogastric tube feeds and may be erratic in neonates. Allow at least 2 hours between nasogastric feeding and administration of phenytoin and flush tube with water. Under optimal conditions oral bioavailability is similar to IV.
IV: must be given slowly at a rate not exceeding 1mg/kg/minute to avoid hypotension and/or arrhythmias. Monitor blood pressure and ECG. Should be diluted in NaCl 0.9% injection only, to a concentration not greater than 10mg in 1mL. This dilution may be filtered without loss of activity. An in-line filter (0.22–0.50 microns) should be used. Avoid rapid flushing of IV lines which may deliver a bolus of phenytoin. Do not mix with glucose or other drugs because this can cause precipitation of phenytoin acid.

CONTRA-INDICATIONS & WARNINGS
Caution in porphyria. Warn not to cease therapy without advice and counsel on recognition of blood or skin disorders. Monitor carefully when plasma albumin is reduced or plasma protein binding altered such as in renal failure.

INTERACTIONS
Phenytoin is a potent enzyme inducer and is highly protein bound. Numerous potentially serious interactions, mainly with drugs which inhibit phenytoin metabolism and by acceleration of metabolism of other drugs by phenytoin. Consult appropriate references when changing dose of phenytoin or interacting drugs or when changing drug therapy. Plasma free phenytoin levels may be a useful guide in complex situations.

PREGNANCY
Plasma phenytoin levels may fall. Increased risk of neural tube defects or other malformations especially if more than one antiepileptic used. Specialist counselling, management and screening required. Administer folate supplements before and during pregnancy. Administer vitamin K during last weeks of pregnancy and to newborn to prevent bleeding disorders.

BREAST-FEEDING
Small amounts pass into milk. Breast-feeding appropriate if maternal dose is normal.

SIDE-EFFECTS
Dose dependent adverse effects include nystagmus, ataxia, dyskinesia, lethargy. Chronic adverse effects include gum hypertrophy, hirsutism and coarse facies, cognitive dysfunction, osteomalacia, folate deficiency.

POISONING/TOXICITY
Measure plasma levels. Initially nystagmus, ataxia and dysarthria may be followed by coma, unresponsive pupils, hypotension, respiratory depression, apnoea. Signs may occur at variable blood levels. Consult UK National Poisons Information Service.

PHARMACOKINETIC PROPERTIES
Highly protein bound, metabolised by saturable hydroxylation in the liver exhibiting zero order kinetics at higher plasma levels. Free phenytoin levels are a better guide than total levels. Toxicity more likely over 2mg/L free phenytoin (approximately 20mg/L total). Half-life may be variable and in range 7-42 hours. Target range of 10-20mg/L (40-80 micromol/L); measure trough level 7 days after oral dose change, 2-4 hours after IV loading dose. Phenytoin is poorly absorbed by the rectal route.

EXCIPIENTS
Infatabs® include sucrose and saccharin. Suspension 30mg in 5mL includes sucrose. Contact manufacturers for further details.

LICENSED STATUS
Suspension 90mg in 5mL is a 'special' and as such is unlicensed. All other preparations can be assumed to be licensed for appropriate ages.

FURTHER INFORMATION
Capsules and tablets are available in several generic brands. Prescriptions should include brand name to ensure consistency of drug delivery. Suspension 90mg in 5mL is available from Rosemont.

P

A weak opioid cough suppressant.

USES
Symptomatic treatment of dry or painful coughs.

PRESENTATION
Linctus: 2mg in 5mL (paediatric) – Galenphol®; 5mg in 5mL – non-proprietary; 10mg in 5mL (strong) – non-proprietary.

DOSAGE

Route	Age				Frequency	Notes
	birth–1 month	1 month–2 years	2–12 years	12–18 years	(times daily)	
Oral	Not recommended	1–2 years 2mg	2–5 years 2mg		3	
			6–12 years 2–5mg	5–10mg	3–4	

CONTRA-INDICATIONS & WARNINGS
Contra-indicated in liver disease and ventilatory failure or known hypersensitivity.

INTERACTIONS
Alcohol or other CNS depressants, may lead to greater drowsiness and sedation.

PREGNANCY
No evidence of ill consequence in pregnancy but not to be used unless benefits outweigh risks.

BREAST-FEEDING
There is no information available as to whether pholcodine is excreted in breast milk but it is unlikely to be harmful to the infant.

SIDE-EFFECTS
Constipation, nausea and drowsiness.

POISONING/TOXICITY
Symptoms: nausea, drowsiness, restlessness, excitement, ataxia and respiratory depression.
Treatment: gastric lavage. In severe cases use naloxone. General supportive and symptomatic treatment.

EXCIPIENTS
Some preparations include sucrose; sugar-free preparations are available. Contact manufacturer for further details.

LICENSED STATUS
Licensed for >1 year of age.

FURTHER INFORMATION
Cough suppressants may cause sputum retention and this may be harmful in bronchiectasis.
If sold over the counter, advise patient to visit doctor if symptoms persist for more than 5 days.
Pavacol-D® (sugar-free) can be diluted with Sorbitol Solution BPC and is stable for 14 days.

Phosphates

USES
Hypercalcaemia.
Hypophosphataemia and phosphate deficiency including rickets and osteomalacia (oral route preferred).
Phosphate source in balanced IV feeds (dipotassium phosphate is not recommended as a source of phosphate in PN as it has been shown to be less compatible than both Addiphos® and potassium acid phosphate).

PRESENTATION
Oral solution: may be extemporaneously prepared; neutral sodium phosphate oral solution containing phosphate 1mmol and sodium 1.8mmol in 1mL – manufactured 'special'; potassium acid phosphate solution 1mmol in 1mL – manufactured 'special'.

Tablet: (effervescent) each containing phosphate 16.1mmol, sodium 20.4mmol and potassium 3.1mmol – Phosphate-Sandoz®.
Solution: phosphate 40mmol, potassium 30mmol, sodium 30mmol per 20mL, for addition to IV fluids – Addiphos®.
Injection: potassium acid phosphate 13.6% (1mmol of each potassium and acid phosphate per 1mL), 10mL ampoule – manufactured special.
Injection: dipotassium hydrogen phosphate – 17.42% (2mmol of potassium and 1mmol of phosphate per 1mL), 10mL ampoule – manufactured special.
Injection: disodium hydrogen phosphate – 17.42% (1.2mmol of sodium and 0.6mmol of phosphate per 1mL), 10mL ampoule – manufactured special.
Polyfusor phosphates: infusion containing 50mmol phosphate, 81mmol sodium and 9.5mmol potassium in 500mL.

DOSAGE

Indication	Route	Age				Frequency (times daily)	Notes
		birth–1 month	1 month–2 years	2–12 years	12–18 years		
Hypercalcaemia	Oral	1mmol/kg	up to 3 tablets*	<5 years up to 3 tablets*	up to 6 tablets*	1	Daily dose can be given in two divided doses. *Tablets = Phosphate-Sandoz®.
				>5 years up to 6 tablets*		1	
Hypo-phosphataemia	Oral	1mmol/kg	2-3 tablets*	<5 years 2-3 tablets*	4-6 tablets*	1	Daily dose can be given in divided doses, especially when treating hypophosphataemic rickets. *Tablets = Phosphate-Sandoz®.
				>5 years 4-6 tablets*		1	
	IV	1 mmol/kg/day	0.7 mmol/kg/day	◄— 0.4mmol/kg/day —►		1	

ADMINISTRATION
Oral: Phosphate-Sandoz® tablets should be dissolved in one third to half a glass of water.
IV: dilute ampoules before use in NaCl 0.9% or glucose 5%; administer by slow IV infusion (maximum rate 0.05mmol/kg/hour). As part of an IV feeding regimen – check compatibility with calcium source. Should not be administered undiluted.

CONTRA-INDICATIONS & WARNINGS
Caution in impaired renal function, cardiac disease, diabetes mellitus and in patients who are dehydrated. renal failure. Infusion can also cause thrombophlebitis and calcification at infusion site.
With oral administration nausea and diarrhoea can occur (more common after IV administration).

SIDE-EFFECTS
Hyperphosphataemia leading to hypocalcaemia, hypocalcaemic tetany, hypotension, oedema and acute

PHARMACOKINETIC PROPERTIES
Mainly excreted in urine, also small amount in faeces.

LICENSED STATUS
Addiphos® is licensed for use in all ages. Phosphate-Sandoz® licensed in children and adults.
Potassium acid phosphate, disodium hydrogen phosphate and dipotassium phosphate injections are 'specials' and as such are unlicensed. Oral solutions extemporaneously prepared or available as 'specials' unlicensed.

FURTHER INFORMATION
'Specials' are available from manufacturers such as Martindale Pharmaceuticals Ltd.

Sodium glycerophosphate

Glucose-1-phosphate

USES
Additional supplementation of phosphorous in PN to avoid the problem of calcium and phosphate precipitation associated with inorganic phosphate.

PRESENTATION
Injection: sodium glycerophosphate (as anhydrous sodium glycerophosphate 216mg per 1mL, providing 2mmol of sodium and 1mmol of phosphate), 10mL – manufactured 'special'.
Injection: glucose-1-phosphate (as disodium salt 125.4mg per mL, providing 6.6mmol sodium, 3.3mmol phosphate and 3.3mmol glucose), 10mL – Phocytan manufactured 'special'.

DOSAGE
Dosage depends on biochemical results, usually 0.1–1mmol/kg/day (although more may be required in infants).

ADMINISTRATION
IV: as part of a PN solution. Compatibility in a particular PN regimen should be assessed by a suitably qualified pharmacist. Organic phosphates generally allow much higher levels of calcium and phosphate to be present in a PN regimen.

CONTRA-INDICATIONS & WARNINGS
Preparations must not be administered undiluted. Use under routine clinical and biochemical monitoring. May cause hyperphosphataemia. Always take into account sodium content.

SIDE-EFFECTS
Hypocalcaemia if the infusion rate is too rapid or the dose is excessive.

POISONING/TOXICITY
See phosphates monograph.

LICENSED STATUS
Sodium glycerophosphate and glucose-1-phosphate are 'specials' and as such are not licensed.

FURTHER INFORMATION
Sodium glycerophosphate injection is manufactured under manufacturers licence by South Devon Healthcare and Queens Medical Centre, Nottingham. Glucose-1-phosphate injection is available from Oxford Nutrition.

Phosphates (rectal)

USES
Pre- and post-operative bowel cleansing in obstetrics and prior to proctoscopy, sigmoidoscopy or X-ray examination.

PRESENTATION
Fleet® Ready-to-use Enema: 118mL self-contained disposable enema containing the equivalent of sodium acid phosphate 21.4g (18.1% w/v) and sodium phosphate 9.4g (8% w/v).
Fletchers' Phosphate Enema®: 128mL enema containing: sodium acid phosphate 12.8g (10% w/v), sodium phosphate 10.24g (8% w/v).

DOSAGE

Route	Age			Frequency (times daily)	Notes
	1 month–2 years	2–12 years	12–18 years		
Rectal	Not recommended	3–7 years $\frac{1}{3} - \frac{1}{2}$ enema 7–12 years $\frac{1}{2} - \frac{3}{4}$ enema	$\frac{3}{4}$ – 1 enema (depending on patient size)	single dose	Do not repeat within 24 hours.

ADMINISTRATION
Rectal: use as directed on container. Squeeze container until the required volume has been expelled. May be warmed in water before use or administered at room temperature.

CONTRA-INDICATIONS & WARNINGS
Contra-indicated in inflammatory or ulcerative conditions of the bowel, congenital megacolon, Hirschsprung's disease, imperforate anus, congestive heart failure and acute gastro-intestinal problems. Caution in patients with renal disease, heart disease, colostomy or pre-existing electrolyte disturbances. Contra-indicated in children <3 years of age.

INTERACTIONS
Caution in patients on *calcium-channel blockers*, *diuretics* or other medications which affect electrolyte levels.

PREGNANCY/BREAST-FEEDING
Contact local Medicines Information Centre for advice.

SIDE-EFFECTS
Fluid and electrolyte imbalance including hyperphosphataemia, hypocalcaemia, hypernatraemia and acidosis may occur. Prolonged use may lead to irritation of the anal canal.

POISONING/TOXICITY
In the event of occurrence, monitor electrolyte levels and restore balance where appropriate.

PHARMACOKINETIC PROPERTIES
Poorly and slowly absorbed following rectal administration. Under normal usage, only minimal absorption likely to occur.

EXCIPIENTS
See manufacturers SPC for further details.

LICENSED STATUS
Licensed for ≥3 years of age.

Phosphocysteamine

USES
Management of nephropathic cystinosis and eye symptoms from cystine crystals in cystinosis. Reduces cystine accumulation in some cells of nephropathic cystinosis patients and, when started early delays the development of renal failure.

PRESENTATION
Capsules: may be extemporaneously prepared.

DOSAGE

| Route | Age | | | Frequency | Notes |
	1 month-2 years	2-12 years	12-18 years	(times daily)	
Oral	←	6mg/kg	→	4	Initial dose. Increase dose every 2-3 weeks by 25mg/kg/day to a maintenance dose of 125mg/kg/day.

ADMINISTRATION
Oral: the powder should be sprinkled onto food or mixed in a strongly flavoured drink. Phosphocysteamine has a very unpleasant taste and smell.

CONTRA-INDICATIONS & WARNINGS
Hypersensitivity to any phosphocysteamine or mercaptamine (cysteamine) salt or to penicillamine.

INTERACTIONS
None known.

PREGNANCY
No safety data available on use during pregnancy. Phosphocysteamine is not recommended during pregnancy. The effect of untreated cystinosis on pregnancy is also unknown.

BREAST-FEEDING
Phosphocysteamine must not be used during breast-feeding.

SIDE-EFFECTS
Phosphocysteamine causes an unpleasant smell on the breath and body odour but less than mercaptamine (cysteamine). It can also cause nausea, vomiting, diarrhoea, lethargy, fever and rash. It may also cause anaemia, leucopenia, raised liver enzymes and rarely gastrointestinal ulceration and bleeding.

LICENSED STATUS
Unlicensed for use.

FURTHER INFORMATION
25mg phosphocysteamine is approximately equivalent to 10mg mercaptamine.

POISONING/TOXICITY
Symptoms would include nausea and vomiting. Seizures and lethargy have been reported at high doses. *Treatment* is symptomatic and supportive.

PHARMACOKINETIC PROPERTIES
Phosphocysteamine is the phosphorothioester prodrug of mercaptamine which reacts with cystine to form cysteine and a cysteine-mercaptamine mixed disulphide. The disulphide complex structurally resembles lysine and uses its lysosome transport system for removal.

Pimozide

Diphenylbutylpiperidine antipsychotic.

USES
Schizophrenia and tic disorders including Tourette syndrome.

PRESENTATION
Tablet: 4mg (scored) – Orap®.

DOSAGE

Indication	Route	Age		Frequency (times daily)	Notes
		2-12 years	12-18 years		
Schizophrenia	Oral	-	1-20mg	1	Normally given as single daily dose,
Tourette syndrome	Oral	1-4mg	2-10mg	1	but may be given in divided doses. Need annual ECG to monitor QT interval.

CONTRA-INDICATIONS & WARNINGS
History of cardiac arrhythmias or pre-existing congenital QT prolongation. It is recommended that a baseline ECG is carried out in all patients prior to commencing treatment and repeated annually (or earlier if clinically indicated). Avoid concurrent use of other cardioreactive medication (see interactions for details).
Electrolyte disturbances, notably hypokalaemia, should be considered a risk factor for ventricular arrhythmias; check plasma potassium before commencing treatment and avoid concurrent use of drugs which cause electrolyte disturbances. Caution is advised in patients with hepatic or renal dysfunction, epilepsy and conditions predisposing to epilepsy. May be relatively high risk of extrapyramidal movement disorders.

INTERACTIONS
Concurrent use with the following is not recommended – *macrolide antibiotics, tricyclic antidepressants,* *other antipsychotic drugs* as potentially an increased risk of arrhythmias. Drugs which may prolong the QT interval such as *quinine, mefloquine, amiodarone, bretylium, disopyramide, procainamide, quinidine, sotolol, terfenadine, astemizole.* Drugs causing electrolyte imbalance (including *diuretics,* but if necessary, a *potassium-sparing diuretic* is preferred). The dosage of *antiepileptic drugs* may need to be increased to take into account the lower seizure threshold.

PREGNANCY
Safety in human pregnancy not established. Animal studies have not demonstrated teratogenic effects. Avoid, if possible.

BREAST-FEEDING
Contra-indicated. Contact local Medicines Information Centre for advice.

SIDE-EFFECTS
As chlorpromazine but less sedative. Cardiotoxic (see above).

POISONING/TOXICITY
Signs and symptoms could include extrapyramidal symptoms, hypotension or sedation. Consider the risks of cardiac arrhythmias. The patient may appear comatose with respiratory depression and hypotension which could be severe enough to produce a shock-like state. No specific antidote. ECG monitoring should be undertaken. Supportive treatment including IV fluids for hypotension and circulatory collapse, which may also require vasopressor agents. In cases of severe extrapyramidal symptoms anti-parkinsonism medication should be administered. Overdose patients should be observed for at least 4 days.

PHARMACOKINETIC PROPERTIES
Half-life is highly variable but is shorter in children than adults at approximately 66 hours.

EXCIPIENTS
See manufacturers SPC for further details.

LICENSED STATUS
Not licensed for <12 years of age.

Piperacillin with tazobactam

A bactericidal ureidopenicillin with a beta-lactamase inhibitor – has a broad spectrum of activity similar to the carbapenems.

USES
Used to treat a range of susceptible organisms, particularly *Pseudomonas aeruginosa*. In cystic fibrosis patients – treatment of early *Pseudomonas aeruginosa* infections not cleared by oral ciprofloxacin plus nebulised colistin and of moderate to severe exacerbations, in combination with an aminoglycoside.

PRESENTATION
Injection: 2.25g (2g piperacillin with 0.25g tazobactam) and 4.5g (4g piperacillin with 0.5g tazobactam) vials – Tazocin®.

DOSAGE
Newborn infant (birth-1 month)

Route	Age birth–1month	Frequency (times daily)	Notes
IV	90mg/kg	3	

Child

Route	Age			Frequency (times daily)	Notes
	1 month–2 years	2–12 years	12–18 years		
IV	← 90mg/kg →			4	Maximum single dose is 4.5g.

Dose adjustment in renal impairment
Reduce dose in moderate impairment. In haemodialysis ensure dose is given post dialysis and given as 45mg/kg three times daily.

Creatinine clearance (mL/minute/1.73m²)	Dose	Frequency (times daily)
40–80	90mg/kg (maximum 4.5g)	4
20–40	90mg/kg (maximum 4.5g)	3
<20	90mg/kg (maximum 4.5g)	2

ADMINISTRATION

IV: displacement value is 1.58mL for 2.25g and 3.15mL for 4.5g. For IV bolus, reconstitute to 225mg in 1mL and give over 3-5 minutes. Reconstitute with Water for Injections or NaCl 0.9%. The reconstituted solution may be further diluted with at least another 50mL of NaCl 0.9% or glucose 5% and given as an infusion over 20 minutes.

Do not mix with aminoglycosides or sodium bicarbonate; do not administer through the same line without adequate flushing in-between.

CONTRA-INDICATIONS & WARNINGS

Allergy to penicillins or hypersensitivity to any ingredients of the preparation.

INTERACTIONS

Possible prolonged prothrombin time with *warfarin*. May prolong the action of *neuromuscular blocking agents* e.g. *vecuronium*. May reduce excretion of *methotrexate*.

PREGNANCY

No evidence of teratogenicity. Contact local Medicines Information Centre for advice.

BREAST-FEEDING

Excreted in low concentrations in breast milk avoid if possible. Contact local Medicines Information Centre for advice.

SIDE-EFFECTS

Serious and occasionally fatal anaphylactic reactions have occurred. Rarely liver disorders, blood dyscrasias and dermatological manifestations have been reported. Rarely renal failure may occur.

POISONING/TOXICITY

General supportive treatment is given in overdose. Serum levels may be reduced by dialysis.

PHARMACOKINETIC PROPERTIES

Rapidly excreted unchanged by glomerular filtration and tubular secretion with a plasma half-life of around 1 hour. Penetrates CSF in the presence of meningitis and binding to protein is low.

EXCIPIENTS

Each 1g of powder contains approximately 2mmol of sodium. See manufacturers SPC for further details.

LICENSED STATUS

Licensed for use in all ages, but only licensed <12 years for sepsis in neutropenia and licensed for appendicitis complicated by rupture with peritonitis and/or abscess formation in children aged 2-12 years. The doses quoted reflect use in severe sepsis in neutropenia.

Piperazine

Anthelmintic.

USES

Eradication of enterobiasis (pinworm, threadworm) and ascariasis (roundworm).

PRESENTATION

Powder: 4g piperazine phosphate and sennosides 15.3mg per sachet – Pripsen®.

DOSAGE

Indication	Route	Age			Frequency	Notes
		1 month–2 years	2-12 years	12-18 years	(times daily)	
Threadworm Roundworm	Oral	3 months–1 year 2.5mL of powder 1–2 years 5mL of powder	2–6 years 5mL of powder 6–12 years 1 sachet	1 sachet	single dose	In <1 year of age use on medical advice only. When treating thread-worm, repeat after 14 days. When treating roundworm, repeat at monthly intervals for up to 3 months if there is a risk of infection.

ADMINISTRATION
Oral: stir Pripsen® powder into small glass of milk or water and drink immediately. Dose to be taken in the morning by children and at bedtime by adults. Note: 1 sachet ≡ 7.5mL powder.

CONTRA-INDICATIONS & WARNINGS
Liver disease, impaired renal function, epilepsy.

INTERACTIONS
Pyrantel embonate antagonises the mode of action of piperazine and therefore should not be administered concurrently.

PREGNANCY
No clinical evidence of harm, but avoid in first trimester if possible.

BREAST-FEEDING
Piperazine is excreted in breast milk but no adverse effects in the infant have been recorded. To minimise the amount of piperazine ingested by the baby, feed infant immediately before dose then allow 8 hours before resuming feeding. Discard expressed breast milk during this 8 hour period.

SIDE-EFFECTS
Nausea, vomiting, colic, diarrhoea, allergic reactions, dizziness, muscular inco-ordination ('worm wobble'), drowsiness, confusion and clonic contractions in patients with neurological or renal abnormalities.

POISONING/TOXICITY
Symptoms of overdose similar to side effects. Treatment consists of general supportive measures including maintenance of adequate fluids and if necessary anticonvulsant therapy. IV diazepam or a short-acting barbiturate may control convulsions.

PHARMACOKINETIC PROPERTIES
Piperazine is readily absorbed from the gastrointestinal tract. It is almost completely excreted in the urine within 24 hours, partly as metabolites.

EXCIPIENTS
Pripsen® powder contains saccharin and is sugar free. See manufacturers SPC for further details.

LICENSED STATUS
Licensed for use in children and adults.

Piroxicam

Non-steroidal anti-inflammatory drug (NSAID).

USES
Pain and inflammation in rheumatic disease including juvenile idiopathic arthritis (JIA) and musculoskeletal disorders.

PRESENTATION
Capsules: 10mg and 20mg – Feldene® and non-proprietary.
Gel: 0.5% – Feldene®.
Injection: 20mg in 1mL – Feldene®.
Suppository: 20mg – Feldene®.
Tablet: (dispersible) 10mg and 20mg – Feldene®.
Tablet: 20mg – Feldene Melt®.

DOSAGE

Route	Weight				Frequency (times daily)	Notes
	≤15 kg	16–25 kg	26–45 kg	≥46kg		
Oral/rectal	5mg	10mg	15mg	20mg	1	

ADMINISTRATION
Oral: take with or after food.
IM: can be given by deep IM injection into the upper outer quadrant of the buttock, for initial treatment of acute conditions using the same dose as for the oral route. This is not however recommended in children.

P

CONTRA-INDICATIONS & WARNINGS
Should not be given to patients with active peptic ulceration, and should be used with extreme caution in patients with a history of peptic ulceration. Also contra-indicated in patients who have previously shown hypersensitivity reactions (asthma, rhinitis, urticaria) to aspirin or other NSAIDs. Use with caution in renal, cardiac or hepatic impairment. The topical preparations should not be applied to broken skin or mucosal surfaces; keep away from the eyes. The rectal route should not be used in patients with any inflammatory lesions of the rectum or anus, or patients with a recent history of rectal or anal bleeding.

INTERACTIONS
May decrease the elimination of *methotrexate*. Increased risk of nephrotoxicity when given with *ciclosporin (cyclosporin)*. The antihypertensive effects of *beta-blockers* may be reduced by piroxicam; the *beta-blocker* dose may need to be increased.

PREGNANCY
NSAIDs should be avoided in the third trimester as they may cause constriction of the ductus arteriosus in utero leading to persistent pulmonary hypertension in the newborn. In addition, these drugs may inhibit labour if used close to delivery. The interaction between piroxicam and *beta-blockers* (see above) is likely to be of particular importance in the management of pre-eclampsia, when this combination should be avoided.

BREAST-FEEDING
Piroxicam is excreted into breast milk, but the amount of the drug ingested by the infant is likely to be insignificant.

SIDE-EFFECTS
Gastrointestinal discomfort, nausea, diarrhoea and occasionally bleeding and ulceration. Headache, dizziness, vertigo, fluid retention, hypersensitivity reactions e.g. bronchospasm, rashes. Local discomfort, burning or itching and occasionally bleeding may occur with NSAID suppositories.
When given by the IM route, burning sensations and tissue damage (sterile abscess formation, fatty tissue necrosis) may occasionally occur at the site of injection.

POISONING/TOXICITY
There is no specific antidote. The stomach may be emptied by either lavage or inducing emesis. Activated charcoal may markedly reduce the absorption of the drug. Further treatment is symptomatic.

PHARMACOKINETIC PROPERTIES
The plasma half-life of piroxicam is around 50 hours in adults, and 30 hours in children. This allows once daily administration. Although oral absorption will be slowed down by the presence of food, piroxicam is rapidly absorbed via any route.

EXCIPIENTS
Feldene Melt® tablets contain aspartame (equivalent to 0.14mg phenylalanine). Feldene® IM injection contains benzyl alcohol. See manufacturers SPC for further details.

LICENSED STATUS
Feldene® dispersible tablets licensed for JIA, in children ≥6 years of age.

FURTHER INFORMATION
The once daily dosage makes piroxicam particularly useful when compliance is a problem, and the 'Melt' formulation is palatable to young children.

Pizotifen

An antihistamine (histamine-1 antagonist) and serotonin (5-HT$_2$) antagonist structurally related to the tricyclic antidepressants.

USES
Migraine prophylaxis.

PRESENTATION
Tablet: 500 microgram, 1.5mg – Sanomigran® and non-proprietary.
Elixir: 250 microgram in 5mL – Sanomigran®.

DOSAGE

Route	Age		Frequency (times daily)	Notes
	2–12 years	**12–18 years**		
Oral	5–10 years 10–12 years 500 microgram 1mg	1.5mg	1	Starting dose Preferably at night.
	≥5 years up to 500 microgram	up to 1.5mg	3	Maintenance dose adjusted according to response. Maximum single dose at night <12 years is 1mg and maximum single dose 12–18 years is 3mg. Maximum **total daily** dose <12 years is 1.5mg and 12–18 years is 4.5mg.

ADMINISTRATION

Oral: the dosing schedule may be changed to twice daily or once daily (at night).

CONTRA-INDICATIONS & WARNINGS

CNS stimulation may occur in children. Patients should be cautioned about drowsiness. The elixir contains a hydrogenated glucose syrup sweetener with a significant absorbable carbohydrate content which should be considered if the patient has diabetes. Caution is required in the presence of closed angle glaucoma and in patients with a predisposition to urinary retention due to anticholinergic activity.

INTERACTIONS

Antagonism of hypotensive effect of *adrenergic neurone blockers*. Potentiation of central effects of *sedatives, hypnotics, antihistamines.*

PREGNANCY

Limited data available – to be used only under compelling circumstances.

BREAST-FEEDING

Amount in breast milk unlikely to be significant but not recommended.

SIDE-EFFECTS

The most commonly occurring are drowsiness, increased appetite which may lead to increase in body weight. Others include dry mouth, nausea and constipation. Rarely, sleep disorders, depression and other mood disturbances have occurred.

POISONING/TOXICITY

Symptoms of overdosage may include drowsiness, dizziness, hypotension, dryness of the mouth, confusion, excitatory states, ataxia, nausea, vomiting, dyspnoea, cyanosis, tachycardia, convulsions, coma and respiratory paralysis.

Treatment with activated charcoal is recommended and gastric lavage should be considered if intake is very recent. Severe hypotension must be corrected (*adrenaline (epinephrine)* may produce paradoxical effects) and convulsions treated with short-acting *benzodiazepines*. Cardiovascular and respiratory systems should be monitored.

PHARMACOKINETIC PROPERTIES

Absorption is fast (absorption half-life 0.5-0.8 hours) and nearly complete (80%). Metabolised with a half-life of about 1 hour. 91% protein bound.

EXCIPIENTS

Contact manufacturers for details.

Elixir includes methyl- and propyl-hydrobenzoate, lycasin 80/55 (hydrogenated glucose syrup), ethyl alcohol; sugar-free. The sweetening agent Lycasin 80/55 has a concentration of 4g in 5ml and contains 45% readily absorbable carbohydrate.

LICENSED STATUS

The elixir and 500 microgram tablets are licensed in children and adults; the 1.5mg tablets are not licensed for use in children.

P

USES
This vaccine was licensed for use in the UK in early 2001. The licence only covers use in children <2 years old. At the time of writing (May 2003), the JCVI has issued preliminary guidance on its use in high-risk children in this age group and is considering whether it should be used as part of the routine infant immunisation schedule. The Royal College of Paediatrics and Child Health (RCPCH) recommends that its use should include all at risk children >2 months old, not just those <2 years old.

The vaccine is indicated to provide active protection against invasive pneumococcal disease in high-risk groups. These include those children with functional asplenia, including sickle cell disease, coeliac disease and prior to elective splenectomy; chronic renal disease or nephrotic syndrome; immunodeficiency or immunosuppression, including HIV infection; chronic heart disease, including congenital cyanotic heart disease; chronic lung disease, including children with severe asthma; chronic liver disease; diabetes mellitus. The vaccine should also be given to those who have had, or are about to have, a cochlear implant as these patients may be at increased risk of invasive pneumococcal disease.

Children >2 years old who fall into the above risk categories should be offered the plain polysaccharide vaccine in addition to the conjugate vaccine. See the monograph for details of dosage.

PRESENTATION
Injection: (single dose suspension) – Prevenar®.
Each 0.5ml contains 2 micrograms of each capsular polysaccharide derived from the following 7 pneumococcal seroytpes – 4, 6B (4 micrograms), 9V, 14, 18C, 19F and 23F – conjugated to CRM_{197}.

DOSAGE/ADMINISTRATION
Deep SC or IM injection: 0.5ml. The number of doses for a primary course depends on the age of the child. For these high-risk groups, RCPCH recommends three doses at monthly intervals for children <2 years old and two doses at a month apart for those ≥2 years. The course should then be followed by a single dose of the plain polysaccharide vaccine to increase the breadth of cover. This should be administered at ≥2 years with a minimum interval of 8 weeks after the conjugate vaccine.

CONTRA-INDICATIONS AND WARNINGS
As for vaccines generally, bearing in mind it is a diphtheria conjugate.

INTERACTIONS
The limited data available suggest that a minimum of 8 weeks should be left between administering the conjugate and then polysaccharide vaccines. There are no other known interactions.

PREGNANCY/BREAST-FEEDING
No information is available, but there are no grounds to believe it would be harmful.

SIDE-EFFECTS
Erythema, slight induration and tenderness at the site of injection. Fever may occur. Major adverse effects are rare.

POISONING/TOXICITY
No information available.

LICENSED STATUS
The vaccine is licensed only for children <2 years old and the dose schedule in the licence is different from that recommended here.

EXCIPIENTS
Sodium chloride.

FURTHER INFORMATION
The use of the vaccine is not a substitute for prophylactic penicillin. If possible the vaccine should be given at least 2 weeks before an elective splenectomy.
The vaccine reduces nasal carriage of vaccine serotypes for at least 18 months.
Material of bovine origin is used in the manufacturing process. There should be none of the original material present in the final product however, all such material is obtained from sources known to be free of BSE.
Store at 2-8°C, and inspect before use to ensure there are no suspended particles visible.

USES

Active protection against invasive pneumococcal disease in high-risk groups, aged ≥2 years. These include those children and adults with functional asplenia, including sickle cell disease, coeliac disease and prior to elective splenectomy; chronic renal disease or nephrotic syndrome; immunodeficiency or immunosuppression, including HIV infection; chronic heart disease, including congenital cyanotic heart disease; chronic lung disease, including children with severe asthma; chronic liver disease; diabetes mellitus. The vaccine should also be given to those who have had, or are about to have, a cochlear implant as these patients may be at increased risk of invasive diseases.

Children >2 months old who fall into the above risk categories should be offered the conjugate vaccine in addition to the plain polysaccharide vaccine. See the monograph for details of dosage.

PRESENTATION

Injection: (single dose suspension) – Pneumovax® II; Pnu-Imune®.
Each dose contains 25 micrograms of each capsular polysaccharide derived from the 23 most prevalent pneumococcal serotypes – 1, 2, 3, 4, 5, 6B, 7F, 8, 9N, 9V, 10A, 11A, 12F, 14, 15B, 17A (Pnu-Imune® – 17F in Pneumovax® II), 18C, 19A, 19F, 20, 22F, 23F, 33F.

DOSAGE/ ADMINISTRATION

Deep SC or IM: 0.5ml. Booster doses of the plain polysaccharide vaccine are not normally recommended and should certainly not take place within 3 years of the first dose as marked local reactions can occur. As the vaccine is likely to be used in conjunction with the conjugate vaccine in children, it is not known whether boosters will be required.

CONTRA-INDICATIONS AND WARNINGS

As for vaccines generally: also should not be given to someone who has had a dose within the last 3 years.

INTERACTIONS

It can be given simultaneously with, or at any interval before or after, any other vaccine.

PREGNANCY

Limited experience of administering the vaccine to women in pregnancy (predominantly in the last trimester) has revealed no adverse effects on the mother, fetus or neonate. However, until more research has taken place, its use in pregnancy cannot be recommended.

BREAST-FEEDING

No information is available, but there are no grounds to believe it would be harmful.

SIDE-EFFECTS

Erythema, slight induration and tenderness at the site of injection may occur. Fever is much less common. Other adverse effects are rare.

POISONING/TOXICITY

No information available.

PHARMACODYNAMIC PROPERTIES

Protection is usually present within 3 weeks of the injection. The duration of immunity is unknown, but the vaccine does not induce immunological memory.

LICENSED STATUS

Licensed for use as described above.

EXCIPIENTS

Pneumovax® II: phenol and sodium chloride.
Pnu-Imune®: thiomersal and sodium phosphate buffer.

FURTHER INFORMATION

A conjugate vaccine is licensed for use in children between 2 months and 2 years old. Where a pneumococcal vaccine would normally be indicated, but the child is between 2 months and 2 years old, it would be appropriate to use the conjugate vaccine. In older children, both vaccines should be used. The use of either vaccine is not a substitute for prophylactic penicillin in individuals with functional asplenia. If possible the vaccine should be given at least 2 weeks before an elective splenectomy.
Store at 2-8°C and inspect before use to ensure there are no suspended particles visible.

Inhibits cell division and causes necrosis of epidermal cells.

USES
Treatment of warts especially genital warts.

PRESENTATION
Paint: 15% in compound benzoin tincture – Podophyllin Paint, Compound, BP: 5mL to be dispensed.

DOSAGE/ADMINISTRATION
Topical: applied weekly by trained nurse. Leave on affected area for not more than 6 hours then wash off. Protect surrounding area with soft paraffin.

CONTRA-INDICATIONS & WARNINGS
Only a few warts to be treated at any one time due to severe toxicity. Avoid normal skin and open wounds. Keep away from face. Very irritant to eyes. Flammable.

PREGNANCY/BREAST-FEEDING
Contra-indicated.

SIDE-EFFECTS
Skin irritation.

POISONING/TOXICITY
Following accidental spillage, wash the skin well with soap and water. In the event of ingestion treatment should be symptomatic. In severe oral overdose ensure the airway is clear, give fluids, check and correct electrolyte balance, monitor blood gases and liver function. Monitor blood count for at least 5 days.

LICENSED STATUS
The preparation from William Ransom & Sons PLC is licensed for use >5 years of age for the treatment of plantar warts. It is licensed for the treatment of anal or genital warts in adults only. The preparation from Nova Laboratories is a 'special' and as such is unlicensed.

FURTHER INFORMATION
Available from William Ransom & Sons PLC and from Nova Laboratories Ltd.

Poliomyelitis vaccine (enhanced inactivated) (eIPV or IPV)

USES
Use in place of oral poliomyelitis vaccine (OPV) when the latter is contra-indicated.

PRESENTATION
Injection: (single dose solution) – Inactivated Poliomyelitis Vaccine (Diploid Cell Origin) – IPV.
Each dose contains types 1, 2 and 3 polio virus which have been grown in human diploid (MRC-5) cell cultures, concentrated, purified and inactivated with formaldehyde.
A vaccine containing DTaP/IPV is also available on a named patient basis.

DOSAGE/ADMINISTRATION
IM or deep SC: 0.5 mL.
Each dose of 0.5mL replaces a single dose of OPV. A basic course consists of 3 injections at monthly intervals. OPV and IPV are interchangeable and the same schedule should be followed whichever vaccine is used. It is not necessary to use the same vaccine throughout the course.

CONTRA-INDICATIONS & WARNINGS
As for vaccines generally.

INTERACTIONS
It can be given simultaneously with, or at any interval before or after, any other vaccine.

PREGNANCY
The evidence available suggests it is not hazardous. It should not be withheld if it is clinically indicated.

BREAST-FEEDING
There is no evidence available, but no reason to believe it would be hazardous. It should not be withheld if it is clinically indicated.

SIDE-EFFECTS
A mild local erythematous reaction or fever may occur.

POISONING/TOXICITY
No data available.

EXCIPIENTS
May contain small quantities of 2-phenoxyethanol, human albumin, formaldehyde, polymixin B, neomycin, bovine serum and Tween 80.

LICENSED STATUS
Not licensed for use in UK, but its use is supported by the Department of Health, if used as recommended in their book *Immunisation against Infectious Disease 1996*. It is available from Farillon on a named patient basis.

FURTHER INFORMATION
Individual protection from IPV is as good as that from OPV. There is debate as to how well it protects against carriage of live polio virus. Some countries use it for all or part of the routine schedule. It is likely that it will replace OPV in the UK schedule in the not too distant future.

Store at 2–8°C, do not freeze.

A quadrivalent preparation (Tetravac®) containing diphtheria, tetanus, acellular pertussis and inactivated polio vaccines is available for use in the UK on a named patient basis (see separate monograph).

Material of bovine origin is used in the manufacturing process. Trace amounts of the original material may be present in the final product, however, all such material is obtained from sources known to be free of BSE.

Poliomyelitis vaccine, live oral (OPV)

USES
Active protection against poliomyelitis as part of the routine childhood immunisation schedule. It is interchangeable with inactivated polio vaccine (IPV) and can be used to complete a course started with IPV if there are no contra-indications.

PRESENTATIONS
Liquid: (single or 10 dose liquid for oral administration).

Each dose contains not less than 10^6 $TCID_{50}$ poliovirus type 1 (LS-c, 2ab), 10^5 $TCID_{50}$ poliovirus type 2 (P712, Ch, 2ab) and $10^{5.5}$ $TCID_{50}$ poliovirus type 3 (Leon 12a1b) live attenuated Sabin strains of polio virus grown in monkey kidney cell culture or human diploid cells.

DOSAGE/ADMINISTRATION
Oral: 3 drops (0.135 mL). The primary course is usually given at 8, 12 and 16 weeks of age. This is followed by a booster 3 years later and another at 13–18 years of age. Boosters every 10 years are only necessary if there is continuing risk of infection, e.g. travel to endemic areas.

CONTRA-INDICATIONS & WARNINGS
As for vaccines generally; also should be postponed when recipient has diarrhoea or vomiting. Where a child or household contact may be immunosuppressed by reason of disease or treatment, inactivated polio vaccine should be used instead. The Joint Committee on Vaccination and Immunisation recommends OPV use in patients who are HIV positive but asymptomatic, whereas symptomatic individuals may be given IPV. Many clinicians recommend that IPV should be used when an individual or household member is HIV positive, whether symptomatic or not. It is recommended that IPV, rather than OPV, should be used in babies in neonatal units. Alternatively, OPV can be given at the time of discharge.

INTERACTIONS
Should not be given at the same time as oral typhoid vaccine.

PREGNANCY
Early case reports have suggested that OPV may cause fetal damage in rare cases. However, extensive experience in Finland and Israel has shown no evidence of harm to the fetus, irrespective of the stage in pregnancy at which the vaccine was given. If a pregnant woman is at significant risk of being exposed to polio, a very rare occurrence unless travelling to one of the few remaining endemic areas in the world, consideration should be given to the use of the inactivated preparation.

BREAST-FEEDING
Although it may be excreted in breast milk, this is not a contra-indication unless the suckling baby or another member of the household is immunosuppressed.

SIDE-EFFECTS
Paralytic poliomyelitis is the only significant adverse reaction. The risk of vaccine-associated paralysis to a

recipient of the vaccine is reported to be 1.46 per million doses after the first dose, 0.49 per million after the second dose, zero after the third and fourth doses and 0.33 per million after the fifth dose. More recently it has been suggested that the risk after the first dose is 0.42 cases per million and 0.08 cases per million overall.

POISONING/TOXICITY
No adverse effects have been noted, even when 10 times the normal dose was administered.

PHARMACODYNAMIC PROPERTIES
Produces humoral and gut immunity.

PHARMACOKINETIC PROPERTIES
Live virus may be excreted from the gut for up to 6 weeks after administration.

EXCIPIENTS
Magnesium chloride, arginine and polysorbate 80. May contain very small amounts of penicillin, neomycin and streptomycin.

LICENSED STATUS
Licensed for use as described.

FURTHER INFORMATION
If any household members have not been fully immunised against polio, they should be immunised at the same time, assuming there are no contra-indications. Inactivated polio vaccine is likely to replace OPV in the UK in the near future. Store at 2–8°C and protect from light.

Potassium acetate

Potassium acetate is metabolised to bicarbonate in vivo (1mmol of acetate ≡ 1mmol of bicarbonate).

USES
As a potassium supplement as part of a balanced PN regimen where the level of chloride needs to be limited to 3mmol/kg (hyperchloraemic acidaemia)and where the patient is becoming acidotic.

PRESENTATION
Injection: 490mg in 1mL (providing 5mmol K$^+$ and 5mmol acetate), 10mL vial; 785mg in 1mL (providing 8mmol K$^+$ and 8mmol acetate), 10mL vial; – manufactured 'specials'. Other strengths available.

DOSAGE
2-3mmol/kg/day, depending on plasma level of K$^+$ and acid base balance. For hypochloraemic patients dose is usually started at 1mmol/kg/day of acetate and should not exceed 2mmol/kg/day of acetate; the rest of the potassium/sodium is given as chloride. Adjust dose in renal impairment.

ADMINISTRATION
IV: dilute at least 50 times before use as part of a balanced PN regimen.

CONTRA-INDICATIONS & WARNINGS
Metabolic or respiratory alkalosis, hypocalcaemia or hypochlorhydria. Caution in renal or adrenocortical disease, cardiac disease, patients receiving potassium sparing diuretics, ACE inhibitors or digoxin.

INTERACTIONS
ACE inhibitors, digoxin and *diuretics.*

SIDE-EFFECTS/POISONING & TOXICITY
Excessive administration may lead to metabolic alkalosis and hyperkalaemia.

LICENSED STATUS
Unlicensed product; manufactured under manufacturers Licence by South Devon Healthcare.

Potassium canrenoate

Potassium canrenoate is rapidly metabolised to canrenone, a metabolite of spironolactone.

USES
To induce diuresis in congestive cardiac failure.
Short-term parenteral treatment in patients for whom oral treatment with spironolactone is difficult or impossible.

PRESENTATION
Injection: 200mg vial – Soldactone®.

DOSAGE
SHOULD ONLY BE GIVEN WITH POTASSIUM SUPPLEMENTS OR DRUGS LIKELY TO INCREASE POTASSIUM PLASMA
LEVELS WHEN POTASSIUM PLASMA LEVELS ARE BEING CLOSELY MONITORED.

Route	Age				Frequency (times daily)	Notes
	birth-1 month	1 month-2 years	2-12 years	12-18 years		
Slow IV injection or IV infusion	←	1–2mg/kg	→	100–200mg	2	See below for administration details.

ADMINISTRATION
IV: either by slow IV injection or by infusion following dilution in a suitable vehicle. To avoid irritation or pain at the site
of injection, undiluted injection should be administered slowly over 3 minutes. For slow IV infusion the injection may be
diluted to 1mg in 1mL with glucose 5% or NaCl 0.9% or up to 2mg in 1ml in glucose 5%. No other drugs or nutrients
may be added.
To convert to the equivalent oral spironolactone dose in mg multiply potassium canrenoate dose in mg by 0.7.

**CONTRA-INDICATIONS & WARNINGS, INTERACTIONS,
SIDE-EFFECTS**
See spironolactone monograph.

PREGNANCY
Potassium canrenoate and its metabolites may cross the
placental barrier. Contact local Medicines Information
Centre for advice.

BREASTFEEDING
Potassium canrenoate is detected in breast milk, an
alternative method of feeding should be arranged.

PHARMACOKINETIC PROPERTIES
Potassium canrenoate is 85-90% protein bound. The
major site of biotransformation is thought to be the liver
and excretion is mainly in the urine. Plasma half-life in
adults ranges from 17-22 hours.

EXCIPIENTS
See manufacturers SPC for further details.

LICENSED STATUS
Not licensed in the UK.

FURTHER INFORMATION
Available via Idis World Medicines.
Diuresis normally commences within the first 24 hours although long latent periods have been reported in refractory cases.

Potassium chloride

USES
Prevention and treatment of hypokalaemic states.

PRESENTATION
Injection: 15% (2mmol in 1mL each of K^+ and Cl^-), 10mL ampoule – Potassium Chloride Concentrate, Sterile –
non-proprietary.
IV fluid: with added potassium – see IV fluids guidance section page G54 for details.
Liquid: 7.5% (1mmol in 1mL each of K^+ and Cl^-) – Kay-Cee-L®.

Tablet: (modified release) 600mg (8mmol each of K$^+$ and Cl$^-$) – Slow-K$^®$.
Tablet: (effervescent) betaine hydrochloride, potassium benzoate, bicarbonate and chloride equivalent to potassium chloride 500mg (6.7mmol each of K$^+$ and Cl$^-$) – Kloref$^®$.
Tablet: (effervescent) potassium bicarbonate and chloride equivalent to potassium 470mg (12mmol K$^+$) and chloride 285mg (8mmol Cl$^-$) – Sando-K$^®$.

DOSAGE

Indication	Route	Age			Frequency	Notes
		1 month–2 years	2–12 years	12–18 years	(times daily)	
Potassium supplement	Oral/IV	←	0.5–1mmol/kg	→	2	IV administration should be in a suitable infusion fluid or as part of a suitable IV feeding regimen.
Acute hypokalaemia	IV infusion	←	0.08–0.2mmol/kg/hour	→	continuous	Always check the dose carefully, an overdose can be rapidly fatal. Recheck the potassium level after 3 hours.

ADMINISTRATION

Oral: give with feeds to neonates/infants. Take with or after food. Modified release tablets should not be crushed but swallowed whole, with fluid, whilst sitting or standing. Total daily dose can be given in three or more divided doses, especially in neonates to minimise gastric irritation.
IV: dilute injection before use with not less than 50 times its volume of IV fluid and mix well. The pre-mixed bags should be used in preference whenever practicable (see Further Information).
Usual maximum concentration for peripheral infusion is 40mmol K$^+$/L given at a rate not exceeding 0.2mmol/kg/hour (a higher rate of up to 0.5mmol/kg/hour may rarely be justified e.g. if patient is fluid restricted and being monitored by ECG). Higher concentrations and rates require special care. Monitor electrolyte status and ECG.

CONTRA-INDICATIONS & WARNINGS

Plasma potassium concentrations >5mmol/L. Avoid routine use in moderate renal impairment – high risk of hyperkalaemia. All solid forms of potassium medication are contra-indicated in the presence of obstructions in the digestive tract. Inadequately treated Addison disease. Acute dehydration. Extreme care should be exercised when calculating infusion doses.

INTERACTIONS

Increased risk of hyperkalaemia with *ACE inhibitors, NSAIDs, ciclosporin (cyclosporin), digoxin, heparin* and *potassium-sparing diuretics*.

PREGNANCY/BREAST-FEEDING

No clinical problems have been encountered.

SIDE-EFFECTS

Abdominal discomfort, diarrhoea, nausea and vomiting. Concentrated solutions can cause thrombophlebitis and pain at the injection site, while extravasation can cause tissue necrosis.

POISONING/TOXICITY

Hyperkalaemia. Absolute toxicity is dependent on other electrolytes and acid-base levels. Hyperkalaemic symptoms include paraesthesia of the extremities, listlessness, mental confusion, weakness, paralysis, hypotension, cardiac arrhythmias, heart block and cardiac arrest.
Treatment: raised serum potassium levels respond to administration of glucose, glucose and insulin or sodium bicarbonate solution. Severe cardiac toxicity may be treated with calcium gluconate. Cation-exchange resins may be used or in some cases peritoneal or haemodialysis may be necessary. Caution should be exercised in patients who are digitalised and who may experience acute digitalis intoxication in the course of potassium removal.

PHARMACOKINETIC PROPERTIES

Potassium is excreted mainly by the kidneys. Capacity of the kidneys to conserve K$^+$ is poor and renal losses continue to occur even in severe depletion. Some K$^+$ excreted in faeces, saliva, sweat, bile and pancreatic juice.

EXCIPIENTS

Kay-Cee-L$^®$ liquid includes sorbitol. Kloref$^®$ tablets include saccharin calcium. Slow-K$^®$ and Sando-K$^®$ include sucrose. Contact manufacturers for further details.

LICENSED STATUS

Slow-K$^®$ tablets are not licensed for use in children; other preparations licensed for use in children and adults.

FURTHER INFORMATION
The National Patient Safety Agency (NPSA) alert re: potassium chloride concentrate solutions (see www.npsa.org.uk for further details) sets out action, including the following:
1. Potassium chloride concentrate solutions are restricted to Critical Care areas only and should be stored in a separate locked cupboard. Documentation should follow the pattern for controlled drugs and the concentrate should not be transferred between clinical areas.
2. Commercially prepared, ready to use, diluted solutions should be prescribed and used wherever possible.
3. A second practitioner check is required for any IV solution prepared from the concentrate.

Potassium permanganate

P

USES
Skin cleansing agent; useful if the skin is infected e.g. weeping eczema, weeping impetigo.

PRESENTATION
Solution tablet: 400mg – Permitabs®.
Solution: potassium permanganate 0.1% (1 in 100) in water – Potassium Permanganate Solution.

DOSAGE/ADMINISTRATION
Topical: pour a pint of very warm water into a heat-resistant container. Add required number of tablets, stirring occasionally. Add this solution to calculated volume of warm water. See table.

STRENGTH	LARGE VOLUMES		SMALL VOLUMES	
	Tablets	Volume of water	Tablets	Volume of water
1:2000			4	2.6l (4.5 pints)
1:4000			2	2.6L (4.5 pints)
1:6000	20	48L (10.5 gallons)	1	1.8L (3 pints)
1:8000	16	51L (11 gallons)	1	2.6L (4.5 pints)
1:10,000 *	13	52L (11.4 gallons)	1	3.4L (6 pints)
1:12,000	11	53L (11.6 gallons)	1	4.2L (7.5 pints)

*This is the usual strength used.
Average bath contains 52L.

CONTRA-INDICATIONS & WARNINGS
Not for oral use. Use with particular care in patients with extensive erosive or ulcerated skin lesions, especially if they have renal failure, due to theoretical risk of absorption. Irritant to mucous membranes. Stains skin and clothing. Do not use in ceramic basin or bath as staining will occur.

POISONING/TOXICITY
If solution is swallowed accidentally, wash out mouth with water and give glass of milk to drink.
If splashed in eye – irrigate with cold water.
Ingestion of substantial quantities of tablets requires immediate medical assistance.

LICENSED STATUS
Permitabs® are unlicensed.

Povidone–iodine

Broad-spectrum antiseptic.

USES
Skin antiseptic.

P

PRESENTATION
Alcoholic solution: 10% Betadine®.
Alcoholic tincture: 10% Videne.
Antiseptic paint: 10% in an alcoholic solution – Betadine®.
Antiseptic solution: 10% in aqueous solution, Betadine®, Videne®.
Dry powder spray: 2.5% – Betadine®.
Ointment: 10% in water miscible basis – Betadine®.
Powder spray: 1.14% – Savlon® Dry Antiseptic.
Skin cleanser solution: 4% in a surfactant basis – Betadine®.
Shampoo solution: 4% in a surfactant solution – Betadine®.
Surgical scrub: 7.5% in non-ionic surfactant basis – Betadine®.
Surgical scrub: 7.5% in aqueous solution – Videne®.

DOSAGE/ADMINISTRATION
Antiseptic paint: apply twice daily.
Dry powder: use for minor wounds and infections.
Ointment: apply once or twice daily for up to 14 days.
Shampoo: use as shampoo twice weekly until improvement noted then once weekly.
Skin cleanser: retain on infected skin for 3-5 minutes before rinsing. Repeat twice daily.
Solutions, tinctures and scrub: use undiluted for skin disinfection.

CONTRA-INDICATIONS & WARNINGS
Most products not licensed to be used <2 years (see licensed status below). Hypersensitivity. Avoid in patients with thyroid disorders or on lithium therapy. Exercise special care when applying to broken skin and in patients with renal insufficiency.

INTERACTIONS
May interfere with *thyroid function tests*.

PREGNANCY/BREAST-FEEDING
Avoid regular use.

SIDE-EFFECTS
Skin irritation. Application to large wounds may produce metabolic acidosis, hypernatraemia and impairment of renal function.

POISONING/TOXICITY
Symptomatic and supportive treatment if accidentally ingested. Special attention to electrolyte balance, renal and thyroid function.

EXCIPIENTS
Contact manufacturers for further details.

LICENSED STATUS
Ointment, dry powder sprays, skin cleanser, shampoo: licensed for use >2 years.
Solutions, tinctures and scrubs: not recommended for regular use in neonates, and contra-indicated in low birth weight infants <1.5kg (although it is sometimes used).

Pravastatin sodium

A 3-hydroxy-3-methylglutaryl coenzyme A (HMG CoA) reductase inhibitor.

USES
Hypercholesterolaemia, including familial hypercholesterolaemia in patients who have not responded adequately to diet therapy and with a total cholesterol >7.7mmol/L (300mg/dL).

PRESENTATION
Tablet: 10mg, 20mg and 40mg – Lipostat®.

DOSAGE

Route	Age		Frequency (times daily)	Notes
	2–12 years	12–18 years		
Oral	5mg	10mg	1 (at night)	Starting dose; if necessary increase dose over 6-12 weeks. Consult specialist advice as little information on dosing in children.

CONTRA-INDICATIONS & WARNINGS, INTERACTIONS, PREGNANCY, BREAST-FEEDING, SIDE-EFFECTS, POISONING/TOXICITY   See simvastatin monograph.

EXCIPIENTS
See manufacturers SPC for further details.

LICENSED STATUS
Not licensed for use in children.

Praziquantel

Anthelmintic.

USES
Anthelmintic with broad spectrum of activity against:
  Trematodes (flukes) – including schistosomiasis, liver flukes, lung flukes, intestinal flukes.
  Cestodes (tapeworms) – adult or intestinal stage, larval or tissue stage (neurocysticercosis).
  Echinococcus – as an adjunct to surgery and in inoperable cases.

PRESENTATION
Tablet: 150mg – Cesol® (imported).
Tablet: 600mg (film coated) – Biltricide® (imported).

DOSAGE
Safety in children <4 years of age has not been established.

Indication	Route	Age		Frequency (times daily)	Notes
		2-12 years	12-18 years		
Schistosomiasis haematobium, S. mansoni	Oral	← ≥4 years 20mg/kg → OR		2	For 1 day. The intervals between doses should be between 4-6 hours. Take doses with food.
		← 40mg/kg →		single dose	Can be given as 2 equally divided doses as single dose therapy has been reported to have a higher incidence of side-effects.
S. japonicum	Oral	← ≥4 years 20mg/kg →		3	For 1 day. The intervals between doses should be between 4-6 hours. Take doses with food.
Liver flukes Clonorchiasis and Opisthorchiasis	Oral	← ≥4 years 30mg/kg →		2	For 3 days.
Lung flukes *Paragonimus westermani*	Oral	← ≥4 years 25mg/kg →		3	For 3 days.

DOSAGE continued

Indication	Route	Age		Frequency (times daily)	Notes
		2–12 years	12–18 years		
Intestinal flukes *Fasciolopsis buski*	Oral	⟵ ≥4 years 25mg/kg ⟶		3	For 1 day.
Beef, pork and fish tapeworm	Oral	⟵ ≥4 years 10–20mg/kg ⟶		single dose	Take after a light breakfast.
Dwarf tapeworm	Oral	⟵ ≥4 years 25mg/kg ⟶		single dose	Take after a light breakfast.
Tapeworm larval or tissue stage (neuro-cysticercosis)	Oral	⟵ ≥4 years 17mg/kg ⟶		3	For 15–21 days. NB: expert advice required on management. A corticosteroid should be given concurrently to reduce the severity of adverse effects e.g dexamethasone 600 microgram/kg/**day** in divided doses (maximum 16mg/**day**) or prednisolone 1.5mg/kg daily (maximum 60mg/**day**).
Hydatid disease (*Echinococcus*)	Oral	⟵ ≥4 years 40mg/kg ⟶		once a week	In combination with albendazole as an adjunct to surgery and for inoperable cysts.

Renal impairment
Dosage adjustment not necessary.

Hepatic impairment
Dosage recommendations for patients with liver disease are controversial. Some clinicians recommend dosage adjustment in severe hepatic impairment, while others do not.

ADMINISTRATION
Oral: administer tablets with food; not to be chewed due to bitter taste; can be halved or quartered to allow administration of individualised doses. Swallow dose immediately with a sufficient amount of liquid during meals since retention of tablets/segments in the mouth may cause gagging/vomiting due to the bitter taste.

CONTRA-INDICATIONS & WARNINGS
Contra–indications: hypersensitivity, ocular cysticercosis, spinal cysticercosis.
Warnings: may impair ability to perform tasks requiring mental alertness, therefore avoid driving/operating machinery etc. on day of and day after treatment.
Caution in severe hepatic disease and patients with a history of seizures.

INTERACTIONS
Phenytoin, carbamazepine, phenobarbital (phenobarbitone) – may reduce serum levels of praziquantel. *Dexamethasone:* may reduce praziquantel serum levels by half. *Chloroquine:* reduces bioavailability of praziquantel. *Cimetidine:* hepatic enzyme inhibitor – may increase serum levels of praziquantel. *Alcohol:* potentiates CNS effects of praziquantel.

PREGNANCY
Animal studies have not shown a fetal risk but no controlled studies in pregnant women. Therefore the drug should be used in pregnancy only if benefit outweighs possible risks to fetus.

BREAST-FEEDING
Praziquantel is excreted into breast milk. It is recommended women do not nurse on the day of treatment or for 72 hours after administration of the last dose of the drug.

SIDE-EFFECTS
Common but usually mild and transient.
CNS: drowsiness, malaise, headache, dizziness, seizures.
Gastrointestinal: abdominal discomfort, nausea, vomiting, anorexia, diarrhoea.
Dermatological: urticarial and pruritic skin rashes.

Hepatic: raised liver enzymes (rarely).
Other: pyrexia.

POISONING/TOXICITY
No experience to date of acute praziquantel overdose. However, manufacturer recommends administration of a fast-acting laxative following acute ingestion of an overdose of the drug.

PHARMACOKINETIC PROPERTIES
Oral absorption is about 80%. Extensive first pass metabolism – metabolised by liver to hydroxylated and conjugated metabolites. CSF concentration is 14-20% of plasma concentration. Protein binding is about 80%. Half-life of 0.8-1.5 hours; metabolite half-life of 4-5 hours (adult). Time to peak serum concentration is 1-3 hours. Drug and metabolites are excreted mainly in urine (99% as metabolites).

LICENSED STATUS
Not licensed for use in the UK.

FURTHER INFORMATION
Available from IDIS World Medicines.

P

Prazosin

Alpha-blocker, vasodilator.

USES
Hypertension, congestive heart failure.

PRESENTATION
Tablet: 500 microgram, 1mg, 2mg and 5mg – Hypovase® and non-proprietary.
Liquid: may be extemporaneously prepared.

DOSAGE

Indication	Route	Age			Frequency	Notes
		1 month–2 years	2–12 years	12–18 years	(times daily)	
Hypertension	Oral	← 10–15 microgram/kg →			2–4	Initial dose. Increase dose gradually to
				500 microgram	2–3	a maximum of 500 microgram/kg/day if <12 years and 20mg/day if >12 years.
Congestive heart failure	Oral	← 5 microgram/kg →			2	Initial dose. Increase dose gradually to
				500 microgram	2–4	a maximum of 100 microgram/kg/day if <12 years and 20mg/day if >12 years.

ADMINISTRATION
Tablets may be dispersed in water

CONTRA-INDICATIONS, WARNINGS & MONITORING
Hypersensitivity to prazosin or related quinazolines. Not recommended for congestive heart failure due to mechanical obstruction. When giving first dose monitor for excessive hypotension or give at bedtime.

INTERACTIONS
Calcium-channel blockers, diuretics and *beta-blockers* – enhanced hypotensive effect; increased risk of first-dose hypotensive effect. Enhanced hypotensive effect also with *ACE inhibitors, anaesthetics, antidepressants, antipsychotics, anxiolytics* and *hypnotics. NSAIDs* – antagonise the hypotensive effect.

PREGNANCY
No evidence of teratogenicity, although studies to date are inadequate to establish the safety of prazosin in pregnancy. Contact local Medicines Information Centre for advice.

BREAST-FEEDING
Excreted in small amounts in breast milk; probably too small to be harmful. Contact local Medicines Information Centre for advice.

POISONING/TOXICITY
Should overdosage lead to hypotension, support of the

cardiovascular system is of first importance. Restoration of blood pressure and normalisation of heart rate may be accomplished by keeping the patient in the supine position. If this measure is inadequate, shock should first be treated with volume expanders. If necessary, vasopressors should then be used. Renal function should be monitored and supported as needed.

Laboratory data indicate prazosin is not dialysable because it is protein bound.

PHARMACOKINETIC PROPERTIES
Highly plasma protein bound. Extensively metabolised and excreted mainly via bile and faeces.

EXCIPIENTS
See manufacturers SPC for further details.

LICENSED STATUS
Licensed ≥12 years of age.

Prednisolone

Corticosteroid.

USES
Acute severe asthma, suppression of inflammatory and allergic disorders, croup, nephrotic syndrome, solid organ graft rejection, autoimmune hepatitis, inflammatory bowel disease, infantile spasms, generalised tonic-clonic and focal seizures, intractable myoclonic seizures and absence seizures, life-threatening systemic disease associated with juvenile idiopathic arthritis (JIA) or disease unresponsive to other therapies, vasculitis, connective tissue diseases (including juvenile dermatomyositis), uveitis, as part of chemotherapy regimens for Hodgkin's and non-Hodgkin's lymphomas, B-cell lymphoma/leukaemias, acute lymphoblastic leukaemia.

PRESENTATION
Injection: (as acetate) 25mg in 1mL – Deltastab®.
Retention enema: (as sodium phosphate) 20mg, 100mL – Predsol®; (as sodium metasulphobenzoate) 20mg, 100mL – Predenema®.
Rectal foam: (as sodium metasulphobenzoate) 20mg per metered application, 25g (14 applications) – Predfoam®.
Suppository: (as sodium phosphate) 5mg – Predsol®.
Tablet: 1mg, 5mg and 25mg – non-proprietary.
Tablet: (soluble) (as sodium phosphate) 5mg – non-proprietary.
Tablet: (enteric coated) 2.5mg and 5mg – non-proprietary.

DOSAGE

Indication	Route	Age			Frequency	Notes
		1 month–2 years	2–12 years	12–18 years	(times daily)	
Acute asthma	Oral	← 1-2mg/kg (maximum dose 40mg) →			1	Treat for 1–5 days and then stop (no need to taper dose).
Suppression of inflammatory and allergic disorders	Oral	← 1-2mg/kg →			1	The daily dose can be given in 2–3 divided doses if necessary. Consider alternate day treatment in long-term.
Croup requiring intubation	Oral	← 1mg/kg →		–	2	Start within 24 hours of intubation continuing until 24 hours after extubation.
Nephrotic syndrome	Oral	← 60mg/m² (maximum dose 80mg) → then ← 40mg/m² (maximum dose 60mg) →			1 (morning) 1 (alternate days)	Initial dose (on presentation) for 4-6 weeks. Then (providing proteinuria has has been absent for 3 days) maintenance. Maintenance dose for 4 weeks then stop. Repeat course for any relapses.

DOSAGE continued

Indication	Route	Age			Frequency	Notes
		1 month–2 years	2–12 years	12–18 years	(times daily)	
Replacement	Oral	–		2.5mg/m²	2	In some cases, could be used as a 5mg/m² once daily dose.
Autoimmune hepatitis	Oral	← 2mg/kg (maximum dose 40mg) →			1	
Inflammatory bowel disease	Oral	–	← 1–2mg/kg → (maximum 60mg daily)		1	Give as a reducing regimen and wean off over a few weeks if possible.
JIA, connective tissue disease, vasculitis	Oral	← up to 2mg/kg →			1 (morning) (or alternate days)	Use the lowest dose that controls the disease without unacceptable side-effects.
	IM/IA	← dose must be individualised →			single dose	Dose depends on condition being treated and its severity.
Local treatment of ulcerative colitis and Crohn's disease	Rectal (enema)	–	–	1 enema	1	At bedtime for 2–4 weeks, continued if good response.
Proctitis and distal ulcerative colitis	Rectal (foam)	–	–	1 metered dose	1–2	For 2 weeks, continued for a further 2 weeks if good response.
Proctitis. Rectal complications of Crohn's disease	Rectal (suppository)	–	← 1 suppository →		2	Night and morning after bowel movement.
Epileptic seizures	Oral	← 2mg/kg →			1	Higher doses have been used in infantile spasms.

Dosage in chemotherapy regimes
Always follow the dosage recommended in the protocol.

Dosage in renal transplant immunosuppression
Contact individual transplant units for details of their own protocol.

ADMINISTRATION

Intra-articular/peri-articular: prednisolone should not be given via these routes when the joint or surrounding tissues are infected.
Oral: the uncoated tablets are scored and can be halved. These and the dispersible tablets should be taken with or after food in order to minimise gastrointestinal side-effects. The enteric coated tablets should be swallowed whole, but must not be used in cystic fibrosis.
Rectal: follow the administration instructions given with individual products.

CONTRA-INDICATIONS & WARNINGS

Use is contra-indicated in patients with systemic infection, unless specific anti-infective therapy is used. Also contra-indicated in patients vaccinated with live vaccines. Administration of live vaccines should be postponed for at least 3 months after immuno-suppressive treatment has been stopped or 3 months after levels have been reached that are not associated with immunosuppression. If starting prednisolone following the administration of vaccinations, the time lag varies depending on the individual vaccination and you are advised to contact the individual manufacturers for further information.
Steroids should not be injected directly into tendons or into spinal or other non-diarthrodial joints.
Caution is necessary when using corticosteroids in patients with any of the following conditions: X-ray indicative of or history of tuberculosis, hypertension, congestive cardiac failure, hepatic or renal failure,

diabetes mellitus, osteoporosis, glaucoma. Rectal use contra-indicated in local conditions where infection might be masked or healing impaired. Patients who encounter stresses and who are at risk of adrenal insufficiency should receive systemic corticosteroid cover during these periods.

Withdrawal of corticosteroids
In patients who have received systemic corticosteroids for greater than 3 weeks, withdrawal should not be abrupt. However, abrupt withdrawal is appropriate in some patients treated for up to 3 weeks if it is considered that the disease is unlikely to relapse or that the dose has been such that abrupt withdrawal is unlikely to lead to clinically relevant hypothalmic-pituitary-adrenal-axis suppression.
Gradual withdrawal of therapy should be considered in some patient groups even after courses lasting 3 weeks or less, for example: patients who have had repeated courses; when a short course has been prescribed within 1 year of cessation of long-term therapy (months or years); patients who may have reasons for adrenocortical insufficiency other than exogenous corticosteroid therapy; patients repeatedly taking doses in the evening.

INTERACTIONS
Drugs which induce liver enzymes (such as *rifampicin, rifabutin, carbamazepine, phenobarbital (phenobarbitone), phenytoin, aminoglutethimide*) will increase the metabolism of corticosteroids and may decrease their effects. Corticosteroids antagonise the effects of *hypoglycaemic agents*, including *insulin;* increased doses of the *hypoglycaemic agents* may be required. The hypokalaemic effects of *acetazolamide, loop diuretics* and *thiazide diuretics* are enhanced. Increased risk of gastrointestinal bleeding and ulceration with *aspirin* and *NSAIDs*; corticosteroids reduce plasma salicylate concentrations. *Oestrogens* are likely to potentiate the effects of corticosteroids, which may necessitate dosage adjustment of the steroid. *Live vaccines* should not be given to patients taking immunosuppressive doses of steroids, as severe infections may develop. The antibody response to other vaccines may also be diminished. Drugs which inhibit liver enzymes (such as *ketoconazole*) may decrease the metabolism of corticosteroids and may increase their effects.

PREGNANCY
Corticosteroids vary in their ability to cross the placenta; betamethasone and dexamethasone cross the placenta readily while 88% of prednisolone is inactivated as it crosses the placenta.
Administration of corticosteroids to pregnant animals can cause abnormalities of fetal development including cleft palate/lip and effects on brain growth and development. However, in humans there is no convincing evidence that systemic corticosteroids cause an increased incidence of congenital abnormalities, such as cleft palate or lip. When administered for prolonged periods during pregnancy,

systemic corticosteroids significantly increase the risk of intra-uterine growth retardation (IUGR), but there is no evidence for an increased incidence of IUGR following short-term treatment, such as prophylactic treatment for neonatal respiratory distress syndrome. There is a theoretical risk of adrenal suppression in the neonate following pre-natal corticosteroid exposure. However, this usually resolves spontaneously after birth and is rarely clinically important. The available evidence supports the use of corticosteroids to control various maternal diseases during pregnancy when their use is essential.

BREAST-FEEDING
Prednisolone is excreted in small amounts into breast milk. However, doses of up to 40mg of prednisolone daily or equivalent are unlikely to cause systemic effects in the infant. Infants of mothers taking higher doses than this should be monitored for signs of adrenal suppression. No data are available on the transfer of other systemic corticosteroids into breast milk.

SIDE-EFFECTS
Side-effects can be minimised by using the lowest effective dose for the minimum period possible.
Immunosuppression: immunosuppressive effects may result in an increased severity of infectious diseases such as chickenpox, measles. If chickenpox exposure occurs, *varicella zoster immunoglobulin (VZIG)* or *aciclovir (acyclovir)* should be given immediately. If measles exposure occurs give pooled human gammabulin.
Gastrointestinal: dyspepsia, peptic ulceration, oesophageal ulceration, acute pancreatitis, oesophageal candidiasis.
Musculoskeletal: osteoporosis, fractures.
Fluid and electrolyte disturbance: sodium and water retention, hypertension.
Endocrine/metabolic: growth suppression, menstrual irregularity, amenorrhoea, hirsutism, increased appetite, precipitation of diabetes or loss of glucose control in diabetes.
Neuropsychiatric: euphoria, depression, insomnia, increased intracranial pressure and papilloedema (pseudotumour cerebri) in children.
Ophthalmic: increased intra-ocular pressure and glaucoma.
Dermatological: bruising and impaired skin healing.
General: thromboembolism, hypersensitivity including anaphylaxis.

POISONING/TOXICITY
There is no specific antidote. Treatment is symptomatic. Plasma electrolytes should be monitored.

PHARMACOKINETIC PROPERTIES
Prednisolone is eliminated by hepatic metabolism. When administered rectally the action of the drug is predominantly local although systemic absorption can occur (especially if the bowel is inflamed). Peak plasma levels are significantly lower with rectal prednisolone 21-sodium metasulphobenzoate than prednisolone 21-phosphate.

EXCIPIENTS
Deltastab® includes benzyl alcohol. Contact manufacturers for further details.

LICENSED STATUS
Injection and tablets licensed for use in children. Suppositories are the only rectal product licensed for use in children.

FURTHER INFORMATION
Equivalent anti-inflammatory doses of corticosteroids*

Betamethasone	750 microgram
Deflazacort	6mg
Dexamethasone	750 microgram
Hydrocortisone	20mg
Methylprednisolone	4mg
Prednisolone	5mg
Triamcinolone	4mg

*Applies only to oral or IV administration; relative potencies may differ greatly when injected IM or into joint spaces.

Prilocaine hydrochloride

Local anaesthetic.

USES
For dental local anaesthesia.

PRESENTATION
Injection: prilocaine hydrochloride 4% (40mg in 1mL), 2mL cartridge – Citanest®. Prilocaine hydrochloride 3% (30mg in 1mL) and felypressin (0.03 international units in 1mL), 2mL cartridge – Citanest with Octapressin®.

DOSAGE
Citanest®: children <10 years usual dose is 1mL; ≥10 years 1-2mL.
Citanest with Octapressin®: children <10 years usual dose is approximately 1-2mL; ≥10 years 1-5mL.

ADMINISTRATION
May be used by infiltration or dental nerve block techniques.

CONTRA-INDICATIONS & WARNINGS
Know hypersensitivity to amide-type anaesthetics. Should be avoided in patients with anaemia or methaemoglobin. Avoid intravascular administration, particularly in susceptible groups of patients. Avoid injection into deep tissue of patients with a bleeding disorder. Avoid administration into inflamed or infected areas. Patients and parents must be strongly warned against any behaviour likely to traumatise anaesthetised tissue.

SIDE-EFFECTS
Hypersensitivity reactions (extremely rarely). Cutaneous lesions, urticaria, oedema, anaphylactic shock (detection of sensitivity by skin testing is of doubtful value).

POISONING/TOXICITY
Significant levels of methaemoglobinaemia may occur when (adult) doses of prilocaine exceed 600mg. This may be treated by the IV administration of a 1% solution of methylthioninium chloride (methylene blue) in a dose of 1mg/kg.
Also see the lidocaine (lignocaine) hydrochloride monograph.

EXCIPIENTS
See manufacturers SPC for further details.

LICENSED STATUS
Licensed for use in children (no lower age limit) and adults.

8-aminoquinoline derivative; an antimalarial agent.

USES
Adjunct in the treatment of *P. vivax* and *P. ovale* malaria; eradication of the parasites in the liver and to produce a radical cure.

PRESENTATION
Tablet: equivalent to 7.5mg base (as phosphate) – named patient.

DOSAGE
All doses given as primaquine base.

Route	Age			Frequency (times daily)	Notes
	1 month–2 years	2–12 years	12–18 year		
Oral	← 250 microgram/kg →		15mg	once daily	For 14 days, or for 21 days for infections contracted in south east Asia or western Pacific.
	← 500–750 microgram/kg →		30mg	once weekly	For 8 weeks. Patients with G6PD deficiency.

>1 year (top dose row), >1 year (bottom dose row)

ADMINISTRATION
Oral: take after food as abdominal pain and cramps are common if taken on an empty stomach.

CONTRA-INDICATIONS & WARNINGS
Acutely ill patients who have systemic diseases associated with granulocytopenia, e.g. rheumatoid arthritis, lupus erythematosus; patients with an underlying condition compromising bone marrow function or taking medication capable of depressing the myeloid elements of bone marrow; children aged <1 year. Use with caution and follow the weekly dosing regimen in patients with G6PD deficiency, as acute haemolytic anaemia can occur.

PREGNANCY
Safe use in pregnancy has not been established. Placental transfer to a G6PD deficient fetus potentially could result in life -threatening haemolytic anaemia in utero. As relapse of *P.vivax* does not usually occur for 6–12 months after the initial infection, treatment can be delayed until after delivery.

BREAST-FEEDING
Primaquine passes into breast milk and mothers taking the drug should not breast-feed. Alternatively, primaquine therapy should be delayed until breast-feeding has been completed.

SIDE-EFFECTS
Generally well tolerated at the doses used for treatment of recurrent malaria although nausea, vomiting, abdominal cramps and gastric distress can occur. Methaemoglobinaemia may occur occasionally and haemolytic anaemia can occur in persons with G6PD deficiency. Headache, pruritus, and interference with visual accommodation have been reported and rarely hypertension, cardiac arrhythmias and leucopenia.

POISONING/TOXICITY
Features of acute overdose include anorexia, nausea, vomiting, weakness, cyanosis, bone marrow depression, and methaemoglobinaemia. There is no specific antidote and treatment is symptomatic.

PHARMACOKINETIC PROPERTIES
Well absorbed from the gastrointestinal tract but has poor bioavailability due to pre-systemic metabolism and enterohepatic circulation. Following oral administration, peak plasma concentrations are generally attained within 6 hours. Widely distributed in the tissues. Rapidly metabolised in the liver and only a small amount is excreted unchanged in the urine.

LICENSED STATUS
Not licensed for use in the UK.

FURTHER INFORMATION
Tablets can be obtained from Durbin.

Methylhydrazine derivative; a cytostatic agent with weak monoamine-oxidase inhibitor properties.

USES
In combination therapy for Hodgkin lymphoma and gliomas.

PRESENTATION
Capsule: 50mg – Cambridge.

DOSAGE
** Always consult the current treatment protocol for details of dosage and scheduling. **

ADMINISTRATION
Oral: in divided doses throughout the day. Administration with food may reduce the incidence of nausea and vomiting.

CONTRA-INDICATIONS & WARNINGS
Full blood count should be satisfactory before commencing treatment. Decrease in dose should be considered in renal/hepatic impairment.

INTERACTIONS
Procarbazine may exacerbate respiratory depression if taken in conjunction with *CNS depressants*. Procarbazine has weak MAOI activity and may precipitate hypertensive crisis, agitation and tremors if taken in conjunction with *some antidepressants* and *sympathomimetics*. Avoid *tyramine-containing foods e.g. cheese, marmite etc.* In general though, it is not considered that procarbazine is a sufficiently potent inhibitor of MAO to make the standard precautions associated with MAOIs necessary. A disulfiram-type reaction may occur if taken with *alcohol* and CNS depression may be accentuated.

PREGNANCY
Should not be administered to patients who are pregnant unless considered essential.

BREAST-FEEDING
Should not be given to breast-feeding mothers.

SIDE-EFFECTS
Common side-effects include myelosuppression, nausea and vomiting in first few days of treatment, diarrhoea and CNS toxicity manifested as paraesthesia, ataxia, dizziness, headaches, nightmares, depression and insomnia. Hallucinations are common in up to 30% of patients. Occasional toxicities include tremors, convulsions and coma and an influenza-like syndrome of fever, chills and myalgia. Rarely, pulmonary toxicity, possibly a result of a hypersensitivity reaction; nystagmus, diplopia, papilloedema and photophobia. Dermatological reactions occur in up to 3% of patients.

POISONING/TOXICITY
Full supportive measures for correction of protracted myelosuppression and CNS complications.

PHARMACOKINETIC PROPERTIES
Rapidly and completely absorbed from the gastrointestinal tract with peak plasma levels at 0.5-1 hour. Peak CSF levels at 0.5-1.5 hours. Extensively metabolised in the liver to several active (cytotoxic) metabolites. Over 75% of dose administered excreted in the urine.

LICENSED STATUS
Licensed for use in children and adults.

FURTHER INFORMATION
The brand name Natulan® was formerly used for procarbazine capsules.

Prochlorperazine

Dopamine agonist that acts centrally by blocking the chemoreceptor trigger zone.

USES
Prophylaxis and treatment of nausea and vomiting associated with chemotherapy or radiotherapy. Intractable vomiting of known cause.

PRESENTATION
Injection: (as mesilate) 12.5mg in 1mL ampoule – Stemetil®.
Suppository: (as maleate) 5mg and 25mg – Stemetil®.
Syrup: (as mesilate) 5mg in 5mL – Stemetil®.
Tablet: 5mg (as maleate) – Stemetil® and non-proprietary.

DOSAGE

Route	Age			Frequency (times daily)	Notes
	1 month–2 years	2–12 years	12–18 years		
Oral		DOSE BY WEIGHT			
	>1 year ←	100–250 microgram/kg	→	single dose	May be repeated up to 2–3 times daily.
		DOSE BY AGE			
	1–2 years (>10kg) 1.25–2.5mg	2–4 years 1.25–2.5mg	5–10mg	single dose	May be repeated up to 2–3 times daily.
		5–12 years 2.5–5mg		single dose	May be repeated up to 2–3 times daily.
Rectal	1–2 years (>10kg) 2.5mg	2–4 years 2.5mg	12.5–25mg	single dose	May be repeated up to 2–3 times daily.
		5–12 years 5–10mg		single dose	May be repeated up to 2–3 times daily.
IM	1–2 years (>10kg) 1.25–2.5mg	2–4 years 1.25–2.5mg	12.5mg	single dose	May be repeated up to 3 times daily.
		5–12 years 5–6.25mg		single dose	May be repeated up to 3 times daily.

ADMINISTRATION
IM: deep IM injection.

CONTRA-INDICATIONS & WARNINGS
Contra-indicated in pregnancy. Not recommended for use in children less than 10kg or one year of age. Reduce dose in renal impairment. Caution in liver disease (may precipitate coma). Avoid in patients with epilepsy. Prochlorperazine has been associated with dystonic reactions particularly after a cumulative dosage of 500 micrograms/kg, it should be used cautiously in children.

INTERACTIONS.
Increased extrapyramidal side-effects with *metoclopramide* and *lithium*. Decreased effect of *antiepileptics*. Decreased levels with *antacids*. Enhanced sedative effects with *anxiolytics* and *hypnotics*. Avoid with *desferrioxamine*.

PREGNANCY
Contra-indicated in pregnancy as inadequate evidence of the safety in human pregnancy. It has been widely used, though for many years without apparent ill consequence. There is evidence of harmful effects in animals. Avoid unless essential.

BREAST-FEEDING
May be excreted in breast milk, so should avoid if breast-feeding unless essential. Although the amount excreted in breast milk is probably too small to be harmful, animal studies with antipsychotics indicate possible adverse effects on the developing nervous system.

SIDE-EFFECTS
Nasal stuffiness, dry mouth, insomnia and agitation. Extrapyramidal symptoms (especially in seriously ill children, those less than 10kg or one year of age). May rarely cause neuroleptic malignant syndrome. Respiratory depression may occur in susceptible patients. Postural hypotension.

POISONING & TOXICITY
Symptoms include drowsiness or loss of consciousness, hypotension, tachycardia, ECG changes, ventricular arrhythmias and hypothermia. Severe extrapyramidal dyskinesias may occur.

EXCIPIENTS
Stemetil® syrup includes sucrose. Contact manufacturer for further details.

LICENSED STATUS
Not licensed for use in children <10kg, or one year of age and for the rectal or parenteral route.

Procyclidine

An anticholinergic drug which exerts an atropine-like action. It is a competitive inhibitor of the peripheral actions of acetylcholine at muscarinic sites.

USES
Treatment of acute dystonic reactions.

PRESENTATION
Tablet: 5mg – Kemadrin® and non-proprietary.
Syrup: 2.5mg in 5ml and 5mg in 5ml – Arpicolin®.

DOSAGE
Child

Route	Age			Frequency (times daily)	Notes
	1 month–2 years	2–12 years	12–18 years		
Oral	-	7-12 years 1.25mg	2.5mg	3	Less severe extrapyramidal symptoms can be controlled with oral doses.

Care is advised when using in children with hepatic dysfunction.

ADMINISTRATION
Oral: tablets – may be crushed and are physically compatible with Keltrol® suspending agent; syrup – further dilution not recommended.

CONTRA-INDICATIONS & WARNINGS
Contra-indicated in tardive dyskinesia as procyclidine will not help and may make it worse. Caution advised in patients predisposed to obstructive disease of the gastrointestinal tract and in hepatic and renal impairment.

INTERACTIONS
The anticholinergic effects may be increased by other drugs which also have anticholinergic properties e.g. *antihistamines, tricyclic antidepressants*. The absorption of *ketoconazole* may be reduced by concomitant administration of procyclidine.

PREGNANCY/BREAST-FEEDING
No information is available. Contact local Medicines Information Centre for advice.

SIDE-EFFECTS
Dry mouth, blurred vision, constipation and urinary retention.

POISONING/TOXICITY
Procyclidine alone is unlikely to cause serious effects. Toxicity is mainly due to anticholinergic effects at autonomic nerve endings and in the brain. Systemic features of toxicity include flushing, dilated pupils, dry mouth and tongue, hot dry skin, sinus tachycardia, ataxia, nystagmus, drowsiness and delirium with confusion, agitation and visual hallucinations. Treatment is symptomatic.

PHARMACOKINETIC PROPERTIES
When given orally acts approximately within 1-2 hours. The therapeutic half-life is 8-18 hours. Procyclidine is rapidly absorbed from the gastrointestinal tract. It is metabolised to several metabolites and appears to be excreted renally. Only a very small fraction of the dose administered appears in the urine as parent compound.

EXCIPIENTS
Syrup is sucrose free. See manufacturers SPC for further details.

LICENSED STATUS
Not licensed for use in children.

Proguanil

A pro-drug which acts through its main metabolite cycloguanil which is effective against the tissue forms of some strains of *P. falciparum*.

P

USES
Malaria prophylaxis (usually with chloroquine; occasionally alone).

PRESENTATION
Tablet: 100mg (scored) – Paludrine®.

DOSAGE

Route	Age	Weight	Dose mg	Dose tablets	Frequency (times daily)	Notes
Oral	0–12 weeks	<6kg	25mg	1/4 tablet	1	Start 1 week before
	12 weeks –11 months	6–9.9kg	50mg	1/2 tablet	1	arriving in endemic
	1–3 years	10–15.9kg	75mg	3/4 tablet	1	area, and continue for
	4–7 years	16–24.9kg	100mg	1 tablet	1	4 weeks after return.
	8–12 years	25–44.9kg	150mg	1 1/2 tablets	1	
	≥13 years	≥45kg	200mg	2 tablets	1	

ADMINISTRATION
Oral: take with or after food; tablets may be crushed and mixed with milk or jam where necessary.

CONTRA-INDICATIONS & WARNINGS
Renal impairment: no data in children – suggest half dose if creatinine clearance is below $60mL/min/1.73m^2$; quarter recommended dose on alternate days if creatinine clearance is below $20mL/min/1.73m^2$.

INTERACTIONS
Antacids may reduce absorption – separate dosing by 2-3 hours. May enhance anticoagulant effects of *warfarin* – monitor INR.

PREGNANCY
Proguanil has been widely used for over 40 years and a causal connection between its use and any adverse effect on mother or fetus has not been established. Folic acid 5mg daily should be taken by the mother.

BREAST-FEEDING
Excreted in breast milk in amount insufficient to be harmful and inadequate for reliable protection against malaria.

SIDE-EFFECTS
Mild gastric upset; occasional stomatitis and mouth ulcers; rarely skin rash and reversible hair loss. Haematological changes have been reported in patients with severe renal impairment.

POISONING
Gastric irritation and vomiting; haematuria. No antidote; symptomatic treatment.

PHARMACOKINETIC PROPERTIES
Peak concentrations of the active metabolite at approximately 5 hours. Steady-state concentrations achieved at 4 days. Half-life of approximately 20 hours. On stopping treatment, little effect after 3 days.

EXCIPIENTS
See manufacturers SPC for further details.

LICENSED STATUS
Licensed for use in children and adults.

Promethazine hydrochloride

Antihistamine with sedative effects.

USES
Night sedation, sedation for procedures and maintenance sedation on Intensive Care Units. Antihistamine. Nausea.

PRESENTATION
Elixir: 5mg in 5mL – Phenergan®.
Injection: 25mg in 1mL, 1mL ampoule – Phenergan®; 1mL and 2mL ampoules – available from Antigen.
Tablet: 10mg and 25mg – Phenergan®.

DOSAGE

Indication	Route	Age			Frequency (times daily)	Notes
		1 month–2 years	2–12 years	12–18 years		
Symptomatic relief of allergy	Oral	<1 year 2.5–5mg	<6 years 5–10mg	10–20mg	2–3	When 3 doses in 24 hours are given, use the lower stated amount.
		>1 year 5–10mg	>6 years 10–15mg		2–3	
Sedation	Oral	DOSE BY WEIGHT ◄— 1–2mg/kg —►		–	single dose	Give at bedtime for night sedation, or for daytime sedation give once, or twice daily using the lower dose.
		DOSE BY AGE				
		<1 year 5–10mg	2–5 years 10–20mg	25–50mg	single dose	
		>1 year 10–20mg	6–10 years 20–25mg		single dose	
			>10 years 25–50mg		single dose	
Sedation on Intensive Care Units	IV slow bolus/oral/ deep IM	500 microgram – 1mg/kg (maximum 25mg)		25–50mg	4	Start at low dose and adjust according to response. May be used in conjunction with chloral hydrate (up to 50mg/kg).

ADMINISTRATION
Injection: for slow IV injection dilute the 2.5% solution (25mg in 1mL) to 10 times its volume with Water for Injections immediately prior to use and give over at least 5 minutes.

CONTRA-INDICATIONS & WARNINGS
Neonates, premature infants or those hypersensitive to phenothiazines; porphyria; patients in coma or suffering CNS depression of any cause; those who have taken MAOIs in the last 14 days. Caution in use <1 year because of a possible association with sudden infant death syndrome.

INTERACTIONS
Potentiates sedative effects of other drugs; avoid alcohol.

PREGNANCY
There is epidemiological evidence for the safety of promethazine in pregnancy, and animal studies have shown no hazard. Nevertheless it should not be used in pregnancy unless the physician considers it essential. Use is not recommended in the 2 weeks prior to delivery in view of the risk of irritability and excitement in the neonate.

BREAST-FEEDING
Available evidence suggests that the amount excreted in milk is insignificant. However, there are risks of neonatal irritability and excitement.

SIDE-EFFECTS
Occasionally produces irritable or excitable behaviour. Some antimuscarinic effects, drowsiness, dizziness, restlessness, headaches, disorientation.

POISONING/TOXICITY
Symptoms of severe overdosage are variable. They are characterised in children by various combinations of excitation, ataxia, inco-ordination, athetosis and hallucinations, while adults may become drowsy and lapse into coma. Convulsions may occur in both adults and children; coma or excitement may precede their occurrence. Cardiorespiratory depression is uncommon. Treatment is supportive with attention to maintenance of adequate respiratory and circulatory status. Convulsions should be treated with diazepam or other suitable anticonvulsant.

PHARMACOKINETIC PROPERTIES
Well absorbed after oral dosing and slowly excreted via urine and bile. It is distributed widely in the body. Half-life is approximately 12 hours.

EXCIPIENTS
Contact manufacturers for further details.

LICENSED STATUS
Licensed for use >2 years.

Propafenone hydrochloride

An antiarrhythmic agent (Class Ic), with some beta-blocking activity.

USES
Supraventricular and ventricular tachyarrhythmias; junctional ectopic tachycardias.

PRESENTATION
Tablet: 150mg and 300mg (scored) – Arythmol®; 10mg – named patient.
Injection: 70mg in 20mL – named patient.

DOSAGE
Propafenone should be used under guidance of the paediatric cardiologist.

Route	Age				Frequency (times daily)	Notes
	birth–1 month	1 month–2 years	2–12 years	12–18 years		
Oral	←	5–10mg/kg		→	2	Start at the lowest dose. If 70kg or over, use adult dose as in the SPC.
IV bolus followed by IV infusion	← 200 microgram/kg repeated every 15 minutes to a total of 2mg/kg followed by IV infusion of 4 microgram/kg/minute increasing to 8 microgram/kg/minute (if necessary) →				single dose then continuous	Slow IV bolus over 10 minutes followed by infusion with ECG monitoring.

Hepatic impairment
Propafenone is metabolised extensively in the liver. The dose of propafenone administered to patients with impaired hepatic function should be approximately 20–30% of the dose given to patients with normal hepatic function.

ADMINISTRATION
Oral: tablets should be swallowed with a drink after food. If crushed the tablets may have a local anaesthetic effect and a bitter taste. They may be crushed and suspended in water with sugar added to mask the taste. This should be taken immediately and the mouth rinsed afterwards.
IV: treatment should be started at the lowest dose. ECG and blood pressure should be closely monitored, for arrhythmias and hypotension. Administer by slow IV bolus over 10 minutes followed by short-term (1-3 hours) or long-term infusion. Compatible with glucose 5%. DO NOT MIX with NaCl 0.9% due to risk of precipitation.

CONTRA-INDICATIONS & WARNINGS
Uncontrolled congestive heart failure, cardiogenic shock (except arrhythmia – induced), severe bradycardia, uncontrolled electrolyte disturbances, severe obstructive pulmonary disease, marked hypotension. Propafenone may worsen myasthenia gravis. Unless patients are adequately paced, propafenone should not be used in the presence of sinus node dysfunction, atrial conduction defects, second degree or greater AV block, bundle branch block or distal block. Hypersensitivity to propafenone. The weak negative inotropic effect may assume importance in patients predisposed to cardiac failure. Propafenone has been known to alter sensitivity and pacing threshold. Care should be exercised in patients with obstructive airways disease or asthma. Patients with structural heart disease may be predisposed to serious adverse effects.

INTERACTIONS

Potentiation of action may be observed if given in combination with other *local anaesthetic agents* or *agents which depress myocardial activity*. Propafenone has been shown to increase plasma levels of *digoxin*. Monitor *digoxin* levels and reduce dose as necessary. Propafenone has been shown to increase the plasma levels of *warfarin* – monitor prothrombin time. Plasma levels of propafenone may be increased by concurrent administration of *quinidine* or *cimetidine*. Increased *propranolol* and *metoprolol* levels have been observed during concurrent use of propafenone. Cases of possible interaction with *ciclosporin (cyclosporin)* (levels increased with deterioration in renal function), *theophylline* (levels increased), *desipramine* (levels increased) have been reported. Monitor patients and adjust doses as necessary. Concurrent administration of *amiodarone* and propafenone has resulted in additive effects; a reduced dose of propafenone may be necessary.

PREGNANCY/BREAST-FEEDING

Animal studies have not shown any teratogenic effects but manufacturers have no experience in human pregnancy or during lactation. Contact local Medicines Information Centre for advice.

SIDE-EFFECTS

Occasionally and particularly with higher doses: gastrointestinal disturbances, dizziness, fatigue, headache, blurred vision, allergic skin reactions. *Rarely:* cardiac – bradycardia, atrioventricular, sinoatrial, or intraventricular block, small risk of pro-arrhythmic effects; blood – very rarely a reversible decrease of white cell, granulocyte and platelet counts. Isolated cases of agranulocytosis.

POISONING/TOXICITY

There is no known antidote. The usual emergency measures for acute cardiovascular collapse should be applied. Hypotension may require inotropic support. Convulsions should be treated with *IV diazepam*.

PHARMACOKINETIC PROPERTIES

Following oral administration of one dose, bioavailability is about 50%; this increases to 100% when steady state is reached in 3-4 days. Propafenone is extensively metabolised in the liver and excreted almost exclusively as metabolites in the faeces and urine. Plasma half-life in adults is 2.4-10 hours. In adults, plasma propafenone concentrations of approximately 500 microgram/L-1.5mg/L have produced a satisfactory clinical response.

EXCIPIENTS

Contact manufacturer for further details.

LICENSED STATUS

Not licensed for use in children or infants.

Propantheline bromide

Anticholinergic.

USES

Adjunctive in gastrointestinal disorders characterised by smooth muscle spasm; enuresis and unstable bladder.

PRESENTATION

Tablet: 15mg – Pro-Banthine®; 2.5mg – manufactured 'special'.
Oral Suspension: may be extemporaneously prepared.

DOSAGE

Route	Age			Frequency	Notes
	1 month–2 years	2–12 years	12–18 years	(times daily)	
Oral	← 300 microgram/kg →		–	3–4	Maximum dose is 2mg/kg/day. Large dose may be required in enuresis.
	–		15mg and 30mg	before meals at bedtime	

P

ADMINISTRATION

Oral: food has been reported to reduce the bioavailability of propantheline. Take tablets at least one hour before meals.

CONTRA-INDICATIONS & WARNINGS

Contra-indicated in patients with obstructive diseases of gastrointestinal or urinary tract, intestinal atony, pyloric stenosis, severe ulcerative colitis and toxic megacolon. Also contra-indicated in patients with myasthenia gravis or glaucoma. Caution in patients with severe heart disease in whom an increase in heart rate is undesirable. Caution in ulcerative colitis due to suppression of gastrointestinal motility which may produce paralytic ileus.

INTERACTIONS

Anticholinergics delay gastric emptying therefore may alter absorption of other medication given concomitantly. Risk of additive effect with other drugs with anticholinergic effects.

PREGNANCY

Avoid unless considered essential.

BREAST-FEEDING

Unknown whether propantheline bromide is excreted in breast milk. Do not use unless essential.

SIDE-EFFECTS

Anticholinergic side-effects – dryness of mouth, dilatation of pupils, increased intra-ocular pressure, flushing, dryness of skin, decreased sweating, heat stroke, arrhythmias (bradycardia followed by tachycardia), urinary retention.

POISONING/TOXICITY

Intensification of usual side-effects. Severe intoxication – disturbances of CNS – convulsions, circulatory failure, respiratory depression, delirium. Toxic doses may produce non-depolarising muscle blockade with paralysis of involuntary muscle. Give activated charcoal and supportive therapy as necessary.

In severe cases (convulsions, hyperpyrexia, respiratory depression) the use of intravenous physostigmine should be considered.

PHARMACOKINETIC PROPERTIES

Extensively metabolised. Some enzymatic hydrolysis of drug may occur in gastrointestinal tract prior to its absorption. Peak plasma levels reached within 2 hours of a dose; elimination half-life 2-3 hours; 1-10% excreted in urine as unchanged drug.

EXCIPIENTS

Tablets contain sucrose and saccharin sodium.

LICENSED STATUS

Not licensed for use in children.

Propofol

Short-acting intravenous anaesthetic agent.

USES

Induction and maintenance of general anaesthesia.

NB. The CSM does not recommend use in patients under age 16 years for sedation for procedures or in intensive care and has received reports of convulsions following anaesthesia.

PRESENTATION

Injection: 10mg in 1mL; 20mL ampoule, 50mL and 100mL bottle – Propofol-®Lipuro 1% and non-proprietary; 20mL ampoule and 50mL vial – Diprivan® 1%.

Injection: 20mg in 1mL, 50mL vial – non-proprietary; 50mL vial and 50mL prefilled syringe – Diprivan® 2%.

DOSAGE

Newborn infant (birth to 1 month) – not recommended.

Indication	Route	Age			Frequency (times daily)	Notes
		1 month–2 years	2–12 years	12–18 years		
Induction of general anaesthesia	IV bolus	≥1 month 2.5mg/kg	2.5mg/kg	1.5-2.5mg/kg	single dose	Adjust dose according to response. Large doses are often required for children <8 years of age. Lower doses recommended for children of ASA grades 3 and 4.
Maintenance of general anaesthesia	IV infusion	9–15mg/kg/hour with Propofol-Lipuro 1%	<3 years see 1 month-2 years		continuous	Only the Propofol-Lipuro 1% is licensed for >1 month-3 years of age for maintenance of general anaesthesia.
			≥3 years 9–15mg/kg/hour	4-12mg/kg/hour	continuous	Adjust dose according to response.

Renal/hepatic impairment
The pharmacokinetics of propofol do not appear to be altered by chronic hepatic cirrhosis or chronic renal impairment.

ADMINISTRATION
IV: inject slowly, or infuse undiluted. If required propofol can be diluted in glucose 5% only. Dilutions must not exceed 1 in 5 (2mg in 1mL). Administer diluted solutions using PVC giving sets. Discard any diluted solution after 6 hours. 2% emulsion should be used for infusion only.

CONTRA-INDICATIONS & WARNINGS
Cautions: administer with caution to patients with hypovolaemia, epilepsy, lipid metabolism disorders, or severe cardiac or respiratory disease. Delayed convulsions have been associated with the use of propofol, therefore special care should be taken when it is used for day case procedures. Abrupt discontinuation may provoke rapid awakening, anxiety and agitation. *Contra-indications:* not recommended in patients with raised intracranial pressure or impaired cerebral circulation, hypersensitivity to propofol or any excipients.

INTERACTIONS
When given concurrently with other *CNS depressant drugs* sedative effects may be intensified and the possibility of severe respiratory and cardiovascular depression should be considered. *Theophylline* may antagonise effects, serum concentrations of *alfentanil* may be increased, serious bradycardias have been seen when used with *suxamethonium* and inadequate anticholinergic premedication. *ACE inhibitors, angiotensin II antagonists, antihypertensives* and *antipsychotics* may increase the hypotensive effects of propofol.

PREGNANCY
Propofol rapidly crosses the placenta and distributes in the fetus. The manufacturer states that it should not be used in pregnancy or for obstetric anaesthesia.

BREAST-FEEDING
Propofol is excreted in breast milk; effects on the nursing infant are unknown; safety has not been established. Breast-feeding is not recommended by the manufacturer.

SIDE-EFFECTS
Respiratory: respiratory acidosis and depression, apnoeas, pulmonary oedema, anaphylaxis.
Cardiovascular: hypotension and bradycardia are frequent following rapid induction of anaesthesia, myocardial depression, asystole.
CNS: fever, headache, dizziness, excitement.
Skin: rash, pruritis, pain on injection.
Endocrine/metabolic: hyperlipidaemia, fatal metabolic acidosis.
Gastrointestinal: nausea and vomiting, abdominal cramping.
Genito-urinary: green discolouration of urine.
Neuromuscular: myalgia, twitching, clonic, myoclonic movements, convulsions.

POISONING/TOXICITY
Children who have received propofol for prolonged sedation in intensive care have suffered severe metabolic acidosis and cardiac failure. There have been fatalities. The CSM has received reports of neurological, cardiac and renal effects, hyperlipidaemia, hepatomegaly, convulsions (sometimes delayed), anaphylaxis and delayed recovery from anaesthesia. Propofol should not be used for intensive care sedation of children age <16 years.

P

P

PHARMACOKINETIC PROPERTIES

Onset of action is approximately 30 seconds; duration is 3-10 minutes depending on the dose and rate of administration. Recovery is usually rapid and clear headed with low incidence of headache and post-operative nausea and vomiting. The drug is highly lipophilic which accounts for its large volume of distribution and rapid onset of CNS effects. Extensively distributed with two distribution phases, the first being a rapid equilibration (2-4 minutes) between the plasma and the highly perfused brain tissue accounting for the rapid onset of anaesthesia. Plasma levels then rapidly decline as a result of the second distribution phase (30-60 minutes) and rapid clearance from the body mainly by the liver to form inactive sulphate and glucuronide conjugates which are excreted in the urine. Total body clearance is high and exceeds liver blood flow suggesting an extrahepatic clearance method. It is 95% bound to plasma proteins. Terminal half-life is 3-12 hours. Accumulates in tissues after prolonged use (about 10 days) and redistributes into plasma resulting in a prolonged duration of action.

EXCIPIENTS
See manufacturers SPC for further details.
Contains no preservatives therefore strict aseptic technique must be maintained during handling, as it is capable of supporting rapid growth of bacteria.

LICENSED STATUS
Licensed for the induction of anaesthesia in children >1 month of age. Licensed for the induction and maintenance of anaesthesia in children >3 years, except Propofol-®Lipuro 1% which is licensed from >1 month of age.
Not recommended for sedation in intensive care or for sedation for procedures in children, since although no causal relationship is established, serious adverse reactions including fatalities have been reported. These have usually been seen in children with respiratory tract infections given doses greater than those recommended for adults. A recent unpublished study has confirmed a higher mortality in a Paediatric Intensive Care Unit (PICU) population age <16 years. See manufacturers SPCs for further details.

Propranolol

Propranolol is a non-selective beta-adrenergic blocking agent. It has no agonist effect but may have a negative inotropic effect on cardiac tissue.

USES
Control and prophylaxis of supraventricular tachycardia, ventricular tachycardia and ventricular ectopics.
Fallot's Tetralogy – management and prevention of cyanotic spells. Management of hypertrophic cardiomyopathy.
Hypertension.
Hyperthyroidism with prominent autonomic symptoms (plus carbimazole); thyrotoxicosis.
Migraine prophylaxis. Treatment of essential tremor.

PRESENTATION
Tablet: 10mg, 40mg, 80mg – Inderal® and non-proprietary; 160mg – non-proprietary.
Capsule: 80mg (slow release) – Half-Inderal LA® and non-proprietary; 160mg (slow release) – Inderal LA® and non-proprietary.
Oral solution: 5mg in 5mL, 10mg in 5mL, 50mg in 5mL – non-proprietary.
Injection: 1mg in 1mL – Inderal®.

DOSAGE

Indication	Route	Age				Frequency (times daily)	Notes
		birth–1 month	1 month–2 years	2–12 years	12–18 years		
Dysrhythmias	Oral	←— 250–500 microgram/kg —→			10–40mg	3–4	Repeat the injection as needed up to 4 times daily. Adults may receive repeated doses up to 10mg in total. Give injection slowly (over 5 minutes) under ECG control.
	IV bolus	←— 25-50 microgram/kg —→			1mg	single dose	

DOSAGE continued

Indication	Route	Age				Frequency (times daily)	Notes
		birth– 1 month	1 month– 2 years	2–12 years	12–18 years		
Tetralogy of Fallot	Oral	◄— 250 microgram/kg-1mg/kg —►			-	2 (neonate) 3-4 (>1 month)	Give the injection slowly (over 5 minutes) under ECG control and repeat as necessary:
	IV bolus	◄— up to 100 microgram/kg —►			-	single dose	2 times daily in neonates, 4 times daily in child >1 month.
Hypertrophic obstructive cardio-myopathy	Oral	◄— 250-500 microgram/kg —►			10-40mg	3-4	This dose may be increased up to 2mg/kg four times daily with monitoring of heart rate and serum level.
Hypertension	Oral	250–500 microgram/kg	250 microgram/kg - 1mg/kg		-	3	Increase if necessary to maximum of 2mg/kg/dose in neonates. In children, increase at weekly intervals as required, usual dose is 1-5mg/kg/**day**.
		-	-		80-160mg	2	
Hyper-thyroidism including neonatal thyrotoxicosis.	Oral	◄— 250–750 microgram/kg		—►		3	Increase dose according to response. May need up to 1mg/kg three times a day.
Migraine prophylaxis	Oral	-	-	20mg	20–40mg	2–3	Licensed in all ages but evidence for efficacy at licensed dose is in >6 years. Lower doses used in comparative trial which included children of 3 years.
Essential tremour	Oral	-	-	20mg	20–40mg	2–3	

ADMINISTRATION

Oral: the tablets may be crushed but oral suspensions are available. The capsule shells contain spheroids which have a sustained release coating. Do not crush or chew spheroids.

Injection: give by slow IV bolus over at least 3-5 minutes. Compatible with NaCl 0.9% and glucose 5%; incompatible with bicarbonate.

CONTRA-INDICATIONS & WARNINGS

Contra-indications: history of bronchial asthma or bronchospasm, hypersensitivity to propranolol, bradycardia, cardiogenic shock, hypotension, metabolic acidosis, severe arterial circulatory disorders, second or third degree heart block, sick sinus rhythm, untreated phaeochromocytoma, uncontrolled heart failure.

Warnings: since the half-life may be increased in patients with significant hepatic or renal impairment, caution must be exercised when starting treatment and selecting doses. Caution is necessary in patients with poor cardiac reserve or controlled heart failure, first degree heart block and in cases of decompensated cirrhosis. May modify tachycardia of hypoglycaemia; may mask signs of thyrotoxicosis; may increase the risk of hepatic encephalopathy in cases of portal hypertension.

INTERACTIONS

With *verapamil* and *other calcium antagonists* with a negative inotropic effect, take care to avoid excessive bradycardia, severe hypotension and cardiac failure. Do not administer IV within 48 hours of each other. In association with *digitalis glycosides*, may increase AV conduction time.

With *adrenaline (epinephrine)* marked increases in blood pressure and severe bradycardia may occur following administration of *adrenaline (epinephrine)* to patients taking beta-blockers.

Anaesthesic drugs used concurrently with beta-blockers may result in attenuation of the reflex tachycardia and increase the risk of hypotension. *Anaesthetic agents* causing myocardial depression are best avoided.

Concurrent use of *chlorpromazine* may lead to increased blood levels of both drugs. Concurrent use with *cimetidine* or *hydralazine* will result in elevated beta-blocker levels.

P

Indometacin (indomethacin) and other *NSAIDs* may reduce the hypotensive effects of beta-blockers.
Beta-blockers may prolong the hypoglycaemic response to *insulin* or modify the tachycardia of hypoglycaemia.
Diuretics or *other antihypertensives* may increase the hypotensive effect of beta-blockers.
Other antiarrhythmics may have additive or antagonistic effects.
May potentiate the effects of *neuromuscular blockers*. Administration of propranolol during infusion of *lidocaine (lignocaine)* may increase the plasma concentration of the latter (by up to 30%).

PREGNANCY
No evidence of teratogenicity. However, propranolol reduces placental perfusion, which may result in intra-uterine death, immature and premature deliveries. In addition, neonatal hypoglycaemia and bradycardia may occur.

BREAST-FEEDING
Beta-blockers pass into breast milk to a variable extent and symptoms of beta-blockade could occur in nursing infants. However, the American Academy of Pediatrics considers propranolol to be compatible with breast-feeding.

SIDE-EFFECTS
Cardiovascular: bradycardia, heart failure deterioration, postural hypotension, precipitation of heart block, intermittent claudication, Raynaud's phenomenon.
Respiratory: bronchospasm.
CNS: confusion, dizziness, mood changes, nightmares, hallucinations, sleep disturbances.
Endocrine: hypoglycaemia.
Haematological: purpura, thrombocytopenia.
Neurological: paraesthesia.
Other: gastrointestinal disturbances, visual disturbances, fatigue, lassitude, alopecia, skin reactions, dry eyes.

POISONING/TOXICITY
Manifestations include bradycardia, hypotension, acute cardiac insufficiency and bronchospasm. Treatment is symptomatic and supportive.

PHARMACOKINETIC PROPERTIES
Oral absorption is >95%. Pre-systemic metabolism by the liver removes up to 95% of an oral dose. Widely and rapidly distributed throughout the body and is highly lipid-soluble. Highly protein bound (80-95%). Undergoes extensive hepatic biotransformation with only 1-4% excreted unchanged in urine and faeces. In infants >7 months the half-life appears to be similar to that in adults i.e. 3-6 hours.

EXCIPIENTS
See manufacturers SPC for further details.

LICENSED STATUS
Licensed for use in children and adults; except Inderal LA® and Half-Inderal LA® which are not licensed for use in children.

Propylthiouracil

Antithyroid drug.

USES
Hyperthyroidism.

PRESENTATION
Tablet: 50mg – non-proprietary.
Oral suspension: may be extemporaneously prepared.

DOSAGE

Route	Age				Frequency (times daily)	Notes
	birth–1 month	1 month–2 years	2–12 years	12–18 years		
Oral		DOSE BY WEIGHT				Initial dosage.
		<u><1 year</u>	<u>2–4 years</u>			
		2.5mg/kg	25mg	100mg	3	
	2.5mg/kg	DOSE BY AGE				Dose may be gradually
		<u>1-2 years</u>	<u>5-12 years</u>			reduced once patient is
		25mg	50mg		3	euthyroid.

CONTRA-INDICATIONS & WARNINGS
Previous hypersensitivity reaction.

INTERACTIONS
Increased sensitivity to *warfarin* has been observed in hyperthyroidism and careful control of dosage is required as the patient is rendered euthyroid. Changes in thyroid state may affect response to *digoxin, theophylline, beta-blockers* and *insulin.*

PREGNANCY
Crosses placenta less than carbimazole, but may still cause fetal goitre and hypothyroidism. Contact local Medicines Information Centre for advice.

BREAST-FEEDING
Monitor infants thyroid function but amounts in milk probably too small to affect infant.

SIDE-EFFECTS
Nausea, headache, rashes, pruritus, arthralgia; rarely alopecia and jaundice – if jaundice develops withdraw propylthiouracil and consider an alternative treatment.

Agranulocytosis: patients should be asked to report symptoms and signs suggestive of infection, especially sore throat (a white cell count should be performed if there is clinical evidence of infection and propylthiouracil should be stopped if there is evidence of neutropenia). Rarely, a tendency to haemorrhage associated with hypoprothrombinaemia, which may be controlled by the administration of phytomenadione.

POISONING/TOXICITY
Acute overdosage may present as vomiting, epigastric distress, headache, fever, arthralgia, pruritus and pancytopenia. It may also be associated with minor and transient changes in thyroid hormone levels. Supportive therapy should be given.

PHARMACOKINETIC PROPERTIES
Oral bioavailability is approximately 75% and peak levels occur about 1 hour after administration. It is actively concentrated in the thyroid and metabolised by the liver, approximately 85% is excreted in 24 hours. It has a half-life of approximately 0.6 hours in adults.

LICENSED STATUS
Licensed for use >6 years of age.

FURTHER INFORMATION
Following initial control of hyperthyroidism, dosage may be reduced to a level able to sustain euthyroid state, or maintained at high dose in combination with replacement levothyroxine (block and replace strategy). 10mg propylthiouracil is approximately equivalent to 1mg carbimazole.

Protamine sulphate

A basic protein that combines with heparin to form a stable, inactive complex.

USES
Antidote to heparin overdose.

PRESENTATION
Injection: 10mg in 1mL, 5mL ampoule – Prosulf® and non-proprietary; 10ml ampoule – non-proprietary.

DOSAGE
All ages: 1mg (0.1mL) for each 100 units mucous heparin (or low molecular weight heparin (LMWH)) or 80 units lung heparin given at last dose. Maximum dose 50mg.
Administer within 15 minutes – if the delay is longer less protamine is required, as heparin is rapidly excreted (after 30 minutes give approximately half dose).

ADMINISTRATION
IV: give by slow IV bolus over 10 minutes.

CONTRA-INDICATIONS/WARNINGS
NOT suitable for reversal of oral anticoagulants; excess protamine is itself anticoagulant. Protamine will completely inhibit the anticoagulant effect of LMWHs but only partially neutralises the anti-Factor Xa activity. Increased risk of allergic reactions if patient has had previous protamine therapy, protamine insulin or an allergy to fish.

PREGNANCY
Use only when clearly needed. Contact local Medicines Information Centre for advice.

BREAST-FEEDING
Use with caution during lactation. Contact local Medicines Information Centre for advice.

SIDE-EFFECTS
Nausea, vomiting, lassitude, flushing, hypotension, bradycardia, dyspnoea.

POISONING/TOXICITY
Acts itself as an anticoagulant. If bleeding continues, use fresh frozen plasma (FFP) or whole blood. Overdose may cause hypotension, bradycardia and dyspnoea.

LICENSED STATUS
Not licensed for use in children.

Protirelin (thyrotrophin releasing hormone; TRH)

USES
Assessment of thyroid function and thyroid stimulating hormone reserve.

PRESENTATION
Injection: 100 microgram in 1mL, 2mL ampoule – non-proprietary.

DOSAGE

Route	Age				Frequency (times daily)	Notes
	birth–1 month	1 month–2 years	2–12 years	12–18 years		
IV	← 7 microgram/kg → (to a maximum of 200 microgram)			200 microgram	1	

ADMINISTRATION
IV: take a blood sample for control thyroid stimulating hormone (TSH), give dose by rapid IV injection over 30 seconds, take a blood sample after 20 minutes for peak TSH; if necessary a further sample may be taken 60 minutes after injection to detect a delayed TSH response. Ampoule should not be diluted.

CONTRA-INDICATIONS & WARNINGS
There are no absolute contra-indications. Caution should be observed in patients with severe hypopituitarism, myocardial ischaemia, bronchial asthma and obstructive airways disease.

INTERACTIONS
TSH response to protirelin may be reduced by *thyroid hormones, phenothiazines, salicylates, carbamazepine,* pharmacological doses of *corticosteroids*. An increased response may be seen in patients taking *metoclopramide, amiodarone* or *theophylline*.

PREGNANCY
Animal studies have shown no hazard. Contact local Medicines Information Centre for advice.

BREAST-FEEDING
Breast enlargement and leaking of milk have been reported. Contact local Medicines Information Centre for advice.

SIDE-EFFECTS
Following rapid IV injection side-effects of a mild and transient nature may be experienced. They comprise of nausea, the desire to micturate, flushing, slight dizziness, a metallic taste, increase in pulse rate and blood pressure.

POISONING/TOXICITY
No symptoms of overdose have been observed in patients receiving up to 1mg IV.

EXCIPIENTS
Contact manufacturer for further details.

LICENSED STATUS
Licensed for use in children and adults.

FURTHER INFORMATION
Prolactin release is also stimulated by TRH.

Pseudoephedrine hydrochloride

A sympathomimetic agent with direct and indirect effects on adrenergic receptors.

USES
Decongestion of the mucous membranes of the upper respiratory tract, especially nasal mucosa and sinuses. Symptomatic relief of allergic rhinitis, vasomotor rhinitis and the common cold.

PRESENTATION
Tablet: 60mg – Galpseud®, Sudafed®.
Linctus: 30mg in 5mL – Galpseud®.
Elixir: 30mg in 5mL – Sudafed®.

DOSAGE

Route	Age				Frequency (times daily)	Notes
	birth–1 month	1 month–2 years	2–12 years	12–18 years		
Oral	not recommended	7.5mg	2-5 years 15mg	60mg	3	
			6-12 years 30mg		3	

CONTRA-INDICATIONS & WARNINGS
Contra-indicated in patients with severe hypertension or severe coronary artery disease. Patients who are taking MAOIs (or have taken MAOIs within last 2 weeks). Use with caution in children <2 years of age.

INTERACTIONS
Other *sympathomimetics e.g. decongestants, tricyclic antidepressants, appetite suppressants, amphetamine-like psychostimulants* and *MAOIs* may cause a rise in blood pressure. *Antihypertensive agents e.g. bretylium, methyldopa* and *guanethidine* may have effect partially reversed by pseudoephedrine.

PREGNANCY
No specific data. Use with caution.

BREAST-FEEDING
Excreted into breast milk in small amounts – effect on infant unknown.

SIDE-EFFECTS
Central nervous system excitation, including sleep disturbance and rarely, hallucinations. Rashes.

POISONING/TOXICITY
Symptoms: irritability, restlessness, tremor, convulsions, palpitations, hypertension, difficulty in micturition.
Treatment: perform gastric lavage if indicated.

PHARMACOKINETIC PROPERTIES
Oral absorption is >95%. Half-life is 5-8 hours.

EXCIPIENTS
Sudafed® elixir has raspberry flavouring, and is Syrup BP based (>80% sucrose). Galpseud® linctus is sugar-free.

LICENSED STATUS
Licensed for >2 years of age.

FURTHER INFORMATION
Substantially less potent than ephedrine in producing tachycardia and raised blood pressure and less potent in stimulating the CNS. Hallucinations have occurred, especially in children with fever.

Pyrantel embonate

Anthelmintic – depolarising neuromuscular blocking agent which promotes release of acetylcholine and inhibits cholinesterase causing neuromuscular paralysis of susceptible helminths.

USES
Anthelmintic effective against *Ascaris lumbricoides* (roundworm), *ancylostomiasis* (hookworm) and *Enterobius vermicularis* (threadworm).

P

PRESENTATION
Tablet: 125mg pyrantel base (imported).
Suspension: 50mg in 1mL pyrantel base (imported).

DOSAGE
Dosage of the pyrantel embonate is expressed in terms of pyrantel base.

Indication	Route	Age		Frequency (times daily)	Notes
		2–12 years	12–18 years		
Roundworm	Oral	← 5–11mg/kg → (maximum 1g)		single dose	The lower dose of 5mg/kg may suffice in infections of *Ascaris* alone.
Threadworm	Oral	← 10–11mg/kg → (maximum 1g)		single dose	Repeat dose after 2–3 weeks.
Hookworm	Oral	← 10–11mg/kg → (maximum 1g)		daily	For 3 days. Repeat dose after 2 weeks if necessary.

ADMINISTRATION
Oral: can be mixed with milk or fruit juice. Administer with or after food.

CONTRA-INDICATIONS & WARNINGS
Known allergy to pyrantel; pre-existing myasthenia gravis. Caution in pre-existing liver dysfunction and in patients with severe malnutrition or anaemia.

INTERACTIONS
Piperazine and pyrantel have antagonistic modes of action and therefore these drugs should not be administered together. There has been a single case report of increased serum *theophylline* levels in an 8 year old child given pyrantel embonate. Significance is not known. Further studies are needed.

PREGNANCY
No congenital defects or postnatal effects observed in pregnant rats. No information in human pregnancy.

BREAST-FEEDING
Contact local Medicines Information Centre for advice.

SIDE-EFFECTS
Generally mild and transient.
Gastrointestinal: nausea, vomiting, anorexia, abdominal pain and diarrhoea.
Dermatological: rash.
CNS: dizziness, drowsiness, insomnia, headache, fever.
Hepatic: raised liver enzymes.

POISONING/TOXICITY
Pyrantel embonate does not appear to be associated with substantial risk of toxicity following acute oral overdosage (from animal data).

PHARMACOKINETIC PROPERTIES
Oral absorption is poor. Undergoes partial hepatic metabolism. Time to peak serum concentration is within 1–3 hours. Eliminated in faeces (50% as unchanged drug) and urine (7% as unchanged drug and metabolites).

EXCIPIENTS
Contact manufacturer for further details.

LICENSED STATUS
Not licensed for use in the UK.

FURTHER INFORMATION
Available from IDIS World Medicines.

Antituberculous drug.

USES
Treatment of tuberculosis, in combination with other drugs.

PRESENTATION
Tablet: (scored) 500mg – Zinamide®.
Oral liquid: may be extemporaneously prepared.

DOSAGE
Treatment should always be given in collaboration with a specialist experienced in tuberculosis.

Route	Age				Frequency (times daily)	Notes
	birth–1 month	1 month–2 years	2–12 years	12–18 years		
Oral	← 35mg/kg →			<50kg 1.5g	1	In children the dose may be rounded to the nearest 125mg to facilitate administration of an easily given amount of liquid or solid dosage form (i.e. tablet or half a tablet). This is for standard unsupervised TB treatment for 6 months, where pyrazinamide is given for the first 2 months only.
				>50kg 2g	1	

CONTRA-INDICATIONS & WARNINGS
Caution with use in children due to hepatotoxicity. Monitor liver function before and during treatment. Baseline and regular monitoring of liver function is required in patients with known chronic liver disease and in those known to be hepatitis B or C antigen positive. In such patients surveillance should be particularly frequent in the first 2 months of treatment (weekly liver function tests for the first 2 weeks, and then at 2 weekly intervals). Use with caution in patients with renal failure or gout.

INTERACTIONS
Antagonises the effect of *probenecid* and *sulfinpyrazone (sulphinpyrazone)*.

PREGNANCY
There have been no well controlled studies in pregnant women; however the Joint Tuberculosis Committee (JTC) of the British Thoracic Society state that standard tuberculosis therapy should be given to pregnant women.

BREAST-FEEDING
The subcommittee of the JTC state that mothers can breast-feed normally while taking pyrazinamide, although the manufacturers state that breast-feeding should be stopped. It is probably excreted into breast milk but the amounts administered to the infant are likely to be small.

SIDE-EFFECTS
A hepatic reaction is the most common side-effect of pyrazinamide. This varies from a symptomless abnormality of hepatic cell function, through a mild syndrome of fever, anorexia, malaise, liver tenderness, hepatomegaly and splenomegaly, to more serious reactions such as clinical jaundice and rare cases of progressive fulminating acute yellow atrophy and death. Patients and their carers should be told how to recognise signs of liver disorder and to seek medical attention if symptoms such as persistent nausea, vomiting, malaise or jaundice develop. Other side-effects include active gout, sideroblastic anaemia, arthralgias, anorexia, nausea and vomiting, dysuria, malaise, fever, urticaria, aggravation of peptic ulcer.

PHARMACOKINETIC PROPERTIES
Readily and extensively absorbed from the gastrointestinal tract. Peak concentrations appear about 2 hours after an oral dose. Serum concentrations then decline with a half-life of about 9-10 hours. About 30% of the dose is excreted in the urine as pyrazinoic acid and 4% as unchanged pyrazinamide within 24 hours.

POISONING/TOXICITY
Liver toxicity and hyperuricaemia may occur with overdose. There is no specific antidote. The stomach should be emptied by gastric lavage if necessary. Liver function should be monitored closely.

EXCIPIENTS
See manufacturers SPC for further details.

LICENSED STATUS
Not licensed for use in children.

FURTHER INFORMATION
Dosage is that given in the 1998 recommendations for chemotherapy and management of tuberculosis in the UK, produced by a subcommittee of the JTC.

P

Pyridostigmine bromide

A potent reversible inhibitor of acetylcholinesterase.

USES
Myasthenia gravis.

PRESENTATION
Tablet: 60mg (quarter-scored) – Mestinon®.
Oral liquid: may be extemporaneously prepared.

DOSAGE

Route	Age				Frequency (times daily)	Notes
	birth–1 month	1 month–2 years	2–12 years	12–18 years		
Oral	← (maximum dose 10mg)	1-1.5mg/kg (maximum dose 30mg)	→ (maximum dose 60mg)	-	single dose	Initial dose, increased in increments of 25-50% daily, until maximum improvement is obtained. **Total daily** requirements are usually in the range of 30-360mg, given in divided doses at suitable intervals throughout the day.
	-	-	-	30–120mg	single dose	Taken at suitable intervals throughout the day. **Total daily** dose is usually in the range of 300mg to 1.2g.

Dose reduction in renal impairment; reduce to 50% in mild, 35% in moderate and 20% in severe renal impairment.

ADMINISTRATION
Oral: newborn infants (birth to 1 month) give 30 minutes to 1 hour before feeds.

CONTRA-INDICATIONS & WARNINGS
Pyridostigmine should not be given to patients with mechanical gastrointestinal or urinary obstruction. Do not use in conjunction with depolarising muscle relaxants (e.g. *suxamethonium*) due to prolonged apnoea. Extreme caution is needed when administered to patients with bronchial asthma, bradycardia, recent coronary occlusion, hypotension, peptic ulceration or epilepsy. Post-thymectomy patients may have a reduced dose requirement.

INTERACTIONS
Effects of pyridostigmine are antagonised by *aminoglycosides, chlorpromazine, clindamycin, colistimethate (colistin), imipenem/cilastatin, lithium, procainamide, quinidine* and *quinolone antibiotics*. Drugs that may worsen myasthenia are *acetazolamide, ampicillin, aspirin, chloroquine, dipyridamole, erythromycin, hydroxychloroquine, ketoprofen, penicillamine* and *propafenone*. *Beta-blockers* can worsen bradycardia. Effect of

suxamethonium is enhanced but that of *atracurium, tubocurarine, pancuronium* and *vercuronium* are antagonised. The use of *steroids* or *immunosuppressants* can increase the response to pyridostigmine.

PREGNANCY
Safety in pregnancy has not been established. Experience in pregnant patients with myasthenia gravis has revealed no untoward effect of the drug on the course of the pregnancy. As severity of myasthenia gravis often fluctuates considerably, particular care is required to avoid cholinergic crisis, due to overdosage of the drug, but otherwise management is no different from that in non-pregnant patients.

BREAST-FEEDING
Safety during lactation has not been established but only negligible amounts of drug are excreted in breast milk and adverse effects have not been noted.

SIDE-EFFECTS
May include nausea and vomiting, increased salivation, diarrhoea and abdominal cramps and bradycardia.

POISONING/TOXICITY
Signs of overdosage due to muscarinic effects may include abdominal cramps, increased peristalsis, diarrhoea, nausea and vomiting, increased bronchial secretions, salivation, sweating, involuntary defaecation and urination, bradycardia, hypotension and miosis. Nicotinic effects consist of involuntary twitching, muscular cramps, and general weakness. Artificial respiration should be instituted if respiration is severely depressed. *Atropine sulphate* (20-40 microgram/kg in a child, 1-2mg in an adult) given IV is an antidote to the muscarinic effects.

PHARMACOKINETIC PROPERTIES
Oral absorption is poor (approximately 10-20%). The onset of action is approximately 30 minutes with peak plasma levels at 1-2 hours. Absorption is delayed by food by up to 90 minutes. There is a large variation, seven fold differences, between dose and plasma levels achieved in different patients. Half-life after an oral dose is 3-4 hours and duration of action 3-6 hours. Elimination is via the kidney as metabolites and unchanged drug. It has a slower onset and longer duration of action than neostigmine.

EXCIPIENTS
See manufacturers SPC for further details.

LICENSED STATUS
Licensed for use in all ages.

FURTHER INFORMATION
Extemporaneous formulation e.g. Nova Laboratories using Suspension Diluent A (xanthan gum 1%) as a suspending agent has a shelf life 1 month stored at room temperature.

Pyridoxine

USES
Pyridoxine responsive cystathionase deficiency (cystathioninuria).
Pyridoxine responsive cystathionine ß-synthase (CBS) deficiency (homocystinuria).
Pyridoxine dependent seizures. Isoniazid neuropathy, prophylaxis.
Pyridoxine supplement to prevent deficiency secondary to penicillamine e.g. in Wilson's disease.

PRESENTATION
Injection: 50mg in 2mL – manufactured 'special'.
Oral solution: 300mg in 5mL – manufactured 'special'.
Tablet: 20mg and 50mg – non-proprietary.

DOSAGE

Indication	Route	Age				Frequency (times daily)	Notes
		birth–1 month	1 month–2 years	2–12 years	12–18 years		
Metabolic indications*	Oral	←	50-250mg		→	1 or 2	Higher doses may help in partially responsive cases. *Use the same doses for Wilson Disease.

Indication	Route	Age				Frequency (times daily)	Notes
		birth– 1 month	1 month– 2 years	2–12 years	12–18 years		
Pyridoxine dependent seizures	Oral	50–100mg	-	-	-	1 or 2	Test: may be repeated on 2 more days.
		25–100mg	-	-	-	2	Usual maintenance dose.
		-	← 20–50mg →			1 or 2	Usual maintenance dose, but up to 500mg twice daily may be required.
	IV bolus	50–100mg	← 25–100mg →		-	single dose	Test: may be repeated on 2 more days. If seizures cease, change to oral.
Prevention of isoniazid neuropathy	Oral	5mg	← 5–10mg →		10mg	1	Neurological side-effects of isoniazid are less common in children. Pyridoxine is given as prophylaxis if considered necessary; risk factors are malnutrition, diabetes, and chronic renal failure.

ADMINISTRATION
IV: injection given over at least 5 minutes, dilute with NaCl 0.9%.
Resuscitation facilities must be available when given IV. Monitor EEG while injecting.

INTERACTIONS
Isoniazid: causes pyridoxine deficiency.
Penicillamine: causes pyridoxine deficiency.
Levodopa: pyridoxine reduces the effect of levodopa but not if a dopa decarboxylase inhibitor is also given.
Oral contraceptives: efficacy of pyridoxine reduced.

PREGNANCY
Pyridoxine crosses the placenta; it may be taken in pregnancy at doses up to 10 times the recommended daily amount (RDA); no adverse effects have been reported at this level.

BREAST-FEEDING
Pyridoxine appears in breast milk; but it may be taken during lactation in doses up to 10 times the RDA. No adverse effects have been reported at this level.

SIDE-EFFECTS
Peripheral neuropathy (doses higher than 1,000mg daily).

POISONING/TOXICITY
At toxic doses, patients have become unresponsive and apnoeic.

PHARMACODYNAMIC PROPERTIES
Constituent of co-enzymes for decarboxylation, transamination, transulfuration; fatty acid metabolism.

EXCIPIENTS
Contact manufacturers for further details.

LICENSED STATUS
Injection and oral solution are 'specials' and as such are unlicensed. Indications outlined in the monograph are unlicensed indications for the tablets.

FURTHER INFORMATION
Oral solution available from Martindale Pharmaceuticals Ltd.

Pyrimethamine

Antiprotozoal.

USES
Toxoplasmosis. Treatment of malaria (only as combined preparation with sulfadoxine; see pyrimethamine with sulfadoxine monograph).

PRESENTATION
Tablet: 25mg (scored) – Daraprim®.
Oral suspension: may be extemporaneously prepared.

DOSAGE
Toxoplasmosis in pregnancy and congenital infection.
Mother: if *Toxoplasma* infection is diagnosed in early pregnancy and the fetus is not infected, spiramycin is given (see spiramycin monograph). If the fetus is found to be infected then pyrimethamine, sulfadiazine (sulphadiazine) and calcium folinate (folinic acid) are given as outlined below.

Route	Drug	Dose	Frequency (times daily)	Notes
Oral	Pyrimethamine	50mg	1	Until delivery.
Oral	Sulfadiazine (sulphadiazine)	1g	3	Until delivery.
Oral	Calcium folinate (folinic acid)	15mg	three times per week	Until delivery.

Infant: if infection is confirmed in the infant, pyrimethamine, sulfadiazine and calcium folinate are given for a total of 12 months. At 6 months pyrimethamine is reduced to 3 times weekly and sulfadiazine is continued daily until completion of the course. At the commencement a loading dose of pyrimethamine should be given.
Prednisolone 500 microgram/kg twice daily is also given until signs of CNS inflammation (CSF protein ≥10g/L) or active chorioretinitis have settled and is then tailed off.

Route	Drug	Dose	Frequency (times daily)	Notes
Oral	Pyrimethamine	Loading Dose 1mg/kg then	2	For 2 days.
		1mg/kg then	1	For 6 months.
		1mg/kg	three times per week	For 6 months.
Oral	Sulfadiazine (sulphadiazine)	50mg/kg	2	For 12 months.
Oral	Calcium folinate (folinic acid)	15mg	three times per week	For 12 months.

Ocular toxoplasmosis, reactivation of toxoplasmosis during HIV infection, toxoplasmosis in immunocompromised patients with protracted or incapacitating illness.

Route	Age			Frequency (times daily)	Notes
	1 month-2 years	2-12 years	12-18 years		
Oral	← 2mg/kg → then		-	1	Loading dose for 2 days.
	← 1mg/kg →		25-100mg	1	Usually for 6 weeks to prevent relapse in HIV infected patients. This is followed by maintenance dose of a quarter to a half of the stated dose, indefinitely.

ADMINISTRATION
Oral: tablets may be crushed and given in juice or with food.

CONTRA-INDICATIONS & WARNINGS
History of pyrimethamine sensitivity. Avoid large loading doses in patients with a history of seizures.

INTERACTIONS
The antifolate properties of pyrimethamine may exacerbate those of other *antifolates* such as *co-trimoxazole, trimethoprim, methotrexate* and *phenytoin*. Sequential blockade of folate pathways by *sulphone* or *sulphonamide* plus pyrimethamine results in considerable potentiation in the treatment of malaria and toxoplasmosis.

PREGNANCY
While there is a theoretical risk of fetal abnormality with all folate inhibitors during pregnancy, no such adverse-effects have been reported. A folate supplement such as calcium folinate (folinic acid) should be given to pregnant women receiving pyrimethamine.

BREAST-FEEDING
The amount excreted is insufficient to contra-indicate its use in breast-feeding mothers but the infants should not receive any other anti-folate agents.

SIDE-EFFECTS
These can include gastrointestinal symptoms, such as atrophic glossitis, abdominal pain and vomiting; haematological effects such as megaloblastic anaemia, leucopenia, thrombocytopenia and pancytopenia and CNS effects, including headache, dizziness, and insomnia. Calcium folinate (folinic acid) should be given concurrently to prevent the haematological effects.

POISONING/TOXICITY
Symptoms: can include vomiting, cyanosis, respiratory distress, convulsions and tachycardia.
Treatment: symptomatic and supportive, including maintenance of a clear airway and control of convulsions. Adequate fluids should be given to ensure optimal diuresis. To counteract possible folate deficiency, calcium folinate (folinic acid) (5-15mg daily, although doses vary depending on the regime used; need an expert opinion) should be given until the signs of toxicity have subsided. There may be a delay of 7–10 days before full leucopenic side-effects become evident and therefore calcium folinate should be continued for the period at risk. Blood transfusions may be needed to counteract blood dyscrasias.

PHARMACOKINETIC PROPERTIES
Well absorbed after oral administration, although absolute bioavailability is unknown. Plasma concentrations peak at 2-6 hours in healthy human subjects with a mean elimination half-life of 85 hours. It undergoes extensive hepatic metabolism and is slowly excreted by the kidney.

EXCIPIENTS
See manufacturers SPC for further details.

LICENSED STATUS
Not licensed for use in toxoplasmosis.

Pyrimethamine with sulfadoxine

USES
Treatment of *Plasmodium falciparum* malaria as an adjunct to quinine. Not recommended for prophylaxis by UK malaria experts.

PRESENTATION
Tablet: 25mg pyrimethamine + 500mg sulfadoxine (scored) – Fansidar®.

DOSAGE

Route	Age				Frequency
	1 month–2 years	2–12 years		12–18 years	
Oral	>2 months 1/2 tablet	≤4 years 1/2 tablet	7–9 years 1 1/2 tablets	12–14 years 2 tablets	Single dose following quinine therapy.
		5–6 years 1 tablet	10–12 years 2 tablets	>14 years 3 tablets	

ADMINISTRATION
Oral: swallow tablets with plenty of fluid after a meal.

CONTRA-INDICATIONS & WARNINGS
Contra-indications: sulphonamide hypersensitivity, severe renal or hepatic failure, blood dyscrasias. Treatment must be discontinued immediately upon the appearance of any mucocutaneous signs or symptoms. Premature babies and during the first 2 months of life. *Precautions:* excessive exposure to the sun should be avoided. Regular blood counts if used for over 3 months (but it is not recommended for prophylaxis).

INTERACTIONS
Avoid other preparations containing *folate antagonists* (e.g. *co-trimoxazole, trimethoprim, methotrexate, anticonvulsants*).

PREGNANCY
The preparation is not contra-indicated during pregnancy but there is a possibility that Fansidar® during pregnancy may produce kernicterus in the neonate.

BREAST-FEEDING
Contra-indicated. Small risk of kernicterus in jaundiced infants and of haemolysis in G6PD deficient infants (due to sulfadoxine).

SIDE-EFFECTS
Skin reactions, gastrointestinal reactions, haematological changes.

POISONING/TOXICITY
Symptoms include headache, anorexia, nausea, vomiting, excitation, convulsions and haematological changes (megaloblastic anaemia, leucopenia, thrombocytopenia). Treatment includes forced diuresis, gastric lavage, alkalinisation of the urine. Hypersensitivity reactions may require treatment with steroids. Calcium folinate (folinic acid) may be given to counteract the effects of pyrimethamine on haemopoiesis.

PHARMACOKINETIC PROPERTIES
After an oral dose, peak plasma levels are reached after about 4 hours. A long elimination half-life is characteristic of both components (96 hours for pyrimethamine and 184 hours for sulfadoxine); excreted mainly via the kidneys.

EXCIPIENTS
See manufacturers SPC for further details.

LICENSED STATUS
Licensed for use >2 months of age.

Quinine

Antiprotozoal drug.

USES
Treatment of *P. falciparum* malaria.

PRESENTATION
Tablet: quinine sulphate 200mg, 300mg; quinine bisulphate 300mg – non-proprietary.
Injection: quinine dihydrochloride 300mg in 1mL; 1mL and 2mL ampoules – non-proprietary.

DOSAGE

Route	Age				Frequency (times daily)	Notes
	birth–1 month	1 month–2 years	2–12 years	12–18 years		
Oral	←	10mg/kg (sulphate)	→	600mg (sulphate)	3	For 7 days. Doses may need to be rounded to the nearest tablet size or given less frequently to achieve a suitable total daily dose.
	←	14mg/kg (bisulphate)	→	900mg (bisulphate)	3	

DOSAGE continued

Route	Age				Frequency (times daily)	Notes
	birth–1 month	1 month–2 years	2–12 years	12–18 years		
IV infusion over at least 4 hours	←	20mg/kg (maximum 1.4g)		→	single loading dose	For seriously ill patients or those unable to take tablets.
	←	then 10mg/kg (maximum 700mg)		→	then after 8–12 hours maintenance dose	Maintenance dose can be repeated every 8–12 hours, but change to oral therapy as soon as possible.
	←	then 5–7mg/kg		→	maintenance dose after 48 hours IV therapy	If IV therapy is required after 48 hours, use this maintenance dose every 8 hours.

ADMINISTRATION
Quinine base 100mg ≡ quinine sulphate 121mg ≡ quinine bisulphate 169mg ≡ quinine dihydrochloride 122mg.
IV: do not give loading dose if patient has received quinine, quinidine or mefloquine during the previous 24 hours. Give by infusion over at least 4 hours. Dilute to 2mg in 1mL with NaCl 0.9% or glucose 5%.
Fluid restricted patients – maximum concentration of 30mg in 1mL can be used.

CONTRA-INDICATIONS & WARNINGS
Caution in reduced liver function (more significant adverse effects) and in patients with cardiac conduction defects and optic neuritis.

INTERACTIONS
Increased risk of arrhythmias with *amiodarone, flecainide, halofantrine, cisapride* and certain *antipsychotics*. Increased risk of convulsions with *mefloquine* – separate administration by 12 hours. Increased plasma-quinine concentration with *cimetidine*. Plasma concentration of *digoxin* increased.

PREGNANCY
High doses are teratogenic, but in malaria benefit of treatment outweighs risks.

BREAST-FEEDING
Sensitivity (wheezing; thrombocytopenia) only problem – uncommon.

SIDE-EFFECTS
Expect symptomatic adverse effects – called 'cinchonism' (tinnitus, headache, nausea, visual disturbances). Sometimes effects are more marked – vertigo, reduced hearing, blurred vision, diplopia, night blindness, visual field defects; but most are reversible. Cardiac side-effects include prolonged QT interval, AV block, sinus arrest, ventricular tachycardia. Hypoglycaemia as quinine stimulates insulin secretion – monitor blood glucose levels.

POISONING
'Cinchonism', loss of hearing, allergic thrombocytopenia, CNS toxicity, cardiotoxicity and asthma. Treatment is mostly symptomatic with attention being given to maintaining blood pressure, respiration and renal function; and treating arrhythmias. Contact UK National Poisons Information Service for full details.

PHARMACOKINETIC PROPERTIES
Similar bioavailability of oral preparations. Peak concentration after 1-3 hours. Steady-state in 3 days. Elimination is 80% via liver and 20% via kidneys.

EXCIPIENTS
Contact manufacturer for further details.

LICENSED STATUS
This varies depending on the generic brand used and therefore should be checked accordingly; the Cox brand is licensed for use in both children and adults.

FURTHER INFORMATION
Quinine dihydrochloride injection is available from Martindale as a 'special' order.

USES
For post exposure passive prophylaxis of those unimmunised or incompletely immunised and who have suffered a high-risk exposure (see section on rabies vaccine). **It should only be used under the guidance of an expert in the field**.

PRESENTATION
Injection: vials of 500 international units. 1mL contains not less than 150 international units of rabies antibody.

DOSAGE
20 international units/kg.
Current guidelines for treatment are outlined below.

	Status of biting animal (irrespective of any earlier vaccination)		Recommended treatment
	At time of exposure	During next 10 days[1]	
Contact, but no lesions; indirect contact; non contact	Healthy		None.
	Suspected as rabid[2]	Healthy	None.
		Rabid	None.
Licks of the skin, scratches or abrasions, minor bites (covered areas of arms, trunk and legs)	Healthy	Healthy	None.
		Rabid	Start vaccination schedule[3].
	Suspected as rabid[2]	Healthy	Start vaccination schedule; stop treatment if animal remains healthy for 15 days.[1,4]
		Rabid	Start vaccination schedule; upon positive diagnosis, complete the course of vaccine.
	Rabid; wild animal[5] or animal unavailable for observation		Give complete course of vaccine.
Licks of mucosa; major bites (multiple or on face, head, neck or finger)	Suspect[2] or confirmed rabid domestic or wild[5] animal, or animal unavailable for observation.		Immunoglobulin and vaccine. Stop treatment only in the case of domestic animal under observation[1] which remains healthy for 15 days.

1 This observation period only applies to dogs and cats. Other domestic animals suspected as rabid should be killed and examined using the fluorescent antibody techniques.
2 All unprovoked bites in endemic areas should be considered suspect unless proved negative by laboratory examination of the animal's brain.
3 During the usual period of 10 days, begin treatment with vaccine at first sign of rabies in a dog or cat that has bitten someone. The symptomatic animal should be killed immediately and examined using the fluorescent antibody technique.
4 Or if the animal's brain is found to be negative by fluorescent antibody examination.
5 In general, exposure to rodents, rabbits and hares seldom, if ever, requires specific anti-rabies treatment.

ADMINISTRATION
IM & infiltration: half infiltrated around wound with the rest IM. Give at a different site to the vaccine.

CONTRA-INDICATIONS & WARNINGS
None.

INTERACTIONS
May reduce the efficacy of *measles, mumps* and *rubella* (MMR) vaccines and so their administration should be delayed for 3 months after HRIG has been given.
Administration of any *immunoglobulin* may raise antibody levels to a number of micro-organisms and this must be borne in mind when interpreting antibody assays within 2–3 months of such administration.

PREGNANCY/BREAST-FEEDING
No data available, but must not be withheld if its use is indicated.

SIDE-EFFECTS
Reactions such as pain at the site of injection and fever may occur. Serious adverse effects have not been reported.

POISONING/TOXICITY
None reported.

R

PHARMACOKINETIC STUDIES
Measurable antibody levels are present 20 minutes after injection. Peak levels are achieved after 2-3 days. Half-life is 21–22 days.

EXCIPIENTS
Sodium chloride, glycine, sodium acetate trihydrate and sodium hydroxide.

LICENSED STATUS
Fully licensed for use as indicated above.

FURTHER INFORMATION
Should only be used on the advice of an appropriate expert.
Protect from light and store at 2–8°C.
The immunoglobulin is sourced from donors in countries where BSE does not occur.
Available from Public Health Laboratory Service, BPL and SNBTS.

Rabies vaccine

USES
Active protection against rabies. It is optimally given pre-exposure to high-risk groups. In children, the main indication would be for those living or travelling in enzootic areas who may be exposed to unusual risk of being infected or are undertaking especially long journeys in remote areas where medical treatment may be delayed.
The vaccine can also prevent disease if given post-exposure but before the development of symptoms. In such instances it may need to be given with specific immunoglobulin.

PRESENTATION
Injection: (single dose suspension) – Rabies Vaccine BP.
Rabies Vaccine BP (Rab/Vac) contains Wistar rabies virus strain PM/WI 38 1503-3M cultured in human diploid cells (MRC5) and inactivated with beta-propiolactone.
Injection: (single dose of lyophilised powder to be reconstituted to 1mL) – Rabipur®.
Rabipur® contains rabies virus strain Flury LEP cultured in purified chick embryo cells and inactivated with beta-propiolactone.
Each 1mL of both reconstituted vaccines has a potency of at least 2.5 international units.

DOSAGE
Pre-exposure
1mL on days 0, 7 and 28 (Rabipur® – day 21 or 28). Two doses 4 weeks apart may be adequate in those not expecting to handle animals if post-exposure treatment will be readily available. In this case, if exposure continues, a further dose after 6-12 months will be necessary. Boosters may be given every 2-3 years if there is continuing risk and post-exposure treatment is not readily available. After 2-3 boosters, expert advice should be sought before giving more.
Post-exposure
When an individual has been exposed via a break in the skin or contamination of a mucosal surface to a potentially rabid animal, consideration should be given to post-exposure treatment. Advice should always be sought before starting treatment. In England and Wales this would be from the Health Protection Agency Virus Reference Division, London (0208 200 4100); in Scotland from the Scottish Centre for Infection and Environmental Health (0141 300 1100) and in Northern Ireland from the Public Health Laboratory, Belfast City Hospital (028 9032 9241). Treatment will depend on the risk of rabies in the country where the incident occurred (for further information on the categorisation of countries see the *Immunoglobulin Handbook*, PHLS, 2002. http://www.phls.org.uk/advice/ImmunoglobulinHandbook.pdf).

Rabies risk in country of incident	Unimmunised or incompletely immunised individual*	Fully immunised individual
No risk	None	None.
Low risk	1mL on days 0, 3, 7, 14 and 30.	1mL on day 0 and a further dose between days 3 and 7.
High risk	1mL on days 0, 3, 7, 14 and 30. Specific immunoglobulin 10 international units/kg infiltrated in and around the wound and 10 international units/kg intramuscularly.	1mL on day 0 and a further dose between days 3 and 7.

*Individuals who have been immunised by the intradermal route, or who have had fewer than three doses of vaccine, or whose last dose of vaccine was given more than 2 years previously.

ADMINISTRATION

IM or deep SC: the intradermal route, using 0.1mL, instead of 1mL, should only be used by those competent at the technique and never for post-exposure treatment. This route would rarely, if ever, be justified in children. Chloroquine suppresses the antibody response and so the intradermal route should not be used in patients taking it. The vaccine should not be given in the gluteal region as the antibody response may be reduced.

CONTRA-INDICATIONS & WARNINGS
There are no absolute contra-indications to post-exposure use of the vaccine. Individuals who have had an anaphylactic reaction to a previous dose or to *neomycin* should not receive the vaccine for pre-exposure prophylaxis.

INTERACTIONS
Chloroquine may reduce the antibody response.

PREGNANCY
No evidence of harm to the fetus has been recorded. The vaccine must be used for post-exposure treatment in pregnancy. If the risk of exposure is high, it can also be used for pre-exposure prophylaxis.

BREAST-FEEDING
No evidence of harm to the suckling infant has been recorded. The vaccine must be used for post-exposure treatment even when a mother is breast-feeding. If the risk of exposure is high, it can also be used for pre-exposure prophylaxis.

SIDE-EFFECTS
Local reactions such as redness, swelling and tenderness have been recorded within 48 hours after the injection. Mild fever, malaise and 'flu-like symptoms may also occur.

POISONING/TOXICITY
No data available.

EXCIPIENTS
Rabies Vaccine BP (Rab/Vac): neomycin and human albumin.
Rabipur®: sucrose, triomethamine (TRIS), sodium chloride, disodium edetate, potassium glutamate, Haemoccel 35. Trace amounts of amphoteracin B, chlortetracycline, neomycin and beta-propriolactone.

LICENSED STATUS
Licensed for use as described except for administration by the intradermal route.

FURTHER INFORMATION
The vaccine would rarely be necessary for children on holiday.
Store at 2–8°C and use within 1 hour of reconstitution.
Always seek advice on the treatment of potential rabies.
The human albumin used in the vaccine is derived from donors in countries where BSE does not occur.

Ranitidine

H$_2$ receptor antagonist.

USES
Treatment of oesophagitis, gastric hyperacidity and gastritis.

Prophylaxis against bleeding from oesophageal and gastric varices, upper gastrointestinal bleeding/perforation in infants receiving high dose steroids for bronchopulmonary dysplasia.
Treatment of peptic ulcer.
Gastro-oesophageal reflux related respiratory disease.
Reduction of degradation of pancreatic enzymes in cystic fibrosis.
Zollinger-Ellison syndrome.
Persistant fat malabsorption despite optimal use of enzyme replacement in cystic fibrosis.

PRESENTATION
Effervescent tablet: 150mg and 300mg – Zantac® and non-proprietary.
Injection: 25mg in 1mL, 2mL ampoule – Zantac®.
Oral solution: 75mg in 5mL – non-proprietary.
Syrup: 75mg in 5mL – Zantac®.
Tablet: 150mg and 300mg – Zantac® and non-proprietary.

DOSAGE
Newborn infant (birth to 1 month)

Route	Age	Frequency	Notes
	birth–1 month	(times daily)	
Oral/IV bolus	1mg/kg	3	Oral experience very limited in newborn infants.
IV infusion	30–60 microgram/kg/hour	continuous	Neonate in intensive care unit – limited data. Maximum 3mg/kg/day.

Child

Route	Age			Frequency	Notes
	1 month–2 years	2–12 years	12–18 years	(times daily)	
Oral	<6 months as for neonates >6 months as for 2–12 years	2–4mg/kg (maximum 150mg)	150mg	2	Doses of up to 9mg/kg/day have been used.
IV bolus	← 1mg/kg →			2–4	Doses of up to 3mg/kg have been used - anecdotal. Standard adult dose is 50mg 3 times a day.
IV infusion	← 125–250 microgram/kg/hour →			continuous	Patients in ITU.

Dosage in renal impairment
Reduce by approximately 50% in severe renal failure.

ADMINISTRATION
Oral: dissolve effervescent tablets in a minimum of 75mL of water. Absorption of oral dose forms is not significantly affected by food or antacids. In cystic fibrosis give 1-2 hours before food.
IV: dilute to 2.5mg in 1mL with NaCl 0.9% or glucose 5% and give as IV bolus over at least 3 minutes, or further dilute and give as an infusion.

CONTRA-INDICATIONS & WARNINGS
Hypersensitivity to ranitidine or any excipient. Acute porphyria. Treatment with ranitidine may mask the symptoms of other gastric disease. Raised liver enzymes may occur with high doses. Effervescent tablets should be avoided in patients with a restricted sodium intake, and in those with phenylketonuria.

PREGNANCY
Crosses the placenta. No reported adverse effect on labour, delivery or neonatal progress.

BREAST-FEEDING
Excreted in breast milk, with concentrations approximately equal to those in plasma. No adverse effects likely.

SIDE-EFFECTS
Hypersensitivity reactions, including urticaria, angioneurotic oedema, fever, bronchospasm, hypotension and anaphylactic shock, are reported, sometimes after a single dose. Transient and reversible changes in liver function tests. Rarely, acute

pancreatitis, leucopenia and thrombocytopenia, bradycardia and AV block. Mental confusion, depression and hallucination, skin rash, including erythema multiforme, have been reported.

POISONING/TOXICITY

Due to specificity of action no particular problems are expected in overdosage. Note sodium content of effervescent tablets and injection, and ethanol content of liquid. Symptomatic and supportive treatment should be given as appropriate. Ranitidine is removed by haemodialysis.

PHARMACOKINETIC PROPERTIES

Oral bioavailability is greater than 50%, with no effect due to food. Plasma half-life of 2-3 hours. Volume of distribution is 1-2L/kg. Plasma protein binding of approximately 15%. Ranitidine is not extensively metabolised, with 30-70% excreted unchanged after oral dosing and 70-86% after IV administration. Elimination is principally by renal tubular secretion.

EXCIPIENTS

Effervescent tablets include aspartame and a high level of sodium. See manufacturers SPC for further details.

LICENSED STATUS

The parenteral route is unlicensed for use in children.
Oral treatment of peptic ulceration is the only licensed indication in children.

Ribavirin (tribavirin)

Has antiviral inhibitory activity *in vitro* against respiratory syncytial virus (RSV), influenza virus and herpes simplex virus.

USES

Treatment of infants and children with severe respiratory syncytial virus (RSV) bronchiolitis.
Life-threatening virus infections in immunocompromised children.

PRESENTATION

Powder for inhalation: 6g when reconstituted – Virazole®.
Injection: 1.2 g in 12mL – named patient.

R

DOSAGE

Route	Age				Frequency (times daily)	Notes
	birth–1 month	1 month–2 years	2–12 years	12–18 years		
Nebulisation	←— 6g (in 300mL) —→		–	–	1	Nebulise via a small particle aerosol generator (SPAG) for 12–18 hours per day for at least 3 but no more than 7 days.
IV Infusion over 15 minutes	←	Day one 8mg/kg then	—→		3	Dose given is based on limited clinical experience in immunocompromised children with life- threatening viral infections.
	←	Days 2–10 5mg/kg	—→		3	
				33mg/kg then	single dose	Loading dose.
				16mg/kg then	4	For 4 days.
				8mg/kg	3	For 3 days.

ADMINISTRATION
IV: dilute in glucose 5% or NaCl 0.9%. There are no specific requirements for the volume of diluent.
Solution for nebulisation: by aseptic technique. Dissolve 6g powder in at least 75mL Water for Injections and shake well. Transfer to a sterilised 500mL flask and dilute to a final volume of 300mL with Water for Injections. Administer into a head box. May be administered into a ventilator circuit by experienced personnel. Use oxygen, air or an oxygen/air mixture as carrier gas, as appropriate. Ventilator circuits must be protected with appropriate filters.

NB. In cases where the patient cannot cope with the headbox/mask for a continuous 12-18 hour period, the following has been done: 6g in 100mL nebulised by administering for 2 hours on, 6 hours off, 3 times a day for 3 days.

CONTRA-INDICATIONS & WARNINGS
Contra-indicated in women who are, or may become pregnant. Healthcare workers and others who are, or expect to become pregnant should be advised not to come into direct contact with ribavirin. Turn SPAG device off for 5-10 minutes prior to prolonged contact with patient. Avoid wearing contact lenses when supervising administration of inhalation. Hypersensitivity to ribavirin.

INTERACTIONS
No known interactions.

PREGNANCY/BREAST-FEEDING
Contra-indicated. Ribavirin is teratogenic and embryo-lethal.

SIDE-EFFECTS
Worsening of respiratory status, bacterial pneumonia and pneumothorax have occurred in infants with severe underlying disease. Anaemia (haemolytic) has occurred with IV administration. Deposition of powder on the skin may irritate or produce conjunctivitis. Wipe off with water or NaCl 0.9%.

POISONING/TOXICITY
No poisoning/toxicity reported.

PHARMACOKINETIC PROPERTIES
Ribavirin administered by inhalation is absorbed systemically. It is likely that the ribavirin concentrations in respiratory tract secretions are much higher than plasma concentrations. Plasma half-life is 9.5 hours, following inhalation. Bioavailability of ribavirin is unknown and may depend on the mode of aerosol delivery. There are no pharmacokinetic studies in children treated with IV ribavirin.

EXCIPIENTS
See manufacturers SPC for further details.

LICENSED STATUS
Licensed for use in infants and children by nebulisation for treatment of RSV only. IV preparation is unlicensed.

FURTHER INFORMATION
Reconstituted solution for inhalation should be used within 24 hours. Ribavirin injection contains no preservatives and should be administered within 24 hours of dilution. The injection can be obtained on a named patient basis from ICN Pharmaceuticals Ltd (UK), telephone 01256 707 744.

Riboflavin (riboflavine)

USES
Glutaric acidaemia type I and glutaric acidacmia type II.
Congenital lactic acidosis. Cytochrome oxidase deficiencies.

PRESENTATION
Capsule: 50mg.
Injection: 5mg in 1mL, 2mL.
Powder.
Tablet: 10mg, 50mg and 100mg.

DOSAGE

Route	Age				Frequency (times daily)	Notes
	birth–1 month	1 month–2 years	2–12 years	12–18 years		
Oral	←		50mg	→	1	The total daily dose may be given as more frequent smaller doses. Doses of 300–400mg/day have been used in some instances.

CONTRA-INDICATIONS & WARNINGS/INTERACTIONS
No information available.

PREGNANCY/BREAST-FEEDING
Riboflavin crosses the placenta; but administration in pregnancy would appear to be safe at normal doses from the limited information available. Riboflavin passes into breast milk; but breast-feeding should be safe at normal doses. The doses used for metabolic disorders are much higher than 'normal' doses given, for example, as part of multivitamin treatment for deficiency states.

SIDE-EFFECTS
Large doses result in bright yellow discolouration of urine, which may interfere with some laboratory tests.

PHARMACODYNAMIC PROPERTIES
Coenzyme for glutaryl CoA dehydrogenase, electron transfer flavoprotein (ETF) and ETF dehydrogenase.

LICENSED STATUS
Injection, powder and tablet not licensed for use in the UK.

FURTHER INFORMATION
Capsule available from Lambert Healthcare. Injection and tablet available from IDIS World Medicines. Powder available from Warner Jenkinson Europe.

R

Rifampicin

USES
Treatment of tuberculosis and serious staphylococcal infections (in combination with other drugs) and meningococcal prophylaxis.
In cystic fibrosis patients – reserve for methicillin-resistant *Staphylococcus aureus* (MRSA) infection or serious *Staphylococcus aureus* infections that do not respond to other anti-staphylococcal antibiotics (in combination with other drugs).
Pruritus due to cholestasis.

PRESENTATION
Capsule: 150mg and 300mg – Rifadin®, Rimactane® and non-proprietary.
IV infusion: 300mg – Rimactane®; 600mg – Rifadin®.
Syrup: 100mg in 5mL – Rifadin® and Rimactane®.

DOSAGE

Route	Age				Frequency (times daily)	Notes
	birth–1 month	1 month–2 years	2–12 years	12–18 years		
Oral or IV infusion over 2–3 hours	10mg/kg	← 10mg/kg (maximum 600mg) →		≤50 kg 450mg	1	*Tuberculosis, in combination with other drugs. Treatment should always be given in collaboration with a specialist experienced in tuberculosis treatment. See guidelines.
				>50 kg 600mg	1	

DOSAGE continued

Route	Age				Frequency (times daily)	Notes
	birth–1 month	1 month–2 years	2–12 years	12–18 years		
Oral	5mg/kg	<1 year 5mg/kg >1 year 10mg/kg	← 10mg/kg (maximum 600mg) →		2 2	Prophylaxis in contacts of patients with meningococcal infection or elimination of nasal carriage. Administer for 2 days. Treatment of staphylococcal infection for 10-14 days.
	10mg/kg	<3 months 10mg/kg >3 months 20mg/kg	← 20mg/kg (maximum 600mg) →		1 1	Prophylaxis in contacts of patients with invasive *Haemophilus influenzae* type B infection. Administer for 4 days.
IV infusion over 2-3 hours	-	← 20mg/kg (maximum 600mg) →			1	Treatment of tuberculous meningitis.
Oral	-	← 5–10mg/kg (maximum dose 600mg) →			1	Pruritus due to cholestasis.
Oral for cystic fibrosis patients	-	← 10-20mg/kg →			1	Reserved for MRSA infection or serious *S. aureus* infection that does not respond to other anti-staphylococcal drugs. Maximum dose of 1.2g.

Dose adjustment in liver failure
Avoid altogether, or reduce doses for tuberculosis and prophylaxis to 8mg/kg daily.

ADMINISTRATION
Oral: take oral preparations at least 30–60 minutes before or 2 hours after food.
IV infusion: infuse over 2-3 hours in glucose 5%, 10% or NaCl 0.9% at a concentration of 1.2mg in 1mL. Discard infusion after 6 hours. Displacement value is 0.48mL per 600mg.

R

CONTRA-INDICATIONS & WARNINGS
Patients who are hypersensitive to rifamycins. Although not recommended for use in patients with jaundice, the therapeutic benefit should be weighed against the possible risks.

INTERACTIONS
Induces liver enzymes reducing plasma levels of many drugs e.g. *anticoagulants, ciclosporin (cyclosprorin), phenytoin, phenobarbital (phenobarbitone), theophylline, digoxin,* most *benzodiazepines, fluconazole* and dose adjustment of these may be necessary if they are given concurrently with rifampicin.

PREGNANCY
Risk of neonatal bleeding when used late in third trimester; administer vitamin K.

BREAST-FEEDING
Amounts excreted too small to be harmful.

SIDE-EFFECTS
Gastrointestinal: these include anorexia, nausea, vomiting, abdominal discomfort, diarrhoea; pseudo-membranous colitis has been reported.
Skin: flushing, urticaria, rash.
Haematological: thrombocytopenia with or without purpura, leucopenia, eosinophilia. Reactions occurring mainly on intermittent therapy and probably of immunological origin include 'flu-like symptoms (with chills, fever, dizziness, bone pain), shortness of breath and wheezing, acute haemolytic anaemia, acute renal failure and thrombocytopenic purpura, alterations of liver function. Other side-effects have included oedema, muscular weakness, and menstrual disturbances.

POISONING/TOXICITY
In the case of overdose, treatment should be symptomatic and supportive.

PHARMACOKINETIC PROPERTIES
Readily absorbed when given orally. It is highly protein bound (80%) and undergoes enterohepatic recirculation. Up to 30% may be excreted in the urine, with about half being unchanged but metabolites are excreted in urine and bile.

EXCIPIENTS
Syrup contains sucrose, IV solvent for 600mg vial contains polysorbate 81. Contact manufacturers for further details.

LICENSED STATUS
Licensed for use in all ages; however, pruritus due to cholestasis is not a licensed indication.

FURTHER INFORMATION
Rifampicin colours urine and other secretions red. Soft contact lenses may be permanently stained.

*The dose stated for treatment of tuberculosis is that given in the 1998 recommendations for chemotherapy and management of tuberculosis in the UK, produced by a subcommittee of the Joint Tuberculosis Committee of the British Thoracic Society.

Risperidone

Benzisoxazole derivative. Neuroleptic/antipsychotic.

USES
Treatment of schizophrenia. Aggressive behaviour, especially in the presence of attention-deficit hyperactivity disorder (ADHD).

PRESENTATION
Tablet: 500 micrograms, 1mg, 2mg, 3mg, 4mg and 6mg – Risperdal®.
Liquid: 1mg in 1mL – Risperdal®.

DOSAGE

Indication	Route	Age		Frequency (times daily)	Notes
		2–12 years	12–18 years		
Aggressive behaviour. Tourette Syndrome	Oral	500 microgram - 2mg	1–4mg	1	May be given in 2 divided doses.
Schizophrenia	Oral	–	500 microgram – 8mg	1	May be given in 2 divided doses. Dosage should usually be increased to 6mg/**day**, gradually over 3 days. From then the dose can be increased as necessary to a maximum of 16mg/**day**, although doses >10mg/**day** do not generally provide additional efficacy over lower doses.

ADMINISTRATION
Oral: liquid can be mixed with mineral water or orange juice and used immediately.

CONTRA-INDICATIONS & WARNINGS
See chlorpromazine monograph. Lower doses in co-existent hepatic and renal disease.

INTERACTIONS
See chlorpromazine monograph.

PREGNANCY
The safety of risperidone for use during human pregnancy has not been established. Animal studies did not show teratogenic effect. Contact local Medicines Information Centre for advice.

BREAST-FEEDING
Risperidone has been shown to be excreted in human milk and breast-feeding should be avoided. Contact local Medicines Information Centre for advice.

SIDE-EFFECTS
See chlorpromazine monograph; but more subjective dysphoria and gastrointestinal side-effects. Appetite increase and weight gain. Extrapyramidal effects.

POISONING/TOXICITY
In general reported signs and symptoms have been

those resulting from an exaggeration of the drugs known pharmacological effects, including drowsiness, sedation, tachycardia, hypotension and extrapyramidal symptoms. Administration of activated charcoal should be considered. ECG monitoring should be carried out to detect possible arrhythmias. No specific antidote, therefore treatment is supportive.

EXCIPIENTS
See manufacturers SPC for further details.

LICENSED STATUS
Not licensed for <15 years of age.

PHARMACOKINETIC PROPERTIES
Rapidly absorbed following oral administration, peak plasma concentrations being reached within 1-2 hours. It undergoes hydroxylation to its main active metabolite, 9-hydroxyrisperidone. Excretion is mainly in the urine, and to a lesser extent in the faeces.

Ropivacaine hydrochloride

Local anaesthetic of the amide type.

USES
Surgical anaesthesia and analgesia in acute pain management.

PRESENTATION
Injection: 2mg in 1mL, 10mL ampoule; 7.5mg in 1mL, 10mL ampoule and 10mg in 1mL, 10mL ampoule – Naropin®.
Infusion (epidural): 2mg in 1mL, 100mL and 200mL bags – Naropin®.

DOSAGE

Route	Age			Frequency (times daily)	Notes
	1 month–2 years	2–12 years	12–18 years		
Epidural injection (intermittant)	← 1–3mg/kg →		20–200mg	single dose	The dose required will depend on the site of injection and the procedure used. See also under ADMINISTRATION.
Epidual infusion	← 400 microgram/kg/hour →		18–20mg/hour	continuous	Use 60 minutes after bolus dose of 1mg/kg.
Local infiltration	-		2–200mg	single dose	Duration 2-6 hours.

ADMINISTRATION
Epidural administration should be carried out by, or under the supervision of, a consultant anaesthetist. A test dose of lidocaine (lignocaine) with adrenaline (epinephrine) should be given before commencing epidural block with ropivacaine to detect inadvertent intravascular administration.

Liver disease: as ropivacaine is metabolised in the liver repeated doses may need to be reduced due to delayed elimination.

Renal disease: there is not normally any requirement to modify the dose in patients with renal impairment.
In alkaline solutions (>pH 6) precipitation may occur.

CONTRA-INDICATIONS & WARNINGS
Contra-indications: intravenous regional anaesthesia, hypovolaemia, obstetric paracervical anaesthesia, known hypersensitivity to local anaesthetics of the amide type.
Cautions: liver disease, partial or complete heart conduction block.
Warnings: acidosis and reduced plasma protein concentration may increase the risk of systemic toxicity; accidental intravascular injection may cause immediate toxic effects (see poisoning/toxicity). IV access should always, therefore, be established before commencing major blocks with ropivacaine.

INTERACTIONS
Fluvoxamine, verapamil may reduce metabolism of ropivacaine; increased risk of adverse effects with *general anaesthetics, opioid analgesics* or other *amide type local anaesthetics* and structurally related medicines.

PREGNANCY
Ropivacaine crosses the placenta but its use at recommended doses during childbirth has not shown any harmful effects.

BREAST-FEEDING
Contact local Medicines Information Centre for advice.

SIDE-EFFECTS
Accidental intrathecal injection can lead to very high spinal anaesthesia possibly with apnoea, severe hypotension and loss of consciousness. Systemic adverse effects are likely to occur following accidental IV administration or following excessive dosage. See poisoning/toxicity below.

POISONING/TOXICITY
In the event of overdose, peak plasma concentrations may not be reached for 1-2 hours depending on the site of the injection. Signs of toxicity may therefore be delayed. *CNS:* symptoms escalate in severity from visual or hearing disturbances, perioral numbness, dizziness, light-headedness, tingling and parathesia to dysarthria, muscular rigidity and twitching which may precede the onset of generalised convulsions and finally unconsciousness and grand mal convulsions.

Treatment: in the event of convulsions oxygen must be given and ventilation assisted. An IV anticonvulsant should be given if the convulsions do not stop spontaneously after 15-20 seconds. *IV thiopental (thiopentone)* or *diazepam* may also be used. *Suxamethonium* will stop muscle convulsions rapidly but controlled ventilation and tracheal intubation will be necessary.
Cardiovascular: symptoms – hypotension, bradycardia, arrhythmias which lead to cardiac arrest in severe cases; treatment – if hypotension or bradycardia occurs, IV ephedrine should be given and repeated, if necessary, after 2-3 minutes. If circulatory arrest occurs cardiopulmonary resuscitation should be initiated.

PHARMACOKINETIC PROPERTIES
Plasma concentration depends on dose, route of administration and vascularity of the injection site. In adults it has a total plasma clearance of the order of 440mL per minute and terminal half-life of 1.8 hours. It shows a complete biphasic absorption from the epidural space, the slow phase, which is the rate limiting factor in the elimination of ropivacaine. Ropivacaine is 94% bound to plasma proteins. Peak plasma levels will be reached within 1-2 hours. It is extensively metabolised in the liver, mediated by the cytochrome P450 ISO enzyme CYP1A.

EXCIPIENTS
See manufacturers SPC for further details.

LICENSED STATUS
Licensed for >12 years of age.

R

Rubella vaccine, live

At the time of writing (May 2003), single antigen rubella vaccine was no longer being produced for use in UK and priority for its use should be given to susceptible women of childbearing age. Once supplies have been exhausted and if no other source becomes available, the combined MMR vaccine should be used in its place.

USES
Active prophylaxis against rubella infection. Usually given combined with measles and mumps vaccine as 'MMR'. Rubella vaccine may be given separately to women known to be rubella seronegative, but other indications are rare.

PRESENTATION
Injection: (single dose freeze-dried pellet which is reconstituted to 0.5mL) – Ervevax®. Also available as MMR vaccine. Each dose of Ervevax® contains not less than 1000 $TCID_{50}$ of the live attenuated Wistar RA 27/3 strain of rubella virus grown on MRC5 human diploid cells. This cell line originates from cells taken from a fetus aborted for medical reasons in 1966. The virus itself originates from a fetus aborted because the mother had rubella infection during pregnancy.

DOSAGE/ADMINISTRATION
IM or deep SC: 0.5mL. Booster doses of single antigen rubella vaccine are not recommended.

CONTRA-INDICATIONS & WARNINGS
As for vaccines generally; also, should not be given to anyone who is immunosuppressed. Single antigen rubella vaccine is not indicated in an HIV positive child, but MMR vaccine may be given.

INTERACTIONS

As it is a live vaccine it may be given at the same time as other live vaccines or after a minimal interval of 3 weeks. It should not be given within a period of 3 weeks before and 3 months after human immunoglobulin and blood or plasma transfusions. The vaccine should not be given to children <1 year old as maternal antibodies may interfere with the response.

The vaccine may temporarily convert someone who would have had a positive response to a tuberculin test to a non-responder. A tuberculin test should be postponed until 4 weeks have elapsed since immunisation.

PREGNANCY

While there is evidence of fetuses becoming infected with rubella virus after inadvertent rubella vaccination during pregnancy, no cases of congenital rubella syndrome have been reported. As immunisation is likely to be an elective procedure, immunisation with a rubella containing vaccine should not be carried out during pregnancy and pregnancy should be avoided for a month after the vaccine has been administered.

BREAST-FEEDING

No information is available, but there are no grounds to believe it would be harmful and it has been used extensively in breast-feeding women.

SIDE-EFFECTS

Local reactions, such as tenderness and redness may occur. Mild transient symptoms of rubella may occur 1-3 weeks after immunisation. These include fever, sore throat, lymphadenopathy, arthralgia and arthritis. Joint symptoms are less common in children than adults. Thrombocytopenic purpura, usually self-limiting, has been shown to be caused by MMR at a frequency of approximately 1 in every 32,000 doses. It has also been reported after single antigen rubella vaccine.

POISONING/TOXICITY

No data available.

PHARMACODYNAMIC PROPERTIES

Immunity is related to the production of circulating antibodies.

EXCIPIENTS

Neomycin sulphate, lactose, sorbitol, amino acids for injection, dextran 10, and human albumin.

LICENSED STATUS

Licensed for use as described.

FURTHER INFORMATION

Protect from light and store at 2-8°C. Should be used within 1 hour of reconstitution. The human albumin in the vaccine originates from countries with no BSE.

Salbutamol

A selective beta-2 agonist providing short-acting (4-6 hours) bronchodilation, with a fast onset (within 5 minutes) in reversible airways obstruction.

USES

Asthma and other conditions associated with reversible airways obstruction, renal hyperkalaemia, vasodilator in intensive care.

PRESENTATION

Injection: 500 micrograms in 1mL, 1mL ampoule – Ventolin®.
Injection for infusion: 1mg in 1mL, 5mL ampoule – Ventolin®.
Syrup: 2mg in 5mL – Ventolin® and non-proprietary.
Tablet: 2mg and 4mg – non-proprietary.
Tablet: (modified release) 4mg and 8mg – Volmax®, Ventmax®.
Aerosol inhaler: 100 microgram/actuation – Ventolin®, Asmasal® Spacehaler, non-proprietary.
Aerosol inhaler CFC free: 100 microgram/actuation – Ventolin Evohaler®, Salamol® Airomir®.
Breath-actuated inhaler: 100 microgram/actuation - Salamol® Easi-breathe, Aerolin Autohaler®, Airomir Autohaler®.
Dry powder device: 200 microgram and 400 microgram – Ventodisks®; 200 microgram – Accuhaler®, 95 microgram/actuation Asmasal® Clickhaler.
Nebuliser solution: 2.5mg in 2.5mL and 5mg in 2.5mL – Ventolin Nebules®, Salamol Steri-Neb®.
Respirator solution: 5mg in 1mL – Ventolin®.

DOSAGE

Route	Age				Frequency	Notes
	birth–1 month	1 month–2 years	2–12 years	12–18 years	(times daily)	
Oral	–	100 microgram/kg	2–6 years 1mg 6–12 years 2mg	2–4mg	3–4 3–4	Asthma: reliever for symptom relief only.
Oral (modified release)	–	–	>3 years 4mg	8mg	2	
Aerosol inhaler	–	← up to 1mg →			single dose	Asthma: reliever given as required. 1–2 hourly initially then reduce frequency to 4–6 hourly.
	–	← 100–200 microgram →			single dose	Asthma: reliever, on demand, routine use.
Inhaled Ventodisks®	–	–	>5 years ← 200–400 micrograms →		single dose	Asthma: reliever, on demand, routine use.
Inhaled Accuhaler®	–	–	>5 years ← 200 microgram →		single dose	Asthma: reliever, on demand, routine use.
Nebuliser solution	1.25–2.5mg	← 2.5–5mg →			single dose	Asthma: reliever given as required.1–2 hourly initially then reduce frequency to 4–6 hourly in hospital with monitoring. In severe acute asthma half hourly doses may be given in hospital.. NB. only licensed for use up to 4 times daily.
IV bolus over 5 minutes	5 microgram/kg		15 microgram/kg (maximum 250 microgram)		single dose	Status asthmaticus
IV infusion	← 1–5 microgram/kg/minute →				continuous	Status asthmaticus or vasodilation in intensive care: doses up to 10 microgram/kg/minute have been used.
IV bolus	← 4 microgram/kg →				single dose	Renal hyperkalaemia: – repeat if necessary.
Nebuliser	← 2.5–5mg →				single dose	Renal hyperkalaemia: – repeat if necessary.

S

ADMINISTRATION

Oral: modified release tablets should not be crushed. Normal release tablets can be dispersed in water. Syrup can be diluted with purified water BP (protect from light and give 28 days expiry). Do not dilute syrup with syrup BP or sorbitol solutions.

Inhaled: nebules can be mixed with ipatropium bromide, budesonide nebuliser solutions and NaCl 0.9%. Use oxygen driven nebuliser if saturation <92%.

Aerosol inhaler: Volumatic® spacer may be used with Volumatic® mask for infants and young children. Other spacers are available for use with salbutamol inhaler e.g. Aerochamber®, Babyhaler® (not on NHS prescription). An Autohaler® can be used for children >5 years.

IV: IV solution is compatible with potassium, incompatible with aminophylline. IV bolus must be given over 5 minutes (EMERGENCY USE ONLY). The 500 microgram in 1mL injection should be diluted with Water for Injections to produce a solution of 50 microgram in 1mL. Use the appropriate volume for the dose to be given. IV infusion 5mg in 5mL should ideally be diluted to 10 micrograms in 1mL, in glucose 5%, NaCl 0.9% or glucose 4%/NaCl 0.18%, although it may, if necessary, be given undiluted via a central line in intensive care. NB. some units are using 200 micrograms in 1mL (peripherally) and others 500 microgram in 1mL (centrally) in fluid restricted patients.

CONTRA-INDICATIONS & WARNINGS
IV administration should be undertaken with caution to diabetics, as ketoacidosis has been reported.

INTERACTIONS
Corticosteroids increase the risk of hypokalaemia if high dose *corticosteroids* are given with high doses of salbutamol. *Diuretics* increase the risk of hypokalaemia if *acetazolamide, loop diuretics,* and *thiazides* are given with high doses of salbutamol. *Theophylline* increases the risk of hypokalaemia if given with high doses of salbutamol. *Beta-blockers* may partially or totally inhibit the effects of salbutamol.

PREGNANCY
Most adverse effects on the fetus are with IV infusions. Usual dose in asthma should not be problematic.

BREAST-FEEDING
Salbutamol is probably excreted in breast milk; but is unlikely to be problematic.

SIDE-EFFECTS
These are usually dose related, and occur more frequently with systemic therapy; hypokalaemia, tremor, nervousness, mild tachycardia.

POISONING/TOXICITY
The preferred antidote for overdose with salbutamol is a cardio-selective beta-blocking agent. However, beta-blocking drugs should be used with caution in patients with a history of bronchospasm. Hypokalaemia may occur following overdose with salbutamol, and serum potassium levels should be monitored.

EXCIPIENTS
See manufacturers SPC for further details.

LICENSED STATUS
All presentations except for the injection are licensed for use in children and adults, but some of the doses given are higher than that recommended by the manufacturer's. Nebules are not licensed for use in renal hyperkalaemia.

Salicylic acid

S

Keratolytic with irritant action.

USES
Treatment of warts.

PRESENTATION
Various preparations of varying strengths are available in gel, ointment and paint presentations.
Application: salicylic acid 26% in polyacrylic solution – Occlusal®.
Gel: salicylic acid 12%, lactic acid 4% – Salatac®; salicylic acid 11%, lactic acid 4% – Cuplex®.
Ointment: salicylic acid 50% in paraffin base – Verrugon®.
Paint: salicylic acid 16.7%, lactic acid 16.7% – Salactol®, Duofilm®.

DOSAGE/ADMINISTRATION
Topical: remove dead skin by gentle rubbing with pumice stone or emery board before applying daily.

CONTRA-INDICATIONS & WARNINGS
Protect surrounding skin and avoid broken skin. Do not apply to face, anogenital region or large areas.

INTERACTIONS
None known.

PREGNANCY/BREAST-FEEDING
No specific precautions.

SIDE-EFFECTS
Skin irritation.

POISONING/TOXICITY
Treat accidental oral ingestion immediately by gastric lavage with 2–5% aqueous sodium bicarbonate solution. Monitor fluid and electrolyte balance and provide appropriate supportive measures. Symptoms include headache, nausea, vomiting, diarrhoea and respiratory depression.

EXCIPIENTS
Consult manufacturers for further details.

LICENSED STATUS
Licensed for use in adults and children, but not in infants.

FURTHER INFORMATION
Paint is extremely flammable; avoid inhaling vapour.

Salmeterol

A direct acting beta-2 receptor stimulant which has a long duration of action.

USES
Prevention of reversible airways obstruction where long-term regular bronchodilator treatment is required.

PRESENTATION
Aerosol inhalation: (as xinafoate) 25 microgram per actuation – Serevent®.
Dry powder for inhalation: (as xinafoate) 50 microgram per blister – Serevent® Accuhaler® and Diskhaler®.

DOSAGE

Route	Age		Frequency (times daily)	Notes
	2–12 years	12–18 years		
Inhaled	≤4 years 25 microgram		2	Preventor for regular use.
	≥ 4 years 50 microgram	50–100 microgram	2	

ADMINISTRATION
Inhalation: aerosol inhaler can be used with Volumatic® spacer.

CONTRA-INDICATIONS & WARNINGS
Hypersensitivity to any ingredient of the preparation. Should not be started in patients with significantly worsening or acutely deteriorating asthma. Not designed to relieve acute asthma symptoms.

INTERACTIONS
Corticosteroids increase the risk of hypokalaemia if high dose corticosteroids are given with salmeterol. *Diuretics* increase the risk of hypokalaemia if *acetazolamide, loop diuretics,* and *thiazides* are given with salmeterol. *Theophylline* increases the risk of hypokalaemia if given with salmeterol. *Beta-blockers* may partially or totally inhibit the effects of salmeterol.

PREGNANCY
Does not appear to be a problem in pregnancy.

BREAST-FEEDING
Low levels of salmeterol are excreted into breast milk; unlikely to be problematic.

SIDE-EFFECTS
Tremor, subjective palpitations, and headache (these tend to be transient and reduce with regular therapy). Tachycardia, hypokalaemia, paradoxical bronchospasm with aerosol inhaler (responds to a fast-acting inhaled bronchodilator). The patient should be reassessed, and changed to the Diskhaler® or Accuhaler® device, or alternative therapy. Skin reactions, muscle cramps, non-specific chest pain, local irritation and arthralgia have been reported.

POISONING/TOXICITY
Signs of toxicity are tremor, headache, and tachycardia. A beta-blocking agent can be used, but should be used with caution in patients with a history of bronchospasm.

S

PHARMACOKINETIC PROPERTIES
Onset of action of 10-20 minutes; duration of action of about 12 hours. Plasma concentrations of salmeterol are negligible at therapeutic inhaled doses.

EXCIPIENTS
Accuhaler® and Diskhaler® blisters contain lactose. See manufacturers SPC for further details.

LICENSED STATUS
All presentations are licensed for use in patients ≥4 years of age.

Secobarbital (quinalbarbitone) (controlled drug)

Barbiturate used as hypnotic and sedative.

USES
Sedation for procedures e.g. magnetic resonance imaging (MRI) and computerised tomography (CT) scans.

PRESENTATION
Capsules: 50mg and 100mg – Seconal Sodium®; 25mg – manufactured 'special'.
Powder: may be extemporaneously prepared.

DOSAGE

Route	Age				Frequency (times daily)	Notes
	birth–1 month	1 month–2 years	2–12 years	12–18 years		
Oral	not recommended	← 7.5–10mg/kg → (maximum 200mg)		200mg	single dose	Round <u>down</u> to the nearest increment of 25mg.

ADMINISTRATION
Oral: administer in e.g. neat blackcurrant juice to disguise very bitter taste if whole capsules cannot be swallowed. Powders can be prepared from the capsule contents if needed.

CONTRA-INDICATIONS & WARNINGS
Contra-indications: hypersensitivity to barbiturates, pre-existing CNS depression or coma, porphyria. *Cautions:* severe hepatic disease, renal insufficiency or respiratory disease particularly where dyspnoea or obstruction is present. Caution should be taken with patients in pain in whom secobarbital can provoke a paradoxical excitatory reaction unless an analgesic is given concurrently. Co-administration with opiates can lead to respiratory depression. Induces hepatic enzymes, which in turn affect the metabolism of many other drugs. Monitoring should be started from the time of administration according to national and local guidelines.

INTERACTIONS
Sedation or respiratory depression may be enhanced by other drugs with CNS depressant properties e.g. *opiates, antidepressants, antiepileptics.* Reduced plasma concentrations of *anti-arrhythmics, antibacterials, antivirals, warfarin, calcium-channel blockers, corticosteroids, ciclosporin (cyclosporin)* and *theophylline.* This is unlikely to be a problem with single dose therapy.

PREGNANCY
Secobarbital crosses the placenta producing detectable concentrations in the neonate. Congenital malformations have been reported in children born of women taking barbiturates during pregnancy, but the causal role is some matter of debate. Neonatal intoxication, drug dependence and symptoms resembling vitamin K deficiency have been reported in infants born to mothers who received barbiturates in pregnancy. Barbiturate withdrawal symptoms including hyperactivity, jitteriness, tremulousness, twitching of extremities and shallow respiration have been reported in new-born infants following *in utero* exposure to secobarbital. Use in pregnancy is not recommended.

BREAST-FEEDING
Secobarbital is excreted into breast milk. Reports state that it can be detected in breast milk for up to 24 hours following a single dose. Due to the relatively long half-life, chronic ingestion by a nursing mother could result in significant accumulation with corresponding accumulation in the nursing infant. Therefore it is advisable for a mother who must continue treatment with secobarbital to avoid breast-feeding.

SIDE-EFFECTS
CNS: drowsiness, sedation and ataxia are the most frequent adverse effects and are a consequence of dose related CNS depression. Some reports say that performance is impaired after therapeutic doses for up to 22 hours. Other side-effects include respiratory depression, headache. Agitation and hyperkinesia have been reported. Paradoxical excitement and irritability may occur, especially in children.
Cardiovascular: hypotension, arrhythmias.
Other: gastrointestinal disturbance, hypersensitivity reactions (rare) including skin rash, hepatitis, cholestasis and photosensitivity.

POISONING/TOXICITY
Nystagmus, miosis, slurred speech and ataxia may occur with excessive doses of barbiturates. Toxic effects of overdosage result from profound central depression. They include coma, respiratory and cardiovascular depression with hypotension, hypothermia and shock leading to renal failure and death.

PHARMACOKINETIC PROPERTIES
Well absorbed from gastrointestinal tract following oral doses with onset of action of 10-30 minutes. Peak plasma concentrations reached 2-4 hours after oral ingestion with 90% of drug being absorbed. Duration of action is 3–8 hours. Protein binding is 46-70%. Hepatic metabolism mainly by hydroxylation is followed by renal elimination of metabolites and only a small amount of unchanged drug. Elimination half-life is reported to be 19-34 hours, less in children 2-13 years (2.7-13.5 hours).

EXCIPIENTS
Contact manufacturers for further details.

LICENSED STATUS
Not licensed for use in children. Licensed in adults only for the short-term treatment of severe intractable insomnia resistant to other drug therapy.

Selenium

USES
As a selenium supplement as part of a complete PN regimen (long-term PN). Selenium deficiency.

PRESENTATION
Tablet: selenium 100 microgram, vitamin A 1500 international units, vitamin C 90mg, vitamin E 45 international units – Selenium Ace®.
Oral solution: (as sodium selenite pentahydrate) selenium 0.2 micromol in 1mL – may be extemporaneously prepared.
Injection: (as selenite) 0.2 micromol selenium in 1mL – manufactured 'special'.
Injection: 100 microgram in 10mL – manufactured 'special'.
Note: Peditrace® and Additrace⁰⁰ contain maintenance amounts of selenium.

DOSAGE
IV: maintenance dose 0.025 micromol/kg/day rising to 0.126 micromol/kg/day in deficiency (2 microgram/kg/day rising to 10 microgram/kg/day) depending upon plasma selenium and glutathione peroxidase levels.
Oral: there is very little information available on oral doses in children but doses in the range 0.024-0.048 micromol/kg/per day have been used. Monitor plasma selenium and glutathione peroxidase levels.

CONTRA-INDICATIONS & WARNINGS
Impaired renal function.

INTERACTIONS
Ascorbic acid at high levels may precipitate out selenium by reducing the selenite salt – not been shown in practice to be a problem.

SIDE-EFFECTS
See toxicity – unlikely at doses suggested. Even though selenium is very toxic there is a big order of magnitude difference in the doses necessary to produce these effects.

POISONING/TOXICITY
Toxic symptoms – fatigue, gastrointestinal disturbances, nail and hair change, peripheral neuropathy.

LICENSED STATUS
Oral solution prepared extemporaneously and as such is unlicensed.
Sodium selenite injection produced under Specials Licence – by Queens Medical Centre, Nottingham.
Selenium injection produced in France; certificates of analysis available – Laboratoire Aguettant.

S

FURTHER INFORMATION
1 micromol selenium ≡ 79 microgram selenium and therefore
1 microgram selenium ≡ 0.0126 micromol selenium.

Selenium sulphide

Antiseborrhoeic agent.

USES
Dandruff and seborrhoeic dermatitis of scalp.

PRESENTATION
Shampoo: 2.5% Selsun®.

ADMINISTRATION
Use as shampoo twice weekly for 2 weeks then once weekly for 2 weeks then as necessary.

CONTRA-INDICATIONS & WARNINGS
Hypersensitivity to any of ingredients. Do not use on broken or inflamed skin. May discolour metallic jewellery. Do not use 2 days before or after dyeing, tinting or waving hair.

PREGNANCY/BREAST-FEEDING
Avoid during first 3 months of pregnancy. Not recommended during lactation as effect unknown.

SIDE-EFFECTS
Irritation or sensitisation of skin, increase in hair loss. Discolouration of hair minimised by thorough washing of hair after treatment. Oiliness or dryness of hair and scalp.

POISONING/TOXICITY
If accidental ingestion occurs, nausea and vomiting may present as symptoms. Treat by provoking vomiting or perform gastric lavage. General supportive measures. A purgative may be given to hasten elimination.

EXCIPIENTS
Fragrance.

LICENSED STATUS
Licensed for >5 years of age. Unlicensed for use in pityriasis versicolor.

S Senna

Stimulant laxative which is virtually colon specific.

USES
Constipation. Effective in opioid-induced constipation, often combined with magnesium hydroxide.

PRESENTATION
Tablet: standardised senna ≡ 7.5mg total sennosides (calculated as sennoside B) – Senokot® and non-proprietary.
Syrup: 5mL spoonful contains standardised senna extract ≡ 7.5mg total sennosides (calculated as sennoside B) – Senokot®.
Granules: 5mL level spoonful (2.7g) contains standardised senna ≡ 15mg total sennosides (calculated as sennoside B) – Senokot®.

DOSAGE

Route	Age			Frequency	Notes
	1 month–2 years	2–12 years	12–18 years		
Oral (tablets)	–	≤6 years Not recommended 6–12 years 1–2 tablets	2–4 tablets	1	

DOSAGE continued

Route	Age			Frequency	Notes
	1 month–2 years	2–12 years	12–18 years		
Oral (liquid)	0.5mL/kg	2–6 years 2.5–5mL	10–20mL	1	
		6–12 years 5–10mL		1	
Oral (granules)	–	<6 years Not recommended			
		6–12 years 2.5–5mL	5–10mL	1	

ADMINISTRATION
Oral: correct dose is the smallest required to produce a comfortable soft-formed motion. Varies between individuals. Usually taken as a single dose at bedtime. May be taken in the morning by children. Tablets can be taken with a drink, the granules can be stirred into hot milk, sprinkled on food or eaten as they are. Once regularity achieved, reduce dosage.

CONTRA-INDICATIONS & WARNINGS
Should not be given when any undiagnosed acute or persistent abdominal symptoms are present. Diabetic patients should use the tablets as they have a negligible sugar content.

PREGNANCY/BREAST-FEEDING
Suitable to use.

SIDE-EFFECTS
Griping may occur.

POISONING/TOXICITY
Griping, severe diarrhoea. Conservative measures: generous amounts of fluid especially fruit drinks should be given.

EXCIPIENTS
Granules include sucrose. Syrup includes 3.3g sucrose in 5mL and 7% v/v alcohol. Contact manufacturers for further details

LICENSED STATUS
Syrup is licensed for ≥2 years of age. Tablets and granules licensed ≥6 years of age.

Sermorelin

S

An analogue of growth hormone releasing hormone (somatorelin, GHRH).

USES
Evaluation of the functional capacity and response of the somatotrophs of the anterior pituitary.

PRESENTATION
Injection: (as acetate) 50 microgram per ampoule, with solvent – Geref 50®.

DOSAGE

Route	Age		Frequency (times daily)	Notes
	2–12 years	12–18 years		
IV bolus	← 1 microgram/kg →		single dose	In the morning following an overnight fast.

ADMINISTRATION
IV: reconstitute immediately before administration with at least 0.5mL of the accompanying sterile diluent (NaCl 0.9%). Venous blood samples should be drawn 15 minutes before and immediately prior to administration and then at 15, 30, 45 and 60 minutes following injection.

CONTRA-INDICATIONS & WARNINGS
Patients already on growth hormone should have their therapy discontinued 1-2 weeks pre-test. Known hypersensitivity to sermorelin or any of the excipients. The test should be conducted in the absence of any drugs which directly affect the pituitary secretion of somatotropin. Untreated hypothyroidism may affect the response to sermorelin. The test should be carried out with particular caution in patients with epilepsy, obesity and hyperglycaemia.

INTERACTIONS
Somatotropin levels may be transiently elevated by *clonidine, levodopa* or *insulin-induced hypoglycaemia*. The response to sermorelin may also be blunted by a*nti-muscarinic agents* such as *atropine*. It is possible that *beta-adrenoceptor agonists* and *blockers* may affect the response to sermorelin.

PREGNANCY/BREAST-FEEDING
Contra-indicated.

SIDE-EFFECTS
Facial heat, facial flush and injection site pain occasionally occur and usually disappear within a few minutes.

POISONING/TOXICITY
No data available.

EXCIPIENTS
See manufacturers SPC for further details.

LICENSED STATUS
No lower age limit stated in the manufacturers SPC.

Sertraline

Selective serotonin re-uptake inhibitor (SSRI).

USES
Depression. Obsessive-compulsive disorder (OCD). Anxiety conditions including social phobia.

PRESENTATION
Tablet: 50mg (scored) and 100mg – Lustral®.

DOSAGE

Route	Age		Frequency	Notes
	2–12 years	**12–18 years**	**(times daily)**	
Oral	≥6 years 25mg	50mg	1	Initial dose. 6–12 years of age dose can be increased if necessary by increments of 25mg daily over several weeks to a maximum of 100mg daily. >12 years of age dose can be increased if necessary by increments of 50mg daily over several weeks to a maximum of 200mg daily. Once optimal therapeutic response is achieved the dose should be reduced to the lowest effective level.

ADMINISTRATION
Tablets taste bitter but can be dispersed in water, orange juice or blackcurrant squash. Tablets can be crushed and mixed with soft food.

CONTRA-INDICATIONS & WARNINGS, INTERACTIONS
See fluoxetine monograph.

PREGNANCY
No adequate well controlled studies in pregnant women. Contact local Medicines Information Centre for advice.

BREAST-FEEDING
Unknown effects but see fluoxetine monograph. Contact local Medicines Information Centre for advice.

SIDE-EFFECTS
See fluoxetine monograph. Somewhat more sedative. Hepatic transaminases and serum uric acid levels may be raised.

POISONING/TOXICITY
Somnolence, nausea, vomiting, anxiety, dilated pupils. Treat as for fluoxetine poisoning.

PHARMACOKINETIC PROPERTIES
Following oral administration, sertraline is only slowly absorbed, peak plasma concentration occurring at about 4.5-8.4 hours after dosing. It undergoes extensive presystemic elimination. The average plasma half-life is 26 hours. It is highly plasma protein-bound (approximately 98%). Sertraline is extensively metabolised and only a small amount (<0.2%) is excreted unchanged in the urine.

EXCIPIENTS
See manufacturers SPC for further details.

LICENSED STATUS
Licensed for ≥6 years of age for OCD. Not licensed for use in children for other indications.

FURTHER INFORMATION
The onset of therapeutic effect may be seen within 7 days, although 2-4 weeks are usually necessary for full antidepressant activity.

Silver nitrate

Caustic agent.

USES
Removal of granulation tissue, warts and verrucae.

PRESENTATION
Caustic applicator: 75% potassium nitrate 25% – AVOCA® (box containing 100 single applicators).
Caustic pencil: 95% potassium nitrate 5% – AVOCA® (treatment pack contains pencil, emery file, 6 adhesive dressings and protector pads).

ADMINISTRATION
Applicators: moisten medicated end of applicator and apply to affected tissue.
Pencil: apply moistened caustic pencil tip for 1-2 minutes. Repeat after 24 hours up to maximum of 3 applications for warts or 6 for verrucae. Cover with dressing afterwards.
The caustic activity depends directly on the contact time. To stop action wash with NaCl 0.9%.

CONTRA-INDICATIONS & WARNINGS
Protect surrounding skin and avoid broken skin. Do not use on face or large areas. Not for use on genital warts. Continued application to mucous membranes and open wounds leads to argyria.

PREGNANCY/BREAST-FEEDING
No specific precautions.

POISONING/TOXICITY
If ingested treat with repeated stomach washouts with sodium chloride solution 1% followed by 250ml of sodium sulphate solution 12% to remain in stomach. Supportive treatment for pain, special attention to renal function and fluid balance.

LICENSED STATUS
Licensed for use in children and adults. Medical supervision recommended.

FURTHER INFORMATION
Protect from moisture and light.

S

USES
Indicated for the prophylaxis and treatment of infection in burn wounds, and also for an aid to the short-term treatment of infection in leg ulcers and pressure sores. It can be used as prophylaxis of infection in skin graft donor sites and extensive abrasions, and for conservative management of finger-tip injuries where pulp and nail loss and/or partial loss of the distal phalanx has occurred.

PRESENTATION
Cream: 1% – Flamazine®.

DOSAGE/ADMINISTRATION
Burns: after cleaning the wound apply over all affected areas to a depth of 3-5mm, using a sterile gloved hand or sterile spatula. Where necessary, re-apply to any area from which it has been removed by patient activity. Re-apply at least every 24 hours or more frequently if the volume of exudate is large.

Hand burns: apply to the burn and enclose the whole hand in a clear plastic bag or glove which is then closed at the wrist. The patient should be encouraged to move the hand and fingers and the dressing should be changed when an excessive amount of exudate has accumulated in the bag.

Leg ulcers/pressure sores: the cavity of the ulcer should be filled with cream to a depth of at least 3-5mm, followed by application of an absorbent pad or dressing, with further application of pressure bandaging as appropriate. Dressings should be changed daily, but if less exudate every 48 hours may be sufficient.

Finger-tip injuries: haemostasis of the injury should be achieved prior to the application of a 3-5mm layer of cream, and then the finger covered with a finger dressing or the finger of a plastic glove. Dressings should be changed every 2-3 days.

In all cases, use the contents of the tube or pot on one person only. Discard 50g tubes 7 days after opening. Discard 250g and 500g pots 24 hours after opening.

CONTRA-INDICATIONS & WARNINGS
Should not be used at or near term pregnancy, on premature infants or newborn infants during the first month of life, due to the risk of causing kernicterus. Patients who are hypersensitive to silver sulfadiazine (sulphadiazine) or to components of the preparation. Concurrent use of enzymatic debriding agents. Leg or pressure ulcers that are very exudative.

INTERACTIONS
Should not be used with *enzymatic debriding agents* as they can be inactivated by silver. In large-area burns where serum sulfadiazine levels may approach therapeutic levels, it should be noted that the effects of systemically administered drugs might be altered. This can especially apply to *oral hypoglycaemic agents* and to *phenytoin*. It is recommended that phenytoin blood levels are monitored as its effects can be potentiated.

PREGNANCY
Contra-indicated at or near term pregnancy, since it can cause kernicterus.

BREAST-FEEDING
Safety not established. Caution is required since all sulphonamides increase the possibility of kernicterus.

SIDE-EFFECTS
Local reactions such as burning, itching and skin rash may occur in about 2% of patients. Leucopenia has been reported in 3-5% of burns patients treated with silver sulfadiazine. Systemic absorption of silver sulfadiazine may very rarely result in any of the adverse reactions attributable to systemic sulphonamide therapy.

POISONING/TOXICITY
There is evidence that in large area wounds and/or after prolonged application, systemic absorption of silver can cause clinical argyria.

EXCIPIENTS
See manufacturers SPC for further details.

LICENSED STATUS
Licensed in all ages after the first few months of life.

Simple linctus BP (adult and paediatric)

Demulcent cough preparation.

USES
Symptomatic relief of dry, irritating cough.

PRESENTATION
Linctus: Simple Linctus BP (contains 2.5% citric acid monohydrate); Simple Linctus Paediatric BP (contains 0.625% citric acid monohydrate) – non-proprietary.

DOSAGE

Route	Age				Frequency (times daily)	Notes
	birth–1 month	1 month–2 years	2–12 years	12–18 years		
Oral	–	← 5–10mL → (paediatric preparation)		5–10mL (adult preparation)	3–4	

CONTRA-INDICATIONS & WARNINGS, INTERACTIONS, SIDE-EFFECTS	None reported.

EXCIPIENTS
Some preparations include sucrose, although sugar-free preparations are also available.

LICENSED STATUS
Licensed for use in children (appropriate preparation) and adults.

Simvastatin

A 3-hydroxy-3-methylglutaryl coenzyme A (HMG CoA) reductase inhibitor.

USES
Hypercholesterolaemia, including familial hypercholesterolaemia in patients who have not responded adequately to diet therapy and with a total cholesterol >7.7mmol/L (300mg/dL).

PRESENTATION
Tablet: 10mg, 20mg, 40mg and 80mg – Zocor®.

DOSAGE

Route	Age		Frequency (times daily)	Notes
	2–12 years	12–18 years		
Oral	<10 years 5mg >10 years 10mg	10mg	1 (at night) 1 (at night)	Starting dose; if necessary increase to 20mg (<10 years) and 40mg (>10 years), daily, over 6-12 weeks.

CONTRA-INDICATIONS & WARNINGS
Active liver disease, renal impairment, unexplained increase in transaminases. Liver function tests should be carried out before and during treatment. Discontinue treatment if serum transaminase concentrations rise to, and persist at, three times the upper limit of normal.

INTERACTIONS
Immunosuppressive therapy including *ciclosporin (cyclosporin)* and *prednisolone* may increase plasma statin concentration and the risk of muscle toxicity. Concomitant use of *fibrates* or *nicotinic acid, erythromycin, clarithromycin* may also be associated with an increased risk of serious muscle toxicity. *Itraconazole* and *ketoconazole* increase risk of myopathy with simvastatin. Anticoagulant effects of *warfarin* increased by simvastatin.

PREGNANCY
Avoid as congenital anomalies reported; decreased synthesis of cholesterol possibly affects fetal development.

BREAST-FEEDING
Some statins are excreted in small amounts in human milk. Contact local Medicines Information Centre for advice.

S

SIDE-EFFECTS
Reversible increases in liver enzymes and creatine kinase. Minor gastrointestinal disturbances-nausea, diarrhoea, constipation; skin rash; peripheral neuropathy; rarely rhabdomyolysis (see interactions), also increased risk with renal impairment; patients should be advised to report unexplained muscle pain.

POISONING/TOXICITY
A few cases of overdose have been reported; no patient had any specific symptoms; symptomatic treatment if necessary.

PHARMACOKINETIC PROPERTIES
Undergoes extensive first pass metabolism in the liver, its primary site of action. Less than 5% of an oral dose has been reported to reach the circulation as active metabolites. Simvastatin and its active metabolites are approximately 95% plasma protein bound.

EXCIPIENTS
See manufacturers SPC for further details.

LICENSED STATUS
Not licensed for use in children.

Sodium acetate

Sodium acetate is metabolised to bicarbonate *in vivo* (1mmol acetate ≡ 1mmol bicarbonate).

USES
As a sodium supplement as part of a balanced PN regimen where the level of chloride needs to be limited to 3mmol/kg (hyperchloraemic acidaemia) and where the patient is becoming acidotic.

PRESENTATION
Injection: 30% (providing per 1mL, 2.2mmol of sodium and acetate), 5mL and 10mL ampoules – manufactured 'specials'. A 4mmol in 1mL strength is also available.

DOSAGE/ADMINISTRATION
IV: 2mmol/kg as part of a PN regimen.

CONTRA-INDICATIONS AND WARNINGS
Impaired renal function, metabolic or respiratory alkalosis, hypocalcaemia or hypochlorhydria. Because of Na^+ content caution also in renal and cardiac impairment, oedema and hypertension.

SIDE-EFFECTS/POISONING & TOXICITY
Excessive administration may lead to metabolic alkalosis and hypernatraemia.

LICENSED STATUS
Available as a 'special' and as such is unlicensed.

FURTHER INFORMATION
5mL ampoules are available from South Devon Healthcare.
10mL ampoules are available from Martindale Pharmaceuticals Ltd; as is the 4mmol in 1mL strength.

Sodium benzoate

USES
Hyperammonaemia due to urea-cycle enzyme defects, non-ketotic hyperglycinaemia.

PRESENTATION
Capsule: 50mg, 250mg, 400mg and 500mg.
Injection: 1g in 5mL.
Oral liquid: 500mg in 5mL, 1g in 5mL and 3g in 10mL.
Powder.
Tablet: 500mg.

DOSAGE

Indication	Route	Age				Frequency (times daily)	Notes
		birth–1 month	1 month–2 years	2–12 years	12–18 years		
Hyper-ammonaemia	Oral	← up to 62.5mg/kg →				4	
	IV	← 250mg/kg →				single dose	IV infusion over 90 minutes Acute loading dose.
	IV	← 250mg/kg/day →				continuous	Neonates. Prompt haemodialysis is needed in severe cases.
	IV	← up to 500mg/kg/day →				continuous	Older patients.
Non-ketotic hyper-glycinaemia	Oral	62.5mg/kg	← 125mg/kg →			4	

ADMINISTRATION
Oral: can be made more palatable by mixing with milk, fruit juice or feeds. Freely soluble in water.
IV infusion: dilute to 20mg in 1mL with glucose 5% or 10%, maximum concentration 50mg in 1mL.
IV compatibilities: can be infused at Y-site with arginine, carnitine, and sodium phenylbutyrate (no data to support this, but has been done in practice).

CONTRA-INDICATIONS & WARNINGS
High sodium content (500mg sodium benzoate contains 3.5mmol sodium) therefore use in caution in patients with congestive heart failure or severe renal insufficiency and in clinical states where there is sodium retention with oedema.
Caution in neonates due to the increased risk of kernicterus and metabolic acidosis.

PREGNANCY/BREAST-FEEDING
No information available. Contact local Medicines Information Centre for advice.

SIDE-EFFECTS
Vomiting is the most common adverse effect. It can be helped by giving smaller doses more frequently or giving with food/feed. Anorexia, irritability, lethargy and coma can occur when high doses are given. Toxicity is more likely in neonates due to incomplete conjugation.

PHARMACODYNAMIC PROPERTIES
Sodium benzoate forms hippurate with glycine; this is readily excreted in the urine. Each mole of sodium benzoate removes one mole of ammonia.

EXCIPIENTS
Contact manufacturers for further details.

LICENSED STATUS
Not licensed for use in the UK.

FURTHER INFORMATION
The tablets, injection, powder and 500mg in 5mL sugar-free oral liquid can be obtained from Special Products Ltd. The capsules, all strengths of oral liquid and powder can be obtained from Martindale Pharmaceuticals Ltd.

Sodium bicarbonate

USES
Metabolic acidosis, renal acidosis, renal hyperkalaemia.

PRESENTATION
Capsule: 500mg (6mmol sodium and bicarbonate) – non-proprietary.
Infusion: 1.26% (0.15mmol sodium and bicarbonate in 1mL), 500mL.
Infusion: 4.2% (0.5mmol sodium and bicarbonate in 1mL), 10mL.
Infusion: 8.4% (1mmol sodium and bicarbonate in 1mL), 200mL – Polyfusor®; 10mL and 50mL – Min-I-Jet®.
Powders: may be extemporaneously prepared.
Solution: may be extemporaneously prepared.
Tablet: 600mg (7.14mmol sodium and bicarbonate) – non-proprietary.

DOSAGE

Indication	Route	Age				Frequency (times daily)	Notes
		birth–1 month	1 month–2 years	2–12 years	12–18 years		
Metabolic acidosis	IV	← to correct acidosis → see intravenous fluid therapeutic section					
Renal acidosis	Oral	1–2mmol/kg/day		70mmol/m²/day		1	Dose adjusted according to plasma bicarbonate level.
Renal hyperkalaemia	Slow IV	← 1mmol/kg →				single dose	
Resuscitation	Slow IV	← 1mL/kg of 8.4% initially, followed by 0.5mL/kg of 8.4% if needed →					

ADMINISTRATION

Oral: injection may be given orally.

IV: 1.26% may be given undiluted peripherally. Dilute other strengths with glucose 5%, glucose 10% or NaCl 0.9%. For peripheral administration dilute the 8.4% 1 in 10 and for central administration 1 in 5. Caution is needed with renal patients – do not dilute with NaCl 0.9% due to the potential for hypernatraemia. Only used undiluted in an arrest or other emergency situations via a central line.

CONTRA-INDICATIONS & WARNINGS

Metabolic and/or respiratory alkalosis. Hypokalaemia, hyperosmolar states – use should be carefully considered.

Significant respiratory acidosis is almost always more appropriately managed by providing adequate respiratory support than by administration of sodium bicarbonate.

INTERACTIONS

Calcium: precipitant haze will occur if sodium bicarbonate is added to parenteral solutions containing calcium.

Diuretics: hyperchloraemic alkalosis may occur if used in conjunction with potassium depleting diuretics such as *bumetanide, furosemide (frusemide)* or *thiazides*. Urinary alkalinisation will increase renal clearance of *tetracyclines,* especially *doxycycline. Sodium bicarbonate* increases the half-lives and duration of action of basic drugs such as *quinidine, ephedrine* and *pseudoephedrine* by alkalinising the urine.

SIDE-EFFECTS

Sodium supplements may increase blood pressure or cause fluid retention and pulmonary oedema in those at risk; hypokalaemia may be exacerbated. Extravasation may cause a chemical cellulitis, with tissue necrosis, ulceration or sloughing.

POISONING/TOXICITY

Overdosage may occur due to excessive or too rapid administration and will result in a metabolic alkalosis. Severe alkalotic states will be accompanied by hyperirritability and/or tetany.

Management is to discontinue administration of sodium bicarbonate. Symptoms may be temporarily alleviated by rebreathing expired air or, if more severe, by the administration of calcium gluconate.

PREGNANCY

Safe use during pregnancy has not been established. Contact local Medicines Information Centre for advice.

BREAST-FEEDING

Patients requiring IV infusions of sodium bicarbonate are unlikely to be in a fit condition to breast-feed. In receiving the drug orally, no harm is likely to come to the infant.

EXCIPIENTS

Contact manufacturers for further details.

LICENSED STATUS

Licensed for use in children and adults.

FURTHER INFORMATION

1.26% is an isotonic infusion.

Sodium chloride is the principal salt involved in maintaining the osmotic tension of blood and tissues.

USES
Oral: salt replacement for patients at risk of salt depletion e.g. CF patients; oral supplement in neonates or others who require sodium.
IV: sodium supplementation, treatment of hyponatraemia.
Nebulised: hypertonic saline is nebulised in cystic fibrosis (CF) patients to promote mucus secretion, enhance mucocillary clearance and to augment the volume of sputum produced. It is not routinely used in paediatric patients.
Intranasal: nasal congestion.

PRESENTATION
Capsule: 300mg, 500mg, 600mg and 1g – manufactured 'specials'.
Oral solution: 1mmol in 1mL, 2mmol in 1mL and 5mmol in 1mL (30%) – manufactured 'specials'.
Tablet: (modified release) 600mg (10mmol each of Na^+ and Cl^-) – Slow Sodium®.
Injection: 0.9% (0.15mmol each of Na^+ and Cl^- in 1mL) – non-proprietary.
Injection: 30% (5mmol each of Na^+ and Cl^- in 1mL), 10mL ampoules – non-proprietary.
Hypertonic solutions for nebulisation: several strengths – manufactured 'specials'.
Nasal drops: 0.9% – manufactured 'special'.

DOSAGE
Sodium supplementation
Dosage should be adjusted to individual needs, according to serum levels. As a guide:-
Oral: daily in divided doses

<1 year	500mg
1-7 years	1g
>7 years	2-4g

IV: usual requirements as part of an IV feeding regimen are 2–5mmol/kg/day. Hyponatraemia: adjust the dose according to serum levels.

Chronic renal loss
Oral: 1–2mmol Na^+/kg/day.

Nasal congestion in babies with rhinitis
Instill 1-2 drops of NaCl 0.9% into each nostril before feeds.

Supplementation for cystic fibrosis
CF patients may require sodium chloride supplements from April to September each year to replace losses in body fluids during warmer summer months. Patients should be supplemented if making trips abroad to warmer climates or if showing symptoms of salt depletion. Newly diagnosed infants may need regular sodium chloride supplements until the age of 1 year (then as above).

To enhance mucocilary clearance in CF
Nebulised: 3-4mL of a 3-7% solution twice daily before physiotherapy.

ADMINISTRATION
Oral: injection solution can be given orally, but it is preferable to use a preparation specifically designed for oral use.
IV: NaCl 30% is hypertonic and should be diluted in a suitable infusion fluid of glucose, sodium chloride or PN before administration.
Nebulised: hypertonic solutions nebulised via an ultrasonic nebuliser. Advise giving nebulised salbutamol first because of bronchoconstriction.

S

CONTRA-INDICATION & WARNINGS
Any situation where salt retention is undesirable such as oedema, heart disease, cardiac decompensation and primary or secondary aldosteronism. The modified release tablets should not be given to patients with Crohn disease or other intestinal conditions where strictures or diverticulae may form, because the tablet matrix is often eliminated intact and there could be a risk of obstruction.

PREGNANCY/BREAST-FEEDING
No problems to be expected.

SIDE-EFFECTS
No adverse effects expected at the recommended dosages. Hypernatraemia can occur with excessive dosages.

POISONING/TOXICITY
In the event of significant overdose serum sodium tests should be evaluated as soon as possible and appropriate steps taken to correct any abnormalities.

PHARMACOKINETIC PROPERTIES
Sodium is excreted by the kidney but there is extensive renal re-absorption. Small amounts of sodium are lost in the faeces and sweat.

EXCIPIENTS
Contact manufacturers for further details.

LICENSED STATUS
Slow Sodium® tablets, the 0.9% injections and infusions are licensed for use in children and adults. Other preparations are 'specials' or prepared extemporaneously and as such are unlicensed.

FURTHER INFORMATION
Unpreserved oral solutions should be given a short shelf life, e.g. 7 days. Cochrane review reports there is insufficient evidence to support the routine use of hypertonic saline in patients with CF.
Capsules are available from Martindale Pharmaceuticals Ltd.
Hypertonic solutions for nebulisation are available from some hospital manufacturing units. Nasal drops are available from Lagap Pharmaceuticals Ltd.

Sodium citrate

Osmotic laxative.

USES
Relief of occasional constipation.
Pre- and post-operative bowel cleansing in obstetrics and prior to proctoscopy, sigmoidoscopy or X-ray examination.

PRESENTATION
Micolette Micro-enema®: sodium lauryl sulphoacetate 45mg, sodium citrate 450mg and glycerol 625mg per 5mL enema.
Microlax Micro-enema®: sodium citrate 450mg, sodium alkylsulphoacetate 45mg and sorbic acid 5mg per 5mL liquid.
Relaxit Micro-enema®: sodium citrate 450mg, sodium laurylsulphate 75mg, sorbic acid 5mg per 5mL liquid.

DOSAGE

Route	Age			Frequency (times daily)	Notes
	1 month–2 years	2–12 years	12–18 years		
Rectal	←	1 enema	→	single dose	When used in children <3 years of age, insert only half the nozzle length.

CONTRA-INDICATIONS & WARNINGS
Contra-indicated in inflammatory or ulcerative bowel disease, acute gastrointestinal conditions.

PREGNANCY/BREAST-FEEDING
Under medical supervision.

SIDE-EFFECTS
Slight cramp may occur. Prolonged use may lead to irritation of the anal canal.

POISONING/TOXICITY
Excessive use may cause diarrhoea and fluid loss. Discontinue therapy and give supportive treatment if required.

EXCIPIENTS
See manufacturers SPC for further details.

LICENSED STATUS
Licensed for >3 years of age: Micolette Micro-enema® and Microlax Micro-enema®. No lower age limit on use of Relaxit®.

A bisphosphonate.

USES
Sodium clodronate may be useful in the following conditions: steroid-induced osteoporosis, immobilisation osteoporosis e.g. high-spinal injury and cerebral palsy, idiopathic juvenile osteoporosis, juvenile idiopathic arthritis and osteogenesis imperfecta.

PRESENTATION
Capsule: 400mg – Bonefos® and Loron®.
Tablet: (scored) 520mg – Loron®; (scored) 800mg – Bonefos®.
IV solution: 60mg in 1mL, 5mL ampoule – Bonefos®.

DOSAGE
Experience in the use of bisphosphonates in children is limited. Seek specialist advice.

Dosage in renal impairment
Creatinine clearance >10mL/minute/1.73m^2 and <30mL/minute/1.73m^2 – give half the normal dose.
Creatinine clearance <10mL/minute/1.73m^2 - avoid.

ADMINISTRATION
Oral: capsules/tablets should be taken 1 hour before or after food with some fluid, but not milk – see interactions.
IV: single infusion over a period of 4 hours, diluted to a concentration of approximately 3mg in 1mL. Compatible with NaCl 0.9% and glucose 5%. Multiple infusions may be given over several successive days. Consult product literature for details.

CONTRA-INDICATIONS & WARNINGS
Hypersensitivity to sodium clodronate or other bisphosphonates. Caution should be exercised in patients with renal impairment – see above. Adequate hydration should be maintained during treatment. Serum calcium should be monitored at regular intervals.

INTERACTIONS
Concurrent use of other *bisphosphonate drugs* is contra-indicated. Concurrent use of *NSAIDs* may precipitate renal dysfunction. *Aminoglycosides* should be used with caution since they may cause hypocalcaemia. Bisphosphonate drugs form complexes with *divalent metal ions* and oral absorption may be impaired if they are given at the same time as *calcium rich food (including milk), antacids* and *mineral supplements*.

PREGNANCY
Avoid during pregnancy due to risk of adverse effects on bone formation in the fetus.

BREAST-FEEDING
In the absence of appropriate studies avoid during breast-feeding due to risk of adverse effects on bone formation in the infant.

SIDE-EFFECTS
Gastrointestinal upset, including nausea and vomiting, may occur but is usually mild. Hypersensitivity reactions, including pruritus, urticaria and exfoliative dermatitis. Bronchospasm has occurred rarely in patients with and without a history of asthma. Renal dysfunction, including renal failure, has been reported. Transient proteinuria has been reported in patients receiving parenteral therapy. Reversible elevations of serum parathyroid hormone, creatinine, lactic acid dehydrogenase, transaminase and alkaline phosphatase have been reported. Asymptomatic hypocalcaemia is rare, but more likely to occur with parenteral therapy.

POISONING/TOXICITY
Theoretical risk of hypocalcaemia up to 3 days after an overdose. Serum calcium should be monitored and calcium supplements administered orally or parenterally as appropriate. Calcium salts and/or antacids may be used to bind sodium clodronate after oral ingestion.

PHARMACOKINETIC PROPERTIES
Adults: oral absorption 1-4%; plasma half-life is 1.8-2.3 hours; plasma protein binding 2-7%.

EXCIPIENTS
See manufacturers SPC for further details.

LICENSED STATUS
Not licensed for use in children.

Sodium cromoglicate (cromoglycate)

An anti-allergic agent that acts mainly by inhibiting the release of inflammatory mediators.

USES
Prevention of allergic rhinitis; treatment of food allergy.

PRESENTATION
Capsule: 100mg – Nalcrom®.
Aqueous nasal spray: 4% – Rynacrom®.
Nasal spray: 2% – Vividrin®.

DOSAGE

Route	Age			Frequency (times daily)	Notes
	1 month–2 years	2–12 years	12–18 years		
Intra-nasal	←	>1 year 1 spray into each nostril	→	2–4 (4%) 4–6 (2%)	Allergic rhinitis. Frequency of administration depends on strength of product (%).
Oral	–	100mg	12–14 years 100mg >14 years 200mg	4 4	Food allergy. May be increased after 2–3 weeks to a maximum of 40mg/kg/day and then reduced according to response.

ADMINISTRATION
Oral: capsules may be swallowed whole or the contents dissolved in hot water and diluted with cold water before administration.

CONTRA-INDICATIONS & WARNINGS
Known hypersensitivity to sodium cromoglicate.

INTERACTIONS
None known.

PREGNANCY
Experience with sodium cromoglicate suggests that it has no adverse effects on fetal development.

BREAST-FEEDING
It is not known whether sodium cromoglicate is excreted in breast milk, however based on physico-chemical properties this is considered unlikely.

SIDE-EFFECTS
Capsules: occasional nausea, rashes and joint pain.
Nasal spray: occasional irritation of the nasal mucosa in the first few days of use.

POISONING/TOXICITY
No action except medical observation should be necessary.

EXCIPIENTS
See manufacturers SPC for further details.

LICENSED STATUS
Nalcrom® licensed for >2 years of age. Rynacrom® and Vividrin® licensed for use in children and adults.

Sodium fusidate/fusidic acid

An anti-staphylococcal agent with ability to penetrate tissue, including bone and necrotic tissue. It is active against *Staphylococcus epidermidis* and methicillin-resistant Staphylococci.

USES
Treatment of all staphylococcal infections due to susceptible organisms, such as osteomyelitis, pneumonia, septicaemia, wound infections, endocarditis, superinfected cystic fibrosis and cutaneous infections.
In severe or deep-seated infections and when prolonged therapy may be required, systemic sodium fusidate should generally be given concurrently with other anti-staphylococcal antibiotic therapy.

In cystic fibrosis patients – second-line treatment of asymptomatic *Staphylococcus aureus* isolates or minor exacerbations. Topical application of fusidic acid is also effective against Streptococci, Corynebacteria, Neisseria and certain Clostridia.

PRESENTATION

IV infusion: sodium fusidate 500mg (≡ 480mg fusidic acid) with buffer – Fucidin®.
Suspension: 250mg fusidic acid in 5mL – Fucidin®.
Tablet: 250mg sodium fusidate – Fucidin®.
Cream: fusidic acid 2% – Fucidin®.
Gel: fusidic acid 2% – Fucidin®.
Ointment: sodium fusidate 2% – Fucidin®.

DOSAGE

Route	Age				Frequency (times daily)	Notes
	birth–1 month	1 month–2 years	2–12 years	12–18 years		
Oral	15mg/kg or 0.3mL/kg (fusidic acid)	<1 year 15mg/kg or 0.3mL/kg (fusidic acid) 1–2 years 250mg (5mL) (fusidic acid)	2–5 years 250mg (5mL) (fusidic acid) 5–12 years 500mg (10mL) (fusidic acid)	750mg (15mL) (fusidic acid) or 500mg (2 tablets) (sodium fusidate)	3 3	For cutaneous infections 12–18 years 1 tablet twice daily is the standard treatment Treatment of asymptomatic *S. aureus* isolates or minor exacerbations in cystic fibrosis patients.
IV infusion	← 6–7mg/kg (sodium fusidate) →			DOSE BY WEIGHT <50kg 6–7mg/kg (sodium fusidate) DOSE BY AGE >50kg 500mg (sodium fusidate)	3 3	Doses may be doubled in severe infections.
Topical	← Apply to the affected area →				3–4	Uncovered lesions; less frequent application may be adequate for covered lesions.

ADMINISTRATION

IV infusion: to reconstitute, dissolve the contents of one vial containing 500mg sodium fusidate powder (equivalent to 480mg of fusidic acid) in the 10mL buffer provided. Further dilute to 1mg in 1mL with NaCl 0.9% or another suitable infusion fluid.* The diluted fluid should be infused over at least 6 hours if a superficial vein is employed or over 2 hours via a central venous line.

If additional antibacterial therapy is to be employed, it is recommended that for parenteral administration, separate infusion fluids be used.

*Sodium fusidate reconstituted to 50mg in 1mL in buffer solution is physically and chemically compatible for at least 24 hours at room temperature with the following infusion solutions: NaCl 0.9%, glucose 5%, compound sodium lactate ('Ringer-Lactate Solution'), sodium lactate, NaCl 0.18%/glucose 4%, KCl 0.3%/glucose 5%; it is physically incompatible with infusion fluids containing 20% or more of glucose, lipid infusions and peritoneal dialysis fluids. Precipitation may occur in dilutions which result in a pH of less than 7.4.

Oral: absorption orally is good and IV therapy is only indicated for patients unable to take or absorb oral medication.

Renal impairment

Since sodium fusidate is excreted in the bile, no dosage modifications are needed in renal impairment. The dosage in patients undergoing haemodialysis needs no adjustment as it is not significantly dialysed.

Liver disease

Impaired biliary excretion; may be increased risk of hepatotoxicity; carry out periodic liver function tests.

S

CONTRA-INDICATIONS & WARNINGS
IV sodium fusidate should not be infused with amino acid solutions or in whole blood. Due to local tissue injury, sodium fusidate should not be administered IM or SC. Periodic liver function tests should be carried out when high oral doses are used, when the drug is given for prolonged periods and in patients with liver dysfunction. Sodium fusidate displaces bilirubin from its albumin binding site in vitro. The clinical significance of this finding is uncertain and kernicterus has not been observed in neonates receiving sodium fusidate. However, this observation should be borne in mind when the drug is given to preterm, jaundiced, acidotic or seriously ill neonates.

Bacterial resistance has been reported to occur with the use of fusidic acid applied topically. As with all topical antibiotics, extended or recurrent application may increase the risk of contact sensitisation and the development of antibiotic resistance.

Sodium fusidate has been shown to cause conjunctival irritation and the ointment should not be used in or near the eye. Fusidic acid does not appear to cause conjunctival irritation in experimental animals. Caution should, however, still be exercised when using Fucidin® cream or gel near the eye.

INTERACTIONS
Caution should be exercised with other antibiotics which have similar biliary excretion pathways e.g. *rifampicin.*

PREGNANCY
There is inadequate evidence of safety in human pregnancy. However, animal studies and many years of clinical experience suggest that fusidic acid is devoid of teratogenic effects. Contact local Medicines Information Centre for advice.

BREAST-FEEDING
Safety in nursing mothers has not been established, although there is no evidence to suggest that breast-feeding is contra-indicated. Contact local Medicines Information Centre for advice.

SIDE-EFFECTS
In some patients, particularly the young, a reversible jaundice has been reported, most frequently in patients receiving intravenous therapy in high dosage, or where the drug has been infused too rapidly. If the jaundice persists treatment should be withdrawn, following which the serum bilirubin will invariably return to normal. Other reported reactions are gastrointestinal upsets and, rarely, skin rashes.

Topical treatment: hypersensitivity reactions to the active ingredient in the form of skin rashes and mild stinging and irritation on application have been reported rarely.

POISONING/TOXICITY
There is no experience of overdose with sodium fusidate/fusidic acid. Treatment should be symptomatic and supportive. Dialysis is of no benefit as the drug is not significantly dialysed.

PHARMACOKINETIC PROPERTIES
The plasma half-life in adults is approximately 10-15 hours. The half-life in children and neonates is less certain. Using direct equivalance, 250mg of sodium fusidate is equivalent to 240mg of fusidic acid. However, due to the reduced oral bioavailability of fusidic acid; 250mg of fusidic acid is equivalent to 175mg of sodium fusidate when used therapeutically.

EXCIPIENTS
Suspension contains liquid glucose and saccharin sodium content 35mg; disodium hydrogen phosphate. Infusion includes 3.1mmol sodium and 1.1mmol phosphate in 10mL when reconstituted.

LICENSED STATUS
Licensed for use in all ages.

Sodium nitroprusside

Vasodilator.

USES
Hypertensive crisis.

PRESENTATION
Injection: 50mg vial – non-proprietary.

DOSAGE

Route	Age				Frequency (times daily)	Notes
	birth–1 month	1 month–2 years	2–12 years	12–18 years		
IV infusion	←	500 nanogram/kg/minute		→	continuous	Initial dose. Increase in increments of 200 nanogram/kg/minute as necessary to a maximum of 8 microgram/kg/minute.

ADMINISTRATION

IV: reconstitute the contents of each 50mg vial with 2mL-3mL of glucose 5%. Then further dilute to a concentration of 50-200 microgram in 1mL with glucose 5%. Protect from light; use amber giving sets if possible. Discard after 24 hours or if solution changes from pale orange to dark brown or blue. Do not mix with any other infusion fluid or drugs.

Infusion rate to be determined by continuous monitoring of blood pressure.

Terminate infusion slowly over 15-30 minutes to avoid any rebound effects.

If treatment continues beyond 72 hours or patient in renal impairment, measure thiocyanate levels (should be <1.7mmol/L or 100 microgram/mL).

CONTRA-INDICATIONS & WARNINGS

Severe hepatic impairment, severe vitamin B_{12} deficiency, Leber's optic atrophy. Caution in renal impairment, if patient is hypothermic, impaired cerebral circulation and hypothyroidism.

INTERACTIONS

As for hydralazine.

PREGNANCY

Crosses the placenta and produces fetal cyanide concentrations higher than maternal levels in animals. Use only if benefits outweigh risks. Monitor plasma cyanide, red blood cell cyanide and methaemoglobin.

BREAST-FEEDING

Contact local Medicines Information Centre for advice.

SIDE-EFFECTS

Headache, dizziness, nausea, retching, abdominal pain, sweating, palpitations, apprehension, retrosternal discomfort are associated with over rapid reduction in blood pressure – reduce the infusion rate.

POISONING/TOXICITY

side-effects caused by excessive plasma concentration of the cyanide metabolite include tachycardia, sweating, hyperventilation, arrhythmias, marked metabolic acidosis. Discontinue and give antidote – see poisoning section under cyanide/contact a National Poisons Information Service.

LICENSED STATUS

Not licensed for use in children.

S

Sodium perborate

An oxidising agent, similar in effect to hydrogen peroxide.

USES

As a mouthwash and, either alone or in conjunction with hydrogen peroxide, as a bleaching agent for non-vital permanent teeth.

PRESENTATION

Mouthwash: sodium perborate monohydrate 68.6% (buffered), 1.7g sachet – Bocasan®.

DOSAGE

For oral hygiene measures 1 sachet to be dissolved in 30mL water 3 times daily after meals.

As a bleaching agent, a small quantity of granules to be mixed to a thick paste with a few drops of 30 vols hydrogen peroxide.

ADMINISTRATION
DO NOT SWALLOW.
Mouthwash: rinse around the mouth, after meals and expectorate.
Bleaching agent: as above, inserted into a previously prepared pulp chamber for a limited period and preferably double-sealed with gutta percha and a non-eugenol based dental cement.

CONTRA-INDICATIONS AND WARNINGS
Not recommended in renal impairment.

SIDE-EFFECTS/INTERACTIONS
None known.

POISONING/TOXICITY
Avoid prolonged use (>2 weeks) because of the likelihood of borate poisoning.

EXCIPIENTS
Contact manufacturer for further details.

LICENSED STATUS
Licensed for >5 years of age. Not licensed for use as a bleaching agent.

Sodium phenylbutyrate

USES
Hyperammonaemia due to disorders of the urea cycle.

PRESENTATION
Injection: 1g in 5mL – manufactured 'special'.
Powder: Ambutyrate®.
Suspension: 500mg in 1mL – Ambutyrate®.
Tablet: 500mg – Ammonaps® and Ambutyrate®.
Taste-masked granules: Ammonaps® and Ambutyrate®.

DOSAGE

Route	Age				Frequency (times daily)	Notes
	birth–1 month	1 month–2 years	2–12 years	12–18 years		
Oral	←	62.5–150mg/kg		→	4	Maximum dose 20g/day
IV infusion	←	250mg/kg		→	single dose	Acute loading dose. IV infusion over 90 minutes.
IV infusion	←	250–600mg/kg/day		→	continuous	

ADMINISTRATION
Oral: give with meals. Can be given in infant formula or milk, yoghurt, fruit juice or soft foods. Less soluble in fruit drinks, especially if acidic. Soluble in water. Injection can be given orally. Reconstituted granules will normally produce a milky white suspension. Ammonaps® granules are supplied with dosage spoons – one level measure is equivalent to: small 0.95g, medium 2.9g and large 8.6g.
IV infusion: dilute to 20mg in 1mL with glucose 10% or 5%, maximum concentration is 50mg in 1mL.
IV compatibilites: can be infused at Y-site with arginine, carnitine and sodium benzoate (no data to support this but has been done in practice).

CONTRA-INDICATIONS & WARNINGS
High sodium content (500mg of sodium phenylbutyrate contains 2.7mmol Na$^+$) therefore use with caution in patients with congestive heart failure or severe renal insufficiency and in clinical states where there is sodium retention with oedema. Hypersensitivity to sodium phenylbutyrate or sodium phenylacetate.

Effectiveness of therapy depends on renal excretion as phenylactylglutamine. In anuric states dialysis will be necessary to treat hyperammonaemia.

INTERACTIONS
Haloperidol, sodium valproate and *steroids* can increase ammonia levels. *Probenecid* can decrease renal excretion of phenylbutyrate and metabolites.

PREGNANCY/BREAST-FEEDING
No information available. Contact local Medicines Information Centre for advice.

SIDE-EFFECTS
Anorexia, gastrointestinal disturbances, rash, bad taste, taste aversion, body odour, headache, syncope, aplastic anaemia, leucopenia, renal tubular acidosis and depression have all been reported.Neurotoxicity observed with phenylacetate (metabolite of phenylbutyrate).

PHARMACODYNAMIC PROPERTIES
Sodium phenylbutyrate is converted to phenylacetate which conjugates with glutamine to form phenylacetylglutamine which is readily excreted in the urine. Each mole of sodium phenylbutyrate removes 2 moles of ammonia.

EXCIPIENTS
Each 500mg of drug contains 2.7mmol sodium. Contact manufacturers for further details.

LICENSED STATUS
Ammonaps® (Orphan Europe) is licensed for use in children.
Ambutyrate® (Special Products Ltd) is an unlicensed preparation.

FURTHER INFORMATION
All preparations available as 'specials'.
Granules and tablets available from Orphan Europe and Special Products Ltd.
Injection available from Martindale Pharmaceuticals Ltd and Special Products Ltd. Powder and suspension available from Special Products Ltd.

Sodium picosulfate (picosulphate)

Stimulant laxative.

USES
Constipation, recent or chronic, effective in opioid-induced constipation; bowel clearance before surgery, labour or radiological investigations.

PRESENTATION
Elixir: 5mg in 5mL – Laxoberal® and Dulco-Lax®.

DOSAGE

Route	Age			Frequency	Notes
	1 month–2 years	2–12 years	12–18 years		
Oral	–	2-5 years 2.5mL	5-15mL	1	Take at night.
		5-10 years 2.5-5mL		1	
		>10 years 5-15mL		1	

ADMINISTRATION
Oral: may be diluted with purified water.

CONTRA-INDICATIONS & WARNINGS
Contra-indicated in patients with undiagnosed abdominal pain or where intestinal obstruction is suspected.

Should not be given to patients being prepared for barium enema examinations where inflammatory bowel disease is suspected.

INTERACTIONS
As sodium picosulfate is broken down by bacteria in the large intestine, it is possible that in patients taking *broad-spectrum antibiotics* there may be some loss of laxative action.

PREGNANCY
No evidence of adverse consequences during human pregnancy.

BREAST FEEDING
Contact local Medicines Information Centre for advice.

SIDE-EFFECTS
Occasional reports of mild abdominal discomfort.

POISONING/TOXICITY
Colicky lower abdominal pain and possible signs of dehydration. Adequate hydration must be maintained and serum potassium measured. Antispasmodics may be of value.

PHARMACOKINETIC PROPERTIES
Sodium picosulfate is a synthetic laxative which is broken down by bacteria in the large intestine to the active substance, bis-(p-hydroxyphenyl)-2-pyridylmethane. Onset of action 10-14 hours after administration.

EXCIPIENTS
Includes saccharin and is sugar-free.

LICENSED STATUS
Licensed for use in children and adults.

Sodium stibogluconate

Pentavalent antimony compound.

USES
Leishmaniasis.

PRESENTATION
Injection: sodium stibogluconate ≡ 100mg pentavalent antimony in 1mL; 100mL multidose bottle – Pentostam®.

DOSAGE

Route	Age			Frequency	Notes
	1 month-2 years	2-12 years	12-18 years		
IV/IM	←	20mg/kg (maximum dose 850mg)	→	1	For 20-30 days. The total daily dose may be given as two divided doses of 10mg/kg 12 hourly.

ADMINISTRATION
IV: undiluted, by slow injection over at least 5 minutes. By infusion in up to 50mL glucose 5% over 15-30 minutes.

CONTRA-INDICATIONS & WARNINGS
Severe renal or hepatic dysfunction. Should not be given to any patient who has experienced a serious adverse reaction to a previous dose. Use with caution in mild to moderate renal or hepatic impairment. Some abnormalities of liver function may be expected in cases of visceral leishmaniasis and in such patients the benefit of treatment outweighs the risk. Use cautiously in patients with heart disease. Intercurrent infections such as pneumonia should be sought and treated concomitantly. IM injection is painful.

INTERACTIONS
None reported.

PREGNANCY
Although no effects on the fetus have been reported, only use during pregnancy if the potential benefits to the patient outweigh any possible risk to the fetus.

BREAST-FEEDING
Contact local Medicines Information Centre for advice.

SIDE-EFFECTS
Side-effects include nausea, vomiting and/or diarrhoea, abdominal pain, anorexia, myalgia, headache and lethargy. If coughing, vomiting or substernal pain occurs administration should be discontinued immediately. IV injection may cause transient pain along the course of the vein and eventually thrombosis of that vein. ECG changes (T, ST and QT prolongation) can occur but are unlikely in courses of treatment up to 30 days. Monitor ECG twice weekly.

POISONING/TOXICITY
Symptoms: the main symptoms are gastrointestinal (nausea, vomiting, severe diarrhoea); haemorrhagic nephritis and hepatitis may also occur.
Treatment: dimercaprol (2.5–3mg/kg IM, 4 hourly for 2 days, 8 hourly on day 3 and then daily until recovery).

PHARMACOKINETIC PROPERTIES
Following IV or IM administration of sodium stibogluconate, antimony is excreted rapidly via the kidneys, reflected by a fall in serum or whole blood antimony levels to 1–4% of the peak level by 8 hours after an IV dose.

EXCIPIENTS
See manufacturers SPC for further details.

LICENSED STATUS
Licensed for use in the UK. No lower age stated in the SPC.

Sodium valproate

Antiepileptic.

USES
Epilepsy; drug of first or second choice in generalised (tonic-clonic, absence, atonic, myoclonic) seizures. Effective for photosensitive epilepsy. Mania.

PRESENTATION
Capsule: (enteric coated) (as valproic acid) 150mg, 300mg and 500mg – Convulex®.
Injection: 400mg powder (with 4mL Water for Injections) – Epilim® Intravenous.
Liquid: 200mg in 5mL – Epilim® and non-proprietary.
Syrup: 200mg in 5mL – Epilim®.
Suppository: 300mg – named patient.
Tablet: (crushable) 100mg – Epilim®.
Tablet: (enteric coated) 200mg and 500mg – Epilim® and non-proprietary.
Tablet: (modified release) 200mg, 300mg and 500mg – Epilim Chrono®.

DOSAGE

Route	Age				Frequency (times daily)	Notes
	*birth–1 month	1 month–2 years	2–12 years	12–18 years		
Oral	20mg/kg	–		–	1	Starting dose.
	–	← 5–7.5mg/kg →		300mg	2	
	10–20mg/kg	← 12.5–15mg/kg →		500mg–1g	2	Usual target maintenance dose up to 20mg/kg twice daily (doses have been used up to 30mg/kg twice daily in the treatment of infantile spasms).
Oral MR tablets	–	← 10–15mg/kg →		600mg	1	Starting dose.
	–	← 25–30mg/kg →		1–2g	1	Usual target maintenance dose.

DOSAGE continued

Route	Age				Frequency (times daily)	Notes
	*birth–1 month	1 month–2 years	2–12 years	12–18 years		
IV bolus over 3–5 minutes	← 10mg/kg →				2	Introduction, if oral not possible. For established therapy substitute IV for oral at same dose.
IV infusion	-	← 20–40mg/kg/day →		maximum 2.5g/day	continuous	Following a bolus of 10mg/kg.
Rectal	← as for oral →					

* Experience with the neonatal use of sodium valproate is extremely limited.

Dose adjustment
Increase from starting dose by 5mg/kg per week. There is no correlation between blood level and seizure control so routine levels are not advised. Reduce dose in severe renal failure.

ADMINISTRATION
Oral: crushable tablets are scored and may be halved and/or crushed. Enteric coated and Chrono® tablets and capsules must be swallowed whole. Avoid indigestion medicines at same time as enteric coated tablets or capsules.
Rectal: liquid has been administered rectally, retained for 15 minutes, in doses similar to oral route. May require dilution with water to avoid rapid expulsion.
IV: adding 4mL Water for Injections to 400mg powder produces 95mg in 1mL. Administer by direct injection or diluted in glucose 5%, or NaCl 0.9% or glucose/saline. Dilutions stable for 24 hours.

CONTRA-INDICATIONS & WARNINGS
Contra-indicated in active liver disease and family history of liver dysfunction, especially if drug related. Porphyria. Counsel on recognition of haematological and liver adverse effects. If doses greater than 40mg/kg/day are required monitor biochemistry and blood counts.

INTERACTIONS
Synergy with *ethosuximide* in absences (typical and atypical) and myoclonic seizures and with *lamotrigine* in absences (typical and atypical), tonic-clonic and myoclonic seizures. Inhibits metabolism of *lamotrigine* increasing risk of rash, ataxia and tremor (see *lamotrigine* monograph for further advice). May increase free *phenytoin* levels. Anticonvulsant effect may be antagonised by *antidepressants, antipsychotics, chloroquine* and *mefloquine*. *Carbamazepine* often lowers plasma concentration of sodium valproate. Many other interactions possible.

PREGNANCY
Significantly increased risk of neural tube defects, other malformations and also the fetal valproate syndrome (dysmorphic facies and developmental delay) especially if more than one antiepileptic used. Specialist counselling, management and screening required. Administer folate supplements before and during pregnancy.

BREAST-FEEDING
Passes in to breast milk in insignificant amounts. Breast-feeding is appropriate.

SIDE-EFFECTS
Dose dependent adverse effects include drowsiness, nausea, diarrhoea, tremor. Chronic adverse effects include thrombocytopenia, weight gain (increased appetite), rarely weight loss, hair loss (usually transient within first 6 months).
The risk of hepatotoxicity with sodium valproate appears to be greatest in children <3 years of age with severe epilepsy, other neurological problems and/or receiving at least one other antiepileptic. Use with caution in these patients and advise parents to contact the hospital immediately if they notice yellow sclera. Measure pre-treatment liver function and monitor liver function and blood tests of patients during therapy if clinically indicated. Full blood count advised before surgery. Pancreatitis has also, very rarely, been reported. For more information refer to SPC.

POISONING/TOXICITY
In massive overdose (plasma levels 10-20 times greater than normal) signs and symptoms involve CNS and respiratory systems. Seizures may occur. Consult UK National Poisons Information Service. Measure blood levels.

PHARMACOKINETIC PROPERTIES
Routine plasma levels are not a useful guide to efficacy and should not be monitored routinely. An increase in adverse effects may be associated with doses above 40mg/kg/day or a trough level above 100mg/L. Modified release preparations produce less fluctuation in plasma

levels but are bioequivalent to liquid and enteric coated tablets. Absorption from suppositories may be increased but dosage may not need to be reduced.

EXCIPIENTS
Epilim® liquid includes sorbitol and saccharin. Epilim® syrup contains sorbitol, saccharin and sucrose. Contact manufacturers for further details.

LICENSED STATUS
Suppositories are not licensed for use in the UK. Epilim Chrono® is licensed for use in children ≥20kg. Rectal use of liquid is unlicensed. All other preparations licensed for all ages.

FURTHER INFORMATION
Suppositories available from IDIS World Medicines.
Manufacturer of Convulex® advises there is a 1:1 relationship with products containing sodium valproate, but nevertheless care is needed in making changes.

Solivito N®

Lyophilised mixture of water-soluble vitamins.

USES
Water soluble vitamin supplement to IV nutrition (Vitlipid N® preparations provide fat soluble vitamins).

PRESENTATION
Solution: powder for reconstitution – Solivito N®.
Each vial contains:

Biotin	60 microgram
Cynanocobalamin	5 microgram
Folic Acid	400 microgram
Nicotinamide	40mg
Pyridoxine hydrochloride	4.9mg
Riboflavin sodium phosphate	4.9mg
Sodium ascorbate	113mg
Sodium pantothenate	16.5mg
Thiamine mononitrate	3.1mg

DOSAGE
Newborn infant (birth to 1 month)
1mL/kg/24 hours.

Child
<10kg body weight – 1mL/kg/24 hours.
≥10kg body weight – 10mL/24 hours.

ADMINISTRATION
IV: reconstitute with Vitlipid N® adult or infant or Intralipid® and add to 10%, 20% or 30% Intralipid® solution for IV infusion **OR** reconstitute with Water for Injections or glucose infusion 5%-60% and add to glucose infusion or water based amino acid solution or Intralipid® 10%, 20% or 30% solution. Infuse 1 vial over not less than 2-3 hours.

CONTRA-INDICATIONS AND WARNINGS
Hypersensitivity to any individual component. For complete range of vitamin supplementation it must be used with Vitlipid N®.

INTERACTIONS
Pyridoxine may reduce the effectiveness of *levodopa*.

Folic acid may lower serum concentrations of *phenytoin* and obscure pernicious anaemia.

PREGNANCY
The solution is a supplement in PN regimens, providing water soluble vitamins. No hazard is expected if used in pregnancy in the recommended doses.

EXCIPIENTS
See manufacturers SPC for further details.

LICENSED STATUS
Licensed for use in all ages.

FURTHER INFORMATION
Dry powder: store in a fridge at 2-8°C and protect from light.

Somatropin

Synthetic human growth hormone produced using recombinant DNA technology.

USES
Treatment of growth hormone insufficiency, in Turner syndrome, Prader-Willi syndrome, chronic renal insufficiency in children, Noonan syndrome and intra-uterine growth retardation (IUGR).

PRESENTATION

Genotropin®
Injection: 5.3mg and 12mg cartridges for use with *Genotropin® Pen*.
MiniQuick® injection: 0.2mg, 0.4mg, 0.6mg, 0.8mg, 1mg, 1.2mg, 1.4mg, 1.6mg, 1.8mg and 2mg single dose syringe.

Humatrope®
Injection: 1.33mg and 5.33mg powder in vials; 6mg, 12mg and 24mg cartridge for use with *Humatro-Pen®II*.

Norditropin®
Simple Xx injection: 5mg, 10mg and 15mg cartridges for use with *Nordipen®*.

Saizen®
Injection: 1.33mg and 3.33mg vial.
Easyject®: 8mg vial for use with *Easyject® device*.

Zomacton®
Injection: 4mg vial for use with *ZomaJet® 2* or *Auto-Jector®*.

DOSAGE

Indication	Route	Age				Frequency (times daily)	Notes
		birth–1 month	1 month–2 years	2–12 years	12–18 years		
GH insufficiency	SC	←	25-35 microgram/kg		→	1	
Turner syndrome	SC	←	50 microgram/kg		→	1	See guidelines for oestrogen replacement.
Chronic renal failure	SC	←	50 microgram/kg		→	1	
Prader-Willi syndrome	SC	←	35 microgram/kg		→	1	
Noonan syndrome	SC	←	35 microgram/kg		→	1	
Intra-uterine growth retardation	SC	←	70 microgram/kg		→	1	

ADMINISTRATION
SC: the total weekly dose may be divided into 6-7 SC injections; vary the injection site to prevent lipoatrophy.

CONTRA-INDICATIONS & WARNINGS
Evidence of tumour activity; growth promotion in children with closed epiphyses. Patients with diabetes mellitus may require adjustment of their insulin dose when growth hormone therapy is instituted. Caution in patients with relative deficiencies of other pituitary hormones – periodic thyroid function tests recommended.

INTERACTIONS
Insulin dose adjustment may be necessary. Clearance of medicines metabolised by cytochrome p450 3A4 e.g. *anticonvulsants* and *ciclosporin (cyclosporin)* may be increased.

PREGNANCY
No clinical experience; in most instances treatment with growth hormone should be interrupted if pregnancy occurs. Contact local Medicines Information Centre for advice.

BREAST-FEEDING
No information available as to whether peptide hormones pass into milk, but absorption of intact protein from the gastrointestinal tract of the infant is extremely unlikely. Contact local Medicines Information Centre for advice.

SIDE-EFFECTS
Common side-effects include transient local skin reactions at injection site, symptoms of fluid retention (peripheral oedema), carpal tunnel syndrome, arthralgia, myalgia, hypothyroidism and hyperglycaemia. In cases of severe or recurrent headache, visual problems, nausea and/or vomiting, a fundoscopy for papilloedema is recommended and if confirmed a diagnosis of benign intracranial hypertension considered and, if appropriate growth hormone treatment stopped.

POISONING/TOXICITY
Acute overdose could lead initially to hypoglycaemia and subsequently to hyperglycaemia. Long-term overdosage could result in signs and symptoms of acromegaly consistent with the known effects of excess human growth hormone.

EXCIPIENTS
Contact manufacturers for further details.

LICENSED STATUS
All products are licensed for treatment of short stature due to inadequate secretion of growth hormone, for use in Turner syndrome and chronic renal insufficiency. Genotropin® is also licensed for use in Prader-Willi syndrome; none of the other indications are licensed.

FURTHER INFORMATION
3 units ≡ 1mg of growth hormone.

Sotalol

S

A non-selective beta-blocker which also has Class III antiarrhythmic properties.

USES
Ventricular arrhythmias, life-threatening ventricular tachyarrhythmias and supraventricular arrhythmias.

PRESENTATION
Tablet: (scored) 40mg, 80mg and 200mg – Beta-Cordone®; 80mg and 160mg – Sotacor®; 40mg, 80mg and 160mg – non-proprietary.
Suspension: may be extemporaneously prepared.

DOSAGE

Route	Age				Frequency (times daily)	Notes
	birth–1 month	1 month–2 years	2–12 years	12–18 years		
Oral	–	← 1–4mg/kg → (maximum 40–80mg)		40mg up to 80-160mg	2	ECG monitoring is recommended especially when initiating therapy. Adjust dose gradually allowing 2-3 days between dose increments in order to attain steady state.

Before starting treatment or changing the dose, the corrected QT interval should be measured and renal function, electrolyte balance and concurrent medications assessed. Caution should be exercised if the QTc exceeds 500 milliseconds, dose should be reduced or therapy discontinued if the QTc exceeds 550 milliseconds.

Renal impairment
Sotalol is excreted mainly in the urine and dosage should be reduced when the creatinine clearance is less than 60mL/minute/1.73m^2 as indicated in the table below.

Creatinine clearance (mL/minute/1.73m^2)	Dosage
30–60	One half of the usual dose.
10–30	One quarter of the usual dose.
<10	Not recommended.

ADMINISTRATION
Oral: tablets may be crushed and dissolved in water. Absorption may be reduced when administered with food.

CONTRA-INDICATIONS & WARNINGS
Sick sinus syndrome, second and third degree AV block (unless pacing is available); congenital or acquired long QT syndromes, torsades de pointes, symptomatic sinus bradycardia, uncontrolled congestive heart failure, cardiogenic shock, anaesthesia which produces myocardial depression, untreated phaeochromocytoma, Raynaud phenomenon and severe peripheral circulatory disorders; bronchial asthma, metabolic acidosis or diabetic ketoacidosis, renal failure (creatinine clearance <10mL/minute/1.73m^2) and hypersensitivity.
Precautions for use include abrupt withdrawal, electrolyte disturbances, congestive heart failure, ECG changes, anaphylaxis, anaesthesia, diabetes mellitus, thyrotoxicosis, renal impairment and psoriasis (see manufacturers SPC for full details).

INTERACTIONS
Antiarrhythmics: class Ia antiarrhythmics (e.g. *disopyramide, quinidine and procainamide*), amiodarone will prolong refractoriness. *Beta-blockers:* concomitant administration with other beta-blockers may result in additive Class III effect. Caution with other drugs which also prolong QT interval e.g. *calcium-channel antagonists of verapamil type*, or *tricyclic antidepressants. Potassium sparing diuretics* increase potential for torsades de pointes. *Clonidine* may potentiate rebound hypertension after discontinuation of clonidine, beta-blocker should be withdrawn gradually. *Digitalis glycosides* – proarrhythmic events more common. *Tubocurarin* – neuromuscular blockade prolonged.

PREGNANCY
Animal studies have shown no evidence of teratogenicity. However, beta-blockers may reduce placental perfusion which can result in intrauterine fetal death, immature and premature deliveries. Adverse effects may occur in the fetus and newborn infant. Contact local Medicines Information Centre for advice.

BREAST-FEEDING
Sotalol passes into breast milk and symptoms of beta-blockade could occur in nursing infants. However, the American Academy of Pediatrics considers sotalol to be compatible with breast-feeding.

SIDE-EFFECTS
Cardiovascular: bradycardia, dyspnoea, chest pain, palpitations, oedema, ECG abnormalities, hypotension, proarrhythmia, syncope, heart failure, presyncope.
Dermatological: rash.
Gastrointestinal: nausea, diarrhoea, dyspepsia, abdominal pain.
Musculoskeletal: cramps.
Nervous/psychiatric: fatigue, dizziness, asthenia, light-headedness, headache, sleep disturbance, depression, paresthesia, mood changes, anxiety.
Respiratory: bronchospasm.
Other: visual disturbances, taste abnormalities, hearing disturbances, fever.

POISONING/TOXICITY
The most common signs of overdose are bradycardia, congestive heart failure, hypotension, bronchospasm and hypoglycaemia and in massive overdose other cardiac arrhythmias. There is no specific antidote. Treatment is symptomatic.

PHARMACOKINETIC PROPERTIES
Oral bioavailability is essentially complete (>90%). Absorption is reduced by approximately 20% when administered with a standard meal, in comparison to fasting conditions. Approximate time to steady state is 2-3 days. Therapeutic range is 0.04-2mg/L. Take trough sample immediately prior to next dose.
Sotalol does not bind to plasma proteins. First pass hepatic metabolism and metabolic destruction are negligible. The primary route of elimination is renal excretion, with approximately 80–90% of a dose excreted unchanged in the urine. The plasma half-life in adults ranges from 10-20 hours.

EXCIPIENTS
Contact manufacturers for further details.

LICENSED STATUS
Not licensed for use in children.

Spiramycin

Macrolide antibiotic.

USES
Toxoplasmosis; toxoplasmosis in pregnancy and chemoprophylaxis in newborns/infants with subclinical congenital toxoplasma infection.

PRESENTATION
Tablet: 750,000 international units, 1.5 million international units, 3 million international units – named patient (imported).
Syrup: 375,000 international units in 5mL – named patient (imported).

DOSAGE/ADMINISTRATION
Pregnant women with suspected or confirmed toxoplasma infection: 1.5g (4.5 million international units) orally twice daily until term if the fetus is not infected.
Chemoprophylaxis in newborns/infants with subclinical infection: 50mg (150,000 international units)/kg orally twice daily, for 6 months.

CONTRA-INDICATIONS & WARNINGS
Previous sensitivity to spiramycin. Use with caution in: patients with a hypersensitivity to other macrolide antibiotics as cross-sensitivity between erythromycin and spiramycin has been reported (cutaneous reactions); liver disease as spiramycin is potentially hepatotoxic; those with gastrointestinal disorders as these may be exacerbated; cardiac disease as spiramycin may be capable of inducing adverse cardiovascular effects, including QT interval prolongation.

INTERACTIONS
None of significance.

PREGNANCY
Not teratogenic.

BREAST-FEEDING
Spiramycin is distributed into breast milk. Contact local Medicines Information Centre for advice.

SIDE-EFFECTS
Relatively infrequent and include nausea, vomiting, diarrhoea, epigastric pain, dizziness, headache, and cutaneous hypersensitivity reactions. Hepatotoxicity, thrombocytopenia, vasculitis, colitis, and QT prolongation have been reported, rarely.

POISONING/TOXICITY
No specific treatment; symptomatic and supportive.

PHARMACOKINETIC PROPERTIES
Incompletely absorbed (bioavailability 35%) from the gastrointestinal tract and widely distributed in the tissues. Relatively high levels are achieved in most tissues and these levels persist longer than those in plasma. It does not diffuse into the CSF to any appreciable extent. Metabolised to some degree in the liver; main route of excretion is biliary; up to 20% excreted unchanged in the urine.

S

LICENSED STATUS
Not licensed for use in the UK.

FURTHER INFORMATION
Available from IDIS World Medicines.
1mg spiramycin ≡ approximately 3000 international units.

Aldosterone antagonist, potassium-sparing diuretic.

USES
To induce diuresis in congestive cardiac failure. Prophylaxis of diuretic (thiazide or loop) or amphotericin-induced hypokalaemia. Oedema and ascites; nephrotic syndrome and primary hyperaldosteronism.

PRESENTATION
Oral suspension: 5mg in 5mL, 10mg in 5mL, 25mg in 5mL, 50mg in 5mL and 100mg in 5mL – manufactured 'specials'.
Tablet: 25mg, 50mg and 100mg – Aldactone® and non-proprietary.

There is no IV preparation of spironolactone. Potassium canrenoate is the IV equivalent.

DOSAGE

Route	Age				Frequency (times daily)	Notes
	birth–1 month	1 month–2 years	2–12 years	12–18 years		
Oral	← 500 microgram/kg –1.5mg/kg →			25–50mg	2	Dose should be adjusted on the basis of response and tolerance. The total daily dose may, if necessary, be given as one dose or divided into more than 2 doses. Plasma potassium levels should be monitored. In children doses up to 9mg/kg/**day** have been used with careful monitoring in resistant ascites.

Spironolactone should not routinely be administered concurrently with potassium-sparing diuretics or potassium supplements as hyperkalaemia may be induced.

Renal/hepatic impairment
Contra-indicated in patients with creatinine clearance <30mL/minute/1.73m^2.
Use with caution – fluid and electrolyte status should be regularly monitored in those with significant renal and hepatic impairment. Although the dose of spironolactone does not generally need to be reduced in hepatic dysfunction such patients should be carefully monitored as hepatic coma may be precipitated in susceptible patients.

ADMINISTRATION
Oral: tablets may be crushed and taken with food or drink.
To convert to IV potassium canrenoate dose multiply spironolactone dose by 1.43.

CONTRA-INDICATIONS & WARNINGS
Hyperkalaemia, hyponatraemia, severe renal impairment, acute renal failure, anuria, Addison's disease, hypersensitivity to spironolactone. *Precautions:* fluid and electrolyte balance should be regularly monitored especially if there is significant renal or hepatic impairment. Hyperkalaemia may occur if there is impaired renal function or excessive potassium intake which may cause fatal cardiac irregularities. Should hyperkalaemia develop, spironolactone should be discontinued and if necessary active measures taken to reduce serum potassium to normal.

Hyponatraemia may be induced, especially if administered in combination with other diuretics. Reversible increases in blood urea have been reported particularly if renal function impaired.

INTERACTIONS
High risk of hyperkalaemia with *ACE inhibitors, NSAIDs, ciclosporin (cyclosporin), potassium salts* and *other potassium-sparing diuretics*. Increased risk of nephrotoxicity and reduced diuretic effect with *NSAIDs*. Potentiation of the effects of *antihypertensive drugs* and *other diuretics* may occur. Spironolactone has been reported to increase serum *digoxin* concentration and to interfere with certain *digoxin* assays. Therefore when used concurrently, the *digoxin* levels should be interpreted in conjunction with clinical presentation.

PREGNANCY
Animal teratogenicity studies have shown evidence of feminisation of the male fetus. No reports linking it with congenital defects have been located. However,

S

some investigators consider diuretics in general contra-indicated in pregnancy except for patients with cardiovascular disorders. Contact local Medicines Information Centre for advice.

BREAST-FEEDING
Metabolites of spironolactone have been detected in breast milk. The American Academy of Pediatrics considers spironolactone to be compatible with breast-feeding.

SIDE-EFFECTS
Hyperkalaemia, hyponatraemia, deterioration in renal function, gynaecomastia, menstrual irregularities, gastrointestinal disturbances, drowsiness, headache, lethargy, mental confusion, skin rashes.
A reversible increase in plasma urea and creatinine may occur; and mild acidosis has been reported.

POISONING/TOXICITY
Acute overdose may be manifested by drowsiness, mental confusion, nausea, vomiting, dizziness or diarrhoea. Hyponatraemia or hyperkalaemia may be induced but these effects are unlikely to be associated with acute overdosage. ECG changes are the earliest specific signs of potassium disturbances. No specific antidote has been identified. General supportive measures including replacement of fluids or electrolytes may be indicated. Hyperkalaemia may be treated with potassium-excreting diuretics, oral ion-exchange resins or IV glucose with insulin.

PHARMACOKINETIC PROPERTIES
Oral absorption of spironolactone is variable depending on its formulation. Current formulations are reported to provide a bioavailability of about 90%. There is improved absorption if the drug is taken after food. Protein binding $\geq 90\%$. The major site of biotransformation of spironolactone is thought to be the liver, and excretion is mainly in the urine. Plasma half-life in adults ranges from 1.3-2 hours (active metabolite up to 11 hours).

EXCIPIENTS
Contact manufacturers for further details.

LICENSED STATUS
Licensed for use in children and adults but the suspensions are 'specials' and therefore unlicensed.

FURTHER INFORMATION
Spironolactone has a gradual and prolonged action, with maximal response usually being obtained after 2–3 days. Combination with a conventional more proximally acting diuretic e.g. furosemide (frusemide) usually enhances diuresis without excessive potassium loss. Spironolactone is usually prescribed at the same dose as furosemide on a mg/kg basis. Oral suspensions available from Rosemont.

Sterculia

S

Bulk-forming laxative.

USES
Normacol Plus®
Treatment of constipation. Initiation and maintenance of bowel action after rectal and anal surgery.
Normacol®
As for Normacol Plus®.
Management of colostomies and ileostomies.
High residue diet management of diverticular disease and other conditions requiring a high fibre regimen.
Administration after ingestion of sharp foreign bodies to provide a coating and reduce the possibility of intestinal damage during transit.

PRESENTATION
Granules: sterculia 62% – Normacol®.
Granules: sterculia 62% and frangula standardised 8% – Normacol Plus®.

DOSAGE

Preparation	Route	Age			Frequency (times daily)	Notes
		1 month–2 years	2–12 years	12–18 years		
Sterculia (Normacol®)	Oral	← 1/2 - 1 sachet → or 1/2 - 1 heaped 5mL spoonful		1–2 sachets or 1–2 heaped 5mL spoonfuls	1–2	After meals. <6 years only at the discretion of the doctor.
Sterculia/ frangula (Normacol Plus®)	Oral	–	6–12 years 1/2 - 1 sachet or 1/2 - 1 heaped 5mL spoonful	1–2 sachets or 1–2 heaped 5mL spoonfuls	1–2	6-12 years only at the discretion of the doctor.

ADMINISTRATION

Oral: place granules on tongue and swallow immediately without chewing or crushing. Take with plenty of cool liquid. May be sprinkled onto and taken with soft food e.g. yoghurt. Must still be followed by plenty of liquid.

CONTRA-INDICATIONS & WARNINGS

Contra-indicated in intestinal obstruction, faecal impaction and total atony of colon. Do not take immediately before bed. Maintain adequate fluid intake. Caution in ulcerative colitis. Do not take Normacol Plus® for more than 4 days if no movement of bowels.

PREGNANCY/BREAST-FEEDING

Normacol® is recommended for constipation during pregnancy and in lactating mothers.

SIDE-EFFECTS

Occasionally mild abdominal distension. Oesophageal obstruction possible if in overdosage or if not adequately washed down with fluid.

POISONING/TOXICITY

Intestinal obstruction is possible in overdosage particularly in combination with inadequate fluid intake. Management is as for intestinal obstruction from other causes.

EXCIPIENTS

Coating of granules contains sucrose. Gluten-free. Each 7g sachet contains 1.72g available carbohydrate 6.75kcal.

LICENSED STATUS

Normacol® licensed for >6 years of age; children <6 years only at discretion of doctor.
Normacol Plus® licensed for ≥12 years of age; 6–12 years only at discretion of doctor.

Streptokinase

Acts as a thrombolytic by activating plasminogen to plasmin which degrades fibrin.

USES

Fibrinolytic – treatment of thrombosis.

PRESENTATION

Injection: powder for reconstitution; 100,000 unit vial – non proprietary; 250,000, 750,000 and 1.5 million unit vials – Streptase® and non-proprietary.

DOSAGE

Route	Age				Frequency (times daily)	Notes
	birth–1 month	1 month–2 years	2–12 years	12–18 years		
IV infusion (over 30 minutes) then IV infusion	3000 units/kg then 500–1000 units/kg/hour	◄— 2500–4000 units/kg —► then ◄— 500–1000 units/kg/hour —►		250,000 units then 100,000 units/hour	single dose then continuous	Loading dose then continue until vascular flow returns, but not beyond 3 days. Check fibrinogen levels frequently and if level <1g/L stop streptokinase and change to heparin infusion until levels reach 1g/L again, strepto-kinase can then be restarted.

ADMINISTRATION
Reconstitute according to manufacturers product information.

CONTRA-INDICATIONS & WARNINGS
All conditions that are likely to be associated with existing or very recent haemorrhage e.g. recent trauma or surgery, coagulation defects, history of cerebrovascular disease, parturition within the last 10 days, heavy vaginal bleeding, oesophageal varices, peptic ulceration. Also, severe hypertension, known intracranial neoplasm, severe liver disease, acute pancreatitis and previous severe allergic reactions to streptokinase or streptokinase-containing products.
There is an increased risk of haemorrhage in patients who are receiving or who have recently been treated with anticoagulants or antiplatelet drugs. Streptokinase should not be given to patients who have had a recent streptococcal infection or who have received streptokinase more than 5 days and less than 12 months previously, due to formation of antibodies.

INTERACTIONS
Simultaneous treatment with *anticoagulants, antiplatelet drugs* and *dextrans* increases the risk of haemorrhage.

PREGNANCY
Contra-indicated in pregnancy (risk of placental separation) but has been used before. Contact local Medicines Information Centre for advice.

BREAST-FEEDING
Contact local Medicines Information Centre for advice.

SIDE-EFFECTS
Pyrexia, nausea and vomiting, bleeding (usually limited to site of infusion), but may occur from other sites including intracerebral. Allergic/anaphylactic reactions have been reported, as has low back pain and hypotension.

POISONING/TOXICITY
Tranexamic acid (10mg/kg slow IV, repeatable after 8-12 hours) may counteract bleeding. Cryoprecipitate may be used to correct haemostatic deficiency.

EXCIPIENTS
Streptase® contains human albumin. See manufacturers SPC for further details.

LICENSED STATUS
Licensed for use in children and adults.

S

Sucralfate

Mucosal protectant.

USES
Treatment or prophylaxis of stress ulceration. Prophylaxis against bleeding from oesophageal and gastric varices.
Adjunct in the treatment of: oesophagitis with evidence of mucosal ulceration, gastric or duodenal ulceration, upper gastrointestinal bleeding of unknown cause.

PRESENTATION
Suspension: 1g in 5mL – Antepsin®.
Tablet: 1g – Antepsin® and non-proprietary.

DOSAGE

Route	Age				Frequency (times daily)	Notes
	birth–1 month	1 month–2 years	2–12 years	12–18 years		
Oral	–	250mg	500mg	1g	4–6	

ADMINISTRATION
Oral: tablets may be crushed or dispersed in water. Sucralfate oral suspension blocks fine bore feeding tubes. Doses should be taken before meals and spread throughout the waking hours.

CONTRA-INDICATIONS & WARNINGS
Hypersensitivity to sucralfate or any excipient. Should not be used in cases of ileus or perforation. Caution should be exercised in patients with renal impairment due to risk of increased absorption of aluminium. In severe renal impairment extreme caution should be used, and other aluminium-containing medication avoided. In preterm neonates, use may lead to bezoar formation and sub-acute obstructive symptoms and is probably best avoided.

INTERACTIONS
Sucralfate may reduce the oral bioavailability of the following: *ciprofloxacin, digoxin, H$_2$- antagonists, ketoconazole, norfloxacin, phenytoin, sulpiride* and *warfarin*. Administration of these drugs, and others where normal bioavailability is critical, and sucralfate should be separated by 2 hours. *Antacids* should be avoided 30 minutes before or after a dose. Administration of sucralfate and *enteral feeds* should be separated by 1 hour – bezoar formation is reported.

PREGNANCY
Safety in pregnant women is not established. Contact local Medicines Information Centre for advice.

BREAST-FEEDING
Excretion into breast milk is not established, but unlikely to be problematic.

SIDE-EFFECTS
Hypersensitivity reactions, including pruritus, oedema and urticaria. Adverse effects are usually minor but the following are reported: constipation, nausea, vomiting, diarrhoea, gastric discomfort, indigestion, flatulence, dry mouth, back pain, dizziness, headache, vertigo and drowsiness. Hypophosphataemia, particularly in patients with renal failure, is a risk due the binding of phosphate in the gastrointestinal tract.

POISONING/TOXICITY
Risk in overdosage should be minimal.

PHARMACOKINETIC PROPERTIES
Sucralfate is minimally absorbed from the gastrointestinal tract (3-5%). The small amounts absorbed are excreted primarily in urine. Absorption of aluminium from sucralfate may be significant in patients on dialysis or with renal impairment.

EXCIPIENTS
Suspension includes sodium saccharin.

LICENSED STATUS
Not licensed for use in children.

S

Sulconazole nitrate

Broad-spectrum antifungal.

USES
Fungal skin infections.

PRESENTATION
Cream: 1% – Exelderm®.

DOSAGE/ADMINISTRATION
Apply 1–2 times daily continuing for 2–3 weeks after lesions have healed.

CONTRA-INDICATIONS & WARNINGS
Avoid contact with eyes.

PREGNANCY/BREAST-FEEDING
Only use if essential. Contact local Medicines Information Centre for advice.

SIDE-EFFECTS
Occasional skin irritation or sensitivity.

POISONING/TOXICITY
Oral ingestion, toxicity unlikely, treat symptomatically.

EXCIPIENTS
See manufacturers SPC for further details.

LICENSED STATUS
Licensed for use in children and adults.

Sulfadiazine (sulphadiazine)

Short-acting sulphonamide.

USES
Toxoplasmosis (with pyrimethamine).

PRESENTATION
Tablet: 500mg – non-proprietary.

DOSAGE
Toxoplasmosis in pregnancy and congenital infection – see pyrimethamine monograph.

Dose for toxoplasmosis in other situations

Route	Age			Frequency (times daily)	Notes
	1 month–2 years	2–12 years	12–18 years		
Oral	← 75mg/kg →		2–4g	single dose	Loading dose.
	← 25–50mg/kg →		1–1.5g	4	Usually for 6 weeks: to prevent relapse in HIV infected patients this is followed by a maintenance dose of a quarter to a half of the stated dose indefinitely.

Pyrimethamine and calcium folinate (folinic acid) also given; see pyrimethamine monograph.

ADMINISTRATION
Oral: take with plenty of water.

CONTRA-INDICATIONS & WARNINGS
Patients with a history of sulphonamide sensitivity; those with G6PD deficiency as it may precipitate haemolysis; acute porphyria; renal or hepatic failure. Caution in hepatic and renal impairment. Avoid sun exposure. Give calcium folinate (folinic acid) during long-term therapy.

INTERACTIONS
Warfarin effects enhanced. *Phenytoin* antifolate effect and plasma concentration increased. *Methotrexate* displaced from albumin binding sites; increases the risk of methotrexate toxicity. Avoid *ascorbic acid* as the likelihood of crystalluria and renal damage is increased when the urine is acid. *Pyrimethamine* antibacterial action potentiated by sulfadiazine. *Ciclosporin (cyclosporin)* plasma concentration possibly reduced.

PREGNANCY
Epidemiological studies in humans have not revealed an association between sulfadiazine and fetal malformations. Fear of increased risk of kernicterus in neonates appears to be unfounded.

S

BREAST-FEEDING
Although only small concentrations appear in breast milk, there is still a danger of precipitation of haemolysis in G6PD deficient babies.

SIDE-EFFECTS
Nausea, vomiting, rash (including rarely Stevens-Johnson syndrome; discontinue if rash occurs), liver damage, blood disorders – discontinue therapy, nephrotoxicity including crystalluria – maintain high fluid intake, serum-sickness type of reaction (3–17 days after start of therapy), headache, dizziness.

POISONING/TOXICITY
Overdose causes crystalluria, the symptoms of which include loin pain, haematuria and anuria if total obstruction of the renal pelvis or ureters occurs. Large volumes of fluid should be administered, by IV infusion if necessary. Sodium bicarbonate should be given to render the urine alkaline. Cystoscopy and ureteric catheterisation may be required with irrigation of warm sodium bicarbonate 2.5% solution with the catheters left in situ for 24-48 hours or until renal function has been restored.

PHARMACOKINETIC PROPERTIES
Rapidly absorbed following oral administration, with peak plasma concentrations reached 3–6 hours after a single dose. Mean plasma half-life is 10 hours. Widely distributed throughout the body and penetrates into CSF. Sulfadiazine is excreted slowly, 50% of an oral dose excreted in 24 hours. Both sulfadiazine and its metabolites are excreted via the kidney with only small amounts excreted in bile.

LICENSED STATUS
Not licensed for use in toxoplasmosis.

Sulfasalazine (sulphasalazine)

Aminosalicylate.

USES
Juvenile idiopathic arthritis (JIA); ulcerative colitis and Crohn's disease.

PRESENTATION
Enema: 3g in 100mL – Salazopyrin®.
Suppository: 500mg – Salazopyrin®.
Suspension: 250mg in 5mL – Salazopyrin®.
Tablet: 500mg – Salazopyrin® and non-proprietary.
Tablet: (enteric coated) 500mg – Salazopyrin EN® and non-proprietary.

DOSAGE

Indication	Route	Age		Frequency	Notes
		2–12 years	12–18 years	(times daily)	
JIA	Oral	← 5mg/kg →		2	1st week.
		← 10mg/kg →		2	2nd week.
		← 20mg/kg →		2	3rd week.
		← 20–25mg/kg →		2	Maintenance dose.
		Maximum 2g/day	Maximum 3g/day		
Ulcerative colitis/ Crohn disease	Oral	10–15mg/kg Maximum dose 60mg/kg/day	1–2g	4–6 4	Acute attack. Reduce dose by 50% for maintenance treatment.

DOSAGE continued

Indication	Route	Age		Frequency	Notes
		2–12 years	12–18 years	(times daily)	
Ulcerative colitis/ Crohn disease	Rectal suppository	2–4 years 1/3 adult dose 5–7 years 1/2 adult dose 8–12 years 1/2- 3/4 adult dose	2 suppositories	2	In the morning and at bedtime, preferably after defaecation. 5–7 years use 1 suppository twice daily 8–12 years use 1 suppository in the morning and 2 in the evening, or vice versa.
	Rectal enema	2–7 years 1/3 - 1/2 adult dose 7–12 years 1/2 - 3/4 adult dose	One enema	1	Preferably at bedtime. A proportion of the enema may be used to administer the smaller doses.

Full blood counts and liver function tests should be performed when treatment is initiated and monthly thereafter. An immediate blood count should be carried out if neutropenia or thrombocytopenia are suspected due to symptoms such as a sore throat, glossitis, buccal ulceration, easy bruising or bleeding. If any abnormal results are found, treatment should be withheld and discussed with the clinician responsible for the child's care. Severe nausea or dizziness may necessitate dosage reduction or drug withdrawal.

Patients with renal or hepatic disease should be treated with caution. In patients with G6PD deficiency, monitor for signs of haemolytic anaemia.

ADMINISTRATION

Oral: the enteric coated tablets should not be broken or crushed. Non enteric-coated tablets may be crushed.

CONTRA-INDICATIONS & WARNINGS

Contra-indicated in children <2 years of age and patients with a history of sensitivity to sulphonamides and salicylates. Caution in patients with G6PD deficiency.

INTERACTIONS

Do not take enteric-coated tablets with *antacids* – may cause premature dissolution. May reduce gastrointestinal absorption of *digoxin* and *folic acid*. *Antibiotics that alter intestinal flora* may interfere with conversion of sulfasalzine to sulfapyridine and 5-aminosalicylic acid (5-ASA) decreasing its effectiveness.

PREGNANCY

Both sulfasalazine and its metabolite, sulfapyridine, cross the placenta to the fetal circulation. Long-term clinical usage and experimental studies have failed to prove any teratogenic effects. Contact local Medicines Information Centre for advice.

BREAST-FEEDING

The amounts of drug present in milk should not present a risk to a healthy infant.

SIDE-EFFECTS

Nausea, vomiting, loss of appetite, headache, rash, haematological side-effects, including leucopenia, neutropenia, agranulocytosis, anaemia. Reversible oligospermia, discolouration of urine, discolouration of soft contact lenses, raised temperature, tinnitus, vertigo, haematuria.

POISONING/TOXICITY

There is no specific antidote and treatment is supportive.

PHARMACOKINETIC PROPERTIES

Sulfasalazine is poorly absorbed from the gastrointestinal tract after oral administration. About 80% is transported to the colon where it is metabolised to 5-ASA (anti-inflammatory) and sulfapyridine (antibacterial) which exert their effects locally. Sulfapyridine is absorbed from the colon; 5-ASA is not. Both compounds are metabolised in the liver. Primary excretion is in the urine.

EXCIPIENTS

Salazopyrin® suspension includes sucrose. Contact manufacturers for further details.

LICENSED STATUS

Plain tablets, suspension and suppositories are licensed for ≥2 years of age for ulcerative colitis and Crohn's disease but not for arthritis. Salazopyrin EN® is licensed for rheumatoid arthritis in adults but not licensed in children for this indication. Salazopyrin EN® is licensed for ulcerative colitis and Crohn's disease in children. The enema is not licensed for use in children.

Substituted benzamide, antipsychotic/neuroleptic.

USES
Treatment of schizophrenia and tic disorders including Tourette syndrome.

PRESENTATION
Oral liquid: 200mg in 5mL – Sulpor®.
Tablet: 200mg – Dolmatil® (scored), Sulpitil® (scored) and non-proprietary, 400mg – Dolmatil® (scored) and non-proprietary.

DOSAGE

Route	Age		Frequency (times daily)	Notes
	2–12 years	12–18 years		
Oral	50–200mg	50mg–1.2g	2	Higher doses necessary for predominantly positive symptoms. Predominantly negative symptoms respond to lower doses.

CONTRA-INDICATIONS & WARNINGS
See chlorpromazine monograph. Reduce dose in hepatic or renal insufficiency. Acute porphyria.

INTERACTIONS
As with other psychotropic compounds, sulpiride may increase the effect of *antihypertensives and CNS depressants or stimulants.*

PREGNANCY
Animal studies and widespread clinical use have not shown teratogenic effects. Contact local Medicines Information Centre for advice.

BREAST-FEEDING
Passes into breast milk. Contact local Medicines Information Centre for advice.

SIDE-EFFECTS
See chlorpromazine monograph but not associated with jaundice or skin reactions.

POISONING/TOXICITY
See chlorpromazine monograph.

PHARMACOKINETIC PROPERTIES
Slowly absorbed after oral dosing with peak serum levels reached 2-6 hours after a dose. Half-life of 6-8 hours.

EXCIPIENTS
Contact manufacturers for further details.

LICENSED STATUS
Not licensed for <14 years of age.

Sumatriptan

A 5-HT$_1$ agonist.

USES
Treatment of acute migraine attack.

PRESENTATION
Tablet: 50mg, 100mg – Imigran.
Injection: (as succinate) 12mg in 1mL, 0.5mL pre filled syringe and auto-injector – Imigran.
Nasal Spray: 20mg in 0.1mL unit-dose spray device – Imigran.

DOSAGE

Route	Age		Frequency	Notes
	2–12 years	12–18 years		
Oral	6–10 years 25mg 10–12 years 50mg	50–100mg	single dose	Dose may be repeated if migraine recurs. Maximum of 300mg in 24 hours. If patient does not respond, they should not take a second dose for the same attack.
SC	10–12 years 6mg	6mg	single dose	Dose may be repeated once, after not less than 1 hour, if migraine recurs. Maximum of 12mg in 24 hours. If patient does not respond, they should not take a second dose for the same attack.
Intranasally	–	20mg	single dose	Dose may be repeated once, after not less than 2 hours, if migraine recurs. Maximum of 40mg in 24 hours. If patient does not respond, they should not take a second dose for the same attack.

Note: 3mg doses have been used SC but due to preparation available it is difficult to administer less than 6mg.

ADMINISTRATION

Oral: 50mg tablet can be halved, however, it has a very bitter taste. The remaining unused half should be discarded.
Intranasal: 1 spray into 1 nostril; can give a bitter taste by this route.

CONTRA-INDICATIONS & WARNINGS
Contra-indications: ischaemic heart disease; coronary vasospasm; uncontrolled hypertension.
Cautions: conditions which predispose to coronary artery disease; hepatic impairment.
Warnings: may cause drowsiness.

INTERACTIONS
CNS toxicity with *St. John's Wort;* and also with *MAOI* and *SSRI antidepressants.* Avoid concomitant use and avoid for 2 weeks after stopping *MAOI.*
Increased risk of vasospasm with *ergotamine.* Avoid *ergotamine* for 6 hours after sumatriptan. Avoid sumatriptan for 24 hours after *ergotamine.*

PREGNANCY
Avoid unless potential benefit outweighs risk. Insufficient data available to assess risk.

BREAST-FEEDING
Excreted into breast milk. Withhold breast-feeding for 24 hours after treatment.

SIDE-EFFECTS
Usually none but the following may occur in some patients.
General: transient sensation of tingling, heat, heaviness, pressure or tightness on any part of body, which may be intense.

CSM advice: discontinue if intense pain in chest – may be due to coronary vasoconstriction or anaphylaxis.
Also flushing, dizziness and weakness; burning sensation in nose and throat with nasal spray; stinging, burning, erythema, bruising and bleeding at injection site with SC administration.
Cardiovascular: hypotension, bradycardia, tachycardia, palpitations.
Gastrointestinal: nausea and vomiting.
CNS: rare reports of seizures.
Skin: hypersensitivity reactions, rarely anaphylaxis.

POISONING/TOXICITY
Side-effects as above. No known antidote, supportive treatment, monitor blood pressure and ECG for at least 10 hours.

PHARMACOKINETICS
Rapidly absorbed after oral and SC dosing. High first-pass metabolism. Oral bioavailability 14%, nasal 16% and SC 96%. Peak plasma levels occur 5–25 minutes after SC administration, 30 minutes – 5 hours (high variability) after oral dosing and 60-90 minutes after nasal administration. Extensively metabolised (80%). Metabolites excreted in urine. Also eliminated via active tubular secretions. Elimination half-life is 2 hours.

S

EXCIPIENTS
See manufacturers SPC for further details.

LICENSED STATUS
Not licensed for use in <18 years old.

Suramin

Antiparasitic agent.

USES
Trypanosomiasis: early (haematolymphatic) stage of trypanosomiasis due to *T. brucei rhodesiense* (African trypanosomiasis; sleeping sickness). Late stage trypanosomiasis prior to dosing with melarsoprol.

PRESENTATION
Injection: 10% – named patient (imported).

DOSAGE

Indication	Route	Age			Frequency	Notes
		1 month–2 years	2–12 years	12–18 years		
Test dose	IV	← 10–20mg →		100–200mg	single dose	
Early stage Trypanosomiasis due to *T. brucei rhodesiense*	IV	← 20mg/kg →		1g	single dose	On days 1, 3, 7, 14 and 21.
Late stage Trypanosomiasis due to *T. brucei gambiense* or *T. brucei rhodesiense*	IV	Day 1: 5mg/kg Day 3: 10mg/kg Day 5: 20mg/kg then ← 20mg/kg →			single dose single dose single dose weekly for 4 further doses	Pre-melarsoprol dosing.

ADMINISTRATION
IV: give as a slow IV injection of a 10% solution. Because of the dangers of severe reactions give a test dose as indicated in the dosage table.

CONTRA-INDICATIONS & WARNINGS
Use with caution in renal impairment; administration to patients with significant hepatic dysfunction may result in toxic serum levels. Use with caution in malnourished or debilitated patients. Persistent, heavy albuminuria or casts in the urine may necessitate discontinuation.

INTERACTIONS
May interfere with serum calcium measurements.

PREGNANCY
Suramin has been given to women for more than 60 years with no reports of infant malformation. Teratogenic effects have been seen in mice. Should be used during pregnancy only if there is no suitable alternative.

BREAST-FEEDING
No information available.

SIDE-EFFECTS
Immediate hypersensitivity reactions can occur although uncommon. The injection is immediately followed by vomiting, shock and collapse and thus a test dose is recommended.
CNS: headache, paraesthesias, peripheral neuropathy, palmar or plantar hyperaesthesia.
Gastrointestinal: nausea and vomiting are common but subside with continued treatment. Diarrhoea and abdominal pain occur infrequently.
Renal toxicity: see contra-indications and warnings.
Ocular: keratopathy, photophobia, lachrymation, optic atrophy, blepharitis and conjunctivitis have all been reported.

Skin: rashes, urticaria, pruritus.
Blood: leucopenia, agranulocytosis, thrombocytopenia.
Endocrine: adrenal insufficiency.
Other: fever, chills; generally subside with continued therapy.

POISONING/TOXICITY
No reports of overdose in the literature. Poorly absorbed orally. Overdose effects IV would be expected to be extensions of therapeutic effects. Long half-life, therefore, effects may extend over a lengthy period of time. No specific antidotes; treatment is symptomatic and supportive. Monitor liver enzymes, renal function and blood parameters.

PHARMACOKINETIC PROPERTIES
Following IV administration suramin is rapidly distributed, becomes bound to plasma proteins and is eliminated unchanged very slowly in the urine; terminal elimination half-life is approximately 50 days. CSF penetration appears to be poor.

LICENSED STATUS
Not licensed for use in the UK.

FURTHER INFORMATION
Can usually be obtained via IDIS World Medicines but clinician/pharmacist should check with one of the Schools of Tropical Medicine if the need to use arises.

Surfactants (natural)

Surfactant lowers surface tension at the air/liquid interface of the alveoli preventing collapse at end expiration.

USES
To improve lung compliance in preterm babies suffering from surfactant deficiency.

PRESENTATION
Injection: poractant alfa 120mg in 1.5mL vial and 240mg in 3mL vial – Curosurf®.
Injection: beractant 200mg in 8mL vial – Survanta®.

DOSAGE
Newborn infant (birth to 1 month)

Product	Route	Age birth–1 month	Frequency (times daily)	Notes
Poractant alfa	Intra-tracheal	200mg/kg (2.5mL/kg)	single bolus	Initial dose. Followed by two further doses of 100mg/kg after 12 and 24 hours if necessary.
Beractant	Intra-tracheal	100mg/kg (4mL/kg)	single bolus	Up to 3 further doses of 100mg/kg can be given, at intervals of not less than 6 hours, within next 48 hours.

ADMINISTRATION
Intra-tracheal: pre-oxygenate before administration. Ventilate during administration.

CONTRA-INDICATIONS & WARNINGS
Stabilise the baby before administration. Be prepared to make early adjustments to ventilation to take account of possible rapid improvement in lung compliance following surfactant administration.

SIDE-EFFECTS
Pulmonary haemorrhage has been reported.

POISONING/TOXICITY
If an excessively large dose is given, observe infant for signs of acute airway obstruction. Treatment should be symptomatic and supportive.

EXCIPIENTS
Both products contain sodium chloride. Curosurf® contains sodium bicarbonate. See manufacturers SPC for further details.

LICENSED STATUS
Licensed for use in preterm infants >700g birth weight.

FURTHER INFORMATION
Vials are for single use only. Used vials with residual drug should be discarded. They should be stored in a refrigerator between 2-8°C and should not be used >8 hours after they reach room temperature. Warmed vials should not be returned to the refrigerator. Evidence is beginning to accumulate suggesting that natural surfactants have a marginally improved survival particularly in smaller babies. They have a quicker onset of action.

Surfactants (synthetic)

Surfactant lowers surface tension at the air/liquid interface of the alveoli preventing collapse at end expiration.

USES
To improve lung compliance in preterm babies suffering from surfactant deficiency.

PRESENTATION
Injection: colfosceril palmitate 108mg vial and 8mL of Water for Injections – Exosurf®.

DOSAGE
Newborn infant (birth to 1 month)

Route	Age	Frequency	Notes
	birth–1 month	(times daily)	
Intra-tracheal	67.5mg/kg	single dose	Give over 4 minutes. A further dose of 67.5mg/kg can be given after 12 hours if the baby is still ventilated.

ADMINISTRATION
Intra-tracheal: pre-oxygenate before administration. Ventilate during administration. See manufacturers SPC for further detail.

CONTRA-INDICATIONS & WARNINGS
See natural surfactants monograph.

SIDE-EFFECTS
Pulmonary haemorrhage. Occasionally obstruction of the endotracheal tube by mucous secretions has occurred.

POISONING/TOXICITY
In cases of accidental overdosage observe infant for signs of acute airways obstruction. Treatment should be symptomatic and supportive.

EXCIPIENTS
See manufacturers SPC for further detail.

LICENSED STATUS
Exosurf® licensed in newborn infants.

FURTHER INFORMATION
Exosurf® should be stored below 30°C. Use within 8 hours of reconstitution.

USE
Short-term depolarising muscle relaxant prior to tracheal intubation.

PRESENTATION
Injection: 50mg in 1ml; 2ml ampoule – Anectine® and non-proprietary.

DOSAGE
Newborn infant (birth to 1 month)

Route	Age	Frequency	Notes
	birth–1 month	(times daily)	
IV	2mg/kg	single dose	Provides 5-10 minutes of muscular paralysis.
IV	3mg/kg	single dose	Provides full neuromuscular blockade.
IM	4mg/kg	single dose	Provides 10-30 minutes paralaysis after a 2-3 minute delay.

Child

Route	Age			Frequency	Notes
	1 month–2 years	2–12 years	12–18 years	(times daily)	
IV	← initially 1-2mg/kg →		–	single dose	Maximum dose 2.5mg/kg.
			1mg/kg	single dose	Dose range of 300 microgram/kg – 1.1mg/kg, but usually 20-100mg. Maximum 500mg/hour.
IM	≤1 year up to 4-5mg/kg >1 year up to 4mg/kg	up to 4mg/kg	–	single dose single dose	Maximum dose of 150mg.

CONTRA-INDICATIONS AND WARNINGS
Suxamethonium should not be used in patients with a family history of malignant hyperthermia or low plasma cholinesterase activity; hyperkalaemia. Suxamethonium should be given after anaesthetic induction because paralysis is usually preceded by painful muscle fasiculations.

PREGNANCY
Single doses of 1mg/kg during pregnancy have not produced any harmful effects to the fetus. Case report describes prolonged neuromuscular block after a single dose. Decreased pseudocholinesterase levels persist in the early puerperium. Normal levels are reached 6 weeks after delivery.

BREAST-FEEDING
It is not known whether suxamethonium is excreted in breast milk. Contact local Medicines Information Centre for advice.

INTERACTIONS
Some drugs may prolong the action of suxamethonium, including: *neostigmine, pyridostigmine, physostigmine, edrophonium, cyclophosphamide, thiotepa (thiopentone), phenelzine, chlorpromazine, ketamine, morphine and morphine antagonists, pethidine, pancuronium, magnesium salts, lithium, azathioprine, quinine, aminoglycosides, clindamycin, quinidine, procainamide, verapamil, beta-blockers, lidocaine (lignocaine), procaine, halothane, enflurane, isoflurane.* Other drugs which affect plasma cholinesterase activity include *aprotinin, diphenhydramine, promethazine, oestrogens, oxytocin, high-dose steroids, oral contraceptives, terbutaline* and *metoclopramide*. See manufacturers SPC for further details.

SIDE-EFFECTS
Tachycardia occurs after a single dose in adults but bradycardia may occur after single or multiple doses in children. Premedication with atropine reduces bradycardia and hypersalivation. Post-operative muscle pain, myoglobinaemia, arrhythmias, hypertension, hypotension, bronchospasm, apnoea, prolonged respiratory depression, hyperkalaemia (a rise of 0.5mmol/L), hyperthermia.

S

POISONING/TOXICITY
Apnoea and prolonged muscle paralysis are the main serious effects of overdose. Reversed by atropine (20 microgram/kg) followed by neostigmine (80 microgram/kg).

PHARMACOKINETIC PROPERTIES
Rapidly hydrolysed by plasma pseudocholinesterase. 10% excreted unchanged in the urine. Half-life is 2-3 minutes.

EXCIPIENTS
Contact manufacturers for further details.

LICENSED STATUS
Licensed for use in all ages.

Tacalcitol

Vitamin D3 derivative which inhibits keratinocyte hyper-proliferation and induces differentiation of these cells.

USES
Psoriasis vulgaris.

PRESENTATION
Ointment: 4 microgram per gram (as monohydrate) – Curatoderm®.

DOSAGE
Child

Route	Age	Frequency	Notes
	12–18 years	(times daily)	
Topical	Apply sparingly	1 preferably at bedtime	Do not exceed 10g of ointment per day. Duration of treatment to be decided by physician. Both continuous and intermittant treatment have been used up to 12 months.

ADMINISTRATION
Topical: preferably apply at bedtime.

CONTRA-INDICATIONS & WARNINGS
Hypersensitivity. Disorders of calcium metabolism; monitor serum calcium in patients at risk of hypercalcaemia and renally impaired patients. Increased risk of hypercalcaemia in patients with generalised pustular or erythrodermic exfoliative psoriasis.

INTERACTIONS
Patients may take up to 500 international units of vitamin D in multivitamin preparations. Ultra-violet light including sunlight may degrade tacalcitol, hence apply at bedtime.

PREGNANCY
Safety not established. Avoid unless no safer alternative available.

BREAST-FEEDING
Not known if excreted in milk. Do not apply to breast area during lactation.

SIDE-EFFECTS
Local skin reactions, itching, erythema, burning, paraesthesia. Usually mild and transient.

POISONING/TOXICITY
Monitor for hypercalcaemia.

PHARMACOKINETIC PROPERTIES
Less than 0.5% drug systematically absorbed after single or repeated application.

EXCIPIENTS
See manufacturers SPC for further details.

LICENSED STATUS
Not licensed for children as not included in clinical trials.

FURTHER INFORMATION
Avoid contact with eyes. Patients should wash hands after applying ointment to avoid inadvertent transfer.

Tacrolimus

Tacrolimus is a macrolide immunosuppressant.

USES
Primary immunosuppression in liver and renal transplantation.
Secondary immunosuppression in patients resistant to conventional immunosuppressive regimens.
Treatment of moderate to severe atopic dermatitis that has not responded adequately to conventional therapies (dermatologists and physicians with extensive experience in atopic eczema treatment only).

PRESENTATION
Capsule: 500 micrograms, 1mg and 5mg – Prograf®.
Concentrate for intravenous infusion: 5mg in 1mL – Prograf®.
Ointment: 0.03% and 0.1%, 30g and 60g – Protopic®.
Suspension: 2.5mg in 5ml – manufactured 'special'.

DOSAGE
Use the oral route, rather than IV where possible.

Indication	Route	Age			Frequency	Notes
		1 month-2 years	2-12 years	12-18 years	(times daily)	
Liver transplantation	IV infusion	← 75-150 microgram/kg/24 hours →			continuous	Initial dose: only IV if clinical condition does not allow use of oral route. Then adjust according to trough levels, which should be 10–15 nanogram/mL in the early phase of treatment.
	Oral	150 microgram/kg (as a start dose) then 75 microgram/kg	<5 years as for 1 month-2 years >5 years 150 microgram/kg		2	Doses are level dependent and vary from unit to unit.
Renal transplantation	IV infusion	← 75-200 microgram/kg/24 hours →			continuous	Adjusted to achieve a trough level of 10–15 nanogram/mL in the early phase of treatment.
	Oral	← 110–400 microgram/kg →			2	Doses are level dependent and vary from unit to unit.

Topical
≥2 years of age: apply thin layer of 0.03% twice daily to affected areas for 3 weeks reducing to once a day until clearance of the lesion.
≥16 years of age: apply thin layer of 0.1% twice daily for up to 3 weeks then reduce to 0.03% twice daily. Reduce to once daily until clearance of lesion.

Dosage in renal impairment
No dose adjustment required. Plasma concentration is not reduced by dialysis.

ADMINISTRATION

Oral: should be taken with fluid, preferably water. Administration should be 1 hour before, or 2–3 hours after meals in order to maximise absorption. Patients should be encouraged to take the capsule without opening or crushing it.

IV: required dose is administered as a 24 hour infusion diluted to a concentration in the range 4–100 microgram in 1mL with glucose 5% or NaCl 0.9%. Administer for not more than 7 days. Tacrolimus is incompatible with PVC. Ensure that all syringes, tubing and other IV administration equipment does not contain PVC.

Topical: wash hands before and after application. Avoid emollient application 2 hours before and after use of tacrolimus. Do not occlude.

CONTRA-INDICATIONS & WARNINGS

Pregnancy. Hypersensitivity to tacrolimus, other macrolides or any excipient, particularly polyoxyethylene hydrogenated castor oil. Patients with known sensitivity to similar compounds, or who are atopic should be monitored closely on commencing treatment (see below).

Particular care required in children <2 years of age who are initially EBV-sero-negative – therefore monitor EBV serology before starting and during treatment with tacrolimus. Concurrent anti-lymphocyte therapy should be avoided in patients switched to tacrolimus rescue therapy. Visual and neurological disturbance. Routine monitoring of cardiovascular, visual, endocrine, renal, haematological and hepatic function is mandatory on commencement of treatment. Dose should be adjusted where clinically relevant changes are identified. Hypertrophic cardiomyopathy has been reported, usually associated with trough level >25 nanogram/mL with most cases reported in children <5 years. Usually reversible on dose reduction or discontinuation. Predisposing factors include cardiac disease, hypertension, fluid overload, hepatic and/or renal dysfunction and concurrent corticosteroid administration.

Topical: avoid exposure to sun. Treat clinical infections at treatment site prior to tacrolimus application. Monitor any lymphadenopathy.

INTERACTIONS

Ciclosporin (cyclosporin) half-life is increased in patients also receiving tacrolimus. Care is required in changing patients from *ciclosporin* to tacrolimus. Risk of enhanced effects of *ciclosporin,* particularly nephrotoxicity; concurrent use is not recommended. Tacrolimus can be initiated 12-24 hours after discontinuation of *ciclosporin,* with continued *ciclosporin* monitoring. Interactions resulting in changes to blood/plasma levels of tacrolimus or the following have been reported: *clotrimazole, danazol, dexamethasone,* and *methylprednisolone.*

Nephrotoxicity may be enhanced by concurrent administration of: *aminoglycosides, amphotericin B, co-trimoxazole, gyrase inhibitors, NSAIDs* and *vancomycin.* Avoid *potassium-sparing diuretics* – risk of hyperkalaemia. *Vaccinations* may be less

effective. *Live attenuated vaccines* should be avoided. Care should be taken with the concurrent administration of any drug metabolised by the cytochrome P450 system, as tacrolimus is extensively metabolised by, and may have both inducing and inhibitory effects on, this system.

On theoretical or experimental grounds the following may be anticipated to influence tacrolimus metabolism: *amphotericin B, barbiturates, bromocriptine, carbamazepine, corticosteroids, cortisone, ciclosporin, diltiazem, ergotamine, erythromycin, ethinyloestradiol, fluconazole, gestodene, isoniazid, ketoconazole, miconazole, midazolam, nifedipine, omeprazole, phenytoin, prednisolone, rifampicin, tamoxifen* and *verapamil.*

May inhibit the metabolism of *ciclosporin, cortisone, testosterone, phenobarbital, antipyrine,* and *oral contraceptives.* Extensively bound to plasma proteins. Interactions with other drugs with a similarly high level of binding to plasma protein, such as *warfarin* and *phenytoin* should be considered likely.

PREGNANCY

Contra-indicated. Tacrolimus crosses the placenta and has been shown to be teratogenic in animal studies. Pregnancy should be excluded before commencing tacrolimus therapy. Due to possible interaction with *oral contraceptives,* other methods of contraception should be used.

BREAST-FEEDING

Tacrolimus is excreted into breast milk. Breast-feeding is not recommended.

SIDE-EFFECTS

See also contra-indications and warnings.

The most common side-effects reported include: tremor, headache, infection, paraesthesia, impaired renal function, hypertension and hyperglycaemia. However, the adverse effect profile is difficult to establish due to the patient's underlying condition and the multiplicity of concurrent drug therapy.

Susceptibility to bacterial, viral, fungal and/or protozoal infection is increased. EBV-associated lympho-proliferative disorders may occur.

Impaired renal function, renal failure, haemolytic uraemic syndrome (HUS) and tubular necrosis have been reported. In renal transplant recipients it is important to distinguish tacrolimus toxicity from signs of acute rejection. CNS and sensory disorders are reported and cover a wide spectrum. Psychiatric adverse effects have also been reported. Diarrhoea, insomnia, diabetes mellitus, chest pain and nausea are reported, in decreasing order of frequency. Haematological effects include anaemia, coagulation disorders, thrombocytopenia, leucocytosis, leucopenia, pancytopenia. Biochemical abnormalities include acidosis, hyper- and hypokalaemia, hyperuricaemia, hypocalcaemia, hypomagnesaemia, hypophosphataemia and hyponatraemia. Other reported adverse effects affect the gastrointestinal tract, skin, cardiovascular, respiratory and musculo-skeletal systems.

Topical: skin irritation, folliculitis, acne, herpes simplex, increased sensitivity to hot and cold, alcohol intolerance (flushing).

POISONING/TOXICITY
Toxicity is likely to produce glucose intolerance, renal, neurological and cardiac disorders, hyperkalaemia and hypertension. There is no specific antidote, and symptomatic treatment should be given as necessary. It is unlikely that tacrolimus is dialysable.

Topical: general supportive measures. Do not induce vomiting or gastric lavage.

PHARMACOKINETIC PROPERTIES
Oral absorption is poor and erratic. Absolute bioavailability is 27% (range 5-67%). Peak plasma levels occur after 0.5-8 hours. Volume of distribution is 1300L. Half-life is variable (average of 12.4 hours).

Erythrocytes sequester tacrolimus such that whole blood levels are 10-30 times greater than those in plasma. Plasma protein binding is 88%. Tacrolimus is almost completely metabolised by cytochrome P450, subtypes Ia and IIIa, in the liver, with <1% being excreted unchanged in urine, bile and faeces up to 48 hours after administration. Of nine identified metabolites, two exhibit significant immuno-suppressant activity.

Topical: systemic levels low and, when measurable, transient.

EXCIPIENTS
Concentrate for infusion includes polyoxyethylene hydrogenated castor oil. See manufacturers SPC for further details.

LICENSED STATUS
Tacrolimus is licensed for use in children and adults. The suspension is a 'special' and as such is unlicensed.
Topical: 0.03% ointment licensed for ≥2 years of age. 0.1% ointment licensed for ≥16 years of age.

FURTHER INFORMATION
Tacrolimus capsules are contained in an aluminium wrapper and should be used within 3 months of opening the wrapper. The suspension is available e.g. from BCM as a 'special'.

Teicoplanin

Glycopeptide antibiotic active against aerobic and anaerobic Gram-positive bacteria.

USES
Potentially serious Gram-positive infections. In cystic fibrosis patients – reserve for methicillin-resistant *Staphylococcus aureus* (MRSA) infection or serious *Staphylococcus aureus* infections that do not respond to other anti-staphylococcal antibiotics.

PRESENTATION
Injection: 200mg and 400mg vials (each vial contains overage – 200mg vial contains 220mg and 400mg vial contains 460mg) – Targocid®.

DOSAGE
Newborn infant (birth to 1 month)

Route	Age	Frequency	Notes
	birth-1month	(times daily)	
IV	16mg/kg	single dose	Loading dose, then 24 hours later
	8mg/kg	1	start the maintenance dose.

DOSAGE continued

Child

Route	Age			Frequency (times daily)	Notes
	1 month–2 years	2–12 years	12–18 years		
IV	←	10mg/kg	→	2	Give this dose for 3 doses then as outlined below for moderate or severe infections. Maximum single dose 400mg.
IM/IV	←	10mg/kg	→	1	Severe infections, neutropenic patients and cystic fibrosis patients. Maximum single dose 400mg.
	←	6mg/kg	→	1	Moderate infections. Maximum single dose 200mg.
Oral	←	10mg/kg	→	2	Unlicensed route in treatment of pseudo-membranous colitis.
Intra–ventricular	5mg	10mg	20mg	1 initially	Frequency of administration may reduce to alternate days if there is a good response. Unlicensed route; very limited experience. Administer in appropriate volume of NaCl 0.9%.
Intra–peritoneal	Concentration of 20mg/L per bag for first week then alternate bags for second week then overnight only during third week.				Treatment of peritonitis in CAPD. Use single IV loading dose first.

Renal impairment
Dose reduction is not required until fourth day of treatment.
Mild impairment – reduce daily dose to 50% of dose.
Moderate to severe impairment – reduce daily dose to one third of dose. Monitor urea and creatinine.

ADMINISTRATION
IV/IM: the injection vial should be reconstituted with the 3.2mL Water for Injections ampoule supplied. This will provide a solution of 400mg or 200mg in 3mL as excess is included in the vial. Roll the vial gently until the powder is completely dissolved. Excessive agitation may lead to foaming. If this occurs allow to stand for 15 minutes. Give as an IM, slow IV injection or by IV infusion over 30 minutes. Further dilute if required in NaCl 0.9%, glucose 5% or 0.18% NaCl/4% glucose.

CONTRA-INDICATIONS & WARNINGS
Previous hypersensitivity reaction to teicoplanin. Cross hypersensitivity to vancomycin may occur but vancomycin-induced 'red man syndrome' is not a contra-indication to teicoplanin.

INTERACTIONS
No specific interactions known. No evidence of synergistic toxicity with other neurotoxic or nephrotoxic agents. However, monitoring of renal and auditory function is advised when such combinations are used.

PREGNANCY
High doses in rats increased incidence of stillbirth. Contact local Medicines Information Centre for advice.

BREAST-FEEDING
No information on excretion into breast milk. Contact local Medicines Information Centre for advice.

SIDE-EFFECTS
Local irritation on injection is the most frequent side effect. Allergic and anaphylactic reactions such as rash and fever. Transient increase in serum creatinine and liver enzymes. Thrombocytopenia (especially at higher than recommended doses) and other blood dyscrasias rarely reported.

POISONING/TOXICITY
Not removed by haemofiltration – treatment should be symptomatic. Anecdotal reports suggest no serious consequences despite plasma levels up to 300mg/L.

PHARMACOKINETIC PROPERTIES
Pharmacokinetics are best described by a three-compartment model. Slow release back into the central compartment following peripheral distribution is the limiting step in excretion.

Oral: not absorbed orally but may be if gastrointestinal tract inflamed. IM: bioavailability is greater than 90% of IV. Peak IM levels achieved about 2 hours after dosing. 90–95% protein bound to albumin with weak affinity.

Only minute metabolites identified accounting for <3% of total elimination. Penetrates well into most body fluids achieving therapeutic concentrations in body compartments. It does not cross the blood-brain barrier. Does not distribute into red cells but does penetrate leucocytes and may cause intraphagocyte anti-bacterial activity. It concentrates in white cells and, unlike vancomycin, may retain anti-bacterial activity. This may be important in patients with impaired phagocytic killing capacity. Determination of teicoplanin serum concentrations may optimise therapy; trough should not be less than 10mg/L, peak concentrations 1 hour after dose should be in the range 25-50mg/L. Measurements may be difficult to arrange – contact manufacturer for details.

EXCIPIENTS
See manufacturers SPC for further details.

LICENSED STATUS
Licensed for use in all ages; however only licensed in newborn infants for administration by infusion over 30 minutes.

Temazepam

Short-acting benzodiazepine with sedative, hypnotic and anxiolytic properties.

USES
Sedation prior to procedures e.g. dressing changes; premedication.

PRESENTATION
Gel-filled capsule: 10mg, 15mg, 20mg and 30mg – non-proprietary.
Oral solution: 10mg in 5mL – non-proprietary.
Tablet: 10mg and 20mg – non-proprietary.

DOSAGE

Route	Age				Frequency	Notes
	birth–1 month	1 month–2 years	2–12 years	12–18 years		
Oral	–	← 1mg/kg →		20-30mg	single dose	Administer one hour prior to surgery.

Renal/hepatic impairment
Caution in severe liver disease, may precipitate coma. Reduce doses in severe renal impairment (increased cerebral sensitivity).

CONTRA-INDICATIONS & WARNINGS
Contra-indications: pre-existing CNS depression or coma, acute pulmonary insufficiency, myasthenia gravis and sleep apnoea syndrome.
Caution: monitoring of cardiorespiratory function is generally recommended when benzodiazepines are used for sedation and should follow national and local guidelines.

INTERACTIONS
Sedation or respiratory and cardiovascular depression may be enhanced by other drugs with CNS depressant properties including *anaesthetics, opioid analgesics, antihistamines, baclofen, nabilone,* and *CNS depressants. Macrolide antibiotics* may inhibit the hepatic enzymes responsible for benzodiazepine metabolism resulting in decreased clearance, increased plasma concentration, increased half-life and volume of distribution. *Theophyllines* antagonise the action of benzodiazepines resulting in decreased effectiveness of temazepam.

PREGNANCY
The manufacturers of temazepam do not recommend its use in pregnancy. This is due to a variety of findings involving other benzodiazepines, such as severe dysmorphism, malformations, intra– and extra-uterine growth retardation and CNS dysfunction which have been described in infants of mothers who have taken benzodiazepines during pregnancy. More recent evaluations of these agents have failed to support these associations.

T

Administration to mothers prior to delivery is likely to cause signs such as hypothermia, hypotonia, difficulties in sucking and respiratory difficulties which may require assisted ventilation in the neonate within the first hours or days after delivery. Infants born to mothers taking temazepam chronically in the later stages of pregnancy may have developed physical dependence and may be at some risk of developing withdrawal symptoms in the postnatal period.

BREAST-FEEDING
Temazepam is excreted into breast milk. The repeated use of benzodiazepines by nursing mothers has not been recommended because they may accumulate in exposed infants, causing poor suckling or somnolence. The WHO Working Group on Drugs and Human Lactation concluded that mothers receiving occasional small doses of benzodiazepines could safely breast-feed.

SIDE-EFFECTS
CNS: drowsiness is the most commonly reported adverse effect; others include confusion, fatigue, muscle weakness, ataxia, vertigo, double vision, hangover, headache, lethargy, slurred speech, agitation. Paradoxical reactions such as restlessness, aggression, nightmares, hallucinations and inappropriate behaviour occur with increased frequency in children.
Gastrointestinal: nausea, abdominal discomfort, diarrhoea
Other: urinary retention, hypersensitivity reactions have been seen.

POISONING/TOXICITY
Symptoms: generally low order toxicity unless ingested with other depressant drugs. CNS depression ranging from drowsiness to coma and respiratory depression are the primary clinical concerns. Deaths from overdose are rare. Hypothermia, hypotension, bradycardia and cardiac arrest have been reported in overdose. Paradoxical excitement has been reported.
Treatment: respiratory depression should be treated aggressively with basic and advanced life support, ventilatory support and flumazenil. The dose of flumazenil may need to be repeated if resedation occurs, or a continuous infusion of flumazenil may be used.

PHARMACOKINETIC PROPERTIES
Fairly readily absorbed from gastrointestinal tract although the exact rate of absorption depends on the formulation used. Peak serum levels occur 0.8–1.4 hours after a single oral dose. Onset of action is within approximately 30 minutes; duration of action is about 4 hours. Approximately 96% bound to plasma proteins. Completely metabolised in the liver prior to excretion in the urine in the form of inactive glucuronide conjugate together with a small amount of the derivative oxazepam also in conjugated form. Elimination is biphasic with early studies reporting a terminal half-life of 8 hours. More recent studies suggest a longer half-life of about 15 hours.

EXCIPIENTS
Contact manufacturers for further details.

LICENSED STATUS
Not licensed for use in children. Gel-filled capsules are not available for NHS prescription.

Terbinafine

Broad-spectrum antifungal agent.

USES
Treatment of fungal infection, especially nails.

PRESENTATION
Tablet: 250mg (scored) – Lamisil®.
Cream: 1% – Lamisil®.

DOSAGE/ADMINISTRATION

Route	Age			Frequency (times daily)	Notes
	1 month–2 years	2–12 years	12–18 years		
Oral		DOSE BY WEIGHT			Maximum dose 250mg.
		≥1 year			Treat for:
	←	3–6mg/kg	→	1	2–6 weeks tinea pedis.
		DOSE BY AGE			2–4 weeks tinea cruris.
	<20kg	20–40kg	≥40kg		4 weeks tinea corporis.
	62.5mg	125mg	250mg	1	6 weeks – 3 months for nail infection.
Topical	←	Apply thinly	→	1–2	Treat for:
					1 week tinea pedis.
					1–2 weeks tinea corporis .
					1-2 weeks tinea cruris.
					2 weeks in cutaneous conditions.
					Review after 2 weeks.

Renal/liver impairment
Patients with pre-existing stable chronic liver dysfunction or impaired renal function (creatinine clearance less than 50mL/minute) should receive half the oral dose.

CONTRA-INDICATIONS & WARNINGS
Cream: avoid contact with eyes.
Tablets: caution in renal and hepatic impairment.

INTERACTIONS
Terbinafine plasma concentration reduced by *rifampicin*, increased by *cimetidine*.

PREGNANCY
Not recommended.

BREAST-FEEDING
Excreted in breast milk; contact local Medicines Information Centre for advice.

SIDE-EFFECTS
Oral use: *gastrointestinal* – loss of appetite, nausea, diarrhoea, mild abdominal pain; *other* – rash, urticaria, arthralgia and myalgia.
Topical use: redness, itching or stinging; rarely allergic reactions.

POISONING/TOXICITY
Supportive treatment.

EXCIPIENTS
See manufacturers SPC for further details.

LICENSED STATUS
Not licensed for use in children.

Terbutaline

T

A selective beta-2 adrenergic agonist.

USES
Relief of bronchospasm in bronchial asthma.

PRESENTATION
Aerosol inhalation: 250 microgram – Bricanyl®.
Dry powder inhaler: 500 microgram – Bricanyl® Turbohaler®.
Injection: 500 microgram in 1mL; 1mL and 5mL ampoules – Bricanyl®.
Nebuliser solution: 2.5mg in 1mL, 2mL – Bricanyl® Respules and non-proprietary; 10mg in 1mL, 20mL – Bricanyl® Respirator solution.

Syrup: 1.5mg in 5mL – Bricanyl® and Monovent®.
Tablet: 5mg (scored) – Bricanyl®.
Tablet: 7.5mg (modified release, scored) – Bricanyl SA®.

DOSAGE

Route	Age			Frequency	Notes
	1 month–2 years	2–12 years	12–18 years	(times daily)	
Oral	75 microgram/kg	DOSE BY WEIGHT ≤7 years 75 microgram/kg DOSE BY AGE >7 years 2.5mg	2.5–5mg	3 2–3	
Oral (modified release tablets)	–	–	7.5mg	2	
Aerosol inhaler	←	250–500 microgram	→	4–6	Reliever: doses are given as required. Higher doses have been used in acute asthma.
Turbohaler	–	← >5 years → 500 microgram		4	Reliever.
Nebulised	2.5–5mg	≤5 years 2.5–5mg >5 years 5–10mg	10mg	single dose single dose	Reliever: doses are given as required; up to 8 times daily if necessary or 12 times daily under hospital supervision.
Injection SC/IM/ slow IV bolus	–	10 microgram/kg (maximum 300 microgram dose)	250–500 microgram	single dose	Emergency use if nebuliser not available. Repeat up to 4 times daily.
IV infusion (loading dose)	←	2–4 microgram/kg	→	single dose	The optimum therapeutic dose in children is still empiric. The doses vary considerably depending on the reference source. Doses up to 5 times those given here have been used.
IV infusion (maintenance)	←	1–10 microgram/kg/hour	→	continuous	

ADMINISTRATION

Oral: tablets are scored, and can be halved.
Inhaled: nebulised solution can be mixed with NaCl 0.9%, ipratropium bromide and budesonide nebuliser solutions. Single dose plastic units in an opened foil envelope must be used within 3 months.
pH of Bricanyl® respules is 3-4.5. pH of Bricanyl® respirator solution is 2.5-3.5.
Aerosol inhaler can be used with Nebuhaler® spacer and mask for infants and young children.
Turbohaler® can be used in children >5 years.
IV: for infusion the recommended infusion fluid is glucose 5%. Using a syringe pump the concentration of drug should be 100 microgram in 1mL; 5mg (10mL of 500 microgram in 1mL) of terbutaline should be diluted to 50mL with glucose 5%.

CONTRA-INDICATIONS & WARNINGS
IV administration should be given with caution to diabetic patients.

INTERACTIONS
Corticosteroids: increases the risk of hypokalaemia.
Theophylline: increases the risk of hypokalaemia.
Diuretics: increases the risk of hypokalaemia.

Beta-blockers: may partially or totally inhibit the effects of terbutaline.

PREGNANCY
Terbutaline is not associated with congenital defects, but may potentially cause maternal and fetal tachycardia, hypotension, and maternal hyperglycaemia.

BREAST-FEEDING
Terbutaline is excreted in breast milk, but effect on infants is unlikely at therapeutic doses.

SIDE-EFFECTS
At the recommended doses the frequency of side-effects is low, and is associated more with systemic therapy. These can include tremor, headache, tonic cramp, palpitations and hypokalaemia.

POISONING/TOXICITY
Terbutaline will cause headache, anxiety, tremor, tonic cramp, palpitations, arrhythmias. Occasionally, it causes a fall in blood pressure, hypokalaemia, hyperglycaemia and lactic acidosis.
Treatment of mild/moderate cases: reduce the dose.

Severe cases: determine acid-base balance, blood sugar and electrolytes. Monitor heart rate, rhythm, and blood pressure. Correct any metabolic changes. Treat arrhythmias that cause haemodynamic deterioration with a cardio-selective beta- blocker. Use beta-blockers with care because of the possibility of bronchoconstriction. Use a volume expander if the beta-2 mediated reduction in peripheral vascular resistance significantly contributes to the fall in blood pressure.

PHARMACOKINETIC PROPERTIES
The bronchodilating effect of terbutaline begins within 5 minutes, and lasts for 3-4 hours after inhalation. The onset of action after oral administration is about 30 minutes, and has a duration of action of 8 hours, with maximal effect 2-3 hours after the dose.

EXCIPIENTS
Syrups include ethanol and are sugar-free. See manufacturers SPC for further details.

LICENSED STATUS
All presentations are licensed for use in all ages, however, as discussed some are only suitable for older children. Some doses and dosage intervals stated are higher than recommended by the manufacturer.

Terlipressin

Terlipressin is triglycyl-lysine-vasopressin. It may be considered as a circulating depot which releases lysine vasopressin at a constant rate. It has both pressor and antidiuretic activity.

USES
Treatment of bleeding oesophageal varices.

PRESENTATION
Injection: 1mg (with 5mL of diluent) – Glypressin®.

DOSAGE

Route	Age			Frequency (times daily)	Notes
	1 month–2 years	2–12 years	12–18 years		
IV bolus	500 microgram	<7 years 500 microgram	2mg	single dose	Initial dose: the children's dose given is purely anecdotal. There is no published data on dosages in children. Dose can be repeated.
		7–12 years 1mg		single dose	≥7 years old a maximum of 4–6 hourly administration has been used.

CONTRA-INDICATIONS & WARNINGS
Contra-indications: pregnancy, vascular disease.
Warnings: terlipressin reduces liver blood flow and may adversely affect hepatic function.
Cautions: patients with hypertension, advanced atherosclerosis, cardiac dysrhythmias or coronary insufficiency due to pressor and antidiuretic effects (which are less than those of arginine vasopressin).

Severe cardiac complications, including bradycardia, cardiac failure and myocardial infarction are well recognised. However, actual incidence may be low due to slow release of lysine-vasopressin from terlipressin and the relatively low doses used.

INTERACTIONS
None identified. However, the likely additive effect of

concurrent administration of other *pressor agents* should be recognised.

PREGNANCY
Use in pregnancy should be avoided, due to contraction of uterine smooth muscle, unless the potential benefit outweighs the risk to the fetus.

BREAST-FEEDING
No information is available.

SIDE-EFFECTS
Abdominal cramps, angina and cardiac arrhythmias. Glyceryl trinitrate, administered sublingually, is likely to be of benefit if anginal pain occurs, and may further lower portal pressure. Skin pallor, feeling of facial warmth, nausea, headache and feeling of weakness occur in approximately 15% of patients, fluid retention, tremor, sweating, vertigo, belching.

POISONING/TOXICITY
Hypertension is likely to be the most common acute effect, with or without cardiac ischaemia, and water retention. IV clonidine has been successfully used in the treatment of hypertension, but calcium antagonists may be more appropriate.

PHARMACOKINETIC PROPERTIES
Terlipressin is not absorbed from the gastrointestinal tract due to its high molecular weight and low lipid solubility. Plasma half-life (mean) of 24 minutes. Volume of distribution 0.7L/kg. Plasma protein binding is not known. Approximately 5-10% of administered terlipressin is converted to lysine-vasopressin over 2-10 hours. Only small quantities (<0.1% terlipressin; <0.05% lysine-vasopressin) are excreted as unchanged drug. Monitoring of serum sodium, potassium and fluid balance is essential.

EXCIPIENTS
See manufacturers SPC for further details.

LICENSED STATUS
Not licensed for use in children.

Testolactone

A derivative of testosterone.

USES
Precocious puberty; McCune-Albright syndrome (MAS); familial male precocious puberty (testotoxicosis).

PRESENTATION
Tablet: 50mg – named patient.

DOSAGE/ADMINISTRATION
Oral: starting dose in some references is 5mg/kg four times daily, increasing to a maximum of 10mg/kg four times daily; combined with spironolactone in testotoxicosis. However, since experience is limited, a paediatric endocrinologist should be consulted.

CONTRA-INDICATIONS & WARNINGS
History of sensitivity to testolactone.

INTERACTIONS
Oral anticoagulants; effects may be increased; monitor and adjust dose accordingly.

PREGNANCY
No adequate studies to date in pregnant women and safety has not been established; not recommended.

BREAST-FEEDING
No data available.

SIDE-EFFECTS
Paraesthesia, aches and oedema of the extremities, glossitis, anorexia, hot flushes, nausea, vomiting and diarrhoea, have occurred in patients receiving testolactone but have not been definitely attributed to the drug. Maculopapular erythema and an increase in blood pressure have been reported rarely as have alopecia alone or with associated growth disturbance but these subsided with continued therapy.

POISONING/TOXICITY
No data.

PHARMACOKINETIC PROPERTIES
Appears to be well absorbed from the gastrointestinal tract. It is metabolised in the liver and excreted in the urine.

LICENSED STATUS
Not licensed for use in the UK.

FURTHER INFORMATION
A German product is available via IDIS World Medicines.

Testosterone and esters

USES
Androgen deficiency; delayed puberty; priming of the pituitary for testing growth hormone secretion.

PRESENTATION
Capsule: (as undecanoate) 40mg in oily solution – Restandol®.
Implant: testosterone 100mg and 200mg – non-proprietary.
Injection (oily): (as enanthate) 250mg in 1mL, 1mL ampoule – non-proprietary.
Injection (oily): (as propionate) 50mg in 1mL, 2mL ampoule – Virormone®.
Injection (oily): testosterone propionate 20mg, testosterone phenylpropionate 40mg and testosterone isocaproate 40mg in 1mL – Sustanon 100®.
Injection (oily): testosterone propionate 30mg, testosterone phenylpropionate 60mg, testosterone isocaproate 60mg and testosterone decanoate 100mg in 1mL – Sustanon 250®.
Patch: releasing testosterone approx. 2.5mg per 24 hours and 5mg per 24 hours – Andropatch®.

DOSAGE/ADMINISTRATION
Androgen replacement
Orally: testosterone undecanoate starting dose 40mg alternate days, increasing slowly up to 120mg daily.

Delayed puberty
Dose/dose schedule depends on the product. An example is given but expert advice should be sought from a paediatric endocrinologist.
IM injection: 1mL of Sustanon 100® by deep IM injection every month for 3 doses.

Priming
IM injection: Sustanon 100® – 1mL by deep IM injection 3–5 days before the test of growth hormone secretion.

CONTRA-INDICATIONS & WARNINGS
Hypersensitivity to any of the ingredients.

INTERACTIONS
Enzyme-inducing agents may exert increasing or decreasing effects on testosterone levels. Therefore adjustment of the dose, and/or intervals between doses may be required.

PREGNANCY/BREAST-FEEDING
Contra-indicated; although not applicable to the indications discussed here.

SIDE-EFFECTS
In prepubertal boys, precocious sexual development, priapism, premature epiphyseal closure; water and sodium retention can also occur.

POISONING/TOXICITY
Acute muscular toxicity is very low and if overdose is given IM, toxic symptoms are not expected to be seen.

EXCIPIENTS
Contact manufacturers for further details.

LICENSED STATUS
Sustanon® and Virormone® are licensed for use in children, other preparations are not.

T

USES

For passive protection against tetanus after tetanus-prone injuries where active tetanus immunisation is incomplete or the wound is highly tetanus prone, or in the treatment of tetanus itself.

PRESENTATION

Human Tetanus Immunoglobulin (BPL) Injection: (solution containing 250 international units of tetanus antitoxin prepared from pooled plasma containing specific antibodies against *Clostridium tetani* toxin in each vial).
Each mL contains not less than 100 international units of tetanus antibody and 40-180mg of human protein of which at least 95% is gammaglobulin.

Human Tetanus Immunoglobulin: (for intravenous use) (Scottish National Blood Transfusion Service [SNBTS]) – injection for intravenous use containing 3g of plasma protein, of which ≥97% is IgG (potency of each vial is stated on the label). For use in treatment of confirmed or suspected tetanus disease.

Tetabulin®: injection (1mL solution containing 250 international units of tetanus antitoxin).
Each mL of solution contains 250 international units of tetanus antitoxin and 100-170mg of protein of which over 90% is gammaglobulin.

DOSAGE

Prevention: a single dose of 250 international units. If there is a risk of heavy contamination or following burns, or more than 24 hours have elapsed since injury, 500 international units should be given.

Tetanus immunisation following injuries

Immunisation Status	Clean Wound	Tetanus Prone Wound*	
	Vaccine	Vaccine	Human tetanus immunoglobulin
Fully immunised i.e. has received a total of 5 doses of tetanus vaccine at appropriate intervals as single antigen or in a combined vaccine	None required.	None required.	Only if risk especially high (e.g. contaminated with stable manure).
Primary immunisation (3 doses) complete and boosters incomplete but up to date	None required (unless next dose due soon and convenient to give now).	None required (unless next dose due soon and convenient to give now).	Only if risk especially high (as above).
Primary immunisation incomplete or boosters not up to date	A reinforcing dose of combined tetanus/diphtheria vaccine and further doses as required to complete the recommended schedule (to ensure future immunity).	A reinforcing dose of combined tetanus/diphtheria vaccine and further doses as required to complete the recommended schedule (to ensure future immunity).	Yes: one dose of human tetanus immunoglobulin in a different site.
Not immunised or immunisation status unknown or uncertain	An immediate dose of vaccine followed, if records are unavailable or confirm this is needed, by completion of a full 3 dose course of combined tetanus/diphtheria vaccine (to ensure future immunity).	An immediate dose of vaccine followed, if records are unavailable or confirm this is needed, by completion of a full 3 dose course of combined tetanus/diphtheria vaccine (to ensure future immunity).	Yes: one dose of human tetanus immunoglobulin in a different site.

*A tetanus prone wound is defined as:
☐ Any wound or burn sustained more than six hours before surgical treatment of the wound or burn.

☐ Any wound or burn at any interval after injury that shows one or more of the following characteristics:
- a significant degree of devitalised tissue
- puncture-type wound
- contact with soil or manure likely to harbour tetanus organisms
- clinical evidence of sepsis.

Treatment of tetanus: 150 international units/kg given IM in multiple sites or IV by infusion. Seek expert advice.

ADMINISTRATION
IM injection: Human Tetanus Immunoglobulin (BPL) and Tetabulin®.
IV injection: Human Tetanus Immunoglobulin (for intravenous use) (SNBTS).

CONTRA-INDICATIONS & WARNINGS
As the immunoglobulin is only indicated in someone at high risk of developing tetanus, which still has a high mortality, there are no absolute contra-indications. If a potential recipient has had an anaphylactic reaction to a previous dose of immunoglobulin, expert advice should be sought.

INTERACTIONS
Live viral vaccines, in particular *measles, mumps and rubella (MMR)*, given within the period 3 weeks before or 3 months after the immunoglobulin may be rendered ineffective. In such circumstances, once a period of 3 months has elapsed since administration of the immunoglobulin, either specific antibody levels should be measured or a repeat dose of the relevant vaccine(s) given. False positive results may occur with some serological testing due to the presence of antibodies other than those directed against tetanus toxin.

PREGNANCY
There are no systematic data, but there is no reason to believe it would harm the fetus. Pregnancy is not a contra-indication.

BREAST-FEEDING
There is no systematic data, but there is no reason to believe it would harm the suckling infant. Breast-feeding is not a contra-indication.

SIDE-EFFECTS
Pain at the site of intramuscular injection can be reduced by using multiple sites. Fever, cutaneous reactions and chills may occur. Nausea, vomiting, hypotension, tachycardia and allergic reactions have been reported rarely. Anaphylactic reactions are extremely rare.

POISONING/TOXICITY
Not known.

PHARMACOKINETIC PROPERTIES
After IM injection, measurable antibody levels are present at 20 minutes and peak levels are achieved after 2–3 days. Half-life is 21–22 days.

EXCIPIENTS
Human Tetanus Immunoglobulin (BPL): sodium chloride, glycine, sodium acetate trihydrate and sodium hydroxide.
Human Tetanus Immunoglobulin (for intravenous use) (SNBTS): sucrose, sodium chloride and trace amounts of porcine pepsin.
Tetabulin®: glycine.

LICENSED STATUS
Licensed for use as described.

Tetanus vaccine (adsorbed)

This vaccine is now extremely rarely indicated as a single antigen. It is usually given as part of a combination containing, at a minimum, diphtheria vaccine.

USES
Active protection against tetanus as part of the routine childhood immunisation schedule. It should be administered at the same time as the other indicated vaccines. The primary course is usually given at 8, 12 and 16 weeks of age. This is followed by a booster 3 years later and another at 13–18 years of age.

Subsequent boosters are only necessary under the following circumstances:
- ☐ If a highly tetanus prone wound is sustained or
- ☐ For travellers to areas where medical attention may not be available and where the last dose of a tetanus containing vaccine was given more than 10 years previously.

When tetanus vaccine is given in these above circumstances, it should usually be as a combination with diphtheria.

For indications for adsorbed tetanus vaccine and immunoglobulin in the management of wounds, see separate monograph for tetanus immunoglobulin.

Tetanus vaccine, as a single antigen, is only indicated when a potential recipient is thought to be hypersensitive to diphtheria vaccine.

PRESENTATIONS

Injection: (single dose suspension) – Adsorbed Tetanus Vaccine BP; Clostet®.
Each dose of vaccine contains not less than 40 international units of tetanus formol toxoid adsorbed on an aluminium carrier.

DOSAGE
0.5mL.

ADMINISTRATION
Deep SC or IM injection.

CONTRA-INDICATIONS & WARNINGS
As for vaccines generally; however, if the individual has suffered a tetanus prone wound and a dose of tetanus vaccine is indicated (see monograph on tetanus immunoglobulin), the vaccine should be given regardless of any intercurrent illness.

INTERACTIONS
It can be given simultaneously with (or at any interval before or after) any other vaccine. When a patient suffers a tetanus prone injury and both tetanus vaccine and immunoglobulin are indicated they can be given simultaneously but at different sites.

PREGNANCY
Tetanus toxoid is given to many pregnant women, predominantly in the second and third trimesters, in less developed countries to protect their newborn babies against tetanus. No fetal or neonatal problems have been reported, but it is not recommended in the UK.
If indicated in the management of a tetanus prone wound, the vaccine should be given.

BREAST-FEEDING
No information is available, but there are no grounds to believe it would be harmful. If indicated in the management of a tetanus prone wound, the vaccine should be given.

SIDE-EFFECTS
Local reactions such as pain, redness and swelling at the injection site may last for several days. Systemic reactions, including headache, lethargy, malaise, myalgia and pyrexia are much less common. Acute anaphylaxis and urticaria are rare. Although peripheral neuropathy has been reported to follow tetanus vaccination on rare occasions, it has not been convincingly shown to be a result of the vaccination. The incidence of reactions is greater with successive doses. Injection site granuloma, due to the aluminium component, are more likely to occur when the vaccine is not injected deep enough.

POISONING/TOXICITY
Doses of tetanus given more frequently than recommended are likely to give rise to an increased incidence and severity of local and systemic reactions.

PHARMACODYNAMIC PROPERTIES
Tetanus vaccine produces humoral immunity due to the stimulation of antibodies to tetanus toxin.

EXCIPIENTS
Clostet®: aluminium hydroxide and sodium thimerfonate.

LICENSED STATUS
Licensed for use as described.

FURTHER INFORMATION
Protect from light and store at 2–8°C.
Material of animal origin is used in the manufacturing process. There should be none of the original material present in the final product however, all such material is obtained from sources known to be free of BSE.

Tetracaine (amethocaine)

Local anaesthetic of the ester type which acts by reversibly blocking nerve conduction.

USES
Local topical anaesthesia of skin prior to venepuncture or venous cannulation.

PRESENTATION
Gel: tetracaine 4%, 1.5g tube – Ametop®.

DOSAGE

Route	Age				Frequency	Notes
	birth–1 month	1 month–2 years	2–12 years	12–18 years		
Topical	Not recommended	← the contents of one tube (approximately 1g) →			single application	This quantity is sufficient to anaesthetise an area up to 30cm² (6 x 5cm). Smaller areas of anaesthetised skin may be adequate in infants and small children.

ADMINISTRATION
The required amount of gel is applied to the centre of the area to be anaesthetised and covered with an occlusive dressing. Anaesthesia will be adequate for venepuncture after 30 minutes and for venous cannulation after 45 minutes. Anaesthesia remains for 4–6 hours in most patients after a single application.

CONTRA-INDICATIONS & WARNINGS
Contra-indicated in patients with known hypersensitivity to local anaesthetics of the ester type. Use with caution in children <1 month of age as metabolic pathways may not be fully developed. Tetracaine should not be applied to inflamed, traumatised or highly vascular areas, the eyes or ears. It is rapidly absorbed from mucous membranes and should never be used to provide anaesthesia for bronchoscopy or cystography. If blistering occurs, the gel should be removed immediately and the affected area treated symptomatically.

PREGNANCY
Topical application during pregnancy is unlikely to be a risk.

BREAST-FEEDING
Contact local Medicines Information Centre for advice.

SIDE-EFFECTS
Erythema, oedema and itch at the site of application. Very rarely blistering may occur.

POISONING/TOXICITY
Systemic toxicity is unlikely to be seen after application to intact skin but may occur if accidentally ingested or following absorption from mucous membranes, broken skin or highly vascular areas. Symptoms include light-headedness followed by sedation, circumoral paraesthesia and twitching, convulsions and cardiovascular collapse.

PHARMACOKINETIC PROPERTIES
Tetracaine is rapidly metabolised in the blood by plasma pseudocholinesterase.

EXCIPIENTS
See manufacturers SPC for further details.

LICENSED STATUS
Licensed for use ≥1 month of age. Not recommended for premature infants and infants <1 month of age.

Tetracosactide (tetracosactrin)

Tetracosactide is a synthetic polypeptide which consists of the first 24 of the 39 amino acids in the naturally occurring corticotropin (corticotrophin) (ACTH) and displays the same physiological properties. It is immunologically much less active than corticotropin.

USES

Synacthen Depot® – infantile spasms.
Synacthen® – testing the pituitary-adrenal axis (the low dose test has a higher reliability for confirming established adrenal failure).

PRESENTATION

IV/IM injection: (as acetate) 250 micrograms – Synacthen®.
IM depot injection: 1mg in 1mL – Synacthen Depot®.

DOSAGE

Indication	Route	Age				Frequency	Notes
		birth–1 month	1 month–2 years	2–12 years	12–18 years	(times daily)	
Infantile spasms	IM (depot injection)	–	500 microgram	–	–	1	Initial dose. Frequency of administration and duration of treatment are individually determined.
Standard dose test	IV (IM)	62.5 microgram	< 6 months 62.5 microgram ◄—— 250 microgram ——►			single dose	Do NOT use the depot injection. Plasma samples to be taken immediately before, 30 and 60 minutes after administration.
			> 6 months 125 microgram			single dose	
Low dose test	IV	◄—— 500 nanogram/1.73m² ——►				single dose	

ADMINISTRATION

IM: depot injection into the buttock.
IV: low test dose add 125 micrograms to 500mL of NaCl 0.9% to give 1 microgram in 4mL.

CONTRA-INDICATIONS & WARNINGS

History of hypersensitivity to tetracosactide or corticotropin. Depot injection contains benzyl alcohol so contra-indicated in neonates. Use with caution in patients with allergic disorders e.g. asthma. Also see the corticotrophin monograph.

PREGNANCY/ BREAST-FEEDING

Contra-indicated. Contact local Medicines Information Centre for advice.

SIDE-EFFECTS

Hypersensitivity reactions: in patients suffering from or susceptible to allergic disorders (e.g. asthma), this may take the form of anaphylactic shock. Hypersensitivity may be manifest as skin reactions at the injection site, dizziness, nausea, vomiting, urticaria, pruritus, flushing, malaise, dyspnoea, angioneurotic oedema and Quinke's oedema.

POISONING/TOXICITY

Overdose may lead to fluid retention and signs of hypercortisolism – symptomatic management only.

PHARMACOKINETIC PROPERTIES

Tetracosactide is absorbed onto a zinc phosphate complex which ensures the sustained release of the active substance from the IM injection site. After IM injection levels detectable by radioimmunoassay may persist for 12 hours. In the plasma, tetracosactide is broken down by serum endopeptidases into inactive oligopeptides and then by aminopeptidases into free amino acids, which are in turn excreted in the urine.

EXCIPIENTS

Synacthen Depot® includes benzyl alcohol. See manufacturers SPC for further details.

LICENSED STATUS

Synacthen® licensed for use in children as a diagnostic test for the investigation of adrenocortical insufficiency.
Synacthen Depot® not licensed for infantile spasms. Licensed for ≥3 years of age.

FURTHER INFORMATION

Tetracosactide should be stored in the refrigerator (2-8°C).
500 microgram tetracosactide depot injection is approximately equivalent to 40 units of corticotropin gel.

Antibiotic.

USES
Severe recurrent aphthous ulceration; acne (both indications >12 years only).
Oral use not discussed as tetracyclines are contra-indicated in children.

PRESENTATION
Capsule: 250mg – non-proprietary.
Tablets: 250mg – non-proprietary.
Topical solution: 2.2mg in 1mL, in 40% alcohol after reconstitution – Topicycline®.

DOSAGE/ADMINISTRATION

Indication	Route	Age	Frequency	Notes
		12–18 years	(times daily)	
Acne	Topical (skin)	Apply generously to entire affected area	2	Maximum duration of treatment is 10–12 weeks. May be repeated after interval of 12 weeks.
Aphthous ulceration	Local (mouthwash)	Contents of one 250mg capsule in a small amount of water	3–4	For 3 days. Hold in the mouth for 2–3 minutes. Do not swallow.

CONTRA-INDICATIONS & WARNINGS
Hypersensitivity. Avoid in renal impairment. Tetracycline is contra-indicated in children <12 years of age.

PREGNANCY
No data available when used topically or as a mouthwash. Oral administration contra-indicated.

BREAST-FEEDING
When used topically in acne, serum level of tetracycline is less than 0.1 microgram per mL, some of which may be excreted in milk. Avoid breast-feeding.

SIDE-EFFECTS
Topical preparation: some patients may experience stinging or tingling sensations, skin rashes and skin discolouration.
Mouthwash: fungal super-infection.

EXCIPIENTS
Contact manufacturers for further details.

LICENSED STATUS
Topical preparation is licensed for use >12 years. Mouthwash is unlicensed.

FURTHER INFORMATION
Topical preparation may stain skin and clothing yellow. Advise patient to lightly wash affected area 1 hour after application. Use within 8 weeks of reconstitution.

Tetrahydrobiopterin

USES
Control of phenylalanine levels in defects of tetrahydrobiopterin synthesis. Given in conjunction with amine precursors.

PRESENTATION
Tablet: 10mg.

DOSAGE

Route	Age				Frequency (times daily)	Notes
	birth–1 month	1 month–2 years	2–12 years	12–18 years		
Oral	←	1–3mg/kg		→	1	Some patients may respond to larger doses (5-20mg/kg/day) as it may increase CSF amine metabolites and produce an improvement in symptoms. May remove the need to treat with amines.

Note: in some patients, large doses (5-20mg/kg/**day**) increase CSF amine metabolites, occasionally removing the need to treat with amines.

ADMINISTRATION
Oral: the tablets may be dissolved in a little water or orange juice immediately before use. They may become slightly coloured but if dark yellow spots appear they should not be used.

CONTRA-INDICATIONS & WARNINGS, INTERACTIONS, PREGNANCY, BREAST-FEEDING
No information available.

SIDE-EFFECTS
No side-effects reported.

PHARMACODYNAMIC PROPERTIES
Decreases phenylalanine levels as tetrahydrobiopterin is a proton donor in the conversion of phenylalanine to tyrosine. Does not penetrate the brain well.

EXCIPIENTS
Contact manufacturer for further details.

LICENSED STATUS
Not licensed for use in the UK.

FURTHER INFORMATION
Tetrahydrobiopterin is not recommended in dihydrobiopterin reductase deficiency; though high doses (20mg/kg/**day**) can lower phenylalanine levels, dietary treatment is preferable. Tablets are stored in the freezer. They can be stored at room temperature for up to 2 months. Available from IDIS World Medicines.

THAM (trometamol) (tris(hydroxymethyl) aminomethane)

An organic amine base which when infused intravenously causes an increase in urinary pH and an osmotic diuresis.

USES
Correction of metabolic acidosis when sodium bicarbonate is unsuitable; also used during cardiac bypass surgery.

PRESENTATION
Injection: 3.6% (0.3M, 0.3mmol per 1mL), 5mL ampoule – manufactured 'special; 7.2% (0.6M, 0.6mmol per 1mL), 5mL ampoule – manufactured 'special'.

DOSAGE
Blood gases should be checked before, during and after administration.
The total number of mmol of alkali required is calculated using the equations outlined in the table.
Only half the base deficit should be corrected initially. Blood gases should be checked before further correction.

Age	Total mmol of alkali (bicarbonate)	Notes
Premature neonate	0.5–0.6 x base deficit (mmol/L) x weight (kg)	
Full term neonate	0.4 x base deficit (mmol/L) x weight (kg)	Do not exceed a total dose
1 month–2 ycars	0.3 x base deficit (mmol/L) x weight (kg)	of 10mmol/kg in 12 hours.
2–12 years	0.3 x base deficit (mmol/L) x weight (kg)	
12–18 years	0.25–0.3 x base deficit (mmol/L) x weight (kg)	

NB 1mL of 7.2% THAM is equivalent to 1mmol of bicarbonate (alkali).

ADMINISTRATION
IV: dilute to at least 3.6% with glucose 5% or Water for Injections. In fluid restricted patients 7.2% can be given undiluted via a long line or central line. DO NOT exceed a rate of 0.5mL/kg/minute (7.2% solution); or 1mL/kg/minute (3.6% solution). The 7.2% solution is hyperosmolar and the 3.6% solution is isosmotic (unless prepared by dilution of the 7.2% with 5% glucose).

CONTRA-INDICATIONS & WARNINGS
Contra-indicated in anuria and should be used with caution in renal impairment. It is also contra-indicated in patients with chronic respiratory acidosis.

INTERACTIONS
No data available.

PREGNANCY
Hypoglycaemic effect in the mother could be detrimental to the fetus. Contact local Medicines Information Centre for advice.

BREAST-FEEDING
Contact local Medicines Information Centre for advice.

SIDE-EFFECTS
Respiratory depression and hypoglycaemia may occur and respiration may need assistance especially in patients with respiratory acidosis. Hyperkalaemia has been reported in patients with renal impairment. Haemorrhagic liver necrosis has been reported in neonates with respiratory distress syndrome who had hypertonic THAM administered via the umbilical vein. Local inflammation, phlebitis and vasospasm have been reported following IV administration. Extreme care should be taken to avoid extravasation.

POISONING/TOXICITY
Over rapid or full correction of acidosis may result in increased CSF acidosis and apnoea.

LICENSED STATUS
Unlicensed for use in all ages.

FURTHER INFORMATION
Injections available from several NHS manufacturing units.

Theophylline

A methylxanthine. It has a bronchodilation effect in asthma.

USES
Prophylaxis and treatment of reversible bronchospasm associated with asthma.

PRESENTATION
Capsule (modified release): 60mg, 125mg and 250mg – Slo-Phyllin®.
Liquid: 60mg in 5mL – Nuelin®.
Tablet: 125mg (scored) – Nuelin®.
Tablet (modified release, all scored): 175mg and 250mg – Nuelin SA®; 200mg and 300mg – Theo-dur®; 200mg, 300mg and 400mg – Uniphyllin Continus®.

DOSAGE
Child

Indication	Route	Age			Frequency	Notes
		1 month–2 years	2–12 years	12–18 years	(times daily)	
Asthma	Oral/normal release preparations	>6 months 5mg/kg	← 5mg/kg →		3–4	Starting dose. Adjust dose according to clinical response and plasma levels.
	Oral/ modified release preparations	>6 months 12mg/kg	2–7 years 12mg/kg	8mg/kg	2	Maximum 500mg per dose. Starting dose. Adjust dose according to clinical response and plasma levels.
			8–12 years 10mg/kg		2	

ADMINISTRATION
Oral: modified release preparations may need to be given 3 times daily in young children (maintain the same total daily dose as outlined in table above). Theo-dur® Nuelin® SA and Uniphyllin® continus tablets MUST NOT be crushed or chewed, but should be swallowed whole or as a half. All strengths of Theo-dur®, Uniphyllin® and the 250mg strength of Nuelin® SA are scored and can be halved. Nuelin® tablets are scored, and can be halved. They are soluble in water. Ideally tablets and liquid should be taken after food. The pellets inside Slo-phyllin® capsules can be sprinkled onto a spoonful of soft food. Do not suck or chew the pellets.

CONTRA-INDICATIONS & WARNINGS
Should not be given concurrently with ephedrine in children. Hypersensitivity to theophylline or other xanthines. Seizures can be exacerbated in patients taking theophylline preparations. Theophylline clearance is reduced in liver disease (increases theophylline levels); reduce dose. Bioequivalence of different brands of oral theophylline cannot be guaranteed. Patients should not change brands once stabilised, unless plasma level monitoring is carried out. Brand names should be stated on prescriptions. Porphyria.

INTERACTIONS
Increased levels with *cimetidine, erythromycin, ciprofloxacin, thiabendazole, mexiletine, norfloxacin* and possibly *fluconazole, isoniazid, diltiazem* and *verapamil.*
Reduced levels with *rifampicin, carbamazepine, phenobarbital (phenobarbitone), phenytoin, primidone* and *sulfinpyrazone.*
There is an increased risk of hypokalaemia with high dose *salbutamol, salmeterol,* and *terbutaline.*

PREGNANCY
There are no reports linking theophylline with congenital defects. Theophylline crosses the placenta and newborn infants may have therapeutic levels. Transient tachycardia, irritability, and vomiting have been reported in newborns of mothers on theophylline and may indicate toxic doses.

BREAST-FEEDING
Theophylline is excreted in breast milk and has been

shown to cause irritability in infants. It is therefore recommended that a mother feeds her baby just prior to taking her next dose, when plasma theophylline levels are expected to be low.

SIDE-EFFECTS
Tachycardia, palpitations, arrhythmias, nausea, gastrointestinal disturbances, headache and convulsions. Introducing theophylline gradually will help minimise side-effects. If adverse effects do occur then the next dose should be missed and subsequent doses reduced to the minimum required to maintain control of symptoms. Significant side-effects can occur in the newborn when the plasma levels exceeds 14mg/L and in older children when the level exceeds 20mg/L.

POISONING/TOXICITY
Symptoms: nausea, vomiting, electrolyte imbalance, gastrointestinal irritation, tachycardia, convulsions and hypotension.
Treatment: repeated doses of activated charcoal should be considered. Charcoal haemoperfusion may be necessary. Blood glucose, electrolytes, arterial gases, and pH should be monitored. Intensive support may be required to maintain respiration and cardiovascular function. Convulsions may be controlled by diazepam. Serum theophylline levels should be measured 4 hours after ingestion and at 4-12 hourly intervals thereafter if symptoms are severe. Modified release preparations may show a slow onset and prolonged effects.

T

PHARMACOKINETIC PROPERTIES

Rapidly and completely absorbed from liquid preparations, capsules and uncoated tablets. The rate of absorption is decreased by the presence of food.

Sustained release preparations have variability in their absorption, and in the effect of food. If patients are to be transferred from one brand to another then the dose should be retitrated.

Approximately 40% bound to plasma proteins, but in neonates, or in the presence of liver disease, protein binding is reduced. Metabolised in the liver, and the metabolites are excreted in the urine; partly metabolised to caffeine in the liver in the neonatal period. In adults about 10% of a dose is excreted unchanged in urine, however, in neonates this can be up to 50%. The serum half-life in children is about 3-5 hours, but in neonates and premature infants it is about 15-58 hours.

Optimum serum concentration of theophylline is 10-20mg/L when used to treat asthma. For sustained release preparations blood samples should be taken 4-6 hours after a dose and at least 3 days after any dosage adjustment. For liquid preparation, and standard release preparation, samples should be taken 1-2 hours after dose. Measure levels 5 days after starting therapy.

The following table is a guide as to how to interpret theophylline levels when using it in the treatment of asthma.

Plasma level	Result	Directions
<10mg/L	Too low	Increase dose by 25%
10-20mg/L	Correct	Maintain dose
21-25mg/L	Too high	Decrease dose by 10%
26-30mg/L	Too high	Miss next dose and decrease subsequent doses by 25%
>30mg/L	Too high	Miss next 2 doses and decrease subsequent doses by 50%

EXCIPIENTS

See manufacturers SPC for further details.

LICENSED STATUS

Nuelin® liquid is licensed for >2 years of age.
Nuelin® tablets, Nuelin® SA and Uniphyllin Continus® are licensed for >6 years of age.
Slo-Phyllin® capsules are licensed for >2 years of age.
Theo-dur® is licensed for use in children and adults.

Thiamine

A water-soluble vitamin; an essential co-enzyme for carbohydrate metabolism in the form of the diphosphate.

USES

Maple syrup urine disease (MSUD) (thiamine responsive variants).
Anecdotal reports of use in congenital lactic acidosis.
Anecdotal reports of use in defects of the mitochondrial respiratory chain (usually with other substances and almost always without success).

PRESENTATION

Tablet: 25mg, 50mg, 100mg and 300mg – non-proprietary.
Injection: 100mg in 1ml -named patient.

DOSAGE

Indication	Route	Age				Frequency (times daily)	Notes
		birth–1 month	1 month–2 years	2–12 years	12–18 years		
Congenital lactic acidosis	Oral	←	100–300mg		→	1	

T

DOSAGE continued

Indication	Route	Age				Frequency (times daily)	Notes
		birth–1 month	1 month–2 years	2–12 years	12–18 years		
MSUD	Oral	←	10–300mg		→	1	A wide range of doses have been used. A trial of thiamine therapy for at least 3 weeks is advisable in every newly diagnosed MSUD patient to determine thiamine responsiveness.

CONTRA-INDICATIONS & WARNINGS, INTERACTIONS, PREGNANCY, BREAST-FEEDING, POISONING/TOXICITY
No information available.

SIDE-EFFECTS
Seldom occur; hypersensitivity reactions have occurred following parenteral administration.

PHARMACOKINETIC PROPERTIES
Small amounts of thiamine are well absorbed from the gastrointestinal tract but absorption of doses larger than 5mg is limited. Well distributed to most body tissues. Amounts in excess of the body's requirements are excreted in the urine as unchanged thiamine or as metabolites.

LICENSED STATUS
Not licensed for metabolic indications.

FURTHER INFORMATION
Injection available John Bell & Croydon.

Thiopental (thiopentone) sodium

Short-acting barbiturate.

USES
IV induction of general anaesthesia; control of prolonged status epilepticus.

PRESENTATION
Injection: 500mg for reconstitution with Water for Injections to 2.5% solution – non-proprietary.

DOSAGE

Route	Age				Frequency	Notes
	birth–1 month	1 month–2 years	2–12 years	12–18 years		
IV bolus	←		4mg/kg	→	single dose	Status epilepticus. Ventilation facilities must be available. Up to 10mg/kg has been used.
IV infusion	2.5mg/kg/hour	←	2–8mg/kg/hour	→	continuous	For ventilated patients.

Only to be given by a trained anaesthetist/intensivist.

Reduce dose in severe hepatic disease.

ADMINISTRATION
For IV infusion dilute in NaCl 0.9%. Stable for 24 hours. Avoid rapid IV injection as causes hypotension and reduced cardiac output. Fractional administration provides closer control, greater flexibility and helps prevent overdosage.

CONTRA-INDICATIONS & WARNINGS

Contra-indications: porphyria, dyspnoea or respiratory obstruction e.g. acute severe asthma.

Cautions: should only be used by a trained anaesthetist or intensivist. Ventilation must be available when used to treat status epilepticus. Use should not generally be for more than 48 hours as delayed recovery of consciousness has been encountered with prolonged use. Avoid intra-arterial injection and extravasation as tissue necrosis may result due to the alkaline pH of 10.6. Caution in patients with asthma or pharyngeal infection as can cause cough, larnygospasm and bronchospasm. Caution in hypotension, hypovolaemia, shock, severe anaemia, hyperkalaemia, severe cardiovascular disease, hepatic and renal dysfunction, myasthenia gravis, muscular dystrophy, adrenocortical insufficiency, raised intracranial pressure, metabolic disorders.

INTERACTIONS

Thiopental is an inducer of liver enzymes and may reduce blood levels of many drugs metabolised by the liver including *antiepileptics*. *Sulphonamides* may potentiate the effects of thiopental. *ACE inhibitors, angiotensin II antagonists, antihypertensives* and *anti-psychotics* may increase the hypotensive effects of thiopental. Some *phenothiazines*, especially *promethazine*, can increase excitatory phenomena produced by thiopental, *cyclizine* may have a similar effect. *Opiates* can potentiate CNS depression.

PREGNANCY

There is epidemiological and clinical evidence of safety in pregnancy. Thiopental readily crosses the placenta and the dose in pregnant women should not exceed 250mg. May depress neonatal respiration if used during labour.

BREAST-FEEDING

Very little appears in breast milk after use during routine operative anaesthesia. It should, however be used with caution in breast-feeding mothers as it can reduce milk flow and small amounts in the milk may cause enzyme induction in the infant.

SIDE-EFFECTS

Cardiovascular: hypotension, reduced cardiac output, myocardial depression, cardiac arrhythmias.
Respiratory: respiratory depression. Cough, sneeze, hiccup, laryngospasm, bronchospasm and apnoea can occur especially at induction. Hypersensitivity reactions can occur.
CNS: hypothermia, post-op shivering, cerebral shutdown. Vertigo, disorientation, amnesia and sedation may be prolonged post-op.
Local: pain and necrosis from extravasation of alkaline injection solution, headache.
Neuromuscular: muscle twitching, jerking – especially at induction.

POISONING/TOXICITY

Symptoms: thiopental has a narrow therapeutic margin, overdosage may occur with respiratory depression, circulatory failure, hypothermia, hypotension and cardiac arrhythmias.
Treatment: ventilate with oxygen and use supportive measures including fluids, inotropes and vasopressors as required.

PHARMACOKINETIC PROPERTIES

Highly lipid soluble, rapidly penetrates the CNS within 30 seconds, then rapid redistribution into fat stores. Duration of action after IV bolus is 5-30 minutes. About 80% plasma protein bound. Metabolised by the liver slowly due to slow release from fat stores. In neonates, liver elimination is slower, elimination half-life at birth is 20-30 hours, double that found in adults, in children it is around 6 hours. Metabolism is primarily to inactive metabolites, but a small amount is converted to pentobarbital. Repeated or continuous administration can lead to accumulation in fatty tissue and this can result in prolonged anaesthesia and respiratory and cardiovascular depression. Accumulation in the neonate is almost inevitable if infusion is continued for more than a few hours.

LICENSED STATUS

Licensed for use in children and adults by bolus injection by a trained anaesthetist or intensivist only. Infusion is not a licensed route of administration.

T

Thiotepa

Alkylating agent.

USES

High dose therapy with progenitor cell support in the treatment of recurrent CNS primitive neuroectodermal tumours.

PRESENTATION

Injection: powder for reconstitution, 15mg – Goldshield.

DOSAGE
** Always consult the current treatment protocol for details of dosage and scheduling. **

ADMINISTRATION
IV: reconstitute the contents of a vial with 1.5mL Water for Injections to provide a solution containing thiotepa 10mg in 1mL (consult current protocol for infusion details).

CONTRA-INDICATIONS & WARNINGS
Previous spinal irradiation increases myelosuppression. Renal or hepatic impairment.

INTERACTIONS
No specific interactions reported.

PREGNANCY/BREAST-FEEDING
Should not normally be administered unless the benefit outweighs the risk to the fetus or child.

SIDE-EFFECTS
Myelosuppression (sometimes late), particularly thrombocytopenia and neutropenia.

POISONING/TOXICITY
Full supportive measures.

PHARMACOKINETIC PROPERTIES
No specific data for children. Following IV injection, thiotepa is metabolised to tepa, which is also an active alkylating agent. Clearance is biphasic with an initial half-life between 8-20 minutes and a terminal half-life between 1.3-2 hours. Thiotepa has excellent CSF penetration.

LICENSED STATUS
Not licensed for use in children.

Tiabendazole (thiabendazole)

Anthelmintic.

USES
Strongyloidiasis, cutaneous larva migrans, dracunculiasis (guinea worm), visceral larva migrans, trichinosis.
Second-line treatment of *Necator americanus* and *Ancylostoma duodenale* (hookworm) and trichuriasis (whipworm).

PRESENTATION
Tablet: 500mg (chewable) – Mintezol® (imported).
Syrup: 500mg in 5mL – Mintezol® (imported).
Suspension: 312.5mg in 5mL – Triasox® (imported).
Topical preparation: 10% – may be extemporaneously prepared.

DOSAGE
Dosage depends on the body weight of the patient and is independent of the condition being treated. Duration of therapy depends on the particular nematode infection.

Indication	Route	Age			Frequency (times daily)	Notes
		1 month–2 years	2–12 years	12–18 years		
Trichinosis	Oral	←	25mg/kg (maximum dose 1.5g)	→	2	For 2–4 days and up to 7 if necessary.
Trichuriasis	Oral	←	25mg/kg (maximum dose 1.5g)	→	2	For 2 days.
Toxocariasis (visceral larva migrans)	Oral	←	25mg/kg (maximum dose 1.5g)	→	2	For 7 days. Limited efficacy.

DOSAGE continued

Indication	Route	Age			Frequency (times daily)	Notes
		1 month– 2 years	2–12 years	12–18 years		
Strongyloidiasis	Oral	←	25mg/kg (maximum dose 1.5g)	→	2	For 2 days. In disseminated infection give for 5-7 days.
Dracunculiasis	Oral	←	25mg/kg (maximum dose 1.5g)	→	2	1 day (1-2 visible worms).
		←	50mg/kg (maximum dose 1.5g)	→	2	1 day (3-9 visible worms).
		←	50mg/kg (maximum dose 1.5g)	→	2	1 day, repeat once after 5-8 days (>9 visible worms).
Cutaneous larva migrans (Ancyclostoma spp and uncinariasis)	Oral	←	25mg/kg (maximum dose 1.5g)	→	2	For 2 days. Repeat course if active lesions still present 2 days after completion.
	Topical	← 10% syrup or ointment →			2 (under occlusive dressing) OR 4-6	Apply 5cm around advancing end and to worm track for 1-14 days after lesion inactivation. Use as alternative or adjunct to oral route.

ADMINISTRATION
Tablets can be crushed although not recommended by the manufacturer. Take with meals and chew before swallowing. Syrup/suspension has been used topically for cutaneous larva migrans in place of an extemporaneously prepared cream. Topical preparation is prepared extemporaneously by crushing a 500mg tablet and triturating into 5g petroleum jelly or aqueous cream. Apply over the track of the worm.

CONTRA-INDICATIONS & WARNINGS
Tiabendazole is not suitable for the treatment of mixed infections with ascaris because it may cause these worms to migrate to other body organs causing serious complications.
Contra-indicated if any hypersensitivity reactions occur. Therapy should be discontinued immediately and not resumed (fatal cases of Stevens-Johnson syndrome have been associated with therapy). Contra-indicated in pregnancy or lactation.
Caution in renal or hepatic impairment, anaemic patients, dehydrated or malnourished patients.

INTERACTIONS
Plasma concentration of *theophylline* may be increased. Monitor effects of concurrent use and reduce *theophylline* dose accordingly. A 50% *theophylline* dosage reduction may be necessary.

PREGNANCY
Contra-indicated due to teratogenesis in animal studies. However, no reports of human teratogenesis have been located. Use only if parasite is causing clinical disease or may cause public health problems.

BREAST-FEEDING
Contact local Medicines Information Centre for advice.

SIDE-EFFECTS
Anorexia, nausea, vomiting, dizziness, diarrhoea, headache, pruritus, drowsiness, hypersensitivity reactions (including fever, chills, angioedema, rashes, erythema multiforme and Stevens-Johnson syndrome). Rarely tinnitus, collapse, parenchymal liver damage and visual disorders.

POISONING/TOXICITY
Toxic disturbance of the gastrointestinal and CNS systems: treat symptomatically and supportively. No known antidote.

PHARMACOKINETIC PROPERTIES
Readily absorbed from the gastrointestinal tract. Peak plasma concentrations after 1-2 hours. Metabolised in liver and excreted principally as glucuronide or sulphate conjugates. 90% recovered in urine within 48 hours of ingestion but only 5% in faeces. Absorption may occur from preparations applied to skin or eyes.

T

EXCIPIENTS
Contact manufacturer for further details.

LICENSED STATUS
Not licensed for use in the UK. Cream is an extemporaneous preparation and as such is unlicensed.

FURTHER INFORMATION
Tablets, syrup and suspension available from IDIS World Medicines.

Tiagabine

Antiepileptic.

USES
For adjunctive treatment of partial seizures with or without secondary generalisation.

PREPARATION
Tablet: (scored) 5mg, 10mg and 15mg – Gabitril®.

DOSAGE

Route	Age		Frequency	Notes
	12–18 years		**(times daily)**	
Oral	← 5mg →		2	Initial dose. Increase at weekly intervals in steps of 5-10mg daily.
	← 15mg →		2-3	Adjunctive therapy *with enzyme inducers.* Usual maintenance dose. Doses above 30mg must be given in three divided doses.
	← 7.5-15mg →		2	Adjunctive therapy *with non-enzyme inducers.* Usual maintenance dose. Doses above 30mg/day can be given in three divided doses.

Dose adjustment in hepatic impairment
In mild to moderate hepatic impairment the initial daily maintenance dosage should be 5-10mg given once or twice daily. Tiagabine should not be used in patients with severely impaired hepatic function.

CONTRA-INDICATIONS & WARNINGS
Avoid in severe liver or renal impairment. Avoid abrupt withdrawal. If spontaneous bruising occurs check full blood count including platelets. May aggravate idiopathic generalised epilepsy and has precipitated absence seizures.

INTERACTIONS
Antiepileptic agents that induce hepatic enzymes (such as *phenytoin, carbamazepine, phenobarbital (phenobarbitone)* and *primidone)* enhance the metabolism of tiagabine.

PREGNANCY /BREAST-FEEDING
Lack of data so manufacturer advises to avoid unless benefits outweigh risks. Contact local Medicines Information Centre for advice.

SIDE-EFFECTS
Gastrointestinal: diarrhoea.
CNS: dizziness, tiredness, nervousness, tremor. Visual field defects have been reported.

POISONING/TOXICITY
Symptoms of overdosage include somnolence, dizziness, ataxia or inco-ordination and, in more severe instances, mute and withdrawn appearance of the patient. Give supportive therapy and contact UK National Poisons Information Service.

PHARMACOKINETICS
Food decreases rate but not extent of absorption. Rapidly absorbed by the oral route and 96% bound to plasma protein. Extensively metabolised in the liver to inactive metabolites. Elimination half-life is 7-9 hours but 2-3 hours when enzymes induced.

EXCIPIENTS
See manufacturers SPC for further details.

LICENSED STATUS
Licensed for ≥12 years of age.

Tick-borne encephalitis (TBE) vaccine

USES
To provide active immunity to tick-borne encephalitis. Recommended for travellers ≥1 year old who will be walking, camping or working in late spring and summer in warm heavily forested parts of Central and Eastern Europe and Scandinavia.

PRESENTATION
Injection: (single dose suspension in pre-filled syringe) – Encepur® children.
Each dose of 0.25mL contains 0.75 micrograms of the inactivated TBE (virus strain K23) virus grown in chick fibroblast cell culture and inactivated with formaldehyde.

Injection: (single dose suspension in pre-filled syringe) – Encepur®.
Each dose of 0.5mL contains 1.5 micrograms of the inactivated TBE (virus strain K23) virus grown in chick fibroblast cell culture and inactivated with formaldehyde.

Injection: (single dose suspension in pre-filled syringe) – FSME-IMMUN 0.25mL Junior®.
Each dose of 0.25mL contains 1-1.38 micrograms of TBE virus antigen. (Neudoerfl) derived from virus grown on chick embryo cells and inactivated with formaldehyde.

Injection: (single dose suspension in pre-filled syringe) – FSME-IMMUN 0.5mL®.
Each dose of 0.5mL contains 2-3.5 micrograms of TBE virus antigen (Neudoerfl) derived from virus grown on chick embryo cells and inactivated with formaldehyde.

Encepur® children and FSME-IMMUN 0.25mL Junior® are licensed for use in children ≥1 year old and <12 years old. Encepur children® and FSME-IMMUN® are for use in those ≥12 years of age.

DOSAGE
There are a number of possible regimens.
Encepur® children.
(a) 0.25mL at 0, 1-3 months and then another after a further 9-12 months. A booster dose may be given after 18 months if there is continuing exposure.
(b) 0.25mL at days 0,7 and 21 days, and 12-18 months.
The same regimen, but with a dose of 0.5mL is suitable for those ≥12 years of age.
A booster dose may be given after 18 months if there is continuing exposure.

Encepur®.
As for Encepur® children, except each dose is 0.5mL.

FSME-IMMUN 0.25mL Junior®.
(a) 0.25mL at 0, 1-3 months and then another after a further 9-12months.
This regimen may be accelerated if the course is started in summer. A booster dose may be given after 3 years if there is continuing exposure.

FSME-IMMUN 0.5mL®.
As for FSME-IMMUN 0.25mL Junior®, except each dose is 0.5mL.

ADMINISTRATION
IM or deep SC.

T

CONTRA-INDICATIONS & WARNINGS
As for vaccines generally.

INTERACTIONS
None reported.

PREGNANCY/BREAST-FEEDING
No data available.

SIDE-EFFECTS
These are uncommon. Reactions at the site of the

injection, local lymphadenopathy, fatigue, limb pain, fever, nausea and headache may occur. Fever is reported in children, particularly after the first dose. A transient pruritic rash may rarely occur. Neurological symptoms have occurred on rare occasions following administration of the vaccine.

POISONING/TOXICITY
No data available.

EXCIPIENTS
Encepur® and Encepur® children: aluminium hydroxide, formaldehyde, salts, sucrose, and trace amounts of chlortetracycline, gentamicin and neomycin.
FSME-IMMUN 0.25mL Junior® and FSME-IMMUN 0.5mL®: aluminium hydroxide, human albumin (prepared from donors resident in BSE-free areas), formaldehyde, protamine sulphate, neomycin sulphate, gentamicin sulphate, sodium chloride, disodium phosphate dihydrate, potassium dihydrogenphosphate.

LICENSED STATUS
Not licensed in UK, but it is recommended in the Department of Health book *Immunisation against Infectious Disease 1996*. Encepur® is available on a named patient basis from Chiron Vaccines Limited and FSME-IMMUN® from Baxter Healthcare Limited.

FURTHER INFORMATION
Store at 2–8°C and do not freeze.
At the time of writing (May 2003), the launch of a licensed preparation for children and adults, 'Tico Vac', had been delayed due to concerns about the frequency and severity of febrile reactions. Professionals considering the use of a tick borne encephalitis vaccine should consult with their local travel health specialist as the situation is in a state of flux.

Tinidazole

5-nitroimidazole derivative which has antimicrobial actions against *Giardia lamblia*, *Entamoeba histolytica* and *Trichomonas vaginalis*, and against most obligate anaerobic bacteria.

USES
Amoebiasis; intestinal disease (colitis). Giardiasis. *Trichomonas vaginalis*.

PRESENTATION
Tablet: 500mg (film coated) – Fasigyn®.

DOSAGE

Route	Age			Frequency (times daily)	Notes
	1 month–2 years	2–12 years	12–18 years		
Oral	← 50–60mg/kg →		2g	1	Single dose for *Trichomonas vaginalis* and giardiasis, repeated once if necessary. Amoebiasis: give for 3 days for intestinal disease and 5 days for liver abscess. Follow with a luminal amoebicide (diloxanide furoate).

ADMINISTRATION
Oral: take during or after a meal. The cut surface of the tablet has a very bitter taste and so it is difficult for children to take less than a whole tablet.

CONTRA-INDICATIONS & WARNINGS
Contra-indicated during the first trimester of pregnancy, in patients with organic neurologic disorders and in those with known hypersensitivity to tinidazole.

INTERACTIONS
Alcohol: disulfiram-like reaction is possible.

PREGNANCY
Tinidazole crosses the placental barrier. Since the effects on fetal development are unknown use during the first trimester is contra-indicated. There is no evidence that it is harmful during the latter stages of pregnancy but potential benefits to the mother should be weighed against possible hazards to the fetus if used in the second or third trimesters.

BREAST-FEEDING
Tinidazole is excreted into breast milk and may continue to appear for more than 72 hours after administration. Women should not breast-feed until 3 days after stopping treatment.

SIDE-EFFECTS
Generally infrequent, mild and self-limiting and can include nausea, vomiting, anorexia, diarrhoea, metallic taste, abdominal pain, and rarely headache, tiredness and hypersensitivity reactions (occasionally severe with rash, urticaria, pruritus and angioneurotic oedema).

POISONING/TOXICITY
No specific antidote; treatment is symptomatic and supportive. Tinidazole is easily dialysable.

PHARMACOKINETIC PROPERTIES
Rapidly and almost completely absorbed following oral administration with peak levels occurring 30 minutes to 2 hours after ingestion. 100% bioavailability; rapidly distributed through body tissues with good penetration into CSF. Elimination half-life is 12-14 hours. Unchanged drug and metabolites are excreted in the urine and, to a lesser extent, in the faeces.

EXCIPIENTS
Includes sucrose.

LICENSED STATUS
Licensed for use in children and adults for the indications stated.

Tinzaparin sodium

A low molecular weight heparin (LMWH).

USES
Prophylaxis and treatment of thromboembolic disease.

PRESENTATION
Injection: 10,000 units in 1mL; 2500 units in 0.25mL, 3500 units in 0.35mL, 4500 units in 0.45mL prefilled syringes and 2mL vial – Innohep®.
Injection: 20,000 units in 1mL; 10,000 units in 0.5mL, 14,000 units in 0.7mL, 18,000 units in 0.9mL prefilled syringes and 2mL vial – Innohep®.

DOSAGE

Indication	Route	Age			Frequency (times daily)	Notes
		1 month– 2 years	2–12 years	12–18 years		
Prophylaxis of venous thrombo-embolism	SC	←	50 units /kg	→	1	
Treatment of deep vein thrombosis and pulmonary embolism	SC	←	175 units/kg	→	1	Used for at least 6 days. Tinzaparin therapy does not require routine monitoring in patients with normal renal and hepatic function.

Experience of the use in children is very limited.

T

Renal impairment
Patients with severe renal impairment may require reduced doses. Both trough and peak anti-Factor Xa activity must be monitored on a daily basis. Take a trough immediately prior to the next dose and a peak level 3-4 hours after the dose. Trough values should be around 0.2 units/mL and peak values should be between 0.8-1 unit/mL.

CONTRA-INDICATIONS & WARNINGS
Contra-indications include generalised haemorrhagic tendency, uncontrolled severe hypotension, active peptic ulcer, septic endocarditis and thrombocytopenia in patients with a positive *in vitro* aggregation test in the presence of tinzaparin. Care should be taken when administered to patients with severe liver or kidney insufficiency who are to undergo surgery, also if patient has recently suffered from cerebral haemorrhage, trauma and/or had recent surgery to the central nervous system. Tinzaparin is to be used with caution in patients with known hypersensitivity to heparin or to other low molecular weight heparins. The presence of sulphites in the 20,000 unit/mL preparations may (especially in patients with asthma) lead to hypersensitivity (with bronchospasm and shock).

INTERACTIONS
It is recommended that agents which affect platelet function or aggregation or blood coagulation should be used with caution in patients receiving tinzaparin.

PREGNANCY
Animal studies show no embryotoxic or teratogenic effects but tinzaparin should not be used in pregnant patients unless no safer alternative is available. There is no evidence that tinzaparin crosses the placental barrier during the second trimester of pregnancy. Contact local Medicines Information Centre for advice.

BREAST-FEEDING
It is not known whether tinzaparin is excreted in human breast milk. The oral absorption of tinzaparin is unlikely. Contact local Medicines Information Centre for advice.

SIDE-EFFECTS
Systemic allergic reactions have been reported extremely rarely. Skin rashes and mild bruising may follow subcutaneous injection, skin necrosis has also been reported and if it occurs treatment must be withdrawn immediately. Thrombocytopenia and hyperkalaemia may also occur.

POISONING/TOXICITY
Accidental overdose following parenteral administration may produce haemorrhagic complications. This can be reversed by intravenous administration of 1% protamine sulphate solution. As a rule, 1mg of protamine sulphate neutralises the effect of 100 anti-Factor Xa international units of tinzaparin. The anti-Factor Xa activity of tinzaparin is only partially neutralised by protamine and the anti-Factor Xa and anti-Factor IIa (APTT) activities are seen to return after its reversal.

PHARMACOKINETIC PROPERTIES
Tinzaparin is around 90% bioavailable after a SC injection. The absorption half-life is 200 minutes, peak plasma activity occurs after 4-6 hours and the elimination half-life is about 90 minutes.

EXCIPIENTS
Some injections contain benzyl alcohol. See manufacturers SPC for details.

LICENSED STATUS
Not licensed for use in children.

Tioconazole

Broad-spectrum imidazole antifungal agent.

USES
Treatment of fungal nail infections.

PRESENTATION
Nail solution: 28% – Trosyl®.

DOSAGE/ADMINISTRATION
Children and adults: apply to nails and surrounding skin twice daily for up to 6 months, using the applicator brush provided.

CONTRA-INDICATIONS & WARNINGS
Avoid contact with eyes.

PREGNANCY
There is insufficient evidence as to safety in human pregnancy, although absorption after topical administration is negligible. Contact local Medicines Information Centre for advice.

SIDE-EFFECTS
Local irritation usually during first week; discontinue if sensitivity develops.

POISONING/TOXICITY
In the event of excessive oral ingestion, gastrointestinal symptoms may occur. Treatment is symptomatic.

EXCIPIENTS
See manufacturers SPC for further details.

LICENSED STATUS
Licensed for use in children and adults.

Tioguanine (thioguanine)

Antineoplastic – a purine antimetabolite.

USES
Acute lymphoblastic leukaemia/lymphoma, acute myeloid leukaemia, chronic granulocytic leukaemia.

PRESENTATION
Tablet: 40mg (scored) – Lanvis®.
Capsule: 10mg – manufactured 'special'.
Oral suspension: 50mg in 5mL – manufactured 'special'.

DOSAGE
** Always consult the current treatment protocol for details of dosage and scheduling. **

ADMINISTRATION
Oral: as a single daily dose.

CONTRA-INDICATIONS & WARNINGS
Contra-indications: there are no absolute contra-indications to its use.
Cautions: if halving a tablet, care should be taken not to contaminate the hands or inhale the drug. The enzyme hypoxanthine guanine phosphoribosyl transferase is responsible for the conversion of tioguanine to its active metabolite. It is possible that patients deficient in this enzyme (e.g. Lesch-Nyhan syndrome) may be resistant to the drug. Consideration should be given to reducing the dosage in patients with impaired hepatic or renal function.
Warnings: tioguanine is an active cytotoxic agent for use only under the direction of physicians experienced in the administration of such agents.

INTERACTIONS
The combination of *busulphan* and tioguanine has resulted in the development of hepatic nodular degenerative hyperplasia, portal hypertension and oesophageal varices. As there is *in vitro* evidence that *aminosalicylate derivatives* (e.g. *olsalazine, mesalazine or sulfasalazine* (*sulphasalazine*)) inhibit the thiopurine s-methyltransferase (TPMT) enzyme, they should be administered with caution to patients receiving concurrent tioguanine therapy.

PREGNANCY
Tioguanine is potentially teratogenic and should be avoided whenever possible during pregnancy, particularly during the first trimester. In any individual case the potential hazard to the fetus must be balanced against the expected benefit to the mother.

BREAST-FEEDING
It is recommended that mothers receiving tioguanine should not breast-feed.

SIDE-EFFECTS
Gastrointestinal: stomatitis, gastric-intestinal intolerance, intestinal necrosis and perforation, associated with veno-occlusive disease (VOD).
Haematological: bone marrow suppression.
Neurological: loss of vibration sense and unsteady gait.
Hepatobiliary system: liver function abnormalities and

T

jaundice (which may be reversible if withdrawn) and VOD of the liver (which in most cases was reversible on withdrawal of chemotherapy).

POISONING/TOXICITY

Symptoms: the principal toxic effect is on the bone marrow and haematological toxicity is likely to be more profound with chronic overdose rather than a single ingestion.

Treatment: there is no antidote and supportive measures e.g. blood transfusion, growth factors etc. may be required.

PHARMACOKINETIC PROPERTIES

Tioguanine is extensively metabolised *in vivo*. There are two principal catabolic routes: methylation to 2-amino-6-methyl-thiopurine and deamination to 2-hydroxy-6-mercaptopurine, followed by oxidation to 6-thiouric acid. Studies with radioactive tioguanine show that peak blood levels of total radioactivity are achieved about 8-10 hours after oral administration and decline slowly thereafter. Later studies using high performance liquid chromatography (HPLC) have shown 6-tioguanine to be the major thiopurine present for at least the first 8 hours after IV administration. Plasma levels decay biexponentially with initial and terminal half lives of 3 and 5.9 hours respectively. Following oral administration peak levels as measured by HPLC occur at 2-4 hours. Levels are reduced by concurrent food intake (as well as vomiting).

EXCIPIENTS

Contact manufacturer for further details.

LICENSED STATUS

Lanvis® tablets 40mg are licensed for use in children and adults. The oral suspension and capsules are available as 'specials' and as such are unlicensed.

FURTHER INFORMATION

Store below 25°C. Keep dry. Protect from light.

Capsules or a 50mg/5mL oral suspension are available as 'specials' from Nova Laboratories (manufacturing unit Leicester Royal Infirmary (tel: 0116 2230 100). Other suspension strengths are available on request.

Tobramycin

An aminoglycoside especially active against *Pseudomonas aeruginosa*.

USES

In cystic fibrosis patients – treatment of early *Pseudomonas aeruginosa* infections not cleared by oral ciprofloxacin plus nebulised colistin and treatment of moderate to severe exacerbations, in combination with other antibiotics (e.g. third generation cephalosporins, anti-pseudomonal penicillins, beta-lactam antibiotics and polymixins). Note tobramycin is preferred to gentamicin because it is more active against *Pseudomonas aeruginosa*. Usually used nebulised for the treatment of *Pseudomonas aeruginosa* infections.

PRESENTATION

Injection: (as sulphate) 40mg in 1mL, 1mL, 2mL and 6mL vials – non-proprietary; 10mg in 1mL, 2mL vial – Nebcin®; 40mg in 1mL, 2mL vial – Nebcin®.

Nebuliser solution: 60mg in 1mL, 5mL unit – Tobi®.

Oral solution: may be extemporaneously prepared.

DOSAGE

Newborn infant (birth to 1 month)

Route	*Postconceptional age	Dose	Dose frequency	Notes
IV	<32 weeks	4–5mg/kg	36 hourly	Plasma samples usually taken around the third dose aiming for a 1 hour post dose (peak) of 5–10mg/L and a pre dose (trough) level of <2mg/L. If there is no change in the dosage regimen or renal function repeat levels every 3-4 days.
	>32 weeks	4–5mg/kg	24 hourly	

*Postconceptional age = gestational plus postnatal age.

Neonates presenting with patent ductus arteriosus (PDA), prolonged hypoxia or treated with indometacin (indomethacin) may have impaired elimination of tobramycin due to reduced glomerular filtration rate (GFR) and increase in dosage interval may be necessary.

Child
Divided daily dose regimen

Route	Age			Frequency (times daily)	Notes
	1 month–2 years	2–12 years	12–18 years		
IV/IM	← 2.5mg/kg →		1–2mg/kg	3	Severe infection. Plasma samples usually taken around the third or fourth dose aiming for a pre dose (trough) level of <2mg/L and a 1 hour post (peak) level of 5-10mg/L.
IV	← 4mg/kg →			3	Starting dose in cystic fibrosis. Monitor levels after third dose. Aim for trough <2mg/L and 1 hour post dose (peak) of 8-12mg/L.
Nebulised for cystic fibrosis patients	–	>6 years 300mg	300mg	2	TOBI preservative-free solution. Alternating 28 days on and 28 days off. Licensed product is nebulised treatment of choice.
	40mg	<8 years 80mg >8 years 160mg	160mg	2 2	Injection – not licensed for nebulisation. Seek advice from pharmacy department before prescribing. Intravenous preparations must be preservative-free (phenol-free) solutions. Dilute to 4mL with NaCl 0.9%.
Oral	20mg	<5 years 20mg 5–12 years 40mg	80mg	4 4	Selective decontamination of digestive tract (with colistin and amphotericin). Unlicensed and limited experience of use.

Renal impairment
Monitor levels and increase the dosing interval, keeping the dose the same as normal, or adjust dose and dosing interval. Two sample regimens are outlined below.
Regimen 1

Degree of renal impairment	Dose adjustment
Mild	75% of a dose 12 hourly
Moderate	50% of a dose 12 hourly
Severe	50% of a dose 24 hourly

Regimen 2

Creatinine clearance (mL/minute/1.73m^2)	Dosage interval (hours) (dose stays the same)
40–70	12
20–40	18
10–20	24
5–10	36
<5	48

T

Child
Single daily dose regimen

Route	Age			Frequency (times daily)	Notes (monitoring)
	1 month–2 years	2–12 years	12–18 years		
IV	←	7mg/kg	→	1	Plasma samples are usually taken at 18–24 hours after the first dose aiming for a level <1mg/L. If the levels are >1mg/L then the dosing interval is normally increased by 12 hours. 1 hour post dose (peak) levels can be taken with a target range of 16–20mg/L If there is no change in the dosage regimen or in renal function repeat levels every 3–4 days.

Pre-dose levels must be monitored in children with impaired renal function.

ADMINISTRATION
IV: slow IV injection over 3-5 minutes injected neat or diluted in NaCl 0.9% or glucose 5%. IV infusion over 30-60 minutes for high dose 'Child – single daily dose regimen' in an appropriate volume of NaCl 0.9% or glucose 5%. Avoid mixing with penicillins, cephalosporins or erythromycin.

Nebulised: after physiotherapy and bronchodilators. For the TOBI® nebuliser solution administer over 15 minutes using a hand held PARI LC Plus nebuliser and suitable compressor (to deliver a flow rate of 4-6L/minute or a back pressure of 110-217KPa). If nebulising the injection solution optimum nebulisation volume is 4mL – make up to volume with NaCl 0.9%; use with an active venturi nebuliser system with outlet so exhaled antibiotic can be discharged via a window, otherwise an effective filter system should be used. Tobramycin must not be mixed in the nebuliser with other antibiotics as precipitation occurs.

CONTRA-INDICATIONS & WARNINGS
Patients with known hypersensitivity to tobramycin. Bronchospasm may occur when nebulised – treat with a beta-agonist. Hearing tests are recommended for cystic fibrosis patients receiving repeated courses of aminoglycosides. Monitor baseline renal function when on regular nebulisation and then every 6 months.

INTERACTIONS
Negligible when nebulised or given orally as systemic absorption very low. For details of interactions when given parenterally, see gentamicin monograph.

PREGNANCY
Contra-indicated as risk of damage to fetus with parenteral use, but tobramycin has been nebulised in pregnant patients when benefits outweigh the risks. Monitor plasma levels if given parenterally. Contact local Medicines Information Centre for advice.

BREAST-FEEDING
Excreted in breast milk if administered parenterally and breast-feeding should be avoided (not known if excreted into milk when nebulised). Contact local Medicines Information Centre for advice.

SIDE-EFFECTS
Bronchospasm can occur if nebulised. Impaired renal function and ototoxicity can occur if optimum blood levels are exceeded. Minimal risk of these effects if nebulised or given orally.

POISONING/TOXICITY
Unlikely if nebulised or given orally. Severity of the manifestations of a parenteral overdose depends on the dose, the patient's renal function, state of hydration, age, and whether concurrent medication with similar toxicity is being given. Nephrotoxicity and ototoxicity can occur. Neuromuscular blockade or respiratory failure can follow rapid IV administration. Neuromuscular blockade can be reversed by giving calcium salts. Fluid balance, creatinine clearance and tobramycin levels should be carefully monitored until the tobramycin levels fall below 2mg/L. Haemodialysis or peritoneal dialysis will aid removal from the blood.

PHARMACOKINETIC PROPERTIES
The plasma half-life of a parenteral dose is 2-3 hours in adults with normal renal function. The half-life is >8 hours in neonates weighing <1.5kg, 6-8 hours in those 1.5-2.5kg and 4 hours in those >2.5kg. Following parenteral administration, little, if any, metabolic transformation occurs and tobramycin is eliminated almost exclusively by glomerular filtration. Absorption is negligible when nebulised or given orally and therefore serum drug monitoring is not necessary with these routes of administration.

EXCIPIENTS
Contact manufacturers for further details.

LICENSED STATUS
Not licensed for oral administration. Parenteral routes licensed in all ages. Nebulisation licensed >6 years of age (the injection is not licensed for administration by this route).

Tolazoline

Tolazoline is an alpha adrenergic receptor antagonist that produces both systemic and pulmonary vasodilation.

USES
A vasodilator used to improve pulmonary blood flow in ventilated babies.

PRESENTATION
Injection: 1mg in 1mL, 1mL ampoules; 10mg in 1mL, 5mL ampoules and 25mg in 1mL, 1mL ampoules – manufactured 'specials'; other strengths are available.

DOSAGE
Newborn infant (birth to 1 month)

Route	Age	Frequency	Notes
	birth–1 month		
IV bolus	1mg/kg	single dose	Anecdotally it only works well when blood pH >7.2.
IV infusion	200 microgram/kg/hour	continuous	

ADMINISTRATION
IV bolus: give over 1-5 minutes. Watch for systemic hypotension. If there is a satisfactory response this can be maintained by infusion.
IV infusion: dilute in NaCl 0.9% or glucose 5%. Diluted solution is stable for 24 hours. Can be co-infused with dopamine and/or dobutamine.

CONTRA-INDICATIONS & WARNINGS
Cardiotoxic accumulation can occur quite rapidly in babies with renal failure when tolazoline is given by continuous infusion. Babies given a continuous tolazoline infusion must have their blood pressure measured periodically, but any sustained systemic hypotension should be rare as long as the dose given does not exceed 300 microgram/kg/hour.

INTERACTIONS
The vasodilator effect of tolazoline is blocked by H_2 *antagonists* such as *ranitidine*.

PREGNANCY
Experience in pregnancy is limited and a conclusion as to safety in pregnancy cannot be made.

BREAST-FEEDING
No data available.

SIDE-EFFECTS
Tolazoline will cause both pulmonary and systemic vasodilatation. Tachycardia due to sympathomimetic action and increased gastric secretion due to a histamine like action. Severe side-effects such as hypotension, haemorrhage from any major organ and renal failure may occur particularly if doses higher than 300 microgram/kg/hour are used.

POISONING/TOXICITY
See adverse effects above.

PHARMACOKINETIC PROPERTIES
Tolazoline is not metabolised but is actively renally excreted. Plasma half-life exceeds 6 hours and therefore continuous infusion is probably not as necessary as was once thought.

EXCIPIENTS
Contact manufacturers for further details.

LICENSED STATUS
Available as 'specials' and as such are unlicensed.

FURTHER INFORMATION
Available as 'specials' from several NHS manufacturing units.

Tolterodine

Antimuscarinic agent.

USES
Urgency, urinary frequency and incontinence.

PRESENTATION
Tablet: 1mg and 2mg – Detrusitol®.

DOSAGE

Route	Age			Frequency (times daily)	Notes
	1 month–2 years	2–12 years	12–18 years		
Oral	–	← 1mg →		1	Initial dose. Increase to 2mg twice daily according to response. Effect usually seen within 4 weeks.

CONTRA-INDICATIONS & WARNINGS
Significant bladder outflow obstruction, urinary retention, myasthenia gravis, glaucoma, toxic megacolon, severe ulcerative colitis. Caution in liver and renal impairment.

INTERACTIONS
Avoid use with *macrolide antibiotics, imidazole* and *triazole anti fungals* and *anti proteases* as enzyme inhibition may result in increased tolterodine concentrations.

PREGNANCY/BREAST-FEEDING
Contact local Medicines Information Centre for advice.

SIDE-EFFECTS
Dry mouth, constipation, dyspepsia, blurred vision, nausea, abdominal discomfort, drowsiness, paraesthesia, dry skin, facial flushing, headache, dizziness.

POISONING/TOXICITY
The symptoms of overdose progress from intensification of usual side-effects of CNS disturbances, circulatory changes (flushing, fall in blood pressure, circulatory failure etc.), respiratory insufficiency.
Benzodiazepine by IV injection for pronounced restlessness, excitation or convulsions. Physostigmine for CNS symptoms. Tachycardia may need treatment with beta-blockers and urinary retention managed by bladder catheterisation.

EXCIPIENTS
See manufacturers SPC for further details.

LICENSED STATUS
Not licensed for use in children.

Topiramate

Antiepileptic.

USES
Drug of second or third choice in partial, generalised tonic-clonic, absence, tonic and atonic seizures and Lennox-Gastaut syndrome.

PRESENTATION
Tablet: 25mg, 50mg, 100mg and 200mg – Topamax®.

Capsules: 15mg, 25mg and 50mg – Topamax® Sprinkle.

DOSAGE

Route	Age				Frequency (times daily)	Notes
	birth–1 month	1 month–2 years	2–12 years	12–18 years		
Oral	–	← 500 microgram/kg →		25mg	1	Usual starting dose.
	–	← 2–4.5mg/kg →		100–200mg	2	Usual target maintenance dose. Doses up to 6mg/kg twice daily have been used.

Dose adjustment
Use starting dose for 2 weeks then increase dose every 2 weeks taking at least 6 weeks to reach maintenance dose. Use with caution in renal failure, titrating dose and intervals between dose adjustments to efficacy and side-effects. Supplemental doses required after dialysis.

ADMINISTRATION
Oral: can be taken with or without food. Crushed tablets are very bitter but can be mixed with strong tasting food or liquid. Capsules may be opened and beads mixed with soft food. Beads should not be chewed.

CONTRA-INDICATIONS & WARNINGS
Warn patients of drowsiness and not to stop therapy abruptly. Ensure adequate hydration to avoid nephrolithiasis. Acute myopia and glaucoma may occur rarely.

INTERACTIONS
May increase plasma *phenytoin* levels. May decrease *digoxin* levels. May decrease the effectiveness of *oral contraceptives*, advise patients to use other measures. *Carbamazepine* and *phenytoin* may decrease topiramate levels.

PREGNANCY/BREAST-FEEDING
Little data, manufacturer advises avoid. Contact local Medicines Information Centre for advice.

SIDE-EFFECTS
Dose dependent side-effects include anorexia, somnolence, fatigue, ataxia. Chronic adverse effects include reduced appetite, anorexia and behavioural changes (including psychosis and depression) but currently there are inadequate long-term data. Renal calculi have been reported in adults.

POISONING/TOXICITY
Supportive therapy, contact UK National Poisons Information Service.

PHARMACOKINETIC PROPERTIES
Well absorbed orally, unaffected by food. Elimination half-life is approximately 21 hours in adults but shorter in children. Plasma level monitoring not advised routinely. Eliminated by the kidney. Blood reference range 6-74 micromol/L.

EXCIPIENTS
Capsules include sugar. See manufacturers SPC for further details.

LICENSED STATUS
Only licensed for adjunctive therapy in >2 years of age.

T

Trace element and mineral preparations

Metabolic Mineral Mixture®

A trace element and mineral mixture. It is unflavoured. It is ACBS prescribable for mineral and trace element supplementation in restrictive therapeutic diets. It is gluten-, sucrose- and lactose-free.
Contains per 100g: sodium (172mmol), potassium (212mmol), chloride (50.8mmol), calcium (205mmol), phosphorus (192mmol), magnesium (39.9mmol), iron (63mg), zinc (48mg), iodine (760 microgram), manganese (5.7mg), copper (13mg), molybdenum (150 microgram).

DOSAGE

The recommended dosage is dependent on the age, bodyweight and medical condition of the patient. Suggested guide:

Infants up to 5.5kg	1.5g/kg/day
>5.5kg until 3 years of age	8g/day
>3 years of age	12g/day

This dosage may need to be adjusted if minerals and trace elements are provided in the diet from other sources. It is advisable to check the total intake against the reference nutrient intakes (RNI) for that age group (see page G75).

ADMINISTRATION

Oral: infants – weigh out the required amount of metabolic mineral mixture and add to daily infant feeds. Ensure it is evenly distributed between all feeds. Children >1 year – Metabolic Mineral Mixture® can be given as a concentrated drink or paste; water or diluted drinks should be offered at the same time. It is better to give in 3 dosages, with meals throughout the day. The powder should be weighed or measured using an SHS scoop *(1 SHS yellow scoop = 5g).

CONTRA-INDICATIONS & WARNINGS

Not suitable for PN. This product does not contain selenium or chromium. If it is inadequately diluted, symptoms of hyperosmolality may occur and the serum electrolytes should be checked.

LICENSED STATUS

It is not licensed.

FURTHER INFORMATION

SHS scoop is the scoop measure provided by the product manufacturers Scientific Hospital Supplies (SHS). Once reconstituted, Metabolic Mineral Mixture® should be stored in a refrigerator and must not be kept longer than 24 hours from the time of preparation.

Aminogran mineral mixture®

A trace element and mineral mixture. It is unflavoured. It is ACBS prescribable for mineral and trace element supplementation in restrictive therapeutic diets. It is gluten-, sucrose- and lactose- free.
Contains per 100g: sodium (170mmol), potassium (210mmol), phosphorus (190mmol), magnesium (40mmol), iron (63mg), zinc (48mg), copper (13mg), manganese (4mg), iodine (trace), aluminium (trace), cobalt (trace), molybdenum (trace).

DOSAGE

The recommended dosage is dependent on the age, bodyweight and medical condition of the patient. Suggested guide:

Weight
Infants <5.5 kg – 1.5g/kg/day
Infants >5.5kg – 8g/day

This dosage may need to be adjusted if minerals and trace elements are provided in the diet from other sources. It is advisable to check the total intake against the RNI for that age group (see page G75).

ADMINISTRATION

Oral: infants – weigh out the required amount of metabolic mineral mixture and add to daily infant feeds. Ensure it is evenly distributed between all feeds. Each 1g powder should be diluted with at least 100mL of fluid.
Children over 1 year – Aminogran Mineral Mixture® can be given as a drink or paste; water or diluted drinks should be offered at the same time. If preferred, the unflavoured drink or paste may be flavoured with a suitable flavouring such as milk shake syrup or concentrate. It is better to give in 3 dosages, with meals throughout the day. The powder should be weighed or measured using an Aminogran Mineral Mixture® scoop (1 yellow scoop = 2.7g; 3 levels scoops = 8g).

CONTRA-INDICATIONS & WARNINGS

Aminogran Mineral Mixture® is not suitable for PN. It is unsuitable where trace element supplementation only is required. If used for infants <5.5kg, the total dose should not exceed 1.5g/kg/day. This product does not contain selenium or chromium and unspecified trace quantities of molybdenum and iodine. If it is inadequately diluted, symptoms of hyperosmolality may occur.

SIDE-EFFECTS

Mineral solutions with high osmolarity may cause vomiting, abdominal pain and diarrhoea.

LICENSED STATUS

It is not licensed.

Paediatric Seravit®

A vitamin, trace element and mineral mixture containing only trace amounts of sodium and potassium on a carbohydrate base; available unflavoured and pineapple flavour. It is ACBS prescribable for vitamin and mineral supplementation in restrictive therapeutic diets in infants and children. It is lactose and gluten free.

Contains per 100g: energy (268kcal, 1139kJ), carbohydrate (67g), vitamin A (4.2mg), vitamin D (55.5 microgram), vitamin E (31.9 units), vitamin C (400mg), vitamin K (166 microgram), thiamin (3.2mg), riboflavin (4.4mg), niacin (35mg), vitamin B6 (3.4mg), folacin (303 microgram), vitamin B12 (8.6 microgram), biotin (214 microgram) pantothenic acid (17mg), choline (350mg), inositol (700mg), sodium (<0.9mmol), potassium (<0.8mmol), chloride (<0.6mmol), calcium (2.57g), phosphorus (1.714g), magnesium (357mg), iron (69mg), copper (4.6mg), zinc (46mg), manganese (4.6mg), iodine (332 microgram), molybdenum (351 microgram) selenium (137 microgram), chromium (137 microgram).

DOSAGE
The recommended dosage is dependent on the age, bodyweight and medical condition of the patient. Suggested guide:

0-6 months	14g/day
6-12 months	17g/day
1-7 years	17-25g/day
7-14 years	25-35g/day

This dosage may need to be adjusted if vitamins, minerals and trace elements are provided in the diet from other sources. It is advisable to check the total intake against the recommended nutrient intakes (RNI) for that age group (see page G75).

ADMINISTRATION
Oral: infant – weigh out the required amount of unflavoured Paediatric Seravit® and add to daily infant feeds. It is important to ensure it is evenly distributed between all feeds. Children >1 year – Paediatric Seravit® can be given as a drink or paste; water or diluted drinks should be offered at the same time. If preferred, the unflavoured drink or paste may be flavoured with a suitable flavouring such as milkshake concentrate. It is better to give in 2-3 dosages throughout the day. The powder should be weighed or measured using a SHS* scoop (1 SHS yellow scoop = 5g).

CONTRA-INDICATIONS & WARNINGS
Not suitable for parenteral nutrition. Flavoured Paediatric Seravit® is not recommended for infants <6 months old. This product does not contain sodium or potassium. If it is used as part of a modular feed in infancy, additional sodium and potassium may be needed to provide maintenance requirements. It contains fish gelatin and is unsuitable for vegetarians and vegans.

LICENSED STATUS
It is not licensed.

FURTHER INFORMATION
Once reconstituted, store in a refrigerator and do not keep longer than 24 hours from the time of preparation.

Forceval®

Forceval Junior Capsules: gelatin capsules containing 22 vitamins, minerals and trace elements. Lactose-, sucrose- and gluten-free.

Contains per capsule: biotin (50 micrograms), vitamin A (1250 units), vitamin D (200 units), vitamin E (5mg), vitamin K (25 microgram), thiamine (1.5mg), riboflavin (1mg), vitamin B6 (1mg), vitamin B12 (2 microgram), vitamin C (25mg), nicotinamide (7.5mg), pantothenic acid (2mg), folic acid (100 microgram), iron (5mg), copper (1mg), magnesium (1mg), zinc (5mg), iodine (75 microgram), manganese (1.25mg), selenium (25 microgram), chromium (50 microgram) and molybdenum (50 microgram). Does not contain calcium, sodium, potassium, and chloride. Contains only minimal quantities of magnesium.

USES
Vitamin and mineral deficiency and as a supplement with synthetic diets for children >5 years.

DOSAGE
Children >5 years: 2 capsules per day. This dosage may need to be adjusted if vitamins, minerals and trace elements are provided in the diet from other sources. It is advisable to check the total intake against the RNI for that age group (see page G75). Not recommended for adults.

ADMINISTRATION
Oral: not to be given to children <5 years because of difficulty in swallowing capsules. They should not be taken on an empty stomach.

CONTRA-INDICATIONS & WARNINGS
Hypercalcaemia, haemochromatosis and other iron storage disorders.

EXCIPIENTS
See manufacturers SPC for further details.

Forceval Capsules: gelatin capsule containing 24 vitamins, minerals and trace elements. Prescribable for vitamin and mineral deficiency and as a supplement to synthetic diets for children >12 years and adults. Lactose, sucrose and gluten free. Contains per capsule: vitamin A (2500 units), vitamin D (400 units), vitamin E (10mg), thiamin (1.2mg), riboflavin (1.6mg), vitamin B6 (2mg), vitamin B12 (3 microgram), vitamin C (60mg), biotin (100 microgram), nicotinamide (18mg), pantothenic acid (4mg), folic acid (400 microgram), calcium (100mg), iron (12mg), copper (2mg), phosphorus (77mg), magnesium (30mg), potassium (4mg), zinc (15mg), iodine (140 microgram), manganese (3mg), selenium (50 microgram), chromium (200 microgram) and molybdenum (250 microgram). Contains only small quantities of calcium, phosphorus and magnesium compared with RNI. Does not contain sodium, chloride or vitamin K.

DOSAGE
>12 years: 1 capsule per day.
<12 years: not recommended for children

ADMINISTRATION
Oral: capsules should not be taken on an empty stomach.

CONTRA-INDICATIONS & WARNINGS
Hypercalcaemia, haemochromatosis and other iron storage disorders.

EXCIPIENTS
See manufacturers SPC for further details.

Tranexamic acid

An antifibrinolytic agent that inhibits the breakdown of fibrin clots.

USES
Antifibrinolytic (prevention of bleeding after dental extraction in haemophilia & von Willebrand disease). Hereditary angioneurotic oedema. Menorrhagia. Counteracts thrombolytic overdose. In palliative care, for epistaxis and surface bleeding from mucous membranes.

PRESENTATION
Injection: 100mg in 1mL, 5mL ampoule – Cyklokapron®.
Liquid: 500mg/5mL (10%) – manufactured 'special'.
Mouthwash: 500mg/10mL (5%) – may be extemporaneously prepared.
Tablet: 500mg – Cyklokapron®.

DOSAGE

Route	Age			Frequency (times daily)	Notes
	1 month–2 years	2–12 years	12–18 years		
Oral	←	25mg/kg	→	3	
Oral		–	1–1.5g	3–4	Menorrhagia, for 3–4 days (initiated when heavy bleeding has started).
Slow IV bolus	←	10mg/kg	→	3	Give over at least 10 minutes.
IV infusion	←	45mg/kg over 24 hours	→	continuous	Infuse in glucose 5% or NaCl 0.9%.

ADMINISTRATION

IV: can be mixed with heparin. DO NOT mix with blood or penicillins.

Renal failure

Reduce the dose in renal failure, according to serum creatinine. Transexamic acid is removed by haemodialysis therefore give post dialysis.

Serum creatinine	Dose (IV/Oral)	Frequency (times daily)
120–250 micromol/L	As above	2
250–500 micromol/L	As above	1
>500 micromol/L	Half the above dose	1

CONTRA-INDICATIONS & WARNINGS

Should not be used in the presence of massive haematuria (risk of ureteric obstruction). For long term treatment of hereditary angioedema, regular eye examinations and LFTs are recommended although some consider eye examinations unnecessary.

PREGNANCY

Consider increased risk of thromboembolic disease in pregnancy when assessing benefits versus risks. Contact local Medicines Information Centre for advice.

BREAST-FEEDING

Levels in breast milk are very low. An antifibrinolytic effect in the infant is unlikely. Contact local Medicines Information Centre for advice.

SIDE-EFFECTS

Nausea and vomiting, diarrhoea (decrease dose), disturbances in colour vision (discontinue drug). Rapid IV injection may cause dizziness with or without hypotension.

POISONING/TOXICITY

Symptoms may be nausea and vomiting with or without hypotension. High fluid intake will promote renal excretion.

PHARMACOKINETIC PROPERTIES

Excreted largely unchanged in urine. Plasma half-life approximately 2 hours in adults. Absorption from the gastrointestinal tract is 30-40%.

LICENSED STATUS

Cyklokapron® is licensed for use in children. The oral liquid manufactured 'special' and extemporaneously prepared mouthwash are unlicensed.

Tretinoin

USES

Treatment of acne.

PRESENTATION
Cream: 0.025% – Acticin®, Retin-A®.
Gel: 0.01% – Retin-A®: 0.025% – Acticin®, Retin-A®.
Lotion: 0.025% – Retin-A®.

DOSAGE/ADMINISTRATION
Topical: apply 1-2 times daily thinly. The skin should be thoroughly washed first. Cream is recommended for dry or fair skin, gel for oily or dark skin.

CONTRA-INDICATIONS & WARNINGS
Avoid contact with eye, nostrils, mouth and mucous membranes. Do not use simultaneously with peeling agent. Do not use ultraviolet lamps (minimise exposure to sunlight).

INTERACTIONS
Concurrent topical medications and *toiletry preparations* should be used with care.

PREGNANCY
Avoid using during pregnancy – teratogenic.

BREAST-FEEDING
Not known if excreted in breast milk.

SIDE-EFFECTS
Irritation, erythema and peeling. Changes in pigmentation. Photosensitivity.

POISONING/TOXICITY
Oral ingestion symptoms are pruritus, dry skin, arthralgias, anorexia, vomiting (vitamin A excess). Accidental ingestion – perform gastric emptying as soon as possible.

EXCIPIENTS
See manufacturers SPC for further details.

LICENSED STATUS
Not licensed for use in children.

FURTHER INFORMATION
Therapeutic effects not observed for 6-8 weeks. An early temporary exacerbation may occur.

Triamcinolone

Glucocorticoid.

USES
Local intra-articular corticosteroid injections in inflammatory arthritis.

PRESENTATION
Intra-articular injection: (as triamcinolone hexacetonide) 20mg in 1mL and 40mg in 2mL – named patient (Hexatrione®).
Intra-articular/intradermal injection: (as triamcinolone acetonide) 10mg in 1mL, 1mL ampoule and 5mL vial – Adcortyl® Intra-articular/Intradermal.
Intra-articular/IM injection: (as triamcinolone acetonide) 40mg in 1mL, 1mL vial, 1mL and 2mL prefilled syringe – Kenalog® Intra-articular/Intramuscular.

DOSAGE

Route	Age			Notes
	1 month–2 years	2–12 years	12–18 years	
Intra-articular	>1 year as for 2-18 years	← 1mg/kg (large joints) →		Dosages are approximate. Maximum 40mg for large joints.
		← 0.5mg/kg (smaller joints) →		Maximum 20mg for small joints. Maximum 10mg for finger and toe joints.

The hexacetonide salt is preferred for intra-articular administration as it produces more prolonged effects than the acetonide.

ADMINISTRATION
Intra-articular/peri-articular: triamcinolone should not be given via these routes when the joint or surrounding tissues are infected. Repeated intra-articular injections should be as infrequent as possible. The vial should be gently agitated to achieve uniform suspension before use.

IM: to avoid subcutaneous fat atrophy, deep IM injections should be administered into the gluteal site. Alternate sides should be used for subsequent doses. The deltoid muscle should not be used.

CONTRA-INDICATIONS & WARNINGS
Although active, latent or questionably healed tuberculosis, ocular herpes simplex, and acute psychoses are generally considered to be absolute contra-indications to corticosteroid therapy, the minimal systemic activity of triamcinolone hexacetonide following local injection might permit cautious use when indicated. Not to be injected directly into tendons or into spinal or other non-diarthrodial joints. Despite optimal technique, leakage into subcutaneous tissues can occur following intra-articular injection, leading to atrophy of subcutaneous tissue.

PREGNANCY/BREAST-FEEDING
Very little data specifically relating to triamcinolone has been found, although available evidence supports the use of corticosteroids to control various maternal diseases during pregnancy when their use is essential. Absorption following intra-articular administration is complete, but very slow. Contact local Medicines Information Centre for advice.

SIDE-EFFECTS
An exacerbation or 'flare-up' of symptoms can occur. Local atrophy, burning, flushing, pain and swelling may occur. Other local effects include abscess, erythema, skin discolouration or depigmentation and necrosis at injection site.

Absorption of triamcinolone following intra-articular injection is rare, so systemic side-effects are not to be expected when this route of administration is used.

POISONING/TOXICITY
Overdosage or excessive frequency of intra-articular injections into the same site may produce local subcutaneous atrophy.

EXCIPIENTS
Adcortyl® and Kenalog® injections include benzyl alcohol. Contact manufacturers for further details.

LICENSED STATUS
Triamcinolone acetonide 10mg in 1mL (Adcortyl®) is licensed via the intra-articular and intradermal routes >6 years of age, in appropriately reduced doses. Triamcinolone acetonide 40mg in 1mL (Kenalog®) is licensed for deep IM use ≥6 years of age but is not licensed for use in children via the intra-articular route. The 1mL and 2mL prefilled syringes are licensed for IM use only. The 1mL vials are licensed for IM use in children and adults, or for intra-articular use in adults. Triamcinolone hexacetonide is not licensed for use in the UK.

FURTHER INFORMATION
Hexatrione® is available from IDIS World Medicines.

Triclofos sodium

USES
Sedation for painless procedures. Night sedation.

PRESENTATION
Oral solution: 500mg in 5mL – non-proprietary.

DOSAGE

Route	Age		Frequency	Notes
	2–12 years	12–18 years	(times daily)	
Oral	← 30–50mg/kg →		single dose	Doses up to 100mg/kg have been used when sedation level 4 is required prior to a procedure. Chloral hydrate is generally used >12 years.

T

CONTRA-INDICATIONS & WARNINGS, INTERACTIONS, SIDE-EFFECTS, PREGNANCY, BREAST-FEEDING, POISONING/TOXICITY	See chloral hydrate monograph. Triclofos causes less gastric irritation than chloral hydrate.

EXCIPIENTS
Oral solution includes granulated sugar.

LICENSED STATUS
Licensed for insomnia (short-term use). Not licensed for sedation for painless procedures.

Trientine dihydrochloride

Produces a cupriuresis through the mobilisation of the copper deposits which are characteristic of Wilson's Disease.

USES
Treatment of Wilson Disease, in patients intolerant of penicillamine.

PRESENTATION
Capsule: 300mg.

DOSAGE

Route	Age			Frequency (times daily)	Notes
	1 month–2 years	2–12 years	12–18 years		
Oral	–	← 300–750mg →		2	Initial dose may be increased to a maximum of 1.5g/**day** (<12 years) and 2g/**day** (≥12 years). Anecdotal as little information about paediatric use.

ADMINISTRATION
Oral: the total daily dose can be given in 2-4 divided doses if necessary. It is best given 30 minutes to 1 hour before meals and other drugs; or 2 hours after food, milk feed and other drugs. In view of a possible teratogenic effect in those with normal serum copper levels, patients should be encouraged to take the capsule without opening or crushing it. If it is impossible to administer the capsule without opening it, gloves and a mask should be worn by the nurse, parent or other carer.
Increase dose if serum copper is persistently >20 microgram/mL. Monitor maintenance dose at 6-12 month intervals.

CONTRA-INDICATIONS & WARNINGS
Hypersensitivity to trientine. Trientine is not indicated as an alternative to penicillamine treatment for rheumatoid arthritis or cystinuria. It should not be used in the treatment of conditions where free copper levels are not elevated. Reduces serum iron levels, possibly by reducing absorption. Iron supplementation may be required.

INTERACTIONS
Although there is no evidence that *calcium* or *magnesium* containing *antacids* affect the efficacy of trientine, it is considered desirable to separate administration if the two therapies are administered concurrently. Do not administer *iron preparations* at the same time of day.

PREGNANCY
Trientine has been shown to be teratogenic in rats and may be teratogenic in humans, particularly when administered to patients with normal free copper levels. However, there is also evidence that high serum copper levels may themselves be fetotoxic. Experience in human pregnancy is limited and it should only be used if the potential benefit justifies the potential risk to the fetus. If trientine is administered, it is recommended that serum copper levels be closely monitored.

BREAST-FEEDING
Excretion into breast milk is not established.

SIDE-EFFECTS
Nausea, epigastric pain, muscle spasm, joint pain, tiredness, anaemia, dystonia, myasthenia gravis, systemic lupus erythematosus (SLE), fever, skin eruptions.

POISONING/TOXICITY
It is reported that a patient has taken 30g without adverse effect. Symptomatic treatment only is indicated.

T

LICENSED STATUS
Licensed for use in children.

Trihexyphenidyl (benzhexol)

A tertiary amine antimuscarinic agent with actions similar to those of atropine. It also has a direct antispasmodic action on smooth muscle.

USES
Antispasmodic. Treatment of extrapyramidal symptoms, particularly dystonia.

PRESENTATION
Tablet: 2mg (scored), 5mg (scored) – non-proprietary.
Syrup: 5mg in 5mL – Broflex®.
Elixir: 2mg in 5mL – manufactured 'special'

DOSAGE

Indication	Route	Age			Frequency (times daily)	Notes
		1 month–2 years	2–12 years	12–18 years		
Extrapyramidal symptoms, dystonia	Oral	←	2mg	→	1	May be given as 2 divided doses.
Antispasmodic	Oral	500 microgram	2-7 years 500 microgram 7-12 years 2mg	2mg	1 1	Initial dose. Increased by 500 microgram – 2mg a day, every 10 days until there is a clinical effect. The daily maintenance dose is usually given as 3 or 4 divided doses.

ADMINISTRATION
Give before food if patient experiences excessive dry mouth and after food if nausea is experienced. If taken after meals thirst can be allayed by peppermint, chewing gum or water.

CONTRA-INDICATIONS & WARNINGS
Caution must be observed in patients with: hypertension, cardiac, liver or kidney dysfunction, glaucoma, gastrointestinal or genito-urinary obstruction. Not recommended for use in patients with tardive dyskinesia. Trihexyphenidyl (benzhexol) may be the subject of abuse, due to hallucinogenic or euphoriant properties, if given in sufficient amounts.

INTERACTIONS
Drug interactions include increased antimuscarinic effects (blurred vision, dry mouth, constipation and urinary retention) with *nefopam, disopyramide, tricyclic antidepressants, MAOIs, antihistamines* and *phenothiazines. MAOIs, amantadine* and some *tricyclic antidepressants* may also cause excitation, confusion and hallucinations. Reduces absorption of *ketoconazole* and *levodopa.* Antagonises *cisapride.*

PREGNANCY
Avoid if at all possible, especially during the first trimester.

BREAST-FEEDING
There is no information available on the presence or absence of trihexyphenidyl (benzhexol) in breast milk.

SIDE-EFFECTS
These are anticholinergic and antimuscarinic.
Cardiovascular: tachycardia.
Digestive: constipation, paralytic ileus, dry mouth, nausea, vomiting.
Nervous system: confusion, psychosis, visual hallucinations, memory impairment, depression.
Special senses: blurred vision, dilated pupils.
Urogenital: urinary retention, dysuria.
Others: hypersensitivity.

T

POISONING/TOXICITY
No specific antidote but gastric lavage, emetics and high enemas are recommended. Forced fluid intake and general supportive measures are necessary.

PHARMACOKINETIC PROPERTIES
Completely absorbed following oral administration. Plasma half-life range 3-7 hours. Excreted in the urine in the form of metabolites. Begins to act within 1 hour, peak effects last 2-3 hours and duration of action 6-12 hours.

EXCIPIENTS
Broflex® syrup includes sucrose. Elixir is sugar-free. Contact manufacturers for further details.

LICENSED STATUS
Not licensed for use in children.

FURTHER INFORMATION
Elixir is available as a "special" e.g. from Rosemont.

Trimethoprim

Antibacterial active *in vitro* against most Gram-positive and Gram-negative aerobic organisms.

USES
Used most commonly in the treatment of urinary and respiratory tract infections and for the prophylaxis of recurrent urinary tract infections, particularly if ureteric reflux or a structural renal tract abnormality is present.

PRESENTATION
Suspension: 50mg in 5mL – Monotrim® and Trimopan®.
Tablet: 100mg and 200mg – Monotrim® and non-proprietary.

DOSAGE
Newborn infant (birth to 1 month)

Route	Age	Frequency	Notes
	birth–1month	(times daily)	
Oral	3mg/kg	loading dose	Treatment dose.
	then	then	
	2mg/kg	2	
Oral	2mg/kg	once	Prophylaxis dose.
		(in the evening)	

Child

Route	Age			Frequency	Notes
	1 month–2 years	2–12 years	12–18 years	(times daily)	
Oral	←	4mg/kg	→	2	Treatment dose. Maximum single dose 200mg.
Oral	←	2mg/kg	→	once (at night)	Prophylaxis dose.

Renal impairment – reduce dose frequency.
Moderate impairment: normal dose for 3 days then 50% of dose twice a day.
Severe impairment: 50% of dose 12 hourly.
Should not be given to dialysis patients unless plasma concentration can be measured.

CONTRA-INDICATIONS & WARNINGS

Avoid in children with fragile X chromosome as folate depletion may worsen psychomotor regression. Avoid in porphyria as may produce clinical exacerbation. Discontinue if skin rash appears. Use cautiously in severe hepatic impairment as absorption may be altered. Caution in use in patients with actual or potential folate deficiency. Avoid particularly in megaloblastic anaemia secondary to folate deficiency and in other haematological abnormalities. If any change in haematopoiesis or if folate deficiency occurs consider supplementation with folinic acid.

INTERACTIONS

May inhibit hepatic metabolism of *phenytoin* leading to increased *phenytoin* concentrations. Theoretical increased risk of folate deficiency with *phenytoin*. May potentiate *warfarin* effects by stereoselective inhibition of *warfarin* metabolism. May potentiate effects of *digoxin* and reduce renal excretion of *lamivudine*. Increased potential for nephrotoxicity when used concurrently with *ciclosporin (cyclosporin)* and may also decrease plasma levels of *ciclosporin*. Potential for increased myelosuppression when used together with other bone marrow depressants particularly with folate inhibitors such as *pyrimethamine* or *methotrexate* when megaloblastic anaemia is a risk. *Rifampicin* may decrease trimethoprim concentrations.

PREGNANCY

Crosses placenta producing similar levels in maternal and fetal blood and in amniotic fluid. Avoid in first trimester as animal studies have shown teratogenic potential and it is a folate antagonist.

BREAST-FEEDING

Appears in breast milk in low concentrations but insufficient to prevent breast-feeding.

SIDE-EFFECTS

Most frequent are rash, pruritus and gastrointestinal symptoms. More serious skin reactions have occurred (Stevens-Johnson syndrome, exfoliative dermatitis and toxic epidermal necrolysis). Severe hypersensitivity reactions reported rarely. Depression of bone marrow resulting in thrombocytopenia, neutropenia, megaloblastic anaemia and leukaemia. Generally mild and reversible but risk increased in folate depletion, concurrent folate antimetabolites, haemolysis, impaired renal function or prolonged high dose. Folinic acid may resolve haematological abnormalities.

POISONING/TOXICITY

Acute overdose may produce nausea, vomiting, headache, diarrhoea, mental depression, confusion, facial swelling and bone marrow depression. Acidification of urine may enhance elimination. Moderately removed by haemodialysis but not by peritoneal dialysis.

PHARMACOKINETIC PROPERTIES

Rapidly and completely absorbed from gastrointestinal tract. Peak concentration in plasma appears after 1-2 hours for liquid and 2-4 hours after tablet administration. Widely distributed in body fluid and tissues including CSF. 42-46% plasma protein bound. Primarily renally excreted by glomerular filtration and tubular secretion with 40-60% excreted in urine within 24 hours. 10-20% of dose hepatically metabolised. Half-life reported as 18-19 hours in newborn neonates, dropping to 4-7 hours in children and rising again to 8-11 hours in adults. Prolonged in premature neonates and renal failure.

EXCIPIENTS

Contact manufacturers for further details.

LICENSED STATUS

Licensed for >6 weeks of age. In neonates licence states 'use under careful medical supervision'.

FURTHER INFORMATION

May interfere with Guthrie test, some methotrexate assays and the Jaffe reaction for creatinine.

Trimipramine

Tricyclic antidepressant.

USES

Depression when sedative effects also required.

PRESENTATION
Tablet: 10mg and 25mg – Surmontil®.
Capsule: 50mg – Surmontil®.

DOSAGE

Indication	Route	Age		Frequency (times daily)	Notes
		2–12 years	12–18 years		
Depression	Oral	>6 years 50–100mg	75–300mg	1 (at night)	

CONTRA-INDICATIONS & WARNINGS, INTERACTIONS, PREGNANCY, BREAST-FEEDING, POISONING/TOXICITY
See imipramine monograph.

SIDE-EFFECTS
As imipramine but markedly sedative. Does not suppress rapid eye movement (REM) sleep.

PHARMACOKINETIC PROPERTIES
Absorption following oral administration is about 80% with extensive pre-systemic metabolism. The mean plasma elimination half-life is in the range 7-23 hours. Trimipramine is highly plasma protein bound (95%). It is extensively metabolised in the liver.

EXCIPIENTS
See manufacturers SPC for further details.

LICENSED STATUS
Not licensed for use in children.

Tryptophan (L-Tryptophan)

USES
Anecdotal evidence of use in non-ketotic hyperglycinaemia.

PRESENTATION
Tablet: 500mg – Optimax®.
Powder.

DOSAGE

Route	Age			Frequency (times daily)	Notes
	1 month–2 years	2–12 years	12–18 years		
Oral	←	33.3mg/kg	→	3	

ADMINISTRATION
Nausea can be minimised by giving tryptophan with food.

CONTRA-INDICATIONS & WARNINGS
Eosinophilia-myalgia syndrome has been reported with tryptophan-containing products and therefore close and regular surveillance is required; monitor eosinophil count, haematological changes and muscle symptomatology.

INTERACTIONS
Antidepressants: CNS excitation and confusion with *MAOIs* (reduce tryptophan dose); agitation and nausea with *SSRIs*.

PREGNANCY/BREAST-FEEDING
Safety has not been established.

SIDE-EFFECTS
Drowsiness, nausea, headache, light-headedness. Eosinophilia-myalgia syndrome (see contra-indications & warnings section).

POISONING/TOXICITY
Drowsiness and vomiting may occur. Supportive measures should be employed.

PHARMACODYNAMIC PROPERTIES
Tryptophan administration increases kynurenic acid, which is an endogenous antagonist of the NMDA receptor.

EXCIPIENTS
See manufacturers SPC for further details.

LICENSED STATUS
Not licensed for use in children and not licensed for non-ketotic hyperglycinaemia.

FURTHER INFORMATION
Powder available from Scientific Hospital Supplies.

For supply of tablets, patient and prescriber must be registered with the Optimax® Information and Clinical Support (OPTICS) unit. A safety questionnaire is sent to the prescriber after 3 and 6 months of treatment and every 6 months thereafter. The information is reviewed by the CSM.

Tuberculin purified protein derivative (PPD)

At the time of writing (May 2003) the supply of PPD is uncertain. It is essential to consult the manufacturers literature as the protocol is different for different preparations.

USES
To assess hypersensitivity to tubercle bacilli. Mainly used prior to BCG in adults and children >3 months old, and in those suspected of having tuberculosis (TB) and their contacts.

PRESENTATION
Injection: (solution).

Contains tuberculin PPD prepared from the heat-treated products of growth and lysis of the appropriate species of mycobacterium. Available in a number of strengths; 10 units in 1mL, 100 units in 1mL, 1000 units in 1mL and 100,000 units in 1mL. A control solution for the Mantoux test is also available.

DOSAGE & ADMINISTRATION
For both the Mantoux and Heaf tests, the volar surface of the left forearm is used.

For the Mantoux test, **0.1mL** of the appropriate solution is given by intradermal injection. For the Heaf test, enough solution is applied to an area of skin larger than that covered by the needles of the apparatus.

Strength of PPD solution (units/ml)	Dilution of PPD	Main use	Route of injection
100,000	–	Multiple puncture Heaf test	Percutaneous.
1000	1 in 100	Mantoux test – special circumstances	Intradermal.
100	1 in 1000	Mantoux test – routine	Intradermal.
10	1 in 10,000	Mantoux test – when TB is suspected	Intradermal.

Interpretation of Test Results

Heaf test. This is best read at 7 days after the test has been performed, but between 3-10 days is acceptable. Depending on the degree of induration, the reaction is graded 0–4 as follows:

Grade 0   No induration at the puncture sites.
Grade 1   Discrete induration at 4 or more needle sites.
Grade 2   Induration around each needle site merging with the next, forming a ring of induration with a clear centre.
Grade 3   The centre of the reaction becomes filled with induration to form one uniform disc of induration 5-10mm wide.
Grade 4   Solid induration over 10mm wide. Vesiculation or ulceration may also occur.

In practice it is useful to have a visual representation available when reading the test. Grades 0–1 are considered 'negative' and grades 2-4 'positive'.

Mantoux test. The test is ideally read at 48-72 hours after being performed, but an interval of 96 hours may be acceptable. A positive test is one where there is an area of induration of at least 5mm across after an injection of **0.1mL** of 100 units/mL PPD.

A positive test indicates tuberculin hypersensitivity which may result from a previous BCG vaccination, previous TB infection or active TB. Depending on whether they have received BCG vaccination in the past, children with a positive result may require further investigation. They should not be given BCG.

CONTRA-INDICATIONS & WARNINGS
The correct strength solution must be used. If a strong solution is used in a child who is tuberculin sensitive, an exaggerated response, possibly with ulceration, may occur.

INTERACTIONS
The following may produce a false negative result: infectious mononucleosis and other viral infections, *live viral vaccines*, Hodgkin disease, sarcoidosis, immunosuppression, e.g. *corticosteroid treatment,* HIV infection, etc.
The test should be postponed until 3 weeks elapse after recovery from a viral infection or administration of a *live viral vaccine* (4 weeks for MMR).

PREGNANCY
It is not recommended in pregnancy unless there is a clear indication, but there are no data to indicate that it may be harmful.

BREAST-FEEDING
It is not recommended, but there are no data to indicate that it may be harmful and it should not be withheld if its performance is important for diagnostic purposes.

SIDE-EFFECTS
Exaggerated reactions such as ulceration and regional lymphadenopathy can rarely occur. Fever, nausea, headache and rashes have also been reported. Lymphangitis and anaphylaxis are very rare. Contact with open cuts, mouth or eyes can cause a severe local reaction needing treatment with topical corticosteroid.

POISONING/TOXICITY
See contra-indications and warnings.

EXCIPIENTS
Polysorbate 80, potassium dihydrogen phosphate, disodium hydrogen phosphate and sodium chloride. The 100,000 unit in 1mL preparation also contains phenol (0.25%w/v) and glycerol.

LICENSED STATUS
Fully licensed for use as described above.

FURTHER INFORMATION
Storage: protect from light and store at 2-8°C, do not freeze. Once reconstituted, it should be used within 1 hour.
Glycerol and polysorbate 80 are of bovine, caprine, ovine and/or porcine origin from EU countries other than UK, Portugal and Switzerland. The sources of these materials are kept under constant review.

Typhoid (strain Ty21a), live (oral)

T

USES
To provide active protection against typhoid to those ≥6 years old travelling to countries where typhoid is endemic. It may not be necessary if the standards of hygiene in the accommodation where the traveller is staying are good and the length of stay is short.

PRESENTATION
Capsule: enteric coated – Vivotif®.
Each capsule contains not less than $2x10^9$ viable organisms of the attenuated *Salmonella typhi* strain Ty21a. Each pack contains 3 capsules.

DOSAGE
One capsule administered on alternate days until all three have been taken. When exposure is repeated or continuous, protection is likely to last for at least 3 years. For those normally living in non-endemic areas and travelling to endemic areas infrequently, the course should be repeated if more than a year has elapsed since the previous course.

ADMINISTRATION
Oral: one hour before a meal with a cold or lukewarm drink. Capsules should be swallowed whole and not chewed.

CONTRA-INDICATIONS & WARNINGS
As for vaccines generally; also, the vaccine should not be given to anyone who is immunosuppressed (including patients with HIV infection). It should not be taken during persistent diarrhoea or vomiting.

INTERACTIONS
Human normal immunoglobulin does not interfere with the action of the vaccine. *Sulphonamides* and *some antibiotics* may interfere with the replication of the salmonella and thus reduce its efficacy. If *mefloquine* is being taken, it should not be given within 12 hours of the vaccine. *Oral polio vaccine* and *oral typhoid vaccine* should be given at least 3 weeks apart. This recommendation is based on theoretical grounds alone, but until there is practical experience to the contrary, it should be followed.

PREGNANCY
There are no data available and so it should not be used in pregnancy.

BREAST-FEEDING
There is no data available and so it should not be used while breast-feeding.

SIDE-EFFECTS
Transient mild nausea, vomiting, abdominal cramps, diarrhoea and urticaria have been reported uncommonly.

POISONING/TOXICITY
Five times the recommended dose given to adults produced no adverse reactions.

PHARMACODYNAMIC PROPERTIES
Protection commences about 7-10 days after ingestion of the third capsule. In the recommended dose, the organism is not excreted in the stools. It may be excreted if the dose is exceeded.

EXCIPIENTS
Lactose, sucrose, ascorbic acid, Hy-Case SF and magnesium stearate.

LICENSED STATUS
Licensed for use as described.

FURTHER INFORMATION
An alternative is the polysaccharide vaccine, which is licensed for use in children >18 months.
Protect from light and store at 2–8°C.

Typhoid vaccine (polysaccharide)

USES
To provide active protection against typhoid to those ≥18 months travelling to countries where typhoid is endemic. It may not be necessary if the standard of hygiene in the accommodation where the traveller is staying is good and the length of stay is short.

PRESENTATION
Injection: (single dose solution) – Typherix®; Typhim Vi®.
Each dose contains 25 micrograms of the Vi polysaccharide capsular antigen of *Salmonella typhi*.

DOSAGE/ADMINISTRATION
IM or deep SC: 0.5mL.

CONTRA-INDICATIONS & WARNINGS
As for vaccines generally.

INTERACTIONS
Can be given in any temporal relation to other vaccines and medication.

PREGNANCY/BREAST-FEEDING
There are no data available and so it should not normally be used in pregnancy or during breast-feeding. However, if there is a very high risk of exposure it may be considered.

SIDE-EFFECTS
Transient mild local reactions occur in up to one-fifth of recipients. Mild systemic reactions such as malaise, headache, fever and nausea are less common.

POISONING/TOXICITY
No data available.

T

EXCIPIENTS
Phenol, sodium chloride, disodium phosphate and monosodium phosphate.

LICENSED STATUS
Licensed for use as above. Typherix® is not recommended for children <2 years.

FURTHER INFORMATION
In people >5 years, immunity lasts for at least 3 years. Those at continued risk should be re-vaccinated after 3 years. There is an oral preparation, but it is not licensed for use in those <6 years old.
Store at 2–8°C and do not freeze.
Bovine materials are used in the manufacturing process. Trace amounts of the original material may be present in the final product, however, all such material is obtained from sources known to be free of BSE.

Ubiquinone (coenzyme Q10)

Co-enzyme involved in electron transport in the mitochondria.

USES
Anecdotal evidence of use in congenital lactic acidosis.

PRESENTATION
Capsule: 10mg and 30mg.
Oral solution: 50mg in 10ml.
Tablet: 10mg.

DOSAGE

Route	Age				Frequency (times daily)	Notes
	birth–1 month	1 month–2 years	2–12 years	12–18 years		
Oral	←	10–100mg		→	3	With meals. Some centres use a dose of 5mg daily, initially.

Dosage in renal impairment/liver failure
Moderate to severe liver disease – caution due to potential accumulation.
No information on use in renal impairment.

CONTRA-INDICATIONS & WARNINGS
Hypersensitivity to any component of formulations.
Diabetes mellitus patients may require less insulin.

INTERACTIONS
Oral hypoglycaemic agents inhibit some ubidecarone enzymes. *Simvastatin*: lower plasma levels of endogenous ubiquinone in hyperlipidaemic patients.

PREGNANCY/BREAST-FEEDING
No information available.

SIDE-EFFECTS
Most commonly nausea, epigastric discomfort, diarrhoea, heartburn, loss of appetite. Responds to dose reduction or cessation of therapy. Rarely irritability, agitation, headache and dizziness. Mild increases in serum aminotransferases at high doses only. Skin rash is quite rare.

POISONING/TOXICITY
No information available.

EXCIPIENTS
Capsules contain gelatin. Contact manufacturer for further details.

LICENSED STATUS
Dietary product, unlicensed for treating mitochondrial diseases.

FURTHER INFORMATION
Capsules 10mg available from Lamberts Healthcare; 30mg from Larkhall Green Farm.
Tablets available from Cantassium. Oral solution available from IDIS World Medicines.

Urea cream

Keratolytic agent that hydrates and penetrates the epidermis.

USES
Hydrating agent in scaling conditions.

PRESENTATION
Cream: 10% – Aquadrate®; Eucerin®; Nutraplus®.
Lotion: 10% – Eucerin®.

DOSAGE/ADMINISTRATION
Topical: wash affected area, rinse off all traces of soap and apply sparingly twice daily.

CONTRA-INDICATIONS & WARNINGS
May cause local irritation and oedema when applied to
sensitive skin.

EXCIPIENTS
See manufacturers SPC for further details.

LICENSED STATUS
Licensed for use in children and adults.

FURTHER INFORMATION
Aquadrate® is lanolin and preservative free.

Urokinase

An enzyme derived from human urine that directly converts plasminogen to the proteolytic enzyme plasmin.

USES
Thrombolysis of blocked arteriovenous shunts and IV cannulas/central lines; thromboembolic disease.

PRESENTATION
Injection: 10,000, 50,000, 100,000 and 250,000 international unit vials – named patient.

DOSAGE

Indication	Route	Age				Frequency	Notes
		birth–1 month	1 month–2 years	2–12 years	12–18 years	(times daily)	
Thrombo-embolic disease	IV	← 4400 international units/kg in 15mL of solution →				single dose	Loading dose over 10 minutes.
	then IV infusion	← 4400 international units/kg/hour →				then for 12 hours	Adjust dose if necessary according to response.
Occluded arteriovenous shunts, IV cannulae, central lines	Directly into catheter	← 5000 international units in 2mL → (volume administered dependent on length and lumen size of catheter)				single dose	Instill into the affected catheter and clamp off. Retain for 2–4 hours, and then aspirate the lysate. Repeat (with 10,000 international units if necessary) if 5000 international units single dose fails to clear occlusion.

ADMINISTRATION
IV infusion: reconstitute with Water for Injections as per product information, then further dilute with NaCl 0.9%, glucose 5% or glucose 10% if needed.

CONTRA-INDICATIONS & WARNINGS
Recent bleeding, surgery (within 3 days), severe hypertension, severe hepatic/renal insufficiency. When used in 'local' situations the above contra-indications may not be relevant. Use with caution in patients with peptic ulceration.

INTERACTIONS
In glucose solution there is a measurable (<10%) reduction in the activity of urokinase after 8 hours. Concomitant administration of *dextran sulphate* may prolong the activity of urokinase.

PREGNANCY
Contra-indicated in pregnancy and the immediate post-partum period. Contact local Medicines Information Centre for advice.

BREAST-FEEDING
Contact local Medicines Information Centre for advice.

SIDE-EFFECTS
When used in occluded arteriovenous shunts, warmth, initial severe pain and dull ache in shunt limb have occasionally been reported. When used in thromboembolic disease, pyrexia, bleeding and haemorrhagic complications may occur.

POISONING/TOXICITY
If severe haemorrhage occurs consider using aprotinin, tranexamic acid or whole blood.

EXCIPIENTS
Contact manufacturers for further details.

LICENSED STATUS
German product (which is licensed in adults only) from Medac, available via IDIS World medicines.

FURTHER INFORMATION
As urokinase is of human origin, it is not immunogenic in man.

Ursodeoxycholic acid

A bile acid.

USES
Anecdotal use as additive therapy to cholesterol in Smith-Lemli-Opitz syndrome (in combination with chenodeoxycholic acid). In cystic fibrosis related liver disease, including cholestasis in infants, to improve bile flow. Biliary atresia in infants. Inborn errors of bile acid synthesis. Paediatric liver disease.

PRESENTATION
Tablet: 150mg – Destolit®, Ursogal® and non-proprietary; 300mg – Urdox®.
Capsule: 250mg – Ursofalk®, Ursogal® and non-proprietary
Powder: may be extemporaneously prepared.
Suspension: 250mg in 5mL – Ursofalk®.

DOSAGE

Route	Age				Frequency (times daily)	Notes
	birth–1 month	1 month–2 years	2–12 years	12–18 years		
Oral	←		5–10mg/kg	→	2–3	Maximum total daily dose of 45mg/kg/day.
Oral for cystic fibrosis patients	-	←	10mg/kg	→	2	To improve bile flow in cystic fibrosis patients with liver impairment. **Total daily dose** may be given in three divided doses.

U

ADMINISTRATION
Oral: The last dose of the day should be taken in the late evening to counteract the rise in biliary cholesterol saturation, which occurs in the early hours of the morning. Take with food; this is especially useful with the late evening dose as it helps to maintain bile flow overnight. Starting at a lower dose initially, increasing to the final dose over about 2 weeks can help to prevent initial problems with abdominal discomfort, which may occur.

CONTRA-INDICATIONS & WARNINGS
Active gastric, or duodenal ulcers.

INTERACTIONS
Avoid drugs which bind bile acids such as *colestyramine (cholestyramine)* and certain antacids e.g. *aluminium hydroxide* which may interfere with the absorption of ursodeoxycholic acid. Drugs which increase cholesterol elimination in bile; such as *oestrogenic hormones, oestrogen-rich oral contraceptives* and certain blood cholesterol lowering agents should not be used concurrently with ursodeoxycholic acid. Increases absorption of *ciclosporin (cyclosporin)*.

PREGNANCY
Manufacturers recommend not using during pregnancy. When treating women of childbearing potential, non-hormonal or low oestrogen oral contraceptive measures are recommended. Contact local Medicines Information Centre for advice.

BREAST-FEEDING
Recommended to avoid breast-feeding. Contact local Medicines Information Centre for advice.

SIDE-EFFECTS
Diarrhoea has occurred occasionally.

POISONING/TOXICITY
Serious adverse effects are unlikely to occur. Diarrhoea may occur. Monitor liver function. Ion-exchange resins may be useful to bind bile acids in the intestines.

PHARMACOKINETIC PROPERTIES
Absorbed from the gastrointestinal tract and undergoes first pass metabolism and enterohepatic recycling. It is partially conjugated in the liver before being excreted into bile and undergoing 7-dehydroxylation to lithocholic acid, some of which is excreted directly in the faeces. The rest is absorbed and mainly conjugated and sulphated by the liver before excretion in the faeces.

EXCIPIENTS
Contact manufacturers for further details.

LICENSED STATUS
Not licensed for use in children; except for Ursofalk® which is licensed for use in children and adults, but only for treatment of primary biliary cirrhosis and the dissolution of radiolucent gallstones in patients with a functioning gall bladder.

Vancomycin

A glycopeptide antimicrobial agent with a primarily bactericidal action.

USES
Active against many Gram-positive bacteria; it is used by injection in potentially life threatening infections including methicillin-resistant *Staphylococcus aureus* (MRSA) which cannot be treated with other effective, less toxic antimicrobial drugs.
In cystic fibrosis patients – reserve for MRSA infection or serious *Staphylococcus aureus* infections that do not respond to other anti-staphylococcal antibiotics.
It may be used orally to treat susceptible infections of the gastrointestinal tract (e.g. *Pseudomembranous colitis*) and intrathecally to treat shunt infections in patients with hydrocephalus.

PRESENTATION
Capsule: 125mg and 250mg – Vancocin® and non-proprietary.
Injection: 500mg and 1g vials – Vancocin® and non-proprietary.

DOSAGE
Newborn infant (birth to 1 month)

Route	*Postconceptional age	Dose	Frequency (times daily)
IV	<28 weeks	15mg/kg	1
	29-35 weeks	15mg/kg	2
	>35 weeks	15mg/kg	3
Intrathecal	All newborn infants	2.5 – 5mg	1

*Postconceptional age = gestational plus postnatal age.

Child

Route	Age			Frequency (times daily)	Notes
	1 month–2 years	2–12 years	12–18 years		
Oral	← 10mg/kg →		125mg	4	Not significantly absorbed e.g. *Pseudomembranous colitis.*
IV	← 15mg/kg then 10mg/kg →			loading dose 4	Total daily dose should not exceed 2g/**day**. The total daily dose may be given in 2-3 divided doses (IV or oral).
IV for cystic fibrosis patients	← 10mg/kg →			4	Starting dose. Amend according to levels. Monitor levels after third dose. Trough level of 5-10mg/L is acceptable and up to 15mg/L may be preferred in severe infections. Post dose 1 hour after completion of infusion (peak) level of 18-26mg/L Always check local policy.
Intrathecal	5mg	<4 years 5mg 4–12 years 10mg	≤15 years 10mg >15 years 20mg	1 1	Patients with enlarged ventricles require higher doses. Adjust dose according to CSF levels after 3-4 days. Aim for trough level of<10mg/L.

Dosage in impaired renal function
Avoid parenteral route if possible in renal impairment. Dose is reduced according to blood levels. In anuric patients a loading dose of 15mg/kg then a dose every several days may be sufficient. In peritoneal dialysis add vancomycin to dialysis fluids either as 20mg/L in each bag for 5 days or 100mg/L in one bag only per day for 5 days.

ADMINISTRATION
IV: intermittent infusion is the preferred method of administration though continuous infusion has been used when intermittent infusion is not feasible. Vancocin® on reconstitution 500mg powder displaces 0.3mL; for IV administration add 9.7mL Water for Injections to give a 50mg in 1mL solution. No displacement volume for non-proprietary products; for IV administration add 10mL Water for Injections to give a 50mg in 1mL solution. Further dilute with NaCl 0.9% or glucose 5% to give 5mg in 1mL, which is infused over at least 1 hour. In fluid restricted patients maximum concentration is 10mg in 1mL, infused centrally over at least 1 hour.
The powder should be stored below 25°C. After reconstitution it may be stored in the fridge for 24 hours. Inspect for particulate matter and discolouration prior to administration.
Oral: the injection may be given orally. Common flavouring syrups may be added to the solution at the time of administration. Solutions of the parenteral powder intended for oral use may be stored in a fridge (2-8°C) for 96 hours.

CONTRA-INDICATIONS & WARNINGS
Hypersensitivity to vancomycin. Too rapid infusion may be associated with 'red man' syndrome. Not for IM use.

INTERACTIONS
Concurrent use of other potentially *nephrotoxic drugs*, such as *aminoglycosides* and *amphotericin B* requires

careful monitoring. Concurrent administration of vancomycin and *anaesthetic agents* has been associated with erythema, histamine-like flushing and anaphylactoid reactions.

PREGNANCY
In teratology studies no evidence of harm to the fetus was demonstrated. Vancomycin is found in cord blood and should be given in pregnancy only if clearly needed and blood levels carefully monitored to minimise risk of fetal toxicity. It has been reported that pregnant patients may require higher doses to achieve therapeutic serum concentrations.

BREAST-FEEDING
Vancomycin is excreted in breast milk. Caution should be exercised when administered to nursing mothers. It is unlikely that the nursing infant will absorb significant amounts of vancomycin from the gastrointestinal tract.

SIDE-EFFECTS
Nephrotoxicity; ototoxicity rarely if serum levels are kept below 30mg/L; infusion related events ('red man' syndrome); reversible haematological disorders; miscellaneous – see manufacturers SPC for details.

POISONING/TOXICITY
In cases of overdose, supportive care is advised with maintenance of glomerular filtration. Vancomycin is poorly removed from the blood by haemodialysis or peritoneal dialysis. Haemoperfusion with Amberlite resin XAD-4 has been reported to be of limited use.

PHARMACOKINETIC PROPERTIES
Blood level monitoring - approximate time to steady state is 1–2 days. Suggested sampling times for levels at fourth dose: trough immediately prior to next dose and post dose (peak) 1 hour after completion of infusion. Therapeutic levels: trough 5-10mg/L and peak 18-26mg/L. CSF level monitoring – take trough sample immediately prior to next dose. Level should be <10mg/L.

EXCIPIENTS
Contact manufacturers for further details.

LICENSED STATUS
Licensed for use in all ages except for administration via the intrathecal route, which is unlicensed.

FURTHER INFORMATION
Prolonged use may result in overgrowth of non-susceptible organisms.

Varicella–zoster immunoglobulin (VZIG)

USES
For passive post-exposure prophylaxis in individuals where there has been significant exposure to chickenpox or herpes zoster, and where the development of chickenpox could be very serious and the potential recipient is unlikely to have protective antibodies already. Expert advice should always be sought. Aciclovir may be indicated in some instances where VZIG is not appropriate.

For exposure to be considered significant the following need to be satisfied:

Type of disease
Chickenpox or disseminated zoster.
Exposed lesions in an immunocompetent individual.
Any lesions in an immunosuppressed patient.

Timing of exposure
If chickenpox or disseminated zoster, in the period from 48 hours prior to the onset of the rash to the time when cropping has ceased and all the lesions are crusted over.
If localised zoster, in the period from the day of onset until crusting is complete.

Closeness and duration of contact
(excluding maternal/fetal and continuous home contact).
Contact in the same room e.g. house, classroom or 2–4 bed hospital bay for 15 minutes or more.
Face-to-face contact e.g. while having a conversation.

NB Consideration should be given to the use of VZIG in larger hospital wards where there is a free flow of patients e.g. in paediatric wards.

V

Those children at risk of serious disease are as follows

Immunosuppressed children as defined below:

☐ Those currently being treated for malignant disease with chemotherapy or generalised radiotherapy, or within 6 months of terminating such treatment.

☐ Those currently on immunosuppressive therapy.

☐ Children who have had a bone marrow transplant within the previous 6 months.

☐ Children receiving prednisolone, orally or rectally, at a daily dose (or its equivalent) of 2mg/kg/day for at least 1 week, or 1mg/kg/day for 1 month.

☐ Anyone taking more than 40mg prednisolone per day for more than 1 week should be considered immunosuppressed. Those who have received such therapy in the preceeding 3 months should also be considered immunosuppressed.

☐ Lower doses of corticosteroids given in combination with cytotoxic drugs should be considered immunosuppressive for up to 3 months after cessation.

☐ Patients with impaired cell mediated immunity.

☐ HIV positive individuals, if symptomatic or CD4 count is reduced.

☐ Children with immunoglobulin deficiencies are not at risk. Either the condition will be relatively mild or they will be on replacement therapy.

Neonates

☐ VZIG should be given if the mother has developed varicella or herpes zoster in the 7 days before or after birth.

☐ VZ antibody negative infants exposed to varicella or herpes zoster in the first 7 days of life.

☐ VZIG should also be given if an exposed neonate is less than 30 weeks gestation or the birth weight was under 1kg, even if the mother was immune.

PRESENTATION

Prepared from the plasma of donors with high titres of VZ antibodies. Available as a fluid preparation of about 1.7mL containing 250mg protein and VZ antibodies at a concentration of no less than 100 international units in 1mL. Supplied by Scottish National Blood Transfusion Service and Bio Products Laboratory (via PHLS).

DOSAGE
Depends on age

Age	Dose
0–5 years	250mg (1 vial)
6–10 years	500mg (2 vials)
11–14 years	750mg (3 vials)
≥ 15 years	1000mg (4 vials)

ADMINISTRATION

IM injection. Can be administered SC to those who have clotting disorders.

CONTRA-INDICATIONS & WARNINGS

Should only be used with caution, if at all, in those who have had a hypersensitivity reaction to a previous dose.

INTERACTIONS

Administration of any immunoglobulin may raise antibody levels to a number of micro-organisms and this must be borne in mind when interpreting antibody assays within 2–3 months of such administration. It may reduce the immunogenicity of live vaccines other than those against yellow fever and typhoid. If the immunoglobulin is given first an interval of at least 3 months should pass before giving a live vaccine other than those mentioned above. If the live vaccine is given first, at least 3 weeks should elapse before giving another live vaccine.

PREGNANCY

Has been used in these circumstances and there is no evidence of harm to the fetus. It should not be withheld if its use is indicated.

BREAST-FEEDING

There is little data available. There is reason to believe it would only be beneficial to the suckling infant. It must not be withheld if its use is indicated.

SIDE-EFFECTS
Local reactions such as pain, erythema and tenderness may occur at the site of injection.

POISONING/TOXICITY
Not reported.

PHARMACODYNAMIC PROPERTIES
Peak antibody levels occur 2-3 days after injection and the half life is 2-3 days.

LICENSED STATUS
Licence for use as described.

EXCIPIENTS
Glycine, sodium chloride, sodium acetate trihydrate and sodium hydroxide.

FURTHER INFORMATION
Protect from light and store at 2–8°C; do not freeze. The diluent should be stored at less than 25°C, but not frozen. Once reconstituted the vaccine should be used within 1 hour.

VZIG is in short supply. It should be used only for the indications described above and preferably after discussion with an appropriate expert. It should be given as soon as possible after contact and is not indicated if 10 days or more have elapsed. Many patients develop chickenpox in spite of appropriate use of VZIG. It is, however, milder than if VZIG had not been given. Donors are tested for HIV, hepatitis B and hepatitis C.

Further information is available from *Immunoglobulin Handbook*, PHLS, 2002
http://www.phls.org.uk/advice/ImmunoglobulinHandbook.pdf

Varicella–zoster vaccine, live

USES
Active protection against chickenpox in those >9 months old. In the USA it is recommended for use as part of the routine childhood vaccination schedule. In the UK, the vaccine has only recently been licensed and it is used only in children who are at high risk of developing severe complications if they contract chickenpox. The indications in these children have not been fully formulated. It has been suggested that the vaccine should be given to children with leukaemia in remission.

It has also been used very successfully in children who were candidates for renal transplantation. The incidence and severity of disease were reduced very significantly. It is recommended that use of the vaccine should be considered in all non-immune children prior to any immunosuppressive therapy. Some clinicians suggest that it should be given to household contacts of immunocompromised children.

For more detailed discussion see *Immunisation of the Immunocompromised Child*
http://www.rcpch.ac.uk/publications/recent_publications/Immunocomp.pdf

PRESENTATION
Injection: (single dose freeze-dried powder) – Varilrix®.
Each 0.5mL dose contains not less than $10^{3.3}$ plaque-forming units of live varicella virus of the OKA strain cultured on MRC-5 human diploid cells.

DOSAGE/ADMINISTRATION
SC: 1-12 years a single dose of 0.5mL if immunocompetent, otherwise two doses are required at least 6 weeks apart.
   ≥13 years two doses of 0.5mL given at least 6 weeks apart.

CONTRA-INDICATIONS & WARNINGS
As for vaccines generally; but also detailed advice in SPC. Should only be used on expert advice.

INTERACTIONS
Specific *varicella-zoster immunoglobulin*, if given within a period extending from 3 months before to 3 weeks after the vaccine, may reduce its efficacy.

PREGNANCY
No data available. As the 'wild' varicella virus is known to be teratogenic, the vaccine should not be given in pregnancy.

BREAST-FEEDING
No data available. As the vaccine virus is transmissible and chickenpox in the neonate can be an extremely

serious disease, the vaccine should not be given to a breast-feeding mother.

SIDE-EFFECTS
Mild transient local reactions may occur. A mild chickenpox with vesicopapular rash and a low fever are relatively common after the first injection. The incidence of herpes zoster is equal to, or less than, that after natural chickenpox. It is usually not severe. The vaccine

virus is sensitive to aciclovir which can be used to treat chickenpox if it develops in an immunocompromised individual consequent to vaccination.

POISONING/TOXICITY
Little data available.

PHARMACODYNAMIC PROPERTIES
The virus may be transmitted from the recipient to a close contact.

EXCIPIENTS
Neomycin, amino acids, human albumin (prepared from donors resident in non-BSE areas), lactose, sorbitol and mannitol.

LICENSED STATUS
Licensed for use as above.

FURTHER INFORMATION
The vaccine should only be used after discussion with a specialist. The human albumin comes from countries with no BSE. Store at 2–8°C. It should be used immediately after reconstitution.

Vecuronium bromide

A competitive non-depolarising muscle relaxant. The duration of action is not as long as that provided by a comparable dose of pancuronium.

USES
Neuromuscular blockade for ventilation and surgery.

PRESENTATION
Injection: powder for reconstitution, 10mg vial – Norcuron®.

DOSAGE

Route	Age				Frequency (times daily)	Notes
	birth–1 month	1 month–2 years	2–12 years	12–18 years		
IV bolus	←	80-100 microgram/kg		→	single dose	Initial dose. Subsequent doses – adjust dose and interval as required.* A test dose of 10–20 microgram/kg should be considered in neonates and infants up to 4 months.
IV infusion	–	← 50–80 microgram/kg/hour		→	continuous	

*The duration of action is longer in neonates and infants than in children and adults, and so fewer supplementary doses may be needed.

ADMINISTRATION
IV injection: reconstitute a vial with 5mL Water for Injections to give a 2mg in 1mL solution.
IV infusion: infuse in glucose 5% or NaCl 0.9% at a suggested concentration of 1mg in 1mL, maximum concentration of 4mg in 1mL.

CONTRA-INDICATIONS & WARNINGS

Since vecuronium causes relaxation of the respiratory muscles, respiration must be assisted in all patients. Only limited changes of pharmacodynamic parameters were reported with vecuronium when administered to patients with renal failure.

INTERACTIONS

Enhanced effect with *aminoglycosides, metronidazole, polymyxins, suxamethonium, nifedipine, verapamil, propranolol, procainamide, quinidine, lithium and parenteral magnesium, high doses of thiopental (thiopentone), ketamine, fentanyl, beta-blockers* and *diuretics*. Decreased effect with prior chronic administration of *corticosteroids, phenytoin* and *carbamazepine*.

PREGNANCY

There are insufficient data available to assess potential harm to the fetus; placental transfer is limited. Studies have shown its safety for use in caesarian section.

BREAST-FEEDING

Contact local Medicines Information Centre for advice.

SIDE-EFFECTS

Vecuronium has only a weak capacity for inducing local histamine release and produces few or no adverse cardiovascular effects.

PHARMACOKINETIC PROPERTIES

The usual duration of action in children is 15-20 minutes and 30-40 minutes in infants. At steady state the plasma elimination half-life averages 71 +/- 20 minutes but considerably longer than this in infancy. Biliary excretion is the main elimination route with about 30% of the drug renally excreted.

EXCIPIENTS

See manufacturers SPC for further details.

LICENSED STATUS

Licensed for use in all ages although neuromuscular blockade for ventilation is not a licensed indication.

Verapamil hydrochloride

Calcium-channel blocker, with Class IV antiarrhythmic therapy.

USES

Treatment and prophylaxis of supraventricular tachycardia (no longer first-line treatment for cardioversion; adenosine is now recommended first line).
Treatment and prophylaxis of atrial flutter/fibrillation (but not if associated with Wolff-Parkinson-White syndrome).
Treatment of mild to moderate systemic hypertension.

PRESENTATION

Capsule (modified release): 120mg, 180mg and 240mg – Univer®.
Injection: 2.5mg in 1mL, 2mL ampoules – Cordilox® and Securon®.
Oral solution: 40mg in 5mL – non-proprietary. Other strengths may be extemporaneously prepared.
Tablet: 40mg and 120mg – Cordilox®, Securon® and non-proprietary; 80mg and 160mg – Cordilox® and non-proprietary.
Tablet (modified release): 120mg – Half Securon SR®; (scored) 240mg – Securon SR®; 240mg – Verapress MR®.

V

DOSAGE

Route	Age				Frequency (times daily)	Notes
	birth–1 month	1 month–2 years	2–12 years	12–18 years		
Oral	1–2mg/kg	20mg	← 40–120mg →		3	
Slow IV bolus	100–200 microgram/kg (maximum 2mg)	≤ 1 year 100–200 microgram/kg (maximum 2mg) > 1 year 100–300 microgram/kg (maximum 5mg)	← 100–300 microgram/kg → (maximum 5mg)		single dose single dose	ECG monitoring required. Dose may be repeated after 30 minutes if necessary. Many cases are controlled by doses at the lower end of the range.

Renal impairment
Patients with impaired renal function should be monitored for prolongation of the PR interval on ECG, blood pressure changes or other signs of overdose during verapamil therapy.

Hepatic impairment
Since verapamil is extensively metabolised in the liver, careful dose titration is required along with careful patient monitoring in those with liver disease.

ADMINISTRATION
IV: it is recommended that the dose of verapamil be administered by direct IV push over at least 2 to 3 minutes. Intermittent or continuous infusions are not recommended. Patients should be monitored for hypotension and under ECG monitoring. Verapamil is usually physically compatible with solutions of pH ranging from 3-6 e.g. glucose 5% or NaCl 0.9% but may precipitate in solutions having a pH greater than 6 e.g. sodium bicarbonate solutions.
Oral: injection may be given orally. The tablets may be dispersed in glucose 5% to disguise the bitter taste, up to a concentration of 10mg in 1mL.

CONTRA-INDICATIONS & WARNINGS
Cardiogenic shock, second or third degree AV block, sino-atrial block, sick sinus syndrome, uncompensated heart failure, significant bradycardia, hypotension. Combination with beta-blockers is contra-indicated in cardiac failure. Concomitant ingestion of grapefruit juice is also contra-indicated.
Warnings: verapamil may affect impulse conduction and should be used with caution in patients with first degree AV block. The effects of verapamil and beta-blockers or other drugs with cardiodepressive action may be additive. Patients with atrial fibrillation/flutter and an accessory pathway (e.g. Wolff-Parkinson-White syndrome) may develop increased conduction across the anomalous pathway and ventricular tachycardia may be precipitated.
Verapamil may affect left ventricular contractility as a result of its mode of action. This effect is small and normally not important but cardiac failure may be precipitated or aggravated. In patients with incipient cardiac failure, therefore, verapamil should be given only after such cardiac failure has been controlled with appropriate therapy.

INTERACTIONS
Enhanced effect of *digoxin* (AV block and bradycardia). *Beta-blockers, anti-arrhythmic agents* or *inhaled anaesthetics* in combination with verapamil may lead to additive cardiovascular effects (e.g. AV block, bradycardia, hypotension, heart failure). *IV beta-blockers* should not be given to patients on verapamil therapy. *Class I antiarrhythmics* (e.g. *flecainide*) in combination with verapamil may result in profound cardiac depression and requires expert supervision. *Amiodarone* co-administration with verapamil may result in bradycardia, AV block and myocardial depression. *Carbamazepine, ciclosporin (cyclosporin)* or *theophylline* with verapamil has resulted in increased serum levels of these medications which could lead to increased side-effects.
Phenytoin and *phenobarbital (phenobarbitone)* reduce the effect of verapamil. *Cimetidine* can cause an increase in the verapamil serum level. *Rifampicin* decreases levels of verapamil. The effects of *neuromuscular blocking agents* employed in anaesthesia may be potentiated by verapamil. The effects of verapamil may be additive with *other hypotensive agents*. Verapamil increases levels of *quinidine* (extreme hypotension). *Grapefruit juice:* increase in verapamil serum level has been reported.

PREGNANCY

Animal studies have not shown any teratogenic effect but verapamil should not be used in pregnancy unless it is essential for the welfare of the patient. The possibility that verapamil can cause relaxation of the uterine muscle and therefore inhibit labour should be considered at term.

BREAST-FEEDING

Verapamil is excreted into the breast milk in small amounts but is unlikely to be harmful. However, rare hypersensitivity reactions have been reported. The American Academy of Pediatrics considers verapamil to be compatible with breast-feeding.

SIDE-EFFECTS

Constipation, flushing, headaches, nausea and vomiting, ankle oedema. When given in high doses or in the presence of previous myocardial damage, some cardiovascular effects of verapamil may occasionally be greater than therapeutically desired: bradycardic arrhythmias such as sinus bradycardia, sinus arrest with asystole, second or third degree AV block, bradyarrhythmia in atrial fibrillation, hypotension, development or aggravation of heart failure. Rarely: irreversible impairment of liver function; allergic reactions.

POISONING/TOXICITY

The course of symptoms in verapamil intoxication depends on the route of administration, the amount taken, the time taken for treatment initiation and myocardial contractility. The main symptoms are; fall in blood pressure, shock symptoms, loss of consciousness, first and second degree AV block, total AV block with total AV dissociation, escape rhythm, asystole, sinus bradycardia, sinus arrest. The therapeutic measures depend on the type and severity of symptoms. Gastric lavage may be appropriate. Intensive resuscitation measures such as extrathoracic heart massage, respiration, defibrillation and/or pacemaker therapy may be necessary.

Specific measures to be taken: elimination of cardiodepressive effects, hypotension or bradycardia. The specific antidote is calcium. See manufacturers SPC for treatment recommendations of other symptoms.

PHARMACOKINETIC PROPERTIES

Over 90% is absorbed following oral administration. Verapamil is subject to pre-systemic hepatic metabolism with up to 80% of the dose eliminated in this way. The bioavailability is therefore 10-35%. Widely and rapidly distributed, 90% bound to plasma proteins. Plasma half-life is 3-7 hours. Extensively metabolised by the liver. 3-4% of the drug is excreted unchanged and 70% as metabolic products in the urine. 16% is excreted in the faeces.

EXCIPIENTS

Contact manufacturers for further details.

LICENSED STATUS

Plain tablets and injection are licensed for use in children; modified release preparations are not.

Vigabatrin

Antiepileptic.

USES

First or second choice treatment for infantile spasms; adjunctive treatment of partial seizures with or without secondarily generalised tonic-clonic seizures that have been inadequately controlled by other antiepileptic combinations.

PRESENTATION

Tablet: 500mg – Sabril®.
Sachet: 500mg (powder to be dissolved) – Sabril®.

DOSAGE

Route	Age				Frequency (times daily)	Notes
	birth–1 month	1 month–2 years	2–12 years	12–18 years		
Oral	←	15–20mg/kg	→	1g	2	Usual starting dose.
	←	30–40mg/kg	→	1–1.5g	2	Usual target maintenance dose.

DOSAGE continued

Route	Age				Frequency (times daily)	Notes
	birth–1 month	1 month–2 years	2–12 years	12–18 years		
Oral	← 15–25mg/kg →		–	–	2	Infantile spasms. Usual starting dose.
	← 40–50mg/kg →		–	–	2	Infantile spasms. Usual target maintenance dose. Maximum dose of 75mg/kg twice daily.

Dose adjustment
Increase to maintenance dose over 2-3 weeks except for infantile spasms when the maintenance dose should be reached in 5-7 days. Reduce dose in impaired renal function.

ADMINISTRATION
Oral: may be taken before or after food. Dissolve contents of sachet in water or soft drink, a proportion can be measured to obtain smaller doses. Tablets can be crushed and dispersed in liquid or soft food.
Rectal: sachets dissolved in small amount of water have been administered rectally in same dose as oral route.

CONTRA-INDICATIONS & WARNINGS
Warn not to cease therapy without advice, withdraw gradually. Can exacerbate myoclonic and absence seizures. Caution in psychosis or behavioural problems. Effects on neurological function still being assessed. May exacerbate myoclonic seizures. Cautionary use in children with pre-existing visual field defects. Formal assessment of visual fields (perimetry) should be undertaken in all children with a cognitive age of 9 years and above before the drug is started and every 6 months while receiving the drug. Reduce dose in renal failure (<60mL/minute/1.73m^2).

INTERACTIONS
May gradually reduce plasma *phenytoin* levels by 20%.

PREGNANCY
Little data on congenital malformations. Manufacturer recommends use in pregnancy only if clearly necessary. Contact local Medicines Information Centre for advice.

BREAST-FEEDING
Only small quantities will be ingested in breast milk but little data available. Contact local Medicines Information Centre for advice.

SIDE-EFFECTS
Dose dependent side-effects include irritability, hypo– or hypertonia, drowsiness. Chronic adverse effects include increased appetite and weight gain, peripheral constriction of visual fields (about 30% of patients).

POISONING/TOXICITY
No specific antidote, use supportive measures.

PHARMACOKINETIC PROPERTIES
Rapidly and completely absorbed when given orally. Excreted unchanged by the kidney with elimination half-life of 5-8 hours. Plasma levels do not correlate with efficacy or side-effects.

EXCIPIENTS
See manufacturers SPC for further details.

LICENSED STATUS
Licensed for use in all ages as adjunctive therapy and as monotherapy in infantile spasms.

FURTHER INFORMATION
On theoretical grounds vigabatrin should be well absorbed when administered by the rectal route but there is limited clinical experience.

Vinca alkaloid.

USES
In combination therapy for treatment of Hodgkin lymphoma and anaplastic large cell lymphomas.

PRESENTATION
Injection: powder for reconstitution, 10mg – Velbe®.
Injection: 1mg in 1mL; 10mL – non-proprietary.

DOSAGE
** Always consult the current treatment protocol for details of dosage and scheduling. **
Maximum single dose 10mg.
A 50% dose reduction has been suggested in patients with serum bilirubin >50 micromol/L.

ADMINISTRATION
IV: bolus into established venous access at a concentration of 1mg in 1mL.

CONTRA-INDICATIONS & WARNINGS
Vinblastine is a highly vesicant drug; great care must be taken to avoid extravasation. For intravenous administration only.

INTERACTIONS
None recorded.

PREGNANCY
Use in pregnancy only in life-threatening situations or severe disease for which safer drugs cannot be used or are ineffective.

BREAST-FEEDING
No information available. Advise against breast-feeding.

SIDE-EFFECTS
Abdominal pain, constipation and leucopenia. Occasional mild peripheral neuropathy, thrombocytopenia and anaemia. Rarely, nausea and vomiting, alopecia and paralytic ileus.

POISONING/TOXICITY
Full supportive measures – see side-effects.

PHARMACOKINETIC PROPERTIES
No published pharmacokinetic data in children. Adult data suggest vinblastine clearance is greater than that of vincristine, hence need for higher doses. Vinblastine pharmacokinetics in adults are variable and elimination is due to metabolism, urinary and faecal excretion. Kinetics may be non-linear and dependent upon hepatic function.

EXCIPIENTS
Contact manufacturer for further details.

LICENSED STATUS
Licensed for use in children and adults.

FURTHER INFORMATION
It is recommended that extemporaneously prepared syringes of vinca alkaloids be clearly labelled: **WARNING – FOR INTRAVENOUS USE ONLY**. The word 'intrathecal' should not under any circumstances appear on a vinca alkaloid label because this might lead to selection by association. Reference: HSC 2001/022.

Vincristine sulphate

Blocks mitosis with metaphase arrest by binding to tubulin and inhibiting the assembly of microtubules. It is M-phase specific.

USES
Used in combination chemotherapy regimens for the treatment of acute lymphoblastic leukaemia, Hodgkin and non-Hodgkin lymphomas, sarcomas, neuroblastoma and Wilms tumour.

V

PRESENTATION

Injection: 1mg in 1mL; 1mL and 2mL vials – Oncovin®. 1mg in 1mL; 1mL, 2mL and 5mL vials, plus 1mL and 2mL syringes – non-proprietary.

DOSAGE

** Always consult the current treatment protocol for details of dosage and scheduling. **
Maximum dose in adults is 2mg weekly.
Small infants may be unexpectedly sensitive to vincristine. Dosage reductions may be necessary if toxicity is unacceptable.
An increase in the severity of side-effects may be seen in patients with liver disease sufficient to decrease biliary excretion. A 50% dosage reduction is recommended in patients with a serum bilirubin level >50 micromol/L.

ADMINISTRATION

IV: bolus injection either directly into a vein or into the tubing of a fast running IV infusion of NaCl 0.9% or glucose 5%.

CONTRA-INDICATIONS & WARNINGS

Contra-indications: Not for intrathecal use. Patients with the demyelinating form of Charcot-Marie-Tooth syndrome should not be given vincristine.
Cautions: when chemotherapy is being given in conjunction with radiation therapy through portals which include the liver, the use of vincristine should be delayed until radiation therapy has been completed.
Warnings: for IV use only. Highly vesicant so care must be taken to avoid extravasation.

INTERACTIONS

Vincristine may reduce serum levels of *phenytoin*.
Caution should be exercised in patients concurrently taking drugs known to inhibit drug metabolism by hepatic cytochrome P450 isoenzymes in the CYP 3A subfamily.
Vincristine plasma clearance can be reduced by *nifedipine, itraconazole, cimetidine* or *ranitidine* and increased by *phenobarbital (phenobarbitone)*. When vincristine is used in combination with *L-asparaginase*, it should be given 12-24 hours before administration of the enzyme in order to minimise toxicity, since administering *L-asparaginase* first may reduce hepatic clearance of vincristine.
Acute shortness of breath and severe bronchospasm have been reported following the administration of vinca alkaloids. These reactions have been encountered most frequently when the vinca alkaloid was used in combination with *mitomycin* and may be serious when there is pre-existing pulmonary dysfunction. The onset may be within minutes or several hours after the vinca is injected and may occur up to 2 weeks following the dose of *mitomycin*. Progressive dyspnoea, requiring chronic therapy, may occur. Vincristine should not be re-administered.

PREGNANCY

Vincristine can cause fetal harm when administered to pregnant women, although there are no adequate and well controlled studies.

BREAST-FEEDING

It is not known whether vincristine is excreted into human breast milk.
A decision should be made whether to discontinue breast-feeding or the drug, taking into account the importance of the drug to the mother.

SIDE-EFFECTS

Alopecia (uncommon), abdominal pain, pain in jaw, bones and joints, peripheral neuropathy, constipation, autonomic neuropathy.
Neuromuscular (often dose limiting): neuritic pain, sensory loss, paraesthesiae, difficulty in walking, loss of deep tendon reflexes, muscle wasting, ataxia, paresis, foot drop and cranial nerve palsies, especially ocular palsies and laryngeal nerve paralysis. Jaw pain, pharyngeal pain, parotid gland pain, bone pain, back pain, limb pain and myalgias have been reported; pain in these areas may be severe. Convulsions, frequently with hypertension, have been reported in a few patients receiving vincristine.
Haematological: leucopenia, anaemia and thrombocytopenia have been reported.
Gastrointestinal: constipation, abdominal cramps, paralytic ileus, diarrhoea, weight loss, nausea, vomiting, oral ulceration, intestinal necrosis and/or perforation, and anorexia have occurred. The constipation which may be encountered responds well to such usual measures as enemas and laxatives.
Pulmonary: see under interactions.
Other: syndrome of inappropriate antidiuretic hormone secretion (SIADH), urinary retention, hypo and hypertension, rare cases of allergic type reactions including anaphylaxis, fever, headache, injection site reaction.

POISONING/TOXICITY

Supportive care should include the following:
(a) prevention of side-effects resulting from the SIADH (this would include restriction of fluid intake and perhaps the administration of a diuretic affecting the

function of Henle's loop and the distal tubule);
(b) administration of anticonvulsants;
(c) use of enemas or cathartics to prevent ileus (in some instances, decompression of the gastrointestinal tract may be necessary);
(d) monitoring the cardiovascular system;
(e) determining daily blood counts for guidance in transfusion requirements.

Isolated case reports suggest that folinic acid may be helpful in treating humans who have received an overdose. A suggested schedule is to administer 100mg of folinic acid IV every 3 hours for 24 hours and then every 6 hours for at least 48 hours.

Haemodialysis is not likely to be helpful.

PHARMACOKINETIC PROPERTIES
After IV injection it disappears rapidly from the blood. Serum concentrations decline in a triphasic manner. The terminal half-life ranges from 10.5-15.5 hours. It is extensively protein bound and it is reported to be concentrated in blood platelets. It is metabolised in the liver and excreted primarily in the bile-about 70% of a dose is found in faeces, as unchanged drug and metabolites, over 72 hours. Some also appears in the urine. Vincristine does not appear to cross the blood-brain barrier in significant amounts.

EXCIPIENTS
Contact manufacturer for further details.

LICENSED STATUS
Licensed for use in children and adults.

FURTHER INFORMATION
It is recommended that extemporaneously prepared syringes of vinca alkaloids should be clearly labelled; **WARNING – FOR INTRAVENOUS USE ONLY**. The word 'intrathecal' should not under any circumstances appear on a vinca alkaloid label because this may lead to selection by association.

Vitamin A (retinol)

USES
Prevention of vitamin A deficiency.

PRESENTATION
Oral solution: 150,000 international units per mL (5000 international units per drop) – Arovit® (imported).

DOSAGE

Route	Age				Frequency (times daily)	Notes
	birth-1 month	1 month-2 years	2-12 years	12-18 years		
Oral	<1 year 5000 international units		10,000 international units		1	
	>1 year 10,000 international units				1	

ADMINISTRATION
Oral: take with or after meals. Can be taken in a drink e.g. water, fruit juice, iced tea.

CONTRA-INDICATIONS & WARNINGS
Known hypersensitivity to the drug or any of the excipients. Caution should be exercised when using vitamin A in pregnancy. Excessive doses of vitamin A may be teratogenic, especially when taken in the first trimester of pregnancy.

INTERACTIONS
Oral contraceptives may increase plasma vitamin A levels.

PREGNANCY
See contra-indications and warnings.

BREAST-FEEDING
Contact local Medicines Information Centre for advice.

SIDE-EFFECTS
Usually signs of overdose (see below). Discontinue treatment.

Vitamin A (retinol) continued

V

POISONING/TOXICITY

Acute poisoning symptoms include headache, nausea, vomiting, sleepiness, irritability, neurological disorders and itching. Symptoms regress within 72 hours of discontinuation of therapy. Chronic poisoning symptoms include alopecia, nausea, vomiting, premature closure of the epiphysis of long bones in children and protrusion of fontanelles in newborns. In adults asthenia, anorexia, skin scaling, bone and joint pains, oedema, headache and hepatosplenomegaly. Symptoms regress slowly depending on the type of symptoms present.

PHARMACOKINETIC PROPERTIES

Intestinal absorption is nearly complete. Partly binds with glucuronic acid and is oxidised into retinal and retinoic acid via the enterohepatic circulation. Only vitamin A metabolites are usually excreted in the urine.

EXCIPIENTS

Contact manufacturer for further details.

LICENSED STATUS

Not licensed for use in the UK.

FURTHER INFORMATION

Available as Arovit® from IDIS World Medicines. Once opened Arovit® has an expiry date of three months.

Vitamins A and D

USES

Prevention of vitamin A and D deficiency.

PRESENTATIONS

Capsules: vitamin A 4000 units, vitamin D 400 units – non-proprietary.
Emulsion: vitamin A 4600 units, vitamin D 380 units in 5mL – Halycitrol®.

DOSAGE/ADMINISTRATION

Infants 0-6months: 2.5mL of emulsion daily, orally.
6 months-adults: 5mL of emulsion or 1 capsule daily, orally.

CONTRA-INDICATIONS & WARNINGS

Known hypersensitivity (it is a preparation of fish oil). Caution should be exercised when using any vitamin supplement containing vitamin A in pregnancy, as excessive doses of vitamin A may be teratogenic, especially when taken in the first trimester. Large doses of vitamin D in lactating mothers may cause hypercalcaemia in infants. Prolonged excessive ingestion of vitamins A and D can lead to hypervitaminosis states.

PREGNANCY

See above under contra-indications & warnings.

POISONING/TOXICITY

In children prolonged excessive ingestion of vitamins A and D can lead to hypervitaminosis states. *Hypervitaminosis A:* symptoms include dry rough skin, painful joint swellings, anorexia and vomiting. *Hypervitaminosis D:* infants already receiving formula milk, vitaminised margarines and cereals can develop infantile hypercalcaemia from excessive vitamin D intake. In children and adults the symptoms of hypercalcaemia are weakness, anorexia, abdominal pain, constipation, thirst and polyuria with the development of nephrocalcinosis, renal stones and renal failure.

EXCIPIENTS

Emulsion includes sucrose and glucose. Contact manufacturers for further details.

LICENSED STATUS

Licensed for use >6 months of age.

FURTHER INFORMATION

Halycitrol® emulsion is not NHS prescribable.

USES
Prevention and treatment of vitamin B complex deficiency.

PRESENTATION
Syrup: thiamin hydrochloride 5mg, riboflavin 2mg, nicotinamide 20mg, pyridoxine hydrochloride 2mg and pantothenol 3mg per 5mL – Vigranon B®.

DOSAGE/ADMINISTRATION
Prophylactic

Infants	One 5mL spoonful daily.
1-12 years	One 5mL spoonful twice daily.
12 18 years	One 5mL spoonful three times daily.

Therapeutic

Infants	One 5mL spoonful three times daily.
1-12 years	Two 5mL spoonfuls three times daily.
12-18 years	Two to three 5mL spoonfuls three times daily.

CONTRA-INDICATIONS & WARNINGS	PREGNANCY
Known sensitivity to any of the ingredients.	Considered safe during pregnancy.

EXCIPIENTS
Syrup includes sorbitol solution. See manufacturers SPC for further details.

LICENSED STATUS
Licensed for use in all ages.

FURTHER INFORMATION
Not NHS prescribable.

Vitamin C (ascorbic acid)

Water soluble vitamin; essential for the synthesis of collagen and intercellular material; used in mitochondrial disorders to bridge a defect in the electron transport chain.

USES
Prevention and treatment of scurvy. Hawkinsinuria. Tyrosinaemia III (4 hydroxyphenylpyruvate dioxygenase deficiency). Transient tyrosinaemia of the newborn; glutathione synthase deficiency.
Anecdotal evidence of use in congenital lactic acidosis.

PRESENTATION
Tablet: 50mg, 100mg, 200mg and 500mg – non-proprietary.
Injection: 100mg in 1mL; 5mL ampoule – non-proprietary.

DOSAGE

Indication	Route	Age				Frequency (times daily)	Notes
		birth–1 month	1 month–2 years	2–12 years	12–18 years		
Scurvy	Oral	←	500mg then		→	1	Initial dose.
		←	100mg then		→	1	For 1 week.
		←	25mg		→	1	Prophylaxis.

DOSAGE continued

Indication	Route	Age				Frequency (times daily)	Notes
		birth–1 month	1 month–2 years	2–12 years	12–18 years		
Metabolic indications	Oral	←	200–400mg		→	1	Dose depends on the condition being treated; seek expert advice e.g. transient tyrosinaemia of the newborn: 50–200mg/day for 1–2 weeks. Hawkinsuria, Tyrosinaemia III: up to 1g daily, for several weeks until symptoms subside.

ADMINISTRATION
Oral: tablets are chewable.

CONTRA-INDICATIONS & WARNINGS
Hyperoxaluria. Increased intake of ascorbic acid over a long period may result in an increase in renal clearance and deficiency may well result if withdrawn too rapidly.

PREGNANCY
Ascorbic acid crosses the placenta; it can be taken in normal doses by pregnant women but a daily intake of 5g or more has been reported to cause abortion.

BREAST-FEEDING
Ascorbic acid passes into breast milk; it may be taken safely during lactation.

SIDE-EFFECTS
Large doses may cause diarrhoea and other gastrointestinal disturbances. Large doses have resulted in haemolysis in patients with G6PD deficiency.

PHARMACOKINETIC PROPERTIES
Readily absorbed from the gastrointestinal tract following oral administration; widely distributed throughout body tissues.

EXCIPIENTS
Redoxon® 200mg and 500mg tablets contain sorbitol and aspartame. Contact manufacturers for further details.

LICENSED STATUS
Not licensed for metabolic indications.

Vitamin E (alpha tocopheryl acetate)

USES
Correction of vitamin E deficiency occurring in malabsorption disorders e.g. cystic fibrosis, chronic cholestasis and abetalipoproteinaemia. Prevention of vitamin E deficiency.

PRESENTATION
Tablet: 50mg and 200mg – Ephynal®.
Suspension: 500mg in 5mL – Vitamin E Suspension, Cambridge Laboratories.
Injection: 50mg in 1mL; 2mL ampoule – named patient.

DOSAGE
Newborn infant (birth to 1 month)

Route	Age	Frequency (times daily)	Notes
	birth–1 month		
Oral	10mg/kg	once daily	Nutritional deficiency.
Oral	100mg/kg	once daily	Abetalipoproteinaemia.
IM	20mg/kg	single dose	Neonatal prophylaxis, given at birth to babies weighing less than 1kg or 1.5kg in some UK neonatal units.

Child

Route	Age			Frequency	Notes
	1 month–2 years	2–12 years	12–18 years	(times daily)	
Oral	<1 year	100mg	200mg	once daily	Supplement in cystic fibrosis.
	50mg				
	>1 year				
	100mg			once daily	
Oral	←	50–100mg/kg	→	once daily	Abetalipoproteinaemia.
Oral	50–100mg	100mg	200mg	once daily	Initial dose to prevent deficiency secondary to chronic cholestasis. Increase to keep vitamin E/lipid ratio >0.6. May need up to 200mg/kg/day.
IM	←	10mg/kg (maximum 100mg)	→	once a month	

ADMINISTRATION
Oral: for cystic fibrosis patients who are pancreatic insufficient, should administer with food and pancreatic enzymes

CONTRA-INDICATIONS & WARNINGS
Hypersensitivity to vitamin E. Premature infants weighing <1.5kg, treated with oral vitamin E have been noted to have a higher rate of necrotising enterocolitis. Patients susceptible to thrombosis have been reported to be at increased risk if taking vitamin E.
Cystic fibrosis and cholestatic patients should have serum concentrations monitored and supplements adjusted accordingly.

INTERACTIONS
None known. May increase the risk of thrombosis in patients taking oestrogens.

PREGNANCY
Neither deficiency nor excess of vitamin E has been associated with maternal or fetal complications during pregnancy. Advised to avoid during first trimester.

BREAST-FEEDING
Vitamin E is excreted into human breast milk. This may influence calcium metabolism in the infant. Contact local Medicines Information Centre for advice.

SIDE-EFFECTS
Diarrhoea and abdominal pain.

POISONING/TOXICITY
Transient gastrointestinal disturbances have been reported with doses greater than 1g. Where necessary, general supportive measures should be employed.

EXCIPIENTS
Suspension includes sucrose. Tablets include sucrose.

LICENSED STATUS
Tablets and suspension licensed for use in children and adults. Injection is an unlicensed preparation.

FURTHER INFORMATION
The injection is available via John Bell and Croydon.
Pharmacological doses of vitamin E administered IM or IV shortly after birth were used in a range of studies between 1980 and 1990 designed to reduce the risk of intraventricular haemorrhage, bronchopulmonary dysplasia, and retinopathy of prematurity but the parenteral preparations are no longer available as licensed products in the UK. They were removed from general sale because of concern about one of the stabilisation agents used. Early parenteral prophylaxis may reduce the incidence of haemorrhage; it is less clear whether it reduces the amount of parenchymal damage. Mortality was not reduced. No trials of long-term outcome have yet been carried out.

Vitamin K is necessary for the production of blood clotting factors and proteins necessary for the normal calcification of bone.

USES
Vitamin K deficiency and prophylaxis, including haemorrhagic disease of the newborn.

Vitamin K supplementation in fat malabsorption e.g. cystic fibrosis, if evidence of abnormal clotting or hepatosplenomegaly; children with any chronic gastrointestinal disorder and those with very poor diets are also at risk.

Treatment of haemorrhage or threatened haemorrhage associated with a low blood level of the vitamin K dependent factors II, VII, IX and X.

Prevention of bleeding problems in biliary atresia and other liver disease. Antidote to anticoagulant drugs.

PRESENTATION
Phytomenadione (vitamin K₁)
Tablet: 10mg – Konakion®.
Injection: 1mg in 0.5mL – Konakion® Neonatal.
Injection (mixed micelles formulation): 2mg in 0.2mL – Konakion® MM Paediatric; 10mg in 1mL – Konakion® MM.
Capsules: 500 microgram and 1mg – Orakay®.

Menadiol sodium diphosphate (vitamin K analogue)
Tablet: (scored, water soluble) 10mg – non-proprietary.

DOSAGE
Neonates and babies: vitamin K deficiency bleeding.
Prophylaxis: current practice continues to vary widely throughout the UK; please refer to local policy.

Exclusively breast-fed babies are at risk of late onset vitamin K deficiency bleeding in the first 3 months of life. Those with undiagnosed liver disease are at increased risk. If oral prophylaxis is used, repeated dosage throughout this period is probably the wisest course. Bottle-fed babies are not at risk because all formula milks are fortified with vitamin K giving an average dose of 50 micrograms per day.

If IM/IV dose is given at birth usually no further doses are required.

Konakion® Neonatal 1mg can be given IM to healthy neonates ≥36 weeks gestation, at birth or shortly after.

Alternatively Konakion® MM Paediatric can be given as follows:

Healthy neonates ≥36 weeks gestation: 2mg orally at birth and at 4-7 days. Exclusively breast-fed babies should receive a further 2mg oral dose 1 month after birth. Further monthly 2mg oral doses until mixed feeding is introduced have been advised but no safety or efficacy data exist for these additional doses.

Preterm neonates <36 weeks gestation and ≥2.5kg and term neonates at special risk: *1mg IM or IV at birth or soon thereafter. The frequency of further doses should depend on coagulation status.

Preterm neonates <36 weeks gestation and <2.5kg: 400 microgram/kg IM or IV at birth or soon thereafter. The frequency of further doses should depend on coagulation status.

Treatment: 1mg IV repeated at 8 hourly intervals if necessary.
*At risk babies are those at increased risk of haemorrhagic disease e.g. birth asphyxia, bleeding problems, maternal liver disease or mother receiving anticonvulsant or antituberculosis drugs.

Neonates and babies: biliary atresia and liver disease.
1mg daily by mouth.

Child

Indication	Route	Age			Frequency (times daily)	Notes
		1 month–2 years	2–12 years	12–18 years		
Antidote to anticoagulants	IV	← 15–30 microgram/kg →			single dose	Seek expert advice before prescribing. Measure INR (venous) after 2-6 hours and again the next day.
Other indications	Oral/IM	← 300 microgram/kg →		10mg	1	Use water soluble preparation for oral supplementation in fat malabsorption.

ADMINISTRATION

Oral: menadiol tablets may be crushed with food or dissolved in water (NB the excipients are not soluble). Konakion® tablets are to be chewed or allowed to dissolve slowly in the mouth. Konakion® MM Paediatric can be given orally. After breaking the ampoule open, 0.2mL (2mg) of solution should be withdrawn into the syringe and the plunger then depressed to dispense the contents directly into the baby's mouth. Orakay® capsules – only the capsule contents are given by cutting the side tube of the capsule and expressing the contents directly into the baby's mouth or into a feed.

IV or IM: Konakion® Neonatal is for IM injection; not recommended to be given by the IV route and should not be diluted. Konakion® MM Paediatric can be injected neat or into the lower part of an infusion set (of glucose 5%). It should not be mixed with other parenteral medications or diluted (but in practice the small volume may necessitate dilution in order to administer the dose; in which case glucose 5% should be used). Konakion® MM is for IV injection (neat solution) or for IV infusion; when it should be diluted with 55mL of glucose 5%.

INTERACTIONS

No significant interactions are known other than antagonism of *coumarin anticoagulants*.

PREGNANCY

Menadiol sodium diphosphate is known to be associated with a small risk of haemolytic anaemia, hyperbilirubinaemia and kernicterus in the infant if administered to the mother in late pregnancy or during labour. There is no specific evidence regarding the safety of Konakion® in pregnancy.

BREAST-FEEDING

The American Academy of Pediatrics considers maternal use of vitamin K to be compatible with breast-feeding. Natural vitamin K content of breast milk is too low to protect the newborn from vitamin K deficiency and resulting haemorrhagic disease.

SIDE-EFFECTS

May induce haemolysis in erythrocyte glucose-6-phosphate dehydrogenase deficiency or low concentrations of alpha-tocopherol in the blood. Anaphylaxis reported rarely in adults receiving IV vitamin K.

EXCIPIENTS

Konakion® tablets include sucrose. Konakion® Neonatal injection contains polyethoxylated castor oil (which has been associated with anaphylaxis). Orakay® capsules contain fractionated coconut oil.

LICENSED STATUS

Konakion® Neonatal is licensed for IM prophylaxis of haemorrhagic disease of the newborn in healthy neonates ≥36 weeks gestation; and as an antidote to anticoagulant drugs of the coumarin type in infants and babies <1 year of age. Konakion® MM Paediatric is licensed for IM and IV prophylaxis of haemorrhagic disease of the newborn <36 weeks gestation or term neonates at special risk. Licensed orally for prophylaxis of haemorrhagic disease of the newborn in healthy neonates ≥36 weeks gestation. Licensed IV for treatment of haemorrhagic disease of the newborn.
Konakion® MM is licensed >1 year of age IV as an antidote to anticoagulant drugs of the coumarin type.
Konakion® tablets and menadiol tablets are licensed for use in children but not for supplementation in malabsorption.
Orakay® is not licensed for use in the UK.

FURTHER INFORMATION

Vitamin K supplementation is only indicated in cystic fibrosis patients with established liver disease and deranged clotting.

Vitlipid N®

Oil in water emulsion containing fat-soluble vitamins.

USES

Supplement to lipid solutions in intravenous nutrition to cover the daily requirements of vitamins A, D2, E, K1. Use with Solivito N®.

PRESENTATION

Emulsion: 10mL ampoule – Vitlipid N®.
Contents per 1mL:

Vitlipid N® **Adult**

Vitamin A	330 international units
Ergocalciferol	20 international units
Di-alpha tocopherol	1 international unit
Phytomenadione	15 microgram

Vitlipid N® **Infant**

Vitamin A	230 international units
Ergocalciferol	40 international units
Di-alpha tocopherol	0.7 international units
Phytomenadione	20 microgram

DOSAGE/ADMINISTRATION
Newborn infant (birth to 1 month)
4mL/kg/24 hours to a maximum of 10mL of Vitlipid N® Infant, added to Intralipid®.
Child
<11 years: 4mL/kg/24 hours to a maximum of 10mL of Vitlipid N® Infant, added to Intralipid®.
≥11 years: use Vitlipid N® Adult 10mL added to Intralipid®.
Once added to Intralipid® infuse as per PN protocol.

CONTRA-INDICATIONS & WARNINGS
Should not be given undiluted.

INTERACTIONS
Possible interaction with *anticoagulants coumarin*.

PREGNANCY
No hazard is expected if used at the recommended dosage.

EXCIPIENTS
See manufacturers SPC for further details.

LICENSED STATUS
Vitlipid N® Adult is licensed for use ≥ 11 years. Vitlipid N® Infant is licensed for use in infants and children <11 years of age.

FURTHER INFORMATION
Store in a fridge at 2-8°C. Protect from direct light.

Warfarin

A synthetic coumarin anticoagulant that acts by inhibiting clotting factors II, VII, IX, and X.

USES
Anticoagulation; prophylaxis and treatment of thromboembolic disease.

PRESENTATION
Tablet: 500 microgram, 1mg, 3mg and 5mg – non-proprietary.
Suspension: may be extemporaneously prepared.

DOSAGE
Newborn infant (birth to 1 month)
There is very little experience of the use of warfarin in the neonatal period. Always seek expert advice before starting anticoagulation.

Child

The table below merely gives an example of a starting dose regimen. Follow local guidelines/protocols for full details of dosing regimes. Loading period is approximately 3-5 days for most patients before a stable maintenance phase is achieved. Start warfarin on day 1 or 2 of heparin therapy. Heparin should be continued for a minimum of 5 days.

Route	Age			Frequency (times daily)	Notes
	1 month–2 years	2–12 years	12–18 years		
Oral	←	200 microgram/kg (minimum 500 microgram per dose)	→	1	Initial dose. Loading doses may need to be altered according to condition, concomitant interacting drugs and if the INR is >1.3. Monitor INR and adjust dose to nearest 500 microgram to keep within the desired range*.

* The INR ranges are outlined below. Recent British Society for Haematology (BSH) guidelines suggest that target INR are more appropriate than ranges but this is in adults. No BSH guidelines as yet published for children.

Current therapeutic ranges	INR
Prophylaxis of deep vein thrombosis (DVT)	2-2.5
Treatment of DVT (whilst on warfarin) and pulmonary embolism (PE)	2-3
Recurrent DVT, pulmonary embolism and mechanical cardiac prosthetic valves	3-4.5

CONTRA-INDICATIONS & WARNINGS

Contra-indications: peptic ulcer, severe hypertension, bacterial endocarditis.
Cautions: hepatic/renal disease, recent surgery.

INTERACTIONS

Warfarin interacts with many drugs. Monitor INR whenever a drug is added to, or withdrawn from a patient's therapeutic regimen.

Enhanced effect with *aspirin, NSAIDS, dipyridamole, clopidrogel, anti-arrhythmics (amiodarone, propafenone, quinidine), antibiotics (chloramphenicol, ciprofloxacin, cotrimoxazole, erythromycin, metronidazole, ofloxacin and sulphonamides),* possibly other antibiotics *(aztreonam, clarithromycin and some other macrolides, nalidixic acid, neomycin, norfloxacin, tetracyclines, trimethoprim), SSRIs,* antifungals *(fluconazole, itraconazole, ketoconazole, miconazole), proguanil, sodium valproate, ifosfamide, clofibrates, simvastatin, levothyroxine (thyroxine), cimetidine, omeprazole, paracetamol, dextropropoxyphene.*
Reduced effect with *rifampicin, griseofulvin, barbiturates, primidone* and *carbamazepine.* Enhanced or reduced effect with *phenytoin* and *colestyramine (cholestyramine).*

EXCIPIENTS

Contact manufacturers for advice.

LICENSED STATUS

Not licensed for use in children.

PREGNANCY

Seek specialist guidance as warfarin should be avoided in the first and third trimesters due to the risk of teratogenicity or fetal haemorrhage. Heparin may be an alternative in the first and third trimesters.

BREAST-FEEDING

Warfarin appears safe in breast-feeding.

SIDE-EFFECTS

Haemorrhage, hypersensitivity, rash, alopecia, diarrhoea, skin necrosis, jaundice, hepatic dysfunction.

POISONING/TOXICITY

Treatment depends on whether full reversal or partial reversal (in patients who need to be kept anticoagulated). Reversal by using vitamin K. For bleeding complications consider use of coagulation factor concentrate or pathogen inactivated fresh frozen plasma (see BSH guidelines in *BNF*). Seek advice from a haematologist.

PHARMACOKINETIC PROPERTIES

Monitor INR. The anticoagulant effect takes up to 36-48 hours to develop, whilst the antithrombotic effect may take at least 3 days. Since the half-lives of the vitamin K dependent coagulation factors vary from 6-72 hours, changes in the dosage will not be fully reflected by the INR until day 3 or 4.

FURTHER INFORMATION
Counselling points: avoid large changes to diet or alcohol consumption and take at the same time each day. Patient or carers should be able to recognise signs of haemorrhage (nose bleed, bruising etc). Do not take aspirin, unless otherwise advised.

Xylometazoline hydrochloride

Sympathomimetic agent. It constricts nasal blood vessels thereby decongesting the mucosa of the nose and neighbouring areas of the pharynx.

PRESENTATION
Nasal drops: 0.05% children's formula – Otrivine® and non-proprietary.
Nasal drops and spray: 0.1% adult formula – Otrivine® and non-proprietary.

USES
Decongestant for relief from perennial and allergic rhinitis. Sinusitis.

DOSAGE

Route	Age			Frequency (times daily)	Notes
	1 month–2 years	2–12 years	12–18 years		
Intra-nasal	-	-	2–3 drops of 0.1% or 1 spray of 0.1%	2–3	Place drops/spray in each nostril. Maximum duration of use 7 days.
	≥3 months 1–2 drops of 0.05%	1–2 drops of 0.05%	-	1–2	

CONTRA-INDICATIONS & WARNINGS
Hypersensitivity to any ingredients. Trans-sphenoidal hypophysectomy. Not to be used in infants <3 months of age.

INTERACTIONS
No drug interactions have been reported.

PREGNANCY/BREAST-FEEDING
No fetal toxicity or fertility studies have been carried out in animals. In view of its potential vasoconstrictor effect, it is not advisable to use xylometazoline during pregnancy.

SIDE-EFFECTS
Burning sensation in nose and throat. Local irritation, nausea, mucosal dryness. Rebound congestion with prolonged use.

POISONING/TOXICITY
In rare incidences of accidental poisoning in children, acceleration and irregularity of pulse, elevated blood pressure, drowsiness and respiratory depression have occurred. No specific antidote – treatment is supportive.

PHARMACOKINETIC PROPERTIES
Systemic absorption may occur.

EXCIPIENTS
Include benzalkonium chloride and disodium edetate.

LICENSED STATUS
0.05% children's formula licensed for use in >3 months of age.
0.1% adult formula licensed for use in ≥12 years of age.

FURTHER INFORMATION
For reasons of hygiene do not use bottle for more than 28 days after first opening it.

USES
To provide active immunity against yellow fever in the following groups:

☐ Those aged ≥9 months, who are travelling through or living in infected areas and those travelling outside urban areas of countries in the yellow fever endemic zone. If there is an unavoidable high risk of infection, infants <9 months may be considered for immunisation.

☐ Travellers who are required to have an International Certificate of Vaccination for entry into a country.

PRESENTATION
Injection: (single dose powder reconstituted to 0.5mL) – Arilvax®; Stamaril®.
Each dose contains at least 1000 mouse LD_{50} units of live attenuated 17D strain of yellow fever virus grown in chick embryos free of avian leucosis viruses. It is available as single (Arilvax® and Stamaril®) and five (Arilvax®) dose vials.

DOSAGE/ADMINISTRATION
Deep SC: 0.5mL repeated every 10 years while still at risk.

CONTRA-INDICATIONS AND WARNINGS
Should not be given to infants <9 months old unless at high risk of exposure. Most authorities consider 4 months as an absolute lower age limit. It should not be given to someone who has had an anaphylactic reaction to egg or who is immunosuppressed. There is little data on its use in individuals who are HIV positive, therefore it should not be used under these circumstances.

INTERACTIONS
As it is a live vaccine, it should either be given at the same time as *other live vaccines*, but at a different site or separated by an interval of at least 3 weeks. Human normal immunoglobulin (HNIG) as used in the UK does not contain significant amounts of antibody to yellow fever virus and so there will be no interaction with the vaccine, whatever the time interval between them.

PREGNANCY
The balance of the limited evidence to date, suggests that the risk of fetal damage following vaccination in the first trimester is small, if any, but possible fetal infection has been reported. In view of the highly neurotropic nature of the vaccine and the known risk of encephalitis if given to infants, it should only be given to a pregnant woman if there is an unavoidable high risk of exposure to the disease.

BREAST-FEEDING
Should not be given to breast-feeding women unless at high risk of exposure.

SIDE-EFFECTS
Mild headache, myalgia, low-grade fever or soreness at the injection site occurs in 5–10% of recipients 5–10 days after immunisation. Urticaria and anaphylaxis are rare. Encephalitis has occurred, rarely, in young infants, one of whom had some residual effects.

POISONING/TOXICITY
No data available.

PHARMACODYNAMIC PROPERTIES
Immunity does not develop until 7 days after immunisation.

EXCIPIENTS
Arilvax®: sorbitol, gelatin (of porcine origin), disodium hydrogen orthophosphate, potassium chloride and potassium dihydrogen orthophosphate.
Stamaril®: lactose, sorbitol, L-histidine hydrochloride, L-alanine, sodium chloride, potassium chloride, disodium phosphate, monopotassium phosphate, calcium chloride, magnesium sulphate and sodium hydroxide.

LICENSED STATUS
Licensed for use as described above.

FURTHER INFORMATION
The vaccine can only be given in approved centres listed in the Department of Health's book *Health Information for Overseas Travel 1995*. If a traveller for whom the vaccine is contra-indicated has to enter a country where a yellow fever certificate is required, they should obtain a letter of exemption from their medical practitioner.
Immunity may last for life, but boosters have to be given every 10 years to maintain a valid yellow fever certificate.
Protect from light and store at 2–8°C. The diluent should be stored at less than 25°C, but not frozen. Once reconstituted the vaccine should be used within 1 hour (Arilvax®) or 3 hours (Stamaril®) depending on the brand.

A nucleoside reverse transcriptase inhibitor.

USES
Management of human immunodeficiency virus (HIV) infected children. Indicated IV for short-term management of serious manifestations of HIV infection. Also indicated for the prevention of maternal-fetal transmission.

PRESENTATION
Capsule: 100mg and 250mg – Retrovir®.
IV infusion: 10mg in 1mL, 20mL vial – Retrovir®.
Oral solution: 10mg in 1mL – Retrovir®.

DOSAGE
Newborn infant (birth to 1 month)

Route	Age		Frequency	Notes
	Up to 7 days	Over 7 days	(times daily)	
Oral	← 2mg/kg →		4	Prevention of maternal fetal transmission. Begin within 12 hours of birth and continue for 6 weeks.
IV	← 1.5mg/kg →		4	

Child

Route	Age			Frequency	Notes
	1 month–2 years	2–12 years	12–18 years	(times daily)	
Oral	← 180mg/m² →			2	Maximum single dose 250mg.
IV	← 120mg/m² →			4	

Dose adjustment in renal impairment
No specific recommendations. Plasma half-life does not appear to be significantly prolonged in renal failure. Glucuronide metabolite does accumulate. Manufacturer recommends patients with advanced renal failure should receive zidovudine at lower end of dosage range and the dose adjusted based on clinical response and haematological parameters.

Dose adjustment in liver impairment
Reduction in glucuronidation may increase concentration of zidovudine. Adjust dose and frequency using above parameters.

ADMINISTRATION
IV: dilute to concentration between 2-4mg in 1mL and administer over 1 hour. Compatible with glucose 5% and NaCl 0.9%.

CONTRA-INDICATIONS & WARNINGS
Hypersensitivity to zidovudine or components.
Contra-indicated in neonates with hyperbilirubinaemia requiring treatment other than phototherapy or if serum transaminases are more than 5 times normal levels. Avoid if haemoglobin <7.5g/dL or neutrophil counts <0.75 x 10⁹/L.

INTERACTIONS
Alterations in *phenytoin* plasma levels may occur, normally a decrease in levels although increase has been reported; monitor carefully. Increased incidence of neutropenia reported with *paracetamol*, but the mechanism is unclear. It has been suggested that short-term *paracetamol* use is acceptable, but with close monitoring.

Other drugs that inhibit or compete for glucuronidation or inhibit hepatic microsomal enzymes should be used with caution as they may alter the metabolism of zidovudine; use with caution and monitor closely. Concurrent therapy with other *potentially nephrotoxic or myelosuppressive drugs* may have additive effects (*pentamidine, ganciclovir, dapsone, amphotericin, pyrimethamine* and *flucytosine*).
Ribavirin (tribavarin) antagonises zidovudine anti-viral activity *in vitro*. Similar data has been reported for ganciclovir. *Rifampicin* may decrease plasma levels of zidovudine. *Probenecid* increases half-life and area under plasma concentration time curve by decreasing

glucuronidation and reducing renal excretion. *Sodium valproate, fluconazole* or *methadone* may increase plasma concentrations of zidovudine; monitor carefully for zidovudine-related adverse effects.

PREGNANCY

Use of zidovudine in pregnant women over 14 weeks gestation has been shown to reduce the rate of maternal-fetal HIV transmission. Due to limited data and potential risks zidovudine should only be used prior to 14 weeks gestation if benefit outweighs risk.

BREAST-FEEDING

Zidovudine may be excreted in breast milk and it is recommended that breast-feeding is avoided.
HIV infected mothers in the UK are advised not to breast-feed to prevent virus transmission.

SIDE-EFFECTS

Reversible anaemia, neutropenia and leucopenia occur, usually after 4-6 weeks of therapy but potentially earlier. Regular monitoring is advised. Patients with pre-existing bone marrow depression are particularly at risk. Dose reduction or suspension of treatment may be required.
Lactic acidosis and severe hepatomegaly with steatosis have been reported. Although a causal relationship is unclear monitoring of liver enzymes is advised and treatment should be suspended if necessary. Headache, nausea, vomiting and other gastrointestinal effects reported. Myalgia, myopathy or polymyositis have been reported generally after 6-12 months therapy in adults. Hypersensitivity reactions, including anaphylaxis, have occurred rarely. Skin rashes also reported. Capsules swallowed at night while lying down have reportedly caused oesophageal ulceration in some adults.

POISONING/TOXICITY

Observe for toxicity signs. Haemodialysis and peritoneal dialysis have a limited effect on removal of zidovudine but increase elimination of glucuronide metabolite.

PHARMACOKINETIC PROPERTIES

Rapidly absorbed from gastrointestinal tract. Wide individual variation in absorption (55-75%).
Undergoes first pass metabolism with around 65% of an oral dose reaching systemic circulation. Presence of food may affect peak levels achieved but not total amount absorbed.
Zidovudine appears to be well absorbed in neonates. Oral bioavailability may be greater in the first 14 days of life (mean 89%) decreasing to mean 65% after 14 days. Widely distributed in body fluids and tissues. Volume in children ranges from $22\text{-}64L/m^2$. Distributed into CSF. Crosses placenta and appears in amniotic fluid, cord blood, fetal plasma and tissues. Plasma protein binding 34-38%.
Rapidly metabolised via glucuronidation. The metabolite has no antiviral activity. Metabolism is reduced in neonates, but appears to reach adult values by 14 days of age. Zidovudine and its metabolites are eliminated principally in the urine via both glomerular filtration and tubular secretion. Around 20% of the zidovudine dose is excreted as unchanged drug, 72-74% of an oral dose and 45-60% of an IV dose appearing in the urine as the major glucuronide metabolite within 6 hours.
Plasma half-life in children 1.5 hours (range 1-1.7 hours). Prolonged in neonates (up to 3 hours) but by 14 days of age is close to above values.

EXCIPIENTS

Oral solution includes glucose syrup and saccharin. See manufacturers SPC for further details.

LICENSED STATUS

Infusion licensed in all ages but data in children are limited. Capsules and oral solution licensed for use in patients ≥3 months of age.

Zinc sulphate

An essential trace element involved in many enzyme systems.

USES

Wilson's disease; acrodermatitis enteropathica; zinc deficiency.

PRESENTATION

Capsule: 61.8mg (22.5mg zinc) (modified-release) – Z-Span® spansule.
Effervescent tablet: 125mg (45mg zinc) – Solvazinc®.
Oral solution: (as sulphate) 15mg of zinc in 5mL – Zincatest®.

DOSAGE

Indication	Route	Age				Frequency (times daily)	Notes
		birth– 1 month	1 month– 2 years	2–12 years	12–18 years		
Wilson disease	Oral	–	–	25 – 37.5mg	50mg	2-4	Prescribed in terms of elemental zinc. Do not give at the same time as penicillamine.
Acrodermatitis enteropathica	Oral	← 500 micrograms - 1mg/kg →				2	Prescribed in terms of elemental zinc. Total daily dose can be given in 3 divided doses.
Demonstrated zinc deficiency	Oral	1mg/kg	<10kg half a tablet			1	Tablet = Solvazinc®. Capsule = Z-Span®.
			>10kg as 2–12 years	10–30kg half a tablet	1 capsule	1–3	Adjust according to response (short-term treatment only).
				>30kg 1 tablet	or 1 tablet	1–3	

ADMINISTRATION
Oral: take Solvazinc® 1 hour after food, dissolved in water. Z-Span® spansule may be opened and sprinkled on cold food; not to be chewed.

CONTRA-INDICATIONS & WARNINGS
No contra-indications. Accumulation of zinc may occur in cases of renal failure.

INTERACTIONS
Zinc reduces absorption of *iron, penicillamine, ciprofloxacin* and *norfloxacin. Tetracyclines* reduce absorption of zinc and vice versa; when both are being given an interval of at least 3 hours should be allowed. *Calcium salts* and *bran products* reduce the absorption of zinc. In Wilson disease do not give zinc at the same time as *penicillamine* – leave an interval of at least 3 hours.

PREGNANCY
Safety not established; zinc crosses the placenta.

BREAST-FEEDING
Zinc passes into breast milk; no information available on possible effect on the infant.

SIDE-EFFECTS
Abdominal pain and dyspepsia.

POISONING/TOXICITY
Zinc is corrosive in overdose. Symptoms are corrosion and inflammation of the mucous membranes of the mouth and stomach; ulceration of the stomach followed by perforation may occur. Gastric lavage and emesis should be avoided. Demulcents such as milk should be given; chelating agents such as sodium edetate may be useful. Causes copper deficiency and anaemia in large doses.

PHARMACODYNAMIC PROPERTIES
Wilson disease: zinc reduces copper absorption from the gastrointestinal tract. Acrodermatitis enteropathica: autosomal recessive disorder of zinc deficiency – zinc administered to correct.

PHARMACOKINETIC PROPERTIES
Absorbed from the gastrointestinal tract (10-40%) and distributed throughout the body.

EXCIPIENTS
Solvazinc® tablets include sorbitol and saccharin. Z-Span® capsules include sucrose. Contact manufacturers for further details.

LICENSED STATUS
Wilson disease is an unlicensed indication. Solvazinc® is licensed for use in children and adults for zinc deficiency. Z-Span® is not licensed for <12 years of age. Zincatest® is classified as a food supplement.

USES
Additional zinc supplementation as part of a PN regimen.

PRESENTATION
Injection: 50 micromol of elemental zinc in 1mL and 200 micromol of elemental zinc in 1mL, other strengths may be available – manufactured 'special'.
Note: Peditrace® and Additrace® contain maintenance amount of zinc.

DOSAGE
2-5 micromol/kg depending on age and deficiency state.

ADMINISTRATION
By infusion as part of an IV feeding regimen.

INTERACTIONS
May diminish effects of *penicillamine*.

SIDE-EFFECTS
Unlikely at doses indicated.

POISONING/TOXICITY
Causes copper deficiency and anaemia in large doses. Chronic zinc poisoning in man has not been identified with certainty.

PHARMACOKINETIC PROPERTIES
Excreted in faeces with only traces in urine.

LICENSED STATUS
Available as a 'special' and as such is unlicensed.

Zopiclone

A non-benzodiazepine hypnotic, a member of the cyclopyrrolone group of components.

USES
Parasomnias. Short-term night sedation in adolescents.

PRESENTATION
Tablet: 3.75mg – Zimovane LS® and non-proprietary; 7.5mg – Zimovane® and non-proprietary.

DOSAGE

Route	Age		Frequency (times daily)	Notes
	12–18 years			
Oral	3.75mg		1	Dose for adolescents. Take shortly before going to bed.

CONTRA-INDICATIONS & WARNINGS
Contra-indicated in severe hepatic insufficiency, sleep apnoea syndrome, myasthenia gravis or any other condition compromising respiration. A reduced dosage is recommended in hepatic and renal insufficiency.

INTERACTIONS
Potentiates other *sedative medication*.

PREGNANCY
Not recommended. Experience of use during human pregnancy is limited. If used during the last 3 months of pregnancy or during labour, effects on the neonate such as hypothermia, hypnotic and respiratory depression can be expected.

BREAST-FEEDING
Zopiclone is excreted in breast milk and use during breast-feeding should be avoided.

SIDE-EFFECTS
Unusual taste in mouth, light-headedness, nightmares and irritable behaviour the following day; has been reported to cause dependence.

POISONING/TOXICITY
Overdose is usually manifested by varying degrees of CNS depression ranging from drowsiness to coma, depending on the quantity ingested. Symptomatic and supportive treatment in an adequate clinical environment is recommended.

PHARMACOKINETIC PROPERTIES
Rapidly absorbed following oral administration with more than 95% of absorption complete 1 hour after administration. The half-life of zopiclone and its active metabolite ranges from 3.5–6 hours. Zopiclone is very extensively metabolised by three major pathways; only 4-5% is excreted unchanged in the urine.

EXCIPIENTS
See manufacturers SPC for further details.

LICENSED STATUS
Not licensed for use in children.

Z

CONTENTS

Eye

Antimicrobials

Cefuroxime

USES
Broad-spectrum antibiotic, usually effective against *Staphylococcus*. *Pseudomonas* is resistant.

PRESENTATION
Eye drops: preservative free 5%, 10mL – manufactured 'special'.

DOSAGE
Severe infection: 1 drop every 1–2 hours, then reduce frequency as infection is controlled and continue for 48 hours after healing.
Minor infection: 1 drop 4 times daily.

EXCIPIENTS
Contact manufacturer for further details.

LICENSED STATUS
Available as a 'special' and as such is unlicensed.

FURTHER INFORMATION
Available as a 'special' from Moorfields Eye Hospital.
Can be kept frozen for 12 months. Once thawed, stable for 14 days in a refrigerator.

Chloramphenicol

USES
Broad-spectrum antibiotic.

PRESENTATION
Eye drops: 0.5%, 5mL – Chloromycetin®; 10mL – Chloromycetin® and non-proprietary.
Eye drops: preservative free, single use, 0.5%, 0.5mL – Minims® Chloramphenicol.
Eye ointment: 1%, 4g – Chloromycetin® and non-proprietary.

DOSAGE
Eye drops: 1 drop 4–6 times daily (1–2 hourly in severe infection). In addition a small amount of ointment can be applied at night.
Eye ointment: apply 4 times daily (1–2 hourly in severe infection).
Continue treatment for at least 48 hours after eye appears normal.

INTERACTIONS	**CONTRA-INDICATIONS & WARNINGS**
Chymotrypsin will be inactivated if given simultaneously with chloramphenicol.	Rare reports of aplastic anaemia.

EXCIPIENTS
Chloromycetin® eye drops include phenylmercuric acetate.
Minims® Chloramphenicol include borax and boric acid.

LICENSED STATUS
Licensed for use in all age groups.

FURTHER INFORMATION
Store eye drops in a refrigerator.

Eye

Ciprofloxacin hydrochloride

USES
Superficial infection; corneal ulcers.

PRESENTATION
Eye drops: 0.3%, 5mL – Ciloxan®.

DOSAGE
Corneal ulcers: apply throughout the day and night.
Day one: 2 drops every 15 minutes for 6 hours then 2 drops every 30 minutes for the rest of the day.
Day two: 2 drops every hour.
Day three to fourteen: 2 drops every 4 hours.
Superficial infection: usual dose is 1-2 drops 4 times a day.
Continue for 48 hours after healing.
Maximum duration of treatment is 21 days.

> **SIDE-EFFECTS**
> Local burning and itching; lid margin crusting; taste disturbance.

EXCIPIENTS
Include benzalkonium chloride.

LICENSED STATUS
Licensed for ≥1 year of age.

Erythromycin

USES
Superficial eye infections. Broad spectrum antibiotic, usually effective against Streptococcus and Chlamydia.

PRESENTATION
Eye ointment: 0.5%, 3g – manufactured 'special'.

DOSAGE
Apply up to 3 times daily.

EXCIPIENTS
Contact manufacturer for further details.

LICENSED STATUS
Available as a 'special' and as such is unlicensed.

FURTHER INFORMATION
Available as a 'special' from Moorfields Eye Hospital.

Framycetin sulphate

USES
Treatment of bacterial eye infection including conjunctivitis, blepharitis, styes, corneal abrasions, burns and ulcers.
Can be used prophylactically for the removal of ocular foreign bodies.

PRESENTATION
Eye drops: 0.5%, 10mL – Soframycin®.
Eye ointment: 0.5%, 5g – Soframycin®.

Eye

DOSAGE
Eye drops: 1 drop 1–2 hourly reducing gradually as infection is controlled. Continue for 48 hours after healing.
Eye ointment: 3 times daily (or may be added at night if drops are used during the day).

CONTRA-INDICATIONS & WARNINGS
Systemic absorption is possible at high doses; care should be taken in young children with renal or hepatic impairment.

EXCIPIENTS
Soframycin® eye drops include benzalkonium chloride.

LICENSED STATUS
Licensed for use in all age groups.

Fusidic acid

USES
Gram-positive infection especially *Staphylococcus aureus*, but not first choice if *Haemophilus* is suspected.

PRESENTATION
Eye drops modified release: 1% in gel basis (liquifies on contact with the eye), 5g – Fucithalmic®.

DOSAGE
1 drop twice a day.
Continue for at least 48 hours after the eye returns to normal.

EXCIPIENTS
Include benzalkonium chloride and disodium edetate.

LICENSED STATUS
Licensed for use in all ages.

Gentamicin sulphate

USES
Broad-spectrum antibiotic effective against Gram negative infection, including *Pseudomonas aeruginosa*.
Eye drops 1.5% used in the treatment of severe eye infection.
Eye drops 0.3% used in the treatment of superficial eye infection/prevention of infection in trauma of the eye.

PRESENTATION
Ear or eye drops: 0.3%, 10mL – Garamycin®, Genticin®.
Eye drops: preservative free, single use, 0.3%, 0.5mL – Minims® Gentamicin Sulphate.
Eye drops: with or without preservative, 1.5%, 10mL – manufactured 'special'.

DOSAGE
Eye drops 0.3%: 1–2 drops up to 6 times a day: with more severe infection 1 drop every 15–20 minutes, reducing frequency as infection is controlled.
Eye drops 1.5%: 1 drop 4–6 hourly.
Continue for 48 hours after healing.

CONTRA-INDICATIONS & WARNINGS
Systemic absorption is possible at high doses, care should be taken in young children with renal disorder.

SIDE-EFFECTS
Epithelial toxicity can occur with high dosage or prolonged use: dose should be reduced as infection is controlled.

EXCIPIENTS
Garamycin® and Genticin® eye drops include benzalkonium chloride.
Eye drops 1.5% with preservative (Moorfields Eye Hospital) include thiomersal.
Minims® Gentamicin Sulphate include borax.

LICENSED STATUS
Eye drops 0.3% are licensed for use in all age groups.
Eye drops 1.5% are available as 'specials' and as such are unlicensed.

FURTHER INFORMATION
Eye drops 1.5% preservative free available as a 'special' from e.g. Moorfields Eye Hospital.

Neomycin sulphate

USES
Prophylaxis and treatment of bacterial infection.

PRESENTATION
Eye drops: 0.5% (3500 units in 1mL), 10mL – non-proprietary.
Eye drops: preservative free, single use, 0.5%, 0.5mL – Minims® Neomycin Sulphate.
Eye ointment: 0.5% (3500 units in 1g), 3g – non-proprietary.
Eye drops: gramicidin 25 units, neomycin sulphate 1700 units, polymixin B 5000 units in 1mL; 5mL – Neosporin®.

DOSAGE
Superficial eye infection: 1 drop 2-4 times daily.
Severe infection: 1 drop every 15-20 minutes initially, reducing as infection is controlled.
Eye ointment: apply 3-4 times daily.
Treatment should be continued for 48 hours after condition resolved.

> **CONTRA-INDICATIONS & WARNINGS**
> Delayed hypersensitivity reactions may occur. Caution in young children with renal impairment as systemic absorption may cause ototoxicity.

EXCIPIENTS
Neosporin® eye drops include thiomersal.
Minims® Neomycin Sulphate include disodium edetate.

LICENSED STATUS
Licensed for use in all age groups, except Neosporin® licensed for >2 years of age.

FURTHER INFORMATION
Not used frequently in children as high incidence of topical allergy.

Ofloxacin

USES
Treatment of bacterial infection, especially Gram negative organisms.

PRESENTATION
Eye drops: 0.3%, 5mL – Exocin®.

DOSAGE
1 drop every 2–4 hours for the first 48 hours, then 4 times daily.
Continue for 48 hours after healing.
Maximum duration of treatment is 10 days.

> **CONTRA-INDICATIONS & WARNINGS**
> Use with caution if sensitive to other quinolones.

> **SIDE-EFFECTS**
> May cause transient ocular irritation, including photophobia. Side-effects reported with systemic quinolones could possibly occur; dizziness, numbness, nausea and headache.

Eye

EXCIPIENTS
Include benzalkonium chloride.

LICENSED STATUS
Licensed for use in all age groups.

Polymixin B sulphate

USES
Bacterial infection, conjunctivitis, keratitis, corneal ulceration, ulcerative blepharitis, prevention of infection post surgery.

PRESENTATION
Eye drops: polymixin B sulphate 10,000 units in 1mL, trimethoprim 0.1%, 5mL – Polytrim®.
Eye ointment: polymixin B sulphate 10,000 units in 1g, trimethoprim 0.5%, 4g – Polytrim®.
Eye ointment: polymixin B sulphate 10,000 units, zinc bacitracin 500 units in 1g, 4g – Polyfax®.

DOSAGE
Eye drops: 1 drop 4 times daily.
Eye ointment: apply thin film to the affected part or inside the lower lid 2-4 times daily depending on severity. Continue for at least 48 hours after apparent recovery.

EXCIPIENTS
Polytrim® eye drops include thiomersal.

LICENSED STATUS
Licensed for use in all age groups.

Propamidine isetionate

USES
Local treatment of minor eye infection, of value only for the rare but devastating condition of acanthamoeba keratitis.

PRESENTATION
Eye drops: 0.1%, 10mL – Brolene®.
Eye ointment: dibromopropamidine isetionate 0.15%, 5g – Brolene®.

DOSAGE
Eye drops: 1 drop 4 times daily.
Eye ointment: apply 1–2 times daily.
For acanthamoeba seek expert advice and use 1 drop every 30 minutes to 1 hour for 1 week (watching for epithelial toxicity) and then reduce depending on course of the disease. Treatment must be sufficiently long to eradicate cysts.

EXCIPIENTS
Brolene® eye drops include benzalkonium chloride.

LICENSED STATUS
Licensed for use in all age groups.

Tobramycin

USES
Local treatment of infection including *Pseudomonas aeruginosa*.

PRESENTATION
Eye drops: 0.3%, 5mL – manufactured 'special'.

DOSAGE
1 drop every 2 hours then reduce frequency as infection is controlled. Continue for 48 hours after healing.

SIDE-EFFECTS
Epithelial toxicity.

LICENSED STATUS
Available as a 'special' and as such is unlicensed.

FURTHER INFORMATION
Available as a 'special' from Moorfields Eye Hospital.

Antifungals

Clotrimazole

USES
Antifungal normally active against *Aspergillus*, *Candida* and *Acanthamoeba*. A good first line treatment until organism identified.

PRESENTATION
Eye drops: 1%, 10mL – manufactured 'special'.

DOSAGE
Depends on severity of infection. 1 drop every 30 minutes to 1 hour initially and then reduce as condition improves. Continue treatment until healing complete (may take months).

EXCIPIENTS
Include arachis (peanut) oil. Contact manufacturer for further details

LICENSED STATUS
Available as a 'special' and as such is unlicensed.

FURTHER INFORMATION
Available as a 'special' from Moorfields Eye Hospital.

Antivirals

Aciclovir (acyclovir)

USES
Herpes simplex keratitis.

PRESENTATION
Eye ointment: 3%, 4.5g – Zovirax®.

DOSAGE
Apply 1cm of eye ointment 5 times daily.
Continue for at least 3 days after healing is complete.

SIDE-EFFECTS
Epithelial toxicity.

EXCIPIENTS
Includes white petroleum USP.

LICENSED STATUS
Licensed for use in all age groups.

Eye

Trifluorothymidine

USES
Herpes simplex keratitis.

PRESENTATION
Eye drops: 1%, 10mL – manufactured 'special'.

DOSAGE
1 drop 5 times daily (at 4 hourly intervals). Maximum total daily dose 9 drops. Treatment should generally not exceed 21 days.

> **SIDE-EFFECTS**
> Toxic epithelial and stromal keratitis.

EXCIPIENTS
Include benzalkonium chloride.

LICENSED STATUS
Available as a 'special' and as such is unlicensed.

FURTHER INFORMATION
Available as a 'special' from Moorfields Eye Hospital. 2 week expiry when stored in a refrigerator.

Corticosteroids

Betamethasone sodium phosphate

USES
Short-term, local treatment of inflammation (with neomycin as bacterial prophylaxis). Used after glaucoma surgery or after cataract surgery.

PRESENTATION
Ear, eye or nose drops: 0.1%, 10mL – Betnesol®; 5mL and 10mL – Vista-Methasone®.
Ear, eye or nose drops: betamethasone sodium phosphate 0.1% and neomycin sulphate 0.5%, 5mL – Betnesol-N®; 5mL and 10mL – Vista-Methasone N®.
Eye ointment: betamethasone sodium phosphate 0.1% and neomycin sulphate 0.5%, 3g – Betnesol-N®.

DOSAGE
Eye drops: depends on condition being treated:
For uveitis, 1 drop every 1-2 hours until controlled then reduce frequency gradually to avoid rebound inflammation.
Eye ointment: apply 1cm 2-3 times daily or at night when used with drops.

> **CONTRA-INDICATIONS & WARNINGS**
> Prolonged use may lead to adrenal suppression in infants.
> Contra-indicated in bacterial, viral, fungal, tuberculous or purulent conditions of the eye. However, used by ophthalmologists with antibacterial/viral cover to suppress scarring due to infection.
> Contra-indicated if glaucoma is present, may also cause glaucoma.
> Neomycin – caution in young children with renal impairment as systemic absorption may cause ototoxicity.

EXCIPIENTS
Betnesol®, Betnesol N® and Vista-Methasone® eye drops include benzalkonium chloride and disodium edetate
Vista-Methasone N® eye drops include thiomersal.

LICENSED STATUS
Licensed for use in all age groups.

Eye

Dexamethasone

USES
Short-term treatment of steroid responsive conditions; in combination with prophylactic antibiotic treatment if required.

PRESENTATION
Eye drops: preservative free, single use, 0.1%, 0.5mL – Minims® Dexamethasone.
Eye drops: dexamethasone 0.1% and hypromellose 0.5%, 5mL and 10mL – Maxidex®.
Ear or eye drops: dexamethasone sodium metasulphobenzoate 0.05%, framycetin sulphate 0.5% and gramicidin 0.005%, 10mL – Sofradex®.
Eye drops: dexamethasone 0.1% and tobramycin 0.3%, 5mL – Tobradex®.
Eye drops: dexamethasone 0.1%, hypromellose 0.5%, neomycin sulphate 0.35% and polymixin B sulphate 6000 units in 1mL, 5mL – Maxitrol®.
Eye ointment: dexamethasone 0.1%, neomycin 0.35% and polymixin B sulphate 6000 units in 1g, 3.5g – Maxitrol®.
Ear or eye ointment: dexamethasone 0.05%, framycetin sulphate 0.5% and gramicidin 0.005%, 5g – Sofradex®.

DOSAGE
Eye drops: 1 drop every 4–6 hours. Severe conditions, apply every hour until controlled, then reduce frequency.
Eye ointment: apply small amounts of ointment into the conjunctival sac 3–4 times daily or use adjunctively with drops at bedtime.

CONTRA-INDICATIONS & WARNINGS
Contra-indicated in bacterial, viral, fungal, tuberculous or purulent conditions of the eye. However, used by ophthalmologists with antibacterial/viral cover to suppress scarring due to infection.

Contra-indicated if glaucoma is present, may also cause glaucoma.
Systemic side-effects may occur with extensive use.
Neomycin – caution in young children with renal impairment as systemic absorption may cause ototoxicity.

EXCIPIENTS
Maxidex® eye drops include benzalkonium chloride, disodium edetate and polysorbate 80. Maxitrol® eye drops include benzalkonium chloride and polysorbate 20. Maxitrol® eye ointment includes hydroxybenzoates (parabens) and wool fat. Minims® Dexamethasone include disodium edetate. Sofradex® eye drops include polysorbate 80. Tobradex® eye drops include benzalkonium chloride and disodium edetate.

LICENSED STATUS
Licensed for use in all age groups.

Fluorometholone

USES
Inflammation of palpebral and bulbar conjunctiva, cornea and anterior segment of the globe.

PRESENTATION
Ophthalmic suspension (eye drops): fluorometholone 0.1%, polyvinyl alcohol (*Liquifilm*®) 1.4%, 5mL and 10mL – FML®.

DOSAGE
1 drop into the conjunctival sac 2-4 times daily.
This may be increased to 2 drops every hour for the first 24-48 hours.
Check intra-ocular pressure frequently. Do not discontinue prematurely.

CONTRA-INDICATIONS & WARNINGS
Contra-indicated in bacterial, viral, fungal, tuberculous or purulent conditions of the eye.
Contra-indicated if glaucoma is present, may also cause

glaucoma (but less likely than other more potent steroid eye drops).
Systemic side-effects may occur with extensive use.

Eye

EXCIPIENTS
Includes benzalkonium chloride, disodium edetate and polysorbate 80.

LICENSED STATUS
Licensed for use in children >2 years. Not licensed for use in children <2 years, but the above doses have been used 'off-label'.

Hydrocortisone acetate

USES
Short-term local treatment of inflammation.

PRESENTATION
Eye drops: 1%, 10mL – non-proprietary.
Eye ointment: 0.5%, 1% and 2.5%, 3g – non-proprietary.

DOSAGE
Eye drops: 1 drop 4 times daily.
Eye ointment: twice daily or at night.

EXCIPIENTS
Contact manufacturer for further details.

LICENSED STATUS
Licensed for use in all age groups.

Prednisolone

USES
Short-term treatment of local inflammation (with neomycin for bacterial prophylaxis).

PRESENTATION
Ear or eye drops: prednisolone sodium phosphate 0.5%, 5mL and 10mL – Predsol®.
Eye drops: preservative free, single use, 0.5%, 0.5mL – Minims® Prednisolone Sodium Phosphate.
Eye drops: prednisolone acetate 1%, 5mL and 10mL – Pred Forte®.
Ear or eye drops: prednisolone sodium phosphate 0.5% and neomycin sulphate 0.5%, 10mL – Predsol-N®.
Eye drops: with or without preservative – manufactured 'specials'.

DOSAGE
Eye drops: 1 drop every 1–2 hours until controlled then reduce frequency.

CONTRA-INDICATIONS & WARNINGS
Contra-indicated in bacterial, viral, fungal, tuberculous or purulent conditions of the eye. However, used by ophthalmologists with antibacterial/viral cover to suppress scarring due to infection.
Contra-indicated if glaucoma is present, may also cause glaucoma.
Systemic side-effects may occur with extensive use.
Neomycin – caution in young children with renal impairment as systemic absorption may cause ototoxicity.

EXCIPIENTS
Predsol® and Predsol-N® eye drops include benzalkonium chloride and disodium edetate.
Pred Forte® eye drops include benzalkonium chloride, disodium edetate and polysorbate 80.
Minims® Prednisolone Sodium Phosphate include disodium edetate.

LICENSED STATUS
Licensed for use in all age groups.

Eye

FURTHER INFORMATION
Prednisolone acetate has a greater penetration than the sodium phosphate salt. Eye drops with or without preservative available as manufactured 'specials' from Moorfields Eye Hospital.

Anti-allergics

Antazoline and Xylometazoline

USES
Allergic conjunctivitis (combination of a long-acting vasoconstrictor and an antihistamine).

PRESENTATION
Eye drops: antazoline sulphate 0.5% and xylometazoline hydrochloride 0.05%, 10mL – Otrivine-Antistin®.

DOSAGE
Children >5 years: 1 drop 2–3 times daily.

INTERACTIONS
Use of *monoamine-oxidase inhibitors* is not recommended within at least 14 days.

SIDE-EFFECTS
Possible systemic effects.

CONTRA-INDICATIONS & WARNINGS
Rebound congestion can occur with continued use.

EXCIPIENTS
Include benzalkonium chloride and disodium edetate.

LICENSED STATUS
Licensed for >5 years of age.

Levocabastine hydrochloride

USES
Seasonal allergic conjunctivitis.

PRESENTATION
Eye drops: 0.05%, 4mL – Livostin®.

DOSAGE
Adults and children >9 years: 1 drop to each eye twice daily, increased if necessary to 3–4 times daily. Discontinue if no improvement within 3 days.

SIDE-EFFECTS
Local irritation, blurred vision, local oedema, urticaria, dyspnoea, headache, drowsiness.

EXCIPIENTS
Include benzalkonium chloride, disodium edetate, polysorbate 80 and propylene glycol.

LICENSED STATUS
Licensed for >9 years of age.

Lodoxamide (as trometanol)

USES
Non-infectious allergic conjunctivitis.

PRESENTATION
Eye drops: 0.1%, 10mL – Alomide®.

DOSAGE
Adults and children >4 years: 1 drop 4 times daily.

> **SIDE-EFFECTS**
> Mild transient burning, stinging.

EXCIPIENTS
Include benzalkonium chloride and disodium edetate.

LICENSED STATUS
Licensed for >4 years of age.

Nedocromil sodium

USES
Allergic conjunctivitis. Vernal keratoconjunctivitis.

PRESENTATION
Eye drops: 2%, 5mL – Rapitil®.

DOSAGE
Seasonal and perennial conjunctivitis: adults and children >6 years – 1 drop twice daily, increased if necessary to 4 times daily. Maximum of 12 weeks treatment for seasonal conjunctivitis.
Vernal keratoconjunctivitis: adults and children >6 years – 1 drop 4 times daily.

> **SIDE-EFFECTS**
> Mild transient burning, stinging.

EXCIPIENTS
Include benzalkonium chloride and disodium edetate.

LICENSED STATUS
Licensed for >6 years of age.

Sodium cromoglicate (cromoglycate)

USES
Relief and treatment of acute allergic (seasonal) conjunctivitis.

PRESENTATION
Eye drops: 2%, 13.5mL – non-proprietary.

DOSAGE
1 drop into each eye 4 times daily.

> **SIDE-EFFECTS**
> Transient stinging and burning may occur.

EXCIPIENTS
Contact manufacturer for further details.

LICENSED STATUS
Licensed for use in all age groups.

Mydriatics and cycloplegics

Atropine sulphate

USES
Mydriasis and cycloplegia. Anterior uveitis.

PRESENTATION
Eye drops: 0.5%, 10mL – non-proprietary; 1%, 10mL – non-proprietary.
Eye drops: preservative free, single use, 1%, 0.5mL – Minims® Atropine Sulphate.
Eye ointment: 1%, 3g – non-proprietary.
Eye drops: atropine sulphate 1% and hypromellose 0.5%, 5mL – Isopto Atropine®.

DOSAGE
Cycloplegia: 1 drop or ointment applied to the lower fornix twice daily for 3 days prior to procedure.
Uveitis: 1 drop up to 4 times daily.

ADMINISTRATION
To reduce systemic absorption, use ointment if possible or compress the lacrimal sac at the medial canthus by digital pressure for at least 1 minute after instillation of the drops. Wash children's hands after use to avoid oral toxicity/contact dermatitis.

CONTRA-INDICATIONS & WARNINGS	**INTERACTIONS**
Use with extreme caution in infants and children, as risk of systemic absorption. This is manifested by dryness and flushing of the skin; a rash may be present in children and abdominal distension in infants. Action may be prolonged for up to 2 weeks.	Enhanced antimuscarinic effects with other *antimuscarinic drugs*.

EXCIPIENTS
Eye drops include benzalkonium chloride (but not in the preservative free preparation).

LICENSED STATUS
Not recommended in infants <3 months, due to possible association between cycloplegia and the development of amblyopia.
Licensed for refraction in children >3 months.

Cyclopentolate hydrochloride

USES
Production of cycloplegia. Uveitis.

PRESENTATION
Eye drops: 0.5% and 1%, 5mL – Mydrilate®.
Eye drops: preservative free, single use, 0.5% and 1%, 0.5mL – Minims® Cyclopentolate Hydrochloride.

DOSAGE
Cycloplegia: 3–12 months   1 drop of 0.5%
              1–16 years   1 drop of 1%
Uveitis: 1 drop 2–4 times daily (strength as above).

ADMINISTRATION
Instill approximately 30–60 minutes before examination.

CONTRA-INDICATIONS & WARNINGS
Recovery from effects may take up to 1 day.

INTERACTIONS
Enhanced antimuscarinic effects with other *antimuscarinic* drugs.

EXCIPIENTS
Mydrilate® eye drops include benzalkonium chloride.

LICENSED STATUS
Not recommended in infants <3 months due to possible association between cycloplegia and the development of amblyopia. Also there is an increased risk of systemic toxicity in neonates.
However used commonly on the neonatal unit to dilate pupils for retinal examination and following neonatal cataract surgery.

Homatropine hydrobromide

USES
Mydriatic and cycloplegic.

PRESENTATION
Eye drops: 0.125%, 0.25% and 0.5% – manufactured 'specials'; 1% and 2%, 10mL – non-proprietary; preservative free 1% and 2% – manufactured 'specials'.
Eye drops: preservative free, single use, 2%, 0.5mL – Minims® Homatropine.

DOSAGE
<2 years: 1 drop of 0.5% daily or alternate days depending on response and desired effect.
>2 years: 1 drop twice daily depending on response and desired effect.

ADMINISTRATION
To reduce systemic absorption, compress the lacrimal sac at the medial canthus by digital pressure for at least 1 minute after instillation of the drops.

CONTRA-INDICATIONS & WARNINGS
Use with extreme caution in children, as risk of systemic absorption. Children with blond hair and blue eyes more susceptible to side-effects. Contra-indicated where filtration angle is narrow. Not recommended in children <3 months due to possible association between cycloplegia and the development of amblyopia. Also the increased risk of systemic toxicity in neonates.

EXCIPIENTS
Eye drops: 0.125%, 0.25% and 0.5%, from Moorfields Eye Hospital, include chlorhexidine.
Non-proprietary eye drops, 1% and 2%, include benzalkonium chloride.

LICENSED STATUS
Not recommended in children <3 months.
Those available as 'specials' are as such unlicensed.

FURTHER INFORMATION
1% and 2% eye drops also available preservative free as 'specials' from Moorfields Eye Hospital.
Used in preference to atropine as more rapid onset and less prolonged mydriatic action.

Tropicamide

USES
As a mydriatic and cycloplegic.
Fundoscopy and post cataract surgery in small children.

PRESENTATION
Eye drops: 0.5% and 1%, 5mL – Mydriacyl®.
Eye drops: preservative free, single use, 0.5% and 1%, 0.5mL – Minims® Tropicamide.

DOSAGE
Fundoscopy: 1 drop 20 minutes before examination (strength used depends on age and eye colour – use 0.5% in infants).
Post cataract surgery in small children: 1 drop of 0.5% once or twice daily.
Used in combination with cyclopentolate or as an alternative after cataract surgery.

ADMINISTRATION
To reduce systemic absorption, compress the lacrimal sac at the medial canthus by digital pressure for at least 1 minute after instillation of the drops. Wash children's hands after use to avoid oral toxicity/contact dermatitis.

CONTRA-INDICATIONS & WARNINGS
Contra-indicated where filtration angle is narrow.
Use with extreme caution in children, as risk of systemic absorption. This is manifested by dryness and flushing of the skin; a rash may be present in children and abdominal distension in infants.

EXCIPIENTS
Mydriacyl® eye drops include benzalkonium chloride and disodium edetate.

LICENSED STATUS
Licensed for use in all age groups.

Sympathomimetics

Phenylephrine hydrochloride

USES
Mydriatic to dilate the pupil in diagnostic or therapeutic procedures.

PRESENTATION
Eye drops: 10%, 10mL – non-proprietary.
Eye drops: preservative free, single use, 2.5% and 10%, 0.5mL – Minims® Phenylephrine Hydrochloride.

DOSAGE
Fundoscopy: Infants: 1 drop of 2.5%, 30 minutes before examination.
Children: 1 drop of 2.5% or 5%, 30 minutes before examination.
Effect in 60-90 minutes, recovery in 5-7 hours.
Therapeutic: Infants: 1 drop of 2.5%, in combination with cyclopentolate twice daily.
Children: 1 drop of 2.5% or 5%, twice daily.

CONTRA-INDICATIONS & WARNINGS
Caution in neonates, especially premature and patients with cardiovascular disease or hypertension.
The 10% preparations are contra-indicated in children because of the increased risk of systemic toxicity.

INTERACTIONS
Sympathomimetic – may interact with *monoamine-oxidase inhibitors, tricyclic antidepressants* and *antihypertensive agents.*

SIDE-EFFECTS
Systemic side-effects include palpitations and tachycardia – very unlikely to occur.

EXCIPIENTS
Minims® Phenylephrine Hydrochloride include disodium edetate and sodium metabisulphite.

LICENSED STATUS
Minims® Phenylephrine Hydrochloride 2.5% are licensed for use in all age groups. The 10% eye drop preparations are contra-indicated in children.

Dipivefrine

USES
Reduction of elevated intra-ocular pressure in patients with chronic open angle glaucoma.

PRESENTATION
Eye drops: 0.1%, 5mL and 10mL – Propine®.

DOSAGE
1 drop twice daily.

CONTRA-INDICATIONS & WARNINGS
Contra-indicated in closed angle glaucoma as it is a mydriatic. Use with caution in patients with heart disease or hypertension.

EXCIPIENTS
Include benzalkonium chloride and disodium edetate.

LICENSED STATUS
Not licensed for use in children.

FURTHER INFORMATION
Dipivefrine is a pro-drug of adrenaline (epinephrine).

Miotics

Pilocarpine

USES
Treatment of glaucoma; preoperative for goniotomy and trabeculotomy.

PRESENTATION
Eye drops: 0.5%, 1%, 2%, 3% and 4%, 10mL – non-proprietary.
Eye drops: preservative free, single use, 1%, 2% and 4%, 0.5mL – Minims® Pilocarpine Nitrate.

DOSAGE
Glaucoma: <2 years 1 drop of 0.5% or 1%, 3 times daily.
>2 years 1 drop 4 times daily (any strength).
Preoperative: 2–3 drops of 1% or 2%, once daily.

ADMINISTRATION
To reduce systemic absorption, compress the lacrimal sac at the medial canthus by digital pressure for at least 1 minute after instillation of the drops.

CONTRA-INDICATIONS & WARNINGS
Caution in hypertension, asthma and urinary obstruction.

SIDE-EFFECTS
May cause ciliary muscle spasms for up to 2 hours. Browache and headache. Cholinergic reactions affecting gut and cardiovascular system.

EXCIPIENTS
Contact manufacturer for further details.

LICENSED STATUS
Not recommended for use in children, but the above doses have been used.

Eye

Beta-blockers

Betaxolol (as hydrochloride)

USES
Reduction of elevated intra-ocular pressure in patients with ocular hypertension and chronic open angle glaucoma.

PRESENTATION
Eye drops: 0.5%, 5mL – Betoptic®.
Ophthalmic suspension modified release (eye drops): 0.25%, 5mL – Betoptic®; preservative free, single use, 0.25mL – Betoptic®.

DOSAGE
1 drop twice daily.

CONTRA-INDICATIONS & WARNINGS
Contra-indicated in sinus bradycardia; second or third degree heart block; cardiogenic shock or overt cardiac failure. Cardioselective beta-blocker but care in airways disease. Stings on instillation.

INTERACTIONS
Caution if on oral *beta-blockers*.

EXCIPIENTS
Includes benzalkonium chloride and disodium edetate (but not in the preservative free preparation).

LICENSED STATUS
Not licensed in children, but the above dose has been used.

Carteolol (as hydrochloride)

USES
Reduction of elevated intra-ocular pressure in patients with ocular hypertension and chronic open angle glaucoma.

PRESENTATION
Eye drops: 1% and 2%, 5mL – Teoptic®.

DOSAGE
1 drop twice daily.

CONTRA-INDICATIONS & WARNINGS
Contra-indicated in sinus bradycardia; second or third degree heart block; cardiogenic shock or overt cardiac failure; bronchospasm.

EXCIPIENTS
Include benzalkonium chloride.

LICENSED STATUS
Not recommended for use in children, but the above dose has been used.

Levobunolol (as hydrochloride)

USES
Reduction of elevated intra-ocular pressure in patients with ocular hypertension and chronic open angle glaucoma.

PRESENTATION
Eye drops: levobunolol hydrochloride 0.5% and polyvinyl alcohol 1.4% (*Liquifilm*®), 5mL– Betagan®; preservative free, single use, 0.4mL – Betagan®.

DOSAGE
1 drop once or twice daily.

CONTRA-INDICATIONS & WARNINGS
Contra-indicated in sinus bradycardia; second or third degree heart block; cardiogenic shock or overt cardiac failure; bronchospasm.

EXCIPIENTS
Include benzalkonium chloride (but not in the preservative free preparation).

LICENSED STATUS
Not licensed for use in children but the above dose has been used.

Timolol maleate

USES
Reduction of elevated intra-ocular pressure in patients with ocular hypertension and chronic open angle glaucoma.

PRESENTATION
Eye drops: 0.25% and 0.5%, 5mL – Timoptol® and non-proprietary.
Eye drops: preservative free, single use, 0.25% and 0.5%, 0.25mL – Timoptol®.
Ophthalmic gel-forming solution (eye drops): 0.25% and 0.5%, 2.5mL – Timoptol® LA.
Eye gel (eye drops): 0.1%, 5mL – Nyogel®.

DOSAGE
Eye drops: 1 drop twice daily.
Timoptol® LA and Nyogel®: 1 drop once daily.

CONTRA-INDICATIONS & WARNINGS
Contra-indicated in sinus bradycardia; second or third degree heart block; cardiogenic shock or overt cardiac failure; bronchospasm.

EXCIPIENTS
Timoptol® and Nyogel® include benzalkonium chloride (but not in the preservative free preparation). Timoptol® LA include benzododecinium bromide.

LICENSED STATUS
Not licensed for use in children, but the above doses have been used.

Carbonic anhydrase inhibitors and systemic drugs

Acetazolamide

Enzyme inhibitor which acts specifically on carbonic anhydrase.

USES
Open and narrow angle glaucoma.
For details see the acetazolamide monograph in the main section of the book.

Brinzolamide

Topical carbonic anhydrase inhibitor.

USES
Adjunctive to topical beta-blockers.
As monotherapy in patients unresponsive to topical beta-blockers or in whom topical beta-blockers are contra-indicated. In treatment of elevated intra-ocular pressure.

Eye

PRESENTATION
Eye drops: 1%, 5mL – Azopt®.

DOSAGE
1 drop twice daily used alone or with topical beta-blocker.
Some patients respond better with 1 drop 3 times a day.

CONTRA-INDICATIONS & WARNINGS	SIDE-EFFECTS
Contra-indicated in severe renal impairment.	Monitor for sulphonamide hypersensitivity and local
Not recommended in hepatic impairment.	effects.
INTERACTIONS	
Avoid concurrent use of *oral carbonic anhydrase inhibitors (e.g. acetazolamide)*.	

EXCIPIENTS
Include benzalkonium chloride and disodium edetate.

LICENSED STATUS
Not licensed for use in children.

FURTHER INFORMATION
If substituting brinzolamide for another ophthalmic anti-glaucoma agent, discontinue the other agent after proper dosing on one day and start brinzolamide the next day.

Dorzolamide

Topical carbonic anhydrase inhibitor.

USES
Adjunctive to topical beta-blockers.
As monotherapy in patients unresponsive to topical beta-blockers or in whom topical beta-blockers are contra-indicated. In treatment of elevated intra-ocular pressure.

PRESENTATION
Eye drops: dorzolamide hydrochloride 2%, 5mL – Trusopt®.

DOSAGE
1 drop twice daily with topical beta-blocker.
1 drop 3 times daily when used alone.

CONTRA-INDICATIONS & WARNINGS	SIDE-EFFECTS
Contra-indicated in severe renal impairment.	Monitor for sulphonamide hypersensitivity and local
Caution in hepatic impairment (but mostly excreted in urine unchanged).	effects of eye lid inflammation.
INTERACTIONS	
Avoid concurrent use of *oral carbonic anhydrase inhibitors (e.g. acetazolamide)*.	

EXCIPIENTS
Include benzalkonium chloride.

LICENSED STATUS
Not licensed for use in children, but the above doses have been used.

FURTHER INFORMATION
If substituting dorzolamide for another ophthalmic anti-glaucoma agent, discontinue the other agent after proper dosing on one day and start dorzolamide the next day.

Eye

Local anaesthetics

Tetracaine (amethocaine) hydrochloride

USES
Local anaesthetic.

PRESENTATION
Eye drops: 0.5% and 1%, 10mL – non-proprietary.
Eye drops: preservative free, single use, 0.5% and 1%, 0.5mL Minims® Amethocaine Hydrochloride.

DOSAGE
1 drop for eye examination. Repeat at 3 minute intervals if required.

CONTRA-INDICATIONS & WARNINGS
In view of the immaturity of the enzyme system, which metabolises the ester type local anaesthetics in premature babies, tetracaine (amethocaine) should be avoided in these patients. Protect anaesthetised eye from dust and bacterial contamination. Prolonged application may damage cornea.

INTERACTIONS
Should not be used in patients taking *sulphonamides*.

SIDE-EFFECTS
Initial burning sensation.

LICENSED STATUS
Licensed for use in all age groups, except premature babies.

Lidocaine (lignocaine) hydrochloride and Fluorescein

USES
Local anaesthetic and diagnostic stain.

PRESENTATION
Eye drops: lidocaine (lignocaine) hydrochloride 4% and fluorescein sodium; preservative free, single use, 0.25%, 0.5mL – Minims® Lignocaine and Fluorescein.

DOSAGE
1 drop, as required.

CONTRA-INDICATIONS & WARNINGS
In view of the immaturity of the enzyme system which metabolises the ester type local anaesthetics in premature babies, lidocaine (lignocaine) should be avoided in these patients. Protect anaesthetised eye from dust and bacterial contamination. Prolonged application may damage cornea.

SIDE-EFFECTS
Initial burning sensation.

EXCIPIENTS
Include polyvidone.

LICENSED STATUS
Licensed for use in all age groups, except premature babies.

Oxybuprocaine hydrochloride

USES
Local anaesthetic.

PRESENTATION
Eye drops: preservative free, single use, 0.4%; 0.5mL – Minims® Benoxinate (Oxybuprocaine) Hydrochloride.

Eye

DOSAGE
1 drop for eye examination. A second drop can be given after 90 seconds for fitting of hard contact lenses. 3 drops at 90 second intervals provide sufficient anaesthesia after 5 minutes for foreign body removal or incision of a meibomian cyst (use in combination with local anaesthetic to the eye lid).

ADMINISTRATION
To reduce systemic absorption, compress the lacrimal sac at the medial canthus by digital pressure for at least 1 minute after instillation of the drops.

CONTRA-INDICATIONS & WARNINGS
Protect anaesthetised eye from dust and bacterial contamination. Prolonged application may damage cornea.

SIDE-EFFECTS
Initial burning sensation. Corneal sensitivity is normal after about 1 hour.

LICENSED STATUS
Licensed for use in all age groups.

Proxymetacaine hydrochloride

USES
Local anaesthetic.

PRESENTATION
Eye drops: preservative free, single use, 0.5%, 0.5mL – Minims® Proxymetacaine Hydrochloride.
Eye drops: preservative free, single use, proxymetacaine hydrochloride 0.5% and fluorescein sodium, 0.25%, 0.5mL – Minims® Proxymetacaine and Fluorescein.

DOSAGE
1 or 2 drops as required.

CONTRA-INDICATIONS & WARNINGS
In view of the immaturity of the enzyme system which metabolises the ester type local anaesthetics in premature babies, proxymetacaine should be avoided in these patients.

LICENSED STATUS
Licensed for use in all age groups, except premature babies.

Ocular lubricants

Acetylcysteine

USES
Dry eye syndromes associated with deficient tear secretion, impaired or abnormal mucus production (mucolytic & lubricant properties).

PRESENTATION
Eye drops: acetylcysteine 5% and hypromellose 0.35%, 10mL – Ilube®; preservative free – manufactured 'special'.

DOSAGE
1 drop 3–4 times daily.

EXCIPIENTS
Ilube® eye drops include benzalkonium chloride.

LICENSED STATUS
Licensed for use in all age groups, except the preservative free which as available as a 'special' and as such is unlicensed.

Eye

Carbomers (polyacrylic acid)

USES
Dry eyes including keratoconjunctivitis sicca, unstable tear film.

PRESENTATION
Liquid gel (eye drops): carbomer 980 (polyacrylic acid) 0.2%; 10g – GelTears®, Viscotears®; preservative free, single use, 0.6mL – Viscotears®.

DOSAGE
Apply 3-4 times daily or as required.

EXCIPIENTS
GelTears® include benzalkonium chloride. Viscotears® include cetrimide and disodium edetate (but not in the preservative free preparation).

LICENSED STATUS
Not licensed for use in children.

Hydroxyethylcellulose

USES
Relief of dry eyes associated with tear deficiency.

PRESENTATION
Eye drops: preservative free, single use, hydroxyethylcellulose 0.44% and sodium chloride 0.35%, 0.5mL – Minims® Artificial Tears.

DOSAGE
1 or 2 drops 3 or 4 times daily, or as required.

EXCIPIENTS
Include borax and boric acid.

LICENSED STATUS
Licensed for use in all age groups.

Hypromellose

USES
Dry eyes associated with tear deficiency.

PRESENTATION
Eye drops: 0.3%, 10mL – non-proprietary; 0.5%, 10mL – Isopto Plain®; 1%, 10mL – Isopto Alkaline®.
Eye drops: hypromellose 0.3% and dextran '70' 0.1%, 15mL – Tears Naturale®.

DOSAGE
1 drop as frequently as required (up to every 10 minutes).

EXCIPIENTS
Isopto Plain®, Isopto Alkaline® and Tears Naturale® include benzalkonium chloride. Tears Naturale® also include disodium edetate.

LICENSED STATUS
Licensed for use in all age groups.

Eye

Liquid paraffin

USES
Dry eyes associated with tear deficiency.

PRESENTATION
Eye ointment: white soft paraffin 57.3%, liquid paraffin 42.5% and wool alcohol 0.2%; 3.5g, 5g – Lacri-Lube®.
Eye ointment: white soft paraffin 60%, liquid paraffin 30% and wool fat (lanolin) 10%; 5g – Lubri-Tears®.

DOSAGE
Apply as required.

LICENSED STATUS
Licensed for use in all age groups.

Paraffin, yellow soft

USES
Corneal exposure, dry eyes, anaesthetic cornea.

PRESENTATION
Eye ointment: liquid paraffin 10%, wool fat 10% in yellow soft paraffin, 4g – simple eye ointment.

DOSAGE
Apply to the lower fornix up to 2 hourly.

EXCIPIENTS
Include benzalkonium chloride.

LICENSED STATUS
Licensed for use in all age groups.

FURTHER INFORMATION
Available from Dominion and Martindale.

Polyvinyl alcohol

USES
Ocular lubricant.

PRESENTATION
Eye drops: polyvinyl alcohol 1.4%, 10mL – Sno Tears®; 15mL – Liquifilm Tears®.
Eye drops: preservative free, single use, polyvinyl alcohol 1.4% and povidone 0.6%, 0.4mL – Liquifilm Tears®.
Eye drops: polyvinyl alcohol 1% and macrogol '8000' 2%, 15mL – Hypotears®.

DOSAGE
1 drop as frequently as required (up to every 10 minutes).

> **CONTRA-INDICATIONS & WARNINGS**
> Discontinue if irritation increases or persists.

EXCIPIENTS
Include benzalkonium chloride and disodium edetate (but not in the preservative free preparation).

LICENSED STATUS
Licensed for use in all age groups.

Eye

Miscellaneous

Sodium chloride

USES
Irrigation, including first aid removal of harmful substances.

PRESENTATION
Eye drops: preservative free, single use, 0.9%, 0.5mL – Minims® Sodium Chloride.

DOSAGE
Adequate solution should be used to irrigate the eye.

LICENSED STATUS
Licensed for use in all age groups.

Acetylcholine chloride

USES
Cataract surgery, penetrating keratoplasty, iridectomy and other anterior segment surgery requiring rapid complete miosis.

PRESENTATION
Solution for intra-ocular irrigation: acetylcholine chloride 1%, and mannitol 3% when reconstituted, 2mL vial – Miochol-E®.

DOSAGE
Adults : 0.5-2mL into anterior chamber will produce a satisfactory miosis which will last for approximately 20 minutes.

SIDE-EFFECTS
Rarely reported but are indicative of systemic absorption and include: bradycardia, hypertension, flushing, breathing difficulty and sweating.

EXCIPIENTS
Mannitol renders the reconstituted solution isotonic with blood and serum. It is not an active ingredient.

LICENSED STATUS
Not licensed for use in children.

Apraclonidine (as hydrochloride)

USES
Control of intra-ocular pressure.

PRESENTATION
Eye drops: preservative free, single use, 1%, 0.25mL – Iopidine®.
Eye drops: 0.5%, 5mL – Iopidine®.

DOSAGE
1% solution: control or prevention of postoperative elevation of intra-ocular pressure after anterior segment laser therapy. Apply 1 drop 1 hour before laser therapy and 1 drop immediately after completion of the procedure.
0.5% solution: short-term adjunctive treatment of chronic glaucoma in patients not adequately controlled by other drugs (may not provide additional benefit if the patient is already using 2 drugs that suppress the production of aqueous humour). Apply 1 drop 3 times daily usually for a maximum of 1 month.

CONTRA-INDICATIONS & WARNINGS
Caution with a history of angina, severe coronary insufficiency, recent myocardial infarction, cardiac failure, hypertension, cerebrovascular disease, vasovagal attack, chronic renal failure, depression.
Exaggerated reduction in intraocular pressure following perioperative use should be closely monitored. Drowsiness may occur.

INTERACTIONS
Antidepressants: possible risk of hypotension with *tricyclic antidepressant drugs.*
Sympathomimetics: possible risk of hypertension with *adrenaline (epinephrine)* and *noradrenaline (norepinephrine).*

SIDE-EFFECTS
Dry mouth, taste disturbance, hyperaemia, ocular pruritus, discomfort (withdraw if ocular intolerance including oedema of lids and conjunctiva), headache, dry nose, lid retraction, conjunctival blanching and mydriasis reported after perioperative use.

EXCIPIENTS
Iopidine® eye drops 0.5% include benzalkonium chloride.

LICENSED STATUS
Not recommended for use in children.

Sodium hyaluronate

USES
Anterior chamber surgery to maintain the anterior chamber shape.

PRESENTATION
Injection: sodium hyaluronate 10mg in 1mL, 0.5mL, 0.85mL; Healonid®; 0.55mL – Provisc®; 14mg in 1mL, 0.55mL – Healonid® GV.

DOSAGE
Volume given intra-ocularly depends on technique and the procedure. Allow to attain room temperature 30–60 minutes before use. Remove after surgery by aspiration or irrigation. Monitor intra-ocular pressure postoperatively.

CONTRA-INDICATIONS & WARNINGS
Rare inflammatory reactions and remote possibility of idiosyncratic reactions.

INTERACTIONS
Do not use hyaluronidase.
Healonid® may become turbid due to precipitate in the presence of cationic agents such as *benzalkonium chloride.*

EXCIPIENTS
Contact manufacturer for further details.

LICENSED STATUS
Licensed for use in all age groups.

Fluorescein sodium

USES
Detection of lesions and foreign bodies.

PRESENTATION
Eye drops: preservative free, single use, 1% and 2%, 0.5mL – Minims® Fluorescein Sodium.

DOSAGE
Sufficient solution should be applied to stain the damaged areas.
Conjunctival abrasions colour yellow/orange. Corneal abrasions colour bright green and foreign bodies are surrounded by green ring.
Wash excess away with NaCl 0.9%.

> **CONTRA-INDICATIONS & WARNINGS**
> Stains soft contact lenses.

> **SIDE-EFFECTS**
> May cause transient blurring of vision on instillation.

LICENSED STATUS
Licensed for use in all age groups.

Topical non-steroidals

Diclofenac sodium

USES
Inhibition of intraoperative miosis during cataract surgery (but does not possess intrinsic mydriatic properties). Post-operative inflammation.

PRESENTATION
Eye drops: single use, 0.1% – Voltarol® Ophtha.

DOSAGE
Control of postoperative inflammation: 1 drop 4 times daily (maximum of 28 days).
Prophylaxis of perioperative miosis: 1 drop 4 times during the 2 hours pre-surgery.

> **CONTRA-INDICATIONS & WARNINGS**
> Caution in asthma.

SIDE-EFFECTS
Mild to moderate burning sensation; rarely blurred vision immediately after instillation, hypersensitivity reactions.

LICENSED STATUS
Not licensed for use in children, but the above doses have been used.

Flurbiprofen sodium

USES
Inhibition of intraoperative miosis; Management of post-operative and post-laser trabeculoplasty inflammation in the anterior segment of the eye in patients in whom topical corticosteroid therapy is contra-indicated.

PRESENTATION
Eye drops: single use, 0.03%, 0.4mL – Ocufen®.

DOSAGE
Inhibition of intra-operative miosis: 1 drop every 30 minutes starting 2 hours before surgery (the final drops should not be instilled less than 30 minutes before surgery).
Post surgery: beginning 24 hours post surgery 1 drop 4 times daily.
Continue for 1 week after laser trabeculoplasty or 2-3 weeks post other surgery.

> **CONTRA-INDICATIONS & WARNINGS**
> Contra-indicated in epithelial herpes simplex keratitis.

SIDE-EFFECTS
Theoretical risk of prolonged bleeding time. Transient stinging and blurring of eyes on instillation.

LICENSED STATUS
Not licensed for use in children.

Eye

Ketorolac trometamol

USES
Prophylaxis and reduction of inflammation and associated symptoms following ocular surgery.

PRESENTATION
Eye drops: 0.5%, 5mL – Acular®.

DOSAGE
1 drop 3 times daily starting 24 hours preoperatively and continuing for up to 3 weeks.

SIDE-EFFECTS
Theoretical risk of prolonged bleeding time. Transient stinging and blurring of eyes on instillation.

EXCIPIENTS
Include benzalkonium chloride and disodium edetate.

LICENSED STATUS
Not licensed for use in children.

CONTENTS

Nutrition tables

All products ACBS listed for the following indications: short bowel syndrome, intractable malabsorption, pre-operative preparation of patients who are undernourished, dysphagia, bowel fistulas, disease-related malnutrition and/or growth failure.

Name of feed	Fortini	Fortini Multi Fibre
Manufacturer	Nutricia Clinical Care	Nutricia Clinical Care
kcal/100mL	150	150
kJ/100mL	630	630
Protein source	Sodium caseinate, calcium caseinate	Sodium caseinate, calcium caseinate
Protein g/100mL	3.4	3.4
Fat source	Canola oil, sunflower oil	Canola oil, sunflower oil
Fat g/100mL	6.8	6.8
Carbohydrate source	Maltodextrin, sucrose	Maltodextrin, sucrose, arabic gum, inulin, soy polysaccharide, resistant starch, cellulose, oligofructose
Carbohydrate g/100mL	18.8	18.8
Osmolality mOsmol/kg water	485	505
Fibre g/100mL	0	1.5
Special characteristics		
Peanut free	Yes	Yes
Suitable for vegetarians	No, trace of fish gelatin (carrier for vitamin E)	No, trace of fish gelatin (carrier for vitamin E)
Suitable for vegans	No	No
Lactose free	Residual lactose only	Residual lactose only
Gluten free	Yes	Yes
Presentation	Carton: 200mL	Carton: 200mL
ACBS listed	Yes	Yes
Nutritionally complete	Yes	Yes
Caution	Not suitable for children below 8kg or over 20kg	Not suitable for children below 8kg or over 20kg
Other information	-	Due to fibre content, intakes of > 2 cartons per day should be used with caution

All products ACBS listed for the following indications: short bowel syndrome, intractable malabsorption, pre-operative preparation of patients who are undernourished, dysphagia, bowel fistulas, disease-related malnutrition and/or growth failure.

Name of feed	Paediasure	Paediasure Fibre	Paediasure Plus
Manufacturer	Abbott Nutrition	Abbott Nutrition	Abbott Nutrition
kcal/100mL	101	101	151
kJ/100mL	422	422	632
Protein source	Whey protein, sodium and calcium caseinate	Whey protein, sodium and calcium caseinate	Whey protein, sodium and calcium caseinate
Protein g/100mL	2.8	2.8	4.2
Fat source	Sunflower oil, MCT oil*, soya oil	Sunflower oil, MCT oil*, soya oil	Sunflower oil, MCT oil*, soya oil
Fat g/100mL	5	5	7.5
Carbohydrate source	Maltodextrin, sucrose	Maltodextrin, sucrose soy polysaccharide	Maltodextrin. sucrose
Carbohydrate g/100mL	11.2	11.2	16.7
Osmolality mOsmol/kg water	320	340	500
Fibre g/100mL	0	0.5	0
Special characteristics			
Peanut free	Yes	Yes	Yes
Suitable for vegetarians	Yes	Yes	Yes
Suitable for vegans	No	No	No
Lactose free	Residual lactose only	Residual lactose only	Residual lactose only
Gluten free	Yes	Yes	Yes
Presentation	Can: 250mL Tetrapak: 200mL	Can: 250mL Tetrapak: 200mL	Tetrapak: 200mL
ACBS listed	Yes	Yes	Yes
Nutritionally complete	Yes	Yes	Yes
Caution	Not suitable for children below 8kg or over 20kg	Not suitable for children below 8kg or over 20kg	Not suitable for children below 8kg or over 20kg
Suggested dosage	1–3 years: 1 carton 4–6 years: 1–2 cartons	1–3 years: 1 carton 4–6 years: 1–2 cartons	1–3 years: 1 carton 4–6 years: 1–2 cartons
Other information	Tetrapak: strawberry, banana, vanilla, chocolate Can: vanilla	Tetrapak: strawberry vanilla, banana Can: vanilla	Strawberry, vanilla, banana

*MCT = Medium Chain Tryglyceride

Nutrition tables

All products are ACBS listed for use as a necessary supplement for short bowel syndrome, intractable malabsorption, proven inflammatory bowel disease, dysphagia, bowel fistulas, and disease-related malnutrition. All products greater than 6g protein/100mL are excluded as they are unsuitable for children.

Name of feed	Clinutren Iso	Ensure	Fresubin Energy
Manufacturer	Nestlé Clinical Nutrition	Abbott Nutrition	Fresenius Kabi
kcal/100mL	100	100	150
kJ/100mL	420	423	630
Protein source	Milk protein, egg yolk	Caseinates, soya protein isolate	Milk protein
Protein g/100mL	3.8	4	5.6
Fat source	Butter oil, corn oil, soya oil	Corn oil	Vegetable oils, MCT oil*
Fat g/100mL	3.3	3.4	5.8
Carbohydrate source	Glucose syrup, sucrose, milk	Maltodextrin, sucrose	Maltodextrin
Carbohydrate g/100mL	13.8	13.6	18.8
Osmolality mOsmol/kg water	430–460	319	400–480
Fibre g/100mL	< 0.6	0	0
Special characteristics			
Peanut free	Yes	Yes	Yes
Suitable for vegetarians	Yes	Yes	Yes
Suitable for vegans	No	No	No
Lactose free	No	Residual lactose only	Residual lactose only
Gluten free	Yes	Yes	Yes
Presentation	Cup: 200mL	Can: 250mL Can: 400g (vanilla) powder	Tetrapak: 200mL
ACBS listed	Yes	Yes	Yes
Nutritionally complete	Yes	Yes	Yes
Caution	Not to be given to children under 1 year. Use with caution in children 1–5 years	Not to be given to children under 1 year. Use with caution in children 1–5 years	Very high in protein. Do not give to children less than 3 years as a sip feed. Use with caution in children 4–12 years
Suggested Dosage	1–3 years: 1 cup 4–6 years: 1–2 cups 7–12 years: 2–3 cups	1–3 years: 1 can 4–6 years: 1–2 cans 7–12 years: 2–3 cans	3–5 years: 1 carton 6–12 years: 2 cartons
Flavours	Vanilla, chocolate	Vanilla, chocolate, coffee, egg-nog, nut, asparagus, chicken and mushroom	Vanilla, strawberry, banana, orange, chocolate-mint, blackcurrant, vegetable cream, toffee-caramel, pineapple, neutral

*See page 713

Nutrition tables

All products are ACBS listed for use as a necessary supplement for short bowel syndrome, intractable malabsorption, proven inflammatory bowel disease, dysphagia, bowel fistulas, and disease-related malnutrition. Products providing over 6g protein/100mL are excluded, as these are considered unsuitable for use in children.

Name of feed	Clinutren 1.5	Fresubin Original	Resource Shake
Manufacturer	Nestlé Clinical Nutrition	Fresenius Kabi	Novartis Medical Nutrition
kcal/100mL	150	100	170
kJ/100mL	630	420	730
Protein source	Milk protein	Milk protein, soya protein	Low lactose skimmed milk
Protein g/100mL	5.6	3.8	5.1
Fat source	Butter oil, corn oil, soya oil	Soya oil	Rapeseed oil, cream
Fat g/100mL	5	3.4	7
Carbohydrate source	Glucose syrup, sucrose, milk (lactose reduced)	Maltodextrin, sucrose	Low lactose skimmed milk, dried glucose syrup, sucrose
Carbohydrate g/100mL	21	13.8	22.6
Osmolality mOsmol/kg water	680–790	360–380	530–660 (depending on flavour)
Fibre g/100mL	< 0.5	0	0
Special characteristics:			
Peanut free	Yes	Yes, but contains extracts of hazelnut	No
Suitable for vegetarians	Strawberry-raspberry flavour contains cochineal	Yes	No
Suitable for vegans	No	No	No
Lactose free	Residual lactose only	Residual lactose only	No
Gluten free	Yes	Yes	Yes
Presentation	Cup: 200mL	Tetrapak: 200mL	Combi-bloc: 175mL
ACBS listed	Yes	Yes	Yes
Nutritionally complete	Yes	Yes	Yes
Caution	Not to be given to children under 1 year. Use with caution in children 1–5 years	Not to be given to children under 1 year. Use with caution in children 1–5 years	High in protein. Do not give to children less than 3 years as a sip feed. Use with caution in children 4–12 years
Suggested dosage	3–5 years: 1 cup 6–12 years: 2 cups	1–3 years: 1 carton 4–6 years: 2 cartons 7–12 years: 2–3 cartons	3–5 years: 1 carton 6–12 years: 2 cartons
Flavours	Vanilla, banana, chocolate, apricot, strawberry-raspberry, coffee	Vanilla, nut, peach, chocolate, moccha, blackcurrant	Strawberry, chocolate, vanilla, banana, summer fruits, lemon, toffee
Other information	–	–	–

Nutrition tables

Milk based powders ACBS listed for malabsorption states/disease-related malnutrition or other conditions requiring a high fat/carbohydrate supplement.

Name of feed	Calshake powder	Scandishake (analysis for flavoured Scandishake)
Manufacturer	Fresenius Kabi	SHS International
kcal/100g	496	514
kJ/100g	2,078	2,153
Protein source	Skimmed milk powder, sodium caseinate	Skimmed milk powder
Protein g/100g	4.6	4.7
Fat source	Hydrogenated vegetable oil, medium chain triglycerides	Vegetable oil, medium chain triglycerides
Fat g/100g	23.5	24.7
Carbohydrate source	Dried glucose syrup, dextrose monohydrate, maltodextrin	Dried glucose syrup, sugar, maltodextrin
Carbohydrate g/100g	66.5	68.2
Osmolality mOsmol/kg water	No information available	Unflavoured 746 mOsmol/kg
Fibre g/100g	0	0
Special characteristics		
Peanut free	Yes	Yes
Suitable for vegetarians	Yes	Yes - except strawberry contains cochineal
Suitable for vegans	No	No
Lactose free	No	No
Gluten free	Yes	Yes
Presentation	Sachet: 87g	Sachet: 85g
ACBS listed	Yes	Yes
Nutritionally complete	No, not fortified with vitamins or minerals	No, not fortified with vitamins or minerals
Caution	Not to be given to children under 1 year. Use with caution in children 1–5 years. Not intended as a sole source of nutrition	Not to be given to children under 1 year. Use with caution in children 1–5 years. Not intended as a sole source of nutrition
Suggested dosage	1–5 years: 1/2 serving (43g) + 240mL whole milk 6–12 years: 1 serving (87g) + 240mL whole milk	1–5 years: 1/2 serving (43g) + 240mL whole milk 6–12 years: 1 serving (85g) + 240mL whole milk
Flavours	Strawberry, vanilla, chocolate, banana	Strawberry, vanilla, chocolate, unflavoured
Other information	Reconstitution: mix 1 sachet (87g) with 240mL whole milk	Reconstitution: mix 1 sachet (85g) with 240mL whole milk

Nutrition tables

Fibre supplements ACBS listed as a necessary nutritional supplement for short bowel syndrome, intractable malabsorption, proven inflammatory bowel disease, bowel fistulas, disease-related malnutrition.
N.B. Supplements greater than 6g protein/100mL or >2g/100mL (over 2g/100mL) of fibre are excluded as they are unsuitable for children.

Name of feed	Enrich
Manufacturer	Abbott Nutrition
kcal/100mL	103
kJ/100mL	431
Protein source	Soya protein isolate, caseinates
Protein g/100mL	3.8
Fat source	Corn oil
Fat g/100mL	3.5
Carbohydrate source	Maltodextrin, sucrose, non-starch polysaccharides
Carbohydrate g/100mL	14
Osmolality mOsmol/kg water	436
Fibre g/100mL	1.4
Special characteristics:	
Peanut free	Yes
Suitable for vegetarians	Yes
Suitable for vegans	No
Lactose free	Residual lactose only
Gluten free	Yes
Presentation	Can: 250mL
ACBS listed	Yes
Nutritionally complete	Yes
Caution	Not to be given to children under 1 year. Use with caution in children 1–5 years
Suggested dosage	1–3 years: 1 can 4–6 years: 1–2 cans 7–12 years: 2–3 cans
Flavours	Vanilla, chocolate

Nutrition tables

Semi-solid supplements ACBS listed as a necessary nutritional supplement for short bowel syndrome, intractable malabsorption, proven inflammatory disease, bowel fistulas, related malnutrition, continuous ambulatory peritoneal dialysis and haemodialysis.
N.B. Supplements greater than 6g protein/100g are excluded as they are unsuitable for children.

Name of feed	Formance	Resource Energy Dessert
Manufacturer	Abbott Nutrition	Novartis Medical Nutrition
kcal/100g	148	160
kJ/100g	622	671
Protein source	Non-fat dried milk, milk protein isolate	Whole milk, milk protein
Protein g/100g	3.5	4.8
Fat source	Soy oil	Soya oil
g/100g	4.4	6.2
Carbohydrate source	Sucrose, modified starch, fructooligosaccharides	Maltodextrin, sucrose
Carbohydrate g/100g	24	21.2
Osmolality mOsmol/kg water	N/A	873–951 (depending on flavour)
Fibre g/100g	0	0
Special characteristics:		
Peanut free	Yes	No
Suitable for vegetarians	Yes	No
Suitable for vegans	No	No
Lactose free	3.7g/100g	2.25g/100g
Gluten free	Yes	Yes
Presentation	Pot: 113g	Cup: 125g
ACBS listed	Yes	Yes
Nutritionally complete	Yes	No
Caution	Not to be given to children under 1 year. Use with caution in children 1–5 years	Not to be given to children under 1 year. Use with caution in children 1–5 years
Suggested dosage	1–3 years: 1 pot 4–6 years: 2–3 pots 7–12 years: 2–3 pots	1–3 years: 1 cup 4–6 years: 2–3 cups 7–12 years: 2–3 cups
Flavours	Chocolate, butterscotch, vanilla	Caramel, chocolate, vanilla
Other information	Semi-solid supplement	Semi-solid supplement

All non-milk tasting supplements ACBS listed as a nutritional supplement for short bowel syndrome, intractable malabsorption, proven inflammatory bowel disease, bowel fistulas, dysphagia, disease-related malnutrition. Products providing over 6g protein/100mL are excluded, as these are considered unsuitable for use in children.

Name of feed	Clinutren Fruit	Enlive	Fortijuce	ProvideXtra
Manufacturer	Nestlé Clinical Nutrition	Abbott Nutrition	Nutricia Clinical Care	Fresenius Kabi
kcal/100mL	125	125	150	125
kJ/100mL	520	531	630	525
Protein source	Hydrolysed whey	Whey protein isolate	Whey protein hydrolysate	Pea and soya hydrolysate
Protein g/100mL	4	4	4	3.75
Fat source	–	–	–	–
Fat g/100mL	< 0.2	0	0	0
Carbohydrate source	Sucrose, glucose syrup, fruit juice, maltodextrin	Maltodextrin, sucrose	Maltodextrin, sucrose	Maltodextrin, sucrose
Carbohydrate g/100mL	27	27.3	33.5	27.5
Osmolality mOsmol/kg water	750–770	835	900	490–650
Fibre g/100mL	< 0.02	0	0	0
Special characteristics				
Peanut free	Yes	Yes	Yes	Yes
Suitable for vegetarians	No, protein is hydrolysed using porcine trypsin	Yes	Yes	Yes
Suitable for vegans	No	No	No	No, vitamin D from sheep's wool
Lactose free	Residual lactose only	Residual lactose only	Residual lactose only	Yes
Gluten free	Yes	Yes	Yes	Yes
Presentation	Cup: 200mL	Tetrapak: 240mL	Tetrapak: 200mL	Tetrapak: 200mL
Nutritionally complete	Does not contain fat, iron, zinc, selenium, chromium or molybdenum	Does not contain fat	Does not contain fat	Does not contain fat
Caution	Not to be given to children under 1 year. Use with caution in children 1–5 years. Not intended as a sole source of nutrition	Not to be given to children under 1 year. Use with caution in children 1–5 years. Not intended as a sole source of nutrition	Not to be given to children under 1 year. Use with caution in children 1–5 years. Not intended as a sole source of nutrition	Not to be given to children under 1 year. Use with caution in children 1–5 years. Not intended as a sole source of nutrition
Suggested dosage	1–3 years: 1 cup 4–6 years: 1–2 cups 7–12 years: 2–3 cups	1–3 years: 1 carton 4–6 years: 1–2 cartons 7–12 years: 2–3 cartons	1–3 years: 1 carton 4–6 years: 1–2 cartons 7–12 years: 2–3 cartons	1–3 years: 1 carton 4–6 years: 1–2 cartons 7–12 years: 2–3 cartons
Flavours	Raspberry-blackcurrant, grapefruit, orange and pear-cherry	Lemon and lime, apple, pineapple, peach, fruit punch, grapefruit, orange and strawberry	Lemon and lime, peach and orange, apricot, pineapple, blackcurrant, apple and pear, forest fruits	Lemon and lime, citrus-cola, orange-pineapple, melon, cherry, apple and blackcurrant

Nutrition tables

All products ACBS listed for disease-related malnutrition, malabsorption states and other conditions requiring fortification with high energy or readily available carbohydrate supplements. Caution: Flavoured glucose polymer syrups are not suitable for use in children < 12 months of age.
** Liquid preparations should always be diluted at least 50% for children <5 years of age.

Name	Caloreen	Maxijul LE	Maxijul Liquid **	Maxijul Super Soluble
Manufacturer	Nestlé Clinical Nutrition	SHS International	SHS International	SHS International
Presentation	Can: 500g	Can: 200g Container: 2kg	Carton: 200mL	Powder: 200g tin, 4 x 132g sachets, 2.5kg tub, 25kg drum
Osmolality mOsmol/kg water	N/A	315 (1 to 5 dilution)	1,100	420 (1 to 3 dilution)
CHO	Glucose polymer	96% dried glucose syrup powder	50% glucose syrup	95% dried glucose syrup
Energy	390kcal/100g 1,638kJ/100g	384kcal/100g 1,632kJ/100g	200kcal/100mL 850kJ/100mL	380kcal/100g 1,615kJ/100g
Flavours	Unflavoured	Unflavoured	Natural, orange, blackcurrant, lemon and lime	Unflavoured

Name	Polycal Liquid**	Polycal Powder	Polycose Powder	Vitajoule
Manufacturer	Nutricia Clinical Care	Nutricia Clinical Care	Abbott Nutrition	Vitaflo
Presentation	Bottle: 200mL	Can: 400g	Can: 350g	Powder: 125g, 200g, 500g, 2.5kg and 25kg tub
Osmolality mOsmol/kg water	1,470 (undiluted)	300 (20% dilution)	N/A	285 (25% dilution)
CHO	61.5% glucose syrup	1.9% glucose 4.3% maltose 88.8% glucose polymer	94% glucose polymer	96% glucose polymer
Energy	247kcal/100mL 1,050kJ/100mL	380kcal/100g 1,615kJ/100g	376kcal/100g 1,598kJ/100g	380kcal/100g 1,610kJ/100g
Flavours	Neutral, apple, blackcurrant, lemon, orange	Unflavoured	Unflavoured	Unflavoured

All products ACBS listed for disease-related malnutrition, malabsorption states and other conditions requiring fortification with a high-fat supplement, with or without fluid and electrolyte restrictions*. MCT oil and Liquigen also ACBS listed for ketogenic diets in the management of epilepsy and type I hyperlipoproteinaemia.

* NOTE: Caution when using. They may cause diarrhoea if introduced too quickly or given in excessive amounts. MCT = medium chain triglyceride.

Name	Alemical-D* (MCT oil)	Calogen	Liquigen*	MCT oil*	MCT oil*
Manufacturer	Alembic Products	SHS International	SHS International	Mead Johnson Nutritionals	SHS International
Pack size	5kg	250mL 1000mL	250mL 1000mL	950mL	500mL
Fat	Fractionated coconut oil	50% arachis (peanut) oil emulsion	50% fractionated coconut oil emulsion, palm kernel oil	Fractionated coconut oil	Fractionated coconut oil, palm kernel oil
Energy/100mL	833kcal 3,500kJ	450kcal (Unflavoured) 1,850kJ	450kcal 1,850kJ	772kcal 3,230kJ	855kcal 3,515kJ
Characteristics % per 100g fatty acids	C6; <3% C8; 50–65% C10; 35–45% C12; <3%	≤ C14:0:<2% C16; 10% C18:0; 3% C18:1; 58% C18:2; 20% C18:3; <1% >C20; 6%	C6; 0.7% C8; 82.1% C10; 15.9% C12; 1.3%	<C8; <6% C8; 67% C10; 23% >C10; <4%	C6; <2% C8; 58% C10; 38% C12; <2% C14; < 1%
ACBS listed	Yes	Yes	Yes	Yes	Yes
Flavours	–	Unflavoured, strawberry, butterscotch	–	–	–

Energy supplements: combined fat and carbohydrate

All products ACBS listed for disease-related malnutrition, malabsorption states and other conditions requiring fortification with fat/carbohydrate supplement. Duocal MCT Powder should be introduced slowly to minimise diarrhoea. LCT = long chain triglyceride.

Product	Duobar	Duocal Liquid	Duocal Super Soluble Powder	Duocal MCT Powder	VitaBite
Manufacturer	SHS International	SHS International	SHS International	SHS International	Vitaflo
Pack size	45g bar	1 Litre, 250mL	400g	400g	25g bar
Fat	Palm oil, shea fat	Coconut oil, maize oil	Coconut oil, maize oil	Coconut oil, sunflower oil	Soya oil, rape seed oil, palm oil
Carbohydrate	Sucrose	Glucose syrup	Glucose syrup	Glucose syrup	Lactose/sucrose
% energy	Fat 69% CHO 31%	Fat 40% CHO 60%	Fat 41% CHO 59%	Fat 42% CHO 58%	Fat 55% CHO 45%
Energy	648 kcal/100g 2692kJ/100g	158kcal/100mL 661kJ/100mL	492kcal/100g 2061kJ/100g	497kcal/100g 2082kJ/100g	547kcal/100g 2287kJ/100g
Characteristics	Protein free Low phenylalanine Low electrolyte	Fat: 30% MCT 70% LCT Low electrolyte	Fat: 35% MCT 65% LCT Low electrolyte	Fat: 83% MCT 17% LCT Low electrolyte	Low electrolyte Low phenylalanine
Flavour	Natural, strawberry, toffee	–	–	–	Chocolate

Nutrition tables

All products are ACBS listed for disease related malnutrition, malabsorption states and other conditions requiring fortification with a fat and carbohydrate supplement.

Name of feed	Pro–cal	QuickCal
Manufacturer	Vitaflo	Vitaflo
kcal/100g	667	780
kJ/100g	2,788	3,216
Protein source	Sodium caseinate, skimmed milk powder	Sodium caseinate
Protein g/100g	13.5	4.6
Fat source	Palm oil	Palm oil
Fat g/100g	56.2	77
Carbohydrate source	Lactose	Lactose
Carbohydrate g/100g	26.8	17
Fibre g/100g	0	0
Presentation	Sachet: 15g Tub: 510g Tub: 1.5kg, 12.5kg	Sachet: 13g Tub: 520g Tub: 1.5kg, 12.5kg
ACBS listed	Yes	Yes
Nutritionally complete	No	No
Other information	Scoop in tub. 1 scoop powder = 15g. Also contains sodium, potassium, chloride, phosphorus, magnesium	Scoop in tub. 1 scoop powder = 13g. Also contains small quantity of sodium, potassium, chloride, calcium, phosphorus

Protein supplements

All are ACBS listed for biochemically proven hypoproteinaemia.

Product	Casilan 90	Forceval Protein	Maxipro	ProMod	Protifar	Vitapro
Manufacturer	Heinz	Unigreg	SHS International	Abbott Nutrition	Nutricia Clinical Care	Vitaflo
Presentation	Powder: 250g carton	Natural, vanilla, strawberry: 14x30g sachets Chocolate: 14x36g sachets	Powder: 200g tin, 1kg tub	Powder: 275g tin	Powder: 225g tin	Powder: 1kg
Protein	Calcium caseinate	Calcium caseinate	Whey protein + amino acids	Whey protein	Skimmed milk	Whey protein
Characteristics (per 100g)	88.5% protein 1% fat 0.3% lactose	55% protein 1% fat 30% sucrose	75.5% protein 7.5% fat 7.5g lactose	75% protein 6.9% fat 4.5% lactose 7.5% carbohydrate	88.5% protein 1.6% fat <1.5% lactose	75% protein 9% lactose 6% fat
ACBS prescribability	Yes	Yes	Yes (only for >1 year)	Yes	Yes	Yes

*ACBS listed for disease-related malnutrition, malabsorption and growth failure in infancy.

Name of feed	SMA High Energy Formula	Infatrini
Manufacturer	SMA Nutrition	Nutricia Clinical Care
kcal/100mL	91	100
kJ/100mL	382	420
Protein source	60% whey, 40% casein	60% whey, 40% casein
Protein g/100mL	2	2.6
Fat source	Coconut, palm, soya, sunflower oils	Canola, sunflower, coconut, palm oils
Fat g/100mL	4.9	5.4
Carbohydrate source	Lactose	Lactose, maltodextrin
Carbohydrate g/100mL	9.8	10.3
Osmolality mOsmol/kg water	415	325
Special characteristics		
Peanut free	Yes	Yes
Suitable for vegetarians	Yes: 100mL bottle; No: 250mL carton	No, trace of fish gelatin (carrier for vitamin E)
Suitable for vegans	No	No
Lactose free	No	No
Gluten free	Yes	Yes
Presentation	Tetrapaks: 250mL Bottles: 100mL	Bottles: 100mL
ACBS listed	Yes*	Yes*
Nutritionally complete	Yes	Yes
Caution	Designed for infants 0-18 months	Designed for infants 0–12 months or up to 8kg

Nutrition tables

All products ACBS listed for the following indications: short bowel syndrome; intractable malabsorption, pre-operative preparation of patients who are undernourished, dysphagia, bowel fistulas, disease-related malnutrition and/or growth failure. *RTH = ready to hang.

Name of feed	Frebini Original	Nutrini	Paediasure	Sondalis Junior
Manufacturer	Fresenius Kabi	Nutricia Clinical Care	Abbott Nutrition	Nestlé Clinical Nutrition
kcal/100mL	100	100	101	100
kJ/100mL	420	420	422	417
Protein source	Milk protein	Caseinates	Whey protein, sodium caseinate, calcium caseinate	Casein, whey
Protein g/100mL	2.5	2.75	2.8	2.97
Fat source	Sunflower, soya, MCT, linseed and fish oils	Sunflower oil, canola oil	Sunflower oil, soy oil, MCT oil	MCT, corn, rapeseed oil, sunflower oil
Fat g/100mL	4.4	4.4	5	4
Carbohydrate source	Maltodextrin	Maltodextrin	Maltodextrin, sucrose	Maltodextrin (corn syrup in powder only)
Carbohydrate g/100mL	12.5	12.3	11.2	13.3
Osmolality mOsmol/kg water	210	250	320	powder = 308 (at 1kcal/mL) liquid = 200
Special characteristics				
Peanut free	Yes	Yes	Yes	Yes
Suitable for vegetarians	No	No, trace amount of fish gelatin	Yes	Yes
Suitable for vegans	No	No	No	No
Lactose free	Residual lactose only	Residual lactose only	Residual lactose only	Residual lactose only
Gluten free	Yes	Yes	Yes	Yes
Presentation	Bottles: 200mL *RTH: 500mL	Bottles: 200mL, RTH: 500mL, 1,000mL	Cans: 250mL RTH: 500mL	Cans: 400g RTH: 500mL
ACBS listed	Yes	Yes	Yes	Yes
Nutritionally complete	Yes	Yes	Yes	Yes
Caution	Not suitable for children below 8kg or over 20kg			
Other information	-	-	-	Vanilla flavour reconstitution: 22g powder and 85mL water=1kcal/mL

All products ACBS listed for the following indications: short bowel syndrome, intractable malabsorption, pre-operative preparation of patients who are undernourished, dysphagia, bowel fistulas, disease-related malnutrition and/or growth failure. RTH = ready to hang.

Name of feed	Nutrini Extra	Paediasure Plus
Manufacturer	Nutricia Clinical Care	Abbott Nutrition
kcal/100mL	150	151
kJ/100mL	630	632
Protein source	Sodium and calcium caseinates	Sodium and calcium caseinates, whey protein
Protein g/100mL	4.1	4.2
Fat source	Sunflower oil, canola oil	Sunflower oil, MCT oil, soy oil
Fat g/100mL	6.7	7.5
Carbohydrate source	Maltodextrin	Maltodextrin, sucrose
Carbohydrate g/100mL	18.5	16.7
Osmolality mOsmol/kg water	410	350
Fibre g/100mL	0	0
Special characteristics		
Peanut free	Yes	Yes
Suitable for vegetarians	No, trace amount of fish gelatin (carrier for vitamin E)	Yes
Suitable for vegans	No	No
Lactose free	Residual lactose only	Residual lactose only
Gluten free	Yes	Yes
Presentation	Bottle: 200mL RTH: 500mL	RTH: 500mL
ACBS listed	Yes	Yes
Nutritionally complete	Yes	Yes
Caution	Not suitable for children below 8kg or over 20kg	Not suitable for children below 8kg or over 20kg

Nutrition tables

All products ACBS listed for the following indications: short bowel syndrome, intractable malabsorption, pre-operative preparation of patients who are undernourished, dysphagia, bowel fistulas, disease-related malnutrition and/or growth failure. RTH = ready to hang.

Name of feed	Paediasure Fibre	Nutrini Multi Fibre	Paediasure Plus Fibre
Manufacturer	Abbott Nutrition	Nutricia Clinical Care	Abbott Nutrition
kcal/100mL	101	100	150
kJ/100mL	422	420	629
Protein source	Sodium and calcium caseinates, whey protein	Caseinates	Sodium and calcium caseinates, whey protein
Protein g/100mL	2.8	2.75	4.2
Fat source	MCT oil, sunflower oil, soya oil	Canola oil, sunflower oil	MCT oil, sunflower oil, soy oil
Fat g/100mL	5	4.4	7.5
Carbohydrate source	Maltodextrin, sucrose, soy polysaccharide	Maltodextrin, arabic gum, inulin, soy polysaccharide, resistant starch, cellulose, oligofructose	Maltodextrin, sucrose, fructooligosaccharides, oat fibre, soy polysaccharides, gum arabic, carboxymethyl cellulose
Carbohydrate g/100mL	11.2	12.3	16.7
Osmolality mOsmol/kg water	340	255	347
Fibre g/100mL	0.5	0.75	0.75
Special characteristics			
Peanut free	Yes	Yes	Yes
Suitable for vegetarians	Yes	No, trace of fish gelatin (carrier for vitamin E)	Yes
Suitable for vegans	No	No	No
Lactose free	Residual lactose only	Residual lactose only	Residual lactose only
Gluten free	Yes	Yes	Yes
Presentation	Can: 250mL RTH: 500mL	Bottle: 200mL RTH: 500mL	RTH: 500mL
ACBS listed	Yes	Yes	Yes
Nutritionally complete	Yes	Yes	Yes
Caution	Not suitable for children below 8kg or over 20kg	Not suitable for children below 8kg or over 20kg	Not suitable for children below 8kg or over 20kg

All products ACBS listed for use as sole source of nutrition or as a nutritional supplement for short bowel syndrome, intractable malabsorption, proven inflammatory bowel disease, bowel fistulas, dysphagia, disease-related malnutrition, pre-operative preparation of patients who are undernourished.
* Also can be used as a sip feed. RTH = ready to hang.

Name of feed	Ensure	Fresubin Original	Isosource Standard
Manufacturer	Abbott Nutrition	Fresenius Kabi	Novartis Medical Nutrition
kcal/100mL	100	100	105
kJ/100mL	423	420	441
Protein source	Caseinates, soy protein isolate	Milk protein, soya protein	Milk proteins
Protein g/100mL	4	3.8	4.1
Fat source	Corn oil	MCT oil, linseed, sunflower, soya, fish oils	Vegetable oil
Fat g/100mL	3.4	3.4	3.5
Carbohydrate source	Maltodextrin, sucrose	Maltodextrin	Maltodextrin
Carbohydrate g/100mL	13.6	13.8	14.2
Osmolality mOsmol/kg water	319	300	240
Fibre g/100mL	0	0	< 1
Special characteristics			
Peanut free	Yes	Yes	No
Suitable for vegetarians	Yes	No	No
Suitable for vegans	No	No	No
Lactose free	Residual lactose only	Residual lactose only	Residual lactose only
Gluten free	Yes	Yes	Yes
Presentation	Can: 250mL Powder: 400g	Bottle: 500mL RTH: 500mL, 1,000mL RTH: 1,500mL	RTH: 500mL RTH: 1,000mL RTH: 1,500mL
ACBS listed	Yes	Yes	Yes
Nutritionally complete	Yes	Yes	Yes
Caution	Not to be given to children under 1 year. Use with caution in children 1–5 years	Not to be given to children under 1 year. Use with caution in children 1–5 years	Not to be given to children under 1 year. Use with caution in children 1–5 years
Other information	Cans available in vanilla, chocolate, coffee, egg-nog, nut, asparagus. *Chicken and mushroom flavours as sip feeds	-	-

Nutrition tables

Nutrition tables

Name of feed	Modulen IBD	Nutrison Standard	Osmolite	Sondalis Iso
Manufacturer	Nestlé Clinical Nutrition	Nutricia Clinical Care	Abbott Nutrition	Nestlé Clinical Nutrition
kcal/100mL	100	100	100	100
kJ/100mL	420	420	424	420
Protein source	Caseinates	Caseinates	Caseinates, soy protein isolate	Casein, soya
Protein g/100mL	3.6	4	4	3.8
Fat source	Milk fat, MCT oil, corn oil	Canola oil, sunflower oil	Canola oil, sunflower oil, MCT oil	MCT oil, corn oil, rapeseed oil, soya oils
Fat g/100mL	4.7	3.9	3.4	3.9
Carbohydrate source	Glucose syrup, sucrose	Maltodextrin	Maltodextrin	Maltodextrin
Carbohydrate g/100mL	11	12.3	13.6	12.5
Osmolality mOsmol/kg water	370	310	288	290
Fibre g/100mL	0	0	0	< 0.5
Special characteristics				
Peanut free	Yes	Yes	Yes	Yes
Suitable for vegetarians	Yes	No, trace of fish gelatin (carrier for vitamin E)	Yes	Yes
Suitable for vegans	No	No	No	No
Lactose free	Residual lactose only	Residual lactose only	Residual lactose only	Residual lactose only
Gluten free	Yes	Yes	Yes	Yes
Presentation	Can: 400g	Bottle: 500mL RTH: 500mL,1,000mL RTH: 1,500mL	Can: 250mL RTH: 500mL,1,000mL RTH: 1,500mL	RTH: 500mL, RTH: 1,000mL
ACBS listed	Yes	Yes	Yes	Yes
Nutritionally complete	Yes	Yes	Yes	Yes
Caution	Not to be given to children under 1 year. Use with caution in children 1–5 years	Not to be given to children under 1 year. Use with caution in children 1–5 years	Not to be given to children under 1 year. Use with caution in children 1–5 years	Not to be given to children under 1 year. Use with caution in children 1–5 years
Other information	Contains casein which is rich in TGF-B2. Designed for active phase of Crohn's disease. 25% of fat as MCT	–	–	44% of fat as MCT

All feeds >6g protein/100mL are excluded as they are unsuitable for children. RTH = ready to hang.
* Also can be used as a sip feed.
All products listed for use as the sole source of nutrition or as a necessary nutritional supplement for short bowel syndrome, intractable malabsorption, proven inflammatory bowel disease, bowel fistulas, disease-related malnutrition.

Name of feed	Fresubin Energy	Isosource Energy	Osmolite Plus	Sondalis 1.5
Manufacturer	Fresenius Kabi	Novartis Medical Nutrition	Abbott Nutrition	Nestlé Clinical Nutrition
kcal/100mL	150	159	121	150
kJ/100mL	630	666	508	640
Protein source	Milk protein, soya protein	Milk proteins	Sodium and calcium caseinates	Caseinates, soya protein
Protein g/100mL	5.6	5.7	5.6	5.6
Fat source	MCT oil, sunflower oil, fish oils, linseed oil, soya oil	Vegetable oils	Corn oil, canola oil, MCT oil, sunflower oil	MCT oil, corn oil, rapeseed oil, soya oil
Fat g/100mL	5.8	6.2	3.9	6
Carbohydrate source	Maltodextrin	Maltodextrin	Maltodextrin	Maltodextrin
Carbohydrate g/100mL	18.8	20	15.8	18.8
Osmolality mOsmol/kg water	430	390	360	540
Fibre g/100mL	0	< 1	0	< 0.1
Special characteristics				
Peanut free	Yes	No	Yes	Yes
Suitable for vegetarians	No	No	Yes	Yes
Suitable for vegans	No	No	No	No
Lactose free	Residual lactose only	Residual lactose only	Residual lactose only	Residual lactose only
Gluten free	Yes	Yes	Yes	Yes
Presentation	Bottle: 500mL RTH: 500mL RTH: 1,000mL	RTH: 500mL RTH: 1,000mL	RTH: 500mL RTH: 1,000mL RTH: 1,500mL	RTH: 500mL RTH: 1,000mL
ACBS listed	Yes	Yes	Yes	Yes
Nutritionally complete	Yes	Yes	Yes	Yes
Caution	Very high in protein. Do not give to children less than 5 years. Use with caution in children 6–12 years	Very high in protein. Do not give to children less than 5 years. Use with caution in children 6–12 years	Very high in protein. Do not give to children less than 5 years. Use with caution in children 6–12 years	Very high in protein. Do not give to children less than 5 years. Use with caution in children 6–12 years
Other information	*Also available in tetrapaks for sip feeds	-	20% of fat as MCT	48% of fat as MCT

Nutrition tables

All products >6g/100mL of protein or >2g/100mL of fibre are excluded as they are unsuitable for children. All products listed for use as the sole source of nutrition or as a nutritional supplement for short bowel syndrome, intractable malabsorption, proven inflammatory bowel disease, bowel fistulas, disease-related malnutrition. RTH = ready to hang. * Also can be used as a sip feed.

Name of Feed	Enrich	Isosource Fibre	Jevity
Manufacturer	Abbott Nutrition	Novartis Medical	Abbott Nutrition
kcal/100mL	103	100	105
kJ/100mL	431	422	441
Protein source	Caseinates, soy protein isolate	Milk protein	Sodium and calcium caseinates
Protein g/100mL	3.8	3.8	4
Fat source	Corn oil	Vegetable oils	Sunflower/safflower oil and canola oil, MCT oil
Fat g/100mL	3.5	3.4	3.5
Carbohydrate source	Maltodextrin, sucrose, soy polysaccharides	Maltodextrin, soy fibre, inulin, wheat fibre	Maltodextrin, oat fibre, soy fibre, gum arabic, sodium carboxymethyl cellulose, fructooligosaccharides
Carbohydrate g/100mL	14	13.6	14.8
Osmolality mOsmol/kg water	436	275	300
Fibre g/100mL	1.4	1.4	1.1
Special characteristics			
Peanut free	Yes	No	Yes
Suitable for vegetarians	Yes	No	Yes
Suitable for vegans	No	No	No
Lactose free	Residual lactose only	Residual lactose only	Residual lactose only
Gluten free	Yes	Yes	Yes
Presentation	Can: 250mL	RTH: 500mL RTH: 1,000mL RTH: 1,500mL	RTH: 500mL RTH: 1,000mL RTH: 1,500mL
ACBS listed	Yes	Yes	Yes
Nutritionally complete	Yes	Yes	Yes
Caution	Not to be given to children under 1 year. Use with caution in children aged 1–5 years	Not to be given to children under 1 year. Use with caution in children aged 1–5 years	Manufacturer states not to be given to children under 2 years. Use with caution in children aged 1–5 years
Other information	Available in vanilla and chocolate flavours as a sip feed*	-	-

Name of Feed	Nutrison Multifibre	Sondalis Fibre
Manufacturer	Nutricia Clinical Care	Nestlé Clinical Nutrition
kcal/100mL	100	100
kJ/100mL	420	420
Protein source	Caseinates	Soya protein caseinates
Protein g/100mL	4	3.8
Fat source	Canola oil, sunflower oil	Rapeseed and soya oil, corn oil, medium chain triglycerides (49% of fat as MCT)
Fat g/100 mL	3.9	3.9
Carbohydrate source	Maltodextrin, arabic gum, cellulose, soy polysaccharides, resistant starch, inulin, oligofructose	Maltodextrin, inulin, pea fibre
Carbohydrate g/100 mL	12.3	12.5
Osmolality mOsmol/kg water	315	320
Fibre g/100 mL	1.5	1.5
Special characteristics		
Peanut free	Yes	Yes
Suitable for vegetarians	No, trace of fish gelatin (carrier for vitamin E)	Yes
Suitable for vegans	No	No
Lactose free	Residual lactose only	Residual lactose only
Gluten free	Yes	Yes
Presentation	Bottle: 500mL RTH: 500mL, 1,000mL, 1,500mL	RTH: 500mL RTH: 1,000mL
ACBS listed	Yes	Yes
Nutritionally complete	Yes	Yes
Caution	Not to be given to children under 1 year. Use with caution in children aged 1–5 years	Not to be given to children under 1 year. Use with caution in children aged 1–5 years

Nutrition tables

*Infant soya formula ACBS listed for proven lactose intolerance in pre-school children, galactokinase deficiency, galactosaemia and proven whole cow's milk sensitivity.

Name of feed	Prosobee	Wysoy	Farley's Soya Formula	InfaSoy	Isomil
Manufacturer	Mead Johnson Nutritionals	SMA Nutrition	H J Heinz	Cow and Gate	Abbott Nutrition
kcal/100mL	68	67	70	66	68
kJ/100mL	283	280	293	280	285
Protein source	Soya protein isolate	Soya protein isolate	Soya protein isolate	Soya protein isolate	Soy protein isolate
Protein g/100mL	1.8	1.8	1.95	1.8	1.8
Fat source	Coconut oil, palm olein oil, sunflower oil, soya oil	Palm oil, coconut oil, sunflower oil, soya oil, lecithin	Sunflower oil, palm kernel oil, rapeseed oil, palm olein oil	Palm oil, sunflower oil, rapeseed oil, coconut oil	Sunflower oil, coconut oil, soy oil
Fat g/100mL	3.6	3.6	3.8	3.6	3.7
Carbohydrate source	Glucose polymers	Glucose syrup	Glucose syrup	Glucose syrup	Corn syrup solids, sucrose
Carbohydrate g/100mL	6.7	6.9	7.0	6.7	6.9
Osmolality mOsmol/kg water	180	189	210	200	171
Special characteristics					
[1]MCT (% per 100g fatty acids)	12.2%	13.5%	13.8%	11.9%	17.7%
Peanut free	Yes	Yes	Yes	Yes	Yes
Suitable for vegans	No, vitamin D from live sheep's wool	No, vitamin D from live sheep's wool	Yes	No, vitamin D from live sheep's wool	No
Lactose free	Yes	Yes	Yes	Yes	Yes
Sucrose free	Yes	Yes	Yes	Yes	No
Presentation	Can: 400g	Can: 430g, 860g	Can: 450g, 900g	Can: 450g, 900g	Can: 400g
Reconstitution	1 scoop powder + 1oz (30mL) water	1 scoop powder + 1oz (30mL) water	1 scoop powder + 1oz (30mL) water	1 scoop powder + 1oz (30mL) water	1 scoop powder + 1oz (30mL) water
Standard dilution %	13	13.2	13.7	12.7	13.2
ACBS listed	Yes*	Yes*	Yes*	Yes*	Yes*
Nutritionally complete	Yes No added molybdenum or chromium	Yes No added molybdenum or chromium	Yes No added selenium, molybdenum, or chromium	Yes No added molybdenum or chromium	Yes No added selenium, molybdenum or chromium
Caution	Not recommended for the management of glucose intolerance or when there is an intolerance to soya protein				
Other information	Take care to prevent prolonged exposure to teeth				

[1]MCT: fatty acids with a chain length C12 down to C6.

Nutrition tables

Nutramigen is ACBS listed for disaccharide and/or whole protein intolerance where additional medium chain triglycerides are not indicated. Pepti-Junior and Pregestimil are ACBS listed for disaccharide and/or whole protein intolerance or where amino acids or peptides are indicated in conjunction with medium chain triglycerides. RTH = ready to hang.

Name of feed	Casein hydrolysate formula for infants		Whey hydrolysate formulae for infants
	Nutramigen	Pregestimil	Pepti-Junior
Manufacturer	Mead Johnson Nutritionals	Mead Johnson Nutritionals	Cow and Gate
kcal/100mL	68	68	67
kJ/100mL	283	283	280
Protein source	Enzymatically hydrolysed casein	Enzymatically hydrolysed casein	Hydrolysed whey protein
Protein g/100mL	1.9	1.9	1.8
Fat source	Palm olein oil, coconut oil, sunflower oil, soya oil	Corn oil, MCT oil, soya oil, safflower oil	MCT oil, soy bean oil, rapeseed oil, corn oil
Fat g/100mL	3.4	3.8	3.6
Carbohydrate source	Glucose polymer, modified corn starch	Dextrose, glucose polymer, maltodextrin, modified corn starch	Glucose syrup
Carbohydrate g/100mL	7.4	6.9	6.9
Osmolality mOsmol/kg water	290	330	200
Special characteristics			
[1]MCT (% per 100g fatty acids)	12.2%	55%	50%
Peanut free	Yes	Yes	Yes
Suitable for vegans	No	No	No
Lactose free	Residual lactose only	Residual lactose only	Residual lactose only
Sucrose free	Yes	Yes	Yes
Presentation	Can: 425g	Can: 450g	Can: 450g
Reconstitution	1 scoop powder + 1oz (30mL) water	1 scoop power + 1oz (30mL) water	1 scoop powder + 1oz (30mL) water
Standard dilution %	13.5	13.5	12.8
ACBS listed	Yes	Yes	Yes
Nutritionally complete	Yes	Yes	Does not contain molybdenum or chromium
Caution	Should not be used for glucose-galactose malabsorption	Should not be used for glucose-galactose malabsorption	Should not be used for glucose-galactose malabsorption
Other information	Care should be taken to prevent prolonged contact with teeth	Care should be taken to prevent prolonged contact with teeth	Care should be taken to prevent prolonged contact with teeth

[1]MCT: fatty acids with a chain length C12 down to C6.

Nutrition tables

Pepdite and Prejomin are ACBS listed for disaccharide and/or whole protein intolerance where additional medium chain triglycerides are not indicated.
Peptite 1+ ACBS listed for both disaccharide and/or whole protein intolerance where additional medium chain triglycerides are not indicated.

Name of feed	Soya and meat hydrolysate formula for infants		Soya and meat hydrolysate formula for child >1 year
	Pepdite	Prejomin	Pepdite 1+
Manufacturer	SHS International	Milupa	SHS International
kcal/100mL	71	75	88
kJ/100mL	297	315	369
Protein source	Hydrolysed pork and soya, amino acids	Porcine collagen, soya hydrolysate	Hydrolysed pork and soya, amino acids
Protein g/100mL	2.1	2	2.8
Fat source	Coconut oil, safflower oil, soya bean oil	Palm oil, sunflower oil, rape seed oil, coconut oil	Coconut oil, canola oil, safflower oil
Fat g/100mL	3.5	3.6	3.5
Carbohydrate source	Glucose syrup	Glucose syrup, pre-cooked starch	Glucose syrup
Carbohydrate g/100mL	7.8	8.6	11.4
Osmolality mOsmol/kg water	237 (15% concentration)	193	319 (20% concentration)
Special characteristics			
[1]MCT (% per 100g fatty acids)	19.1%	10.4%	35%
Peanut free	No	Yes	No
Suitable for vegans	No	No	No
Lactose free	Yes	Yes	Yes
Sucrose free	Yes	Yes	Yes
Presentation	Can: 400g	Can: 400g	Can: 400g
Reconstitution	1 scoop powder + 1oz (30mL) water	1 scoop powder + 1oz (30mL) water	Weigh out required amount of Pepdite 1+; mix to paste with water; continue stirring whilst adding rest of prescribed water
Standard dilution %	15	15	20
ACBS listed	Yes	Yes	Yes
Nutritionally complete	Yes	Yes	Yes
Caution	Should not be used for glucose-galactose malabsorption	Should not be used for glucose-galactose malabsorption	Should not be given to children under 1 year of age
Other information	Care should be taken to prevent prolonged contact with teeth	Care should be taken to prevent prolonged contact with teeth	-

[1]MCT: fatty acids with a chain length C12 down to C6.

* Galactomin 17 is ACBS listed for proven lactose intolerance in pre-school children, galactosaemia and galactokinase deficiency.
** SMA LF and Enfamil Lactofree are ACBS listed for proven lactose intolerance.

Name of feed	Enfamil Lactofree**	SMA LF **	Galactomin 17 *
Manufacturer	Mead Jonhson Nutritionals	SMA Nutrition	SHS International
kcal/100mL	68	67	70
kJ/100mL	284	281	294
Protein source	Milk protein (isolate)	60% whey 40% casein	Caseinates
Protein g/100mL	1.4	1.5	1.7
Fat source	Palm olein oil, coconut oil, soya oil, sunflower oil	Palm oil, coconut oil, soya oil, sunflower oil	Palm oil, sunflower oil, rapeseed oil, coconut oil
Fat g/100mL	3.6	3.6	3.7
Carbohydrate source	Glucose polymers, trace lactose <0.007	Glucose syrup	Glucose syrup
Carbohydrate g/100mL	7.3	7.2	7.6
Osmolality mOsmol/kg water	200	198	184
Special characteristics [1]MCT (% per 100g fatty acids)	12.2%	13.5%	10.7%
Peanut free	Yes	Yes	Yes
Suitable for vegans	No	No	No
Lactose free	Residual lactose only < 0.005g	Residual lactose only < 0.1g/100g	Residual lactose only
Sucrose free	Yes	Yes	Yes
Presentation	Can: 400g	Can: 430g	Can: 400g
Reconstitution	1 scoop powder + 1oz (30mL) water	1 scoop powder + 1oz (30mL) water	1 scoop powder + 1oz (30mL) water
Standard dilution %	13	13	13.6
Nutritionally complete	Yes	Does not contain molybdenum or chromium	Does not contain molybdenum or chromium
Caution	Not suitable for cow's milk protein intolerance	Not suitable for cow's milk protein intolerance or galactosaemia	Not suitable for cow's milk protein intolerance
Other information	Care should be taken to prevent prolonged contact with teeth	Care should be taken to prevent prolonged contact with teeth	Care should be taken to prevent prolonged contact with teeth

[1]MCT: fatty acids with a chain length C12 down to C6.

Nutrition tables

Specialised formula: MCT infant formula

Caprilon and MCT Peptide are ACBS listed for disorders in which a high intake of MCT is beneficial. Monogen is ACBS listed for long-chain acyl-CoA dehydrogenase deficiency (LCAD), carnitine palmitoyl transferase deficiency (CPTD), primary and secondary lipoprotein lipase deficiency.

MCT infant formula			
Name of feed	Caprilon	MCT Pepdite	Monogen
Manufacturer	SHS International	SHS International	SHS International
kcal/100mL	66	68	74
kJ/100mL	277	286	313
Protein source	Skimmed milk powder, concentrated whey protein	Hydrolysed pork, soya amino acids	Whey protein, amino acids
Protein g/100mL	1.5	2.0	2.0
Fat source	MCT oil, soya oil	Walnut oil, palm kernel oil, coconut oil, maize oil	MCT oil, walnut oil
Fat g/100mL	3.6	2.7	2.1
Carbohydrate source	Glucose syrup	Glucose syrup	Glucose syrup
Carbohydrate g/100 mL	7	8.8	12
Osmolality mOsmol/kg water	233	290	280
Special characteristics			
[1]MCT (% per 100g fatty acids)	75%	77%	90%
Peanut free	Yes	Yes	Yes, but not nut free
Suitable for vegans	No	No	No
Lactose free	No	Yes	No
Sucrose free	Yes	Yes	Yes
Presentation	Can: 420g	Can: 400g	Can: 400g
Reconstitution	1 scoop powder + 1oz (30mL) water	1 scoop powder + 1oz (30mL) water	Weigh out powder. Add a little water to form a paste. Make up to required volume with water
Standard dilution %	12.7	15	17.5
ACBS listed	Yes	Yes	Yes
Nutritionally complete	Yes	Yes	Yes
Caution	Due to the higher osmolality of MCT and its rapid absorption, side-effects may occur in the initial stages of feeding. Introduce feed at lower concentration initially	Due to the higher osmolality of MCT and its rapid absorption, side-effects may occur in the initial stages of feeding. Introduce feed at lower concentration initially	Due to the higher osmolality of MCT and its rapid absorption, side-effects may occur in the initial stages of feeding. Introduce feed at lower concentration initially
Other information	Care should be taken to prevent prolonged contact with teeth	Care should be taken to prevent prolonged contact with teeth	A 5g scoop is provided in the can. Please note full strength feed is made up to a 17.5% concentration. Monitoring of fatty acid profile is recommended. Care should be taken to prevent prolonged contact with teeth

[1]MCT: fatty acids with a chain length C12 down to C6.

*Locasol is ACBS listed for hypercalcaemia and other conditions which require extreme restriction of calcium in the diet. Galactomin 19 is ACBS listed for glucose-galactose intolerance.

Name of feed	Fructose based infant formula Galactomin 19	Low calcium infant formula Locasol*
Manufacturer	SHS International	SHS International
kcal/100mL	69	66
kJ/100mL	288	278
Protein source	Caseinate	Demineralised whey powder, caseinate
Protein g/100mL	1.9	1.9
Fat source	Sunflower oil, palm oil, rapeseed oil, coconut oil	Palm oil, sunflower oil, rapeseed oil, coconut oil
Fat g/100mL	4	3.4
Carbohydrate source	Fructose	Lactose
Carbohydrate g/100mL	6.4	7
Osmolality mOsmol/kg water	407 at 12.9% dilution	310 at 13.1% dilution
Special characteristics		
[1]MCT (% per 100g fatty acids)	10.8%	10.8%
Peanut free	Yes	Yes
Suitable for vegans	No	No
Lactose free	Residual lactose only	No
Sucrose free	Yes	Yes
Presentation	Can: 400g	Can: 400g
Reconstitution	1 scoop powder + 1oz (30mL) water	1 scoop powder + 1oz (30mL) water
Standard dilution %	12.9	13.1
ACBS listed	Yes	Yes
Nutritionally complete	Yes	Very low in calcium and vitamin D
Caution	Should be introduced gradually in infants in acidotic states. Do not use at higher concentrations than recommended due to feed osmolality	Continued monitoring of vitamin D status necessary. Infants fed solely on Locasol for several months may develop low blood levels of calcium and vitamin D
Other information	Galactomin 19 is ACBS listed for glucose-galactose intolerance	Prepare with distilled water as tap water may contain calcium

[1]MCT: fatty acids with a chain length C12 down to C6.

Nutrition tables

Neocate and Neocate Advance ACBS listed for disaccharide or dietary protein intolerance where an elemental formula is specifically indicated.

Name of feed	Infant amino acid formula Neocate	Child amino acid formula Neocate Advance
Manufacturer	SHS International	SHS International
kcal/100mL	71	100
kJ/100mL	298	400
Protein source	L-amino acids	L-amino acids
Protein g/100mL	1.95	2.5
Fat source	Safflower oil, coconut oil, soya oil	Safflower oil, coconut oil, canola oil
Fat g/100mL	3.5	3.5
Carbohydrate source	Glucose syrup	Glucose syrup
Carbohydrate g/100mL	8.1	14.6
Osmolality mOsmol/kg water	360	610 (at 1 to 4 dilution)
Special characteristics		
[1]MCT (% per 100g fatty acids)	19.1%	35%
Peanut free	Yes	Yes
Suitable for vegans	No, may include amino acids of animal origin. Contains fish gelatin	No, may include amino acids of animal origin. Contains fish gelatin
Lactose free	Yes	Yes
Sucrose free	Yes	Yes
Presentation	Can: 400g	Sachets: 100g
Reconstitution	1 scoop powder + 1oz (30mL) water	1 sachet (100g) to 340mL water
Standard dilution %	15	25
Nutritionally complete	Yes	Yes
Caution	Designed for infants 0 – 1 year	Designed for children 1-10 years. Unsuitable for children less than 1 year
Other information	Care should be taken to prevent prolonged contact with teeth	Care should be taken to prevent prolonged contact with teeth

[1]MCT: fatty acids with a chain length C12 down to C6.

All adult amino acid formula are ACBS listed for use as a sole source of nutrition or as necessary nutritional supplement for short bowel syndrome, intractable malabsorption, proven inflammatory bowel disease, bowel fistulas.
*Nutrison Soya is ACBS listed for lactose intolerance and milk protein intolerance. RTH = ready to hang.

Name of feed	Adult amino acid formula				Adult soya formula
	Elemental 028	Elemental 028 Extra	Elemental 028 Extra Liquid	Emsogen	Nutrison Soya*
Manufacturer	SHS International	SHS International	SHS International	SHS International	Nutricia Clinical Care
kcal/100mL	78	89	86	84–88	100
kJ/100mL	328	374	360	351–368	420
Protein source	L–amino acids	L–amino acids	L–amino acids	L–amino acids	Soya protein isolate
Protein g/100mL	2	2.5	2.5	2.5	4
Fat source	Canola oil, safflower oil, coconut oil	Canola oil, safflower oil, coconut oil	Coconut oil, canola oil, safflower oil	MCT oil, maize oil, coconut oil	Canola oil, sunflower oil
Fat g/100mL	1.3	3.5	3.5	3.3	3.9
Carbohydrate source	Glucose syrup, Flavoured: sucrose	Glucose syrup	Glucose syrup , Flavoured: sucrose	Glucose syrup, sucrose	Maltodextrin
Carbohydrate g/100mL	14.4	11.8	11	11–12	12.3
Osmolality mOsmol/kg water	Flavoured: 711 Unflavoured: 496	Flavoured: 636 Unflavoured: 502	673–725	Flavoured: 563 Unflavoured: 539	250
Special characteristics					
[1]MCT (% per 100g fatty acids)	5%	35%	35%	83%	0.2%
Peanut free	Yes	Yes	Yes	Yes	Yes
Suitable for vegans	No, contains fish gelatin and may contain amino acids from animal origin	No, contains fish gelatin and may contain amino acids from animal origin	No, contains fish gelatin and may contain amino acids from animal origin	No, contains fish gelatin and may contain amino acids from animal origin	No, traces of fish gelatin act as a carrier for vitamin E
Lactose free	Yes	Yes	Yes	Yes	Yes
Sucrose free	Unflavoured: Yes Flavoured: No	Unflavoured: Yes Flavoured: No	No	Unflavoured: Yes Flavoured: No	Yes
Presentation	Sachets: 100g	Sachets: 100g	Tetrapak: 250mL	Sachets: 100g	Bottle: 500mL RTH: 1,000mL
Reconstitution	Mix contents of 1 sachet (100g) with water to form a paste. Make up to a final volume of 500mL with water (20%)	Mix contents of 1 sachet (100g) with water to form a paste. Make up to a final volume of 500mL with water (20%)	Ready to use	Mix contents of 1 sachet (100g) with water to form a paste. Make up to a final volume of 500mL with water (20%)	Ready to use
Standard dilution %	20%	20%	–	20%	–
ACBS listed	Yes	Yes	Yes	Yes	Yes

[1]MCT: fatty acids with a chain length C12 down to C6.

Nutrition tables

Name of feed	Adult amino acid formula continued				Adult soya formula
	Elemental 028	Elemental 028 Extra	Elemental 028 Extra Liquid	Emsogen	Nutrison Soya*
Nutritionally complete	Yes	Yes	Yes	No, low in alpha linolenic acid	Yes
Caution	Not suitable for children <1 year. Use with caution in children 1–5 years	Not suitable for children <1 year. Use with caution in children 1–5 years	Not suitable for children <1 year. Use with caution in children 1–5 years	Not suitable for children <1 year. Use with caution in children 1–5 years	Not suitable for children <1 year or people with galactosaemia. Use with caution in children 1–5 years
Other information	Available in orange flavour (beta carotenes/beetroot red) and unflavoured powder. Contains added glutamine, equivalent to whole protein foods and added arginine	Available in orange flavour (beta carotenes/beetroot red) and unflavoured powder. Contains added glutamine, equivalent to whole protein foods and arginine	Available in orange and pineapple; grapefruit and summer fruit flavours. Patients with food intolerance may be intolerant to the colours and flavouring. Does not contain added glutamine, but has arginine added	Available in orange flavour (beta carotene/beetroot red) and unflavoured powder. Contains added glutamine, equivalent to whole protein foods and added arginine. Needs supplementation with additional essential fatty acids if given as sole source of nutrition	Care should be taken to prevent prolonged contact with teeth

All products ACBS listed for short bowel syndrome, intractable malabsorption, proven inflammatory bowel disease and bowel fistulas. RTH = ready to hang.

Name of feed	Peptide based adult formula		
	Peptamen	Peptisorb	Survimed OPD
Manufacturer	Nestlé Clinical Nutrition	Nutricia Clinical Care	Fresenius Kabi
kcal/100mL	100	100	100
kJ/100mL	420	420	420
Protein source	Whey protein hydrolysate	Whey protein hydrolysate	Lactalbumin hydrolysate
Protein g/100ml	4	4	4.5
Fat source	MCT oil, soya oil, soya lecithin	MCT oil, soy oil	MCT oil, vegetable oil, fish oils
Fat g/100mL	3.7	1.7	2.4
Carbohydrate source	Maltodextrin, starch, (sucrose in the vanilla)	Maltodextrin	Maltodextrin, modified starch
Carbohydrate g/100mL	12.7	17.6	15
Osmolality mOsmol/kg water	240 (unflavoured) 340 (vanilla)	520	440
Special characteristics			
[1]MCT (% per 100g fatty acids)	72%	49%	54%
Peanut free	Yes	Yes	Yes
Suitable for vegans	No	No	No
Lactose free	Residual lactose only	0.1g/100mL	Residual lactose only
Sucrose free	Unflavoured: Yes Vanilla: No	Yes	Yes
Presentation	Can: 375mL RTH: 500mL, 1,000mL Cup: 200mL (vanilla)	Bottles: 500mL RTH: 500mL RTH: 1,000mL	RTH: 500mL
Reconstitution	Ready to use	Ready to use	Ready to use
Standard dilution %	-	-	-
ACBS listed	Yes	Yes	Yes
Nutritionally complete	Yes	Yes (liquid) low in fat	Yes
Caution	Not to be given to children under 1 year. Use with caution in children 1–5 years	Not to be given to children under 1 year. Use with caution in children 1–5 years	Not to be given to children under 1 year. Use with caution in children 1–5 years
Other information	Five flavour sachets available to add to Peptamen cans and cups	-	-

[1]MCT: fatty acids with a chain length C12 down to C6.

Nutrition tables

Name of feed	Comminuted Chicken Meat	Hydrolysed Whey Protein Maltodextrin Mix
Manufacturer	SHS International	SHS International
kcal/100 g	51–64	348
kJ/100 g	212–266	1,479
Protein source	Chicken breast meat	Whey protein hydrolysate
Protein g/100g	7–8	49.8
Fat source	Chicken fat	–
Fat g/100g	2.5–3.5	Nil
Carbohydrate source	Nil	Maltodextrin, lactose
Carbohydrate g/100g	0	37.2 (lactose 3.7g/100g)
Osmolality mOsmol/kg water	131	250
Special characteristics [1]MCT (% per 100g fatty acids)	–	No
Peanut free	Yes	Yes
Suitable for vegans	No	No
Lactose free	Yes	No
Sucrose free	Yes	Yes
Presentation	Jars: 150g	Can: 250g
Reconstitution	It should be diluted with water before use and supplemented with a carbohydrate, fat, vitamin and mineral source	It should be diluted with water before use and supplemented with a carbohydrate, fat, vitamin and mineral source
ACBS listed	Yes	No
Nutritionally complete	No	No
Caution	Use only under supervision of a dietitian. Only a source of protein and fat, not suitable as a sole source of nutrition	Use only under supervision of a dietitian. Only a source of protein and carbohydrate, not suitable as a sole source of nutrition
Other information	ACBS listed for carbohydrate intolerance in association with possible or proven intolerance of milk, glucose and galactose intolerance	Indications: intolerance to whole protein, intractable malabsorption, chronic intestinal disease and short bowel syndrome

[1]MCT: fatty acids with a chain length C12 down to C6.

Name of feed	Complete Amino Acid Mix Code 124	Generaid	Hepatamine
Manufacturer	SHS International	SHS International	SHS International
kcal/100g	328	374	360
kJ/100g	1,394	1,586	1,530
Protein source	L–amino acids	Whey protein enriched with branch chain amino acids (33%)	L-amino acids enriched with branch chain amino acids (40%)
Protein g/100g	82	76	25
Fat source	–	No direct fat source. A small amount is supplied by whey protein	–
Fat g/100mL	0	5.5	0
Carbohydrate source	–	Lactose	Dried glucose syrup, sucrose
Carbohydrate g/100g	0	5.0	65
Osmolality mOsmol/kg water	360 at 5% dilution	316 at 1 to 7.5 dilution	669 at 1 to 7 dilution
Special characteristics [1]MCT (% per 100g fatty acids)	No	15%	No
Peanut free	Yes	Yes	Yes
Suitable for vegans	No, may contain amino acids from animal origin	No	No, may contain amino acids from animal origin
Lactose free	Yes	No	Yes
Sucrose free	Yes	Yes	No
Presentation	Can: 200g	Can: 200g	Sachets: 50g
Reconstitution	It should be diluted with water before use and supplemented with a carbohydrate, fat, vitamin and mineral source	It should be diluted with water before use and supplemented with a carbohydrate, fat, vitamin and mineral source	It should be diluted with water before use. Intended to be given as a drink to supplement a low protein diet
ACBS listed	No	Yes	No
Nutritionally complete	No	No	No
Caution	Use only under supervision of a dietitian. Only a source of protein; not suitable as a sole source of nutrition	Use only under supervision of a dietitian. Only a source of protein; not suitable as a sole source of nutrition	Use only under supervision of a dietitian. Only a source of protein; not suitable as a sole source of nutrition
Other information	Indications: conditions where an oligoallergenic diet is indicated, e.g. infants with an intolerance to milk protein or other whole protein, intractable malabsorption, chronic intestinal disease and short bowel syndrome	ACBS listed for the dietary management of patients with hepatic disorders	Indications: in the dietary management of liver disease. Orange flavoured. High in arginine and branch chain amino acids. Low in aromatic amino acids

[1]MCT: fatty acids with a chain length C12 down to C6.

Nutrition tables

* Nutrison MCT is ACBS listed as a nutritional supplement prescribed on medical grounds for short bowel syndrome, intractable malabsorption, pre-operative preparation of patients who are undernourished, proven bowel disease, following total gastrectomy, dysphagia, bowel fistulas and disease related to malnutrition, inflammatory bowel disease.
**MCT Pepdite 1+ is ACBS listed for disorders in which a high intake of medium chain triglycerides is beneficial. RTH = ready to hang.

Name of feed	MCT adult and children formula		Product for liver conditions
	*Nutrison MCT	**MCT Pepdite 1+	Generaid Plus
Manufacturer	Nutricia Clinical Care	SHS International	SHS International
kcal/100mL	100	91	102
kJ/100mL	420	381	428
Protein source	Caseinates	Hydrolysed pork and soya amino acids	Whey protein supplemented with branch chain amino acids
Protein g/100mL	5.0	2.8	2.4
Fat source	MCT oil, sunflower oil, canola oil, soy oil	Coconut oil, walnut oil, palm kernel oil, maize oil	Maize oil, palm kernel oil, coconut oil
Fat g/100mL	3.3	3.6	4.2
Carbohydrate source	Maltodextrin	Dried glucose syrup	Dried glucose syrup
Carbohydrate g/100mL	12.6	11.8	13.6
Osmolality mOsmol/kg water	315	460 (at 20% concentration)	Depends on dilution used. 287 at 1 kcal/mL (22% w/v)
Special characteristics [1]MCT (% per 100g fatty acids)	65%	77%	48.1%
Peanut free	Yes	Yes	Yes
Suitable for vegans	No	No	No
Lactose free	Residual lactose only	Yes.	No
Sucrose free	Yes	Yes	Yes
Presentation	Bottles: 500mL RTH: 1,000mL	Can: 400g	Can: 400g
Reconstitution	Ready to use	Weigh out powder. Add a little water to form a paste. Make up to required volume with water	Weigh out powder. Add a little water to form a paste. Stir in remaining volume of water
Standard dilution %	–	20%	Depends on body weight and requirements of individual patient. 22% dilution for 1kcal/mL
ACBS listed	Yes	Yes	Yes
Nutritionally complete	Yes	Yes	Yes
Caution	Not to be given to children < 1 year. Use with caution in children aged 1–5 years	Not to be given to children < 1 year. Use with caution in children aged 2–5 years	Not suitable for children < 1 year
Other information	See above	See above	ACBS listed for children over 1 year of age with hepatic disorders

[1]MCT: fatty acids with a chain length C12 down to C6.

Nutrition tables

	Products for renal conditions	
Name	Dialamine (analysis per 100g)	Kindergen (analysis per 100mL)
Manufacturer	SHS International	SHS International
kcal/100g or kcal/100mL	360	101
kJ/100g or kJ/100mL	1,530	421
Protein source	Amino acids (essential)	Whey protein, amino acids
Protein g/100mL or g/100g	25	1.5
Fat source	–	Safflower oil, coconut oil, soya oil
Fat g/100mL or g/100g	0	5.3
Carbohydrate source	Maltodextrin, sucrose	Dried glucose syrup
Carbohydrate g/100g or /100mL	65	11.8
Osmolality mOsmol/kg water	947 (20% dilution)	215 (1to 5 dilution)
Special characteristics		
[1]MCT (% per 100g fatty acids)	No	17.9%
Peanut free	Yes	Yes
Suitable for vegans	No, may contain amino acids from animal origin	No
Lactose free	Yes	No
Sucrose free	No	Yes
Presentation	Can: 200g	Can: 400g
Reconstitution	It should be diluted with water before use. It is intended as a supplement to a low protein diet	Weigh out Kindergen. Add a small amount of water and mix to a paste. Stir in remaining volume of water (1 to 5 dilution)
Standard dilution %	1 to 5	20%
ACBS listed	Yes	Yes
Nutritionally complete	No, contains vitamin C, essential amino acids and carbohydrate only	No, low in phosphorus, calcium, chloride, vitamin A and potassium
Caution	Use only under supervision of a dietitian. Only a source of protein, carbohydrate and vitamin C. It is not suitable as a sole source of nutrition	Use only under supervision of a dietitian. Requires monitoring of potassium, chloride, phosphorus, calcium and vitamin A status
Other information	A source of essential amino acids. ACBS listed for chronic renal failure, hypoproteinaemia, wound fistula leakage with protein loss, controlled nitrogen intake, haemodialysis. Orange flavoured. Can be used in certain urea cycle disorders (see page 752)	Suitable for infants and children. ACBS listed for complete nutritional support or supplementary feeding for infants and children with chronic renal failure who are receiving rapid overnight peritoneal dialysis or continuous cycling peritoneal dialysis

[1]MCT: fatty acids with a chain length C12 down to C6.

Nutrition tables

All of these products are ACBS listed for phenylketonuria (PKU). Note: With the exception of the infant formulas, XP Analog, XP Analog LCP, Phlexy-10 bars/capsules and Aminogran PKU tablets, all of these products are designed to be mixed with liquid and given as a paste or drink. They all have a high osmolarity and thus water or diluted drinks should be offered at the same time. The prescribed amount of powder should be introduced gradually over a period of a few days.

A Nutritionally complete Yes/No
B Complete vitamin and mineral supplement needed Yes/No

Phenylketonuria							
Product	Manufacturer	Presentation	Age suitability	Nutrient details	A	B	Comments
XP Analog LCP	SHS International	400g tin	0 – 1 year	Per 100mL: 72kcal (300kJ) 1.95g protein 2.3g amino acids 8.1g CHO 3.5g fat	Yes	No	Infant phenylalanine free protein substitute for PKU. Protein is a mixture of L-amino acids. Contains added LCPs
XP Analog	SHS International	400g tin	0 – 1 year	Per 100mL: 72kcal (300kJ) 1.95g protein 2.3g amino acids 8.1g CHO 3.5g fat	Yes	No	Infant phenylalanine free protein substitute for PKU. Protein is a mixture of L-amino acids
Aminogran Food Supplement	UCB Pharma	500g tub	> 6 months of age	Per 100g: 97% amino acids 400kcal (1675kJ)	No	Yes	Free of phenylalanine
Minaphlex	SHS International	30 x 29g sachets	1 year – 10 years	Per 29g sachet: 10g amino acids (8.4g protein) 11g CHO, 3.9g fat 113kcal (474kJ)	Yes	No	Free of phenylalanine. Contains added CHO and fat. Supplemented with vitamins and minerals. Protein is a mixture of L-amino acids . Pineapple, vanilla and unflavoured
Phlexy –10 Drink Mix	SHS International	30 x 20g sachets	> 1 year of age	Per 20g sachet: 10g amino acids (8.33g protein equivalent) 8.8g CHO 69kcal (291kJ)	No	Yes	Free of phenylalanine. Contains added CHO but no fat. Blackcurrant and apple flavours. Designed to be interchangeable with Phlexy 10 capsules and bars
Phlexy –10 Bar	SHS International	20 x 42g bars	> 1 year but use with caution in children <5 years of age	Per 42g bar: 10g amino acids (8.33g protein equivalent) 20.5g CHO, 4.5g fat 156kcal (657kJ)	No	Yes	Designed to be interchangeable with Phlexy-10 sachets and Phlexy-10 capsules. Free of phenylalanine. Fruit flavoured bars
Phlexy –10 Capsules	SHS International	200 capsules in tub	> 8 years	Per 20 capsules: 10g amino acids (8.33g protein equivalent) CHO nil added 33kcal (142kJ)	No	Yes	Designed to be interchangeable with Phlexy-10 sachets and Phlexy-10 bars. Free of phenylalanine. Does not contain fat, low in CHO

A Nutritionally complete Yes/No
B Complete vitamin and mineral supplement needed Yes/No
* Need to monitor selenium intake

Phenylketonuria continued							
Product	Manufacturer	Presentation	Age suitability	Nutrient details	A	B	Comments
PK Aid 4	SHS International	500g tin	> 6 months of age	Per 100g: 95% amino acids (79% protein equivalent) 4.5% CHO 334kcal (1420kJ)	No	Yes	Free of phenylalanine. Does not contain added carbohydrate or fat
PKU 2	Milupa	500g tin	> 1 year of age	Per 100g: 80.1% amino acids (67g protein equivalent) 8.2% CHO 300kcal (1275kJ)	No	*	Free of phenylalanine. Supplemented with vitamins and minerals. Does not contain selenium. Contains minimum carbohydrate
PKU 3	Milupa	500g tin	> 8 years	Per 100g: 81.6% amino acids (68g protein equivalent) 3.9% CHO 288 kcal (1210 kJ)	No	*	Free of phenylalanine. Supplemented with vitamins and minerals. Does not contain selenium. Contains minimum carbohydrate
PKU - gel	Vitaflo	25 x 20g sachets	> 1 year - 10 years	Per 20g sachet: 10g amino acids (8.4g protein equivalent) 8.6g CHO, 0.03g fat 68kcal (286kJ)	No	No	Free of phenylalanine. Supplemented with vitamins and minerals. Contains added carbohydrate but no fat. Raspberry, orange and unflavoured available
XP Maxamaid	SHS International	500g tin	1–8 years	Per 100g: 30% amino acids (25% protein equivalent) 51% CHO 309kcal (1311kJ)	No	No	Available in orange and unflavoured varieties. Free of phenylalanine. Supplemented with vitamins and minerals. Contains added carbohydrate but no fat
XP Maxamaid Concentrate	SHS International	500g tin	> 1 year	Per 100g: 65% amino acids (53.5% protein equivalent) 5% CHO 239kcal (1013kJ)	No	No	Free of phenylalanine. Supplemented with vitamins and minerals. Low in carbohydrate and contains no fat. Unflavoured
XP Maxamum	SHS International	500g tin	> 8 years	Per 100g: 47% amino acids (39% protein equivalent) 34g CHO 297kcal (1260kJ)	No	No	Available in orange and unflavoured varieties. Free of phenylalanine. Supplemented with vitamins and minerals. Added carbohydrate but no added fat
Aminogran PKU Tablets	UCB Pharma	60 tablets per box	>10 years	Per 100g: 76% amino acids 264kcal (1109kJ) neg CHO, 0.19g fat	No	Yes	Free of phenylalanine. A source of amino acids only. Designed for older patients

Nutrition tables

All of these products are ACBS listed for the conditions indicated
All of the listed products are manufactured by SHS International
A Nutritionally complete Yes/No
B Complete vitamin and mineral supplement needed Yes/No

Nutrition tables

Conditions other than PKU – for infants						
Product	Presentation	Age suitability	Nutrient details	A	B	ACBS listed condititions
MSUD Analog	400g tin	0–1 year	Per 100mL: 72kcal (300kJ), 1.95g protein 2.32g amino acids, 8.1g CHO 3.5g fat	Yes	No	Infant protein substitute formula for maple syrup urine disease. Protein is a mixture of L-amino acids free of valine, leucine and isoleucine
XMET Analog	400g tin	0–1 year	Per 100mL: 72kcal (300kJ), 1.95g protein, 2.32g amino acids, 8.1g CHO, 3.5g fat	Yes	No	Infant protein substitute formula for homocystinuria or hypermethioninaemia. Protein is mixture of L-amino acids free of methionine
XLEU Analog	400g tin	0–1 year	Per 100mL: 72kcal (300kJ), 1.95g protein, 2.32g amino acids, 8.1g CHO, 3.5g fat	Yes	No	Infant protein substitute formula for isovaleric acidaemia. Protein is a mixture of L-amino acids free of leucine
XLYS Analog	400g tin	0–1 year	Per 100mL: 72kcal (300kJ), 1.95g protein, 2.32g amino acids, 8.1g CHO, 3.5g fat	Yes	No	Infant protein substitute formula for hyperlysinaemia. Protein is a mixture of L-amino acids free of lysine
XLYS Low TRY Analog	400g tin	0–1 year	Per 100mL: 72kcal (300kJ), 1.95g protein, 2.32g amino acids, 8.1g CHO, 3.5g fat	Yes	No	Infant protein substitute formula for glutaric aciduria type I. Protein is a mixture of L-amino acids free of lysine and low in trytophan
XMTVI Analog	400g tin	0–1 year	Per 100mL: 72kcal (300kJ), 1.95g protein, 2.32g amino acids, 8.1g CHO, 3.5g fat	Yes	No	Infant protein substitute formula for propionic and methylmalonic acidaemia. Protein is a mixture of L-amino acids free of methionine, threonine, valine; low in isoleucine
XPHEN TYR Analog	400g tin	0–1 year	Per 100mL: 72kcal (300kJ), 1.95g protein 2.32g amino acids, 8.1g CHO, 3.5g fat	Yes	No	Infant protein substitute formula for tyrosinaemia where plasma methionine concentrations are normal. Protein is a mixture of L-amino acids free of phenylalanine and tyrosine
XPTM Analog	400g tin	0–1 year	Per 100mL: 72kcal (300kJ), 1.95g protein, 2.32g amino acids, 8.1g CHO, 3.5g fat	Yes	No	Infant protein substitute formula for tyrosinaemia where plasma methionine is raised. Protein is a mixture of L-amino acids free of methionine, phenylalanine and tyrosine

All of these products are ACBS listed for the conditions indicated. All are manufactured by SHS International
A Nutritionally complete Yes/No
B Complete vitamin and mineral supplement needed Yes/No

Conditions other than PKU – for children over 1 year of age and adults						
Product	Presentation	Age suitability	Nutrient details	A	B	ACBS listed conditions and description of product
MSUD Maxamaid	500g tin	1–8 years	Per 100g: 30% amino acids (25g protein equivalent) 51% CHO, 309kcal (1,311kJ)	No	No	Amino acid protein substitute supplemented with vitamins and minerals. Free of leucine, valine and isoleucine. For children with maple syrup urine disease. No added fat. Contains CHO
MSUD Maxamum	500g tin	> 8 years	Per 100g: 47% amino acids (39g protein equivalent) 34% CHO, 297kcal (1,260kJ)	No	No	Amino acid protein substitute supplemented with vitamins and minerals. Free of leucine, valine and isoleucine. For use in maple syrup urine disease. No added fat. Contains CHO. Unflavoured and orange flavour
MSUD Aid III	500g tin	> 6 months – adulthood	Per 100g: 93% amino acids (77g protein equivalent) 4.5% CHO, 326kcal (1,386kJ)	No	Yes	Concentrated amino acid protein substitute. Free of leucine, valine, isoleucine. For maple syrup urine disease. No added fat or CHO
XMET Maxamaid	500g tin	1–8 years	Per 100g: 30% amino acids (25g protein equivalent) 51% CHO, 309kcal (1,311kJ)	No	No	Amino acid protein substitute supplemented with vitamins and minerals. Free of methionine. For hypermethioninaemia and homo-cystinuria. No added fat. Contains CHO
XMET Maxamum	500g tin	> 8 years	Per 100g: 47% amino acids (39g protein equivalent) 34% CHO, 297kcal (1,260kJ)	No	No	Amino acid protein substitute supplemented with vitamins and minerals. Free of methionine. For hypermethioninaemia and homocystinuria. No added fat. Contains CHO
XMet Homidon	200g tub	Infancy – adulthood	Per 100g: 93% amino acids (77g protein equivalent) 4.5% CHO, 326kcal (1,385 kJ)	No	Yes	Concentrated amino acid protein substitute. Free of methionine. For hypermethioninaemia and homo-cystinuria. No added fat or CHO
XLEU Maxamaid	500g tin	1–8 years	Per 100g: 30% amino acids (25g protein equivalent) 51% CHO, 309kcal (1,311kJ)	No	No	Amino acid protein substitute supplemented with vitamins and minerals. Free of leucine. For isovaleric acidaemia. No added fat. Contains CHO
XLEU Faladon	200g tub	> 6 months – adulthood	Per 100g: 93% amino acids (77g protein equivalent) 4.5% CHO, 326kcal (1,386kJ)	No	Yes	Concentrated amino acid protein substitute. Free of leucine. For isovaleric acidaemia. No added fat or CHO
XLEU Maxamum	500g tin	> 8 years	Per 100g: 47% amino acids (39g protein equivalent) 34% CHO, 297kcal (1,260kJ)	No	No	Amino acid protein substitute supplemented with vitamins and minerals. Free of leucine. For isovaleric acidaemia. No added fat. Contains CHO

Nutrition tables

A Nutritionally complete Yes/No
B Complete vitamin and mineral supplement needed Yes/No

	Conditions other than PKU – for children over 1 year of age and adults continued						
Product	Presentation	Age suitability	Nutrient details	A	B	ACBS listed conditions and description of product
XPHEN TYR Maxamaid	500g tin	1–8 years	Per 100g: 30% amino acids (25g protein equivalent) 51% CHO, 309kcal (1,311kJ)	No	No	Amino acid protein substitute supplemented with vitamins and minerals. Free of phenylalanine and tyrosine. For children with tyrosinaemia where plasma methionine is normal. No added fat. Contains CHO
XPHEN TYR Maxamum	500g tin	> 8 years	Per 100g: 47% amino acids (39g protein equivalent) 34% CHO, 297kcal (1,260kJ)	No	No	Amino acid protein substitute supplemented with vitamins and minerals. Free of phenylalanine and tyrosine. For children with tyrosinaemia where plasma methionine is normal. Contains CHO. Does not contain fat
XPHEN TYR Tyrosidon	200g tin	Infants > 6 months – adulthood	Per 100g: 93% amino acids (77g protein equivalent) 4.5% CHO , 326kcal (1,386kJ)	No	Yes	Concentrated amino acid protein substitute. Free of phenylalanine and tyrosine. For tyrosinaemia where plasma methionine is normal. Does not contain added fat or CHO
XPTM Tyrosidon	200g tub	Infancy – adulthood	Per 100g: 93% amino acids (77g protein equivalent) 4.5% CHO, 326kcal (1,386kJ)	No	Yes	Concentrated amino acid protein substitute. Free of phenylalanine, tyrosine and methionine. For children with tyrosinaemia where plasma methionine is raised. Does not contain added fat or CHO
XPTM Maxamaid	500g tin	1–8 years	Per 100g: 30% amino acids (25g protein equivalent) 51% CHO, 309kcal (1,311kJ)	No	No	Amino acid protein substitute supplemented with vitamins and minerals. Free of phenylalanine, tyrosine and methionine. For children with tyrosinaemia where plasma methionine is raised. Does not contain added fat. Contains CHO

A Nutritionally complete Yes/No
B Complete vitamin and mineral supplement needed Yes/No

			Conditions other than PKU – for children over 1 year of age and adults continued			
Product	Presentation	Age suitability	Nutrient details	A	B	ACBS listed conditions and description of product
XLYS Maxamaid	500g tin	1–8 years	Per 100g: 30% amino acids (25g protein equivalent) 51% CHO, 309kcal (1,311kJ)	No	No	Amino acid protein substitute supplemented with vitamins and minerals. Free of lysine. For children with hyperlysinaemia. Does not contain added fat. Contains CHO
XLYS Hyperlidon	200g tub	> 6 months – adulthood	Per 100g: 95% amino acids (79g protein equivalent) 4.5% CHO, 334kcal (1,420kJ)	No	Yes	Concentrated amino acid protein substitute. Free of lysine. For hyper-lysinaemia. No added fat or CHO
XLYS Low TRY Maxamaid	500g tin	1–8 years	Per 100g: 30% amino acids (25g protein equivalent) 51% CHO, 309kcal (1,311kJ)	No	No	Amino acid protein substitute supplemented with vitamins and minerals. Free of lysine and low in tryptophan. For children with glutaric aciduria type I. No added fat. Contains CHO
XLYS Low TRY Maxamum	500g tin	> 8 years	Per 100g: 47% amino acids (39g protein equivalent) 34% CHO, 297kcal (1,260kJ)	No	No	Concentrated amino acid protein substitute. Free of lysine and low in tryptophan. For glutaric aciduria type I. No added fat. Contains CHO
XLYS TRY Glutaridon	200g tub	> 6 months – adulthood	Per 100g: 95% amino acids (79g protein equivalent) 4% CHO, 331kcal (1,411kJ)	No	Yes	Concentrated amino acid protein substitute supplement. Free of lysine and tryptophan. For children with glutaric aciduria type I. No added fat or CHO
XMTVI Maxamaid	500g tin	1–8 years	Per 100g: 30% amino acids (25g protein equivalent) 51% CHO, 309kcal (1,311kJ)	No	No	Amino acid protein substitute supplemented with vitamins and minerals. Free of methionine, threo-nine, valine and low in isoleucine. For children with methylmalonic/propionic acidaemia. No added fat. Contains CHO
XMTVI Maxamum	500g tin	> 8 years	Per 100g: 47% amino acids (39g protein equivalent) 34% CHO, 297kcal (1,260kJ)	No	No	Amino acid protein substitute supplemented with vitamins and minerals. Free of methionine, threonine, valine and low in isoleucine. For children with methyl malonic/propionic acidaemia. No added fat. Contains CHO
XMTVI Asadon	200g tub	7-6 months– adulthood	Per 100g: 93% amino acids (77g protein equivalent) 4.5% CHO, 326kcal (1,386kJ)	No	Yes	Concentrated amino acid protein substitute powder. Free of methionine, threonine, valine and low in isoleucine. For methylmalonic/propionic acidaemia. No added fat or CHO

Nutrition tables

Nutrition tables

All are ACBS listed for the conditions indicated (except the essential amino acid mix).
All are manufactured by SHS International.
A Nutritionally complete Yes/No
B Complete vitamin and mineral supplement needed Yes/No

			Other metabolic products			
Product	Presentation	Age suitability	Nutrient details	A	B	ACBS listed conditions and description of product
L-Tyrosine	100g tub	Infancy – adulthood but see 'ACBS listed Conditions'	100% L-tyrosine	No	Yes	Only ACBS listed for 'maternal phenylketonuria' but may be used for all individuals with phenylketonuria if plasma tyrosine concentrations are regularly monitored
L-Arginine	100g tub	Infancy – adulthood	100% L-arginine	No	Yes	Use in conjunction with low protein diets for infants, children and adults with urea cycle disorders with the exception of Argininaemia where L-arginine is contra-indicated
Dialamine	200g tub	Infancy – adulthood	Per 100g: 30% essential amino acids (25g protein equivalent) 65g CHO 360kcal (1530kJ)	No	Yes	For oral feeding where essential amino acids are required. Orange flavoured powder (see page 745)
Essential amino acid mix (code 1490)	200g tub	Infancy – adulthood	Per 100g: 94.5% essential amino acids (79g protein equivalent) 316kcal (1343kJ)	No	Yes	Not ACBS listed. For oral feeding of infants with urea cycle disorders where essential amino acids are required to supplement protein intake. Unflavoured
Energivit	400g tin	Infancy	Per 100g: No amino acids/protein free 66.7g CHO 25g fat 492kcal (2059kJ) Per 100mL: No amino acids/protein free 10g CHO 3.8g fat 74kcal (309kJ)	No	No	Protein-free mixture containing CHO, fat, vitamins and minerals. Protein-free feed which can be used in the short term as an emergency regimen or when waiting diagnosis in protein/amino acid disorders. Can be used in conjunction with specific amino acids or natural protein sources. ACBS listed for infants with disorders of amino acid and protein metabolism on a protein restricted diet

Name	Instant Carobel	Nestargel
Manufacturer	Cow and Gate	Nestlé Clinical Nutrition
Ingredients	Endosperm portion of carob or locust bean with maltodextrin and calcium lactate	Carob seed flour and calcium lactate. It contains no metabolisable carbohydrate
Energy kcal/100g	251	38
kJ/100g	1065	158
CHO g/100g	59	0
Sodium mg/100g	8	5
Potassium mg/100g	240	350
Calcium mg/100g	130	640
Phosphorus mg/100g	20	Not declared
Reconstitution	Bottle feed: add 2-3 level scoops of Carobel for every 60-90mL (2-3fl oz) hand warm infant formula. Shake well and leave to thicken for 3-4 minutes. Breast feeds: add 6-7 level scoops of Carobel to 60mL (2fl oz) hand warm water to form a thick gel. Feed in small quantities by spoon before and during the breast feed	Recommended concentration 0.5-1%. Bottle feed: add Nestargel in the quantity of cold water required for the feed; gently bring to the boil, stir and simmer for 1 minute; cool and add the formula powder; mix until smooth. Breast feeds: give 1 tablespoon of thickened Nestargel water (1% concentration) pre-feeds
Comments	An instant thickener 1 scoop = 0.58g Carobel	An effective thickener; produces a smooth and stable thickened liquid. 1 scoop = 1g Nestargel
Presentation	Box: 135g	Can: 125g
ACBS listed	Yes, for thickening feeds in the treatment of vomiting	Yes, for thickening feeds in the treatment of vomiting
side-effects	A minority of infants may develop loose stools. If used in galactosaemia, the red cell galactose 1-phosphate content should be monitored	A minority of infants may develop loose stools. If used in galactosaemia, the red cell galactose 1-phosphate content should be monitored

Nutrition tables

Name	Thick and Easy	Thixo D	Vitaquick
Manufacturer	Fresenius Kabi	Sutherland Health	Vitaflo
Ingredients	Modified food starch (maize), maltodextrin	Modified waxy maize, food starch (E1442)	Modified maize starch, (E1422)
Energy kcal/100g	372	392	380
kJ/100g	1,562	1,635	1,590
CHO g/100g	92.6	97	95
Sodium mg/100g	174	90	115
Potassium mg/100g	Not declared	5	0.4
Calcium mg/100g	4.5	Not declared	Not declared
Phosphorus mg/100g	24	2	20
Reconstitution	No specific instructions given for infants. 1–3% concentration suggested. Ref: Macdonald S (2001) The Gastrointestinal Tract. In Shaw V, Lawson M (eds) *Clinical Paediatric Dietetics*, 2nd edition. Blackwell Science. Oxford		
Comments	An effective thickener. Unsuitable for infants under 1 year, unless failing to thrive		An effective thickener. Unsuitable for infants under 1 year, unless failing to thrive. Each tub contains a 15mL scoop
Presentation	Can: 225g, Sachets: 8g, Catering pack: 4.5kg	Tub: 375g	Tub: 100g, 300g
ACBS listed	Yes, for thickening of foods in the treatment of dysphagia	Yes, for thickening of foods in the treatment of dysphagia	Yes, for thickening of foods in the treatment of dysphagia
side-effects	–	–	–

Product is ACBS listed for use in the management of significant reflux. For use not in excess of a six month period. Do not use in combination with any other feed thickeners or antacid products.

Name of feed	Enfamil AR
Manufacturer	Mead Johnson Nutritionals
kcal/100mL	68
kJ/100mL	283
Protein source	Skimmed milk
Protein g/100mL	1.7
Fat source	Palm olein oil, coconut oil, soya oil, sunflower oil
Fat g/100mL	3.5
Carbohydrate source	Glucose polymers, lactose, rice starch
Carbohydrate g/100mL	7.4
Osmolality mOsmol/kg water	230
Fibre g/100mL	0
Special characteristics	
Peanut free	Yes
Suitable for vegetarians	Yes
Suitable for vegans	No
Lactose free	No
Gluten free	Yes
Presentation	400g tin
Nutritionally complete	Yes, no added molybdenum or chromium
Reconstitution	1 scoop powder + 1oz (30mL) water
Standard dilution %	13.5
Caution	Do not give with other feed thickeners or antacid products
Other	A pre-thickened formula for infants with mild reflux

Nutrition tables

The following food products can be regarded as having the characteristics of drugs if they are used as part of the management of the clinical conditions listed in the 'prescribability' column.

Product	Manufacturer	Description	ACBS Prescribability
Cornflour/cornstarch	Various	Maize Starch BP- maize starch powder	Hypoglycaemia associated with glycogen storage disease
Fructose	Various	Fructose BP Laevulose powder 500g	Glucose-galactose intolerance
Glucose/dextrose	Various	Glucose BP Dextrose monohydrate powder 500g	Glycogen storage disease. Sucrose-isomaltose intolerance
GTE oil	SHS International	89% GTE oil. 801 kcal/100g, 3293kJ/100g, fat 89g/100g. Presentation: 1 litre bottle	Not ACBS prescribable. Indicated for biochemically proven adrenoleukodystrophy
GTO oil	SHS International	91% GTO oil. 819 kcal/100g, 3367kJ/100g, fat 91g/100g. Presentation: 1 litre bottle	Not ACBS prescribable. Indicated for biochemically proven adrenoleukodystrophy
Lorenzo's oil	SHS International	80% glycerol trioleate 20% glycerol trierucate. 806 kcal/100g, 3312kJ/100g, fat 89.5g/100g. Presentation: 500mL bottle	Not ACBS prescribable. May be used in the management of biochemically proven adrenoleukodystropphy
SHS Module Flavour System	SHS International	Blackcurrant, orange, pineapple, tomato, *grapefruit, *cherry vanilla, *lemon and lime. Contains maltodextrin +/- lactose, modified starch, sugar according to flavour. Presentation: 100g tubs or *5g sachets	For flavouring unflavoured amino acid/peptide based products